Handbook of
ASSESSMENT METHODS
for EATING BEHAVIORS and
WEIGHT-RELATED PROBLEMS
Measures, Theory, and Research

SECOND EDITION

Handbook of
ASSESSMENT METHODS
for EATING BEHAVIORS and
WEIGHT-RELATED PROBLEMS
Measures, Theory, and Research

SECOND EDITION

DAVID B. ALLISON ◆ MONICA L. BASKIN

University of Alabama at Birmingham

EDITORS

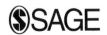

Los Angeles | London | New Delhi
Singapore | Washington DC

For information:

SAGE Publications, Inc.
2455 Teller Road
Thousand Oaks, California 91320
E-mail: order@sagepub.com

SAGE Publications India Pvt. Ltd.
B 1/I 1 Mohan Cooperative Industrial Area
Mathura Road, New Delhi 110 044
India

SAGE Publications Ltd.
1 Oliver's Yard
55 City Road
London EC1Y 1SP
United Kingdom

SAGE Publications Asia-Pacific Pte. Ltd.
33 Pekin Street #02-01
Far East Square
Singapore 048763

Printed in the United States of America

Library of Congress Cataloging-in-Publication Data

Handbook of assessment methods for eating behaviors and weight-related problems : measures, theory, and research / David B. Allison, Monica L. Baskin.—2nd ed.
    p. cm.
Includes bibliographical references and index.
ISBN 978-1-4129-5135-7 (cloth : acid-free paper)
    1. Eating disorders—Diagnosis. 2. Overweight persons—Psychological testing. 3. Eating disorders—Patients—Psychological testing. I. Allison, David B. (David Bradley), 1963- II. Baskin, Monica L. (Monica Loundy), 1970-

RC552.E18H357 2009
616.85'26075—dc22   2009002536

This book is printed on acid-free paper.

09   10   11   12   13   10 9 8 7 6 5 4 3 2 1

Acquisitions Editor:	Kassie Graves
Editorial Assistant:	Veronica K. Novak
Production Editor:	Astrid Virding
Copy Editor:	Gillian Dickens
Typesetter:	C&M Digitals (P) Ltd.
Proofreader:	Dennis Webb
Indexer:	Naomi Linzer
Cover Designer:	Candice Harman
Marketing Manager:	Carmel Schrire

Contents

Introduction   vii
David B. Allison and Monica L. Baskin

Chapter 1. Assessment of General Personality and Psychopathology Among Persons With Eating and Weight-Related Concerns   1
Chi A. Chan, Melissa A. Napolitano, and Gary D. Foster

Chapter 2. Assessment of Health-Related Quality of Life in Obesity and Eating Disorders   33
Ronette L. Kolotkin, Steffany Haaz, and Kevin R. Fontaine

Chapter 3. Methods for Measuring Attitudes About Obese People   79
Todd G. Morrison, Sarah Roddy, and Travis A. Ryan

Chapter 4. Assessment of Body Image   115
Hemal P. Shroff, Rachel M. Calogero, and J. Kevin Thompson

Chapter 5. Measures of Restrained Eating: Conceptual Evolution and Psychometric Update   137
Michael R. Lowe and J. Graham Thomas

Chapter 6. Measures of Physical Activity and Exercise   187
Donna Spruijt-Metz, David Berrigan, Louise A. Kelly, Rob McConnell, Donna Dueker, Greg Lindsey, Audie A. Atienza, Selena Nguyen-Rodriguez, Melinda L. Irwin, Jennifer Wolch, Michael Jerrett, Zaria Tatalovich, and Susan Redline

Chapter 7. Measuring Food Intake in Free-Living Populations: Focus on Obesity   255
Lauren Lissner and Nancy Potischman

Chapter 8. Measuring Food Intake, Hunger, Satiety, and Satiation in the Laboratory   283
John Blundell, Kees de Graaf, Graham Finlayson, Jason C. G. Halford, Marion Hetherington, Neil King, and James Stubbs

Chapter 9. Measuring Food Intake in Field Studies   327
Brian Wansink

Chapter 10. Binge Eating and Purging   347
Giorgio A. Tasca, Valerie Krysanski, Natasha Demidenko, and Hany Bissada

Chapter 11. Assessment of Eating-Disordered Thoughts, Feelings, and Behaviors   397
Drew A. Anderson, Kyle P. De Young, and D. Catherine Walker

Chapter 12. Assessment of Eating and Weight-Related Problems in Children   447
Tanja V. E. Kral, Myles S. Faith, and Angelo Pietrobelli

Chapter 13. Assessment of Human Body Composition   481
Dympna Gallagher and Fahad Javed

Chapter 14. Measurement of Energy Expenditure   529
James A. Levine and Ann M. Harris

Appendices   555

Index   637

About the Editors   689

About the Contributors   691

Introduction

The latest estimates of the prevalence of obesity suggest that one third of adults in the United States are obese (Ogden et al., 2006). Among children and adolescents, the rate of obesity (body mass index [BMI] ≥ 95th percentile [from a prior era] of sex-specific, BMI-for-age growth charts) is 17% (Ogden et al., 2006). These rates reflect substantial increases in the past three decades and are higher than were the case when the first edition of this book was published. Increases have been noted among all age, gender, and racial/ethnic groups. Similarly, the incidence of eating disorders increased significantly through the 1990s (Hoek, 2006; Hoek & van Hoeken, 2003). Not surprisingly, there has been a continued and growing interest in these topics. At the time of the publication of the first edition of this handbook, there were at least three journals devoted to obesity (*International Journal of Obesity, Obesity Research*, and *Obesity Surgery*), and similarly, there were at least three journals devoted to eating disorders (*International Journal of Eating Disorders, Eating Disorders: Journal of Treatment & Prevention*, and *Eating Disorders Review*). New books related to the two topics were also emerging at frequent intervals. Current journals related to obesity and weight-related problems number over 10, while there are at least 5 journals relating to eating disorders. Published books on these topics in the past decade are over 483.

Over the 10 years since *The Handbook of Assessment of Methods for Obesity and Eating Behaviors* was first published, many compliments were received about the book. Colleagues have remarked that it is a highly valuable and unique reference resource enabling them to identify the best tools to accurately and consistently measure concepts critical to obesity and eating disorders. In recent years, several individuals have suggested an updated edition, particularly when the book went out of press. We are pleased that SAGE Publications agreed.

The elevated obesity rates in the United States and most of the developed world have provoked enormously increased interest in the study of obesity across many sectors. The continued need to identify high-quality assessment measures for research and clinical pursuits is apparent. The first edition of this handbook was the first comprehensive reference guide to the measurement of obesity and eating disorders. It provided detailed descriptions of available assessment measures, including a review of the psychometric properties of each measure and a discussion of the advantages and disadvantages of the tool. This second edition of the handbook includes the review of new tools and methodologies as well as the addition of more recent data on measures that may have been included in the original book. This edition also includes increased attention to assessment issues related to the population group(s) being assessed (e.g., racial/ethnic groups, age, gender, disabled). The latter is particularly relevant as we are increasingly aware that obesity, eating disorders, and weight-related problems affect all segments of the population.

Who Is This Book For?

Like the first edition, this book is a *handbook* that is highly useful as a reference. The book should be useful to researchers, graduate students, and clinicians who adhere to the scientist/practitioner model. It will be of value to professionals and students working in the fields of obesity, eating disorders, preventive medicine, and nutrition. Based on past experience, it is likely to be highly used by academics, researchers at pharmaceutical and food companies, and some clinicians. Ultimately, this book is for anyone whose work involves measuring the thoughts, feelings, behaviors, or bodies of persons with obesity, eating disorders, or weight-related concerns and who believes in the value of rigorous measurement.

Changes in This Edition

Like its predecessor, this edition is intended as a reference book (e.g., encyclopedic). It will ideally be a source that readers could easily pick up and review a comprehensive description of the tests and assessment methods available for evaluating obesity, eating disorders, or weight-related issues. With that in mind, there have been some limited changes to original contents to ensure that this updated version is the most comprehensive and complete guide possible. Topics have been eliminated, added, or expanded to capture our current understanding of the most relevant assessment measures in the field. Table 1 describes such changes and the related rationale.

Contents of This Book

Authors of each chapter attempted to locate all available measures pertaining to their chapter topic. Measures were then selected from this larger set on the basis of promise in the case of new instruments or demonstrated quality in the case of more established instruments. In some cases, instruments of lesser quality but wide prominences are reviewed if only to offer readers caveats regarding their use.

Each chapter is written to be self-contained, but all chapters adhere to a similar format. With a few exceptions, each chapter reviews instruments assessing one or a few closely related constructs. Authors provide a brief overview of the area of focus followed by a review of fundamental assessment issues or special concerns in assessing the construct, assessment issues related to specific populations (e.g., racial/ethnic

Table 1   Changes in Topic Areas From the First Edition to the Second Edition of the *Handbook*

First Edition Chapter Topic	Second Edition Chapter Topic	Rationale for Change
Measuring food intake	Measuring food intake in free-living populations	The original chapter was broken into three separate chapters to identify measures related to intake in free-living populations versus laboratory settings versus realistic laboratory analog settings.
	Measuring food intake, hunger, and satiation in the laboratory	
	Measuring food intake in realistic laboratory analog settings	
Motivational readiness to control weight	*Eliminated*	These measures, though intuitively appealing, have not been found to have much utility.
Assessment of specific eating behaviors and eating style	*Eliminated*	Key measures presented in this chapter have been included elsewhere in the text.
Assessment of eating and weight-related problems in children and special populations	Assessment of eating and weight-related problems in children	Issues relevant to the assessment of "special populations" such as minorities, the elderly, and persons with disabilities are included in each chapter.
Identification of psychological problems of patients with eating and weight-related disorders in general medical settings	*Eliminated*	Key measures presented in this chapter have been included elsewhere in the text.
	Measurement of energy expenditure	This chapter was not previously included, but advances have been made in technology, and these measurements are more widely used today.
The big picture	*Eliminated*	This topic was not viewed as essential in a reference guide.

groups, children, elderly, women, persons with disabilities), and an in-depth review (including psychometric properties, availability, and critique) of the "better" instruments in the area. Each chapter is concluded with a discussion of suggestions for future research and additional comments.

A Psychometrics "Refresher"

In this last section of the Introduction, we provide a brief "refresher" on psychometric or measurement issues and techniques. We use the term *refresher* and not *primer* or *introduction* because any piece this short can only serve to remind readers of some key issues, terms, and techniques involved in the development and evaluation of measurement techniques. Readers who truly require an introduction to or in-depth discussion of these issues are referred to one of the major psychometric texts available (Furr & Bacharach, 2007; Kline, 2000).

When evaluating measurement techniques, one needs to consider numerous issues. Does the technique provide consistent answers (reliability)? Does it measure what it purports to measure (validity)? Does it measure equally well in all populations (validity generalization)? Can the subjects understand the questionnaire (readability)?

In the following chapters, authors comment on the following aspects of the tests reviewed (to the extent that the information is available and relevant for specific tests and constructs).

Reliability

The simplest definition of reliability is "consistency." A test is reliable if it measures something consistently. Of course, reliability is not an all-or-none issue. Some tests are very reliable, others are not at all reliable, and still others are "somewhat" reliable. Reliability can be quantified via reliability coefficients, the most common being correlation-based statistics such as the Pearson product-moment correlation coefficient or the intraclass correlation coefficients. These coefficients typically range from 0.0 to 1.0, with higher numbers indicating greater reliability.

Classical test theory postulates that observed scores are a combination of a true score plus an error score. True variance is variation among individuals irrespective of artifacts of measurement. Error variance, however, assesses the degree to which trait-irrelevant variation contaminates an observed score. An index of reliability indicates the proportion of variance in the measure that is true variance rather than error variance. For example, a reliability coefficient of .80 indicates that 80% of the variance in the measure is true variance. Note that reliability coefficients are *not* squared to yield these estimates of true variance. Although there is no fixed rule, reliability coefficients between .70 and .80 are considered "minimally acceptable," between .80 and .90 are "adequate," and above .90 are "excellent." Given the many sources of error that could enter into observed scores, there are many kids of reliability. One can assess whether measurements are consistent across different nontrait factors (e.g., time, raters, instrument forms, or items). Each of these nontrait factors represents a difference source of error.

Internal Consistency. To what degree do the items of the scale intercorrelate with each other and tap a unitary construct? In answering this question, we will typically refer to Cronbach's *alpha* coefficient (of which Kuder-Richardson 21 is a special case)—a measure of internal consistence reliability. Cronbach's α is a function of both the number of items and the intercorrelation of items. To some degree, a high α might reflect high positive correlations among the items, but it can also reflect the number of items. Thus, although α is a good measure of reliability, it should not be construed as a measure of homogeneity per se.

Test-Retest. Test-retest reliability addresses the question of how consistent are the answers a test gives from one time to the next. The assessment of test-retest reliability is of concern when attempting to measure a "trait" rather than a "state."

Interrater. Interrater reliability refers to the extent to which two raters or observers provide similar scores when rating the same subject at the same time. Interrater reliability is crucial when interview and observation methods are used to assess individuals.

Factor Structure

The assessment of factor structure can be seen as an early state of validity assessment. Reliability assessment tells us whether the test is measuring *something* consistently. Assessing factor structure tells us *how many things* (underlying dimensions) the test is measuring and provides some clues as to what those things are. The questions that need to be asked of a test include the following: What are the number and nature of factors? Do they support the proposed structure and the use of the instrument; that is, do they give preliminary evidence of construct validity? Finally, is the factor structure stable across different samples, ethnic groups, genders, age groups, weight and diagnostic categories, and so on?

Validity

If reliability assessment tells us if we are measuring *something* and factor analysis tells us *how many things* (dimensions) we are measuring, then validity assessment tells us *if* (how well) we are measuring what we are trying to measure. It has been argued that all types of validity are subsumed under construct validity. Although this point is well taken, most psychometricians still find it useful to talk about the different "processes" of validation separately.

Convergent and Discriminant Validity. Construct validity refers to the network of relationships (called the nomological net) in which the scale is embedded. Two major types of construct validity are *convergent* and *divergent* or *discriminant* validity. *Convergent validity* refers to the relationship of the present measure with other measures that purportedly measure the same or related constructs. For example, convergent validity would demand that one measure of restrained eating correlate with other measures of restrained eating.

Discriminant validity refers to the degree to which a measure does *not* correlate with measures of traits that it does not purport to measure. For example, discriminant validity would demand that a measure of restrained eating *not* correlate highly with a measure of reading ability—that is, we hope not. If it does, the scale may be measuring something other than restraint. Discriminant validity is obviously important but, unfortunately, infrequently assessed by test developers.

A particularly important form of discriminant validity is freedom from response sets. The problem of response sets has long plagued personality and clinical researchers. A response set can be defined as the tendency to endorse items for some reason other than the content of the items might suggest. Among the response sets frequently mentioned are acquiescence (the tendency to check many positive statements, or "yea-saying," and the tendency to check many negative statements, or "nay-saying"), extreme response set (the tendency to choose extreme Likert scale values rather than use intermediate categories), and social desirability (the tendency to endorse items in terms of their perceived desirability to others rather than in terms of how the person actually feels, believes, or behaves).

Investigators are often especially concerned with social desirability. Edwards originally suggested in 1957 that many scales primarily measure the tendency to respond in a socially desirable manner, and the issue is still very much alive today (Holden, 2007). Alternatively, Crowne and Marlowe (1964) argued that social desirability may not be a "nuisance variable" associated with tests but a characteristic or trait of individuals. Similarly, Campbell and Fiske (1959) asserted that when a measure of another construct (social desirability) is embedded in the nomological net of the construct of theoretical interest, then the evidence of some covariation would strengthen rather than weaken the case for construct validity. Regardless of the interpretation of social desirability, it is clear that if measures are to have discriminant validity, their correlations with measures of social desirability must be lower than their correlation with alternative measures of the construct of interest. This is the essence of Campbell and Fiske's multitrait-multimethod matrix.

Predictive Validity. Predictive validity refers to the extent to which the instrument successfully predicts prognosis, course, response to treatment, or other important endpoints.

Susceptibility to Dissimulation. In testing for susceptibility to dissimulation, we are asking a question similar to but distinct from that of discriminant validity. Here the question is very simple: Can subjects "fake" their responses if they are motivated to do so?

Norms

The final psychometric issues we will consider is a characteristic less of the tests themselves than of the body of data supporting the test. For the results of any test to be interpretable, it is necessary to have some frame of reference for the obtained scores. Two general approaches exist for establishing a frame of reference: (a) norm referencing and (b) criterion referencing.

In norm referencing, one establishes the average score for a group and then places some "range of normality" around this average. Often, the range is selected to be the 95% confidence limits, that is, the mean ± two standard deviations. People within the range are considered "normal" and people out of the range are considered "abnormal" or "unusual." This approach can be refined through the presentation of more refined categorizations such as percentiles. As Babbitt and colleagues (1995) in the first edition of this book pointed out, it is often necessary to have separate norms for different subsections of the population. For example, the normal range of weight will obviously be very different for a 6-foot-tall, 30-year-old man than for a 3-year-old girl.

One limitation of the norm-referenced approach is that it tends to equate "average" with "normal." This is problematic when the average member of the population is not at the optimal point on the trait of interest. Relative body weight is an excellent example of this. In the United States, the average person is too heavy. If we recommended that all people be average, then we would be recommending that people be overweight. Instead, a more objective criterion is sought on which to evaluate an individual's relative weight. The most commonly chosen criterion is death. Specifically, we often set as "normal" the range of body weights that are associated with minimal mortality rate. This use of an objective standard in determining normative values is referred to as criterion referencing.

Conclusion

We hope that this Introduction has succeeded in reaffirming or convincing you of the necessity for rigorously evaluating your measurement instruments as well as of the merits of this book. Good research and clinical practice are built on a strong foundation of measurement. The authors of the following chapters were selected because of their expertise in assessing constructs related to obesity, eating disorders, and/or weight-related problems. Their collective knowledge of measurement in these fields is reflected in the details of the pages that follow. The result is a user-friendly reference for researchers and clinicians to help improve their investigation and treatment of obesity, eating behaviors and weight-related problems.

Finally, we wish to express our gratitude to the chapter authors, who worked so hard to bring you this book; the reviewers, who carefully evaluated each chapter; our wonderful spouses (Stacy and Beth) for their patience and support; and especially Richard Sarver for his exquisite organization skills and dogged determination, which were essential to moving this book to fruition.

The following reviewers are acknowledged:

Richard N. Baumgartner, PhD

France Bellisle, PhD

Tamilane E. Blaudeau, PhD

Mac Buchowski, PhD

Christian Crandall, PhD

Éric Doucet, PhD

Johanna Dwyer, DSc, RD

Anthony Fabricatore, PhD

Richard A. Forshee, PhD

Angela S. Guarda, MD

Ian Janssen, PhD

Kristine L. Lokken, PhD

Jennifer D. Lundgren, PhD

Corby K. Martin, PhD

Richard Mattes, MPH, PhD, RD

Susan Phelan, PhD

Angelo Pietrobelli, MD

Katherine Presnell, PhD

Rebecca M. Puhl, PhD

Christopher B. Scott, PhD

Jennifer Shapiro, PhD

Eric Stice, PhD

Dennis Styne, MD

Beverly J. Tepper, PhD

Patricia van den Berg, PhD

Cortney Warren, PhD

References

Babbitt, R. L., Edlen-Nezien, L., Manikam, R., Summers, J., & Murphy, C. M. (1995). Assessment of eating and weight-related problems in children and special populations. In D. B. Allison (Ed.), *Handbook of assessment methods for eating behaviors and weight related problems: Measures, theory, and research* (pp. 431–492). Thousand Oaks, CA: Sage.

Campbell, D. T., & Fiske, D. W. (1959). Convergent and discriminant validation by the multitrait-multimethod matrix. *Psychological Bulletin, 56,* 81–105.

Crowne, D. P., & Marlowe, D. (1964). *The approval motive.* New York: John Wiley.

Furr, R. M., & Bacharach, V. R. (2007). *Psychometrics: An introduction.* Thousand Oaks, CA: Sage.

Hoek, H. W. (2006). Incidence, prevalence and mortality of anorexia nervosa and other eating disorders. *Current Opinion in Psychiatry, 19,* 389–394.

Hoek, H. W., & van Hoeken, D. (2003). Review of the prevalence and incidence of eating disorders. *International Journal of Eating Disorders, 34,* 383–396.

Holden, R. R. (2007). Socially desirable responding does moderate personality scale validity both in experimental and in nonexperimental contexts. *Canadian Journal of Behavioural Science, 39,* 184.

Kline, P. (2000). *A psychometrics primer.* London: Free Association Books.

Ogden, C. L., Carroll, M. D., Curtin, L. R., McDowell, M. A., Tabak, C. J., & Flegal, K. M. (2006). Prevalence of overweight and obesity in the United States, 1999–2004. *Journal of the American Medical Association, 295,* 1549–1555.

CHAPTER 1

Assessment of General Personality and Psychopathology Among Persons With Eating and Weight-Related Concerns

Chi C. Chan, Melissa A. Napolitano, and Gary D. Foster

Considering the intricate and contiguous relationship between personality, behavior, and physiology, the assessment of persons with obesity and eating disorders would be incomplete without looking at these factors. This chapter focuses on issues and methods in assessing personality and psychopathology in this population. Personality is an individual's unique and long-term experience and behavior, with personality traits being consistent and expected reactions and behaviors (Comer, 2005). Psychopathology is defined as problematic patterns of thought, feeling, or behavior that are disruptive to an individual's well-being or functioning (Kowalski & Westen, 2005). Psychopathology can be viewed as a spectrum of psychological disturbances, ranging from minor abnormalities to personality disorders (rigid patterns of experience and behavior that deviate markedly from the expected norm of the culture) to delusional psychoticism (Kowalski & Westen, 2005).

Early research in the populations with eating and weight concerns suggested that there was an obese personality characterized by dependency, immaturity, and negative affect (Rydén & Danielsson, 1983) but that the obese population does not show greater levels of psychological disturbance than the normal-weight population (Striegel-Moore & Rodin, 1986; Stunkard & Wadden, 1992; Wadden & Stunkard, 1985). Eating disorders have also been thought to be related to certain personalities and mood disorders, such as the need for control and depression (Bruch, 1973; Hudson, Pope, Jonas, & Yurgelun-Todd, 1983; Walsh, Roose, Glassman, Glades, & Sadik, 1985). These conclusions have been abandoned in favor of later research suggesting that personality characteristics associated with obese persons may in fact be a result of being obese rather than its cause (Plante & Rodin, 1990). Cooper (1995) also suggests that depression most likely occurs subsequent to an eating disorder as opposed to being a causal factor. It has then been concluded that there is much heterogeneity in the obese (Friedman & Brownell, 1995) and the eating disorder (Vitousek & Stumpf, 2005) populations. Friedman and Brownell (1995) regarded these findings as "first-generation studies" and suggested that "second-generation studies" should aim at identifying those at risk and consequences within the obese population. Finally, Friedman and Brownell suggested that "third-generation studies" should investigate causality; this model can also be applied to the eating disorder group.

The question of what should be considered "normal" and "abnormal" personality and behavior has long been discussed in the field of psychology (Adams & Cassidy, 1993).

Although there is debate regarding this issue, which is beyond the scope of this chapter, assessment tools consisting of norms within certain populations (e.g., eating disordered, obese) can provide a context for evaluating and comparing different groups.

Fundamental Assessment Issues and Concerns

Cause and Effect

Perhaps the most difficult task in psychological assessment is uncovering the cause and effect of a phenomenon. Assessing personality and psychopathology in persons with obesity and disordered eating is no exception in that it has yet to be clarified whether the eating and weight disorder causes psychological distress or vice versa. Correlational studies have been useful in establishing that there is comorbidity between personality, psychopathology, and eating and weight disorders (e.g., Godt, 2002; Matos et al., 2002;

O'Brien & Vincent, 2003). There are also correlations between the level of psychopathology and the comorbidity of the disorder (e.g., more psychopathology in obese binge eaters than obese nonbingers; Picot & Lilenfeld, 2003) and with the severity of the disorder (Speranza, Corcos, Atger, Paterniti, & Jeammet, 2003). What correlational studies lack is the ability to identify causal relationships. For that purpose, more revealing are study designs where individuals with eating and weight disorders are assessed before treatment and after recovery. These studies have found some significant declines in scores for personality disturbances and psychopathology after recovery from an eating disorder, such as dependency (Ames-Frankel et al., 1992; Bornstein & Greenberg, 1991; Kennedy, McVey, & Katz, 1990) and impulsivity (Ames-Frankel et al., 1992). One study also found significant declines in clinical scale scores of the Minnesota Multiphasic Personality Inventory– (MMPI-2) 6 months to a year following bariatric surgery (Maddi et al., 2001).

In these cases, it is apparent that treatment was associated with improvements, but to identify a causal relationship, we must understand how the treatment worked (i.e., what did it treat?). Several different mechanisms are possible. First, the treatment may have altered the patients' problematic eating patterns, which, in turn, improved their psychological functioning. On the other hand, the treatment may have alleviated their psychological disturbances, which then improved their eating and/or weight disorder. This second conclusion can be argued against with evidence from studies where the personality disturbances improve quite early in therapy (Ames-Frankel et al., 1992; Garner et al., 1990) before the necessary amount of change in personality needed to affect eating habits can take place (Cassin & von Ranson, 2005). Furthermore, bariatric surgery for the obese affects their eating patterns more directly than their personality. More interesting are the results where some personality traits that deviate from the norm persist even after recovery, such as perfectionism, rigidity, obsessiveness (Srinivasagam et al., 1995), novelty seeking, and harm avoidance

(Bloks, Hoek, Callewaert, & van Furth, 2004; Klump et al., 2004), which may point to enduring traits that contributed to the eating and/or weight disorder.

State Versus Trait

An important consideration when assessing personality and psychopathology is the distinction between personality traits and current mental states. Personality assessments are aimed at finding persistent characteristics that exist independently of any current and temporary mental problems, but distinguishing between the two is difficult. This problem is exacerbated in the population with weight concerns and eating disorders. The fundamental issue in this group is food intake and behaviors used to control it—these individuals are tampering with their basic physiological need for nourishment necessary for proper brain and body functions. This will undoubtedly affect their performance on tests and interviews. This issue is most apparent in individuals with the restricting subtype of anorexia nervosa or those who are on severely restricted diets. The Minnesota starvation study by Keys and colleagues in the 1940s revealed stunning changes in previously healthy men who volunteered to be put on a semi-starvation diet. The subjects displayed significant changes in attitude, mood, and behavior, including increased impulsivity, aggression, and irritability. Their personality profile by the end of the semi-starvation period resembled the profile of restricting subtype anorexic patients (Vitousek & Manke, 1994). Other studies with humans and animals have also found that severe caloric restriction alters behavior and thought profoundly (Lore, Gottdiener, & Delahunty, 1986; Rohles & Wilson, 1974; Rowland, 1968; Schiele & Brozek, 1948; Swanson & Dinello, 1970). However, when they resume normal eating, these changes dissipate with increased nourishment (Keys, Brozek, Henschel, Mickelsen, & Taylor, 1950; Robinson & Winnik, 1973; Rowland, 1968; Schiele & Brozek, 1948).

Abnormal mental states resulting from caloric deprivation, or any type of deviation from a healthy eating pattern, can mimic or exaggerate personality disorders and psychopathology. Improvement in assessment after treatment may in fact be due to the normalization of the patients' chaotic eating habit, which then eliminates its state effect on their performance on test and interview (Vitousek & Stumpf, 2005). Researchers should be cautious when assessing this group of individuals and be aware that the assessment can be affected by their current abnormal eating behavior.

Self-Report Inventories Versus Diagnostic Interviews

Self-report inventories and diagnostic interviews are two ways of assessing personality and psychopathology, each with their own advantages and disadvantages. Self-report inventories are cost-effective, easy to administer, and time efficient. They are useful screening tools for psychiatric disorders, can be used to quantify symptom severity, and may be able to reliably distinguish between types of psychopathology (Peveler & Fairburn, 1990). The rating scales and scoring keys available with self-report inventories standardize the evaluation of the results. On the other hand, the cutoff score marking the presence or absence of a disorder can be problematic in their artificiality and arbitrariness (Vitousek & Stumpf, 2005). In comparison to diagnostic interviews, self-report inventories overestimate personality disorders (Cassin & von Ranson, 2005; Fichter & Quadflieg, 2000; O'Brien & Vincent, 2003). A meta-analysis by Cassin and von Ranson (2005) found that self-report measures of personality disorders among individuals with eating disorders were overestimated by up to 35 times.

Diagnostic interviews have been regarded as a superior form of evaluation (Hill, Harrington, Fudge, & Rutter, 1989; Modestin, Erni, & Oberson, 1998). Interviews allow for a more dimensional and accurate assessment

(Vitousek & Stumpf, 2005) and are most helpful when the construct of interest is complex (Hill et al., 1989). Unlike self-report inventories, information can be obtained by directly observing behaviors, reactions, and overall face-to-face interaction (Groth-Marnat, 2003). Still, there are some downfalls to interviews. They can be time-consuming, which may become a problem when an individual needs to be assessed on multiple occasions (Loeb, Pike, Walsh, & Wilson, 1994). Furthermore, for the assessment to be accurate, the evaluation must be conducted by one or more trained interviewers, which raises the cost and limits the type of person who is able to conduct the interview. Finally, the reliability and validity of this method may pose a problem, depending on the extent of the structured natured of the interview (Groth-Marnat, 2003).

Assessment Issues With Populations

Race, Ethnicity, and Culture

Many personality assessment instruments used today were developed and standardized largely on White Americans (e.g., MMPI-2, Temperament and Character Inventory [TCI], Beck Depression Inventory [BDI]; Dana, Aponte, & Wohl, 2000). When assessing individuals from different ethnic or cultural backgrounds, the appropriateness of the instruments is an important consideration. Many tests have been translated to multiple languages for individuals who are unfamiliar with the language of the original test. For example, the MMPI-2 has been translated to more than 150 languages (Butcher, 2004). Although translated versions of tests are readily available, the quality and equivalence of the translation must be considered (Cheung, 2004). Studies on the validity of translated measures have reported mixed results that vary with the combination of measure and cultural group. For instance, the use of translated

versions of the MMPI-2 in various Asian countries has generated different results (see Butcher, Cheung, & Kim, 2003), and differences were found between American Indian and U.S. MMPI-2 norms (Pace et al., 2006), as well as between New Zealand students and SCL-90-R norms (Barker-Collo, 2003). Even beyond the language barrier, general discrepancies in outlook, attitude, and lifestyle can invalidate the extension of measures across cultural groups. Thus, this issue can manifest even in populations with a common language, as is the case with the "melting pot" of the United States. Dana (1996) suggests that "culturally competent assessment includes culture-specific styles of service delivery, use of the client's first language, and an evaluation of the client as a cultural being prior to test administration using cultural orientation categories" (p. 472). This third factor determines whether certain instruments are appropriate for their assessment (Dana, 1996).

Gender

Gender differences in various personality traits and tendencies have been found in a number of previous research studies (e.g., Byrnes, Miller, & Schafer, 1999; Goodwin & Gotlib, 2004; Maier, Lichtermann, Minges, & Heun, 1992). Research on the population with weight-related concerns has predominantly focused on women. Most studies on eating disorders have been conducted with only female subjects (e.g., Blouin et al., 1996; Jiménez-Murcia et al., 2007; Spindler & Milos, 2007). The few studies that have incorporated both sexes have found differences in scores on several traits (e.g., perfectionism, novelty seeking, harm avoidance) for males and females with eating disorders (Fassino et al., 2001; Joiner, Katz, & Heatherton, 2000). However, Fernández-Aranda et al. (2004) found difference only in the Harm Avoidance scale of the TCI. Obese samples have been more diverse, but women still outnumber men (e.g., Ro, Martinsen, Hoffart, Sexton, & Rosenvinge, 2005;

Ryden et al., 2003; Sullivan, Cloninger, Przybeck, & Klein, 2007). In comparing obese men and women, Ryden et al. (2003) found that obese and nonobese women scored higher than men in anxiety, although effect size was small.

Norms

Among cultural and gender differences, many other factors such as socioeconomic status and life situations can affect assessment (Bathurst, Gottfried, & Gottfried, 1997; Rychlak & Boland, 1973). One of the ways to address assessment issues with populations is to develop pertinent norms for comparison. A substantial number of studies have been dedicated to developing applicable norms for different populations (e.g., Bathurst et al., 1997; Hessel, Schumacher, Geyer, & Brähler, 2001; Lucio, Ampudia, Duran, Leon, & Butcher, 2001; Miettunen et al., 2004). Gender differences are addressed in some assessment inventories that have separate normative data for men and women (i.e., MMPI-2, TCI). To clarify relationships between variables, one must find an appropriate comparison group (Vitousek & Stumpf, 2005).

Assessment Instruments

Table 1.1 and Table 1.2 present a list of relevant personality and psychopathology assessment instruments. These measures were selected based on the amount of research on obesity and eating disorders that has used them. A simultaneous search, using the search terms "obes* or binge eat* or anorexi* or bulimi* or eating disorder," along with the name of the instrument, on the PsychINFO, MEDLINE, and PsychARTICLES databases in August 2007 returned the reported number of studies. There are limitations to this data-driven method for instrument inclusion, however, by distilling the most widely used instruments using an objective criterion (i.e., frequency of citations), readers will be able to select the measure most appropriate for their use. For descriptive purposes, we decided to group the instruments into measures of either personality or psychopathology, although there is significant overlap in the categories, and some measures have subscales for both. Due to space limitations, we are not able to provide extensive reviews for all of the measures listed in these tables.

Table 1.1   Overview of Personality Assessment Instruments

Personality Assessment Instruments	Authors	Brief Description	# Citations: Obesity and Binge Eating	# Citations: Eating Disorders
Minnesota Multiphasic Personality Inventory (MMPI-2)[a,b]	Hathaway and McKinley (1942); Butcher, Dahlstrom, Graham, Tellegen, and Kaemmer (1989)	567 true/false questions examine personality to detect a wide variety of psychiatric problems.	150[c]/15	196[c]/18
Rorschach[a]	Rorschach (1921/1942)	Assesses personality and emotional functioning based on subject's response to 10 inkblots.	74	131

(Continued)

Table 1.1 (Continued)

Personality Assessment Instruments	Authors	Brief Description	# Citations: Obesity and Binge Eating	# Citations: Eating Disorders
Temperament and Character Inventory (TCI)[a]	Cloninger, Svrakic, and Przybeck (1993)	226 true/false questions identify the overall personality by assessing seven dimensions of temperament and character.	21	98
Tridimensional Personality Questionnaires (TPQ)	Cloninger (1987)	100 true/false questions that analyze three dimensions of personality: novelty seeking, harm avoidance, and reward dependence.	2	16
Karolinska Scale of Personality (KSP)	Schalling, Åsberg, Edman, and Oreland (1987)	135 items rated on a 4-point scale assess stable personality traits.	9	8
Personality Diagnostic Questionnaire–Revised (TPQ-R)	Hyler and Rieder (1987)	152 true/false items measure the *DSM-III-R* criteria for Axis II personality disorders.	2[c]/6	6[c]/10
NEO Personality Inventory Revised (NEO-PI-R)	Costa and McCrae (1992)	240 items measure personality traits and NEO-PI's Big Five personality factors: neuroticism, extraversion, openness to experience, agreeableness, and conscientiousness.	3	7
Personality Assessment Inventory (PAI)	Morey (1991)	344 items with 22 nonoverlapping scales measure personality and psychopathology.	2	3

a. Extensively reviewed here.

b. Short form reviewed here.

c. Number of studies using original or other revised versions of the instrument.

Table 1.2   Overview of Psychopathology Assessment Instruments

Psychopathology Assessment Instruments	Authors	Brief Description	# Citations: Obesity and Binge Eating	# Citations: Eating Disorders
Beck Depression Inventory Second Edition (BDI-II)[a]	Beck, Ward, Mendelson, Mock, and Erbaugh (1961); Beck, Steer, Ball, and Ranieri (1996)	Total score of 21 items rated on a 3-point scale indicates depression ranging from normal mood to severe depression	250[b]/9	538[b]/12
Symptoms Checklist 90–Revised (SCL-90-R)[a]	Derogatis (1994)	90 items rated on a 5-point scale measure 9 symptom subscales and 3 overall indices	32[b]/38	87[b]/97
Structured clinical interview for *DSM* disorders (SCID)	Spitzer, Williams, Gibbon, and First (1990)	Semi-structured interview for diagnosis of all DSM disorders	50	16[b]
Hamilton Rating Scale for Depression (HAM-D)	Hamilton (1960)	21 items are rated by interviewer during a structured interview to determine severity of depression	32	88
State-Trait Anxiety Inventory (STAI)[a]	Spielberger, Gorsuch, Lushene, Vagg, and Jacobs (1983)	40 items rated on a 4-point scale measures emotional state and underlying trait	46	78
Millon Clinical Multiaxial Inventory (MCMI-III)[a]	Millon (1994)	175 true/false items assess all DSM-IV-R personality disorders and 4 personality styles	14[b]/1	23[b]/3
Profile of Mood States (POMS)[a]	McNair, Lorr, and Droppleman (1992)	65 mood-related adjectives rated on a 5-point scale to assess subject's mood state	23	20
Self-Rating Depression Scale (SDS)	Zung (1965)	20 items rated on a 4-point scale measures severity of depressive symptoms	9	27

a. Extensively reviewed here.

b. Number of studies using original or revised versions of the instrument.

Below are eight extensive reviews of measures that have been used in more than 10 studies (either as original or revised versions) for assessment of both obesity and binge eating as well as eating disorders. The studies mentioned in the research applications section are chosen to represent the use of the instrument in the area as a whole, and readers should note that the section is not by any means comprehensive. The prices are estimates and are subject to change. Although we have suggested that interviews (e.g., Structured Clinical Interview for DSM

Disorders) can provide more accurate and individualized information, we have decided to provide detailed reviews only of self-report inventories as these inventories can be administered to a larger sample size in a cost- and time-efficient manner. In addition, analyzing the stability of interviews is beyond the scope of this chapter. For interested readers, more information on one such structured interview (i.e., the Structured Clinical Interview for DSM Disorders; Spitzer, Williams, Gibbon, & First, 1990) is available online at www.scid4.org.

Personality

The Minnesota Multiphasic Personality Inventory–Second Edition (MMPI-2)

The MMPI-2 (Butcher, Dahlstrom, Graham, Tellegen, & Kaemmer, 1989) is the current revised and standardized version of the original MMPI (Hathaway & McKinley, 1942). The MMPI is one of the most widely used self-report inventories in psychology (Camara, Nathan, & Puente, 2000) and is frequently used in the assessment of populations with weight concerns. It was originally designed to assess a wide range of the more important dimensions of personality with scores that could be quantified (Hathaway & McKinley, 1942). After almost 50 years of use in its original form, the MMPI Restandardization Project (Butcher et al., 1989) introduced the MMPI-2. The revision included rewriting test items and developing new norms for all of the scales. Extensive research has already established the psychometric stability of the original MMPI. Thus, initial research on the MMPI-2 focused on the comparability of the two versions. A host of research generally agrees that they are equivalent (Ben-Porath & Butcher, 1989; Gaston, Nelson, Hart, Quatman, & Rojdev, 1994; Graham, 1990; Harrell, Honaker, & Parnell, 1992; Rojdev, Nelson, Hart, & Fercho, 1994).

The test consists of 567 items that take approximately 60 to 90 minutes to complete. Each item is a short statement to which the subject answers true, false, or cannot say. Results can be interpreted by comparing the subject's answers, scores, and profiles with those of normal and psychiatric groups. The test contains 9 validity scales, 5 superlative self-presentation subscales, 10 clinical scales, 9 restructured clinical (RC) scales, 15 content scales, 27 content component scales, 20 supplementary scales, 31 clinical subscales, and 5 supplementary scales (see Butcher et al., 2001, for a complete list of scales and subscales). An abbreviated format consists of the first 370 items, which is sufficient to obtain scores for the basic validity scales and the clinical scales. Butcher et al. (2001) provide extensive psychometric statistics for MMPI-2 scales and subscales. However, since most research on obesity, eating disorders, and weight concerns have focused and found significant results on the content and clinical scales (Gleaves & Eberenz, 1995; Klinger, 2000; Pryor & Wiederman, 1996; Youssef et al., 2004), and since the new restructured clinical scale (RC scale; Tellegen et al., 2003) has been shown to have better internal consistency and convergent and discriminate validity than the basic clinical scale (Sellbom & Ben-Porath, 2005; Simms, Casillas, Clark, Watson, & Doebbeling, 2005; Tellegen et al., 2003; Wallace & Liljequist, 2005), this section reports statistics on those three scales.

Reliability. Butcher et al. (2001) present reliability statistics separately for men and women of the normative sample. For the content scales, internal consistency coefficient alphas ranged from .72 (Fears and Type A) to .86 (Depression) for men and from .73 (Anger) to .86 (Depression) for women. Test-retest reliability over a 9-day interval ranged from .78 (Bizarre Mentation) to .91 (Social Discomfort) for men and from .79 (Type A) to .91 (Work Interference) for women. For the clinical scales, internal consistency ranged from .34 (Paranoia) to .85 (Psychasthenia and Schizophrenia) for men and from .37 (Masculinity/Femininity) to .87 (Psychasthenia) for women. Test-retest reliability over a 1-week interval ranged from .67 (Paranoia) to .93 (Social Introversion) for men and from .54 (Schizophrenia) to .92 (Social Introversion) for women. For the RC scales, internal consistency ranged from .63 (RC6, Ideas of Persecution) to .87 (RCd, Demoralization) for men and from .62 (RC2, Low Positive Emotions) to .89 (Demoralization) for women. Test-retest reliability over a 1-week interval ranged from .76 (RC2, Low Positive Emotions and RC3, Cynicism) to .91 (RC7, Dysfunctional) for men and from .54 (RC6, Ideas of Persecution) to .90 (RCd, Demoralization) for women. In another study, Matz, Altepeter, and Perlman (1992) studied college students with the MMPI-2 and found that internal consistency alpha coefficients ranging from .39 to .91 and a test-retest interval over a mean of 21 days yielded coefficients ranging from .60 to .90.

Validity. Barthlow, Graham, Ben-Porath, and McNulty (1999) tested the incremental validity of the content scales with a sample of 274 men and 425 women outpatient mental health patients. Hierarchal regression analysis found incremental validity for seven scales for men and three scales for women. Palav, Ortega, and McCaffrey (2001) also found the content scales to be useful in identifying symptoms beyond the clinical scales alone. The clinical scales have been criticized for their overlapping items and lack of discriminate validity (Helmes & Reddon, 1993), which led Tellegen and colleagues to develop the RC scales in 2003. Sellbom and Ben-Porath (2005) compared the RC scales with the Multidimensional Personality Questionnaire (MPQ; Tellegen, 1982) and found that the two scales correlated as expected for different constructs. To further increase validity of the measure as a whole, the validity scales of the MMPI-2 evaluate the extent to which the test taker is answering questions in a way that allows the results to be interpreted accurately. The scores on the other scales are analyzed based on the scores of the validity scales.

Norms. The normative sample is a nationwide adult community group consisting of 2,600 individuals (1,462 men and 1,138 women). The demographics of the normative sample represent that of the U.S. national population, increasing its external consistency. Graham (1990) presents detailed normative sample data.

Availability. Pearson Assessments is the exclusive distributor of the MMPI, MMPI-2, and the adolescent version, the MMPI-A. All materials can be purchased via its Web site at www.pearsonassessments.com. The purchaser must submit a Test User Qualification Form (http://ags.pearsonassessments.com/assessments/test_user_form2.asp). User qualification for the MMPI includes having a licensure to practice psychology independently, being a full member of the American Psychological Association or the National Association of School Psychologists, having a doctoral or master's degree that provided training, or having proof that the individual has been granted permission to administer the test. The manual and 10 test booklets total approximately $90.00. Scoring services include mail-in service or scoring software, ranging from around $42.00 to $89.00. Packages are also available.

Limitations. Although the MMPI-2 is an improvement from the original MMPI, there are still questionable issues regarding the new use of uniform *T* scores versus linear *T* scores, the retention of a large amount of the original test items, and its clinical diagnostic utility (Horvath, 1992). The entirely empirical foundation of the MMPI-2 has also been criticized: Helmes and Reddon (1993) suggest that recent advances in psychological theories should be used in the revision. In terms of evaluating persons with weight and eating disorders, there may be some inconsistencies in the research. Studies using the original MMPI generally found distinctions between patients with anorexia nervosa and bulimia nervosa (Casper, Hedeker, & McClough, 1992; Vitousek & Manke, 1994), yet one study by Scott and Baroffio (1986) assessing anorexia, bulimia, and morbid obesity suggests that there was no clinically significant difference among the overall profiles of the groups, but they did differ from the control group in that the scores were significantly lower in almost all of the clinical scales. Later research with the MMPI-2 (Cumella, Wall, & Kerr-Almeida, 2000; Pryor & Wiederman, 1996) found little or no significant difference between anorexia nervosa and bulimia nervosa. These inconsistent results may be due to studies using different significant *p* values or using inpatient or outpatient groups.

Research Applications. Studies have shown that the MMPI-2 is useful in classifying individual profiles of eating disordered subgroups, even if elevations do not reach the clinical level (Vitousek & Manke, 1994). Restricting subtype anorexics' MMPI-2 scores especially appear to differ from other eating disorders (Cumella et al., 2000; Vitousek & Manke, 1994). Klinger (2000) also found the MMPI-2 useful in predicting weight loss and program completion in obese individuals. The amount of weight loss was correlated with the Hypochondriasis, Hysteria, and Psychopathic Deviant scales (weight loss of 5 body mass index [BMI] in 104 weeks) as well as Depression, Paranoia, and Schizophrenia (weight loss of 8 BMI in 104 weeks). Research on obesity and eating disorders with the MMPI-2 is limited, however, as many studies (e.g., Ragazzoni & Riva, 1996; Valtolina, 1996; Wadden, Foster, Letizia, & Wilk, 1993) have used the original MMPI. More research using the MMPI-2 in patients with eating and weight disorders will be helpful in determining its utility.

MMPI-2 Short Form

Despite its popularity and positive psychometric evaluations, the utility of the MMPI-2 may be compromised by its length. Clinicians may lack the time to administer 567 items that take 60 to 90 minutes, and the test taker may lack the time and/or ability. Therefore, Dahlstrom and Archer (2000) developed a short form of the MMPI-2 by using test records from the restandardization sample of 2,600 men and women as well as a sample of 632 records from persons beginning treatment at a psychiatric service. They found correlations on the basic scales (i.e., the main validity scales L [Lie], F [Infrequency], and K [Correction] and all of the clinical scales) between the scores on the first 180 items and the scores of the entire test to be high, ranging from .78 to .98 for the restandardization sample and .82 to .99 for the psychiatric sample.

A search for the MMPI-2 short form in the literature revealed only six citations, none of which included samples in the population with eating and weight-related concerns. This may be due to the fact that it is relatively new and that psychometric evaluations have found problems with its reliability and validity (Gass & Gonzalez, 2003). Two published evaluations on two different populations (Gass & Luis, 2001; Gass & Gonzalez, 2003) found that although correlations were high between the short form and the abbreviated or original form, when analyzed further, many of the scales of the MMPI-2 short form were unreliable, with scores varying in accuracy with each scale. An area of positive evaluation was in the validity scales, where acceptable reliability and validity have been reported for the L, F, and K items, with a correct classification rate of 77% (Cassisi & Workman, 1992) compared with the full Validity scale of the MMPI-2. Administration of the full MMPI-2 is highly recommended, but the MMPI-2 short form may be of some use in special circumstances.

Rorschach

The Rorschach (1924) is a projective method that was developed to examine personality and psychological functioning. Since the introduction of this measure, there has been much criticism and controversy surrounding its validity, reliability, and standardization for administration, scoring, and interpretation (e.g., Garb, Wood, Lilienfeld, & Nezworski, 2005; Pick, 1956; Weiner, 2001). However, this method has been used frequently in the area of weight concerns and eating disorders (e.g., Bornstein & Greenberg, 1991; Elfhag, Carlsson, & Rossner, 2003; Elfhag, Rossner, & Carlsson, 2004; Salorio et al., 2003). In fact, it was the second most cited measure in our search (see Table 1.1). Therefore, given its popularity, it is important to review the psychometric properties of this measure and its application in this area of research.

The premise of the Rorschach is based on the idea that when presented with an ambiguous stimulus and asked to interpret it, a person will mostly likely project his or her own personality and feelings onto the stimulus or situation (Rorschach, 1924). The Rorschach contains 10 standard inkblots to which the person responds. These inkblots are made by randomly smearing or dripping ink on a paper and folding it in half to make it symmetrical and do not inherently represent anything. Hence, whatever the subject sees within these inkblots is thought to be a projection of his or her own feelings. To address the criticism of the lack of a standard protocol for administering and scoring the test (Pick, 1956), Exner (1991, 1993) created the Comprehensive System (CS) to standardize the assessment and coding procedures. With this new system comes a new line of studies on its psychometric stability (e.g., Acklin, McDowell, Verschell, & Chan, 2000; McGrath et al., 2005; Meyer et al., 2002; Meyer, Mihura, & Smith, 2005; Sultan, Andronikof, Reveillere, & Lemmel, 2006).

Reliability. The "percentage of agreement" approach that Exner (1993) used has been criticized for its validity in determining interrater reliability (Wood, Nezworski, & Stejskal, 1996a). The debate on whether this is a valid method continues. A more recent study of interclinician reliability was performed by Meyer et al. (2005). Three to eight clinicians scored 55 patient protocols over four data sets. The mean interrater aggregated judgment reliability between three clinicians using a rating scale was .88. The mean reliability of individual interpretive judgment was .79. Exner and Weiner (1995) found test-retest correlations above .75 for most of the variables. A meta-analysis by Gronnerod (2003) found a generally high level of temporal stability using the CS.

Validity. Evaluating the validity of the Rorschach and the CS is a difficult task. Few studies clearly report Rorschach CS validity. Garb et al. (2005) reviewed these studies and, based on their criteria that "(1) studies on a score should be methodologically sound, (2) significant results should be replicated by independent investigators, and (3) results should be consistent across studies" (p. 106) concluded that only a handful of indices and variables have been validated by research. It should be noted that these criteria have been criticized for being too stringent (Perry, 2003). Nonetheless, more research is necessary for validation.

Norms. The normative sample has been revised several times due to representative problems, invalidity, and duplications (Exner & Erdberg, 2005). The current published normative sample consists of 600 adult nonpatients, 300 men and 300 women. A new revision has begun due to the need for a more current normative sample as well as discrepancies found between the data in this current version and that of a study with graduate students by Shaffer, Erdberg, and Haroian (1999). This project is still in progress, and current findings can be found in Exner and Erdberg (2005). However, the sample is not yet large enough to be representative.

Availability. The Rorschach inkblots can be purchased from Pearson Assessments at www.pearsonassessments.com. Instructions on administering and scoring are available in Exner and Erdberg (2005). The purchaser must submit a Test User Qualification Form (http://ags.pearsonassessments.com/assessments/test_user_form2.asp). User qualification for the Rorschach includes having a licensure to practice psychology independently, being a full member of the American Psychological Association or the National Association of School Psychologists, having a doctoral or master's degree that provided training, or having proof that the individual has been granted permission to administer the test. Rorschach plates are $110.00, and 100 summary forms are $55.00. A workbook to aid in interpretation using the Comprehensive System by John Exner is $58.00.

Limitations. This measure should be used with caution due to the uncertainty that still surrounds it. Wood, Nezworski, and Stejskal (1996a) critically examined the CS and questioned its theory, and psychometric stability. This led to a heated discussion involving a number of researchers. The debate is beyond the scope of this section, but interested readers should refer to the following articles in order: Wood et al. (1996a); Exner (1996); Wood, Nezworski, and Stejskal (1996b); Meyer (1997a); Wood, Nezworski, and Stejskal (1997); and Meyer (1997b). Furthermore, the CS does not address the fundamental issues with the theory of the test. Questions about the usefulness of projective methods (Lilienfeld, Wood, & Garb, 2000), whether the Rorschach is indeed a perceptual task as the creator's original theory indicates (Leichtman, 1996), and the correct usage of the technique (Wood, Nezworski, & Garb, 2003) still remain.

Research Applications. Despite criticism, the Rorschach and Exner's CS have been used extensively in research on obesity and eating disorders with significant results. For example, Bornstein and Greenberg (1991) found that eating-disordered females display more dependency issues than do obese and normal-weight psychiatric patients. Another study with the Rorschach CS have found that obesity and binge eating were associated with believing that body size has a psychological function (e.g., being part of an identity) and irregular or chaotic eating (Elfhag, Carlsson, & Rossner, 2003). Smith, Hillard, Walsh, and Kubacki (1991) found heightened thought disturbances (SZCI index) in bulimics as well as more ambient (i.e., inconsistent) coping styles (EB scale) in bulimics when compared to controls. Elfhag, Barkeling, Carlsson, and Rossner (2003) used the Rorschach CS to assess the microstructure of eating (i.e., specific eating behaviors) and found that the initial eating rate was higher with more signs of stress overload and more response to external stimuli.

The Temperament and Character Inventory (TCI)

The TCI (Cloninger, Przybeck, Svrakic, & Wetzel, 1994) assesses temperament and character with seven independent dimensions. This measure was developed by adding to the previously established Tridimensional Personality Questionnaire (TPQ; Cloninger, 1987). The TPQ measured temperament and consisted of the Novelty Seeking (NS), Harm Avoidance (HA), and Reward Dependence (RD) dimensions, which were all included in the TCI for the temperament inventory. The Persistence (P) dimension was later identified as a fourth dimension of temperament and was also added to the TCI. Cloninger, Svrakic, and Przybeck (1993) then developed the three dimensions for assessing character, which is based on the idea of self-concept as an individual, as part of humanity, and as part of the universe. These are the Self-Directedness (SD), Cooperativeness (C), and Self-Transcendence (ST) dimensions, respectively. Combining all seven dimensions, the TCI assesses personality with a self-report inventory that consists of 240 true or false items.

Reliability. Cloninger et al. (1994) reported TCI internal consistency coefficients for a community sample ranging from .65 (Persistence) to .89 (Cooperativeness). Coefficients are also available for inpatients, college students, and outpatients, with Persistence repeatedly having the lowest internal consistency. All other dimensions yielded coefficients above .70. Test-retest correlations over a 6-month interval ranged from .54 (Novelty Seeking) to .75 (Self-Transcendence) for psychiatric inpatients and from .71 (Reward Dependence) to .83 (Self-Transcendence) for psychiatric outpatients.

Validity. The TCI has five validity scales and one honesty question that were designed to detect any invalid answers. These scales take into account the number of rare answers, consecutive answers, persistent true answers, and consistent answers to determine their validity. Bayon, Hill, Svrakic, Przybeck, and Cloninger (1996) administered the TCI and the Millon Clinical Multiaxial Inventory (MCMI-II) to 109 psychiatric outpatients and found a strong convergent validity, with the TCI accounting for much of the variance of the MCMI-II. Puttonen, Ravaja, and Keltikangas-Jarvinen (2005) found support for the predictive validity of the TCI with 91 subjects, especially for the Novelty Seeking and Harm Avoidance scales.

Norms. Normative data for the TCI are available for several populations. The community sample consisted of 150 men and 150 women. Mean scores for the seven scales are as follows: Novelty Seeking, $M = 9.7$, $SD = 3.7$; Harm Avoidance, $M = 7.6$, $SD = 4.5$; Reward Dependence, $M = 9.5$, $SD = 3.1$; Persistence, $M = 3.4$, $SD = 1.5$; Self-Directedness, $M = 17.6$, $SD = 5.1$; Cooperativeness, $M = 19.6$, $SD = 4.6$; and Self-Transcendence, $M = 8.3$, $SD = 3.9$ (Cloninger et al., 1994). Data for Norwegian physicians, inpatients, and college students are also available (see Cloninger et al., 1994).

Availability. The TCI can be purchased online at https://psychobiology.wustl.edu from the Washington University in St. Louis. There is no qualification requirement to purchase the TCI. The manual and test booklet is $85.00, and a computerized scoring system with all materials included is $400.00.

Limitations. The TCI has similar limitations to other self-report inventories. This measure lacks psychometric evaluation in the English version; therefore, no specific limitations have been mentioned. However, the TCI has been translated into multiple transcultural versions, including Japanese (Tomita et al., 2000), Spanish (Gutiérrez et al., 2001), and Dutch (Duijsens, Spinhoven, Goekoop, Spermon, & Eurelings-Bontekoe, 2000), and their evaluations have deemed the TCI satisfactory.

Research Applications. Lower scores in Self-Directedness have been found in patients with obesity and binge-eating disorder (Fassino et al., 2002; Sullivan et al., 2007), as well as individuals with anorexia or bulimia (Fassino et al., 2001; Klump et al., 2000) when compared with healthy controls. Higher Harm Avoidance has been found in eating-disordered patients (Fassino et al., 2002) and obese individuals (Fassino et al., 2002; Sullivan et al., 2007). Obese patients have been found to score higher in Novelty Seeking than controls and lower on Cooperativeness (Fassino et al., 2002). Comparing subtypes of obesity, obese binge eaters scored even lower in Self-Directedness than obese nonbingers (Sullivan et al., 2007). Within subtypes of eating disorders, patients with bulimia scored lower in persistence than those with anorexia (Grave et al., 2007). Cognitive-behavioral therapy for patients with both types of eating disorders and eating disorder not otherwise specified has been found to normalize some scores by lowering Persistence and Self-Transcendence and raising Self-Directedness (Grave et al., 2007).

Psychopathology

Beck Depression Inventory–II (BDI-II)

The BDI (Beck, Ward, Mendelson, Mock, & Erbaugh, 1961) is one of the most prominent instruments for assessing depression. Psychometric analysis revealed shortcomings, which led to an amended version, the BDI-IA (Beck & Steer, 1993), and the most current version, the BDI-II (Beck, Steer, & Brown, 1996). The BDI-II is a self-report inventory consisting of 21 items that is rated on a 4-point scale. The items have a heading that is the target of assessment (e.g., sadness, crying) followed by four statements (0–4) varying in intensity of the target assessment that subjects must select based on their feeling during the past week, including the day of the test. The final score is the sum of the score of each item. A total score of 0 to 13 is considered minimal or normal, 14 to 19 is mild, 20 to 28 is moderate, and 29 to 63 is severe (Beck, Steer, & Brown, 1996).

Reliability. Beck, Steer, Ball, and Ranieri (1996) found a high internal consistency coefficient alpha of .92 with a sample of 140 psychiatric outpatients. Arnau, Meagher, Norris, and Bramson (2001) studied 340 primary care patients and found a coefficient alpha of .94. In a sample of college students in 1996, the coefficient alpha was .93 (Beck, Steer, & Brown, 1996) and .90 for a sample in 2004 (Storch, Roberti, & Roth, 2004). Test-retest reliability over a 1-week interval for 26 outpatients was .93 (Beck, Steer, Ball, et al., 1996).

Validity. The BDI-II was found to be more positively correlated with the Hamilton Psychiatric Scale for Depression (Riskind, Beck, Brown, & Steer, 1987), with $r = .71$, than with the Hamilton Rating Scale for Anxiety (Riskind et al., 1987), with $r = .47$ (Beck, Steer, & Brown, 1996). Krefetz, Steer, Gulab, and Beck (2002) reported that the scores for adolescents diagnosed with major depressive disorder (MDD; $M = 30.09$, $SD = 12.80$) is significantly higher than those for adolescents without the diagnosis for MDD ($M = 17.56$, $SD = 11.27$).

Norms. Beck, Steer, and Brown (1996) reports a normative sample consisting of 500 outpatients, 317 women and 183 men. The average age of the sample ranged from 13 to 86 with a mean of 37.20. Whites represented the majority of this sample (91%). There is also a normative sample of 120 undergraduate college students.

Availability. The BDI-II is published by Harcourt Assessments, Inc. Materials can be purchased via its Web site at www.harcourtassessment.com. Qualification requirements include a licensure or certification to practice in the respective state in a related field or a doctorate degree with appropriate training. The BDI-II complete kit, including the manual and 25 record forms, is $99.00.

Limitations. The BDI-II and its predecessors have been subjected to much psychometric scrutiny and have consistently indicated above-satisfactory reliability and validity. However, it is important to note that the authors of the measure did not intend for it to serve as a diagnostic tool. It is meant to detect the presence and severity of depressive symptoms. The cutoff scores provided are designed to serve as general guidelines, and Beck, Steer, and Brown (1996) suggest that the scores be analyzed within the context of the individual case. Furthermore, the BDI has been criticized for its lack of representative norms (Richter, Werner, Heerlein, Kraus, & Sauer, 1998).

Research Applications. A long line of research has associated depressive symptoms with obesity (e.g., Bornstein, Schuppenies, Wong, & Licinio, 2006; Cahill & Mussap, 2007; Moore, 2004) as well as eating disorders (Bravata, Storch, & Storch, 2003; Gee & Troop, 2003; Rejeski et al., 2006). Therefore, the BDI-II is a useful tool in assessing persons with problematic eating behaviors. It is often used in conjunction with other measures to subtype eating disorders (Eipe, 2005; Fontenelle, Mendlowicz, Moreira, & Appolinario, 2005), assess changes in mood and thought after treatment or stimuli (Blouin et al., 1996), or correlate eating behavior and emotions (Bravata et al., 2003).

Symptoms Checklist 90 Revised (SCL-90-R)

The SCL-90-R (Derogatis, 1994) was originally derived from the Hopkins Symptom Checklist (HSCL; Derogatis, Lipman, Rickels, Uhlenhuth, & Covi, 1974) and was revised from its first prototype, the SCL-90. The SCL-90-R is a 90-item self-report questionnaire. The items are 90 descriptions of symptoms that are rated on their severity using a 5-point scale from 0 = *not at all* to 4 = *extremely.* The test takes about 10 to 15 minutes to complete. It is scored on nine different dimensions of symptoms: somatization, obsessive-compulsive, interpersonal sensitivity, depression, anxiety, hostility, phobic anxiety, paranoid ideation, and psychoticism. There are also three global indices: global severity index (assesses the extent of present psychiatric distress), positive symptom index (number of symptoms present), and positive symptom distress index (assesses the intensity of the symptoms).

Reliability. Derogatis (1994) reports internal consistency for psychiatric outpatients ranging from .79 (Paranoid Ideation) to .90 (Depression). Derogatis, Savitz, and Maruish (1999) report internal consistency for symptomatic volunteers ranging from .77 (Psychoticism) to .90 (Depression). A more recent study comparing paper-and-pencil versus computerized administration of mental health questionnaires in a nonpatient sample of 245 found paper-and-pencil internal consistency ranging from .40 (Hostility) to .95 (Psychoneuroticism). Test-retest over a 1-week interval yielded coefficients from .78 (Hostility) to .90 (Phobic Anxiety; Wijndaele et al., 2007).

Validity. Convergent validity of the SCL-90-R has been validated by multiple studies comparing its dimensions with other psychological measures. It has been correlated with appropriate MMPI-2 scales (Green, Handel, & Archer, 2006), and its Depression dimension has been correlated with depression inventories such as the Inventory for Depressive Symptomatology–Self-Rated (IDS-SR; $r = .84$; Corruble, Legrand, Duret, Charles, & Guelfi, 1999; Rush, Gullion, Basco, & Jarrett, 1996) and the Beck Depression Inventory ($r = .80$; Peveler & Fairburn, 1990). It has also been found to perform well in predicting comorbid psychiatric disorders with alcoholism (Benjamin, Mossman, Graves, & Sanders, 2006).

Norms. The SCL-90-R provides four normative groups for comparison. Table 1.3 presents demographic data for the normative groups. Detailed normative data can be found in Derogatis (1994).

Table 1.3 Demographic Data for SCL-90-R Normative Samples

Population	n	Male	Female	Ethnic/Socioeconomic Profile
Norm A: Psychiatric outpatients	1,002	425	577	Approximately 67% White Skewed towards low socioeconomic status (SES)
Norm B: Nonpatients	1,000	494	480	Stratified random sample from a large U.S. eastern state
Norm C: Psychiatric in patients	313	1/3	2/3	55.7% White 43.6% Black. 7% other
Norm D: Nonpatient adolescents	806	40%	60%	Primarily middle-class Whites

SOURCE: Derogatis (1994). Copyright ©1994 by National Computer Systems.

Availability. The SCL-90-R is published by National Computer Systems, Inc. All materials can be purchased at www.pearsonassessments.com. The purchaser must submit a Test User Qualification Form (http://ags.pearsonassessments.com/assessments/test_user_form2.asp). User qualification for the SCL-90-R is level M on its Web site, which includes a specialized degree in the health care field and a licensure or certification, or proof of a granted right to administer tests. The manual and five test booklets are about $47.00.

Limitations. Groth-Marnat (2003) suggested that the SCL-90-R not be regarded as a measurement of personality but more as a measure of current symptoms. While Derogatis and Cleary (1977) found evidence of "theoretical-empirical" agreement, or construct validity, in almost all of the scales, others have suggested that this measure be used as an overall indicator of distress because of concerns with its divergent validity and factor structure (Cyr, McKenna-Foley, & Peacock, 1985; Rauter, Leonard, & Swett, 1996; Vassend & Skrondal, 1999). Many factor-analytic studies attempting to replicate the original nine-factor model of the SCL-90-R have failed, generally reporting fewer factors (many reported only one large factor) as well as factors that are different from the original nine (e.g., Bonynge, 1993; Rauter et al., 1996; Vassend & Skrondal, 1999). Despite problems with factor structure, Rief and Fichter (1992) found that the average hit rate for distinguishing between patients with dysthymia, anxiety disorders, and anorexia nervosa was 67%. Peveler and Fairburn (1990) found the Global Severity Index (GSI) score sensitivity to be 77% and the specificity to be 91% for detecting the presence of bulimia.

Research Applications. Mills and Andrianopoulos (1993) used the SCL-90-R to evaluate obese patients in outpatient treatment and found that patients with early or childhood-onset obesity showed more psychopathology than those who developed obesity later in life ($r = -.40$). Ro et al. (2005) found decreases in SCL-90-R-measured psychopathology after 2 years of treatment for eating disorders. These studies used the GSI to measure an overall level of psychopathology. The GSI is perhaps the most useful global index of the SCL-90-R. It is a combined measure of the severity or extent of all psychiatric distress symptoms, yielding one number that summarizes the test. If the assertion is true that the test measures only one large factor and is best used to assess general distress, then it appears as though the GSI score will be sufficient. Generally, a GSI T-score above 63 is evidence of a clinically significant level of psychopathology (Groth-Marnat, 2003).

State-Trait Anxiety Inventory

The concept of state versus trait was discussed earlier in this chapter—specifically, that it is important to distinguish between the two to assess personality accurately. Cattell and Scheier (1961) initially proposed the idea of differentiating between a state form and a trait form of anxiety. Thereafter, a host of research followed (e.g., Hodges & Spielberger, 1969; Johnson, 1968; Johnson & Spielberger, 1968). These studies generally administered a test of state anxiety (e.g., a checklist of adjectives that the subject fills out based on his or her feeling "at that moment" or physiological measures such as monitoring heart rate and blood pressure) and a test of trait anxiety (e.g., Taylor Manifest Anxiety Scale [TMAS]; Taylor, 1953) before and after a anxiety-provoking situation and found a clear distinction between state and trait anxiety.

The State-Trait Anxiety Inventory (STAI) began as a test with a single set of items with one set of instructions to complete them according to how they felt at the moment (state) and another set of instructions to complete them based on how they generally felt (trait). This was then revised so that the two measures had their own individual items for more accuracy. A final revision took into account psychometrics and a clearer concept of anxiety. The current version of the STAI (Spielberger, 1983) is a 40-item self-report inventory. Twenty items are designated to assess state anxiety and 20 for trait anxiety. Subjects rate items on a 4-point scale from 1 = *not at all* to 4 = *very much so*.

Reliability. Kabacoff, Segal, Hersen, and Van Hasselt (1997) reported an internal consistency coefficient alpha of .92 for the state scale and .90 for trait. Spielberger (1983) reported trait anxiety test-retest reliability for college students ranged from .73 to .86. Coefficients for state anxiety ranged from .36 (females) to .51 (males). This difference is expected given that state anxiety was designed to assess fluctuating states.

Validity. Tanaka-Matsumi and Kameoka (1986) established convergent validity by finding correlations between the STAI and the Zung Self-Rating Anxiety Scale (Zung, 1971) to be .60 for state and .69 for trait anxiety. Correlations with the TMAS (Taylor, 1953) were .53 for state and .79 for trait anxiety. On the other hand, the study did not have evidence for divergent validity. Correlations between the STAI and depression inventories such as the Beck Depression Inventory and Zung Self-Rating Depression Scale (Zung, 1965) were also high, with correlations ranging from .60 to .61 for state anxiety and .73 to .74 for trait anxiety. However, studies of geriatric patients did find that patients with anxiety disorders scored higher on the STAI than did normal controls (Kabacoff et al., 1997; Stanley, Beck, & Zebb, 1996).

Norms. The STAI has a number of normative samples for comparison, including employees of the Federal Aviation Administration, military recruits, university students, and high school students. Detailed normative data can be found in Spielberger (1983).

Availability. The STAI is published by Mind Garden, Inc. All materials can be purchased on its Web site at www.mindgarden.com. There is no qualification requirement to purchase the materials. The manual and a package of 25 inventory booklets are $30.00 each.

Limitations. Psychometric analysis has credited the STAI with the ability to distinguish between state and trait anxiety. However, its ability to assess the anxiety construct alone as it was designed has been questioned. As a long line of research has suggested, depression and anxiety are highly correlated and often comorbid conditions, and differentiating the two constructs is difficult (Clark & Watson, 1991; Lovibond & Lovibond, 1995; Watson, 2000). As was mentioned above, the STAI has been correlated with measures of depression. Bieling, Antony, and Swinson (1998) studied the structure of the STAI and found that it measured not only anxiety but depression and other negative affects as well. Although effective in discriminating between state and trait anxiety, this instrument should be used with the awareness that it may be assessing constructs other than pure anxiety.

Research Application. Matos et al. (2002) found that binge-eating disorder (BED) was more frequent in obese individuals with high trait anxiety than moderate trait anxiety. Other studies using the STAI have found that individuals with eating disorders generally score higher than controls on both the state and trait scales (Mizes, 1988; Pollice, Kaye, Greeno, & Weltzin, 1997; Wagner et al., 2006). Even after treatment, elevated anxiety continued to be found in bulimics (Stein et al., 2002) and anorexics (Wagner et al., 2006). The STAI also helps to associate certain behaviors with either state or trait anxiety. Weltzin, Bulik, McConaha, and Kaye (1995) studied anxiety in bulimics and found that patients who abused laxatives scored higher on the state scale than those who did not, but not on the trait scale.

Profile of Mood States

The Profile of Mood States (POMS; McNair, Lorr, & Droppleman, 1992) is a 65-item self-report inventory that was designed to measures transient or fluctuating mood states. It is often used in clinical, medical, and counseling settings to track treatment changes. Items are affective adjectives (e.g., lively) rated on a 5-point scale from 0 = *not at all* to 4 = *extremely,* referring to how participants have been feeling during the past week, including the day of the test. It identifies six different mood dimensions: tension-anxiety, depression-rejection, anger-hostility, vigor-activity, fatigue-inertia, and confusion-bewilderment. Each dimension consists of 7 to 15 adjectives, which are summed to obtain a score for each dimension.

Reliability. McNair et al. (1992) reported good internal consistency of coefficient alphas ranging from .84 or greater (vigor-activity and confusion-bewilderment) to above .90 for all of the other dimensions. Test-retest reliability over a 20-day interval ranged from .65 to .74. In another study, Salinsky, Storzbach, Dodrill, and Binder (2001) administered the POMS to 72 healthy participants. Test-retest correlations over a 12- to 16-week interval ranged from .39 (Fatigue) to .77 (Confusion).

Validity. McNair et al. (1992) have found the POMS to be significantly correlated with depression and anxiety. Malouff, Schutte, and Ramerth (1985) administered the POMS Depression Scale and the Beck Depression Inventory to 131 adult participants and found a correlation of .81. Nyenhuis, Yamamoto, Luchetta, Terrien, and Parmentier (1999) also found a significant correlation of .69 between the two. Correlation between the POMS Tense Scale and the State-Trait Anxiety Inventory State scale was .72, and the Trait scale was .70 (Nyenhuis et al., 1999). Constructs that were not expected to correlate with each other indeed did not (see Nyenhuis et al., 1999).

Norms. The normative sample was 1,000 outpatients. Normative data are available in McNair et al. (1992). Nyenhuis et al. (1999) developed normative data for nonpatients and a geriatric sample. In the adult sample (*n* = 400), mean scores and standard deviations for women are as follows: Tension, *M* = 8.2, *SD* = 6.0; Depression, *M* = 8.5, *SD* = 9.4; Anger, *M* = 8.0, *SD* = 7.5; Vigor, *M* = 18.9, *SD* = 6.5; Fatigue, *M* = 8.7, *SD* = 6.1; and Confusion, *M* = 5.8, *SD* = 4.6. For men, scores are as follows: Tension, *M* = 7.1, *SD* = 5.8; Depression, *M* = 7.5, *SD* = 9.2; Anger, *M* = 7.1, *SD* = 7.3; Vigor, *M* = 19.8, *SD* = 6.8; Fatigue, *M* = 7.3, *SD* = 5.7; and Confusion, *M* = 5.6, *SD* = 4.1.

Availability. The POMS is published by Multi-Health Systems, Inc., and test materials can be purchased on its Web site at www.mhs.com. Purchasers must complete a Purchaser Qualification

Form at the MHS Web site. Qualifications require that the user has completed graduate-level courses in tests and measurement or documented equivalent training. The POMS standard kit, including a technical manual and 25 POMS Standard Quikscore Forms, is $55.00.

Limitations. Lower test-retest correlations may seem a problem, but since the POMS was designed to assess changing mood states, the test-retest correlation is not expected to be high. The sensitivity of the POMS has been questioned by some researchers. Spielberger (1972) suggested that POMS is helpful in assessing relatively persistent mood states. Other researches indicate that the sensitivity of the POMS may depend on the initial mood state at the baseline of an intervention (Cramer, Nieman, & Lee, 1991; Nieman, Custer, Butterworth, Utter, & Henson, 2000).

Research Application. The POMS is frequently used for keeping track of mood changes during intervention of obesity or eating disorders. Carels, Berger, and Darby (2006) studied postmenopausal, obese, sedentary women and found lower scores in the Tension, Depression, Anger, and Confusion dimensions after graded exercise. Melanson, Dell'Olio, Carpenter, and Angelopoulos (2004) also found changes in POMS scores in obese adults after exercise counseling on the Depression, Vigor, Fatigue, and Confusion dimensions. On the other hand, Nieman et al. (2000) did not find any mood states difference in their study on obese women. The POMS has also been used to measure the effects of certain stimuli on eating moods such as sugar (Reid & Hammersley, 1998) and stress (Malkoff, 1996).

Millon Clinical Multiaxial Inventory–Third Edition

The Millon Clinical Multiaxial Inventory–Third Edition (MCMI-III; Millon, 1994) was developed on a theoretical foundation established by the author (Choca, 2004), unlike many other empirically derived measures reviewed here (e.g., MMPI-2, SCL-90-R). It is a 175-item, true-false self-report inventory with 24 clinical scales clustered into six groups: Validity scale, modifying indices, personality style scales, severe personality scales, clinical syndrome scales, and severe clinical syndrome scales.

Reliability. Test-retest reliability for the MCMI-III, based on the standardization sample, ranged from .82 (Debasement of the modifying indices) to .90 (Somatoform of the clinical syndrome scales). The manual also presents internal consistency coefficient alphas ranging from .66 (Compulsive of the personality style scales) to .90 (Major Depression of the severe clinical syndrome scales). Other studies, however, reported lower internal consistency (R. J. Craig & Olson, 1998; Hyer, Brandsma, Boyd, & Millon, 1997). Hyer et al. (1997) reported a coefficient alpha of .54 for the Posttraumatic Stress scale.

Validity. The Validity scale of the MCMI-III was designed to detect whether test answers were valid enough for proper interpretation. Schoenberg, Dorr, and Morgan (2006) examined whether the MCMI-III could differentiate student dissimulators from psychiatric patients and found an overall hit rate of 76% to 77%. Another test studied whether the MCMI-III could detect random responding and found that 50% of examinees who respond randomly will go undetected (Charter & Lopez, 2002). Since the MCMI-III has been viewed as very similar to the

MMPI-2, many studies have compared the two scales and found generally good convergent validity (Egger, De Mey, Derksen, & van der Staak, 2003; Rossi, Van den Brande, Tobac, Sloore, & Hauben, 2003).

Norms. The developmental sample for the MCMI-III consisted of 600 individuals: 86% were White, 9% African American, 3% Hispanic, and 1% other. The standardized sample was 1,079 psychiatric patients (see Millon, 1994).

Availability. The MCMI-III is published by National Computer Systems, Inc. All materials can be purchased through Pearson Assessments via its Web site at www.pearsonassessments.com. The purchaser must submit a Test User Qualification Form (http://ags.pearsonassessments .com/assessments/test_user_form2.asp). User qualification for the MCMI-III is coded as a level 3 on its Web site, which includes having a licensure to practice psychology independently, being a full member of the American Psychological Association or the National Association of School Psychologists, having a doctoral or master's degree that provided training, or having proof that the individual has been granted permission to administer the test. The manual and 10 test booklets total about $82.00.

Limitations. The divergent validity of the MCMI-III has been found problematic with the Anxiety scale. Blais et al. (2003) found it to be more highly correlated with measures of depression such as the BDI ($r = .56$) and the Hamilton Rating Scale for Depression (HAM-D; $r = .53$) versus a measure of anxiety, the HAM-A ($r = .42$). Góngora (2006) compared the diagnostic accuracy of the MCMI-III and the Structural Clinical Interview II (SCID-II) for personality disorders in patients with bulimia. The study found that the prevalence rate for personality disorders was similar using both instruments (68% for SCID-II and 67.2% for MCMI-III), but the personality disorders diagnosed were different. Furthermore, the fact that the MCMI was developed on a theoretical basis may raise concerns about its empirical properties. It has frequently been compared and contrasted to the MMPI, a solidly empirical instrument. For more information, see Choca (2004), who discusses the advantages and disadvantages of each instrument.

Research Application. The MCMI-III is a relatively new version and has not been used extensively in assessing obesity and eating disorders. S. E. Craig (1997) differentiated eating disorder and personality types with the MCMI-III and reported that anorexics with the restricting subtype and anorexic bulimics tend to display Passive Aggressive, Depressive, Paranoid, Schizoid, and Self-Defeating personality patterns, while bulimics tend to display Histrionic and Narcissistic personality patterns. The MCMI-III has also been used to evaluate the role of relationship attachment to obesity (Marsh, 2006).

Closing Comments and Suggestions

Significant progress has been made over the past century that is allowing us a much better understanding of the population with weight and eating concerns. Research has established some general personality profiles and psychopathology that manifest repeatedly in this group (e.g., perfectionism, obsessiveness). These findings allude to areas where clinicians can begin to focus on when treating these individuals. However, research in this area still has a long way to go and many difficulties to overcome. The assessment instruments mentioned have been invaluable in our advancement so far, but improvements in validity are necessary to further clarify and pinpoint problem areas. Furthermore, researchers should take into account more often the heterogeneity of persons with eating and weight disorders. Eating concerns aside, this group is as diverse as any other population. The appropriate comparison groups will yield priceless information. Past research has been mostly correlational, giving an idea of associations between certain personalities and eating disorders. Now that those certain traits have been established to be prevalent in this population, future research should aim to uncover the direction of causality or at least begin to disentangle the complex relationship between personality, psychopathology, and eating/weight disorders.

References

Acklin, M. W., McDowell, C. J., II, Verschell, M. S., & Chan, D. (2000). Interobserver agreement, intraobserver reliability, and the Rorschach Comprehensive System. *Journal of Personality Assessment, 74*(1), 15–47.

Adams, H. E., & Cassidy, J. F. (1993). The classification of abnormal behavior. In P. B. Sutker & H. E. Adams (Eds.), *Comprehensive handbook of psychopathology* (2nd ed., p. 7). New York: Plenum.

Ames-Frankel, J., Devlin, M. J., Walsh, B. T., Strasser, T. J., Sadik, C., Oldham, J. M., et al. (1992). Personality disorder diagnoses in patients with bulimia nervosa: Clinical correlates and changes with treatment. *Journal of Clinical Psychiatry, 53*(3), 90–96.

Arnau, R. C., Meagher, M. W., Norris, M. P., & Bramson, R. (2001). Psychometric evaluation of the Beck Depression Inventory-II with primary care medical patients. *Health Psychology, 20*(2), 112–119.

Barker-Collo, S. L. (2003). Culture and validity of the Symptom Checklist-90-Revised and Profile of Mood States in a New Zealand student sample. *Cultural Diversity & Ethnic Minority Psychology, 9*(2), 185–196.

Barthlow, D. L., Graham, J. R., Ben-Porath, Y. S., & McNulty, J. L. (1999). Incremental validity of the MMPI-2 content scales in an outpatient mental health setting. *Psychological Assessment, 11*(1), 39–47.

Bathurst, K., Gottfried, A. W., & Gottfried, A. E. (1997). Normative data for the MMPI-2 in child custody litigation. *Psychological Assessment, 9*(3), 205–211.

Bayon, C., Hill, K., Svrakic, D. M., Przybeck, T. R., & Cloninger, C. R. (1996). Dimensional assessment of personality in an out-patient sample: Relations of the systems of Millon and Cloninger. *Journal of Psychiatric Research, 30,* 341–352.

Beck, A. T., & Steer, R. A. (1993). *Manual for the Beck Depression Inventory.* San Antonio, TX: Psychological Corporation.

Beck, A. T., Steer, R. A., Ball, R., & Ranieri, W. (1996). Comparison of Beck Depression Inventories -IA and -II in psychiatric outpatients. *Journal of Personality Assessment, 67,* 588–597.

Beck, A. T., Steer, R. A., & Brown, G. K. (1996). *Beck Depression Inventory—Second Edition Manual.* San Antonio, TX: Psychological Corporation.

Beck, A. T., Ward, C. H., Mendelson, M., Mock, J., & Erbaugh, J. (1961). An inventory for measuring depression. *Archives of General Psychiatry, 4,* 561–571.

Benjamin, A. B., Mossman, D., Graves, N. S., & Sanders, R. D. (2006). Tests of a symptom checklist to screen for comorbid psychiatric disorders in alcoholism. *Comprehensive Psychiatry, 47*(3), 227–233.

Ben-Porath, Y. S., & Butcher, J. N. (1989). The comparability of MMPI and MMPI-2 scales and profiles. *Psychological Assessment, 1,* 345–347.

Bieling, P. J., Antony, M. M., & Swinson, R. P. (1998). The Stait-Trait Anxiety Inventory, Trait version: Structure and content re-examined. *Behaviour Research and Therapy, 36,* 777–788.

Blais, M. A., Holdwick, D. J., Jr., McLean, R. Y. S., Otto, M. W., Pollack, M. H., & Hilsenroth, M. J. (2003). Exploring the psychometric properties and construct validity of the MCMI-III anxiety and avoidant personality scales. *Journal of Personality Assessment, 81,* 237–241.

Bloks, H., Hoek, H. W., Callewaert, I., & van Furth, E. (2004). Stability of personality traits in patients who received intensive treatment for a severe eating disorder. *Journal of Nervous and Mental Disease, 192*(2), 129–138.

Blouin, A. G., Blouin, J. H., Iversen, H., Carter, J., Goldstein, C., Goldfield, G., et al. (1996). Light therapy in bulimia nervosa: a double-blind, placebo-controlled study. *Psychiatry Research, 60*(1), 1–9.

Bonynge, E. R. (1993). Unidimensionality of the SLC-90-R scales in adult and adolescent crises samples. *Journal of Consulting Psychology, 49,* 212–215.

Bornstein, R. F., & Greenberg, R. P. (1991). Dependency and eating disorders in female psychiatric inpatients. *Journal of Nervous and Mental Disease, 179*(3), 148–152.

Bornstein, S. R., Schuppenies, A., Wong, M. L., & Licinio, J. (2006). Approaching the shared biology of obesity and depression: The stress axis as the locus of gene-environment interactions. *Molecular Psychiatry, 11,* 892–902.

Bravata, E. A., Storch, E. A., & Storch, J. B. (2003). Correlations among symptoms of depression and problematic eating patterns in intercollegiate athletes. *Psychological Reports, 93,* 1243–1246.

Bruch, H. (1973). *Eating disorders: Obesity, anorexia, and the person within.* New York: Basic Books.

Butcher, J. N. (2004). Personality assessment without borders: Adaptation of the MMPI-2 across cultures. *Journal of Personality Assessment, 83*(2), 90–104.

Butcher, J. N., Cheung, F. M., & Kim, J. (2003). Use of the MMPI-2 with Asian populations. *Psychological Assessment, 15,* 248–256.

Butcher, J. N., Dahlstrom, W. G., Graham, J. R., Tellegen, A., & Kaemmer, B. (1989). *MMPI-2 manual for administration and scoring.* Minneapolis: University of Minnesota Press.

Butcher, J. N., Graham, J. R., Ben-Porath, Y. S., Tellegen, A., Dahlstrom, W. G., & Kaemmer, B. (2001). *MMPI-2: Manual for administration, scoring and interpretation* (Rev. ed.). Minneapolis: University of Minnesota Press.

Byrnes, J. P., Miller, D. C., & Schafer, W. D. (1999). Gender differences in risk taking: A meta-analysis. *Psychological Bulletin, 125,* 367–383.

Cahill, S., & Mussap, A. J. (2007). Emotional reactions following exposure to idealized bodies predict unhealthy body change attitudes and behaviors in women and men. *Journal of Psychosomatic Research, 62,* 631–639.

Camara, W. J., Nathan, J. S., & Puente, A. E. (2000). Psychological test usage: Implications in professional psychology. *Professional Psychology: Research and Practice, 31*(2), 141–154.

Carels, R. A., Berger, B., & Darby, L. (2006). The association between mood states and physical activity in postmenopausal, obese, sedentary women. *Journal of Aging & Physical Activity, 14*(1), 12–28.

Casper, R. C., Hedeker, D., & McClough, J. F. (1992). Personality dimensions in eating disorders and their relevance for subtyping. *Journal of the American Academy of Child & Adolescent Psychiatry, 31,* 830–840.

Cassin, S. E., & von Ranson, K. M. (2005). Personality and eating disorders: A decade in review. *Clinical Psychology Review, 25,* 895–916.

Cassisi, J. E., & Workman, D. E. (1992). The detection of malingering and deception with a short form of the MMPI-2 based on the L, F, and K scales. *Journal of Clinical Psychology, 48*(1), 54–58.

Cattell, R. B., & Scheier, I. H. (1961). *The meaning and measurement of neuroticism and anxiety.* Oxford, England: Ronald.

Charter, R. A., & Lopez, M. N. (2002). Million Clinical Multiaxial Inventory (MCMI-III): The inability of the validity conditions to detect random responders. *Journal of Clinical Psychology, 58,* 1615–1617.

Cheung, F. M. (2004). Use of Western and indigenously developed personality tests in Asia. *Applied Psychology: An International Review, 53*(2), 173–191.

Choca, J. P. (2004). *Interpretive guide to the Millon Clinical Multiaxial Inventory* (3rd ed.). Washington, DC: American Psychological Association.

Clark, L. A., & Watson, D. (1991). Tripartite model of anxiety and depression: Psychometric evidence and taxonomic implications. *Journal of Abnormal Psychology, 100,* 316–336.

Cloninger, C. R. (1987). A systematic method for clinical description and classification of personality variants: A proposal. *Archives of General Psychiatry, 44,* 573–588.

Cloninger, C. R., Przybeck, T. R., Svrakic, D. M., & Wetzel, R. D. (1994). *The temperament and character inventory (TCI): A guide to its development and use.* St. Louis, MO: Washington University.

Cloninger, C. R., Svrakic, D. M., & Przybeck, T. R. (1993). A psychobiological model of temperament and character. *Archives of General Psychiatry, 50*, 975–990.

Cooper, P. J. (1995). Eating disorders and their relationship to mood and anxiety disorders. In K. D. Brownell & C. G. Fairburn (Eds.), *Eating disorders and obesity: A comprehensive handbook* (pp. 159–164). New York: Guildford.

Comer, R. J. (2005). *Fundamentals of abnormal psychology* (4th ed.). New York: Worth.

Corruble, E., Legrand, J. M., Duret, C., Charles, G., & Guelfi, J. D. (1999). IDS-C and IDS-SR: Psychometric properties in depressed in-patients. *Journal of Affective Disorders, 56*(2–3), 95–101.

Costa, P. T., & McCrae, R. R. (1992). *Professional manual: Revised NEO Personality Inventory (NEO-PI-R) and NEO Five-Factor Inventory (NEO-FFI).* Odessa, FL: Psychological Assessment Resources.

Craig, R. J., & Olson, R. (1998). Stability of the MCMI-III in a substance-abusing inpatient sample. *Psychological Reports, 83*, 1273–1274.

Craig, S. E. (1997). *The comorbidity of eating disorders and substance abuse and their relationship to DSM-IV personality disorders.* Ann Arbor, MI: ProQuest Information & Learning, US.

Cramer, S. R., Nieman, D. C., & Lee, J. W. (1991). The effects of moderate exercise training on psychological well-being and mood state in women. *Journal of Psychosomatic Research, 35*(4–5), 437–449.

Cumella, E. J., Wall, A. D., & Kerr-Almeida, N. (2000). MMPI-2 in the inpatient assessment of women with eating disorders. *Journal of Personality Assessment, 75*, 387–403.

Cyr, J. J., McKenna-Foley, J. M., & Peacock, E. (1985). Factor Structure of the SCL-90-R: Is there one? *Journal of Personality Assessment, 49*, 571–578.

Dahlstrom, W. G., & Archer, R. P. (2000). A shortened version of the MMPI-2. *Assessment, 7*(2), 131–137.

Dana, R. H. (1996). Culturally competent assessment practice in the United States. *Journal of Personality Assessment, 66*, 472–487.

Dana, R. H., Aponte, J. F., & Wohl, J. (2000). *Psychological assessment in the diagnosis and treatment of ethnic group members.* Needham Heights, MA: Allyn & Bacon.

Derogatis, L. R. (1994). *SCL-90-R: Symptom Checklist-90-RL Administration scoring and procedures manual.* Minneapolis: National Computer Systems.

Derogatis, L. R., & Cleary, P. A. (1977). Confirmation of the dimensional structure of the SCL-90: A study in construct validation. *Journal of Clinical Psychology, 33*, 981–989.

Derogatis, L. R., Lipman, R. S., Rickels, K., Uhlenhuth, E. H., & Covi, L. (1974). The Hopkins Symptom Checklist (HSCL): A self-report symptom inventory. *Behavioral Science, 19*(1), 1–15.

Derogatis, L. R., Savitz, K. L., & Maruish, M. E. (1999). *The SCL-90-R, Brief Symptom Inventory, and Matching Clinical Rating Scales.* Mahwah, NJ: Lawrence Erlbaum.

Duijsens, I. J., Spinhoven, P., Goekoop, J. G., Spermon, T., & Eurelings-Bontekoe, E. H. M. (2000). The Dutch Temperament and Character Inventory (TCI): Dimensional structure, reliability and validity in a normal and psychiatric outpatient sample. *Personality and Individual Differences, 28*, 487–499.

Egger, J., De Mey, H., Derksen, J., & van der Staak, C. (2003). MMPI-2 and MCMI-III scores among Dutch inpatient substance abusers: Assessing correspondence and cross-cultural equivalence. *Current Psychology: Developmental, Learning, Personality, Social, 22*(2), 117–124.

Eipe, A. (2005). *A comparison of women in weight loss programs: Differences between those with binge eating disorder and without binge eating disorder on familial, peer, and affective factors.* Ann Arbor, MI: ProQuest Information & Learning, US.

Elfhag, K., Barkeling, B., Carlsson, A. M., & Rossner, S. (2003). Microstructure of eating behavior associated with Rorschach characteristics in obesity. *Journal of Personality Assessment, 81*(1), 40–50.

Elfhag, K., Carlsson, A. M., & Rossner, S. (2003). Subgrouping in obesity based on Rorschach personality characteristics. *Scandinavian Journal of Psychology, 44*, 399–407.

Elfhag, K., Rossner, S., & Carlsson, A. M. (2004). Degree of body weight in obesity and Rorschach personality aspects of mental distress. *Eating and Weight Disorders, 9*(1), 35–43.

Exner, J. E., Jr. (1991). *The Rorschach: A comprehensive system: Vol. 2. Interpretation* (2nd ed.). Oxford, England: John Wiley.

Exner, J. E., Jr. (1993). *The Rorschach: A comprehensive system: Vol. 1. Basic foundations* (3rd ed.). Oxford, England: John Wiley.

Exner, J. E., Jr. (1996). A comment on "The comprehensive system for the Rorschach: A critical examination." *Psychological Science, 7*(1), 11–13.

Exner, J. E., Jr., & Erdberg, P. (2005). *The Rorschach: A comprehensive system* (3rd ed.). Hoboken, NJ: John Wiley.

Exner, J. E., Jr., & Weiner, I. B. (1995). *The Rorschach: A comprehensive system, Vol. 3. Assessment of children and adolescents* (2nd ed.). Oxford, England: John Wiley.

Fassino, S., Abbate-Daga, G., Leombruni, P., Amianto, F., Rovera, G., & Rovera, G. G. (2001). Temperament and character in Italian men with anorexia nervosa: A controlled study with the Temperament and Character Inventory. *Journal of Nervous and Mental Disease, 189*, 788–794.

Fassino, S., Leombruni, P., Piero, A., Daga, G. A., Amianto, F., Rovera, G., et al. (2002). Temperament and character in obese women with and without binge eating disorder. *Comprehensive Psychiatry, 43*, 431–437.

Fernández-Aranda, F., Aitken, A., Badía, A., Giménez, L., Solano, R., Collier, D., et al. (2004). Personality and psychopathological traits of males with an eating disorder. *European Eating Disorders Review, 12*, 367–374.

Fichter, M. M., & Quadflieg, N. (2000). Comparing self- and expert rating: A self-report screening version (SIAB-S) of the Structured Interview for Anorexic and Bulimic Syndromes for DSM-IV and ICD-10 (SIAB-EX). *European Archives of Psychiatry and Clinical Neuroscience, 250*(4), 175–185.

Fontenelle, L. F., Mendlowicz, M. V., Moreira, R. O., & Appolinario, J. C. (2005). An empirical comparison of atypical bulimia nervosa and binge eating disorder. *Brazilian Journal of Medical and Biological Research, 38*, 1663–1667.

Friedman, M. A., & Brownell, K. D. (1995). Psychological correlates of obesity: Moving to the next research generation. *Psychological Bulletin, 117*(1), 3–20.

Garb, H. N., Wood, J. M., Lilienfeld, S. O., & Nezworski, M. T. (2005). Roots of the Rorschach controversy. *Clinical Psychology Review, 25*(1), 97–118.

Garner, D. M., Olmsted, M. P., Davis, R., Rockert, W., Goldbloom, D., & Eagle, M. (1990). The association between bulimic symptoms and reported psychopathology. *International Journal of Eating Disorders, 9*(1), 1–15.

Gass, C. S., & Gonzalez, C. (2003). MMPI-2 short form proposal: CAUTION. *Archives of Clinical Neuropsychology, 18*, 521–527.

Gass, C. S., & Luis, C. A. (2001). MMPI-2 Short Form: Psychometric characteristics in a neuropsychological setting. *Assessment, 8*(2), 213–219.

Gaston, M. F., Nelson, W., Hart, K. J., Quatman, G., & Rojdev, R. (1994). The equivalence of the MMPI and MMPI-2. *Assessment, 1*, 415–418.

Gee, A., & Troop, N. A. (2003). Shame, depressive symptoms and eating, weight and shape concerns in a non-clinical sample. *Eating and Weight Disorders, 8*(1), 72–75.

Gleaves, D. H., & Eberenz, K. P. (1995). Correlates of dissociative symptoms among women with eating disorders. *Journal of Psychiatric Research, 29*, 417–426.

Godt, K. (2002). Personality disorders and eating disorders: The prevalence of personality disorders in 176 female outpatients with eating disorders. *European Eating Disorders Review, 10*(2), 102–109.

Góngora, V. (2006). Personality disorders in bulimic patients: A comparative study between MCMI-III and SCID-II interview. *Acta Psiquiátrica y Psicológica de America Latina, 52*(3), 157–163.

Goodwin, R. D., & Gotlib, I. H. (2004). Gender differences in depression: The role of personality factors. *Psychiatry Research, 126*(2), 135–142.

Graham, J. R. (1990). *MMPI-2: Assessing personality and psychopathology.* New York: Oxford University Press.

Grave, R. D., Calugi, S., Brambilla, F., Abbate-Daga, G., Fassino, S., & Marchesini, G. (2007). The effect of inpatient cognitive-behavioral therapy for eating disorders on temperament and character. *Behaviour Research and Therapy, 45*, 1335–1344.

Green, B. A., Handel, R. W., & Archer, R. P. (2006). External correlates of the MMPI-2 content component scales in mental health inpatients. *Assessment, 13*(1), 80–97.

Gronnerod, C. (2003). Temporal stability in the Rorschach method: A meta-analytic review. *Journal of Personality Assessment, 80*, 272–293.

Groth-Marnat, G. (2003). *Handbook of psychological assessment* (4th ed.). Hoboken, NJ: John Wiley.

Gutiérrez, F., Torrens, M., Boget, T., Martín-Santos, R., Sangorrín, J., Pérez, G., et al. (2001). Psychometric properties of the Temperament and Character Inventory (TCI) questionnaire in a Spanish psychiatric population. *Acta Psychiatrica Scandinavica, 103*, 143–147.

Hamilton, M. (1960). A rating scale for depression. *Journal of Neurology, Neurosurgery, and Psychiatry, 23*, 56–62.

Harrell, T. H., Honaker, L., & Parnell, T. (1992). Equivalence of the MMPI-2 with the MMPI in psychiatric patients. *Psychological Assessment, 4,* 460–465.

Hathaway, S. R., & McKinley, J. C. (1942). *The Minnesota Multiphasic Personality Schedule.* Minneapolis: University of Minnesota Press.

Helmes, E., & Reddon, J. R. (1993). A perspective on developments in assessing psychopathology: A critical review of the MMPI and MMPI-2. *Psychological Bulletin, 113,* 453–471.

Hessel, A., Schumacher, J., Geye, M., & Brähler, E. (2001). Symptom-Checklist SCL-90-R: Validation and standardization based on a representative sample of the German population [in German with English summary]. *Diagnostica, 47,* 27–39.

Hill, J., Harrington, R., Fudge, H., & Rutter, M. (1989). Adult Personality Functioning Assessment (APFA): An investigatory-based standardised interview. *British Journal of Psychiatry, 155,* 24–35.

Hodges, W. F., & Spielberger, C. D. (1969). Digit span: An indicant of trait or state anxiety? *Journal of Consulting and Clinical Psychology, 33,* 430–434.

Horvath, P. (1992). The MMPI-2 considered in the contexts of personality theory, external validity, and clinical utility. *Canadian Psychology Psychologie Canadienne, 33*(1), 79–83.

Hudson, J. I., Pope, H. G., Jr., Jonas, J. M., & Yurgelun-Todd, D. (1983). Phenomenologic relationship of eating disorders to major affective disorder. *Psychiatry Research, 9,* 345–354.

Hyer, L., Brandsma, J., Boyd, S., & Millon, T. (1997). *The MCMIs and posttraumatic stress disorder.* New York: Guilford.

Hyler, S. E., & Rieder, R. O. (1987). *Personality Disorder Questionnaire—Revised.* New York: New York State Psychiatric Institute.

Jiménez-Murcia, S., Fernández-Aranda, F., Raich, R. M., Alonso, P., Krug, I., Jaurrieta, N., et al. (2007). Obsessive-compulsive and eating disorders: Comparison of clinical and personality features. *Psychiatry and Clinical Neurosciences, 61,* 385–391.

Johnson, D. T. (1968). The effects of interview stress on measure of state and trait anxiety. *Journal of Abnormal Psychology, 73,* 245–251.

Johnson, D. T., & Spielberger, C. D. (1968). The effects of relaxation training and the passage of time on measures of state- and trait-anxiety. *J Clinical Psychology, 24*(1), 20–23.

Joiner, T. E., Jr., Katz, J., & Heatherton, T. F. (2000). Personality features differentiate late adolescent females and males with chronic bulimic symptoms. *International Journal of Eating Disorders, 27*(2), 191–197.

Kabacoff, R. I., Segal, D. L., Hersen, M., & Van Hasselt, V. B. (1997). Psychometric properties and diagnostic utility of the Beck Anxiety Inventory and the State-Trait Anxiety Inventory with older adult psychiatric outpatients. *Journal of Anxiety Disorders, 11*(1), 33–47.

Kennedy, S. H., McVey, G., & Katz, R. (1990). Personality disorders in anorexia nervosa and bulimia nervosa. *Journal of Psychiatry Research, 24,* 259–269.

Keys, A., Brozek, J., Henschel, A., Mickelsen, O., & Taylor, H. L. (1950). *The biology of human starvation* (2 vols). Oxford, UK: University of Minnesota Press.

Klinger, W. R. (2000). *The MMPI-2: A predictor of success in weight loss among the obese.* Philadelphia: Pennsylvania State University.

Klump, K. L., Bulik, C. M., Pollice, C., Halmi, K. A., Fichter, M. M., Berrettini, W. H., et al. (2000). Temperament and character in women with anorexia nervosa. *Journal of Nervous and Mental Disease, 188,* 559–567.

Klump, K. L., Strober, M., Bulik, C. M., Thornton, L., Johnson, C., Devlin, B., et al. (2004). Personality characteristics of women before and after recovery from an eating disorder. *Psychological Medicine, 34,* 1407–1418.

Kowalski, R., & Westen, D. (2005). *Psychology* (4th ed.). Hoboken, NJ: John Wiley.

Krefetz, D. G., Steer, R. A., Gulab, N. A., & Beck, A. T. (2002). Convergent validity of the Beck Depression Inventory-II with the Reynolds Adolescent Depression Scale in psychiatric inpatients. *Journal of Personality Assessment, 78,* 451–460.

Leichtman, M. (1996). The nature of the Rorschach task. *Journal of Personality Assessment, 67,* 478–493.

Lilienfeld, S. O., Wood, J. M., & Garb, H. N. (2000). The scientific status of projective techniques. *Psychological Science in the Public Interest, 1*(2), 27–66.

Loeb, K. L., Pike, K. M., Walsh, B. T., & Wilson, G. T. (1994). Assessment of diagnostic features of bulimia nervosa: Interview versus self-report format. *International Journal of Eating Disorders, 16*(1), 75–81.

Lore, R., Gottdiener, C., & Delahunty, M. J. (1986). Lean and mean rats: Some effects of acute changes in the food supply upon territorial aggression. *Aggressive Behavior, 12*, 409–415.

Lovibond, P. F., & Lovibond, S. H. (1995). The structure of negative emotional states: Comparison of the Depression Anxiety Stress Scales (DASS) with the Beck Depression and Anxiety Inventories. *Behaviour Research and Therapy, 33*, 335–343.

Lucio, E., Ampudia, A., Duran, C., Leon, I., & Butcher, J. N. (2001). Comparison of the Mexican and American norms of the MMPI-2. *Journal of Clinical Psychology, 57*, 1459–1468.

Maddi, S. R., Fox, S. R., Khoshaba, D. M., Harvey, R. H., Lu, J. L., & Persico, M. (2001). Reduction in psychopathology following bariatric surgery for morbid obesity. *Obesity Surgery: The Official Journal of the American Society for Bariatric Surgery and of the Obesity Surgery Society of Australia and New Zealand, 11*, 680–685.

Maier, W., Lichtermann, D., Minges, J. R., & Heun, R. (1992). Personality traits in subjects at risk for unipolar major depression: A family study perspective. *Journal of Affective Disorders, 24*(3), 153–163.

Malkoff, S. B. (1996). *Cognitive and affective responsivity to psychological stress in obese women with binge eating disorder.* Pittsburgh: University of Pittsburgh.

Malouff, J. M., Schutte, N. S., & Ramerth, W. (1985). Evaluation of a short form of the POMS-Depression scale. *Journal of Clinical Psychology, 41*, 389–391.

Marsh, G. M. (2006). *The role of attachment to obesity and psychopathology.* Ann Arbor, MI: ProQuest Information & Learning, US.

Matos, M. I. R., Aranha, L. S., Faria, A. N., Ferreira, S. R. G., Bacaltchuck, J., & Zanella, M. T. (2002). Binge eating disorder, anxiety, depression and body image in grade III obesity patients. *Revista Brasileira de Psiquiatria, 24*(4), 165–169.

Matz, P. A., Altepeter, T. S., & Perlman, B. (1992). MMPI-2: Reliability with college students. *Journal of Clinical Psychology, 48*, 330–334.

McGrath, R. E., Pogge, D. L., Stokes, J. M., Cragnolino, A., Zaccario, M., Hayman, J., et al. (2005). Field reliability of comprehensive system scoring in an adolescent inpatient sample. *Assessment, 12*(2), 199–209.

McNair, D. M., Lorr, M., & Droppleman, L. F. (1992). *POMS manual.* North Tonawanda, NY: MHS Inc.

Melanson, K. J., Dell'Olio, J., Carpenter, M. R., & Angelopoulos, T. J. (2004). Changes in multiple health outcomes at 12 and 24 weeks resulting from 12 weeks of exercise counseling with or without dietary counseling in obese adults. *Nutrition, 20*, 849–856.

Meyer, G. J. (1997a). Assessing reliability: Critical corrections for a critical examination of the Rorschach Comprehensive System. *Psychological Assessment, 9*, 480–489.

Meyer, G. J. (1997b). Thinking clearly about reliability: More critical corrections regarding the Rorschach Comprehensive System. *Psychological Assessment, 9*, 495–498.

Meyer, G. J., Hilsenroth, M. J., Baxter, D., Exner, J. E., Jr., Fowler, J. C., Piers, C. C., et al. (2002). An examination of interrater reliability for scoring the Rorschach Comprehensive System in eight data sets. *Journal of Personality Assessment, 78*(2), 219–274.

Meyer, G. J., Mihura, J. L., & Smith, B. L. (2005). The interclinician reliability of Rorschach interpretation in four data sets. *Journal of Personality Assessment, 84*, 296–314.

Miettunen, J., Kantojarvi, L., Ekelund, J., Veijola, J., Karvonen, J. T., Peltonen, L., et al. (2004). A large population cohort provides normative data for investigation of temperament. *Acta Psychiatrica Scandinavica, 110*(2), 150–157.

Millon, T. (1994). *Manual for the MCMI-III.* Minneapolis, MN: National Computer Systems.

Mills, J. K., & Andrianopoulos, G. D. (1993). The relationship between childhood onset obesity and psychopathology in adulthood. *Journal of Psychology, 127*, 547–551.

Mizes, J. S. (1988). Personality characteristics of bulimic and non-eating-disordered female controls: A cognitive behavioral perspective. *International Journal of Eating Disorders, 7*, 541–550.

Modestin, J., Erni, T., & Oberson, B. (1998). A comparison of self-report and interview diagnoses of DSM-III-R personality disorders. *European Journal of Personality, 12*, 445–455.

Moore, T. R. (2004). Adolescent and adult obesity in women: A tidal wave just beginning. *Clinical Obstetrics and Gynecology, 47*, 884–889.

Morey, L. C. (1991). *The Personality Assessment Inventory professional manual.* Odessa, FL: Psychological Assessment Resources.

Nieman, D. C., Custer, W. F., Butterworth, D. E., Utter, A. C., & Henson, D. A. (2000). Psychological response to exercise training and/or energy restriction in obese women. *Journal of Psychosomatic Research, 48*(1), 23–29.

Nyenhuis, D. L., Yamamoto, C., Luchetta, T., Terrien, A., & Parmentier, A. (1999). Adult and geriatric normative data and validation of the Profile of Mood States. *Journal of Clinical Psychology, 55*(1), 79–86.

O'Brien, K. M., & Vincent, N. K. (2003). Psychiatric comorbidity in anorexia and bulimia nervosa: Nature, prevalence and causal relationships. *Clinical Psychology Review, 23*(1), 57–74.

Pace, T. M., Robbins, R. R., Choney, S. K., Hill, J. S., Lacey, K., & Blair, G. (2006). A cultural-contextual perspective on the validity of the MMPI-2 with American Indians. *Cultural Diversity & Ethnic Minority Psychology, 12*, 320–333.

Palav, A., Ortega, A., & McCaffrey, R. J. (2001). Incremental validity of the MMPI-2 Content Scales: A preliminary study with brain-injured patients. *Journal of Head Trauma Rehabilitation, 16*, 275–283.

Perry, W. (2003). Let's call the whole thing off: A response to Dawes (2001). *Psychological Assessment, 15*, 582–585.

Peveler, R. C., & Fairburn, C. G. (1990). Measurement of neurotic symptoms by self-report questionnaire: Validity of the SCL-90R. *Psychological Medicine, 20*, 873–879.

Pick, T. (1956). A critique of current methods of Rorschach scoring. *Journal of Projective Techniques, 20*, 318–325.

Picot, A. K., & Lilenfeld, L. R. R. (2003). The relationship among binge severity, personality psychopathology, and body mass index. *International Journal of Eating Disorders, 34*, 98–107.

Plante, T. G., & Rodin, J. (1990). Physical fitness and enhanced psychological health. *Current Psychology: Research and Reviews, 9*, 3–24.

Pollice, C., Kaye, W. H., Greeno, C. G., & Weltzin, T. E. (1997). Relationship of depression, anxiety, and obsessionality to state of illness in anorexia nervosa. *International Journal of Eating Disorders, 21*, 367–376.

Pryor, T., & Wiederman, M. W. (1996). Use of the MMPI-2 in the outpatient assessment of women with anorexia nervosa or bulimia nervosa. *Journal of Personality Assessment, 66*, 363–373.

Puttonen, S., Ravaja, N., & Keltikangas-Jarvinen, L. (2005). Cloninger's temperament dimensions and affective responses to different challenges. *Comprehensive Psychiatry, 46*(2), 128–134.

Ragazzoni, P., & Riva, G. (1996). Personalita e atteggiamento alimentare in un gruppo di soggetti obesi [Personality and eating habits in a sample of obese subjects]. *Minerva Psichiatrica, 37*, 135–140.

Rauter, U. K., Leonard, C. E., & Swett, C. P. (1996). SCL-90–R factor structure in an acute, involuntary, adult psychiatric inpatient sample. *Journal of Clinical Psychology, 52*, 625–629.

Reid, M., & Hammersley, R. (1998). The effects of sugar on subsequent eating and mood in obese and non-obese women. *Psychology, Health & Medicine, 3*, 299–313.

Rejeski, W. J., Lang, W., Neiberg, R. H., Van Dorsten, B., Foster, G. D., Maciejewski, M. L., et al. (2006). Correlates of health-related quality of life in overweight and obese adults with type 2 diabetes. *Obesity, 14*, 870–883.

Richter, P., Werner, J., Heerlein, A. S., Kraus, A., & Sauer, H. (1998). On the validity of the Beck Depression Inventory: A review. *Psychopathology, 31*(3), 160–168.

Rief, W., & Fichter, M. (1992). The Symptom Check List SCL-90–R and its ability to discriminate between dysthymia, anxiety disorders, and anorexia nervosa. *Psychopathology, 25*(3), 128–138.

Riskind, J. H., Beck, A. T., Brown, G., & Steer, R. A. (1987). Taking the measure of anxiety and depression: Validity of reconstructed Hamilton scales. *Journal of Nervous and Mental Disease, 175*, 474–479.

Ro, O., Martinsen, E. W., Hoffart, A., Sexton, H., & Rosenvinge, J. H. (2005). The interaction of personality disorders and eating disorders: A two-year prospective study of patients with long-standing eating disorders. *International Journal of Eating Disorders, 38*(2), 106–111.

Robinson, S., & Winnik, H. Z. (1973). Severe psychotic disturbances following crash diet weight loss. *Archives of General Psychiatry, 29*, 559–562.

Rohles, F. H., Jr., & Wilson, L. M. (1974). Hunger as a catalyst in aggression. *Behaviour, 48*(1–2), 123–130.

Rojdev, R., Nelson, W. M., III, Hart, K. J., & Fercho, M. C. (1994). Criterion-related validity and stability: Equivalence of the MMPI and the MMPI-2. *Journal of Clinical Psychology, 50*, 361–367.

Rorschach, H. (1924). The application of the interpretation of form to psychoanalysis. *Journal of Nervous and Mental Disease, 60,* 359–379.

Rorschach, H. (1942). *Psychodiagnostics: A diagnostic test based on perception* (3rd ed. rev.). Oxford, England: Grune & Stratton. (Original work published 1921)

Rossi, G., Van den Brande, I., Tobac, A., Sloore, H., & Hauben, C. (2003). Convergent validity of the MCMI-III personality disorder scales and the MMPI-2 scales. *Journal of Personality Disorders, 17,* 330–340.

Rowland, C. V., Jr. (1968). Psychotherapy of six hyperobese adults during total starvation. *Archives of General Psychiatry. 18,* 541–548.

Rush, A. J., Gullion, C. M., Basco, M. R., & Jarrett, R. B. (1996). The Inventory of Depressive Symptomatology (IDS): Psychometric properties. *Psychological Medicine, 26,* 477–486.

Rychlak, J. F., & Boland, G. C. (1973). Socioeconomic status and the diagnostic significance of healthy and unhealthy group Rorschach content. *Journal of Personality Assessment, 37,* 411–419.

Ryden, A., Sullivan, M., Torgerson, J. S., Karlsson, J., Lindroos, A. K., & Taft, C. (2003). Severe obesity and personality: A comparative controlled study of personality traits. *International Journal of Obesity & Related Metabolic Disorders: Journal of the International Association for the Study of Obesity, 27,* 1534–1540.

Rydén, O., & Danielsson, A. (1983). Personality features of grossly obese surgical patients: A preoperative study. *Archives for Psychology (Frankfurt), 135*(2), 115–134.

Salinsky, M. C., Storzbach, D., Dodrill, C. B., & Binder, L. M. (2001). Test-retest bias, reliability, and regression equations for neuropsychological measures repeated over a 12–16-week period. *Journal of the International Neuropsychological Society, 7,* 597–605.

Salorio, P., Ruiz, M., Martinez-Moya, A., Gomez, R., Velo, E., & Onate, A. (2003). Personality and eating disorders: A study with Rorschach test (EXNER). *Anales de Psiquiatria, 19*(1), 1–4.

Schalling, D., Åsberg, M., Edman, G., & Oreland, L. (1987). Markers of vulnerability to psychopathology: Temperament traits associated with platelet MAO activity. *Acta Psychiatrica Scandinavica, 76,* 172–182.

Schiele, B. C., & Brozek, J. (1948). 'Experimental neurosis' resulting from semistarvation in man. *Psychosomatic Medicine, 10,* 31–50.

Schoenberg, M. R., Dorr, D., & Morgan, C. D. (2006). Development of discriminant functions to detect dissimulation for the Millon Clinical Multiaxial Inventory (3rd edition). *Journal of Forensic Psychiatry & Psychology, 17,* 405–416.

Scott, R. L., & Baroffio, J. R. (1986). An MMPI analysis of similarities and differences in three classifications of eating disorders: anorexia nervosa, bulimia, and morbid obesity. *Journal of Clinical Psychology, 42,* 708–713.

Sellbom, M., & Ben-Porath, Y. S. (2005). Mapping the MMPI-2 Restructured Clinical scales onto normal personality traits: evidence of construct validity. *Journal of Personality Assessment, 85*(2), 179–187.

Shaffer, T. W., Erdberg, P., & Haroian, J. (1999). Current nonpatient data for the Rorschach, WAIS–R, and MMPI-2. *Journal of Personality Assessment, 73,* 305–316.

Simms, L. J., Casillas, A., Clark, L. A., Watson, D., & Doebbeling, B. N. (2005). Psychometric evaluation of the restructured clinical scales of the MMPI-2. *Psychological Assessment, 17,* 345–358.

Smith, J. E., Hillard, M. C., Walsh, R. A., & Kubacki, S. R. (1991). Rorschach assessment of purging and nonpurging bulimics. *Journal of Personality Assessment, 56,* 277–288.

Speranza, M., Corcos, M., Atger, F., Paterniti, S., & Jeammet, P. (2003). Binge eating behaviours, depression and weight control strategies. *Eating and Weight Disorders, 8,* 201–206.

Spielberger, C. D. (1972). Review of Profile of Mood States. *Professional Psychology, 3,* 387–388.

Spielberger, C. D. (1983). *Manual for the State-Trait Anxiety Inventory (Form Y).* Palo Alto, CA: Consulting Psychologists Press, Inc.

Spindler, A., & Milos, G. (2007). Links between eating disorder symptom severity and psychiatric comorbidity. *Eating Behaviors, 8,* 364–373.

Spitzer, R. L., Williams, J. B. W., Gibbon, M., & First, M. B. (1990). *User's guide for the structured clinical interview for DSM-III-R: SCID.* Washington, DC: American Psychiatric Association.

Srinivasagam, N. M., Kaye, W. H., Plotnicov, K. H., Greeno, C., Weltzin, T. E., & Rao, R. (1995). Persistent perfectionism, symmetry, and exactness after long-term recovery from anorexia nervosa [see comment]. *American Journal of Psychiatry, 152,* 1630–1634.

Stanley, M. A., Beck, J. G., & Zebb, B. J. (1996). Psychometric properties of four anxiety measures in older adults. *Behaviour Research and Therapy, 34,* 827–838.

Stein, D., Kaye, W. H., Matsunaga, H., Orbach, I., Har-Evan, D., Frank, G., et al. (2002). Eating-related concerns, mood, and personality traits in recovered bulimia nervosa subjects: A replication study. *International Journal of Eating Disorders, 32,* 225–229.

Storch, E. A., Roberti, J. W., & Roth, D. A. (2004). Factor structure, concurrent validity, and internal consistency of the Beck Depression Inventory–Second Edition in a sample of college students. *Depression and Anxiety, 19*(3), 187–189.

Striegel-Moore, R., & Rodin, J. (1986). The influence of psychological variables in obesity. In K. D. Brownell & J. P. Foreyt (Eds.), *Handbook of eating disorders: Physiological, psychological and treatment of obesity, anorexia and bulimia* (pp. 99–121). New York: Basic Books.

Stunkard, A. J., & Wadden, T. A. (1992). Psychological aspects of severe obesity. *American Journal of Clinical Nutrition, 55*(Suppl.), 524S–532S.

Sullivan, S., Cloninger, C. R., Przybeck, T. R., & Klein, S. (2007). Personality characteristics in obesity and relationship with successful weight loss. *International Journal of Obesity (London), 31,* 669–674.

Sultan, S., Andronikof, A., Reveillere, C., & Lemmel, G. (2006). A Rorschach stability study in a nonpatient adult sample. *Journal of Personality Assessment, 87,* 330–348.

Swanson, D. W., & Dinello, F. A. (1970). Severe obesity as a habituation syndrome: Evidence during a starvation study. *Archives of General Psychiatry, 22*(2), 120–127.

Tanaka-Matsumi, J., & Kameoka, V. A. (1986). Reliabilities and concurrent validities of popular self-report measures of depression, anxiety, and social desirability. *Journal of Consulting and Clinical Psychology, 54,* 328–333.

Taylor, J. A. (1953). A personality scale of manifest anxiety. *Journal of Abnormal and Social Psychology, 48,* 285–290.

Tellegen, A. (1982). *Brief manual for the Multidimensional Personality Questionnaire.* Minneapolis: University of Minnesota.

Tellegen, A., Ben-Porath, Y. S., McNulty, J. L., Arbisi, P. A., Graham, J. R., & Kaemmer, B. (2003). *The MMPI–2 restructured clinical (RC) scales: Development, validation, and interpretation.* Minneapolis: University of Minnesota Press.

Tomita, T., Aoyama, H., Kitamura, T., Sekiguchi, C., Murai, T., & Matsuda, T. (2000). Factor structure of psychobiological seven-factor model of personality: A model-revision. *Personality and Individual Differences, 29,* 709–727.

Valtolina, G. (1996). Weight loss and psychopathology: A three-cluster MMPI typology. *Perceptual and Motor Skills, 82,* 275–281.

Vassend, O., & Skrondal, A. (1999). The problem of structural indeterminacy in multidimensional symptom report instruments: The case of SCL-90-R. *Behaviour Research and Therapy, 37,* 685–701.

Vitousek, K. M., & Manke, F. (1994). Personality variables and disorders in anorexia nervosa and bulimia nervosa. *Journal of Abnormal Psychology, 103*(1), 137–147.

Vitousek, K. M., & Stumpf, R. E. (2005). Difficulties in the assessment of personality traits and disorders in eating-disordered individuals. *Eating Disorders, 13*(1), 37–60.

Wadden, T. A., Foster, G. D., Letizia, K. A., & Wilk, J. E. (1993). Metabolic, anthropometric, and psychological characteristics of obese binge eaters. *International Journal of Eating Disorders, 14,* 17–25.

Wadden, T. A., & Stunkard, A. J. (1985). Social and psychological consequences of obesity. *Annals of Internal Medicine, 103*(Pt. 2), 1062–1067.

Wagner, A., Barbarich-Marsteller, N. C., Frank, G. K., Bailer, U. F., Wonderlich, S. A., Crosby, R. D., et al. (2006). Personality traits after recovery from eating disorders: Do subtypes differ? *International Journal of Eating Disorders, 39,* 276–284.

Wallace, A., & Liljequist, L. (2005). A comparison of the correlational structures and elevation patterns of the MMPI-2 restructured clinical (RC) and clinical scales. *Assessment, 12*(3), 290–294.

Walsh, B. T., Roose, S. P., Glassman, A. H., Glades, M. A., & Sadik, C. (1985). Depression and bulimia. *Psychosomatic Medicine, 47,* 123–131.

Watson, D. (2000). *Mood and temperament.* New York: Guilford.

Weiner, I. B. (2001). Advancing the science of psychological assessment: The Rorschach Inkblot Method as exemplar. *Psychological Assessment, 13,* 423–432.

Weltzin, T. E., Bulik, C. M., McConaha, C. W., & Kaye, W. H. (1995). Laxative withdrawal and anxiety in bulimia nervosa. *International Journal of Eating Disorders, 17*(2), 141–146.

Wijndaele, K., Matton, L., Duvigneaud, N., Lefevre, J., Duquet, W., Thomis, M., et al. (2007). Reliability, equivalence and respondent preference of computerized versus paper-and-pencil mental health questionnaires. *Computers in Human Behavior, 23,* 1958–1970.

Wood, J. M., Nezworski, M., & Garb, H. N. (2003). What's right with the Rorschach? *The Scientific Review of Mental Health Practice, 2*(2), 142–146.

Wood, J. M., Nezworski, M., & Stejskal, W. J. (1996a). The comprehensive system for the Rorschach: A critical examination. *Psychological Science, 7*(1), 3–10.

Wood, J. M., Nezworski, M., & Stejskal, W. J. (1996b). Thinking critically about the comprehensive system for the Rorschach: A reply to Exner. *Psychological Science, 7*(1), 14–17.

Wood, J. M., Nezworski, M., & Stejskal, W. J. (1997). The reliability of the Comprehensive System for the Rorschach: A comment on Meyer (1997). *Psychological Assessment, 9,* 490–494.

Youssef, G., Plancherel, B., Laget, J., Corcos, M., Flament, M. F., & Halfon, O. (2004). Personality trait risk factors for attempted suicide among young women with eating disorders. *European Psychiatry: The Journal of the Association of European Psychiatrists, 19*(3), 131–139.

Zung, W. W. (1965). A self-rating depression scale. *Archives of General Psychiatry, 12*(1), 63–70.

Zung, W. W. (1971). A rating instrument for anxiety disorders. *Psychosomatics: Journal of Consultation Liaison Psychiatry, 12,* 371–379.

CHAPTER 2

Assessment of Health-Related Quality of Life in Obesity and Eating Disorders

Ronette L. Kolotkin, Steffany Haaz, and Kevin R. Fontaine

What Is Health-Related Quality of Life (HRQOL)?

Quality of life is a concept very commonly used but rarely well defined. Many may dismiss the need to define it since we all seem to "know what it is." As scientists and consumers of science, however, there are problems that arise when individuals are using the same term to refer to slightly or even drastically different concepts. Since quality of life can describe many domains of one's life and experience (e.g., financial and material resources, educational attainment), the term *health-related quality of life* (HRQOL) has been used to specify the quality of one's life as related to aspects of health.

HRQOL does not have a universal definition but is designed to reflect an individual's subjective response and assessment of his or her health or illness (Fontaine, Cheskin, & Barofsky, 1996; Osterhaus, Townsend, Gandek, & Ware, 1994; Sullivan, Sullivan, & Kral, 1987; Wan, Counte, & Cella, 1997), including physical, mental, and social dimensions (Guyatt, Feeny, & Patrick, 1993). The World Health Organization (WHO) defines health as a state of complete physical, mental, and social well-being and not merely the absence of disease or illness. "HRQOL can include general health, physical functioning, physical symptoms, toxicity, emotional functioning, cognitive functioning, role functioning, social well-being and functioning, sexual functioning and existential issues" (WHO, 1948). Guyatt et al. (1993) explain that "widely valued aspects of life exist that are not generally considered as 'health,' including income, freedom, and quality of the environment" (p. 622). They go on to state, however, that all of these may adversely affect health (and vice versa) and that "when a patient is ill or diseased, almost all aspects of life can become health related."

Because of the many areas of life that are considered when assessing HRQOL, most scientists

AUTHORS' NOTE: We thank Scott Engel, PhD, for his comments on the eating disorder section, Myles Faith, PhD, for his comments on the pediatric section, and the two anonymous reviewers for their insightful comments.

and scholars agree that it is a multidimensional construct. A single question regarding HRQOL would be vague and difficult to interpret (Fayers & Machin, 2000). They do not necessarily agree, however, on which dimensions are most relevant to constitute HRQOL.

For some investigators, the dimensions included in assessment of HRQOL are dependent on their particular investigative focus (Stucki et al., 2006). A scientist examining HRQOL during recovery from gastric bypass surgery, for example, may be interested in different dimensions (e.g., adjustment to new dietary restrictions) than someone who is interested in comparing the HRQOL of obese and nonobese exercisers and may choose, therefore, to use a different scale. Conversely, the measurement tool that an investigator chooses may dictate the focus of the research questions at hand. While it may be unrealistic to suggest a unified theory of HRQOL that is sufficient and appropriate for all applications, it is important for the methods to be as well described and standardized as possible.

Why Is HRQOL Measured?

The patient's perspective is an essential aspect of medical care. Recognition of this within the medical community has shifted toward the inclusion of subjective evaluations, such as HRQOL. This inclusion allows a more comprehensive assessment of a complicated and multifaceted condition such as obesity.

There are many complications from obesity, not all of which are medical. Obesity negatively affects functioning, mood, perceived health, and self-concept thus, having a substantial impact on HRQOL (Fontaine et al., 1996; Sarlio-Lahteen-korva, Stunkard, & Rissanen, 1995; Stewart & Brook, 1983; Sullivan et al., 1987). As such, the effect of obesity on HRQOL might be one of the primary reasons for seeking treatment (Fontaine & Bartlett, 2003). In addition, HRQOL gains are often reported as the most important benefit of weight loss (Kral, Sjöström, & Sullivan, 1992).

Outcomes measurement is necessary to evaluate the efficacy of treatments and the impact that treatments have on all aspects of an individual's life, including HRQOL. HRQOL assessment

allows various study treatment conditions to be compared for expected improvement, prevention of negative impact, and proof of no (or relatively low) harm (Fayers & Machin, 2000). Assessing HRQOL also allows comparison of the same treatments across different populations and between different studies.

While a pharmacological intervention's physiological efficacy can be measured through biomarkers, such as serum cholesterol and blood glucose, the patient may not actually feel better as a result of the treatment. In fact, there can be negative HRQOL consequences of any treatment, including treatments for obesity (e.g., social alienation or physical discomfort). The reverse may also be true, whereby a patient feels marked improvements in many areas of life, but actual changes to his or her body mass index (BMI) or cardiovascular risk are not apparent.

In the arena of public health, HRQOL measurement can help to identify broader psychosocial impact of obesity, beyond the "harder" outcomes of morbidity and mortality. Emphasizing gains in HRQOL as another benefit of small weight loss, and thereby redefining successful weight management, might be motivational for discouraged individuals (Fontaine & Bartlett, 2003). When weight loss does not come easily, knowing that the intervention can improve how a person feels may increase the likelihood of continuing with the program until actual weight loss occurs. Also, understanding obesity's impact on HRQOL for a particular patient could assist in tailoring treatment to his or her life circumstances and challenges. One individual may suffer through dietary change with very negative consequences to his or her personal life, while another may enjoy the change and feel revitalized by the new approach. Last, the inclusion of HRQOL in regular patient evaluation could help guide the development of broad health care policies that recognize the biopsychosocial impact of the growing obesity epidemic. Disregarding this important aspect of health is unfortunately common in policy development and implementation. Assessment of HRQOL in obesity is increasingly recognized as critical to the understanding of obese persons and evaluation of treatment outcomes. Several review papers emphasize the importance of assessing HRQOL in obesity and describe the various types of measures that are available (Duval, Marceau, Perusse, & Lacasse, 2006; Fontaine & Barofsky, 2001; Kolotkin, Meter, & Williams, 2001; Kushner & Foster, 2000).

How Is HRQOL Measured?

It is universally agreed that HRQOL is a subjective concept by nature and can only be assessed via self-report. While overt behaviors and expert opinions can be helpful, they are secondary and serve only as proxies for self-report (Fayers & Machin, 2000). Many instruments have been developed based on the perspective of investigators, resulting in hundreds of measures of different aspects of quality of life (Fallowfield, 1996). Some are generic measures, while others focus on specific diseases, populations, or aspects of life (Guyatt et al., 1993). They also vary greatly in length, scaling, and question format. While each has its unique characteristics, it can be difficult to compare results between different studies when researchers use such a variety of measurement tools. Some of the most widely used instruments of HRQOL for obesity and eating-related conditions are highlighted in this chapter. Determining the most useful methods for assessing HRQOL in an obese population would allow us to better understand and treat the condition (Gill & Feinstein, 1994).

Differences Between Generic and Disease-Specific Measures

There are two basic approaches to HRQOL measurement. The first involves the use of generic instruments that measure broad aspects of HRQOL and are suitable for administration to any population or disease. These instruments are not designed to assess HRQOL relative to a particular medical condition but rather provide a generalized assessment. The major advantage of generic measures is that they allow for comparisons across a variety of conditions. Moreover, generic instruments can be administered to examine the impact of various health care programs on HRQOL. The major limitation of generic HRQOL instruments is that they may not be sensitive enough to detect

subtle condition-specific effects. For example, a generic assessment of an obese patient will not provide information on the specific issues associated with obesity such as the impact of weight on self-esteem, public distress, or sexual activity.

The second approach to HRQOL measurement involves the use of instruments that are specific to a disease (e.g., obesity, asthma), a population (e.g., elderly), or a problem (e.g., sexual function, pain). Measures geared toward specific diseases or populations are likely to have greater relevance to practicing clinicians and patients. In treatment outcome studies, disease-specific instruments are typically more responsive to change than generic measures. The major limitation of specific HRQOL instruments is that it is difficult to compare across diseases.

Generic HRQOL Instruments

Medical Outcomes Study—Short Form 36 (SF-36). The SF-36 (Ware, 1993a) is the most widely used instrument for assessing HRQOL in obesity research. It contains a subset of 36 items from the Medical Outcomes Study (Stewart, Hays, & Ware, 1988). These items constitute eight scales or domains: Physical Functioning, Role Physical, Bodily Pain, General Health, Vitality, Role Emotional, Social Functioning, and Mental Health. To minimize Type I error from multiple statistical testing, a scoring algorithm exists that differentially weighs the eight domain scores to produce two summary scales (Physical Component Summary and Mental Component Summary; Hays, Sherbourne, & Mazel, 1993). Factor-analytic assessments confirm the utility of the two-factor model (Hays et al., 1993).

The SF-36 has been thoroughly assessed, and its psychometric properties are well established (Ware, 1996; Ware & Sherbourne, 1992). All scales were found to have an internal consistency of at least .78 (Hays et al., 1993; Ware, 1993b). The range of reliability coefficients is .63 to .94 in different demographic groups (McHorney, Ware, Lu, & Sherbourne, 1994; Ware, 1993b). The SF-36 has also been shown to discriminate well between groups that differ in disease states or severity (Essink-Bot, Krabbe, Bonsel, & Aaronson, 1997; Kantz, Harris, Levitsky, Ware, & Davies, 1992;

McHorney et al., 1994), representing strong support of its validity.

The SF-36 has been translated into numerous languages, and evaluations of the psychometric properties of these translations are ongoing (Aaronson et al., 1992; Alonso, Prieto, & Anto, 1995; Apolone, Filiberti, Cifani, Ruggiata, & Mosconi, 1998).

The SF-36 has been used in dozens of obesity-related studies in many countries, including observational and longitudinal studies and clinical trials testing a variety of interventions to promote weight reduction (e.g., dietary/lifestyle modification, pharmacotherapy, bariatric surgery). It is beyond the scope of this chapter to provide an exhaustive review of this vast literature. However, we will highlight a selection of these studies to provide a sense of the findings derived from this measure and to assess its value as a generic assessment of HRQOL within the obesity field.

SF-36 Assessment of HRQOL in Obese Populations

The SF-36 has been used to identify an "HRQOL profile" of overweight and obese adults. In one of the earliest of these studies, Fontaine and colleagues (1996)_assessed the HRQOL among 312 obese adults (mean BMI = 38.1) seeking university-based weight loss treatment. After adjusting for sociodemographic factors and various comorbidities, including depression, significant decrements were observed in all eight SF-36 domains. Specifically, relative to SF-36 general population norms, the obese adults scored significantly lower (i.e., reported greater impairment) on Physical Functioning, Role Physical, Bodily Pain, General Health, Vitality, Social Functioning, Role Emotional, and Mental Health. Since depression was statistically controlled, the result with regard to the Mental Health scale primarily reflects anxiety. The largest decrements in HRQOL were found on the Vitality and Bodily Pain SF-36 scales, and the HRQOL impairment observed among these obese persons seeking weight reduction was comparable to that of individuals with chronic diseases such as AIDS and congestive heart failure.

Several population studies have used the SF-36 to evaluate HRQOL across the BMI range.

Among nearly 1,000 French adults who completed the SF-36, Le Pen, Levy, Loos, Banzet, & Basdevant (1998) found that compared to healthy-weight individuals, overweight individuals (BMI = 27 to < 30) reported greater impairment on Physical Functioning, while obese individuals (BMI ≥ 30) reported greater impairment on the Physical Functioning, Role Physical, Bodily Pain, General Health, and Vitality scales. The obese individuals also reported significantly greater impairment on the Physical Functioning scale compared to the overweight group. In a Dutch sample of 4,041 adults, men in the highest waist circumference and BMI tertile reported significantly poorer Physical Functioning and greater Bodily Pain, while women in the highest tertile reported significantly impaired Physical Functioning, General Health, and Bodily Pain (Han, Tijhuis, Lean, & Seidell, 1998). A study of 13,431 Australian women ages 45 to 49 years reported that increased BMI was associated with impaired Physical Functioning, Bodily Pain, General Health, and Vitality (Brown, Dobson, & Mishra, 1998).

In a prospective cohort study of 40,098 women participating in the Nurses' Health Study, Fine and colleagues (1999) found that women who had gained 5 pounds or more over the course of 4 years reported significant impairment (i.e., lower scores) on the SF-36 Physical Functioning, Vitality, and Bodily Pain scales, independent of baseline weight. Those who lost 5 pounds or more reported improved Physical Functioning and Vitality and reduced Bodily Pain.

Apart from the SF-36's use in observational studies as a means of estimating the association of obesity to HRQOL, it is also commonly used to estimate HRQOL among persons seeking weight loss treatment or taking part in a weight loss trial. Specifically, the SF-36 has been used to estimate if HRQOL improves as a function of taking part in weight loss interventions, including diet, exercise, behavior modification, pharmacotherapy, and combinations thereof. Finally, given the large increase in the number of obese people undergoing surgical interventions to reduce their weight (Steinbrook, 2004), the SF-36 has been used extensively in trials of bariatric surgery to determine whether dramatic weight reduction via surgery improves HRQOL.

SF-36 Among Those Seeking Weight Loss

A handful of studies have used the SF-36 to evaluate whether the HRQOL of persons seeking treatment is markedly different from population reference values. In general, these studies suggest that scores are significantly lower among those seeking weight loss treatment compared to population norms. For example, in one such study (Dittmar, Heintz, Hardt, Egle, & Kahaly, 2003), persons seeking a surgical intervention completed the SF-36 scores prior to surgery. These scores were significantly lower than population references values on all eight scales. In another study (Fontaine, Bartlett, & Barofsky, 2000), SF-36 scores among 312 obese persons seeking university-based weight loss treatment were compared to 89 obese adults not seeking weight reduction. Prior to participation, the obese adults who sought weight loss treatment reported significantly more impairment on the Bodily Pain, General Health, and Vitality scales of the SF-36 compared to obese nontreatment seekers.

SF-36 in Weight Loss Intervention Studies

The effect of intentional weight loss on HRQOL has become an increasingly important outcome in clinical weight loss trials, and the SF-36 has been used in studies to evaluate changes in HRQOL associated with weight reduction. For example, in a randomized controlled trial of lifestyle modification (diet, physical activity, group meetings) versus controls among 80 overweight and obese women, Rippe and colleagues (1998) found that a mean weight loss of 6.1 kg was associated with significant improvements in Physical Functioning, Vitality, and Mental Health compared to controls. In a similar study, Fontaine and associates (1999) found that overweight and obese adults who lost an average of 7.8 kg via a low-calorie diet coupled with either traditional aerobic exercise or self-selected lifestyle physical activity produced, relative to baseline, significant improvements in Physical Functioning, Role Physical, Vitality, General Health, and Mental Health scores. At 1-year follow-up, the improvements in General

Health and Vitality remained significant, regardless of whether the weight loss was maintained (Fontaine, Barofsky, Bartlett, Franckowiak, & Andersen, 2004). Among 250 overweight and obese New Zealand adults participating in a randomized weight loss trial, Ni Mhurchu and colleagues (2004) observed that, at baseline, those in the highest BMI tertile group reported significantly more impaired Physical Functioning and Physical Component Summary (PCS) scores than did persons in the lower tertiles. No significant differences were observed at baseline on the Mental Component Summary (MCS) scores among the BMI tertile groups. Perhaps because less than 10% of the sample lost at least 5% of their baseline weight, no differences on the SF-36 as a function of weight loss were obtained.

A nonrandomized study evaluating the effects of cognitive-behavioral therapy among an Italian sample of obese binge and nonbinge eaters found that weight loss (a mean reduction of 9.4 kg) was associated with significant improvements in Role Physical, Role Emotional, Vitality, Mental Health, and Social Functioning compared to the untreated controls. Interestingly, the improvements on SF-36 scale scores were greatest among obese binge eaters (Marchesini et al., 2002).

A growing number of pharmacotherapy trials have used the SF-36 to estimate changes in HRQOL. Samsa, Kolotkin, Williams, Nguyen, and Mendel (2001) conducted a pooled analysis of four double-blind, randomized controlled trials (RCTs) evaluating the short-term (8–12 weeks), medium-term (24–28 weeks), and long-term (52 weeks) effects of sibutramine versus placebo among 555 mildly to moderately obese adults with type 2 diabetes, dyslipidemia, or hypertension. They found that, in the short-term, weight losses of 5% to 10% (regardless of whether achieved with sibutramine or placebo) were associated with improved scores on General Health and PCS score of the SF-36. In the medium term, they observed improvements in all except Social Functioning, Mental Health, and MCS. In the long term, this amount of weight loss was associated with improvements in the Physical Functioning, Role Physical, General Health, and Vitality scores. Although patients in the sibutramine group were more likely to experience weight reduction than patients receiving placebo, patients with similar weight reductions reported similar improvements in HRQOL regardless of treatment.

A randomized controlled trial evaluating the effects of a 12-month treatment with 15 mg sibutramine among 210 obese adults with type 2 diabetes found that, despite the superior weight loss (means for sibutramine vs. placebo = 7.1 kg vs. 2.6 kg, respectively), the sibutramine group did not report benefits on the SF-36 over placebo (Kaukua, Pekkarinen, & Rissanen, 2004). When changes on the SF-36 were examined as a function of weight lost, however, Physical Functioning scores improved with at least a 5% weight loss, and Vitality and General Health scores improved only after at least a 15% weight loss was obtained.

Several studies have used the SF-36 to examine the effects of bariatric surgery on HRQOL. Recently, Hooper, Stellato, Hallowell, Seitz, and Moskowitz (2007) reported findings from a study of 48 patients (47 women, mean age of 44) who underwent gastric banding. The SF-36 was administered before and 6 to 12 months after surgery. Significant improvements were seen in all SF-36 domains ($p < .001$) after an average weight loss of 41 kg. After surgery, mean scores were higher than U.S. norms for Physical Functioning and Mental Health, with no other significant differences, suggesting that postoperatively, patients report HRQOL at least as high as normal reference values.

Looking at longer term outcomes, a study by de Zwaan, Lancaster, et al. (2002) compared SF-36 scores from a postoperative group (averaging 13.8 years postoperatively) of 78 patients to a preoperative control group of 110 patients. Patients in the preoperative group had a mean BMI of 43.8, whereas patients in the postoperative group had a mean BMI of 32.8. Scores from the postoperative group were significantly higher (better HRQOL) than those obtained by the preoperative group on all SF-36 scales except Mental Health. SF-36 scores for the postoperative group were similar to U.S. norms, with the exception of impairment on Bodily Pain and PCS. PCS scores were more impaired for women, those hospitalized since surgery, and those who had lost less weight. Patients who reported binge-eating disorder at follow-up had greater impairment on the MCS.

Carmichael, Sue-Ling, and Johnston (2001) compared patients who underwent a particular type of bariatric surgery (Magenstrasse and Mill [M-M] procedure) to morbidly obese patients considering surgery (MO) and nonobese controls ($n = 82, 35$, and 20, respectively). Assessments were conducted through personal, postal, and telephone survey with postoperative measurement occurring 1 to 8 years later (median = 3 years). Patients in the M-M group lost an average of 37 kg. Significant differences were found between postsurgical M-M patients and MO patients for all SF-36 scales and between M-M patients and nonobese controls on Physical Functioning, General Health, and Bodily Pain. The MO patients also differed from nonobese controls for all SF-36 scales.

Results of some studies have been mixed, however. Examining effects of laparoscopic adjustable gastric banding (LAGB) surgery in a Dutch sample of female patients ($n = 42$), Horchner, Tuinebreijer, and Kelder (2001) found that no preoperative differences existed between surgery candidates and Dutch population norms. However, all scores improved after surgery, with 2-year postoperative scores for Bodily Pain, General Health, and Mental Health being higher than norms ($p \leq .03$). Mean BMI declined significantly from 40.7 preoperatively to 31.3 at 2-year follow-up. A second study by the same group was too small to expect significant results. Scores were lower for some variables before surgery, and a trend was seen toward improvement in Bodily Pain.

Another study of Dutch LAGB patients found poor preoperative HRQOL (retrospectively) on the SF-36 compared to population norms and postoperative evaluations (Schok et al., 2000). At 1 year postsurgery, the average weight reduction was 27 kg. Postoperatively, Physical Functioning, Vitality, and General Health were still below population norms, although other domains were in the normal range. No HRQOL differences were found between patients with varying postoperative evaluations (12–16 months, 17–23 months, and 24–38 months).

Comparing two different surgical methods (laparoscopic vs. open gastric bypass) in 155 randomized patients, Nguyen et al. (2001) found more similarities in HRQOL at 6 months than at shorter follow-up durations. At 1 month, four of eight domains of the SF-36 were higher in the laparoscopic than the open gastric bypass group. After 3 months, all domains had improved in the laparoscopic group and were equivalent to U.S. norms, but Physical Functioning was still impaired for patients who underwent open gastric bypass. (The mean percent of excess body weight lost [%EWL] at 3 months was higher after laparoscopic gastric bypass [37%] than after open gastric bypass [32%].) After 6 months, all domains were comparable to norms, and no differences were seen between groups, although the laparoscopic group reduced excess body weight by 54%, whereas the open group reduced excess body weight by 45%.

Some studies have aimed to determine predictors of change in HRQOL following surgery. Looking at all patients over 3 years ($n = 459$ preoperative, 641 postoperative), Dixon, Dixon, and O'Brien (2001a) found that preoperatively, all domains were lower than community norms, with the PCS being more impaired than MCS (Dixon et al., 2001a). After 1 year (and a mean percent excess weight loss of 46%) and the 3 years following (with %EWL of 52, 50, and 51, respectively), SF-36 scores were closer to population norms. Significant predictors of low preoperative PCS were (a) history of arthritis or joint pain, (b) high preoperative BMI, (c) older age, (d) depression, (e) gastroesophageal reflux, and (f) alcohol consumption. Improvement in PCS was predicted by (a) history of arthritis or joint pain, (b) history of depression, and (c) total weight loss (in kg). Percentage of excess weight lost (%EWL) was not a predictor of improved PCS. For the MCS, predictors of low preoperative scores were (a) history of depression, (b) younger age, (c) weight gain later in life, and (d) gastroesophageal reflux. Improvements in MCS were predicted by (a) younger age and (b) history of arthritis or joint pain. MCS impairment and improvement were not correlated with any measures of weight loss. Domain scores for Vitality, Bodily Pain, and Role Physical dropped after 4 years, although still higher than baseline, and the authors note that these domain scores were higher than norms at 1-year follow-up.

Torquati, Lufti, and Richards (2007) found an inverse correlation between HRQOL and number of comorbidities, both before and after laparoscopic gastric bypass surgery ($r = .29$, $p = .001$; $r = .22$,

$p = .005$, respectively). However, the magnitude of improvement in HRQOL was not related to comorbidities. In the group with least improvement, there was a higher prevalence of men and a lower prevalence of patients with type 2 diabetes. In multivariate analysis, being female and having diabetes led to greater likelihood of HRQOL improvement (6.2 times and 16.1 times, respectively).

Conversely, some aspects of HRQOL have been shown to predict postsurgical outcomes. In a study by Dixon, Dixon, and O'Brien (2001b) of 175 consecutive patients, preoperative PCS was the strongest HRQOL predictor of %EWL at 1 year, after adjusting for age and initial BMI ($r = .20$, $p < .01$). Other significant predictors included Role Physical, Bodily Pain, General Health, and Role Emotional.

Taken together, studies such as these suggest an overall trend of improvements in HRQOL, as assessed by the SF-36, after bariatric surgery. Because of mixed findings, some investigators have questioned the utility of the SF-36 or other generic measures for assessing postsurgical HRQOL changes. Nonetheless, the American Society for Bariatric Surgery (2004) suggests use of the SF-36 as a generic measure of HRQOL.

Comments

The SF-36 is the most extensively used generic measure of HRQOL. It possesses impressive psychometric properties and has been used with virtually every medical population throughout the world. It is responsive to clinically meaningful changes and clinical changes over time and, as such, represents the "gold standard" of generic HRQOL assessment (Garratt, Ruta, Abdalla, & Russell, 1994; Katz, Larson, Phillips, Fossel, & Liang, 1992). It has been used widely by obesity researchers to characterize the HRQOL of obese populations (LePen et al., 1998), as well as to estimate changes on HRQOL as a function of intervention, and its construct validity for use among obese persons has been confirmed recently (Corica et al., 2006). Specifically, among a sample of 1,735 obese Italian adults, the SF-36 items clustered in a consistent fashion around the original eight-domain structure. Moreover, BMI was significantly associated with impairment in all eight scales, suggesting that the SF-36 is robust and can be used with obese persons as a valid generic HRQOL assessment.

Overall, obesity-related studies using the SF-36 indicate that physically oriented domains of functioning tend to be impaired in overweight and obese people compared to population norms. Studies (e.g., Doll, Petersen, & Stewart-Brown, 2000) also suggest a linear association between BMI and SF-36 scores (i.e., greater HRQOL impairment at greater levels of BMI). Intervention studies using the SF-36 generally show that weight reduction, whether promoted by lifestyle modification, pharmacotherapy, or surgery, markedly improves SF-36 scores. In general, greater weight loss appears to promote greater improvement in SF-36 scores (Fine et al., 1999; Fontaine et al., 1999). Although a meta-analysis of RCTs for weight loss interventions (Maciejewski, Patrick, & Williamson, 2005) concluded that HRQOL outcomes were not consistently improved (only 9 of 34 trials showed improvements in generic measures of HRQOL; see Appendix 2.I), results from the broad range of weight loss studies reported above suggest a stronger and more consistent effect with respect to HRQOL. This discrepancy may be accounted for by differences in methodology between controlled and uncontrolled trials, a threshold effect of weight loss above which changes in HRQOL are observed, or some unknown other factors.

Recently, briefer variants of the SF-36 have been developed—specifically, the SF-12 and SF-12, version 2, and the SF-8. Although these questionnaires have not been widely used in obesity research, psychometric evaluations relative to the SF-36 indicate that they possess acceptable levels of reliability, as well as construct and predictive validity (Ware, Kosinski, & Keller, 1996). The reduction in participant burden suggests that the SF-12 and the SF-8 may become increasingly popular as a generic HRQOL assessment in obese populations (Jia & Lubetkin, 2005). The SF-12 contains 12 items from the SF-36 that reproduce the PCS and MCS scales in the general U.S. population (multiple R^2 of .911 and .918 in predictions of the SF-36 PCS and SF-36 MCS scores, respectively). Test-retest correlations of .89 and .76 were reported for the 12-item PCS and the 12-item MCS, respectively, in the general U.S. population. Twenty cross-sectional and longitudinal tests of empirical validity previously published for the 36-item scales and summary measures were replicated for the 12-item PCS and the 12-item MCS. In general, scores for the SF-12 were comparable to those obtained on the SF-36.

Nottingham Health Profile (NHP). There are two parts to the NHP, which was created in the United Kingdom to reflect lay perceptions of health, as distinct from professional evaluation (McEwen, McKenna, & Spilker, 1996). The NHP is completed in a yes versus no response format. There are six sections within Part I, including physical abilities, pain, sleep, social isolation, emotional reactions, and energy level. It is scored from 1 to 100 through weighted values (McKenna, Hunt, & McEwen, 1981). Part II is optional and contains seven items to indicate degree of handicap, as well as measures the impact that health problems have on occupation, household jobs, personal relationships, social life, sex life, hobbies, and holidays. The developers of the NHP no longer recommend the use of Part II (Bowling, 1997). The NHP has not been rigorously evaluated for test-retest reliability, although it has been estimated to be between .71 and .88 (Hunt, McEwen, & McKenna, 1986; Hunt, McKenna, McEwen, Williams, & Papp, 1981). Internal consistency has been reported with a mean greater than .58 (Calder, Anderson, Harper, Jagger, & Gregg, 1995; Essink-Bot et al., 1997; Hunt, McKenna, McEwen, Williams, & Papp, 1981; Lukkarinen & Hentinen, 1998). The NHP has been shown to effectively distinguish between disease states and patient populations (Essink-Bot et al., 1997; Hunt et al., 1981; Jenkinson, Fitzpatrick, & Argyle, 1988; O'Brien, 1988). Use of the NHP in the general population is limited because of the high prevalence of a score of zero. As such, it is not as sensitive as other measures for uncovering minor health problems (Brazier et al., 1992; Hunt, McEwen, & McKenna, 1985).

The NHP is not commonly used in obese populations. There has been report of improvement, however, after weight loss surgery. van Gemert, Adang, Greve, and Soeters (1998) found that greater weight loss and shorter postoperative follow-up were associated with better HRQOL outcome, which did not differ by surgical method or surgical complications, although these changes tended to decrease with time. The NHP has been effective in reflecting changes with treatment of other medical problems (Calder et al., 1995; Lukkarinen & Hentinen, 1998), although there may be some difficulty in using it to discriminate between patients with higher levels of disability (Gater, Kind, & Gudex, 1995).

Sickness Impact Profile (SIP). The SIP (Bergner, Bobbitt, Kressel, et al., 1976) was designed in the mid-1970s to measure how illness influences behavior. It contains 136 items, scored in 12 categories: ambulation, mobility, body care and movement, communication, alertness behavior, emotional behavior, social interaction, sleep and rest, eating, work, home management, and recreation and pastimes. Two underlying dimensions of these categories are physical and psychosocial. Items are scored from 1 to 11, with higher scores indicating greater dysfunction. The scores range from 0 to 100 and are reported as a percent of dysfunction for both dimensions (Bergner, Bobbitt, Pollard, Martin, & Gilson, 1976).

High test-retest reliability of .81 to .97 has been reported for the SIP, as well as internal consistency reliability of .81 to .94 (Bergner, Bobbitt, Carter, & Gilson, 1981; de Bruin, de Witte, Stevens, & Diederiks, 1992). Validity, as determined by correlations with self-assessment, clinician assessment, and other disability indices, is moderate (.30–.69; Bergner et al., 1981). Because the length of the instrument can make it burdensome, a shorter version has been created (de Bruin et al., 1992; de Bruin, Buys, de Witte, & Diederiks, 1994), although it has not been well validated.

The SIP is not often used in obese populations. When compared to healthy subjects, severely obese individuals participating in the Swedish Obese Subjects study showed more functional limitations in most aspects of life (Karlsson, Sjöström, & Sullivan, 1995), though effect sizes were small to moderate (Sullivan, Karlsson, Sjöström, Taft, & Bjorntorp, 2001). The severely obese also had worse functional limitations in most areas when compared to cancer survivors 2 to 3 years postdiagnosis (Sullivan, Cohen, & Branehog, 1988). When compared to disabling conditions such as chronic pain syndrome and rheumatoid arthritis, however,

SIP overall index scores for obesity are substantially lower, suggesting less impairment (Augustinsson, Sullivan, & Sullivan, 1989). With surgical intervention for obesity, functional health improved in several domains, especially leisure activities and social interactions (Sullivan et al., 2001). In a case-controlled study by Karlsson, Sjöström, and Sullivan (1998), low HRQOL was improved after gastric restriction surgery, which peaked at 6 to 12 months postsurgery and decreased slightly at 2 years. Improvements were related to amount of weight lost. Karlsson et al. (1994) also conducted a randomized controlled trial of weight reduction diets (lacto-ovo vegetarian, standard, and controls) and found positive long-term improvements in SIP functional status. Poorer HRQOL at baseline predicted greater weight regain but not overall weight loss.

The SIP has the benefit of being well established and responsive to clinically significant changes (Katz et al., 1992), but it is lengthy to complete. It is also disadvantaged by the absence of eating-related problems in the eating category that are common for obese individuals (Sullivan et al., 2001). In addition, wording may be difficult to comprehend for those with lower education levels, and there is a skew toward healthy responses (Brooks, Jordan, Divine, Smith, & Neelon, 1990; Fisher, Lake, Reutzel, & Emery, 1995).

General Health Questionnaire (GHQ). The GHQ was created in the 1970s by a British psychiatrist (D. P. Goldberg, 1978) and is possibly the most common tool for measuring mental well-being (Jackson, 2007). It is most often used as a screening tool for risk of psychiatric conditions through its four domains of depression, anxiety, somatic symptoms, and social withdrawal. The original version contained 60 items, but three shorter versions have emerged, with the 28-item being the most commonly used (Bowling, 1997). Item responses range from 0 to 3, with 0 being not at all and 3 meaning much more than usual. For the 28-item version, total scores range from 0 to 84, and subscale scores and distributions can also be calculated. A unique aspect of the GHQ is its ability to determine the likelihood of psychiatric caseness (i.e., individuals whose scores would be indicative of a person requiring psychiatric services).

The GHQ focuses primarily on mental well-being and is not as comprehensive as other measures of HRQOL. It is most often used in occupational research with regard to workplace health (Jackson, 2007) and is not widely used in obesity research. The GHQ was used in a cross-sectional study to compare obese patients with a history of gastric bypass (> 5 years) to obese patients who had not experienced the surgery (Sanchez-Santos et al., 2006). The GHQ questionnaire showed statistical differences between the surgical patients and the obese patients who did not have surgery, with symptoms of depression being more frequent in the latter (25% vs. 14%; $p = .007$).

In Japan, the GHQ was administered to evaluate efficacy of a diet and exercise program for obese employees of a particular company. Several indicators of physical functioning seemed to improve with the intervention, and GHQ scores became worse with decreases in diet/exercise lifestyle activities and achievements (Irie et al., 1996). A Brazilian study of university employees examined body weight perceptions in relation to BMI and mental disorders (Veggi, Lopes, Faerstein, & Sichieri, 2004). For women, BMI and perceptions that body weight was substantially above normal were associated with common mental disorders. These relationships were not seen among men in the study.

Quality of Well-Being Scale (QWB). This measure includes preference-weighted values for functioning and symptoms at a given time point (Kaplan, Anderson, Walker, & Rosser, 1988; Kaplan & Bush, 1982). It contains three scales of function (Mobility, Physical, and Social) with a measure of symptoms and problems. These are combined for a total score that ranges from 0 (dead) to 1 (optimal function). The components included in the instrument are life expectancy (mortality), functioning and symptoms (morbidity), preference for observed functional status (utility), and duration of stay in health states (prognosis; Kaplan, Ganiats, Sieber, & Anderson, 1998). Using duration affected and number of people, quality-adjusted life years (QALYs) can be determined (Kaplan, Anderson, & Spilker, 1996), with an attempt to quantify HRQOL in relationship to life expectancy (Kaplan, Ganiats, et al., 1998). Because of this application, the QWB is often used in

cost-effectiveness analysis. It is generally administered by a trained interviewee. A self-administered version was created that shows promise for reducing time and staff burden, but its performance has only been evaluated in one trial to date (Andresen, Rothenberg, & Kaplan, 1998). The QWB weights various aspects of health status, allowing for objective comparison across conditions and populations; however, this eliminates the option for subjective cost-benefit analysis for a specific individual or group (i.e., a treatment that results in increased function but lower energy).

The QWB has not been used often with obese populations, although it has been used for the common comorbidities of arthritis (Kaplan, Kozin, & Anderson, 1988) and diabetes (Kaplan, Hartwell, Wilson, & Wallace, 1987), as well as several other chronic conditions (Kaplan, Ganiats, et al., 1998). Using the QWB, Groessl, Kaplan, Barrett-Connor, and Ganiats (2004) found that obese persons had significantly lower HRQOL than those with normal or overweight BMI, although HRQOL among overweight participants did not differ from those with normal BMI. For a BMI > 30, this represented an incremental loss of QALYs. In 70 adults with diabetes, those completing a diet and exercise program showed greater improvements in HRQOL than diet alone, exercise alone, or control groups, independent of weight change (Kaplan et al., 1987).

Obesity-Specific HRQOL Instruments

A number of obesity-specific measures of HRQOL have been developed in the past decade. Table 2.1 provides a list of these instruments in alphabetical order, plus details such as domains being assessed and each of the instrument's strengths and weaknesses. The most widely used instruments will be discussed below, also in alphabetical order.

Bariatric Analysis and Reporting Outcome System

The Bariatric Analysis and Reporting Outcome System (BAROS) was developed to

(Text continues on page 52)

Table 2.1   Obesity-Specific Instruments

Instrument Name	Number of Items	Country of Origin	Domains/Scales	Strengths	Weaknesses	Comments
Bariatric Analysis and Reporting Outcome System (BAROS; Oria, 1998)	7	United States and Austria	Weight Loss Medical Conditions Quality of Life • Self-Esteem • Physical • Social • Labor • Sexual	Developed for use after bariatric surgery and provides an overall score taking into account weight loss, medical conditions, and quality of life. Very simple to use and applicable across cultures and languages due to graphic images with few words. Used in a large number of bariatric surgery studies.	Designed only for use after weight loss (items ask about how life has changed since weight loss). Cannot isolate the quality of life domain from total score.	Quality of life items are the original Moorehead-Ardelt Quality of Life Questionnaire. Listed in *Suggestions for the Pre-Surgical Psychological Assessment of Bariatric Surgery Candidates* (asbs.org). Accepted as the standard for reporting results after bariatric surgery in Austria, all German-speaking countries, Brazil, and Spain (Oria, 2003).
Bariatric Quality of Life (BQL; Weiner et al., 2005)	19	Germany	Comorbid Conditions/Gastrointestinal Side Effects Quality of Life	Good test-retest reliability. Good internal consistency reliability on the overall score.	The items on the quality of life (QOL) section are a mixture of weight-related items (e.g., "I like my weight"), general quality of life/life satisfaction items (e.g., "All in all, I feel satisfied in my life"), and self-report of moods/activities (e.g., "Sometimes, I feel depressed").	Also available in English, Spanish, and Italian. In a communication with the authors of the BQL, they indicate that they will soon publish a paper that provides a new way of analyzing BQL scores, distinguishing between the QOL and non-QOL scores and identifying four factors.

(Continued)

Table 2.1 (Continued)

Instrument Name	Number of Items	Country of Origin	Domains/Scales	Strengths	Weaknesses	Comments
					Internal consistency reliability for the non-QOL subscale was relatively weak (.548 to .690). Although three factors were derived, only two domains exist.	
Impact of Weight on Quality of Life (IWQOL; Kolotkin, Head, Hamilton, & Tse, 1995; Kolotkin, Head, & Brookhart, 1997)	74	United States	Health Social/Interpersonal Work Mobility Self-Esteem Sexual Life Activities of Daily Living Comfort With Food	Developed in clinical setting by obesity practitioners with input from patients in weight loss/lifestyle change treatment.	Large number of items creates heavy respondent burden. Test-retest reliability of only one day. Developed using homogeneous sample. Comfort With Food Scale is psychometrically weak.	No longer recommend use of IWQOL due to superiority of short form IWQOL-Lite.
Impact of Weight on Quality of Life—Lite (IWQOL-Lite; Kolotkin, Crosby, Kosloski, & Williams, 2001; Kolotkin & Crosby, 2002)	31	United States	Physical Function Self-Esteem Sexual Life Public Distress Work Total score	Excellent psychometric properties (test-retest from .83 to .94; alphas from .90 to .96; good convergent and discriminant validity; sensitive to body mass index [BMI], treatment-seeking status, weight loss, and weight gain). Scale structure verified with confirmatory factor analysis. Samples used for scale development were heterogeneous.	No specific scale to assess vitality or sleep, which are common problem areas reported in obese patients.	Translated or culturally adapted for use in 56 countries. Listed in *Patient-Reported Outcome and Quality of Life Instruments Database (PROQOLID)*, *Compendium of Quality of Life Instruments*, *On-Line Guide to Quality-of-Life-Assessment (OLGA)*, and *Suggestions for the Pre-Surgical Psychological Assessment of Bariatric Surgery Candidates (asbs.org)*.

Instrument Name	Number of Items	Country of Origin	Domains/Scales	Strengths	Weaknesses	Comments
				Different samples used for scale development and cross-validation.		Users of the IWQOL-Lite should note that in early studies, higher scores represented poorer quality of life, whereas current scoring associates higher scores with better quality of life.
Lewin-TAG Health-Related Quality of Life, Health State Preference (Lewin-TAG; Mathias et al., 1997)	55	United States	General Health Comparative Health Overweight Distress Depression Self-Regard Physical Appearance Health-State Preference	Support for construct validity. Scales are internally consistent (.85–.94). Adequate test-retest reliability (.59–.90). Able to detect change during weight loss treatment.	Lengthy. Displayed instability in the weight stable group. Some scales show weak test-retest. Little information available on the item scaling and total score. Some scales are generic and others are obesity specific.	
Moorehead-Ardelt Quality of Life Questionnaire II (MA II; Moorehead, Ardelt-Gattinger, Lechner, & Oria, 2003)	6	U.S. and Austria	General self-esteem Physical Activity Social Contacts Satisfaction Concerning Work	This is an update of the original MA Quality of Life Questionnaire that includes an item about eating behavior, improves wording of items and graphic symbols, allows for	Psychometric properties tested in a homogeneous sample of bariatric surgery candidates.	This instrument was designed as a stand-alone tool and/or to be used in conjunction with BAROS. Listed in *Suggestions for the Pre-Surgical Psychological*

(Continued)

Table 2.1 (Continued)

Instrument Name	Number of Items	Country of Origin	Domains/Scales	Strengths	Weaknesses	Comments
			Pleasure Relating to Sexuality Eating Behavior	assessment of pre- and post-weight loss changes, and makes response scale a 10-point scale. Internal consistency good (alpha = .84) in bariatric surgery sample. Some evidence for construct validity (correlations with SF-36, Beck Depression Inventory, and Three Factor Questionnaire).	Total score shows a negative, significant correlation with SF-36 Bodily Pain and a nonsignificant correlation with Physical Functioning. No individual item correlations reported (e.g., Physical Activity with SF-36 Physical Functioning).	Assessment of Bariatric Surgery Candidates (asbs.org).
Obesity Adjustment Survey–Short Form (OAS-SF; Butler et al., 1999)	20	Canada	Overall obesity adjustment/ psychological distress.	Total score is internally consistent (alpha = .72). Total score shows good test-retest (.87). Support for construct validity. Ability to detect change after bariatric surgery.	Quite a number of items demonstrate poor psychometric properties. Limited to measuring psychological distress. The 20 items were selected after unsuccessful factor analysis of original items. Development sample was predominantly female.	

Instrument Name	Number of Items	Country of Origin	Domains/Scales	Strengths	Weaknesses	Comments
Obesity and Weight Loss Quality of Life Questionnaire (OWLQOL; Patrick, Bushnell, & Rothman, 2004; Niero et al., 2002)	17	United States and Europe	Feelings and beliefs related to obesity and weight loss.	Developed on very large sample of obese persons in the United States and Europe, with the aim of being multicultural. Good internal consistency (alpha > .90). Good test-retest reliability (.95). A principal components analysis across four studies justifies unidimensionality of the construct and use of a single score. Provides evidence for construct validity. Responsive to reductions in body weight ($\geq$ 10% weight loss = effect size of 1.38).	Scores improved also for participants who gained weight.	Intended to be used in conjunction with WRSM.
Obesity-Related Coping Scale (OC; Ryden et al., 2001; Ryden, Karlsson, Sullivan, Torgerson, & Taft, 2003)	16	Sweden	Social Trust Fighting Spirit Wishful Thinking	Scales were derived by factor analysis, as well as developed in one group and tested psychometric properties in another. Good internal consistency reliability (alpha = .69 to .78).	Changes in Coping scores were similar in both surgical and conventional treatment groups despite differing amounts of weight loss.	Also available in English.

(Continued)

Table 2.1 (Continued)

Instrument Name	Number of Items	Country of Origin	Domains/Scales	Strengths	Weaknesses	Comments
				Able to differentiate between surgical candidates and participants seeking conventional treatment (lower Social Trust and Fighting Spirit and higher Wishful Thinking).		
Obesity-Related Distress Scale (OD; Ryden et al., 2001; Ryden et al., 2003)	13	Sweden	Intrusion Helplessness	Scales were derived by factor analysis, as well as developed in one group and tested psychometric properties in another. Good internal consistency reliability (alpha = .83 to .89). Able to differentiate surgical candidates from those seeking conventional treatment (surgical candidates report higher levels of distress).	Changes in Distress scores were similar in both surgical and conventional treatment groups despite differing amounts of weight loss.	Also available in English.

Instrument Name	Number of Items	Country of Origin	Domains/Scales	Strengths	Weaknesses	Comments
Obesity-Related Psychosocial Problems (OP; Karlsson, Sullivan et al., 1993; Taft, Sjöström, Torgerson, & Sullivan, 2003)	8	Sweden	Psychosocial problems related to obesity.	Brief. Good internal consistency (alpha = .92). Developed as part of the Swedish Obese Subjects large-scale studies. Validation data provided from four different samples. Strong support for construct validity. Factor analysis confirmed homogeneity of the construct. Demonstrated responsiveness to change with weight loss treatment. Guidelines are provided for interpretation of scores (< 40 = mild impairment; 40–59 = moderate; > 60 = severe).	Test-retest reliability not conducted.	Also available in English and Finnish.

(Continued)

Table 2.1 (Continued)

Instrument Name	Number of Items	Country of Origin	Domains/Scales	Strengths	Weaknesses	Comments
Obesity-Related Well-being Scale (ORWELL 97; Mannucci et al., 1999)	18	Italy	Psychological Status/Social Adjustment Physical Symptoms	Assesses relevance of symptoms plus occurrence. Total score is internally consistent (alpha = .83). Total score shows good test-retest reliability (.92).	Only physical symptoms correlated with BMI, not psychosocial impact. Little information is available on responsiveness and interpretation.	
Obese Specific Quality of Life (OSQOL; LePen, Levy, Loos, Banzet, & Basdevant, 1998)	11	France	Physical State Vitality/Desire to Do Things Relations With Other People Psychological State	Brief. Developed in a large community sample. Differentiated between obese and nonobese on three domains. Total score is internally consistent (.77).	Not tested on obese patients in treatment. Did not differentiate between obese and nonobese on Relations With Other People. No test-retest reliability conducted. Did not test internal consistency of individual scales. Only a moderate correlation obtained with BMI (r = .40).	

Instrument Name	Number of Items	Country of Origin	Domains/Scales	Strengths	Weaknesses	Comments
Weight-Related Symptom Measure (WRSM; Patrick, Bushnell, & Rothman, 2004; Niero et al., 2002)	20	United States and Europe	Symptoms associated with obesity and weight loss.	Developed on very large sample of obese persons in the United States and Europe, with the aim of being multicultural. Good internal consistency (.87). Good test-retest reliability (.83). Moderate responsiveness to weight reduction ($\geq$ 10% weight loss = effect size of –.47).		Designed to be used in conjunction with OWLQOL.

assess outcomes of bariatric surgery in three areas: percentage of excess weight lost, changes in medical conditions, and HRQOL (Oria & Moorehead, 1998). To develop the BAROS, the authors received survey input from 18 obesity surgeons regarding issues felt to be most important in evaluating bariatric surgery outcomes (Oria, 1996). Although the bariatric surgeons were most interested in assessing amount of weight loss and change in major and minor comorbid conditions, the BAROS authors recognized a need to include a quality of life component to the assessment. The original BAROS included the original Moorehead-Ardelt Quality of Life Questionnaire, (see Appendix 2.E.), which consisted of five items (feelings about self, ability to participate in physical activities, willingness to be involved socially, ability to work, and interest in sex) rated on a 5-point scale with pictures associated with each response category. The original instructions asked respondents to rate themselves with respect to how life had changed after weight loss, and thus this was not constructed as a pre-post weight loss measure. The Moorehead-Ardelt Quality of Life Questionnaire was revised in 2003 to become the Moorehead-Ardelt Quality of Life Questionnaire II (MA II; Moorehead, Ardelt-Gattinger, Lechner, & Oria, 2003), and this version of the instrument should be used with BAROS. In this revision, the wording of the items was changed to make them less suggestive and to allow for administration of the questionnaire pre– and post–weight loss, a sixth item assessing eating behavior was added (ranging from "I live to eat" to "I eat to live"), the number of response options was changed from 5 to 10, and drawings were used to depict the response options. Psychometric evaluation of the MA II was conducted. Although the MA II is part of the BAROS, it is also possible to use as a stand-alone instrument, as some authors have done (Caniato & Skorjanec, 2002). It is important to note that there has been some confusion in the literature regarding the BAROS and the MA II (Oria, 2003), with authors reporting that they used the BAROS when in fact they used the MA II and vice versa. In addition, some studies report BAROS results based on the original 5-point Moorehead-Ardelt Quality of Life Questionnaire, and others use the new MA II as recommended.

The BAROS results define five possible outcomes of bariatric surgery ("failure," "fair," "good," "very good," and "excellent") based on a total score derived from points obtained for percentage of excess weight lost (ranging from –1 for "weight gain" to +3 for "75 to 100% excess weight lost"), medical conditions (ranging from –1 for "aggravated" to +3 for "all major conditions resolved and others improved"), and quality of life (from –3 for "very poor" to +3 for "very good"). Points are deducted for minor complications (.2 points each), major complications (1 point each), and reoperation (1 point).

The BAROS has been used in the evaluation of a number of bariatric surgery studies. Some report results of gastric banding procedures (Caniato & Skorjanec, 2002; Favretti et al., 1998; Kalfarentzos, Kechagias, Soulikia, Loukidi, & Mead, 2001; Kinzl et al., 2007; Martikainen et al., 2004; Steffen, Biertho, Ricklin, Piec, & Horber, 2003; Victorzon & Tolonen, 2001), others report results of vertical banded gastroplasty (Kalfarentzos et al., 2001), and still others compare results of different surgical procedures (Hell, Miller, Moorehead, & Norman, 2000; Kalfarentzos, Skroubis, Kehagias, Mead, & Vagenas, 2006; Wolf, Falcone, Kortner, & Kuhlmann, 2000). Because the BAROS assesses overall bariatric surgery outcome and not quality of life per se, the following discussion is limited to studies that report results of the Moorehead-Ardelt Quality of Life Questionnaire. Nguyen and colleagues compared 3- and 6-month changes in MA quality of life (QoL) scores for U.S. patients randomized to either laparoscopic or open gastric bypass surgery (Nguyen et al., 2001). At 3 months, scores for the sexual and work domains were significantly higher after the laparoscopic procedure than after the open procedure; however, at 6 months, there were no significant differences between the two groups on MA QoL. The average %EWL was higher at both time points for the laparoscopic patients (37% vs. 32% at 3 months and 54% vs. 45% at 6 months). In Finland, Tolonen and Victorzon (2003) compared MA QoL results of 60 patients who received Swedish adjustable gastric banding on average 2 years earlier with a group of 65 patients who were assessed preoperatively. Scores on all domains of the MA QoL were significantly better among the operated patients.

No weight loss results were reported in this study. In a later study by this group (Tolonen, Victorzon, & Makela, 2004), significant improvements were found in all domains of the MA QoL one year after laparoscopic adjustable gastric banding in a prospective sample of 52 patients who experienced an average reduction of 45% EWL. Researchers in the United Kingdom reporting on changes in body weight and MA QoL in 81 patients who received laparoscopic adjustable gastric banding found improved self-esteem, physical activity, social involvement, and work on the MA QoL in 79% of patients, as well as greater than 50% EWL in 64% of patients (Titi, Jenkins, Modak, & Galloway, 2007). Gabriel and colleagues (2005) in Greece reported 2-year changes in %EWL and MA QoL for three groups of patients undergoing different bariatric surgery procedures. At the 2-year follow-up, MA QoL scores were higher in the two groups that underwent biliopancreatic diversion surgery and experienced greater changes in %EWL (99.6% EWL and 79.3% EWL vs. 77.4% EWL for the gastric bypass group). A U.S. study comparing gastric bypass patients with BMIs of > 60 with those having BMIs of < 60 found that both groups reported similar MA QoL scores during a 2-year period following surgery (Gould, Garren, Boll, & Starling, 2006). In a prospective randomized trial of laparoscopic versus open gastric bypass in the United States, no significant differences were observed in the %EWL between groups at the 3-year follow-up (77% for laparoscopic vs. 67% for open), nor were there differences in the amount of improvement shown on the MA QoL (Puzziferri, Austrheim-Smith, Wolfe, Wilson, & Nguyen, 2006). In a French study of two bariatric surgery procedures, MA QoL scores gradually improved over a 5-year period postsurgically, during which time a regular weight loss was also observed (Folope et al., 2008). As weight subsequently increased over the next 5 years, MA QoL scores worsened. MA II data from 67 U.S. laparoscopic adjustable gastric banding patients at an average of 27 months postsurgery revealed improved scores on self-esteem and physical activity and an average %EWL of 53.2% (Myers et al., 2006). A study of obese adolescents undergoing laparoscopic adjustable gastric banding in Austria reported improved MA QoL scores over a mean

follow-up period of 34.7 months, occurring in conjunction with a mean weight loss of 35.2 kg and %EWL of 61.4% (Silberhumer et al., 2006). Thus, a number of studies conducted internationally report improvements in MA QoL scores following various bariatric surgery procedures.

Impact of Weight on Quality of Life

Items for the Impact of Weight on Quality of Life (IWQOL; Kolotkin, Head, & Brookhart, 1997; Kolotkin, Head, Hamilton, & Tse, 1995) were developed to reflect the most commonly expressed concerns by patients in intensive treatment for obesity. Patients, individually and in groups, were asked to describe the effects of being overweight in their everyday lives. Their responses were recorded, rewritten in the form of items, and grouped by category. In addition, clinicians who specialized in the treatment of obese persons wrote and categorized items based on their clinical experience. Items were tested for clarity and modified as needed. Psychometric properties of the IWQOL were adequate. Test-retest reliabilities averaged .75 for single items and .89 for scales (Kolotkin et al., 1995). Scale internal consistency reliability ranged from .68 to .92 in one study (Kolotkin et al., 1995) and from .76 to .95 in another study (Kolotkin et al., 1997). Scores improved after weight loss treatment, demonstrating responsiveness, and scores varied by BMI, demonstrating sensitivity. IWQOL scores correlated highly with similar measures in the expected direction (Kolotkin et al., 1997).

A few published studies report results obtained from the IWQOL. In an RCT of sibutramine versus placebo for patients with type 2 diabetes, IWQOL scores improved over a 24-week period for the treatment group relative to placebo (Fujioka, Seaton, Rowe, & et al., 2000). In a study of pooled data from four RCT sibutramine trials, weight loss was associated with improvements in IWQOL scores on several of the domains at various assessment points up to 1 year (Samsa et al., 2001). Results from an RCT of zonisamide for weight loss indicated improvement in several scales of the IWQOL over 16 weeks (Gadde, Franciscy, Wagner, & Krishnan, 2003). In a study of patients undergoing biliopancreatic diversion (a type of bariatric surgery), improvements were observed on the IWQOL (Adami et al., 2005). A 6-month RCT of sibutramine conducted in Italy reported that participants in the sibutramine group not only lost more weight than those in the placebo group, but their IWQOL scores showed greater improvements (Di Francesco et al., 2007).

Impact of Weight on Quality of Life–Lite

The Impact of Weight on Quality of Life–Lite (IWQOL-Lite; Kolotkin & Crosby, 2002; Kolotkin, Crosby, Kosloski, & Williams, 2001), a short form of the IWQOL, was developed in response to feedback from clinical trial researchers about the potential respondent burden of a 74-item instrument (see Appendix 2.D). Because the IWQOL-Lite is superior psychometrically to the IWQOL (see Table 2.1) and contains only 31 items, the instrument developer (RK) no longer recommends use of the IWQOL. For researchers who have administered the IWQOL items, a simple algorithm for scoring the IWQOL-Lite items and scales is available from the developer.

The IWQOL-Lite contains 31 items, most of which begin with the phrase, "Because of my weight." For each item, there are five response options ranging from *never true* to *always true*. The IWQOL-Lite provides scores on five factor-analyzed scales (Physical Function, Self-Esteem, Sexual Life, Public Distress, and Work), as well as a total score. Scores are transformed to a 0 to 100 scale, with 100 representing the best HRQOL.

In a large sample of individuals, most of whom were seeking weight loss treatment, reliability coefficients (Cronbach's alpha) for individual scales ranged from .90 to .94, with an overall alpha of .96 (Kolotkin, Crosby, Kosloski, & Williams, 2001). In a sample of community volunteers (Kolotkin & Crosby, 2002), Cronbach's alpha for the IWQOL-Lite total score was .96, and alphas for individual scales ranged from .82 to .94. Test-retest reliability ranged from .84 to .91 for scales (average of .89) and was .95 for total score. The IWQOL-Lite has also demonstrated reliability and validity in obese individuals with type 2 diabetes (Kolotkin, Crosby, & Williams, 2003), in individuals with schizophrenia (of whom 64% were obese)

or bipolar disorder (of whom 68% were obese; Kolotkin, Crosby, Corey-Lisle, & Swanson, 2006), and in two Portuguese samples (participants enrolled in a weight loss program and community volunteers; Engel et al., 2005).

Results from confirmatory factor analysis provided strong support for both the scale structure of the IWQOL-Lite and the existence of a higher order factor, presumably weight-related HRQOL. Correlations between IWQOL-Lite and collateral measures (Beck Depression Inventory, Rosenberg Self-Esteem, SCL-90R, global ratings, SF-36, Marlowe-Crowne Social Desirability) supported the construct validity of the IWQOL-Lite (convergent and discriminant validity; Kolotkin & Crosby, 2002). In addition, higher BMIs were also associated with poorer HRQOL on the IWQOL-Lite, further supporting construct validity. In the primarily clinical sample, all five scales and the total IWQOL-Lite score correlated significantly ($p < .001$) with BMI at baseline (Kolotkin, Crosby, Kosloski, & Williams, 2001). Individual correlations were Physical Function = .61, Self-Esteem = .34, Sexual Life = .30, Public Distress = .68, Work = .35, and total score = .59. In the sample of community volunteers, the correlation between BMI and IWQOL-Lite scores ($p < .001$) were as follows: Physical Function = .681, Self-Esteem = .370, Sexual Life = .281, Public Distress = .518, Work = .522, and total score = .615 (Kolotkin & Crosby, 2002).

Other evidence of construct validity was provided by examining 1-year changes in IWQOL-Lite scores for participants in an open-label trial of phentermine-fenfluramine. Changes in IWQOL-Lite scores showed statistically significant correlations with percentage of weight loss for all scales and total score ($r = .370$ total score, .396 Physical Function, .242 Self-Esteem, .294 Sexual Life, .166 Public Distress, and .169 Work; Kolotkin, Crosby, Williams, Hartley, & Nicol, 2001). About 14% of the variance in IWQOL-Lite total score could be accounted for by weight loss. The scales showing the most change at 1 year were Physical Function and Self-Esteem. In a study to evaluate the impact of weight regain on IWQOL-Lite scores over a period of up to 41 months, it was determined that weight regain produces mirror effects on IWQOL-Lite scores (i.e., weight loss is associated with improvements in IWQOL-Lite scores, and weight regain is associated with comparable reductions in IWQOL-Lite scores; Engel et al., 2003).

In addition to reporting pre-post treatment changes in HRQOL using tests of statistical significance, it is beneficial to determine whether the size of these changes is meaningful or clinically significant (Crosby, Kolotkin, & Williams, 2003). Often described as "clinically meaningful change," "minimally important difference," or "clinically important difference," such analyses have practical significance for interpretability of results of clinical trials (Food and Drug Administration [FDA], 2006). An algorithm for determining whether changes in IWQOL-Lite scores are meaningful has been described by Crosby and colleagues (Crosby et al., 2003; Crosby, Kolotkin, & Williams, 2004). This algorithm combines information from anchor-based and distribution-based methods and takes into account baseline severity (none/mild, moderate/severe) and statistical regression to the mean. Baseline severity is determined by comparison to a normative sample of 534 nonobese individuals not enrolled in any weight loss program. The cutoff for determining whether changes in IWQOL-Lite scores are meaningful is 7.8 points for individuals with low baseline impairments in weight-related quality of life and 12 points for those with severe baseline impairments.

Several studies have used the IWQOL-Lite to evaluate HRQOL. In a large, geographically and demographically diverse sample of overweight/obese adults who were or were not seeking obesity treatment, IWQOL-Lite scores were compared across groups to determine if HRQOL varied by treatment-seeking status (Kolotkin, Crosby, & Williams, 2002). Results indicated that overweight/obese individuals not seeking weight loss treatment had higher IWQOL-Lite scores (i.e., better quality of life) than those seeking weight loss treatment. In addition, IWQOL-Lite scores for those seeking weight loss treatment varied by treatment intensity, with the greatest impairment occurring for the group seeking bariatric surgery, followed by the group seeking treatment in an intensive day treatment setting, followed by participants in outpatient weight loss programs/studies, followed by participants in clinical trials. In a different study addressing a similar issue, a group of patients seeking gastric bypass surgery was compared to an obese control sample on IWQOL-Lite scores (Kolotkin, Crosby, Pendleton, et al., 2003). After controlling for BMI, age, and gender, obesity-specific HRQOL was significantly more impaired ($p < .001$) in the surgery-seeking group than in the control group on all five scales and total score of the IWQOL-Lite. For total score, Physical Function, and Sexual Life, there was increasing impairment with increasing number of comorbid conditions. Treatment-seeking status, BMI, gender, and the presence of depression accounted for most of the variance in IWQOL-Lite total score. Another study comparing IWQOL-Lite scores in bariatric surgery patients versus obese patients seeking residential treatment found that despite equivalent BMIs and degree of depressive symptoms, bariatric surgery patients reported greater impairments in IWQOL-Lite scores than patients seeking residential treatment for obesity (Stout, Applegate, Friedman, Grant, & Musante, 2007).

The relationship of gender and race to IWQOL-Lite scores in a sample with extreme obesity seeking bariatric surgery (mean BMI = 53.3) was evaluated by White, O'Neil, Kolotkin, and Byrne (2004). In general, White women reported the most impairment in IWQOL-Lite scores, despite having significantly lower BMIs than other race/gender groups. Compared with previous studies, the observed relationships between BMI and IWQOL-Lite were attenuated in this sample. As in the studies reported above, the deleterious effects of even extreme obesity on weight-related HRQOL are not experienced equally across subgroups of obese persons.

Several studies have evaluated IWQOL-Lite scores in obese individuals with binge-eating disorder (de Zwaan, Mitchell, et al., 2002; de Zwaan et al., 2003; Kolotkin et al., 2004). In two studies by de Zwaan and colleagues (de Zwaan, Mitchell, et al., 2002; de Zwaan et al., 2003), bariatric surgery patients with and without binge-eating disorder (BED) were compared on IWQOL-Lite scores. Patients with BED had lower scores (greater impairment) than patients without BED. Another study compared obese participants with BED enrolled in a multisite RCT of sibutramine for treatment of BED with obese individuals without BED enrolled in an RCT investigating the effectiveness of psychological interventions for weight loss maintenance in children and their parents (Rieger, Willey, Stein, Marino, & Crow, 2005). Results demonstrated that participants with BED had greater impairment on the IWQOL-Lite total score as well as four of the five individual scales (all except Physical Function). In another study, patients with BED who enrolled in an intensive residential lifestyle modification program demonstrated reduced HRQOL compared to participants without BED on total IWQOL-Lite score and all IWQOL-Lite subscales (Kolotkin et al., 2004). However, after controlling for demographic variables, BMI, and psychological symptoms, BED was not independently associated with HRQOL. Thus, the association between BED and impairment in HRQOL previously reported in the literature may largely be accounted for by differences between those with and without BED on demographic variables, BMI, and psychological symptoms.

In a study of individuals referred for weight management at U.K. specialist centers, about a third of individuals demonstrated markedly impaired IWQOL-Lite scores (Tuthill, Slawik, O'Rahilly, & Finer, 2006). Sexual Life, Work, and Public Distress were areas of particular impairment in men; Sexual Life and Self-Esteem were the major areas of impairment in women.

Several studies have examined how weight loss relates to IWQOL-Lite scores. In a cross-sectional study of bariatric surgery patients, Dymek, Le Grange, Neven, and Alverdy (2002) compared a preoperative control group of morbidly obese patients awaiting surgery (T1) with groups of patients at three different postsurgical time points: 2 to 4 weeks postsurgery (T2), 6 months postsurgery (T3), and 1 year postsurgery (T4). Results showed significant differences between T1 and T2 only on the Physical Function scale of the IWQOL-Lite (as well as three of the SF-36 scales—General Health, Vitality, and Mental Health). Significant differences were found between T2 and T3 on all IWQOL-Lite scales (and also all scales of the SF-36). Significant differences were found between T3 and T4 on IWQOL-Lite total score and three of the individual scales (Physical Function, Self-Esteem, and Public Distress) but on none of the SF-36 scales, suggesting greater sensitivity in this study of the obesity-specific measure between 6 and 12 months postsurgery.

In a study of changes in HRQOL after gastric bypass, Boan, Kolotkin, Westman, McMahon, and Grant (2004) found significant improvement in all IWQOL-Lite scores ($p < .0001$) at 6 months following an average weight loss of 26.7%. Mean scores at 6 months were comparable to those obtained by a reference sample of community volunteers, despite a mean follow-up BMI of 38.9 in the surgically treated patients.

In a multicenter randomized clinical trial for weight reduction, Heshka and colleagues (2003) compared treatment outcomes over a 2-year period for participants in a self-help group with participants in a structured commercial program. Mean weight loss in the commercial group was greater than in the self-help group at 1 and 2 years, but no significant differences were observed between groups in HRQOL (IWQOL-Lite and SF-36). Improvement in HRQOL was related to the amount of weight reduction. The IWQOL-Lite scales showing the greatest improvements were Physical Function, Public Distress, and total score.

A German study of a weight reduction program (self-help and counseling) reported that 66% of participants lost at least 5% of their weight and 24% lost at least 10% of their weight. In 80% of the subjects, IWQOL-Lite scores showed improvement (Scholz et al., 2002).

Obesity-Related Psychosocial Problems (OP Scale). The OP Scale (Karlsson, Taft, Sjöström, Torgerson, & Sullivan, 2003; Sullivan et al., 1993) was developed for the Swedish Obese Subjects (SOS) study (Sullivan et al., 1993) as part of a large assessment battery that included generic measures of HRQOL, global measures of quality of life, measures of mental health, and condition-specific complaints regarding daily functioning, eating behavior, and psychosocial problems (see Appendix 2.C). The SOS study was the first large-scale research effort to emphasize the importance of assessing perceived health status and HRQOL in obesity. The OP Scale, which provides a single score assessing psychological problems related to obesity, asks respondents to rate on a 4-point scale if their obesity bothers them in activities such as private gatherings, community activities, and intimate relations. Lower scores indicate better HRQOL. Details on the psychometric properties of the OP Scale are provided in Table 2.1.

Cross-sectional results from the first 1,743 subjects registered in the SOS study showed high levels of obesity-related psychosocial problems in everyday life on the OP Scale, with women experiencing more of these problems than men (Sullivan et al., 1993). In the SOS 2-year follow-up study of bariatric surgical cases (65% vertical banded gastroplasty, 28% gastric banding, and 7% gastric bypass) versus matched controls, significant improvements on the OP Scale were found in the surgical group compared to controls. However, changes in the OP Scale were also significant for women in the control group but not men (Karlsson et al., 1998).

In the 4-year follow-up of the SOS study (Karlsson et al., 2003), greater reductions in body weight were associated with greater improvements on the OP Scale for both the surgical and control groups (the surgical group lost an average of 18.9% of weight and the controls gained an average of 1.1%). Although scores on the OP Scale improved in both surgical and control groups, improvement was markedly higher in the surgical group. Effect sizes for the surgically treated patients were 1.25 and 1.04 for women and men, respectively, whereas for the control group, effect sizes were .39 and .21. For those who lost 15% or more of their body weight, improvements on the OP Scale scores were stable over the 4-year follow-up period. For those who experienced less than 5% weight loss, OP Scale scores tended to return to baseline levels. At 4 years, approximately 20% of the surgical patients had BMIs below the obese range. For these individuals, OP Scale scores were similar to those obtained by the nonobese reference group.

Another study conducted in Sweden (using 6,863 subjects from the SOS cross-sectional study, 2,128 from the SOS intervention study, 1,017 nonobese from the SOS reference study, and 3,305 obese subjects from a randomized clinical trial for a pharmacological agent) reported large differences on the OP Scale between obese and nonobese individuals and greater psychosocial problems for women than for men (Karlsson et al., 2003). In addition, psychological disturbance due to obesity was related to increased anxiety and decreased mood. Intentional weight loss was strongly correlated with changes in the OP Scale, with greater reductions in weight associated with even greater changes in the OP Scale.

In an 8-month randomized trial of a very low-energy diet/behavior modification treatment for men conducted in Finland, the mean weight loss of the treated group was 13.9%, whereas the control group was weight stable (Kaukua, Pekkarinen, Sane, & Mustajoki, 2002). Significant improvements in OP Scale scores were maintained until the end of follow-up for men in the treated group, while scores for the control group remained stable throughout the study. In another Finnish study, changes in weight and HRQOL were assessed at 2 years in 126 obese men and women referred for a 4-month very low-energy diet and behavior modification treatment in an outpatient setting (Kaukua, Pekkarinen, Sane, & Mustajoki, 2003). Improvements in the OP Scale peaked at the end of therapy (when patients had lost 12.5% of baseline weight), and this improvement was maintained up to 2 years despite weight regain (mean weight loss at 2 years was 2.6%). A dose-response effect was demonstrated at 2 years, such that greater weight loss was associated with less obesity-related psychosocial disturbance.

Comments: Obesity-Specific HRQOL Instruments

The OP Scale has generally strong psychometric properties, including sensitivity to BMI and responsiveness to changes in body weight. Women report more psychosocial problems than men on the OP Scale. In addition, greater psychosocial problems on the OP Scale have been associated with increased anxiety/depression and decreased mood. The greatest concern about the OP Scale is in regard to its responsiveness in weight-stable individuals. Scores improved for women (not men) in the control group at the 2-year follow-up, as well as in the control subjects at the 4-year follow-up. Although surgical cases improved more than control subjects, ideally, scores on the OP Scale would be relatively unchanged for control subjects.

The IWQOL is no longer recommended for use due to the psychometric superiority of its short form version (IWQOL-Lite). When the IWQOL has been administered, it is recommended that researchers obtain the scoring algorithm for the IWQOL-Lite.

There is a large body of evidence supporting the strong psychometric properties of the IWQOL-Lite. Widely used in studies, the IWQOL-Lite has been recommended for use in clinical practice and research studies on obesity by major organizations, including the Task Force on Developing Obesity Outcomes and Learning Tools (TOOLS; Wadden & Phelan, 2002), the American Society for Bariatric Surgery (2004), and the European Association for Endoscopic Surgery (Korolija et al., 2004). Moreover, a review paper by Ballantyne (2003), which discusses the importance of assessing HRQOL with standardized instruments following bariatric surgery, indicates that the IWQOL-Lite is one of three instruments that has been tested extensively (the other two are the SF-36 and the BAROS). Stucki and colleagues (2006) compared the content of 12 obesity-specific measures, identifying 413 core concepts and linking these to the International Classification of Functioning, Disability, and Health (ICF). After reviewing each of the instruments, they concluded that only the IWQOL-Lite (and the Bariatric Quality of Life Index [BQL]—see Table 2.1 and Appendix 2.G) contains all of the ICF components (body structures, body function, activity and participation, environmental factors, and personal factors). Thus, the IWQOL-Lite appears to be a reliable, valid, and useful tool for assessment of HRQOL in obesity. In addition, the IWQOL-Lite has been has been translated/adapted for use in 60 countries.

The BAROS, which includes the MA II, is widely used in bariatric surgery studies, particularly in Europe. The BAROS takes into account percentage of excess weight lost, medical conditions, and HRQOL. A potential weakness of the BAROS is that one cannot necessarily isolate the HRQOL score from the total score and/or categorical outcome (five outcomes ranging from *failure* to *excellent*). In addition, the BAROS was designed to assess changes after surgery and thus was not designed as a pre-post measure. The MA II is listed in *Suggestions for the Pre-Surgical Psychological Assessment of Bariatric Surgery Candidates* (American Society for Bariatric Surgery, 2004). The MA II has good internal consistency and some evidence for construct validity. However, no individual item correlations with collateral measures/scales were reported, and total score shows a nonsignificant correlation with SF-36 Physical Functioning as well as a negative correlation with Bodily Pain.

Several of the other obesity-specific instruments listed in Table 2.1 deserve special mention. The Obesity and Weight Loss Quality of Life Questionnaire (OWLQOL—see Appendix 2.A; Patrick, Bushnell, & Rothman, 2004; Niero et al., 2002) and Weight-Related Symptom Measure (WRSM; Patrick, Bushnell, & Rothman, 2004; Niero et al., 2002) are unique in that they were developed using samples from both the United States and Europe, with the aim of being multicultural. In addition, ratings of "bothersomeness" (OWLQOL) have been separated from symptom ratings (WRSM) by creating two separate instruments designed to be used simultaneously. The OWLQOL was developed using sound methodology, and its psychometric properties are good (Patrick et al., 2004). However, there may be some problems regarding its responsiveness. Although weight reductions of at least 10% were associated with improved OWLQOL scores, scores also showed improvement for subjects who gained weight.

Although the BQL (see Table 2.1) in its current form has significant weaknesses, future developments on this instrument look promising. The authors have indicated (personal communication, 2007) that they are developing a new way of analyzing scores that identifies four factors (psychological, social, physical, and weight related), separates a quality of life scale from a non-quality of life scale, and adds new items. However, the instrument may still be scored with only a total score rather than individual domain scores, which may dilute some of the information and is only warranted if confirmed by factor analysis.

An instrument in development may be of interest for use with patients with extreme obesity. Duval, Marceau, Lescelleur, et al. (2006) identified 187 items related to extreme obesity (based on literature reviews, expert opinion, currently available obesity-specific instruments, and semistructured interviews with patients). They asked bariatric surgery candidates to identify the items most significant for them and to rate each item's importance. The impact of each item was determined from the proportion of patients who identified it as important and the mean importance score attributed to the item. Using this system, 46 items were retained and assigned into one of seven domains by clinical judgment (not factor analysis): activity/mobility, symptoms, personal hygiene/clothing, emotions, social interactions, sexual life, and eating behavior. The areas of impairment due to obesity were quite similar for men and women; however, women reported greater overall impact of obesity and rated dissatisfaction with physical appearance as more important (second in importance for women and seventh in importance for men). BMI showed a strong association with the degree of impact of these items (higher BMI associated with greater impact). This new instrument shows some promise for researchers/clinicians assessing individuals with extreme obesity; however, additional research is needed on its psychometric properties, including factor analysis.

Generic HRQOL Instruments for Childhood and Adolescent Obesity

Three measures of generic HRQOL have been used in pediatric populations to study obesity. These are presented below in alphabetical order.

Child Health Questionnaire

The Child Health Questionnaire (CHQ; Waters, Salmon, Wake, Wright, & Hesketh, 2001) is an 80-item generic self-report measure of adolescent HRQOL with 12 domains: Physical Functioning, Role Social–Emotional, Role Social–Behavioral, Role Social–Physical, Bodily Pain, Behavior, Mental Health, Self-Esteem, General Health, Family Activities, Family Cohesion, and Change in Health (Waters et al., 2001). Item responses are made on a 4- to 6-point scale, and scores are transformed to a 0 to 100 scale. The 80-item CHQ is a modification of the original 87-item CHQ, which was developed in the United States for children ages 10 to 16 years. The 80-item CHQ was adapted for use in Australia after pilot testing revealed a need for eliminating some items and changing the recommended age to 12 to 18 years. The psychometric properties of the 80-item CHQ were tested in a large representative population-based sample of

adolescents with a mean age of 15. Internal consistency alphas ranged from .79 to .92 for the nine multi-item scales (the other scales contained one or two items and thus alphas were not computed). Nearly 100% of the items correlated more highly with their own scale than with competing scales (i.e., item-scale discriminant validity). Item-to-scale correlations ranged from .38 to .76; 10% of the items did not meet the recommended .40 criterion. Adolescents with health conditions/concerns reported lower scores, supporting content and construct validity. Ceiling effects were observed on some of the scales, with Role Social–Behavioral and Role Social–Physical exhibiting the greatest ceiling effects (74.3% and 81.6%, respectively).

The large number of items on the CHQ may make administration of this instrument impractical. In addition, the presence of ceiling effects on some of the scales may present some difficulties in assessment.

The CHQ is also available in a 50-item parent form (CHQ-PF50; Landgraf, Abetz, & Ware, 1996). The CHQ-PF50 has been evaluated for psychometric properties across different ages, cultures, education, marital status, and work status and also with children who have various chronic health conditions.

The association between HRQOL (as assessed by CHQ-PF50) and BMI in preadolescent school-aged children (ages 8–11 years) was examined in a community-based sample of 371 children in the United States (Friedlander, Larkin, Rosen, Palermo, & Redline, 2003). Compared with healthy-weight children, children in the overweight group had significantly lower scores on Psychosocial Health Summary, Self-Esteem, Parental Emotional Well-Being, Physical Functioning, Behavior, Global General Health, and Global Behavior. Only Physical Functioning was lower in the at risk for overweight group compared with the healthy-weight children.

Another study examined parent-reported HRQOL using the CHQ-PF50 in a large school-age sample in Australia (Wake, Salmon, Waters, Wright, & Hesketh, 2002). Using logistic regression analyses with "normal weight" as the referent category, obese boys were at greater risk of poor health (< 15th percentile) on 7 of the 12 CHQ scales: Physical Functioning (odds ratio [OR] = 2.8), Bodily Pain (OR = 1.8), General Health

(OR = 3.5), Mental Health (OR = 2.8), Self-Esteem (OR = 1.8), Parent Impact–Emotional (OR = 1.7), and Parent Impact–Time (OR = 1.9). Obese girls were at greater risk of poor health on only two scales: General Health (OR = 2.1) and Self-Esteem (OR = 1.8). Forty-two percent of parents with obese children and 81% with overweight children did not report concern about their child's weight.

KINDL

The KINDL (Ravens-Sieberer & Bullinger, 1998) is a 40-item generic HRQOL instrument for children ages 8 to 16 years developed in Germany (Ravens-Sieberer & Bullinger, 1998). The items cover four conceptual domains: Mental, Physical, Everyday Life, and Social Life. Scores are provided on each of these domains plus total score. Psychometric properties of the KINDL were tested on a group of 45 chronically ill children with diabetes or asthma in comparison to 45 age- and gender-matched healthy children. Cronbach's alpha was .95 for total score and at least .75 for individual scales (from .76–.95 for chronically ill children and from .74–.90 for healthy children). Some support for validity was provided by statistically significant correlations between KINDL scales and particular SF-36 scales (General Health, Mental Health, and Vitality), as well as with a German questionnaire for life satisfaction (FLZ; Henrich & Herschbach, 1995). Intercorrelations among the scales were high (.54–.94). However, the KINDL was unable to differentiate between chronically ill and healthy children, and the scales appear not to have been factor analytically derived.

A revised version of the KINDL, along with a 12-item obesity module, was used in a study of the effects of obesity and obesity treatment on HRQOL in children with a mean age of 12 (Ravens-Sieberer, Redegeld, & Bullinger, 2001). The revised KINDL contained 24 items assessing Physical Functioning, Self-Esteem, Psychological Well-Being, Friends, Family, and School. The KINDL was administered to children, and parents completed a parent proxy form. Scores were significantly lower (poorer HRQOL) for children above the age of 13 on the Physical Functioning, Self-Esteem, and School scales. Girls also had reduced HRQOL relative to boys in Physical Functioning,

Psychological Well-Being, Self-Esteem, and total score. For all scales except Physical Functioning, obese children exhibited greater impairments in HRQOL than children with asthma/atopic dermatitis. Obese children's scores on the KINDL also indicated improvement on all scales except Psychological Well-Being following treatment for obesity.

Pediatric Quality of Life Inventory

The Pediatric Quality of Life Inventory (PedsQL; Varni, Seid, & Kurtin, 2001) is a 23-item generic measure of HRQOL with complementary scales for children (ages 8–12) and adolescents (ages 13–18). There are four core scales (Physical, Emotional, Social, and School), two broad domain scores (Physical and Psychosocial Functioning), and a total score. Scales are standardized, ranging from 0 to 100, with higher scores representing better HRQOL. The PedsQL has been shown to be both reliable and valid, with internal consistency reliability coefficients approaching or exceeding .70. Cronbach's alpha was .88 for the total score, .80 for the Physical Health summary, and .83 for the Psychosocial Health summary. Validity was demonstrated using the known-groups method, as well as correlations with indicators of morbidity and illness burden. In addition, the PedsQL distinguished between healthy children and pediatric patients with acute or chronic health conditions, was related to indicators of morbidity and illness burden, and displayed a factor-derived solution largely consistent with conceptually derived scales. The PedsQL has been translated or culturally adapted for use in 71 countries.

Parent proxy forms of the PedsQL have also been developed and validated for ages 2 to 16 in a sample of over 13,000 children recruited from general pediatric clinics, subspecialty clinics, and hospitals in which their children were being seen for well-child visits, mild acute illness, or chronic illness care, as well as from a state health insurance program (Varni, Limbers, & Burwinkle, 2007). The majority of the parent proxy report scales exceeded the minimum internal consistency reliability standard of .70 required for group comparisons, while the total scale scores across the age subgroups approached or exceeded the reliability criterion of .90 recommended for analyzing individual patient scale scores. Construct validity was demonstrated using known-groups comparisons. For each PedsQL scale and summary score, across age subgroups, healthy children demonstrated better HRQOL than children with known chronic health conditions.

The PedsQL has been used in a number of studies to assess generic HRQOL in overweight and obese youth. Schwimmer, Burwinkle, and Varni (2003) compared PedsQL scores in children/adolescents referred for evaluation of obesity at a hospital with youth who were healthy or diagnosed with cancer. In addition to the self-report PedsQL forms, parent proxy forms were used. Compared with healthy children/adolescents, obese children/adolescents reported significantly reduced HRQOL in all domains on both the self-report and parent proxy forms. Scores for obese children/adolescents were similar to scores obtained by children/adolescents diagnosed with cancer.

Hughes, Farewell, Harris, and Reilly (2007) compared a clinical sample of 126 obese children in the United Kingdom with 71 matched lean controls using the PedsQL (both self-report and parent proxy). With regard to self-reports of HRQOL among children, only Physical Health was significantly lower for obese children compared to lean controls. Parent proxy HRQOL was lower than child self-reports for the clinical sample in all domains except Physical Health and School Functioning. However, parent proxy HRQOL was higher for lean controls than for obese children in all domains.

A study of 166 obese youth referred to a pediatric weight management program indicated that PedsQL self-report scores were impaired relative to published norms for healthy children (Zeller & Modi, 2006). Parents also reported significantly lower scores for their children on most scales of the PedsQL. In addition, depressive symptoms, perceived social support from classmates, degree of overweight, and socioeconomic status were strong predictors of PedsQL scores.

HRQOL was assessed retrospectively using PedsQL self-report and parent proxy forms in 33 adolescents with extreme obesity presenting for bariatric surgery (Zeller, Roehrig, Modi, Daniels, & Inge, 2006). Both self-report and parent proxy HRQOL scores were markedly reduced relative to instrument norms for healthy youth. Results

indicated that females exhibited greater impairments than males for Social Functioning (self-report and parent proxy). Furthermore, scores obtained by this sample were more impaired than those reported in the literature for a less overweight clinical sample of overweight youth (Schwimmer et al., 2003).

A study conducted in Israel compared PedsQL scores (both self-report and parent proxy) of 182 obese children in a hospital setting to children from the community (Pinhas-Hamiel et al., 2006). Obese children reported significantly lower HRQOL in the Physical, Social, and School domains compared with children who were not overweight. There were no differences between obese children from the hospital setting and community-dwelling obese children. Results of the parent proxy forms were similar to the self-report forms among nonoverweight children; however, parents' scores for overweight children were consistently lower than children's self-report.

Another study of HRQOL in overweight and obese youth was conducted in Australia on a large population-based community sample (Williams, Wake, Hesketh, Maher, & Waters, 2005). Both parent proxy and child self-reported PedsQL scores decreased with increasing child weight. However, scores on the PedsQL were less impaired for overweight/obese children in this community sample compared to those obtained by Schwimmer and colleagues (2003) in a clinical sample.

Only two studies could be found that described changes in PedsQL scores in overweight youth following weight loss interventions. Holterman and colleagues (2007) reported short-term results (9 months) of the first 10 obese adolescent girls to participate in a prospective trial of laparoscopic adjustable gastric banding in the United States. Self-reported PedsQL total score showed significant improvements at 6 and 9 months, whereas parent reports showed significant improvements at 3, 6, and 12 months. The mean %EWL was 22%, 30%, and 30%, respectively. In a 6-month prospective randomized trial of an intensive instructor-led weight loss intervention versus self-help in Mexican American children, changes in PedsQL total score, physical HRQOL, and psychosocial HRQOL were evaluated along with changes in zBMI (Fullerton et al., 2007). Children in the instructor-led group reported significantly greater improvements in physical HRQOL than children in the self-help group, and they experienced greater changes in zBMI. Improvements in physical HRQOL were associated with reductions in zBMI. There were no differences between groups on the other aspects of HRQOL.

Disease-Specific HRQOL Instruments for Childhood and Adolescent Obesity

Impact of Weight on Quality of Life–Kids

The Impact of Weight on Quality of Life–Kids (IWQOL-Kids—see Appendix 2.H; Kolotkin, Zeller, et al., 2006), designed for adolescents ages 11 to 19, is the only disease-specific measure of HRQOL for pediatric obesity to date. The IWQOL-Kids is a 27-item instrument consisting of four factor analytically derived domains (Physical Comfort, Body Esteem, Social Life, and Family Relations), with the factors accounting for 71% of the variance. Similar to the IWQOL-Lite for adults, items begin with the phrase, "Because of my weight"; there are five response options ranging from *never true* to *always true;* and scores are transformed to a 0- to 100-scale, with 100 representing the best HRQOL.

The IWQOL-Kids was developed in a large, geographically and ethnically diverse sample that included a range of BMIs as well as both clinical and community samples. Items were created based on a literature review and the clinical experience of obesity and/or pediatric experts. Internal consistency coefficients for the IWQOL-Kids ranged from .88 to .95 for domains and .96 for total score (Kolotkin, Zeller, et al., 2006). Tests of mean group differences among BMI groups and between clinical and community samples provided support for the validity of the IWQOL-Kids (Kolotkin, Zeller, et al., 2006). In addition, correlations with zBMI and scales of the PedsQL were significant and in the hypothesized direction. As expected, the highest correlations between IWQOL-Kids and PedsQL scales were obtained on similar domains, supporting convergent validity of the IWQOL-Kids (e.g., Physical Comfort with

PedsQL Physical). Furthermore, lower correlations were found between dissimilar constructs on the IWQOL-Kids scales and the PedsQL (e.g., IWQOL-Kids Family Relations, PedsQL School), showing evidence of discriminant validity.

The sensitivity of the IWQOL-Kids was compared to the sensitivity of the PedsQL by calculating effect sizes comparing the highest and lowest BMI groups (Kolotkin, Zeller, et al., 2006). For the IWQOL-Kids, effect sizes exceeded 1.00 for all scales except Family Relations (effect size = .59). For the PedsQL, effect sizes ranged from .46 (Emotional) to .95 (Physical).

Gender differences were demonstrated on Body Esteem and total score after adjusting for zBMI, with girls reporting lower scores than boys. After adjusting for zBMI, significant race group differences were demonstrated on all scales except Family Relations, with White, non-Hispanic youth reporting lower scores.

The IWQOL-Kids exhibited responsiveness to change in a sample of participants attending a weight loss camp who reduced their BMI by an average of 3 points (SD = 1.4; Kolotkin, Zeller, et al., 2006). Significant improvements were found on all four IWQOL-Kids scales following treatment. Physical Comfort improved by 9.95 points (effect size = .43), Body Esteem by 17.89 points (effect size = .72), Social Life by 13.54 points (effect size = .60), Family Relations by 9.84 points (effect size = .41), and total score by 13.43 points (effect size = .75). Because there was no control group in this study, it is not possible to evaluate whether changes in IWQOL-Kids scores were a result of BMI changes, camp participation, or some other factors. It is also not possible to know if such changes would have occurred in the absence of changes in BMI.

Comment

To date, the IWQOL-Kids is the only weight-related measure of HRQOL for use in a pediatric population. The IWQOL-Kids is suitable for adolescents ages 11 to 19. Data from the initial development and validation paper provide support for the measure's strong psychometric properties, discrimination among BMI groups and between clinical and community samples, and responsiveness to a weight loss/social support intervention.

Future studies are needed to address test-retest reliability and confirmatory factor analysis.

Generic HRQOL Instruments for Eating Disorders

Generic HRQOL has been assessed in individuals with eating disorders in a few studies using the SF-36 (Ware, Snow, Kosinski, & Gandek, 1993), SF-12 (Ware et al., 1996), and the Nottingham Health Profile (Hunt et al., 1981).

Padierna, Quintana, Arostegui, Gonzalez, and Horcajo (2000, 2002) conducted both a cross-sectional and a longitudinal study of HRQOL in eating-disordered patients in Spain. Patients (98% female) with eating disorders (anorexia nervosa, bulimia nervosa, or binge-eating disorder) showed greater impairment on all scales of the SF-36 than women from the general population (Padierna et al., 2000). In addition, severity of eating disorders symptoms was associated with degree of HRQOL impairment. A prospective study by these authors (Padierna et al., 2002) evaluated 2-year changes in HRQOL after outpatient treatment (psychotherapeutic and psychopharmacologic treatment) for eating disorders (anorexia nervosa and bulimia nervosa). Patients demonstrated improvement in all domains of the SF-36 except Role Emotional. The mean PCS score at follow-up was comparable to that of a general population; however, the mean MCS score was still below that of the general population.

A study conducted in the Netherlands compared SF-36 scores in eating disorder patients, former eating disorder patients, patients with mood disorders, and a normal reference group (de la Rie, Noordenbos, & van Furth, 2005). Eating disorder patients (anorexia, bulimia, and eating disorder not otherwise specified) reported greater impairments in HRQOL than patients with mood disorders and the normal reference group. No differences were found among diagnostic groups. Compared to the normal reference group, former patients had poorer HRQOL.

Results of a study conducted in Australia (Mond et al., 2004) revealed lower SF-12 scores (i.e., greater impairment) for a community sample of individuals with eating disorders as compared to a community sample who did not have eating disorders (as assessed by the Eating Disorders Questionnaire [Fairburn & Beglin, 1994] and the Eating Disorders Examination [Fairburn & Cooper, 1993]). Although both the PCS and MCS of the SF-12 showed differences between these two groups, the difference was greater for the MCS.

In another study conducted in Australia, subgroups of eating disorder patients meeting full criteria (anorexia nervosa–restricting type, anorexia nervosa–purging type, bulimia nervosa, and binge-eating disorder) were compared on the SF-12 with a general population (Mond, Hay, Rodgers, Owen, & Beumont, 2005). The study authors hypothesized that restricting anorexia patients would report less impairment than other patient groups. Significant differences were found in HRQOL between the eating disorder patients as a whole and the general population on both PCS and MCS. As hypothesized, scores on MCS were significantly higher (i.e., less impaired) among restricting anorexia patients than among purging anorexia and bulimia nervosa patients, even after controlling for psychological distress. Scores on the PCS tended to be lower for the binge-eating group than the other patient subgroups, but the differences did not reach statistical significance.

In a representative community sample in Australia, structured interviews were conducted, and three eating disorder behaviors were assessed: binge eating, purging, and strict dieting or fasting (Hay, 2003). Eating disorder behaviors were associated with significantly lower scores on the SF-36.

Researchers using the Nottingham Health Profile to assess HRQOL in the United Kingdom also reported that patients with eating disorders (anorexia nervosa and bulimia nervosa) had more impairment than a healthy control group (Keilen, Treasure, Schmidt, & Treasure, 1994). Eating disorder patients in both diagnostic groups showed significantly more impairment than the healthy controls. The areas most affected were Emotional Reaction, Social Isolation, Energy, and Sleep.

Comments

Results from community studies and clinical studies in Spain, Australia, and the United Kingdom consistently reported reduced generic HRQOL for individuals with eating disorders. Some evidence also exists for an association between symptom severity and HRQOL, differences among subgroups of eating-disordered persons, and improvements after treatment.

Disease-Specific HRQOL Instruments for Eating Disorders

Four measures have been developed to assess disease-specific HRQOL for eating disorders. These will be described below in alphabetical order.

Eating Disorder Quality of Life

The Eating Disorder Quality of Life (EDQOL—see Appendix 2.F; Engel et al., 2006), developed in the United States, is a disease-specific measure of HRQOL for use with women who have eating disorders. The EDQOL is a 25-item instrument, containing four factor analytically derived scales (Psychological, Physical/Cognitive, Work/School, and Financial) and a total score. The methodology used in the development and testing of this instrument was sophisticated and carefully implemented. To ensure that the domains and items covered the content area completely, the developers used the expertise of six highly experienced eating disorder clinicians, a literature search, pilot testing of items in different samples, and cognitive debriefing regarding the item wording and meaning. One of the unique strengths of the EDQOL is that items were selected using a combination of both classical test theory and item response theory (IRT; Anastasi & Urbina, 1997; Weiss & Yoes, 1991). In addition to the usual iterative process of exploratory factor analysis and item reduction, confirmatory factor analysis was also used to support the scale structure of the four domains and the total score. Possible ranges for each scale and the total score are 0 to 4, with lower scores indicating better quality of life.

The psychometric properties of the EDQOL are generally strong. Reliability coefficients (Cronbach's alpha) were as follows: .95 for Psychological, .86 for Physical/Cognitive, .84 for Work/School, .86 for Financial, and .94 for total score. Test-retest intraclass correlations were acceptable for three of the four domain scores (.97 Psychological, .87 Physical/ Cognitive, .90 Financial) and .93 for total score. A weakness of the EDQOL is that the test-retest correlation for the Work/School domain was .14 (Engel et al., 2006). However, IRT analyses showed that the Work/School items are particularly appropriate for individuals with more serious eating pathology. Given that the test-retest reliability was calculated using a heterogeneous sample that included individuals without serious eating pathology, test-retest reliability will likely improve considerably when administered to a sample of eating-disordered individuals.

Support for the validity of the EDQOL was obtained in a number of ways. Convergent and discriminant validity were demonstrated by examining hypothesized relationships between EDQOL scale scores and a number of collateral measures: SF-36 (Ware et al., 1993), Neuroticism (L. R. Goldberg, 1992), Beck Depression Inventory (Beck, Rush, Shaw, & Emery, 1979), Social Adjustment Scale (Weissman & Bothwell, 1976), Financial Global Ratings, and Grade Point Average. In addition, it was demonstrated that the EDQOL is sensitive to group differences between eating-disordered and nondisordered groups and able to differentiate among groups based on symptom severity. Furthermore, the EDQOL was able to explain more symptom severity and group-related variance than a generic HRQOL instrument.

Despite the rigorous design of the EDQOL, there are several limitations. To date, the authors have not demonstrated responsiveness to change, which is an important aspect of clinical research. Since the items were specifically developed for women with eating disorders and only women were used in the testing of the EDQOL, the degree to which the EDQOL is generalizable to men is unknown. In addition, the sample used in the creation and assessment of the EDQOL was primarily White, and thus the EDQOL may not be generalizable to individuals with other ethnic backgrounds. Finally, due to sample size limitations, the authors were unable to make comparisons across the various eating disorder diagnostic groups. Nevertheless, the EDQOL was the first disease-specific instrument to assess HRQOL in eating disorders, and the instrument developers used methods that were sophisticated, as well as carefully executed. More research is needed on this very promising measure of HRQOL in eating disorders. The EDQOL has been translated into French, Spanish, German, Swedish, Portuguese, Chinese, Japanese, and Hebrew.

Eating Disorders Quality of Life Scale

Preliminary work has been done on the development and testing of another HRQOL measure specific for eating disorders. The Eating Disorders Quality of Life Scale (EDQLS; Adair et al., 2007), developed in Canada, contains 40 items assessing 12 theoretical domains: Cognitive Functioning, Education/Vocation, Family and Close Relationships, Relationships With Others, Future/Outlook Appearance, Leisure, Psychological Health, Emotional Health, Values, and Beliefs. There are five response options for each item, ranging from *strongly disagree* to *strongly agree,* and items are balanced for polarity. A separate section allows for importance ratings in each domain, as well as up to two additional domains rated for importance.

The EDQLS was designed to minimize response bias attributable to ego-syntonicity in patients with eating disorders (i.e., to avoid items that describe self-destructive behaviors or attitudes but are viewed as positive by the patient). Items were developed using input from patients in treatment (with anorexia nervosa, bulimia nervosa, or eating disorder not otherwise specified), health professionals, Internet first-person narratives, and a literature review. Content was selected to measure the broader aspects of quality of life confirmed to be important to eating disorder patients, including those specifically affected by the eating disorder. Items were designed to be developmentally appropriate in language and content for young adolescents as well as adults. Item reduction considered responsiveness (expected to show change over time with treatment), universality (captures behaviors/feelings across diagnostic groups and age ranges, including in adolescents), wording, and likeability by focus group participants (who rated their "best three" items in each category based on their perception of the items' relevance to their quality of life and their ability to show change with treatment).

Psychometric analyses were conducted on 171 patients over age 14 from 12 treatment programs (Adair et al., 2007). Analyses focused on items and total scores because of the "preliminary nature of the domains." Although factor analysis revealed up to eight factors accounting for 64.4% of the variance, the authors do not report factor loadings. They state they are deferring thematic interpretation of factors for confirmatory factor analysis in a larger sample.

Cronbach's alpha was .96, but alphas for individual domains ranged from .36 (Family and Close Relationships) to .79 Eating Issues (Adair et al., 2007). Test-retest reliability was not conducted, nor was change assessed longitudinally. At least two of the items were of concern to the authors due to less than optimal findings in analyses.

Some support was obtained for validity of the EDQLS. Moderate to strong correlations were obtained on an item level for hypothesized relationships to items from other measures: SF-12, Quality of Life Inventory (Frisch, Cornell, Villanueva, & Retzlaff, 1992), and 16 D (Apajasalo et al., 1996). The Quality of Life Inventory is a psychometrically sound instrument that assesses general quality of life and life satisfaction in 16 life areas (Frisch et al., 1992). The 16 D assesses general HRQOL in adolescents and has been shown to have known-groups validity and good test-retest reliability (Apajasalo et al., 1996). Scores were predicted to be lower for inpatients as compared to outpatients, but these differences were not significant. Patients in treatment longer reported statistically higher scores, except for the group of patients just beginning treatment. Those with psychiatric comorbidities and greater symptom severity on the Brief Symptom Inventory (Derogatis, 1993) and the Eating Disorder Inventory–2 (EDI-2; Garner, 1991) had lower scores on the EDQLS.

Health-Related Quality of Life in Eating Disorders

The Health-Related Quality of Life in Eating Disorders (HeRQoLED; Las Hayas et al., 2006) is a 50-item measure of HRQOL specific to eating disorders. This instrument was developed in Spain. Like the EDQOL, the methodology used in the development and testing of this instrument was rigorous. The HeRQoLED contains eight factor analytically derived scales (Symptoms, Restrict Behaviors, Body Image, Mental Health, Emotional Role, Physical Role, Personality Traits, and Social Relations). Items contain either five or six response options, ranging from *never* to *a lot* or *always.* Scores for each scale are transformed to 0 to 100 scoring, where higher scores represent lower HRQOL.

Items were developed by beginning with seven focus groups: four groups with eating disorders, two groups with family members of individuals with eating disorders, and one with a multidisciplinary group of experts. The instrument developers also used a literature search, expert opinion, and field testing of the pilot instrument. Although factor analysis was used to select items and scales for the final instrument, unconventional methods were used. For example, items believed to belong to the Symptom and Binge Eating domains were factor analyzed separately due to the deliberate heterogeneity of the Symptom scale and the smaller sample size of the binge eaters. In addition, four items were retained on the final instrument despite psychometric weaknesses due to perceived relevance by the clinicians, and two of the items were retained despite cross-loadings on the factor analysis. One of the hypothesized scales (Binge Eating) did not hold up in the factor analysis and was removed from the final version. In addition to the usual iterative process of exploratory factor analysis and item reduction, confirmatory factor analysis was also used to support the scale structure of the domains and the total score.

The psychometric properties of the HeRQoLED were strong, excluding the above mentioned weaknesses. Reliability coefficients (Cronbach's alpha) were as follows: .85 for Symptoms, .78 for Restrictive Behavior, .92 for Body Image, .90 for Mental Health, .93 for Emotional Role, .95 for Physical Role, .82 for Personality Traits, and .87 for Social Relations. Test-retest intraclass correlations were good, ranging from .87 (Mental Health and Personality Traits) to .96 (Restrictive Behavior).

Support for the validity of the HeRQoLED was obtained using various methods. Convergent validity was demonstrated by confirmation of hypothesized relationships between HeRQoLED domains and collateral measures: SF-12 (Ware et al., 1996), EAT-26 (Castro, Toro, Salamero, & Guimera, 1991), and EDI-2 (Garner, 1998). However, the Social Relations domain had a higher correlation with the dieting concern subscale of the EAT-26 than with the hypothesized mental component of the SF-12. Known-groups validity was demonstrated by comparing scores

obtained by groups differing in symptom severity, as determined separately using results from the Clinical Global Index and the EAT-26. The HeRQoLED was also sensitive to differences between individuals with eating disorders and the general population. (Because the HeRQoLED was designed for individuals with eating disorders, some of the items required wording changes when administered to a general population to test for sensitivity of the instrument.)

Despite rigorous methods used in the development and testing of the HeRQoLED, several limitations exist. One of the domains clearly assesses eating-disordered HRQOL (Social Relations) in that the items evaluate the impact of eating disorders on the quality of social relations. However, other domains assess important aspects of eating disorders but not necessarily HRQOL—for example, symptoms, personality traits, and mood states. It is also unknown whether results will generalize to men with eating disorders because 96% of the sample was female. Furthermore, no tests of responsiveness were conducted, no attempt was made to distinguish among the various eating disorders, and the large number of items may create respondent burden. Finally, despite differences obtained between a general population and an eating-disordered sample on the HeRQoLED, mean scores for the eating-disordered sample appear to be limited in range (approximately 31–59 out of 100).

The Quality of Life for Eating Disorders

The Quality of Life for Eating Disorders (QOL ED; Abraham, Brown, Boyd, Luscombe, & Russell, 2006) is a 20-item measure derived from a larger computer-generated examination of eating and exercise behavior, attitudes, and feelings, the Eating and Exercise Examination (Abraham & Lovell, 1999). The ED QOL, applicable to all eating disorders, provides scores for the domains of body weight, eating behavior, eating disorder feelings, psychological feelings, effects on daily life, effects on acute medical status, and a global score. Although initially designed as a measure of change to be used by health insurance assessors to determine treatment outcomes in an eating disorders unit, the QOL ED is appropriate for use in both clinical and research settings. Scores for domains range from 0 to 4, and global scores range from 0 to 24. The QOL ED was developed in English for use in Australia and also has been translated into German and Hindi.

The QOL ED was tested on a sample of 306 female eating disorder patients treated as inpatients in Australia (109 completed the instrument at both admission and discharge from hospital, 65 at both admission and after 12 months). Patients also completed the Eating Disorder Inventory (EDI; Garner, 1991), Eating and Attitudes Test (EAT; Garner, Olmsted, Bohr, & Garfinkel, 1982), Beck Depression Inventory (BDI; Beck, Steer, & Brown, 1996), State-Trait Anxiety Inventory (Spielberger, Gorusch, & Luschene, 1970), and SF-12 (Ware et al., 1996). Correlations between QOL ED domain scores and collateral measures were in the expected direction. For example, the eating disorder domain correlated .51 with the EDI drive for thinness scale, the eating behavior domain correlated .57 with the EDI bulimia scale, and the psychological feelings correlated .67 with EDI ineffectiveness, .70 with BDI depression, and .64 with trait anxiety. Cronbach's alpha ranged from .58 for eating behavior to .89 for psychological feelings. The scores differed for individuals with anorexia nervosa, bulimia, eating disorder not specified (EDNOS), and a student reference group. In addition, scores were significantly improved between admission and 12-month follow-up.

Comments: Disease-Specific Eating Disorders Instruments

Both the EDQOL and the HeRQoLED are promising new disease-specific measures for eating disorders. In both of these instruments, rigorous methodology was used to develop and test the items/scales. For example, both of these instruments performed confirmatory factor analysis to verify the scale structure of the domains and justify the use of a total score. One of the differences between these measures pertains to how the items were developed. The EDQOL began with eating disorder experts and later brought in patients' opinions, whereas the HeRQoLED started with patients and later sought expert opinion. Second, the EDQOL performed psychometric analysis using both classical test theory and IRT, whereas

the HeRQoLED used only classical test theory for analyses. The advantage of IRT is that it promotes the selection of items across a broad range of functioning, which in turn provides maximal information about HRQOL using the fewest number of items. Indeed, the EDQOL contains 25 items, whereas the HeRQoLED contains 50 items. Another difference between these instruments is in the samples used for instrument development. Whereas the EDQOL assessed eating-disordered patients as well as students without eating disorders and students who used diet and exercise to control weight, the sample used to develop the HeRQoLED used eating-disordered patients only. The developers of the EDQOL argue that inclusion of study participants who do not have the disorder has precedence in the assessment literature and allows assessment across the spectrum of problems, which may in turn facilitate longitudinal evaluation (because prior to treatment, patients are likely to score in the disordered range, but after treatment, they may score in the nondisordered range). Another difference between these two instruments is that the EDQOL was developed in the United States, whereas the HeRQoLED was developed in Spain. Thus, it is unknown how use of each instrument in other cultural contexts may affect results.

The EDQLS and QOL ED appear not to have been tested as thoroughly as the EDQOL and the HeRQoLED. The authors of the EDQLS describe their instrument as promising but recognize that domains may not hold up during further factor analysis, and their small sample size did not allow for use of confirmatory factor analysis and IRT analyses. The only publication available about the QOL ED contains no information on how the items were selected, and there is no discussion of the factor structure of the domains. Because these instruments are so new, additional research is needed to further explore their psychometric properties.

Conclusions

HRQOL assessment has become increasingly integrated within both clinical obesity treatment and research. Such an assessment provides a subjective evaluation of the effects of excess weight on various physical, social, and emotional domains of functioning as perceived and reported by the respondent. Apart from its potential value to the respondent as a means of gauging how their weight influences various aspects of their life, it has become an important outcome in research because it assesses phenomena beyond merely physiological indices related to weight reduction (e.g., weight, body fat, blood pressure). Moreover, assessment of HRQOL underscores that obesity can produce a range of complications beyond medical issues and thereby potentially enlarges the targets for intervention.

HRQOL measures fall into two camps: generic and condition specific. Both have strengths and weaknesses, and as such, the choice of which measure to use depends primarily on the goals in mind. To quote a recent study comparing the content of 12 obesity-specific HRQOL instruments, "As the selection of an appropriate condition-specific health-status measure depends among other considerations on the study question, the population to be studied and the intervention, there is probably no unique ideal obesity-specific measure existing" (Stucki et al., 2006, p. 1798). These authors add that their content comparison based on the international classification of functioning, disability, and health may be useful in guiding clinicians and researchers in their selection of instruments (Stucki et al., 2006). To this end, many investigators (e.g., Fontaine & Bartlett, 1998; Maciejewski et al., 2005) advocate the use of both generic and obesity-specific measures as a means of providing the most comprehensive assessment of HRQOL possible.

Of the measures commonly used with adults in obesity research, the SF-36 and its variants and the IWQOL-Lite are by far those with the best established psychometric properties. Both have consistently demonstrated that they are responsive to change with respect to weight reduction arising from various sorts of interventions. The generic SF-36 indicates that obesity has a devastating impact on HRQOL, especially with respect to physical domains of functioning, and weight reduction can markedly improve HRQOL. The obesity-specific IWQOL-Lite also suggests that obesity can profoundly impair physically oriented domains of HRQOL, as well as self-esteem and public distress, domains that the SF-36 does not capture. Although

the BAROS is widely used in bariatric surgery studies, most of these studies do not use the revised MA II, which appears promising pending further psychometric testing. In addition, the OWLQOL and WRSM (see Appendix 2.B) were developed by experts in the quality-of-life field using sound and rigorous methods and, as such, are worth further investigation. The majority of the other generic and obesity-specific measures reviewed herein appear to require additional studies to further demonstrate and confirm their psychometric properties before they can be highly recommended for use in obesity research. With respect to pediatric populations, the generic PedsQL and the obesity-specific IWQOL-Kids are currently the measures with the best established psychometric properties.

A number of generic and condition-specific measures have been used to assess the HRQOL of individuals with eating disorders. The SF-36, SF-12, and NHP have been used to provide generic assessments, and overall, these measures appear to suggest that HRQOL is impaired among this group and that treatment can improve HRQOL. To date, four eating disorder–specific measures have been developed, two of which, the EDQOL and the HsRQoLED, were developed using rigorous methodologies and appear to provide reasonable HRQOL assessment for this population.

Limitations

An issue that plagues the field has to do with the use of different HRQOL definitions and measures. Use of a vast array of generic and obesity-specific measures limits the development of a definitive understanding of effects of obesity on HRQOL. Although there is an emerging consensus (American Society for Bariatric Surgery, 2004; Wadden & Phelan, 2002) among obesity-related organizations concerning which measures to use, it remains difficult to compare the results of HRQOL across studies that used different measures.

That said, even though obesity-specific measures provide information on domains that are not captured by generic measures, some subgroups of obese individuals may have issues related to HRQOL that even obesity-specific measures do not adequately assess. For example, an obese individual with severe arthritis might have quality of life concerns related to joint pain and fatigue that are not queried in an obesity-specific HRQOL questionnaire. As such, it might be worthwhile to consider the potential value of obesity HRQOL assessments that are tailored toward specific and common comorbidities such as arthritis and diabetes. Such assessments may be of particular value in the clinical setting to help identify issues that might require remediation beyond weight reduction.

Current HRQOL assessments involve the completion of questionnaires that ask people to provide a subjective judgment of their functioning along several domains within a certain time frame (e.g., during the past 4 weeks for the SF-36 and past week for IWQOL-Lite). As such, the individual is asked to recall and provide an estimate along a scale that captures his or her evaluation. What individuals bring to bear when they make this evaluation is unknown as are the cognitive processes they engage in to generate this evaluation. Our current HRQOL instruments are static in that they do not capture the processes involved when one makes a judgment. It may be helpful, especially from a clinical perspective, to develop measurement technologies that are more dynamic and capture the processes involved when people are asked to evaluate their HRQOL. The advent of real-time assessments, used to track symptoms and, for example, physical activity, might be applied to the assessment of HRQOL to provide a greater understanding of how HRQOL judgments are made. Such information might inform intervention efforts and provide insights as to how obesity influences HRQOL.

The dramatic increase in the prevalence of obesity in much of the developed world has made the assessment of HRQOL all the more important because the personal, social, and economic burden imposed by obesity will likely become even more pressing issues in the years to come. Articulating this burden should inform investigators and provide valuable insights that can be used to develop interventions to remediate not only body weight but the impaired HRQOL as well.

References

Aaronson, N. K., Acquadro, C., Alonso, J., Apdone, G., Bucquet, D., Bullinger, M., et al. (1992). International Quality of Life Assessment (IQOLA) project. *Quality of Life Research, 1,* 349–351.

Abraham, S., Brown, T., Boyd, C., Luscombe, G., & Russell, J. (2006). Quality of life: Eating disorders. *Australian and New Zealand Journal of Psychiatry, 40,* 150–155.

Abraham, S., & Lovell, N. (1999). Research and clinical assessment of eating and exercise behaviour. *Hospital Medicine, 60,* 481–485.

Adair, C. E., Marcoux, G. C., Cram, B. S., Ewashen, C. J., Chaffe, J., Cassin, S. E., et al. (2007). Development and multi-site validation of a new condition-specific quality of life measure for eating disorders. *Health and Quality of Life Outcomes, 5,* 23.

Adami, G. F., Ramberti, G., Weiss, A., Carlini, F., Murelli, F., & Scopinaro, N. (2005). Quality of life in obese subjects following biliopancreatic diversion. *Behavioral Medicine, 31,* 53–60.

Alonso, J., Prieto, L., & Anto, J. M. (1995). The Spanish version of the SF-36 Health Survey (the SF-36 health questionnaire): An instrument for measuring clinical results [in Spanish]. *Medical Clinic (Barcelona), 104,* 771–776.

American Society for Bariatric Surgery, Allied Health Section Ad Hoc Behavioral Health Committee. (2004). *Suggestions for the pre-surgical psychological assessment of bariatric surgery candidates.* Gainesville, FL: Author.

Anastasi, A., & Urbina, S. (1997). *Psychological testing.* Upper Saddle River, NJ: Prentice Hall.

Andresen, E. M., Rothenberg, B. M., & Kaplan, R. M. (1998). Performance of a self-administered mailed version of the Quality of Well-Being (QWB-SA) questionnaire among older adults. *Medical Care, 36,* 1349–1360.

Apajasalo, M., Sintonen, H., Holmberg, C., Sinkkonen, J., Aalberg, V., Pihko, H., et al. (1996). Quality of life in early adolescence: A sixteen-dimensional health-related measure (16D). *Quality of Life Research, 5,* 205–211.

Apolone, G., Filiberti, A., Cifani, S., Ruggiata, R., & Mosconi, P. (1998). Evaluation of the EORTC QLQ-C30 questionnaire: A comparison with SF-36 Health Survey in a cohort of Italian long-survival cancer patients. *Annals of Oncology, 9,* 549–557.

Augustinsson, L. E., Sullivan, L., & Sullivan, M. (1989). Chronic pain in functional neurosurgery: Function and mood in various diagnostic groups with reference to epidural spinal electrical stimulation. *Schmertz, Pain, Douleur, 10,* 30–40.

Ballantyne, G. H. (2003). Measuring outcomes following bariatric surgery: Weight loss parameters, improvement in co-morbid conditions, change in quality of life and patient satisfaction. *Obesity Surgery, 13,* 954–964.

Beck, A. T., Rush, A. J., Shaw, B. F., & Emery, G. (1979). *Cognitive therapy of depression.* New York: Guilford.

Beck, A. T., Steer, R. A., & Brown, G. K. (1996). *Manual for Beck Depression Inventory–II.* San Antonio, TX: Psychological Corporation.

Bergner, M., Bobbitt, R. A., Carter, W. B., & Gilson, B. S. (1981). The Sickness Impact Profile: Development and final revision of a health status measure. *Medical Care, 19,* 787–805.

Bergner, M., Bobbitt, R. A., Kressel, S., Pollard, W. E., Gilson, B. S., & Morris, J. R. (1976). The Sickness Impact Profile: Conceptual formulation and methodology for the development of a health status measure. *International Journal of Health Services, 6,* 393–415.

Bergner, M., Bobbitt, R. A., Pollard, W. E., Martin, D. P., & Gilson, B. S. (1976). The sickness impact profile: Validation of a health status measure. *Medical Care, 14,* 57–67.

Boan, J., Kolotkin, R. L., Westman, E. C., McMahon, R. L., & Grant, J. P. (2004). Binge eating, quality of life and physical activity improve after Roux-en-Y gastric bypass for morbid obesity. *Obesity Surgery, 14,* 341–348.

Bowling, A. (1997). *Measuring health: A review of quality of life measurement scales.* Buckingham, UK: Open University Press

Brazier, J. E., Harper, R., Jones, N. M., O'Cathain, A., Thomas, K. J., Usherwood, T., et al. (1992). Validating the SF-36 health survey questionnaire: New outcome measure for primary care. *British Medical Journal, 305,* 160–164.

Brooks, W. B., Jordan, J. S., Divine, G. W., Smith, K. S., & Neelon, F. A. (1990). The impact of psychologic factors on measurement of functional status: Assessment of the sickness impact profile. *Medical Care, 28,* 793–804.

Brown, W. J., Dobson, A. J., & Mishra, G. (1998). What is a healthy weight for middle aged women? *International Journal of Obesity, 22,* 520–528.

Butler, G., Vallis, T., Perey, B., Veldhuyzen van Zanten, S., MacDonald, A., & Konok, G. (1999). The Obesity Adjustment Survey: Development of a scale to assess psychological adjustment to morbid obesity. *International Journal of Obesity and Related Metabolic Disorders, 23,* 505–511.

Calder, S. J., Anderson, G. H., Harper, W. M., Jagger, C., & Gregg, P. J. (1995). A subjective health indicator for follow-up: A randomised trial after treatment of displaced intracapsular hip fractures. *Journal of Bone and Joint Surgery (British), 77,* 494–496.

Caniato, D., & Skorjanec, B. (2002). The role of brief strategic therapy on the outcome of gastric banding. *Obesity Surgery, 12,* 666–671.

Carmichael, A. R., Sue-Ling, H. M., & Johnston, D. (2001). Quality of life after the Magenstrasse and Mill procedure for morbid obesity. *Obesity Surgery, 11,* 708–715.

Castro, J., Toro, J., Salamero, M., & Guimera, E. (1991). The Eating Attitudes Test: Validation of the Spanish version. *Evaluacion Psicologica, 7*(2), 175–189.

Corica, F., Corsonello, A., Apolone, G., Lucchetti, M., Melchionda, N., Marchesini, G., et al. (2006). Construct validity of the Short Form-36 Health Survey and its relationship with BMI in obese outpatients. *Obesity (Silver Spring), 14,* 1429–1437.

Crosby, R. D., Kolotkin, R. L., & Williams, G. R. (2003). Defining clinically meaningful change in health-related quality of life. *Journal of Clinical Epidemiology, 56,* 395–407.

Crosby, R. D., Kolotkin, R. L., & Williams, G. R. (2004). An integrated method to determine meaningful changes in health-related quality of life. *Journal of Clinical Epidemiology, 57,* 1153–1160.

de Bruin, A. F., Buys, M., de Witte, L. P., & Diederiks, J. P. (1994). The Sickness Impact Profile: SIP68, a short generic version: First evaluation of the reliability and reproducibility. *Journal of Clinical Epidemiology, 47,* 863–871.

de Bruin, A. F., de Witte, L. P., Stevens, F., & Diederiks, J. P. (1992). Sickness Impact Profile: The state of the art of a generic functional status measure. *Social Science Medicine, 35,* 1003–1014.

de la Rie, S. M., Noordenbos, G., & van Furth, E. F. (2005). Quality of life and eating disorders. *Quality of Life Research, 14,* 1511–1522.

de Zwaan, M., Lancaster, K. L., Mitchell, J. E., Howell, L. M., Monson, N., & Roerig, J. L., et al. (2002). Health-related quality of life in morbidly obese patients: Effect of gastric bypass surgery. *Obesity Surgery, 12,* 773–780.

de Zwaan, M., Mitchell, J. E., Howell, L. M., Monson, N., Swan-Kremeier, L., Crosby, R. D., et al. (2003). Characteristics of morbidly obese patients before gastric bypass surgery. *Comprehensive Psychiatry, 44,* 428–434.

de Zwaan, M., Mitchell, J. E., Howell, L., Monson, N., Swan-Kremeier, L., Roerig, J. L., et al. (2002). Two measures of health related quality of life in morbid obesity: The role of binge eating, eating-specific and general psychopathology. *Obesity Research, 10,* 1143–1151.

Derogatis, L. R. (1993). *Brief Symptom Inventory (BSI) administration, scoring, and procedures manual.* Minneapolis, MN: NCS Pearson.

Di Francesco, V., Sacco, T., Zamboni, M., Bissoli, L., Zoico, E., Mazzali, G., et al. (2007). Weight loss and quality of life improvement in obese subjects treated with sibutramine: A double-blind randomized multicenter study. *Annals of Nutrition and Metabolism, 51,* 75–81.

Dittmar, M., Heintz, A., Hardt, J., Egle, U. T., & Kahaly, G. J. (2003). Metabolic and psychosocial effects of minimal invasive gastric banding for morbid obesity. *Metabolism, 52,* 1551–1557.

Dixon, J. B., Dixon, M. E., & O'Brien, P. E. (2001a). Preoperative predictors of weight loss at 1-year after Lap-Band surgery. *Obesity Surgery, 11,* 200–207.

Dixon, J. B., Dixon, M. E., & O'Brien, P. E. (2001b). Quality of life after lap-band placement: Influence of time, weight loss, and comorbidities. *Obesity Research, 9,* 713–721.

Doll, H. A., Petersen, S. E. K., & Stewart-Brown, S. L. (2000). Obesity and physical and emotional well-being: Associations between body mass index, chronic illness, and the physical and mental components of the SF-36 questionnaire. *Obesity Research, 8,* 160–170.

Duval, K., Marceau, P., Lescelleur, O., Hould, F. S., Marceau, S., Biron, S., et al. (2006). Health-related quality of life in morbid obesity. *Obesity Surgery, 16,* 574–9.

Duval, K., Marceau, P., Perusse, L., & Lacasse, Y. (2006). An overview of obesity-specific quality of life questionnaires. *Obesity Reviews, 7,* 347–360.

Dymek, M. P., Le Grange, D., Neven, K., & Alverdy, J. (2002). Quality of life after gastric bypass surgery: A cross-sectional study. *Obesity Research, 10,* 1135–1142.

Engel, S. G., Crosby, R. D., Kolotkin, R. L., Hartley, G. G., Williams, G. R., Wonderlich, S. A., et al. (2003). The impact of weight loss and regain on obesity-specific quality of life: mirror image or differential effect. *Obesity Research, 11,* 1207–1213.

Engel, S. G., Kolotkin, R. L., Teixeira, P. J., Sardinha, L. B., Vieira, P. N., Palmeira, A. L., et al. (2005). Psychometric and cross-national evaluation of a Portuguese version of the impact of weight on Quality of Life-Lite (IWQOL-Lite) Questionnaire. *European Eating Disorders Review, 13,* 133–143.

Engel, S. G., Wittrock, D. A., Crosby, R. D., Wonderlich, S. A., Mitchell, J. E., & Kolotkin, R. L. (2006). Development and psychometric validation of an eating disorder-specific health-related quality of life instrument. *International Journal of Eating Disorders, 39,* 62–71.

Essink-Bot, M. L., Krabbe, P. F., Bonsel, G. J., & Aaronson, N. K. (1997). An empirical comparison of four generic health status measures: The Nottingham Health Profile, the Medical Outcomes Study 36-item Short-Form Health Survey, the COOP/WONCA charts, and the EuroQol instrument. *Medical Care, 35,* 522–537.

Fairburn, C., & Beglin, S. (1994). Assessment of eating disorders: Interview or self-report questionnaire? *International Journal of Eating Disorders, 16,* 363–370.

Fairburn, C. G., & Cooper, Z. (1993). The Eating Disorder Examination. In C. G. Fairburn & G. T. Wilson (Eds.), *Binge eating: Nature, assessment and treatment* (pp. 317–360). New York: Guilford.

Fallowfield, L. (1996). Quality of quality-of-life data. *Lancet, 348,* 421–422.

Favretti, F., Cadiere, G. B., Segato, G., Busetto, L., Loffredo, A., Vertruyen, M., et al. (1998). Bariatric Analysis and Reporting Outcome System (BAROS) applied to laparoscopic gastric banding patients. *Obesity Surgery, 8,* 500–504.

Fayers, P. M., & Machin, D. (2000). *Quality of life: Assessment, analysis and interpretation.* New York: John Wiley.

Fine, J. T., Colditz, G. A., Coakley, E. H., Moseley, G., Manson, J. E., Willett, W. C., et al. (1999). A prospective study of weight change and health-related quality of life in women. *Journal of the American Medical Association, 282,* 2136–2142.

Fisher, D. C., Lake, K. D., Reutzel, T. J., & Emery, R. W. (1995). Changes in health-related quality of life and depression in heart transplant recipients. *Journal of Heart and Lung Transplantation, 14,* 373–381.

Folope, V., Hellot, M. F., Kuhn, J. M., Teniere, P., Scotte, M., & Dechelotte, P. (2008). Weight loss and quality of life after bariatric surgery: A study of 200 patients after vertical gastroplasty or adjustable gastric banding. *European Journal of Clinical Nutrition, 62,* 1022–1030.

Fontaine, K. R., & Barofsky, I. (2001). Obesity and health-related quality of life. *Obesity Reviews, 2,* 173–182.

Fontaine, K. R., Barofsky, I., Andersen, R. E., Bartlett, S. J., Wiersema, L., Cheskin, L. J., et al. (1999). Impact of weight loss on health-related quality of life. *Quality of Life Research, 8,* 275–277.

Fontaine, K. R., Barofsky, I., Bartlett, S. J., Franckowiak, S. C., & Andersen, R. E. (2004). Weight loss and health-related quality of life: results at 1-year follow-up. *Eating Behaviors, 5,* 85–88.

Fontaine, K. R., & Bartlett, S. J. (1998). Estimating health-related quality of life in obese individuals. *Disease Management and Health Outcomes, 3,* 61–70.

Fontaine, K. R., & Bartlett, S. J. (2003). Health-related quality of life in obese individuals. In R. E. Andersen (Ed.), *Obesity: Etiology, assessment, treatment and prevention* (pp. 59–72). Champaign, IL: Human Kinetics.

Fontaine, K. R., Bartlett, S. J., & Barofsky, I. (2000). Health-related quality of life among obese persons seeking and not currently seeking treatment. *International Journal of Eating Disorders, 27,* 101–105.

Fontaine, K. R., Cheskin, L. J., & Barofsky, I. (1996). Health-related quality of life in obese persons seeking treatment. *Journal of Family Practice, 43,* 265–270.

Food and Drug Administration (FDA). (2006). *Guidance for industry: Patient-reported outcome measures: Use in medical product development to support labeling claims.* Rockville, MD: Author.

Friedlander, S. L., Larkin, E. K., Rosen, C. L., Palermo, T. M., & Redline, S. (2003). Decreased quality of life associated with obesity in school-aged children. *Archives of Pediatric and Adolescent Medicine, 157,* 1206–1211.

Frisch, M. B., Cornell, J., Villanueva, M., & Retzlaff, P. J. (1992). Clinical validation of the Quality of Life Inventory: A measure of life satisfaction for use in treatment planning and outcome assessment. *Psychological Assessment: A Journal of Consulting and Clinical Psychology, 4,* 92–101.

Fujioka, K., Seaton, T. B., Rowe, E., Jelinek, C. A., Raskin, P., Lebovitz, H. E., et al. (2000). Weight loss with sibutramine improves glycemic control and other metabolic parameters in obese patients with type 2 diabetes mellitus. *Diabetes, Obesity and Metabolism, 2,* 175–184.

Fullerton, G., Tyler, C., Johnston, C. A., Vincent, J. P., Harris, G. E., & Foreyt, J. P. (2007). Quality of life in Mexican-American children following a weight management program. *Obesity, 15,* 2553–2556.

Gabriel, S. G., Karaindros, C. A., Papaioannou, M. A., Tassioulis, A. A., Gabriel, S. G., Sigalas, V. I., et al. (2005). Biliopancreatic diversion with duodenal switch combined with laparoscopic adjustable gastric banding. *Obesity Surgery, 15,* 517–522.

Gadde, K. M., Franciscy, D. M., Wagner, H. R., II, & Krishnan, K. R. (2003). Zonisamide for weight loss in obese adults: A randomized controlled trial. *Journal of the American Medical Association, 289,* 1820–1825.

Garner, D. M. (1991). *Eating Disorder Inventory–2, professional manual.* Odessa, FL: Psychological Assessment Resources.

Garner, D. M. (1998). *Inventory of eating disorders* (TEA ed.). Madrid, Spain: Publicaciones de Psicologia Aplicada.

Garner, D. M., Olmsted, M. P., Bohr, Y., & Garfinkel, P. E. (1982). The Eating Attitudes Test: psychometric features and clinical correlates. *Psychological Medicine, 12,* 871–878.

Garratt, A. M., Ruta, D. A., Abdalla, M. I., & Russell, I. T. (1994). SF 36 health survey questionnaire: II. Responsiveness to changes in health status in four common clinical conditions. *Quality Health Care, 3,* 186–192.

Gater, R. A., Kind, P., & Gudex, C. (1995). Quality of life in liaison psychiatry: A comparison of patient and clinician assessment. *British Journal of Psychiatry, 166,* 515–520.

Gill, T. M., & Feinstein, A. R. (1994). A critical appraisal of the quality of quality-of-life measurements. *Journal of the American Medical Association, 272,* 619–626.

Goldberg, D. P. (1978). *Manual of the General Health Questionnaire.* Windsor, UK: NFER Publishing.

Goldberg, L. R. (1992). The development of markers for the big-five factor structure. *Psychological Assessment, 4,* 26–42.

Gould, J. C., Garren, M. J., Boll, V., & Starling, J. R. (2006). Laparoscopic gastric bypass: risks vs. benefits up to two years following surgery in super-super obese patients. *Surgery, 140,* 524–529; discussion 9–31.

Groessl, E. J., Kaplan, R. M., Barrett-Connor, E., & Ganiats, T. G. (2004). Body mass index and quality of well-being in a community of older adults. *American Journal of Preventive Medicine, 26,* 126–129.

Guyatt, G. H., Feeny, D. H., & Patrick, D. L. (1993). Measuring health-related quality of life. *Annals of Internal Medicine, 118,* 622–629.

Han, T. S., Tijhuis, M. A., Lean, M. E., & Seidell, J. C. (1998). Quality of life in relation to overweight and body fat distribution. *American Journal of Public Health, 88,* 1814–1820.

Hay, P. (2003). Quality of life and bulimic eating disorder behaviors: findings from a community-based sample. *International Journal of Eating Disorders, 33,* 434–442.

Hays, R. D., Sherbourne, C. D., & Mazel, R. M. (1993). The RAND 36-Item Health Survey 1.0. *Health Economics, 2,* 217–227.

Hell, E., Miller, K. A., Moorehead, M. K., & Norman, S. (2000). Evaluation of health status and quality of life after bariatric surgery: Comparison of standard Roux-en-Y gastric bypass, vertical banded gastroplasty and laparoscopic adjustable silicone gastric banding. *Obesity Surgery, 10,* 214–219.

Henrich, G., & Herschbach, P. (1995). Fragen zur Lebenszufriedenheit (FLZ) [Questions about life satisfaction]. In R. Schwartz (Ed.), *Lebenszufriedeneit (FLZ) in der Onkologie II* (pp. 77–93). München, Germany: Zuckschwerdt.

Heshka, S., Anderson, J. W., Atkinson, R. L., Greenway, F. L., Hill, J. O., Phinney, S. D., et al. (2003). Weight loss with self-help compared with a structured commercial program: A randomized trial. *Journal of the American Medical Association, 289,* 1792–1798.

Holterman, A. X., Browne, A., Dillard, B. E., III, Tussing, L., Gorodner, V., Stahl., C., et al. (2007). Short-term outcome in the first 10 morbidly obese adolescent patients in the FDA-approved trial for laparoscopic adjustable gastric banding. *Journal of Pediatric Gastroenterology and Nutrition, 45,* 465–473.

Hooper, M. M., Stellato, T. A., Hallowell, P. T., Seitz, B. A., & Moskowitz, R. W. (2007). Musculoskeletal findings in obese subjects before and after weight loss following bariatric surgery. *International Journal of Obesity (London), 31,* 114–120.

Horchner, R., Tuinebreijer, M. W., & Kelder, P. H. (2001). Quality-of-life assessment of morbidly obese patients who have undergone a Lap-Band operation: 2-year follow-up study. Is the MOS SF- 36 a useful instrument to measure quality of life in morbidly obese patients? *Obesity Surgery, 11,* 212–218; discussion 9.

Hughes, A. R., Farewell, K., Harris, D., & Reilly, J. J. (2007). Quality of life in a clinical sample of obese children. *International Journal of Obesity (London), 31,* 39–44.

Hunt, S. M., McEwen, J., & McKenna, S. P. (1985). Measuring health status: A new tool for clinicians and epidemiologists. *Journal of the Royal College of General Practice, 35,* 185–188.

Hunt, S. M., McEwen, J., & McKenna, S. P. (1986). *Measuring health status.* London: Croom Helm.

Hunt, S. M., McKenna, S. P., McEwen, J., Williams, J., & Papp, E. (1981). The Nottingham Health Profile: Subjective health status and medical consultations. *Social Science Medicine [A], 15*(3 Pt 1), 221–229.

Irie, M., Mishima, N., Nagata, S., Himeno, E., Nanri, H., Ikeda, M., et al. (1996). Psychosomatic effect of a health program on obese employees [in Japanese]. *Sangyo Eiseigaku Zasshi, 38,* 11–16.

Jackson, C.(2007). The General Health Questionnaire. *Occupational Medicine, 57,* 79.

Jenkinson, C., Fitzpatrick, R., & Argyle, M. (1988). The Nottingham Health Profile: An analysis of its sensitivity in differentiating illness groups. *Social Science Medicine, 27,* 1411–1414.

Jia, H., & Lubetkin, E. I. (2005). The impact of obesity on health-related quality-of-life in the general adult US population. *Journal of Public Health (Oxford), 27,* 156–164.

Kalfarentzos, F., Kechagias, I., Soulikia, K., Loukidi, A., & Mead, N. (2001). Weight loss following vertical banded gastroplasty: Intermediate results of a prospective study. *Obesity Surgery, 11,* 265–270.

Kalfarentzos, F., Skroubis, G., Kehagias, I., Mead, N., & Vagenas, K. (2006). A prospective comparison of vertical banded gastroplasty and Roux-en-Y gastric bypass in a non-superobese population. *Obesity Surgery, 16,* 151–158.

Kantz, M. E., Harris, W. J., Levitsky, K., Ware, J. E., Jr., & Davies, A. R. (1992). Methods for assessing condition-specific and generic functional status outcomes after total knee replacement. *Medical Care, 30,* MS240–MS252.

Kaplan, R. M., Anderson, J. P., & Spilker, B. (1996). The general health policy model: An integrated approach. In B. Spilker (Ed.), *Quality of life and pharmacoeconomics in clinical trials* (pp. 309–322). Philadelphia: Lippincott-Raven.

Kaplan, R. M., Anderson, J. P., Walker, S. R., & Rosser, R. (1988). The quality of well-being scale: Rationale for a single quality of life index. In S. R. Walker & R. Rosser (Eds.), *Quality of life: Assessment and application* (pp. 51–77). London: MTP Press.

Kaplan, R. M., & Bush, J. W. (1982). Health-related quality of life measurement for evaluation research and policy analysis. *Health Psychology, 1,* 61–80.

Kaplan, R. M., Ganiats, T. G., Sieber, W. J., & Anderson, J. P. (1998). The Quality of Well-Being Scale: Critical similarities and differences with SF-36. *International Journal of Quality Health Care, 10,* 509–520.

Kaplan, R. M., Hartwell, S. L., Wilson, D. K., & Wallace, J. P. (1987). Effects of diet and exercise interventions on control and quality of life in non-insulin-dependent diabetes mellitus. *Journal of General Internal Medicine, 2,* 220–228.

Kaplan, R. M., Kozin, F., & Anderson, J. P. (1988). Measuring quality of life in arthritis patients (including discussion of a general health-decision model). *Quality of Life and Cardiovascular Care, 4,* 131–139.

Karlsson, J., Hallgren, P., Kral, J., Lindroos, A. K., Sjöström, L., & Sullivan, M. (1994). Predictors and effects of long-term dieting on mental well-being and weight loss in obese women. *Appetite, 23,* 15–26.

Karlsson, J., Sjöström, L., & Sullivan, M. (1995). Swedish Obese Subjects (SOS)—an intervention study of obesity: Measuring psychosocial factors and health by means of short-form question-naires: Results from a method study. *Journal of Clinical Epidemiology, 48,* 817–823.

Karlsson, J., Sjöström, L., & Sullivan, M. (1998). Swedish obese subjects (SOS)—an intervention study of obesity: Two-year follow-up of health-related quality of life (HRQL) and eating behav-ior after gastric surgery for severe obesity. *International Journal of Obesity and Related Metabolic Disorders, 22,* 113–126.

Karlsson, J., Taft, C., Sjöström, L., Torgerson, J. S., & Sullivan, M. (2003). Psychosocial functioning in the obese before and after weight reduction: Construct validity and responsiveness of the Obesity-related Problems scale. *International Journal of Obesity and Related Metabolic Disorders, 27,* 617–630.

Katz, J. N., Larson, M. G., Phillips, C. B., Fossel, A. H., & Liang, M. H. (1992). Comparative measure-ment sensitivity of short and longer health status instruments. *Medical Care, 30,* 917–925.

Kaukua, J., Pekkarinen, T., & Rissanen, A. M. (2004). Health-related quality of life in a randomised placebo-controlled trial of sibutramine in obese patients with type II diabetes. *International Journal of Obesity and Related Metabolic Disorders, 28,* 600–605.

Kaukua, J., Pekkarinen, T., Sane, T., & Mustajoki, P. (2002). Health-related quality of life in WHO Class II-III obese men losing weight with very-low-energy diet and behaviour modification: A randomised clinical trial. *International Journal of Obesity, 26,* 487–495.

Kaukua, J., Pekkarinen, T., Sane, T., & Mustajoki, P. (2003). Health-related quality of life in obese out-patients losing weight with very-low-energy diet and behaviour modification: A 2-y follow-up study. *International Journal of Obesity and Related Metabolic Disorders, 27,* 1072–1080.

Keilen, M., Treasure, T., Schmidt, U., & Treasure, J. (1994). Quality of life measurements in eating disorders, angina, and transplant candidates: Are they comparable? *Journal of the Royal Society of Medicine, 87,* 441–444.

Kinzl, J. F., Schrattenecker, M., Traweger, C., Aigner, F., Fiala, M., & Biebl, W. (2007). Quality of life in morbidly obese patients after surgical weight loss. *Obesity Surgery, 17,* 229–235.

Kolotkin, R. L., & Crosby, R. D. (2002). Psychometric eval-uation of the Impact Of Weight On Quality Of Life-Lite Questionnaire (IWQOL-Lite) in a community sample. *Quality of Life Research, 11,* 157–171.

Kolotkin, R. L., Crosby, R. D., Corey-Lisle, P., Li, H., & Swanson, J. (2006). Performance of a weight-related measure of quality of life in a psychiatric sample. *Quality of Life Research, 15,* 587–596.

Kolotkin, R. L., Crosby, R. D., Kosloski, K. D., & Williams, G. R. (2001). Development of a brief measure to assess quality of life in obesity. *Obesity Research, 9,* 102–111.

Kolotkin, R. L., Crosby, R. D., Pendleton, R., Strong, M., Gress, R. E., & Adams, T. D. (2003). Health-related quality of life in patients seeking gastric bypass surgery vs. non-treatment-seeking con-trols. *Obesity Surgery, 13,* 371–377.

Kolotkin, R. L., Crosby, R. D., & Williams, G. R. (2002). Health-related quality of life varies among obese subgroups. *Obesity Research, 10,* 748–756.

Kolotkin, R. L., Crosby, R. D., & Williams, G. R. (2003). Assessing weight-related quality of life in obese persons with type 2 diabetes. *Diabetes Research and Clinical Practice, 61,* 125–132.

Kolotkin, R. L., Crosby, R. D., Williams, G. R., Hartley, G. G., & Nicol, S. (2001). The relationship between health-related quality of life and weight loss. *Obesity Research, 9,* 564–571.

Kolotkin, R. L., Head, S., & Brookhart, A. (1997). Construct validity of the Impact of Weight on Quality of Life questionnaire. *Obesity Research, 5,* 434–441.

Kolotkin, R. L., Head, S., Hamilton, M. A., & Tse, C. T. J. (1995). Assessing impact of weight on quality of life. *Obesity Research, 3,* 49–56.

Kolotkin, R. L., Meter, K., & Williams, G. R. (2001). Quality of life and obesity. *Obesity Reviews, 2,* 219–229.

Kolotkin, R. L., Westman, E. C., Ostbye, T., Crosby, R. D., Eisenson, H. J., & Binks, M. (2004). Does binge eating disorder impact weight-related quality of life? *Obesity Research, 12,* 999–1005.

Kolotkin, R. L., Zeller, M., Modi, A. C., Samsa, G. P., Quinlan, N. P., Yanovski, J. A., et al. (2006). Assessing weight-related quality of life in adolescents. *Obesity (Silver Spring), 14,* 448–457.

Korolija, D., Sauerland, S., Wood-Dauphinee, S., Abbou, C. C., Eypasch, E., Garcia Caballero, M., et al. (2004). Evaluation of quality of life after laparoscopic surgery: Evidence-based guidelines of the European Association for Endoscopic Surgery. *Surgical Endoscopy, 18,* 879–897.

Kral, J. G., Sjöström, L. V., & Sullivan, M. B. (1992). Assessment of quality of life before and after surgery for severe obesity. *American Journal of Clinical Nutrition, 55,* 611S–614S.

Kushner, R. F., & Foster, G. (2000). Obesity and quality of life. *Nutrition, 16,* 947–952.

Landgraf, J., Abetz, L., & Ware, J. E. (1996). *The CHQ user's manual.* Boston: The Health Institute, New England Medical Center.

Las Hayas, C., Quintana, J. M., Padierna, A., Bilbao, A., Muñoz, P., Madrazo, A., et al. (2006). The new questionnaire Health-Related Quality of Life for Eating Disorders showed good validity and reliability. *Journal of Clinical Epidemiology, 59,* 192–200.

LePen, C., Levy, E., Loos, F., Banzet, M., & Basdevant, A. (1998). 'Specific' scale compared with 'generic' scale: A double measurement of the quality of life in a French community sample of obese subjects. *Journal of Epidemiology and Community Health, 52,* 445–450.

Lukkarinen, H., & Hentinen, M. (1998). Assessment of quality of life with the Nottingham Health Profile among women with coronary artery disease. *Heart and Lung, 27,* 189–199.

Maciejewski, M. L., Patrick, D. L., & Williamson, D. F. (2005). A structured review of randomized controlled trials of weight loss showed little improvement in health-related quality of life. *Journal of Clinical Epidemiology, 58,* 568–578.

Mannucci, E., Ricca, V., Barciulli, E., Di Bernardo, M., Travaglini, R., Cabras, P. L., et al. (1999). Quality of life and overweight: The obesity related well-being (Orwell 97) questionnaire. *Addictive Behavior, 24,* 345–357.

Marchesini, G., Natale, S., Chierici, S., Manini, R., Besteghi, L., Di Domizio, S., et al. (2002). Effects of cognitive-behavioural therapy on health-related quality of life in obese subjects with and without binge eating disorder. *International Journal of Obesity and Related Metabolic Disorders, 26,* 1261–1267.

Martikainen, T., Pirinen, E., Alhava, E., Poikolainen, E., Pääkkönen, M., Uusitupa, M., et al. (2004). Long-term results, late complications and quality of life in a series of adjustable gastric banding. *Obesity Surgery, 14,* 648–654.

Mathias, S., Williamson, C., Colwell, H., Cisternas, M. G., Pasta, D. J., Stolshek, B. S., et al. (1997). Assessing health-related quality-of-life and health state preference in persons with obesity: A validation study. *Quality of Life Research, 6,* 311–322.

McEwen, J., McKenna, S. P., & Spilker, B. (1996). Nottingham Health Profile. In B. Spilker (Ed.), *Quality of life and pharmacoeconomics in clinical trials* (pp. 281–286). Philadelphia: Lippincott-Raven.

McHorney, C. A., Ware, J. E., Jr., Lu, J. F., & Sherbourne, C. D. (1994). The MOS 36-item Short-Form Health Survey (SF-36): III. Tests of data quality, scaling assumptions, and reliability across diverse patient groups. *Medical Care, 32,* 40–66.

McKenna, S. P., Hunt, S. M., & McEwen, J. (1981). Weighting the seriousness of perceived health problems using Thurstone's method of paired comparisons. *International Journal of Epidemiology, 10,* 93–97.

Mond, J., Hay, P. J., Rodgers, B., Owen, C., & Beumont, P. J. (2005). Assessing quality of life in eating disorder patients. *Quality of Life Research, 14,* 171–178.

Mond, J., Rodgers, B., Hay, P., Korten, A., Owen, C., & Beumont, P. (2004). Disability associated with community cases of commonly occurring eating disorders. *Australian and New Zealand Journal of Public Health, 28,* 246–251.

Moorehead, M. K., Ardelt-Gattinger, E., Lechner, H., & Oria, H. E. (2003). The validation of the Moorehead-Ardelt Quality of Life Questionnaire II. *Obesity Surgery, 13,* 684–692.

Myers, J. A., Clifford, J. C., Sarker, S., Primeau, M., Doninger, G. L., & Shayani, V. (2006). Quality of life after laparoscopic adjustable gastric banding using the Baros and Moorehead-Ardelt Quality of Life Questionnaire II. *Journal of the Society of Laparoendoscopic Surgeons, 10,* 414–420.

Nguyen, N. T., Goldman, C., Rosenquist, C. J., Arango, A., Cole, C. J., Lee, S. J., et al. (2001). Laparoscopic versus open gastric bypass: A randomized study of outcomes, quality of life, and costs. *Annals of Surgery, 234,* 279–289; discussion 89–91.

Ni Mhurchu, C., Bennett, D., Lin, R., Hackett, M., Jull, A., & Rodgers, A. (2004). Obesity and health-related quality of life: Results from a weight loss trial. *New Zealand Medical Journal, 117,* U1211.

Niero, M., Martin, M., Finger, T., Lucas, R., Mear, I., Wild, D., et al. (2002). A new approach to multicultural item generation in the development of two obesity-specific measures: the Obesity and Weight Loss Quality of Life (OWLQOL) questionnaire and the Weight-Related Symptom Measure (WRSM). *Clinical Therapeutics, 24,* 690–700.

O'Brien, B. (1988). Assessment of treatment in heart disease. In G. Teeling Smith (Ed.), *Measuring health: A practical approach* (pp. 191–210). Chichester, UK: John Wiley.

Oria, H. E. (1996). Reporting Results in Obesity Surgery: Evaluation of a Limited Survey. *Obesity Surgery, 6,* 361–368.

Oria, H. E. (2003). The BAROS and the Moorehead-Ardelt quality of life questionnaire. *Obesity Surgery, 13,* 965.

Oria, H., & Moorehead, M. (1998). Bariatric Analysis and Reporting Outcome System (BAROS). *Obesity Surgery, 8,* 487–499.

Osterhaus, J. T., Townsend, R. J., Gandek, B., & Ware, J. E., Jr. (1994). Measuring the functional status and well-being of patients with migraine headache. *Headache, 34,* 337–343.

Padierna, A., Quintana, J. M., Arostegui, I., Gonzalez, N., & Horcajo, M. J. (2000). The health-related quality of life in eating disorders. *Quality of Life Research, 9,* 667–674.

Padierna, A., Quintana, J. M., Arostegui, I., Gonzalez, N., & Horcajo, M. J. (2002). Changes in health related quality of life among patients treated for eating disorders. *Quality of Life Research, 11,* 545–552.

Patrick, D. L., Bushnell, D. M., & Rothman, M. (2004). Performance of two self-report measures for evaluating obesity and weight loss. *Obesity Research, 12,* 48–57.

Pinhas-Hamiel, O., Singer, S., Pilpel, N., Fradkin, A., Modan, D., & Reichman, B. (2006). Health-related quality of life among children and adolescents: Associations with obesity. *International Journal of Obesity (London), 30,* 267–272.

Puzziferri, N., Austrheim-Smith, I. T., Wolfe, B. M., Wilson, S. E., & Nguyen, N. T. (2006). Three-year follow-up of a prospective randomized trial comparing laparoscopic versus open gastric bypass. *Annals of Surgery, 243,* 181–188.

Ravens-Sieberer, U., & Bullinger, M. (1998). Assessing health-related quality of life in chronically ill children with the German KINDL: First psychometric and content analytical results. *Quality of Life Research, 7,* 399–407.

Ravens-Sieberer, U., Redegeld, M., & Bullinger, M. (2001). Quality of life after in-patient rehabilitation in children with obesity. *International Journal of Obesity and Related Metabolic Disorders, 25*(Suppl. 1), S63–S65.

Rieger, E., Wilfley, D. E., Stein, R. I., Marino, V., & Crow, S. J. (2005). A comparison of quality of life in obese individuals with and without binge eating disorder. *International Journal of Eating Disorders, 37,* 234–240.

Rippe, J. M., Price, J. M., Hess, S. A., Kline, G., DeMers, K. A., Damitz, S., et al. (1998). Improved psychological well-being, quality of life, and health practices in moderately overweight women participating in a 12-week structured weight loss program. *Obesity Research, 6,* 208–218.

Ryden, A., Karlsson, J., Persson, L. O., Sjöström, L., Taft, C., & Sullivan, M. (2001). Obesity-related coping and distress and relationship to treatment preference. *British Journal of Clinical Psychology, 40,* 177–188.

Ryden, A., Karlsson, J., Sullivan, M., Torgerson, J. S., & Taft, C. (2003). Coping and distress: What happens after intervention? A 2-year follow-up from the Swedish Obese Subjects (SOS) study. *Psychosomatic Medicine, 65,* 435–442.

Samsa, G. P., Kolotkin, R. L., Williams, G. R., Nguyen, M. H., & Mendel, C. M. (2001). Effect of moderate weight loss on health-related quality of life: An analysis of combined data from 4 randomized trials of sibutramine vs placebo. *American Journal of Managed Care, 7,* 875–883.

Sanchez-Santos, R., Del Barrio, M. J., Gonzalez, C., Madico, C., Terrado, I., Gordillo, M. L., et al. (2006). Long-term health-related quality of life following gastric bypass: Influence of depression. *Obesity Surgery, 16,* 580–585.

Sarlio-Lahteenkorva, S., Stunkard, A., & Rissanen, A. (1995). Psychosocial factors and quality of life in obesity. *International Journal of Obesity and Related Metabolic Disorders, 19* (Suppl. 6), S1–S5.

Schok, M., Geenen, R., van Antwerpen, T., de Wit, P., Brand, N., & van Ramshorst, B. (2000). Quality of life after laparoscopic adjustable gastric banding for severe obesity: Postoperative and retrospective preoperative evaluations. *Obesity Surgery, 10,* 502–508.

Scholz, G. H., Flehmig, G., Kahl, Y., Gutknecht, D., Schmidt, U., Tolkmitt, S., et al. (2002). Proper Weight Loss with Intelligence (MIRA): 2 programs for weight reduction in general practice trial [in German]. *MMW Fortschr Med, 144,* 28–32.

Schwimmer, J. B., Burwinkle, T. M., & Varni, J. W. (2003). Health-related quality of life of severely obese children and adolescents. *Journal of the American Medical Association, 289,* 1813–1819.

Silberhumer, G. R., Miller, K., Kriwanek, S., Widhalm, K., Pump, A., & Prager, G. (2006). Laparoscopic adjustable gastric banding in adolescents: The Austrian experience. *Obesity Surgery, 16,* 1062–1067.

Spielberger, C., Gorusch, R., & Luschene, R. (1970). *STAI manual for the State-Trait Anxiety Inventory.* Palo Alto, CA: Consulting Psychologists Press.

Steffen, R., Biertho, L., Ricklin, T., Piec, G., & Horber, F. F. (2003). Laparoscopic Swedish adjustable gastric banding: A five-year prospective study. *Obesity Surgery, 13,* 404–411.

Steinbrook, R. (2004). Surgery for severe obesity. *New England Journal of Medicine, 350,* 1075–1079.

Stewart, A. L., & Brook, R. H. (1983). Effects of being overweight. *American Journal of Public Health, 73,* 171–178.

Stewart, A. L., Hays, R. D., & Ware, J. E., Jr. (1988). The MOS short-form general health survey: Reliability and validity in a patient population. *Medical Care, 26,* 724–735.

Stout, A. L., Applegate, K. L., Friedman, K. E., Grant, J. P., & Musante, G. J. (2007). Psychological correlates of obese patients seeking surgical or residential behavioral weight loss treatment. *Surgery for Obesity and Related Diseases, 3,* 369–375.

Stucki, A., Borchers, M., Stucki, G., Cieza, A., Amann, E., & Ruof, J. (2006). Content comparison of health status measures for obesity based on the international classification of functioning, disability and health. *International Journal of Obesity (London), 30,* 1791–1799.

Sullivan, M., Cohen, J., & Branehog, I. (1988). *A psychosocial study of surviving cancer patients in California, USA and the western region of Sweden: Part II: Response patterns and determinants of adjustment to cancer in Sweden.* Goteborg: Sahlgrenska University Hospital.

Sullivan, M., Karlsson, J., Sjöström, L., Backman, L., Bengtsson, C., Bouchard, C., et al. (1993). Swedish obese subjects (SOS)—an intervention study of obesity: Baseline evaluation of health and psychosocial functioning in the first 1743 subjects examined. *International Journal of Obesity, 1743,* 503–512.

Sullivan, M., Karlsson, J., Sjöström, L., Taft, C., & Bjorntorp, P. (2001). Why quality of life measures should be used in the treatment of patients with obesity. 2001. In P. Björntorp (Ed.), *International textbook of obesity* (pp. 485–510). New York: John Wiley.

Sullivan, M., Sullivan, L. G., & Kral, J. G. (1987). Quality of life assessment in obesity: physical, psychological, and social function. *Gastroenterology Clinics of North America, 16,* 433–442.

Titi, M., Jenkins, J. T., Modak, P., & Galloway, D. J. (2007). Quality of life and alteration in comorbidity following laparoscopic adjustable gastric banding. *Postgraduate Medical Journal, 83,* 487–491.

Tolonen, P., & Victorzon, M. (2003). Quality of life following laparoscopic adjustable gastric banding: The Swedish band and the Moorehead-Ardelt questionnaire. *Obesity Surgery, 13,* 424–426.

Tolonen, P., Victorzon, M., & Makela, J. (2004). Impact of laparoscopic adjustable gastric banding for morbid obesity on disease-specific and health-related quality of life. *Obesity Surgery, 14,* 788–795.

Torquati, A., Lutfi, R. E., & Richards, W. O. (2007). Predictors of early quality-of-life improvement after laparoscopic gastric bypass surgery. *American Journal of Surgery, 193,* 471–475.

Tuthill, A., Slawik, H., O'Rahilly, S., & Finer, N. (2006). Psychiatric co-morbidities in patients attending specialist obesity services in the UK. *QJM—Monthly Journal of the Association of Physicians, 99,* 317–325.

van Gemert, W. G., Adang, E. M., Greve, J. W., & Soeters, P. B. (1998). Quality of life assessment of morbidly obese patients: Effect of weight-reducing surgery. *American Journal of Clinical Nutrition, 67,* 197–201.

Varni, J. W., Limbers, C. A., & Burwinkle, T. M. (2007). Parent proxy-report of their children's health-related quality of life: An analysis of 13,878 parents' reliability and validity across age subgroups using the PedsQL 4.0 Generic Core Scales. *Health and Quality of Life Outcomes, 5,* 2.

Varni, J. W., Seid, M., & Kurtin, P. S. (2001). PedsQL 4.0: Reliability and validity of the Pediatric

Quality of Life Inventory version 4.0 generic core scales in healthy and patient populations. *Medical Care, 39,* 800–812.

Veggi, A. B., Lopes, C. S., Faerstein, E., & Sichieri, R. (2004). Body mass index, body weight perception and common mental disorders among university employees in Rio de Janeiro [in Portuguese]. *Revista Brasileira de Psiquiatria, 26,* 242–247.

Victorzon, M., & Tolonen, P. (2001). Bariatric Analysis and Reporting Outcome System (BAROS) following laparoscopic adjustable gastric banding in Finland. *Obesity Surgery, 11,* 740–743.

Wadden, T. A., & Phelan, S. (2002). Assessment of quality of life in obese individuals. *Obesity Research, 10* (Suppl. 1), 50S–57S.

Wake, M., Salmon, L., Waters, E., Wright, M., & Hesketh, K. (2002). Parent-reported health status of overweight and obese Australian primary school children: A cross-sectional population survey. *International Journal of Obesity and Related Metabolic Disorders, 26,* 717–724.

Wan, G. J., Counte, M. A., & Cella, D. F. (1997). The influence of personal expectations on cancer patients' reports of health-related quality of life. *Psychooncology, 6,* 1–11.

Ware, J. E. (1993a). Measuring patients' views: The optimum outcome measure. *British Medical Journal, 306,* 1429–1430.

Ware, J. E. (1993b). *SF-36 health survey: Manual and interpretation guide.* Boston: Nimrod.

Ware, J. E. (1996). The SF-36 health survey. In B. Spilker (Ed.), *Quality of life and pharmacoeconomics in clinical trials* (pp. 337–345). Philadelphia: Lippincott-Raven.

Ware, J., Jr., Kosinski, M., & Keller, S. D. (1996). A 12-Item Short-Form Health Survey: Construction of scales and preliminary tests of reliability and validity. *Medical Care, 34,* 220–233.

Ware, J., Jr., & Sherbourne, C. D. (1992). The MOS 36-item short-form health survey (SF-36): I. Conceptual framework and item selection. *Medical Care, 30,* 473–483.

Ware, J., Snow, K., Kosinski, M., & Gandek, B. (1993). *SF-36 Health Survey: Manual and interpretation guide.* Boston: The Health Institute, New England Medical Center.

Waters, E. B., Salmon, L. A., Wake, M., Wright, M., & Hesketh, K. D. (2001). The health and well-being of adolescents: A school-based population study of the self-report Child Health Questionnaire. *Journal of Adolescent Health, 29,* 140–149.

Weiner, S., Sauerland, S., Fein, M., Blanco, R., Pomhoff, I., & Weiner, R. A. (2005). The Bariatric Quality of Life index: A measure of well-being in obesity surgery patients. *Obesity Surgery, 15,* 538–545.

Weiss, D. J., & Yoes, M. E. (1991). Item response theory. In R. K. Hambleton & J. Zaal (Eds.), *Advances in education and psychological testing: Theory and applications.* Norwell, MA: Kluwer.

Weissman, M. M., & Bothwell, S. (1976). Assessment of social adjustment by patient self-report. *Archives of General Psychiatry, 33,* 1111–1115.

White, M. A., O'Neil, P. M., Kolotkin, R. L., & Byrne, T. K. (2004). Gender, race, and obesity-related quality of life at extreme levels of obesity. *Obesity Research, 12,* 949–955.

Williams, J., Wake, M., Hesketh, K., Maher, E., & Waters, E. (2005). Health-related quality of life of overweight and obese children. *Journal of the American Medical Association, 293,* 70–76.

Wolf, A. M., Falcone, A. R., Kortner, B., & Kuhlmann, H. W. (2000). BAROS: An effective system to evaluate the results of patients after bariatric surgery. *Obesity Surgery, 10,* 445–450.

World Health Organization. (1948). *Constitution of the World Health Organization.* Geneva, Switzerland: Author.

Zeller, M. H., & Modi, A. C. (2006). Predictors of health-related quality of life in obese youth. *Obesity (Silver Spring), 14,* 122–130.

Zeller, M. H., Roehrig, H. R., Modi, A. C., Daniels, S. R., & Inge, T. H. (2006). Health-related quality of life and depressive symptoms in adolescents with extreme obesity presenting for bariatric surgery. *Pediatrics, 117,* 1155–1161.

CHAPTER 3

Methods for Measuring Attitudes About Obese People

Todd G. Morrison, Sarah Roddy, and Travis A. Ryan

Obesity is a condition of excessive fat accumulation in the body to the extent that health and well-being are adversely affected (World Health Organization [WHO], 2000). It has emerged as a world-wide epidemic (James, 2004; Popkin & Doak, 1998), with about "315 million people world-wide estimated to fall into the WHO-defined obesity category with a body mass index (BMI) of 30 or above" (Caterson & Gill, 2002, p. 595). Furthermore, the prevalence of obesity is increasing among children and adolescents (Jolliffe, 2004; Kumanyika, Jeffrey, Morabia, Ritenbaugh, & Antipatis, 2002; Lobstein & Frelut, 2003) as well as adults (Kumanyika et al., 2002; WHO, 1997). Indeed, in 2007, the British government-funded "Foresight" project revealed that being overweight is the norm in Britain, with citizens gaining weight through a process referred to as *passive obesity*. This term refers to weight accumulation that occurs due to living in an "'obesogenic' environment" characterized by an "abundance of energy dense food, transport and sedentary lifestyles" (Government Office for Science, 2007, p. 2).

Despite being a ubiquitous physical condition, obesity[1] is heavily stigmatized in Western cultures. Puhl and Brownell (2003) assert that, although "research on weight stigma is relatively new . . . [it] is robust enough to show that this bias is powerful, pervasive, and difficult to change" (p. 213). On the dimension of pervasiveness, negative attitudes toward overweight and obese individuals have been reported among samples of psychologists (e.g., Davis-Coelho, Waltz, & Davis-Coelho, 2000; Harvey & Hill,

AUTHORS' NOTE: The second and third authors contributed equally to this manuscript and are listed in alphabetical order. Sarah Roddy's work on this chapter was made possible by funding received from the Irish Research Council for the Humanities and Social Sciences. Travis Ryan's work was made possible by the Lady Gregory Research Fellowship Scheme of the Faculty of Arts, National University of Ireland, Galway.

2001), physicians (e.g., Foster et al., 2003; Hebl & Xu, 2001), health professionals specializing in obesity treatment (e.g., Schwartz, Chambliss, Brownell, Blair, & Billington, 2003; Teachman & Brownell, 2001), nurses (Brown, 2006), exercise science students (e.g., Chambliss, Finley, & Blair, 2004), registered dieticians (e.g., Oberrieder, Walker, Monroe, & Adeyanju, 1995), dietetics students (e.g., Berryman, Dubale, Manchester, & Mittelstaedt, 2006), physical education teachers (e.g., Greenleaf & Weiller, 2005; O'Brien, Hunter, & Banks, 2007) as well as heterogeneous groups of college and university students (e.g., Crandall, 1994; Morrison & O'Connor, 1999), members of the community (e.g., Teachman, Gapinski, Brownell, Rawlins, & Jeyaram, 2003), adolescents (e.g., Greenleaf, Chambliss, Rhea, Martin, & Morrow, 2006; Morrison & O'Connor, 1999), and children (e.g., Latner & Stunkard, 2003; Turnbull, Heaslip, & McLeod, 2000). Importantly, research also indicates that negative attitudes toward obesity (henceforth antifat attitudes) are evident in persons across the weight spectrum (e.g., Kraig & Keel, 2001; Vartanian, Herman, & Polivy, 2005).

Available evidence indicates that, among those categorized as obese, antifat attitudes are associated with various mental and physical health problems (e.g., Friedman et al., 2005; Harris et al., 2006; Meyer, 2003; Ogden & Sidhu, 2006). For instance, using a sample of 93 adults seeking treatment for obesity, Friedman and associates (2005) found that the occurrence of weight-related stigmatizing experiences was positively associated with depression, general psychiatric symptoms, and body image disturbance and negatively associated with self-esteem. The authors also noted that antifat attitudes moderated the association between stigma and body image (i.e., the "effects" of stigma on body image were greatest among participants who evidenced the most negativity toward fatness). According to Puhl and Brownell (2006), the most common stigmatizing situations reported by a sample of 2,449 adult women varying in weight (i.e., normal weight [5%], overweight [17%], obese I [22%], obese II [20%], and obese III [36%]) were others making negative

assumptions (e.g., others having low expectations of an individual because of his or her weight), receiving nasty comments from children, encountering physical barriers and obstacles, and receiving inappropriate comments from doctors and negative comments from family members. Results from a second sample of 222 adults (50% men, 50% women), similarly varying in weight, revealed that men, too, reported such stigmatizing experiences. Indeed, 48% of the situations were reported by at least 50% of the men surveyed.[2]

People subject to weight-related stigma also may experience disadvantages such as economic hardship and social isolation. Researchers have shown that obese people are less likely to be hired, more harshly disciplined on the job, assigned to inferior professional assignments, paid less than their nonobese coworkers, perceived by employers as a liability when it comes to providing health care insurance, penalized through some companies' benefits programs, and even terminated for failure to lose weight at their employer's request (see Fikkan & Rothblum, 2005; Puhl & Brownell, 2001). Studies also have documented that, in comparison to their normal-weight counterparts, obese persons are less "well liked" (e.g., Latner, Stunkard, & Wilson, 2005) and less likely to be selected as prospective sexual partners (e.g., Chen & Brown, 2005).

Given their psychological, physical, and social sequelae, antifat attitudes constitute an important area of psychological inquiry. Eagly and Chaiken (1998) state that an attitude "is a psychological tendency that is expressed by evaluating a particular entity with some degree of favor or disfavor . . . inferred by psychologists from observable responses" (p. 269). Although there is some debate about the elements that constitute an attitude, in the current chapter, a two-dimensional model will be used. This model suggests that affect (i.e., feelings) and cognitions (i.e., beliefs) represent interrelated, yet distinct, attitudinal components (Tropp & Pettigrew, 2005), each of which may be differentially associated with other attitudes and behaviors (e.g., Trafimow & Sheeran, 1998). In addition, a fairly recent development in the psychological study of attitudes concerns their measurement at implicit and explicit levels. According to Gawronski and Bodenhausen (2006), explicit attitudes are "evaluative judgments that are based on syllogistic inferences" (p. 694) while implicit attitudes are "automatic affective reactions" (p. 696).

The purpose of this chapter is to review the various tools that have been used to assess antifat attitudes. In the first section, instruments designed to measure explicit attitudes are discussed. To minimize duplication with a review of the literature conducted by Yuker, Allison, and Faith (1995), we pay attention primarily to measures appearing from the mid-1990s onward. In addition, for the sake of concision, the following selection criteria were employed: (a) The instrument must appear in a minimum of two published articles, (b) the instrument must have been developed and/or validated with English-speaking samples, and (c) the instrument must be designed to assess feelings toward and/or beliefs about obese persons. The review of these measures is stratified by type of sample; specifically, the psychometric properties of instruments designed to measure children's antifat attitudes are outlined followed by research pertaining to adolescents and adults. In the second portion of this chapter, techniques assessing implicit antifat attitudes are discussed.

Before commencing our review, it is important to acknowledge that, while standards can be delineated for best practice in psychometric testing, it is imperative that one be cognizant of the practical constraints in which researchers operate. Thus, asserting that a given measure was not constructed in an "optimal" manner or that it possesses gaps in terms its reliability, validity, and/or dimensionality is not tantamount to regarding the measure or the findings obtained via its use as lacking in value. Furthermore, as psychometric testing is an incremental and ongoing process, any of the limitations we identify might be addressed at some future point. Thus, with the understanding that psychological measurement is an imperfect process, it is our

intention to identify instruments that are the best among the array available currently.

In most cases, the information we present follows the sequence that is typically pursued when developing a scale; that is, we begin by describing the processes that informed item generation and reduction (if the latter is applicable) followed by assessments of dimensionality, reliability, and validity. We then review other published articles that have used the same scale (or a modified version thereof) and thus provide (or in some cases do not provide) further evidence of psychometric soundness. By presenting information in this sequence, we are not prioritizing the various elements of psychometric testing; in other words, we are not arguing that item generation is more important than reliability, which, in turn, is more important than validity. Given the interrelatedness of scale score reliability and scale score validity (i.e., the former establishes the upper limit for the latter—Hoyt, Warbasse, & Chu, 2006), arranging them in a "hierarchy of importance" would make little sense. If the resultant scale is to be optimal, *each* of these elements must be demonstrated.

Measurement of Children's Explicit Antifat Attitudes

Considerable research has been conducted to determine the age at which children become aware of different body builds and shapes. The measurement techniques employed in such investigations are diverse and include (a) ranking tasks in which children indicate their liking of targets that differ on select physical dimensions, (b) adjectival evaluations of line drawings and body silhouettes, (c) attitudinal instruments such as the Attributions of Controllability Scale (Tiggemann & Anesbury, 2000), and (d) peer and friendship nominations and preferences. Each of these techniques will be reviewed briefly.

Ranking Tasks. Richardson, Goodman, Hastorf, and Dornbusch (1961) assessed the attitudes of a large number ($N = 640$) of boys and girls (ages 10–11 years) toward six same-sex images; one depicted a healthy child and one an obese child, while the remaining four showed children with various physical disabilities (e.g., a child with crutches and a brace on the left leg). Rank ordering of preferences was obtained by randomly placing the stimulus pictures in front of the child and asking him or her to select the stimulus that he or she liked best. This stimulus then was removed, and the procedure was repeated until all pictures had been ranked. Surprisingly, in this study, the obese child was rated lower (i.e., selected last) than the children with physical handicaps.

In a recent replication of the Richardson et al. (1961) study, Latner and Stunkard (2003) examined the attitudes of boys and girls ($N = 458$) between the ages of 10 and 12 years, employing the same six images and rank-ordering procedure. Consistent with the results obtained in 1961, the obese child received the lowest mean rating. The relative positions of the highest and lowest ranked drawings remained the same; however, the mean distance between the child ranked the highest (i.e., the healthy child) and the child ranked the lowest (i.e., the overweight child) was 41% greater than the mean distance observed in 1961.

Similar research has been conducted with other populations and cultural groups (e.g., Goodman, Dornbusch, Richardson, & Hastorf, 1963; Latner et al., 2005) employing the same stimuli and procedure. However, modifications also have taken place. For example, in an effort to determine the salience of skin color and physical disability on children's preferences for the six targets, Richardson and Royce (1968) varied skin color and type of handicap (i.e., children were presented with white and colored versions of the stimuli employed by Richardson et al. [1961]).

There have been concerns that line drawings provide inaccurate representations of the body (Swami & Tovée, 2005; Tovée, Reinhardt, Emery, & Cornelissen, 1998) and that the ones used by Richardson et al. (1961) are now dated in terms of clothing and hairstyles (Latner, Simmonds,

Rosewall, & Stunkard, 2007). Using computer technology, Latner, Simmonds, et al. (2007) modified the original pictures to create more realistic and contemporary three-dimensional images. They also employed a modified version of the ranking procedure such that participants were presented with the six pictorial stimuli and were required to circle their preferred stimulus. Following this, the participants were presented with another set of the six stimuli below the first set and, again, asked to circle the stimulus figure they liked second best. This procedure was repeated until the six ranked preferences were obtained. Participants were presented with same-sex targets only. In addition, they were required to check their selections to ensure they had completed the procedure correctly and that all figures had been selected only once. Similar to Richardson et al. (1961), the rankings of the obese stimuli (boy and girl) were used as an indicator of liking for the obese peer in comparison with other peers.

In the final part of the study, participants were presented with the six images originally employed by Richardson et al. (1961), and their preferences were obtained using the modified ranking procedure. To ensure congruency with the earlier research, drawings were matched to the sex of the participants (i.e., girls were presented with female figures and boys were presented with male figures). Results indicated that there was a moderate to large degree of correspondence between the updated and older versions of the stimuli for both males (ρ [77] = .72, $p < .001$) and females (ρ [153] = .68, $p < .001$), demonstrating evidence for the criterion-related validity of the newer measure.

In another study, Latner, Rosewall, and Simmonds (2007) examined the relationship between mass media exposure (television, video games, and magazines) and weight stigmatization. Consistent with previous research, the overweight male and female targets were ranked lowest. Furthermore, self-reported magazine use emerged as a statistically significant predictor of the rankings of obese boys and girls (i.e., children who reported spending more time reading magazines evidenced less liking of the obese targets).

Given the forced-choice nature of the exercise, it is unclear whether those ranked last are disliked or merely less well liked than those receiving a higher ranking.[3] The concern that rankings may be fairly arbitrary also is difficult to dismiss. Furthermore, as this method provides ordinal data, available options for statistical analysis are limited (i.e., parametric statistics should not be used).

Adjectival Evaluations. Currently, the most popular method of measuring children's attitudes toward various body sizes is the adjective attribution task. In one of the earliest studies using this means of assessment, Staffieri (1967) asked boys ages 6 to 11 years to assign a list of 39 positive and negative behavior and personality traits to three body shapes (mesomorphic, ectomorphic, and endomorphic). In general, participants ascribed unfavorable characteristics to the endomorph (e.g., *lazy, sloppy, dirty, naughty, cheats, lies, argues, mean, ugly,* and *stupid*). Staffieri (1972) asked 7- to 11-year-old girls to assign 38 adjectives of various behavior/personality traits to the three body builds depicting female targets. Results, again, demonstrated that the endomorph was assigned adjectives that were consistently unfavorable, whereas the mesomorph received the most favorable ascriptions.

This adjective attribute task has been employed in a wide range of studies, including investigations of the relationship between body build stereotypes and attitudes toward personal body weight and playmate preferences (Cramer & Steinwert, 1998) and investigations of the influence of participant gender and age on adjective attributions (Kirkpatrick & Sanders, 1978). Modified and extended versions of the same basic procedure also have been employed with children as young as 30 months (Turnbull et al., 2000) and in other investigations of weight-based stereotyping (e.g., Tiggemann & Anesbury, 2000; Tiggemann & Wilson-Barrett, 1998).

Bell and Morgan (2000) used a clever variation of this adjective attribution method, in which children (N = 184; 88 boys and 96 girls) were presented with a video of a normal-weight child or the same child in a "fat suit." Videos were approximately 100 seconds in length. Participants were randomly assigned to one of six conditions: (a) average-weight boy, (b) average-weight girl, (c) obese boy, (d) obese girl, (e) obese boy with information that his obesity was due to a medical problem, and (f) obese girl with information that her obesity was due to a medical problem. After watching one of four video segments (obese boy/girl; average-weight boy/girl), participants completed the Adjective Checklist (Siperstein, 1980; Siperstein & Bak, 1977), which contains 32 descriptors (16 positive [e.g., *smart, neat*]/16 negative [e.g., *dumb, sloppy*]). For this task, participants were required to select the adjectives that they associated with the target child. The authors reported a coefficient alpha of .91 for the Adjective Checklist, suggesting good scale score reliability. The checklist also possessed adequate construct validity as it correlated significantly (r = .45) with a measure designed to assess children's willingness to engage in certain activities with the target child: the Shared Activities Questionnaire (SAQ; Morgan, Bieberich, Walker, & Schwerdtfeger, 1998). Thus, children providing more positive adjectival ratings of obese targets also evidenced greater willingness to interact with them.

Questions have been raised concerning the utility of such tasks with younger children who may find it difficult to assign abstract personality traits to pictorial target figures (e.g., Cramer & Steinwert, 1998). Such attribution tasks are limited in that they use a forced-choice procedure in which children have to assign each adjective to only one of the target figures; it is possible that a particular adjective could be equally associated with two body shape figures for some of the children. However, these tasks are easy to administer and appear to capture the interest of children. When reported, this type of task also possesses adequate psychometric properties.

Semantic differential scales are another popular means of assessing children's antifat attitudes (e.g., Irving, 2000; Kraig & Keel, 2001; Musher-Eizenman, Holub, Barnhart Miller, Goldstein, & Edwards-Leeper, 2004). For example, Brylinsky and Moore (1994) presented 368 children, ages 4 to 10 years, with line drawings of thin, average, and chubby same-sex figures. Participants were asked to rate these figures on a 7-point rating scale anchored by 12 pairs of bipolar adjectives; all of which had been previously employed in related research (Lerner & Korn, 1972; Staffieri, 1967; Stager & Burke, 1982; see Appendix 3.A at the end of the book). Results indicated there was a tendency for participants to evaluate the average child as favorable and the chubby build as unfavorable. Interestingly, in this study, assessments of the thin body type reflected a mixture of the positive aspects of the average-weight body shape and the negative aspects of the chubby body build. This finding suggests that the thin stereotype may be more complex than had been assumed in earlier studies.

Research indicates that, when used with children, the semantic differential technique is adequate psychometrically. For instance, Irving (2000) reports internal reliabilities of .81, .68, and .65 for the scales with the thin, average, and heavy figures, respectively. Musher-Eizenman et al. (2004) report an alpha coefficient of .63 for the six adjectives for the chubby figure in their study. In terms of construct validity, research indicates that participants who believe weight is under volitional control provide more negative trait ascriptions for a chubby figure ($r = -.34$, $p < .05$).

Some researchers interested in adjectival evaluations of overweight targets employ visual analog scales (VAS). A VAS is an instrument that measures any characteristic or attitude that is believed to range across a continuum of values. For example, Latner, Simmonds, et al. (2007) presented the children in their study with a questionnaire containing 12 stimulus figures (6 male and 6 female) and attributes such as intelligent and lazy. Questions such as "How smart would you guess this girl (or boy) is?" were responded to on a 100-mm VAS, along which participants drew a line. The scale was anchored on the left by

not at all and on the right by *very much*, with lower scores indicating greater stigmatization. Target drawings were presented to the left of the question itself. The questions for the overweight figures were combined to form an overall 10-item measure of stigmatizing attitudes, referred to by these authors as the Stigmatizing Attitudes Scale (SAS). This scale had moderate scale score reliability, with a Cronbach's alpha of 0.65. Results also indicated that scores for liking on the VAS were related to the rank ordering of overweight figures for both boys (ρ [237] $= -.18$, $p < .005$) and girls (ρ [239] $= -.37$, $p < .001$). In addition, responses on the 10-item SAS were found to be associated with rankings of both male and female overweight figures (ρ [240] $= -.22$, $p < .001$ for girls; ρ [240] $= -.16$, $p < .01$ for boys). Such findings attest to the construct validity of measuring adjectival endorsement with the VAS.

Using a variation of the VAS, Latner, Rosewall, and Simmonds (2007) asked participants the following: (a) How much do you like the girl (or the boy) on the left? (b) How much would you yourself want to be like this girl (or boy)? (c) How smart would you guess that this girl (or boy) is? Again, participants responded by placing a line on the scale. The internal reliability of this six-item measure was .82. Scores on the SAS were significantly, albeit weakly, associated with weekday video game playing ($r = -.13$) and total media use ($r = -.14$); thus, participants who reported greater media utilization tended to evidence less positive attitudes toward overweight persons.

The VAS is a flexible procedure that is easily administered and allows the participant to respond along a continuum when associating characteristics with body builds as opposed to forcing a choice between builds (e.g., Brylinsky & Moore, 1994) as in adjective attribution tasks. However, further research on such measures examining their test-retest reliability, validity, and generalizability is required (Latner, Simmonds, et al., 2007).

None of the adjectival measures we reviewed was demonstrably superior to its counterparts. If this type of assessment is needed, the reader should ensure that details are provided about the applicability of the adjectives to obese persons in general and obese men (boys) and women (girls) in particular. Mindless responding should be controlled either by using a combination of positive and negative adjectives (e.g., Wade, Fuller, Bresnan, Schaefer, & Mlynarski, 2007; Wade, Loyden, Renninger, & Tobey, 2003) or by alternating the response scale (see Barnette [2000] for details about this technique). If composite scores are computed, some indicant of item interrelatedness (e.g., item-total correlations) should be provided. Finally, issues of dimensionality warrant exploration as subsets of adjectives may be differentially associated with other attitudes and behaviors of interest.

Attributions of Controllability Scale (ACS; Tiggemann & Anesbury, 2000). The authors developed the ACS to measure the controllability beliefs of children ages 8 to 12 years. The scale is based on the Willpower subscale of Crandall's (1994) Anti-Fat Attitudes Questionnaire (AFA), Tiggemann and Rothblum's (1988) Perceived Etiology of Obesity Scale, and Sigelman's (1991) controllability manipulations and measures. The original scale consists of 13 items related to weight and obesity, covering both the initial cause of the condition and the possible solutions. For these items, a score of 1 was given to each answer that suggested controllability, .5 indicated a "don't know" answer, and 0 was given to each answer that indicated there was no controllability. Coefficient alpha for this scale was low at .44. Consequently, 4 items were removed from the scale, resulting in a reliability coefficient of .64. Scale scores for this version range from 0 to 9, with higher scores indicating greater perceived controllability. The scale was first employed in an investigation of negative stereotyping and controllability beliefs (Tiggemann & Anesbury, 2000), with results indicating a positive correlation between perceived controllability and negative stereotyping. These researchers also used the scale in a study investigating the effects of an intervention assumed to reduce the controllability beliefs of 74

children ages 9 to 12 years (Anesbury & Tiggemann, 2000). The alpha coefficient for the ACS was .87. Furthermore, scores on the ACS correlated with the measure of negative stereotyping for the female ($r = 0.27$, $p < .05$) and male targets ($r = 0.26$, $p < .05$).

In an attempt to measure children's ($N = 42$, 18 boys and 24 girls, mean age = 5.2 years) beliefs concerning the causes of obesity and how to solve the problem of obesity, Musher-Eizenman et al. (2004) developed a five-item scale based on the Attributions of Controllability Scale. For each item, children were required to respond *yes* or *no*. If a *yes* response was provided, they had to indicate whether this was *definitely* or *maybe*, resulting in a 3-point Likert-type scale (0 = *no*, 1 = *maybe*, 2 = *definitely*). Children were allowed to respond verbally or to point to the correct response. The five-item scale had an alpha coefficient of .56. Participants' control attributions were moderately related ($r = -.34$) to their adjective attributions to the overweight target on the measure of antifat prejudice, providing evidence for the construct validity of this indicant of controllability.

Friendship Measures. Examinations of peer friendship preferences and nominations can serve as a useful way for understanding how overweight children are evaluated and, subsequently, accepted into the social world. Adams, Hicken, and Salehi (1988) conducted two investigations to determine parental socialization processes underlying the transmission of the physical attractiveness stereotype. In their first study, 86 preschool and first-, third-, and fifth-grade students (approximately 4 to 11 years of age) were presented with same-sex sketches of line drawings of boys and girls who are mesomorphic and endomorphic. (Line drawings of boys and girls who are facially attractive, unattractive, and not disabled or disabled also were presented.) Participants completed a social choice task in which they were told, "Each child [from the array of same-sex sketches] has indicated that they would like to play with you." Each participant then was asked to indicate the child with whom he or she would prefer to play. In general, children preferred the mesomorphic target.

Cramer and Steinwert (1998) presented children (N = 83, 3- to 5-year-olds) with same-sex target figures depicting thin, average, and chubby body shapes. These figures were presented in pairs—thin/average, thin/chubby, and average/chubby. For each of the three pairs, children were asked, "Which child would you like to play with?" This was followed by the question, "Which child would you not like to play with?" The thin target was preferred to the chubby target, and this preference was stronger for girls than boys. Similar methods have been employed more recently by Tiggemann and Anesbury (2000), Musher-Eizenman et al. (2004), and Penny and Haddock (2007).

Stimuli can be presented individually or in the context of other stimuli, and children can be asked a variety of questions concerning their willingness to befriend the particular targets. Such a measure may be useful when employed with other techniques to determine the relationship between weight-based stereotyping and behavioral intentions toward overweight children.

Summary. A variety of techniques have been employed to investigate children's antifat attitudes. Based on a review of the available literature, playmate preference tasks are an effective measure for use with younger participants, and

semantic differential tasks permit good flexibility and validity for the assessment of a wide range of stereotypes toward the overweight. With further research, the modified ranking procedure and images employed by Latner and colleagues also may prove useful.

Measurement of Adolescents' and Adults' Explicit Antifat Attitudes

A plethora of measures exist to assess feelings and/or beliefs about obese persons. These include (a) semantic differential scales (e.g., Bacon, Scheltema, & Robinson, 2001; Foster et al., 2003; Ginis & Leary, 2006; Teachman & Brownell, 2001) and (b) rankings of pictures/drawings of normal-weight and overweight targets as well as those with various disabilities (e.g., facial disfigurement) on dimensions of liking (e.g., Latner et al., 2005) and sexual attraction (e.g., Chen & Brown, 2005). In addition, a number of attitudinal scales have been developed to assess antifat prejudice (see Table 3.1).[4] Each of these methods of assessment will be reviewed briefly.

Semantic Differential Measures.[5] Typically, for this type of measure, participants are instructed to evaluate "fat people" and "thin people" on 5- to 7-point scales in which endpoints consist of

Table 3.1   Common Scales Used to Measure Antifat Attitudes

Scale (Acronym)	Author(s)
Anti-Fat Attitudes Questionnaire (AFA)	Crandall (1994)
Anti-Fat Attitudes Scale (AFAS)	Morrison and O'Connor (1999)
Anti-Fat Attitudes Test (AFAT)	Lewis, Cash, Jacobi, and Bubb-Lewis (1997)
Attitudes Toward Obese Persons Scale (ATOP)	Allison, Basile, and Yuker (1991)
Fat Stereotypes Questionnaire (FSQ)	Davison and Birch (2004)

NOTE: Scale items and scoring procedures for all measures (with the exception of the FSQ, which is not recommended) are given in Appendices 3.C through 3.F at the end of the book.

a given adjective (e.g., *smart*) and its antonym (e.g., *stupid*). The number of adjectives that are rated by participants varies. For example, Teachman and Brownell (2001) used 2 adjective pairs (*good/bad* and *lazy/motivated*), whereas, in their modified F-scale, Bacon and colleagues (2001) used 14 (see Appendix 3.B at the end of the book).

This type of instrument appears to be fairly popular (e.g., Gapinski, Schwartz, & Brownell, 2006; Ginis & Leary, 2006; Polinko & Popovich, 2001; Schwartz et al., 2003; Smith, Schmoll, Konik, & Oberlander, 2007). However, when selecting a semantic differential measure of antifat attitudes, researchers are advised to consider the following questions.

First, has the content validity of the adjectives been demonstrated clearly (i.e., are the terms relevant to obese individuals)? On a related note, has sufficient evidence been provided attesting to the comparable applicability of the adjectives to obese men and women? For example, Bacon et al. (2001) generated descriptors on the basis of clinical experience and input from a community sample whereby persons entering a motor vehicles license bureau were asked to list terms "to describe people who are fat" (Robinson, Bacon, & O'Reilly, 1993, p. 470). Notice that the gender-neutral term *people* was used rather than *man* or *woman*. Semantic differential measures that have been developed in reference to generic targets are potentially problematic because they (a) assume that the same trait ascriptions apply to obese men and women and (b) cannot capture beliefs that are perceived as unique to obese members of one sex.

Second, have positive and negative endpoints been alternated to control for mindless responding, or do negative adjectives appear uniformly on one side and positive adjectives on the other side? Third, have the authors provided any evidence attesting to the reliability of their measure? If items are being analyzed individually, then test-retest reliability would serve as a useful indicant of consistency. If composite scores are computed, then the number of items used must be considered. When two adjective pairs are

employed (e.g., *good/bad* and *lazy/motivated*), calculating a correlation coefficient is appropriate; when more than two adjective pairs are used, an index of internal reliability such as Cronbach's alpha should be given. Fourth, and finally, if multiple adjective pairs are used, have the authors provided information about dimensionality? For example, Robinson and associates (1993) conducted a principal components analysis (PCA) of a 50-item semantic differential scale focusing on beliefs about obese persons. A six-component solution was obtained. Underscoring the importance of dimensionality assessment, the effects of a self-esteem/body image program on antifat attitudes differed across components, with scores on some components evidencing greater levels of improvement than scores on other components.

None of the examples we identified in our review of the available literature addressed all of the aforementioned questions. However, while acknowledging extant limitations, we recommend that individuals wishing to use this type of measure employ the 14-item F scale (Bacon et al., 2001). Its internal reliability is good (alphas range from .87 to .91), and it correlates strongly with the original 50-item version published in 1993 (*r*s for two samples were .82 and .90). Some evidence of construct validity is available (i.e., among those who attended a self-esteem/body image program, a statistically significant change occurred in pretest/posttest scores on the F scale); however, additional validation work is needed. At present, the F scale's susceptibility to response artifacts such as social desirability bias is unknown, and the dimensionality of the measure has not been assessed. Finally, given the gender-neutral development of the 50-item Fat Phobia Scale from which the F scale was derived, it is unclear whether the adjectives used adequately sample the domain of trait ascriptions for obese men and women.

Ranking Tasks. For this type of measure, participants are shown drawings depicting various types of men or women (e.g., "healthy," obese, missing a hand, sitting in a wheelchair, having a leg brace, and being facially disfigured—Latner et al., 2005; Latner, Rosewall, & Simmonds, 2007). Typically, six figures are used, and they are matched on key dimensions such as clothing and ethnicity. Participants are instructed to inspect the drawings and then rank order the targets in terms of liking (e.g., Latner et al., 2005; Latner, Rosewall, & Simmonds, 2007) or suitability as a sexual partner (Chen & Brown, 2005). This type of assessment is seldom used with adolescents and adults, and as mentioned earlier, we believe it possesses limitations that compromise its usefulness.

Anti-Fat Attitudes Questionnaire (Crandall, 1994). The AFA (see Appendix 3.C at the end of the book) contains 13 items (e.g., I really don't like fat people much) and uses a Likert-type response format (0 = *very strongly disagree;* 9 = *very strongly agree*). Higher scores denote stronger antifat attitudes. In the original article detailing the measure's construction and validation, Crandall (1994) reported that 26 items were generated initially.[6] A PCA with varimax rotation then was conducted on the 26 items. Three components with eigenvalues greater than 1.0 were retained and labeled Dislike of Fat People (7 items), Fear of Fat (i.e., individuals' concern about weight, 3 items), and Willpower (i.e., individuals' beliefs in the controllability of weight, 3 items). Alpha coefficients ranged from good (.84—Dislike) to adequate (.66—Willpower).

Subsequent validation work indicated that (a) variables representing a personal worldview in which people deserve what they get and get what they deserve (e.g., belief in a just world and the Protestant work ethic) correlated positively with Dislike and Willpower but not Fear of Fat, (b) students who were members of the University of Florida college Democrats evidenced lower Dislike and Willpower scores in comparison to student college Republicans (again, no difference was noted for Fear of Fat), and (c) participants exposed to a persuasive communication emphasizing the genetic and metabolic underpinnings of obesity evidenced lower Dislike and Willpower scores than those in the control condition. No

differences were obtained for Fear of Fat. These findings provide strands of evidence in support of the construct validity of the Dislike and Willpower subscales. However, the absence of statistically significant findings for the Fear of Fat subscale (with the exception of its inverse association with right-wing authoritarianism) is of concern. It also is unclear why Fear of Fat is the only antifat dimension that fails to correlate with *all* components of an ideological system that denotes the "general tendency to make controllable attributions" (Crandall, 1994, p. 884).

It should be noted that some of the statistical decisions that were used in the construction of the AFA may be questioned. First, to assess dimensionality, PCA was employed rather than exploratory factor analysis (EFA). The latter is recommended for structure detection because PCA does not distinguish between common and unique variance (Fabrigar, Wegener, MacCallum, & Strahan, 1999). Second, the use of varimax rotation, which constrains components (or factors) to be orthogonal (Finch & West, 1997), does not appear to be optimal with this scale (i.e., the Dislike and Willpower subscales were moderately intercorrelated: *r*s ranged from .43 [Study 1] to .60 [Study 2]). Oblique rotation would have been a preferable means of rotation. Third, the eigenvalue greater than 1.0 rule, although used commonly, may result in component overextraction and is regarded by some researchers as arbitrary (Hayton, Allen, & Scarpello, 2004). Instead, parallel analysis appears to be a better choice, as it "is one of the most accurate methods for determining the number of factors [or components] to retain" (Hayton et al., 2004, p. 192).

Crandall and Martinez (1996) subsequently tested the AFA among samples of Mexican and American university students (*n*s = 236 and 170, respectively). An unspecified form of factor analysis was conducted (type of rotation not indicated), with three factor solutions emerging for both the English and Spanish versions of the scale (i.e., Dislike, Fear of Fat, and Willpower). Measurement and structural equivalence (see Byrne & Watkins, 2003) were not formally assessed, although the researchers did "correlate the pattern of factor loadings across different solutions" and found correlations ranging from .90 (Dislike) to .71 (Willpower). For this study, indicants of reliability (e.g., alpha coefficients) were not reported. Finally, as hypothesized, the association between social ideology and antifat attitudes was stronger for American participants; that is, statistically significant correlations were observed between Dislike of Fat People, for example, and belief in a just world and political conservatism. These correlations were not significant for Mexican participants. The confirmation of these hypotheses provides additional evidence attesting to the construct validity of the AFA.

Another cross-cultural study was conducted by Crandall and associates (2001) using participants, primarily students, from Australia, the United States, India, Poland, Venezuela, and Turkey (ns range from 98 to 202). Again, the measurement and structural equivalence of the AFA were not examined statistically. Alpha coefficients were .81 (Dislike) and .66 (Willpower). No alpha was provided for Fear of Fat. Additional strands of evidence supporting the AFA's construct validity were obtained (e.g., scores on the Dislike subscale correlated positively with scores on measures assessing the negative cultural value of fatness and the tendency to regard weight as controllable).

Other researchers have examined the psychometric properties of the AFA. Morrison and O'Connor (1999) investigated the dimensionality and scale score reliability of the Dislike subscale using a sample of Canadian university students ($N = 113$). The authors failed to replicate the single-component solution obtained by Crandall (1994) for this subscale and also noted that the component solutions for male and female participants were dissimilar. However, these researchers did not formally test whether this dissimilarity was meaningful. They also used principal components analysis, varimax rotation, and the eigenvalue greater than 1 "rule"—all of which may be regarded as nonoptimal statistical choices. Internal reliability for the Dislike

subscale was .80 (.81 for men and .73 for women). Finally, these authors examined the association between responses on the Dislike subscale and social desirability bias. A statistically significant, though modest, correlation was obtained for women ($r = -.29$) but not for men ($r = -.16$).

Quinn and Crocker (1999) distributed the Dislike and Willpower subscales of the AFA to 257 American female college students. In an effort to increase internal reliability, the authors generated additional scale items (i.e., three items were added to Dislike and five items were added to Willpower). The resultant alpha coefficients were good: .89 (Dislike) and .84 (Willpower). However, no details were provided about the generation of these additional items and whether their inclusion had implications for scale dimensionality. The authors reported that scores on Dislike and Willpower were not associated with respondents' body mass index (BMI) but did correlate with their endorsement of the Protestant work ethic (i.e., the stronger the endorsement, the greater the dislike and the belief that weight is controllable [$rs = .27$ and $.38$, respectively]). It should be noted that Crandall (1994) obtained similar results using the original Dislike and Willpower subscales. The identification of similar correlative patterns among studies conducted by different researchers with different samples provides compelling evidence of construct validity. Finally, Quinn and Crocker reported that self-perceived weight status interacted with scores on the Dislike subscale to predict scores on a composite measure of psychological well-being (i.e., somewhat and very overweight participants who reported greater dislike of fat people evidenced poorer psychological well-being). For Willpower, no statistically significant main effects or interactions were observed.

Butler (2000) distributed copies of the AFA in conjunction with other measures (e.g., right-wing authoritarianism and homonegativity) to 82 American college students. Alpha coefficients for the Dislike, Willpower, and Fear of Fat subscales were .84, .83, and .68, respectively. As predicted, right-wing authoritarianism correlated positively with negative attitudes toward fat people (Dislike) and the belief that weight is controllable (Willpower) but did not correlate with Fear of Fat. Again, these results replicate findings observed by Crandall (1994) in his original validation study of the AFA. Butler also noted that participants' level of ethnocentrism and homonegativity correlated significantly with scores on the Dislike subscale (specific *r*s were not provided).

Recently, O'Brien and colleagues (2007) used the AFA to examine explicit antifat attitudes among a sample of university students in New Zealand ($N = 344$). The researchers modified one of the items from the Fear of Fat subscale (i.e., "One of the worst things that could happen to me would be if I gained 25 pounds" became "One of the worst things that could happen to me would be if I gained 25 pounds of fat"), thereby reducing potential confusion about whether the additional poundage referred to muscle mass or fat.[7] Alpha coefficients were good: .85 (Dislike), .84 (Fear of Fat), and .79 (Willpower). Further corroborating the measure's construct validity, hypothesized associations between scores on the AFA and other variables of interest were confirmed (e.g., scores on the Dislike subscale correlated positively with social dominance orientation for both psychology and year 3 physical education students).

Anti-Fat Attitudes Scale (AFAS; Morrison & O'Connor, 1999). The AFAS (see Appendix 3.D at the end of the book) consists of five items (e.g., "Fat people are less sexually attractive than thin people") and uses a 5-point Likert-type response format (1 = *strongly disagree;* 5 = *strongly agree*). Higher scores denote stronger antifat attitudes. Using samples of Canadian university students and adolescents, Morrison and O'Connor (1999) conducted four studies to test the dimensionality, scale score reliability, and construct validity of the AFAS. Results indicated that the scale was consistently unidimensional, as determined by two principal components analyses; possessed acceptable reliability (i.e., alpha coefficients ranged from .70 to .77); and was construct valid (i.e., scores on the AFAS correlated significantly

with scores on measures of authoritarianism, political conservatism, and homonegativity but, as expected, did not correlate with fear of fat or social desirability bias).

Several limitations pertaining to the construction and validation of the AFAS warrant mention. First, the authors did not provide any details concerning the processes that informed item generation. Second, the authors did not oversample content domain by generating a large number of items and then reducing them through the application of various item reduction criteria. As the AFAS contains only five questions, construct underrepresentation (i.e., failure to include critical facets of a construct—Hubley & Zumbo, 1996) may be problematic. Third, as mentioned previously, the authors' use of principal components analysis and the eigenvalue greater than 1 "rule" to assess dimensionality does not reflect best practice.

Greenleaf and Weiller (2005) used the AFAS to investigate antifat attitudes among 105 American physical educators. Coefficient alpha was acceptable (.69), with a small pilot test suggesting that the scale possesses criterion-related validity (i.e., scores on the AFAS correlated with another psychometrically sound indicant of antifat attitudes, the Anti-Fat Attitudes Test [Lewis, Cash, Jacobi, & Bubb-Lewis, 1997]: $r = .63$). The authors found that participants evidencing higher scores on the AFAS also were more likely to believe that "normal weight youth would perform better than overweight youth, specifically on tasks requiring endurance, coordination, sport competence, physical abilities, reasoning abilities, and social interaction abilities" (p. 419). These associations provide further evidence that the AFAS is construct valid.

Aruguete, Yates, and Edman (2006) used the AFAS to investigate gender differences in attitudes toward fat among a sample of American college students ($N = 196$). Internal reliability was good (Cronbach's alpha = .80). Congruent with findings reported by Morrison and O'Connor (1999), Aruguete and colleagues found that (a) male participants obtained higher scores on the AFAS (suggesting greater dislike of fat people), and (b) individuals' BMI correlated negatively with their AFAS scores (i.e., those who were overweight were less likely to endorse antifat attitudes). Finally, as hypothesized, an inverse correlation was observed between scores on the AFAS and scores on a measure of body dissatisfaction; thus, participants who were more satisfied with their appearance tended to report more negative antifat attitudes. These findings provide additional strands of support for the construct validity of the AFAS.

Anti-Fat Attitudes Test (AFAT; Lewis et al., 1997). The AFAT (see Appendix 3.E at the end of the book) contains 47 items (e.g., "When fat people exercise, they look ridiculous") and uses a 5-point Likert-type scale (1 = *definitely disagree;* 5 = *definitely agree*). Higher scores reflect more negative attitudes toward overweight individuals. The measure is designed to assess "cognitive, affective, and behavioral dispositions toward fat people" (Perez-Lopez, Lewis, & Cash, 2001, p. 687) and consists of three subscales: Social/Character Disparagement (15 items), Physical/Romantic Unattractiveness (10 items), and Weight Control/Blame (9 items). Thirteen additional items are included in the computation of total scale scores, though the rationale for doing so is unclear.

Several issues emerge with respect to the development and validation of the AFAT. First, the stability of the measure's three-dimensional structure is unknown. A confirmatory factor analysis is needed to address this issue. Second, given the length of the scale, the usefulness of the 13 filler items may be questioned. Third, the magnitude of the alpha coefficients for the total scale (α = .95 for both men and women) suggests that some items are redundant and could be eliminated (Streiner, 2003). Fourth, the combination of attitudinal and behavioral items (e.g., "I prefer not to associate with fat people") is regarded by some researchers as problematic (e.g., Morrison, Morrison, Hopkins, & Rowan, 2004).

In a survey of 409 American female university students, Ojerholm and Rothblum (1999) found

that scores on the AFAT correlated significantly with scores on measures of homonegativity, feminist identity, and feminist attitudes (i.e., respondents who were more antifat tended to be more homonegative, less likely to self-identify as feminist, and less likely to evidence positive attitudes toward the feminist movement). The authors did not examine the reliability of the AFAT in terms of alpha or test-retest coefficients, nor were findings reported that could be used as evidence in support of the reliability and validity of the AFAT subscales. Similar to Lewis et al. (1997), Ojerholm and Rothblum obtained a nonsignificant correlation between the AFAT and scores on a measure of social desirability bias.

In a study investigating the extent to which prejudice is a generalized phenomenon, Perez-Lopez and associates (2001) distributed the AFAT in conjunction with measures of racism, sexism, homonegativity, and acceptance of a masculine ideology to 179 American university students. The authors report that alpha coefficients for the AFAT and its subscales ranged from .82 to .95 but do not provide specific details. As predicted, participants who evidenced greater antifat prejudice also tended to be more racist, homonegative, sexist, and more likely to endorse traditional gender-related beliefs. Contrary to earlier studies, moderate correlations were observed between scores on a measure of social desirability bias and scores on the AFAT and its three subscales. Intriguingly, the correlation between social desirability and scores on the Physical/Romantic Unattractiveness subscale was positive, suggesting that the more socially desirable response is to evaluate fat people as unattractive. (Correlations for the total score and the remaining two subscales were negative.) Finally, the authors found that, in comparison to female participants, the men in their study evidenced stronger antifat prejudice. The authors also found that White participants were more antifat than were Black participants.

Chambliss and colleagues (2004) used the AFAT to examine explicit antifat prejudice among a sample of American undergraduate and graduate exercise science students ($ns = 136$ and 110, respectively). No details concerning reliability were provided. However, various statistically significant findings were obtained that attest to the construct validity of the AFAT. For example, (a) individuals who did not have a family history of obesity evidenced significantly higher scores on the AFAT as well as the Social/Character Disparagement and Weight Control/Blame subscales, and (b) individuals who did not have obese friends reported significantly higher scores on the AFAT and all three of its subscales. No association was observed between the AFAT and an implicit measure of antifat prejudice.

Hague and White (2005) used the AFAT to investigate the efficacy of a Web-based intervention designed to promote size acceptance among a sample consisting predominately of American undergraduate students majoring in education ($N = 258$). The authors report that coefficient alpha for the AFAT was .94. (No alphas were given for its subscales.) The AFAT was distributed to participants three times (i.e., pretest, posttest, and 6-week follow-up), thereby providing a useful opportunity to evaluate test-retest reliability. However, no correlations were given. The authors found that scores on the AFAT decreased across all treatment conditions, indicating that the intervention was effective in reducing antifat attitudes.

Attitudes Toward Obese Persons Scale (ATOP; Allison, Basile, & Yuker, 1991). The ATOP (see Appendix 3.F at the end of the book) contains 20 items (e.g., "Obese people tend to have family problems") and uses a 6-point Likert-type response format ($-3 = I$ *strongly disagree;* $+3 = I$ *strongly agree*). Lower scores denote stronger antifat attitudes. The authors report that items were generated on the basis of "face validity and past utility in measuring beliefs about obesity" (p. 602). Alpha coefficients for samples of graduate ($n = 52$) and undergraduate ($n = 72$) psychology students as well as members of the National Association to Advance Fat Acceptance (NAAFA; $n = 514$) were good ($αs = .81$, .80, and .84,

respectively). Principal components analysis was used to assess the dimensionality of the ATOP, with a scree test being used for component retention. Both varimax and oblique rotation were performed; however, as correlations among factors were small and oblique rotation did not provide a "substantially simpler structure" (p. 604), the varimax output was interpreted. A three-component solution was obtained. In terms of construct validity, only one association was statistically significant across the three samples; specifically, individuals who evidenced more positive attitudes toward obese persons were more likely to perceive obesity as operating outside an individual's control.

Several limitations warrant discussion. First, oversampling of content domain did not occur (i.e., the authors did not generate a large number of items and then apply item reduction criteria). Thus, one must assume the authors regarded the 20 items on the ATOP as reflecting the best exemplars of antifat attitudes. Second, the numbers of items loading on each component was not specified, nor were the component loadings provided. Third, indices of reliability for the components were not given; thus, it is unclear whether each component possesses sufficient item interrelatedness and stability to serve as a stand-alone subscale. Fourth, there is an absence of findings that could be used to corroborate the measure's construct validity.

Using data from 255 general practitioners and clinical psychologists in the north of England, Harvey and Hill[8] (2001) reported good internal reliability ($α = .83$) for the ATOP. Principal components analysis with oblique rotation was performed to identify whether scale items could "be grouped in a meaningful way to describe a smaller number of underlying principles or 'latent variables'" (p. 1255). A three-component solution was obtained. However, the authors did not specify (a) the method used to retain components, (b) item loadings, or (c) the reliability of the components. A series of independent samples t tests were conducted to evaluate if participants' responses on each ATOP item differed as a function of whether the question referred to an extremely overweight person versus a moderately overweight person. Statistically significant differences were noted for 14 of the 20 items, with more negative attitudes being evident among those completing the "extremely overweight" version.

Harvey, Summerbell, Kirk, and Hill (2002) administered the ATOP to 187 members of the British Dietetics Association. Again, principal components analysis with oblique rotation was used to assess the dimensionality of the scale. A three-component solution was noted; however, the same limitations observed for the earlier PCA conducted by Harvey and Hill (2001) arise (i.e., no details were given about component retention, component loadings, and whether components denote internally reliable subscales). The latter issue warrants concern as the authors appear to have conducted multiple regression analyses with ATOP components serving as predictor variables (see Harvey et al., 2002, Table 5, p. 338). Finally, in contrast to Harvey and Hill (2001), fewer differences were noted between participants completing the overweight versus obese version of the scale (i.e., statistically significant differences were obtained for 6 of the 20 items, with attitudes toward obese individuals being more negative).

In an experimental study investigating the effects of advertisements on explicit and implicit attitudes toward overweight persons, 59 American female undergraduate students completed the ATOP (Geier, Schwartz, & Brownell, 2003). Results indicated that individuals exposed to either a "before and after" weight loss advertisement or a non-weight-related advertisement featuring the "before" female model evidenced greater negative attitudes toward obese persons in comparison to those exposed to the same non-weight-related advertisement featuring the "after" female model. The authors also noted that ATOP scores correlated positively with belief in the controllability of weight (i.e., those regarding weight as controllable evidenced more negative attitudes) and negatively with life satisfaction (i.e., those with higher levels of satisfaction

reported less negative attitudes toward obese persons). The reliability of the ATOP was not reported. In addition, although the authors measured social desirability bias, they did not examine its association with scores on the ATOP.

Friedman and colleagues (2005) used the ATOP to examine associations between weight-related beliefs, weight-based stigmatization, and psychological functioning in a small sample of adults seeking treatment for obesity ($N = 93$). Details concerning scale reliability were not provided. In terms of construct validity, negative correlations were obtained between scores on the ATOP and scores on the Beck Depression Inventory, the Body Shape Questionnaire, and the Global Severity Index of the Brief Symptom Inventory (rs range from $-.28$ to $-.30$). Thus, individuals who evidenced stronger antifat attitudes (as denoted by lower scores on the ATOP) reported higher levels of depression, greater body image distress, and increased psychiatric symptomatology. A positive correlation was noted between the ATOP and a measure of self-esteem ($r = .31$), suggesting that participants with stronger antifat attitudes also had lower levels of self-esteem. Finally, the authors reported that antifat beliefs served to moderate the association between weight stigma and body image distress (i.e., the stigma/distress correlation was statistically significant only for participants evidencing strong endorsement of antifat attitudes).

In a large-scale Internet survey consisting of 2671 American respondents, Puhl and Brownell (2006)[9] used the ATOP in conjunction with a battery of other measures (e.g., Beck Depression Inventory and the Rosenberg Self-Esteem scale). The alpha coefficient was .76, suggesting adequate internal reliability. For Subsample 1 ($n = 2,449$ women), statistically significant, though very weak, correlations were noted between ATOP scores and beliefs about the controllability of weight ($r = .08$) and binge eating ($r = -.13$). Thus, individuals possessing negative attitudes toward obese individuals were more likely to perceive weight as controllable and more likely to be categorized as binge eaters. For Subsample 2 ($n = 222$

men and women), no systematic pattern of correlations was observed between scores on the ATOP and the other variables examined.

Fat Stereotypes Questionnaire (FSQ; Davison & Birch, 2004). The FSQ consists of 18 statements (9 duplicate items for thin people and fat people—e.g., "It is hard for fat people [thin people] to get to know people"). A 4-point Likert-type response format is used (*really disagree, sort of disagree, sort of agree, really agree*). Difference scores are computed for each attribute and then summed, with higher scores denoting stronger endorsement of negative characteristics for fat people. Among a sample of 178 parents, alpha coefficients for the FSQ were .65 (mothers) and .69 (fathers). For both mothers and fathers, scores on the FSQ correlated significantly with scores on an indicant of social desirability bias ($rs = -.21$ and $-.22$, respectively). Parents' scores on the FSQ also correlated significantly with their beliefs that appearance is central to their self-concept and that social goodness is linked with attractiveness. These various associations provide strands of evidence in support of the FSQ's construct validity.

As noted with most of the other scales described thus far, the sources that informed selection of the fat stereotypes were not outlined. Given that only nine stereotypes are used, construct underrepresentation may be problematic. Indeed, the authors recommend that researchers use a "broader range of stereotypical attitudes" (Davison & Birch, 2004, p. 92) in future studies. The dimensionality of the FSQ also was not examined.

Greenleaf and associates (2006) used the FSQ to investigate weight stereotypes among a sample of American adolescents ($N = 274$). Seven items were added to the scale, the content validity of which was determined by researchers with "expertise in attitudes and weight bias" (p. 547). Thus, this version of the FSQ contained 32 items (16 duplicate stereotypes for fat people and thin people). The method of scoring was changed such that *lower* scores reflected *stronger* endorsement of the attributes for fat people. Internal reliability

was good ($\alpha = .80$), with a pilot study revealing modest test-retest reliability over a 2-week period ($r = .62$). Results indicated that scores on the FSQ emerged as a significant predictor of participants' willingness to engage in general social and recreational activities with an overweight person (i.e., individuals who rejected fat stereotypes appeared to be more willing to interact with an overweight person in these domains).

Summary. For those wishing to use an attitudinal measure, the AFA, AFAS, ATOP, and AFAT appear to be comparable in their psychometric robustness (see Appendices 3.C to 3.F at the end of the book for copies of these instruments). Thus, determining which measure to use should be based, in part, on the goals of the researcher. If brevity is key, then the Dislike and Willpower subscales of Crandall's (1994) AFA or Morrison and O'Connor's (1999) AFAS may be sufficient. If one is interested in the interplay between different elements of antifat prejudice (e.g., character disparagement vs. perceptions of unattractiveness), then a longer measure such as the AFAT may be the measure of choice. Key psychometric findings are provided in Table 3.2.

This literature review indicates clearly that, while various studies provide evidence attesting to the reliability and validity of these measures, future research is needed to fill in extant gaps. In some cases, scale dimensionality is unknown (e.g., FSQ), is unclear (e.g., AFAT and ATOP), or does not reflect best practices in factor analysis (e.g., AFA and AFAS). Alpha coefficients for all measures appear to be satisfactory, though few provide evidence of test-retest reliability. (See Weng [2004] for details concerning why *both* forms of reliability are important.) In some cases, scale components have not been validated (e.g., ATOP), and in other instances, the applicability of specific subscales to antifat prejudice is unclear. For example, the AFA's Fear of Fat subscale reflects personal concerns about gaining weight rather than prejudice toward people who are overweight (Klaczynski, Goold, & Mudry, 2004). The suitability of these measures in non-Western

Table 3.2   Summary of Key Psychometric Findings for Recommended Scales Measuring Antifat Attitudes

Scale	Key Findings
Anti-Fat Attitudes Questionnaire (AFA; Crandall, 1994)	Decision making underlying item generation is unclear.
	Evidence of dimensionality is mixed (i.e., some studies find the expected three-component/factor solution, whereas others do not). To date, no confirmatory factor analysis (CFA) on the entire scale has been conducted.
	Reliability, as measured by Cronbach's alpha, ranges from satisfactory to good.
	Good evidence of construct validity for Dislike of Fat People and Willpower subscales. Poor evidence for Fear of Fat subscale.
Anti-Fat Attitudes Scale (AFAS; Morrison & O'Connor, 1999)	Decision making underlying item generation is unclear.
	A small number of items were generated; therefore, construct underrepresentation may be an issue.
	A single-component/factor solution is consistently obtained. However, to date, no CFA has been conducted.
	Reliability, as measured by Cronbach's alpha, ranges from satisfactory to good.
	Good evidence of construct validity.
Anti-Fat Attitudes Test (AFAT; Lewis, Cash, Jacobi, & Bubb-Lewis, 1997)	Decision making underlying item generation is unclear.
	Dimensionality is unclear (i.e., few studies have attempted to replicate three-factor structure noted by original authors). No CFA has been conducted.
	Reliability, as measured by Cronbach's alpha, is good. However, alpha for total scale suggests item redundancy may be problematic.
	Good evidence of construct validity for total scale but less evidence for subscales.
Attitudes Toward Obese Persons Scale (ATOP; Allison, Basile, & Yuker, 1991)	Rationale for item generation is provided.
	Three-component solution is consistently obtained; however, to date, no CFA has been conducted.
	Reliability, as measured by Cronbach's alpha, is satisfactory.
	Modest evidence of construct validity.

NOTE: These measures are recommended for assessing antifat attitudes, with the understanding that subsequent work is needed to address extant gaps in psychometric testing. Finally, it should be noted that none of these measures uses parallel forms for overweight men and overweight women.

cultural contexts is, at best, ambiguous. For instance, although the AFA has been distributed to participants in countries such as Mexico and Turkey, to date, tests of measurement invariance have not been conducted.

Finally, an important limitation—one that is shared by all of these scales—concerns their reliance on gender-neutral targets. There is no published antifat attitudes scale that adheres to best practices in scale development (e.g., Springer, Abell, & Hudson, 2002) *and* is designed to measure similarities and differences in attitudes toward overweight men versus overweight women. As a stopgap approach, we recommend that researchers use parallel versions of the AFA, AFAS, ATOP, or AFAT, with one focusing on female targets and the other focusing on male targets. Each version could be allocated randomly to participants.

Measurement of Implicit Attitudes

In response to prevailing social norms, the nature of prejudice toward obese individuals has changed in recent times, thus necessitating a shift in measurement. Although antifat attitudes are prevalent in modern society, it is apparent that many individuals are aware of the inappropriateness of the public expression of such attitudes (Brochu & Morrison, 2007; Teachman & Brownell, 2001; Vartanian et al., 2005). This awareness may account for findings suggesting that, on some explicit measures of antifat prejudice, people score at the scale midpoint (e.g., AFAS; Greenleaf & Weiller, 2005) or evidence neutral to positive attitudes (e.g., ATOP; Harvey et al., 2002). Traditional measures such as Likert-type and semantic differential scales also require individuals to consciously consider their evaluation of an attitude object (i.e., an obese target) and thus are unable to capture attitudes that are activated automatically. In addition, such measures depend on the participant's ability and willingness to accurately report his or her evaluations

and judgments (Greenwald et al., 2002). Due to these limitations, the use of explicit measures alone may not be optimal.

Implicit Measures

Greenwald and Banaji (1995) define implicit attitudes as "introspectively unidentified (or inaccurately identified) traces of past experience that mediate favorable or unfavorable feeling, thought or action towards social objects" (p. 8). There has been an upsurge in research focusing on the development of measures that can assess this type of attitude. These indirect or implicit measures, as they are referred to frequently in the literature, circumvent the problems inherent in explicit measures and potentially tap into unique components of attitudes that lie outside of consciousness or even direct control (Cunningham, Preacher, & Banaji, 2001). For the majority of implicit measures, a person's attitude is inferred based on his or her performance on reaction time (RT) tasks, where response latencies indicate the amount of attention required to evaluate particular socially relevant items.

The following implicit techniques are reviewed in this chapter: the Lexical Decision Task and the Implicit Association Test. Each of these methods will be outlined briefly, with their application to antifat attitudes delineated in greater detail.

Lexical Decision Task. This task requires participants to make a judgment, as quickly and accurately as possible, as to whether the letter string presented is a word or a nonword (Gaertner, & McLaughlin, 1983). For example, based on the previous experimental research of Meyer and Schvaneveldt (1971) and Gaertner and McLaughlin (1983), Wittenbrink, Judd, and Park (1997) presented participants with a prime stimulus referring to an ethnic group (either *Black* or *White*), an unrelated prime (e.g., *table*), or a neutral nonword prime (e.g., xxxxx). Primes were presented for 15 milliseconds (i.e., subliminally) and were immediately followed by a masking stimulus (xxxxx) presented for 200 milliseconds. Target stimuli that were stereotypic of White Americans and counterstereotypic of African Americans (e.g., *ambitious*), stereotypic of African Americans and counterstereotypic of White Americans (e.g., *lazy*), irrelevant attributes, or nonwords then were presented. Half of these stereotypic and counterstereotypic attributes were positively valenced, and half were negatively valenced. Subjects were required to make a decision as to whether the target was a word or a nonword. The dependent measure was response latency in making such judgments. Results demonstrated that identification of the target stimulus was significantly facilitated when positively valenced White American items followed the *White* prime and when negatively valenced African American items followed the *Black* prime.

With respect to antifat attitudes, Bessenoff and Sherman (2000) examined the extent to which controlled (explicit) and automatic (implicit) attitudes predicted how far participants chose to sit from an overweight woman. Participants were presented with photographs of overweight and thin women, followed by a Lexical Decision Task (LDT) in which they had to make judgments about words that were negative fat stereotypical (e.g., *insecure*), positive fat stereotypical (e.g., *kind*), negative thin stereotypical (e.g., *selfish*), positive thin stereotypical (e.g., *confident*), negative stereotype irrelevant (e.g., *violent*), and positive stereotype irrelevant (e.g., *musical*). Similar to Wittenbrink and colleagues (1997), the dependent measure was response latency in making word/nonword judgments. In addition, these researchers assessed participants' behavioral intention toward an overweight woman by examining preferred seating distance. Physical distance between a chair that participants were led to believe an overweight woman was to sit on and a chair that participants were instructed to place in the room was measured, with greater seating distance indicating more negative behavioral intent.

Overall, there was greater activation for negative trait words when preceded by the photo of the overweight as opposed to the thin model. There was no effect of trait stereotypicality; therefore, all negative words, regardless of whether they were fat stereotypical, thin stereotypical, or stereotype irrelevant, were associated with faster activation levels following presentation of the overweight prime. Interestingly, automatic evaluations were found to correlate with behavioral intention, such that participants evidencing greater implicit negativity chose to sit father away from the overweight woman. Explicit attitudes did not correlate with behavioral intention, suggesting that the lexical decision task had greater predictive validity.

Implicit Association Test. The Implicit Association Test (IAT; Greenwald, McGhee, & Schwartz, 1998) is the most commonly used measure of implicit attitudes.[10] Each IAT consists of two critical blocks of 60 trials. On a particular trial, a target stimulus is presented center screen (e.g., *tulip, bee, family,* and *rotten*), and participants are required to classify stimuli into one of four categories: pleasant, unpleasant, flower, or insect. Stimuli are categorized using two response keys (typically one toward the left and the other toward the right of the keyboard), with the response labels for these keys being presented toward the top right and left of the screen (Lemm, 2006). Correct categorization of a given stimulus permits the participant to advance to the next trial. Incorrect categorization of a given stimulus results in the automatic presentation of an "X," with participants being unable to advance to the next trial until the stimulus has been categorized correctly.

Stimulus categories are organized such that two categories are assigned to each response key. For example, in one such critical block, flowers + pleasant are assigned to the same response key, and insect + unpleasant are assigned to the other response key. This is referred to as a consistent block as response assignment is likely to be consistent with the participant's preexperimental attitudes. In the other critical block, pleasant + insect are assigned to one response key, and unpleasant + flower are assigned to the other response key. This is referred to as an inconsistent block as response assignment is likely to be inconsistent with the participant's preexperimental attitudes. In a standard IAT, the order of these consistent and inconsistent blocks is counterbalanced. The IAT effect is calculated as the difference in mean response latencies across consistent and inconsistent trials (Greenwald et al., 1998).

A computerized antifat/ pro-thin IAT would involve the presentation of target words related to weight (e.g., *fat, chubby, overweight, thin, slim, slender*) or images of average-weight and overweight male and/or female targets and pairs of evaluative attributes (e.g., *good* vs. *bad, lazy* vs. *motivated, smart* vs. *stupid*). Participants are required to categorize items as they appear on the computer screen through selection of particular response keys (i.e., the "d" or "k" keys on a QWERTY keyboard). Consistent and inconsistent trials are presented in a counterbalanced order across participants. At the start of each block, participants are provided with instructions that describe the category discriminations and the assignments of response keys to categories. Tasks are administered in blocks of 50 trials (on average) with participants being exposed to seven blocks (both practice and critical test blocks). Target category names appear as labels (e.g., *overweight* and *slim*) and are positioned to the left and the right of the screen. Target attributes (e.g., *good, bad,* and *lazy*) appear one at a time in the center of the screen. Figure 3.1 provides a diagrammatic representation of the typical sequence of trials used on a computerized IAT.

Computerized versions of the IAT typically require participants to sort the stimuli into the correct category to progress to the next trial. Response latencies are usually recorded in milliseconds and are compared across consistent and inconsistent trials.

In addition to the computerized IAT, a paper-and-pencil version has been used by researchers investigating antifat attitudes. The underlying rationale is the same; however, the latter involves presenting participants with a sheet of paper

containing target words and attributes (see Figure 3.2). Participants are instructed to examine the words that belong to the target (e.g., *overweight* and *slim*) and attribute groups (e.g., *good* and *bad*). Two category headings are assigned to both the right (e.g., *overweight + bad*) and the left (e.g., *slim + good*) column, and participants are given 20 seconds to complete as many items as possible and are instructed to classify the words as opposed to making judgments about them. Participants complete attitude-consistent and attitude-inconsistent category pairings in counterbalanced order. For the attitude-consistent pairings, participants classify a list of words into their appropriate category by placing a tick in the right or the left column as quickly as possible. Thus, looking at the IAT in Figure 3.2, under the *slim + good* column, participants would tick *thin, cool, skinny, joyful, petite, smart, slender, small, active,* and *disciplined,* whereas under the *overweight + bad* column, participants would select *large, lazy, ugly, obese, heavy, unpopular, stupid, chubby, sloppy,* and *fat.* When completed, participants are provided with a second sheet with the same four groups; however, this time, category-inconsistent headings anchor each column (e.g., *overweight + good, slim + bad*). Again, participants classify words as quickly as possible. Lemm, Lane, Sattler, Khan, and Nosek (2008) note that computation of difference scores between attitude-consistent (i.e., *overweight + bad*) and attitude inconsistent (i.e., *overweight + good*) blocks is inadequate because it does not take into account variations in the speed with which participants complete the task. Thus, these authors recommend that researchers use a *product: square root of difference* scoring method: (X/Y) * SQRT of (X − Y), where X is the greater of Block A (*slim + good*) or Block B (*overweight + good*), and Y is the smaller of A or B. Lemm and colleagues (2008) note that if B is greater than A, resulting values should be multiplied by −1 so as to preserve the directionality of the IAT effect (i.e., in the example provided, if participants classify more items correctly for the *slim + good* block than the *overweight + good* block, it suggests an implicit preference for *slim*).

Sequence					
	1	*2*	*3*	*4*	*5*
Task description	*Initial target-concept discrimination*	*Associated attribute discrimination*	*Initial combined task*	*Reversed target-concept discrimination*	*Reversed combined task*
Task instruction	SLIM OVERWEIGHT	Good Bad	SLIM Good OVERWEIGHT Bad	SLIM OVERWEIGHT	SLIM Good OVERWEIGHT Bad
Sample stimuli	CHUBBY (r) OVERWEIGHT (r) CHUNKY (r) BONY (l) LANKY (l) SLENDER (l)	Bad (r) Unpleasant (r) Negative (r) Good (l) Pleasant (l) Positive (l)	HEAVY (r) Wonderful (l) BONY (l) Nasty (r) OBESE (r) Friendly (l)	CHUBBY (l) OVERWEIGHT (l) CHUNKY (l) BONY (r) LANKY (r) SLENDER (r)	Happy (l) THIN (r) Brave (l) FAT (l) Lazy (r) LEAN (r)

Figure 3.1   Schematic Description and Illustration of the IAT

NOTE: The IAT procedure outlined above involves a series of five discrimination tasks (numbered tasks). A pair of target concepts and an attribute dimension are introduced in the first two steps. Categories for each of these discriminations are assigned to a left or right response, indicated by the (l) or (r) after each stimulus. These are combined in the third step and then recombined in the fifth step, after reversing response assignments (in the fourth step) for the target-concept discrimination.

It should be noted that it is standard practice to include explicit attitudinal measures, thereby permitting comparisons of both types of attitude. Although a recent meta-analysis of IAT studies suggests no effect for order of presentation of implicit and explicit measures (Hofmann, Gawronski, Gschwender, Le, & Schmitt, 2005), Nosek, Greenwald, and Banaji (2007) recommend counterbalancing the order of IAT and self-report measures in the absence of reasons for administering either test before the other.

The IAT has been used to assess antifat attitudes among a variety of groups, including health professionals (e.g., Schwartz et al., 2003; Teachman & Brownell, 2001), college/university students (e.g., Ahern & Hetherington, 2006; Brochu & Morrison, 2007; Chambliss et al., 2004; Gapinski et al., 2006; Geier et al., 2003; O'Brien et al., 2007; Rudman, Feinberg, & Fairchild, 2002; Vartanian et al., 2005), individuals participating in weight loss programs (Wang, Brownell, & Wadden, 2004), and members of the general community (e.g., Grover, Keel, & Mitchell, 2003; Schwartz, Vartanian, Nosek, & Brownell, 2006; Teachman et al., 2003). For example, Teachman and Brownell (2001) employed a paper-and-pencil version of the IAT to investigate antifat bias among a sample of health care specialists ($N = 84$) attending a meeting on obesity. As is typical in most IAT research, both feelings and beliefs toward overweight individuals were assessed. Participants classified more items correctly when "fat people" + bad (denoting the affective component of attitudes) and "fat people" + lazy (denoting the cognitive component of attitudes) were paired together. Poorer performance occurred when the category pairings were inconsistent (i.e., "fat people" + good; "fat people" + motivated). Levels of explicit bias were low, as indicated by 7-point semantic differential scales

Slim Good		Overweight Bad		Overweight Good		Slim Bad
O	Thin	O		O	Skinny	O
O	Cool	O		O	Smart	O
O	Large	O		O	Heavy	O
O	Lazy	O		O	Unpopular	O
O	Skinny	O		O	Slender	O
O	Ugly	O		O	Disciplined	O
O	Obese	O		O	Large	O
O	Joyful	O		O	Ugly	O
O	Heavy	O		O	Petite	O
O	Unpopular	O		O	Active	O
O	Petite	O		O	Fat	O
O	Smart	O		O	Cool	O
O	Slender	O		O	Chubby	O
O	Stupid	O		O	Lazy	O
O	Chubby	O		O	Thin	O
O	Sloppy	O		O	Joyful	O
O	Small	O		O	Obese	O
O	Active	O		O	Sloppy	O
O	Fat	O		O	Stupid	O
O	Disciplined	O		O	Small	O

Figure 3.2   Example of a Pen-and-Paper IAT

NOTE: These tasks are measuring the implicit association between the target categories *slim* and *overweight* and good and bad attributes. The tasks on the left are consistent; thus, participants tend to be faster to categorize these stimuli. The tasks on the right are inconsistent; thus, participants tend to be slower to categorize these stimuli.

assessing positive and negative feelings and beliefs toward "fat people" and "thin people."

Recently, Schwartz and colleagues (2006) assessed implicit and explicit antifat attitudes and obesity stereotypes among a large online sample ($N = 4283$). Using a Web site created specifically for the purposes of the research, subjects performed two computerized IATs, completed three 5-point semantic differential scales, and rated the personal trade-offs they would be willing to make to avoid being overweight. Similar to the results reported by Teachman and

Brownell (2001), participants were faster when "fat people" + bad and "fat people" + lazy were assigned to the same response key. Table 3.3 provides a summary of key findings in other research that has employed the IAT to investigate antifat attitudes.

Researchers also have examined the modifiability of antifat attitudes using the IAT. For example, Gapinski and colleagues (2006) presented American female undergraduate participants ($N = 108$) with either control video clips or ones designed to evoke empathy for overweight individuals, as well as clips that portrayed overweight women either stereotypically (e.g., *unattractive, unintelligent, unprofessional,* and *sluggish*) or counterstereotypically (e.g., *smart, competent, professional,* and *motivated*). Neither the empathy nor the stereotype manipulation reduced implicit or explicit antifat attitudes. Similar findings underscoring the difficulty of changing implicit antifat attitudes have been reported by Grover et al. (2003) and Teachman et al. (2003).[11, 12]

The various studies summarized in Table 3.3 underscore the burgeoning popularity of the IAT as a means of assessing implicit antifat attitudes. However, do these studies provide compelling evidence attesting to the psychometric soundness of this technique?[13] On the basis of the literature we reviewed, the answer to this question is a prudent "not yet." First, none of the studies explicitly report the reliability of the IAT.[14–16] Second, in terms of construct validity, only limited evidence has been accumulated. For example, Teachman and Brownell (2001) hypothesized that the level of implicit antifat bias demonstrated by members of the general population tested in an earlier study would be greater than the level of implicit bias shown by a group of health professionals. Results supported this hypothesis. O'Brien et al. (2007) proposed that (a) physical education (PE) students in their study would demonstrate greater levels of antifat bias than non-PE students, and (b) third-year PE students would demonstrate more bias than first-year PE students. Importantly, the expected differences emerged for the implicit, but not explicit, measure

of prejudice. Both sets of results suggest that the IAT, when applied to the domain of antifat attitudes, possesses known-groups validity.

However, in terms of associations between antifat IATs and other individual difference variables, inconsistent patterns emerge. For instance, O'Brien et al. (2007) noted that social dominance orientation (SDO) correlated with good/bad and smart/stupid but not lazy/motivated IAT scores. Furthermore, these correlations were obtained for just one subsample (third-year PE students). Chambliss and associates (2004) reported a small but statistically significant negative correlation between participants' BMI and good/bad IAT scores (i.e., greater bias was observed among those with a lower BMI). Conversely, Schwartz and colleagues (2003) noted that BMI did not correlate significantly with good/bad, motivated/lazy, or valuable/worthless IAT scores. (For this sample, a significant negative correlation emerged between BMI and smart/stupid IAT scores.) The authors also found that participants who worked directly with obese patients evidenced less implicit antifat prejudice on the lazy/motivated IAT but not on the other measures. A different pattern emerged when the researchers examined participants' friendships with persons who were obese (i.e., having more obese friends was associated with less implicit bias on the smart/stupid IAT measure). It is difficult to provide an interpretative framework that parsimoniously accounts for these idiosyncrasies.

Third, the issue of criterion-related validity is problematic. On one hand, nonsignificant correlations between the IAT and explicit measures of antifat attitudes can be accounted for on the grounds that the two measures assess different constructs (Greenwald & Banaji, 1995; Wilson, Lindsey, & Schooler, 2000) and vary in their susceptibility to response artifacts such as social desirability bias. However, it should be noted that researchers examining the association between implicit and explicit measures often obtain variable findings (e.g., a nonsignificant r between the AFAT and all IAT tasks [Chambliss et al., 2004;

(Text continues on page 106)

Table 3.3   Summary of Published Studies Using the IAT to Examine Antifat Prejudice

Study	Sample	Overweight Stimuli	Thin Stimuli	Attitudes	Stereotypes	Key Findings
Teachman and Brownell (2001)[a]	Health care specialists (N = 84)	Fat Obese Large	Slim Thin Skinny	Good vs. bad	Lazy vs. motivated	1. Strong antifat bias on the two IATs. 2 Explicit biases were low; with the exception that thin people were seen to be more motivated. 3. Small correlation between implicit and explicit measures on lazy/motivated dimension. 4. Inverse correlations between bias, both implicit and explicit, and body mass index (BMI). 5. Level of bias demonstrated by this sample was smaller than that noted previously by members of the general public.
Rudman, Feinberg, and Fairchild (2002)[b]	Students (N = 593)	Fat Overweight Heavy	Slim Thin Skinny	Pleasant vs. unpleasant		1. Overweight individuals demonstrated a strong antifat bias on the IAT and a modest antifat bias on the explicit measure.
Teachman, Gapinski, Brownell, Rawlins, and Jeyaram (2003)[a,b]	Study 1: General community (N = 144) Study 2A: Introductory psychology students and general community (N = 90) Study 2B: General community (N = 63)	Fat Obese Large	Slim Thin Skinny	Good vs. bad	Lazy vs. motivated Worthless vs. valuable	1. Strong antifat bias on the three IATs. 2. Low levels of antifat bias on explicit measure. 3. Moderate correlations between some implicit and explicit measures.

Study	Sample	Overweight Stimuli	Thin Stimuli	Attitudes	Stereotypes	Key Findings
Schwartz, Chambliss, Brownell, Blair, and Billington (2003)[a]	Researchers and health professionals (N = 389)	Obese Large Fat	Slim Thin Skinny	Good vs. bad	Lazy vs. motivated Stupid vs. smart Worthless vs. valuable	1. Strong antifat bias on the four IATs. 2. Participants demonstrated a strong explicit antifat bias. 3. Inverse correlation between BMI and smart/stupid scores on the IAT and explicit good/bad scores.
Gapinski, Schwartz, and Brownell (2006)[a]	Students (N = 108)	Fat people	Thin people	Good vs. bad	Lazy vs. motivated Worthy vs. worthless Competent vs. incompetent Intelligent vs. stupid Blameworthy vs. blameless	1. Strong antifat bias on six IATs. 2. Strong antifat bias at the explicit level (except on bad/good and stupid/intelligent dimensions). 3. Moderate correlations between implicit and explicit attitudes. 4. Empathy manipulation did not successfully reduce implicit or explicit attitudes.
Geier, Schwartz, and Brownell (2003)[b]	Students (N = 59)	Fat	Thin	Good vs. bad	Lazy vs. motivated Ugly vs. beautiful Blameworthy vs. blameless	1. All participants demonstrated strong antifat bias. 2. Participants demonstrated explicit antifat bias. 3. Control beliefs were positively related to antifat attitudes.

(Continued)

Table 3.3 (Continued)

Study	Sample	Overweight Stimuli	Thin Stimuli	Attitudes	Stereotypes	Key Findings
Grover, Keel, and Mitchell (2003)[b]	General community (N = 83)	Overweight Plump Chubby	Under-weight Thin Skinny	Good vs. bad		1. Explicit antifat attitudes demonstrated by normal-weight and overweight males and females. 2. Implicit antifat attitudes demonstrated by normal-weight and overweight males and females. 3. No correlations between implicit and explicit measures.
Wang, Brownell, and Wadden (2004)[a]	Study 1: Overweight Whites and African Americans (N = 68) Study 2: Overweight individuals (N = 48)	Fat people	Thin people	Good vs. bad	Lazy vs. motivated Stupid vs. smart Worthless vs. valuable	1. Strong antifat bias on IAT. 2. Lower levels of explicit antifat bias, with the exception of the lazy/motivated dimension
Chambliss, Finley, and Blair (2004)[a]	Exercise science students (N = 246)	Fat Obese Large	Slim Thin Skinny	Good vs. bad	Lazy vs. motivated	1. Antifat bias was demonstrated on the two IATs. 2. Small negative correlation was found between the lazy/motivated implicit and explicit measures.
Vartanian, Herman, and Polivy (2005)[b]	Study 1: Students (N = 56; females) Study 2: Students (N = 53; females)	Chubby Overweight Chunky Plump Heavy Pudgy Obese Stout	Bony Lanky Slender Lean Slim Willowy Skinny Scrawny	Pleasant vs. unpleasant		1. Implicit antifat attitudes demonstrated by both restrained and unrestrained eaters. 2. Restrained eaters had stronger explicit antifat beliefs than unrestrained eaters.

Study	Sample	Overweight Stimuli	Thin Stimuli	Attitudes	Stereotypes	Key Findings
Schwartz, Vartanian, Nosek, and Brownell (2006)[b]	General community (N = 4,283)	Fat Overweight Large	Slim Thin Skinny	Good vs. bad	Lazy vs. motivated	1. Strong antifat bias on the two IATs. 2. Low levels of explicit antifat attitudes. 3. BMI was inversely correlated with implicit attitudes and stereotypes and explicit attitudes.
Ahern and Hetherington (2006)[b]	Students (N = 86; females)	Images of fat women	Images of thin women	Positive vs. negative		1. Strong antifat bias demonstrated on IAT. 2. No association between implicit and explicit measures
O'Brien, Hunter, and Banks (2007)[a]	Students (N = 344)	Fat Overweight Large	Slim Thin Skinny	Good vs. bad	Lazy vs. motivated Stupid vs. smart	1. Strong antifat bias demonstrated on three IATs. 2. Explicit antifat bias was moderate. 3. Small correlations between implicit and explicit measures.
Brochu and Morrison (2007)[b]	Students (N = 76)	Images of overweight men and women	Images of average-weight men and women	Pleasant vs. unpleasant		1. Antifat bias was demonstrated for the male and female IAT. 2. Implicit attitudes were not found to be a significant predictor of behavioral intention. 3. Correlations between implicit and explicit attitudes were low.

a. Paper-and-pencil version.

b. Computerized version.

Wang et al., 2004]; a significant *r* between the Fat Phobia Scale and a lazy-motivated IAT [Teachman et al., 2003]; significant *rs* between the AFA's Dislike subscale and good/bad and smart/stupid IATs for third-year PE students [O'Brien et al., 2007]). Again, the critical issue is how does one *explain* this variability?

Finally, there is a need for more systematic assessments of the relationship between stereotyping and prejudice, as measured by the IAT, and individual difference variables. The linkages between responses on the IAT and both behavioral intention and behavior toward overweight persons also constitute critical areas of inquiry.

Conclusion

In conclusion, given the prevalence of obesity and the documented negativity that exists, both attitudinally and behaviorally, toward obese persons, it is imperative that social scientists interested in antifat prejudice have access to measures that reflect best practices in scale development and display excellent psychometric properties. In terms of explicit measures, depending on the specific requirements of the researchers, the AFA (Dislike and Willpower subscales; Crandall, 1994), AFAS (Morrison & O'Connor, 1999), AFAT (Lewis et al., 1997), and ATOP (Allison et al., 1991) are reasonable choices. Finally, the most commonly used implicit measure of antifat attitudes is the IAT, which may be used in either computerized or paper form. However, in the interests of triangulation, we would encourage researchers to explore other types of implicit assessment as well (e.g., lexical decision tasks and facial electromyography).

Notes

1. Unless specified, the term *obesity* is being used to denote the possession of excess weight and not a specific BMI cutoff (see Puhl & Brownell, 2003).

2. Despite the chapter's focus on measures used to assess antifat attitudes, Myers and Rosen's

(1999) Stigmatizing Situations Inventory and Coping Responses Inventory deserve mention. The former assesses experiences of weight stigma, and the latter assesses whether and how often participants used different strategies to cope with stigmatizing situations based on their weight. Evidence attesting to the reliability and validity of these measures is provided by numerous researchers (e.g., Friedman et al., 2005; Myers & Rosen, 1999; Puhl & Brownell, 2006). While these measures are not reviewed in this chapter, weight-related stigmatizing experiences and associated coping strategies represent a dynamic area of research that illustrates the effects of antifat attitudes.

3. It should be noted that some researchers employ a modified form of this type of assessment. For example, Tiggemann and Anesbury (2000) showed normal-weight or obese silhouette drawings to 96 children (ranging in age from 8 to 12) and instructed them to indicate which figure was healthier, lazier, smarter, and so on. Importantly, the children were given the option of classifying both targets as being the same on any one of the dimensions tested.

4. Excluded from this list are measures that appear to have been used in single studies (e.g., 16-item Attitude Scale [Crerand et al., 2007]; a feeling thermometer [Gapinski et al., 2006]; untitled 44-item measure [Glenn & Chow, 2002]; 10-item Blame People for Their Fatness scale [Jaffe & Worobey, 2006]; 40-item Obesity Stereotypes Instrument [Klaczynski et al., 2004]; untitled 24-item measure [McArthur, 1995]; untitled 37-item measure [McArthur & Ross, 1997]; 20-item Obese Persons Trait Survey [Puhl, Schwartz, & Brownell, 2005]; and 4-item Attitudes Toward Overweight Persons scale [Thompson & Sargent, 2000]).

5. In some cases, Likert response formats are used (e.g., Regan, 1996), or participants are instructed to circle adjectives that they believe apply to a "fat" target (e.g., Greenleaf et al., 2006).

6. Crandall (1994) does not outline the processes that informed item generation of the AFA.

7. Morrison and O'Connor (1999) also expressed concerns about the wording of specific items. For example, they questioned whether an affirmative response to the statement, "I don't

have many friends who are fat," logically implies an antifat attitude. (In a subsequent study by Jaffe and Worobey [2006], this item was deleted from the Dislike subscale because it attenuated internal reliability.) A confirmatory factor analysis of the Dislike and Willpower subscales (O'Bryan, Fishbein, & Ritchey, 2004) revealed that at least one item was problematic. Although specific details were not provided, on the basis of the output, the authors removed one question. The resultant nine-item version had an alpha coefficient of .80.

8. These authors used a modified version of the ATOP (i.e., the term *obese people* was replaced with either *moderately overweight people* or *extremely overweight people*).

9. A subsample of this data set ($n = 1,013$) was used in another study by Puhl, Moss-Racusin, and Schwartz (2007). The alpha coefficient for the ATOP was again .76.

10. Fiedler, Messner, and Bluemke (2006) contend that "no other recent innovation in testing has [achieved] a comparable degree of popularity in both basic and applied research" (p. 78). The authors' review of the literature identified "166 empirical articles comprising 331 studies that dealt with 495 separate IAT applications" (p. 90).

11. Some researchers have found that participants' weight status has a moderating influence on the efficacy of intervention strategies. For example, Teachman and colleagues (2003) observed that an empathy manipulation reduced implicit antifat attitudes among overweight participants (i.e., those with a BMI > 25) but not among those classified as normal or underweight.

12. Research examining the modifiability of antifat attitudes suggests that, though resistant to eradication, they may be intensified quite easily. Teachman and associates (2003) noted that the provision of information attributing obesity to overeating and lack of exercise increased implicit bias. However, contrary to what was expected, providing information about the genetic underpinnings of obesity did not lessen antifat attitudes either implicitly or explicitly.

13. For detailed conceptual and psychometric critiques of the IAT, the interested reader is

directed to Arkes and Tetlock (2004); Blanton and Jaccard (2006); Blanton, Jaccard, Gonzales, and Christie (2006); and Fiedler et al. (2006).

14. This issue has been addressed explicitly outside the domain of antifat attitudes. For example, in a study conducted by Cunningham and colleagues (2001), 93 American university students completed four IATs designed to assess racial prejudice (i.e., Black and White faces were used in conjunction with "good" and "bad" words such as *love* and *poison*, respectively). The authors reported alpha coefficients ranging from .68 to .88 and test-retest coefficients between .16 and .50. As the latter values were poor, the researchers then computed stability estimates, which reflect the "the proportion of consistent, substantively meaningful variance that [remains] stable over time" (p. 167). For the IAT, this value was .46.

15. Studies that use two attribute categories (e.g., *good/bad* and *lazy/motivated*) and calculate the correlation between them provide an estimate of internal reliability. However, these values tend not to be very high (e.g., for *good/bad* and *lazy/motivated*, $rs = .52$ [Chambliss et al., 2004], .47 [Teachman & Brownell, 2001], and .33 [Teachman et al., 2003—Study 1]).

16. Teachman and associates (2003) calculated split-half reliability across IAT tasks that assessed feelings and beliefs about fat people and used words and pictures as stimuli. The average r was .67.

References

Adams, G. R., Hicken, M., & Salehi, M. (1988). Socialization of the physical attractiveness stereotype: Parental expectations and verbal behaviors. *International Journal of Psychology, 23*, 137–149.

Ahern, A. L., & Hetherington, M. M. (2006). The thin ideal and body image: An experimental study of implicit attitudes. *Psychology of Addictive Behaviors, 20*, 338–342.

Allison, D. B., Basile, V. C., & Yuker, H. E. (1991). The measurement of attitudes toward and beliefs about obese persons. *International Journal of Eating Disorders, 10*, 599–607.

Anesbury, T., & Tiggemann, M. (2000). An attempt to reduce negative stereotyping of obesity in children by changing controllability beliefs. *Health Education Research, 15,* 145–152.

Arkes, H. R., & Tetlock, P. E. (2004). Attributions of implicit prejudice, or "would Jesse Jackson 'fail' the Implicit Association Test?" *Psychological Inquiry, 15,* 257–278.

Aruguete, M. S., Yates, A., & Edman, J. (2006). Gender differences in attitudes about fat. *North American Journal of Psychology, 8,* 183–192.

Bacon, J. G., Scheltema, K. E., & Robinson, B. E. (2001). Fat Phobia Scale revisited: The short form. *International Journal of Obesity, 25,* 252–257.

Barnette, J. J. (2000). Effects of stem and Likert response option reversals on survey internal consistency: If you feel the need, there is a better alternative to using those negatively worded items. *Educational & Psychological Measurement, 60,* 361–370.

Bell, S. K., & Morgan, S. B. (2000). Children's attitudes and behavioral intentions towards a peer presented as obese: Does a medical explanation for the obesity make a difference? *Journal of Pediatric Psychology, 25,* 137–145.

Berryman, D. E., Dubale, G. M., Manchester, D. S., & Mittelstaedt, R. (2006). Dietetics students possess negative attitudes toward obesity similar to non-dietetics students. *Journal of the American Dietetics Association, 106,* 1678–1682.

Bessenoff, G. R., & Sherman, J. W. (2000). Automatic and controlled components of prejudice toward fat people: Evaluation versus stereotype activation. *Social Cognition, 18,* 329–353.

Blanton, H., & Jaccard, J. (2006). Arbitrary metrics in psychology. *American Psychologist, 61,* 27–41.

Blanton, H., Jaccard, J., Gonzales, P. M., & Christie, C. (2006). Decoding the Implicit Association Test: Implications for criterion prediction. *Journal of Experimental Social Psychology, 42,* 192–212.

Brochu, P. M., & Morrison, M. A. (2007). Implicit and explicit prejudice toward overweight and average-weight men and women: Testing their correspondence to behavioral intentions. *Journal of Social Psychology, 147,* 681–706.

Brown, I. (2006). Nurses' attitudes towards adult patients who are obese: Literature review. *Journal of Advanced Nursing, 53,* 221–232.

Brylinsky, J. A., & Moore, J. C. (1994). The identification of body build stereotypes in young children. *Journal of Research in Personality, 28,* 170–181.

Butler, J. C. (2000). Personality and emotional correlates of right-wing authoritarianism. *Social Behavior and Personality, 28,* 1–14.

Byrne, B. M., & Watkins, D. (2003). The issue of measurement invariance revisited. *Journal of Cross-Cultural Psychology, 34,* 155–175.

Caterson, I. D., & Gill, T. P. (2002). Obesity: Epidemiology and possible prevention. *Best Practice & Research Clinical Endocrinology and Metabolism, 16,* 595–610.

Chambliss, H. O., Finley, C. E., & Blair, S. N. (2004). Attitudes toward obese individuals among exercise science students. *Medicine and Science in Sports and Exercise, 36,* 468–474.

Chen, E. Y., & Brown, M. (2005). Obesity stigma in sexual relationships. *Obesity Research, 13,* 1393–1397.

Cramer, P., & Steinwert, T. (1998). Thin is good, fat is bad: How early does it begin? *Journal of Applied Developmental Psychology, 19,* 429–451.

Crandall, C. S. (1994). Prejudice against fat people: Ideology and self-interest. *Journal of Personality and Social Psychology, 66,* 882–894.

Crandall, C. S., D'Anello, S., Sakalli, N., Lazarus, E., Wieczorkowska Nejtardt, G., & Feather, N. T. (2001). An attribution-value model of prejudice: Anti-fat attitudes in six nations. *Personality and Social Psychology Bulletin, 27,* 30–37.

Crandall, C. S., & Martinez, R. (1996). Culture, ideology, and anti-fat attitudes. *Personality and Social Psychology Bulletin, 22,* 1165–1176.

Crerand, C. E., Wadden, T. A., Foster, G. D., Sarwer, D. B., Paster, L. M., & Berkowitz, R. I. (2007). Changes in weight-related attitudes in women seeking weight reduction. *Obesity, 15,* 740–747.

Cunningham, W. A., Preacher, K. J., & Banaji, M. R. (2001). Implicit attitude measures: Consistency, stability and convergent validity. *Psychological Science, 12,* 163–170.

Davis-Coelho, K., Waltz, J., & Davis-Coelho, B. (2000). Awareness and prevention of bias against fat clients in psychotherapy. *Professional Psychology: Research and Practice, 31,* 682–684.

Davison, K. K., & Birch, L. L. (2004). Predictors of fat stereotypes among 9-year-old girls and their parents. *Obesity Research, 12,* 86–94.

Eagly, A. H., & Chaiken, S. (1998). Attitude structure and function. In D. T. Gilbert, S. T. Fiske, & G. Lindzey (Eds.), *The handbook of social psychology* (pp. 269–322). New York: McGraw-Hill.

Fabrigar, L. R., Wegener, D. T., MacCallum, R. C., & Strahan, E. J. (1999). Evaluating the use of exploratory factor analysis in psychological research. *Psychological Methods, 4,* 272–299.

Fiedler, K., Messner, C., & Bluemke, M. (2006). Unresolved problems with the "I," the "A," and the "T": A logical and psychometric critique of the Implicit Association Test (IAT). *European Review of Social Psychology, 17,* 74–147.

Fikkan, J., & Rothblum, E. (2005). Weight bias in employment. In K. D. Brownell, R. M. Puhl, M. B. Schwartz, & L. Rudd (Eds.), *Weight bias: Nature, consequences, and remedies* (pp. 15–28). New York: Guilford.

Finch, J. F., & West, S. G. (1997). The investigation of personality structure: Statistical models. *Journal of Research in Personality, 31,* 439–483.

Foster, G. D., Wadden, T. A., Makris, A. P., Davidson, D., Sanderson, R. S., Allison, D. B., et al. (2003). Primary care physicians' attitudes about obesity and its treatment. *Obesity Research, 11,* 1168–1177.

Friedman, K. E., Reichmann, S. K., Costanzo, P. R., Zelli, A., Ashmore, J. A., & Mustante, G. J. (2005). Weight stigmatization and ideological beliefs: Relation to psychological functioning in obese adults. *Obesity Research, 13,* 907–916.

Gaertner, S. L., & McLaughlin, J. P. (1983). Racial stereotypes: Associations and ascriptions of positive and negative characteristics. *Social Psychology Quarterly, 46,* 23–30.

Gapinski, K. D., Schwartz, M. B., & Brownell, K. D. (2006). Can television change anti-fat attitudes and behaviour? *Journal of Applied Biobehavioral Research, 11,* 1–28.

Gawronski, B., & Bodenhausen, G. V. (2006). Associative and propositional processes in evaluation: An integrative review of implicit and explicit attitude change. *Psychological Bulletin, 132,* 692–731.

Geier, A. B., Schwartz, M. B., & Brownell, K. D. (2003). "Before and after" diet advertisements escalate weight stigma. *Eating and Weight Disorders, 8,* 282–288.

Ginis, K. A. M., & Leary, M. R. (2006). Single, physically active, female: The effects of information about exercise participation and body weight on perceptions of young women. *Social Behavior and Personality, 34,* 979–990.

Glenn, C. V., & Chow, P. (2002). Measurement of attitudes toward obese people among a Canadian sample of men and women. *Psychological Reports, 91,* 627–640.

Goodman, N., Dornbusch, S. M., Richardson, S. A., & Hastorf, A. H. (1963). Variant reactions to physical disabilities. *American Sociological Review, 28,* 429–435.

Government Office for Science. (2007, October). *Tackling obesities: Future choices—Summary of key messages.* Retrieved November 10, 2007, from http://www.foresight.gov.uk/Obesity/obesity_final/20.pdf

Greenleaf, C., Chambliss, H., Rhea, D. J., Martin, S. B., & Morrow, J. R. (2006). Weight stereotypes and behavioral intentions toward fat and thin peers among White and Hispanic adolescents. *Journal of Adolescent Health, 39,* 546–552.

Greenleaf, C., & Weiller, K. (2005). Perceptions of youth obesity among physical educators. *Social Psychology of Education, 8,* 407–423.

Greenwald, A. G., & Banaji, M. R. (1995). Implicit social cognition: Attitudes, self-esteem and stereotypes. *Psychological Review, 102,* 4–27.

Greenwald, A. G., Banaji, M. R., Rudman, L. A., Farnham, S. D., Nosek, B. A., & Mellott, D. S. (2002). A unified theory of implicit attitudes, stereotypes, self-esteem, and self-concept. *Psychological Review, 109,* 3–25.

Greenwald, A. G., McGhee, D. E., & Schwartz, J. L. K. (1998). Measuring individual differences in implicit cognition: The Implicit Association Test. *Journal of Personality and Social Psychology, 74,* 1464–1480.

Grover, V. P., Keel, P., & Mitchell, J. P. (2003). Gender differences in implicit weight identity. *International Journal of Eating Disorders, 34,* 125–135.

Hague, A. L., & White, A. A. (2005). Web-based intervention for changing attitudes of obesity among current and future teachers. *Journal of Nutrition Education and Behavior, 37,* 58–66.

Harris, R., Tobias, M., Jeffreys, M., Waldegrave, K., Karlsen, S., & Nazroo, J. (2006). Racism and health: The relationship between experience of racial discrimination and health in New Zealand. *Social Science and Medicine, 63,* 1428–1441.

Harvey, E. L., & Hill, A. J. (2001). Health professionals' views of overweight people and smokers. *International Journal of Obesity, 25,* 1253–1261.

Harvey, E. L., Summerbell, C. D., Kirk, S. F. L., & Hill, A. J. (2002). Dietitians' views of overweight and obese people and reported management practices. *Journal of Human Nutrition and Dietetics, 15,* 331–347.

Hayton, J. C., Allen, D. G., & Scarpello, V. (2004). Factor retention decisions in exploratory factor analysis:

A tutorial on parallel analysis. *Organizational Research Methods, 7,* 191–205.

Hebl, M. R., & Xu, J. (2001). Weighing the care: Physicians' reactions to the size of a patient. *International Journal of Obesity, 25,* 1253–1261.

Hofmann, W., Gawronski, B., Gschwender, T., Le, H., & Schmitt, M. (2005). A meta-analysis on the correlation between the Implicit Association Test and explicit self-report measures. *Personality & Social Psychology Bulletin, 31,* 1369–1385.

Hoyt, W. I., Warbasse, R. E., & Chu, E. Y. (2006). Construct validation in counseling psychology research. *The Counseling Psychologist, 34,* 769–805.

Hubley, A. M., & Zumbo, B. D. (1996). A dialectic on validity: Where we have been and where we are going. *Journal of General Psychology, 123,* 207–215.

Irving, L. M. (2000). Promoting size acceptance in elementary school children: The EDAP puppet program. *Eating Disorders, 8,* 221–232.

Jaffe, K., & Worobey, J. (2006). Mothers' attitudes toward fat, weight, and dieting in themselves and their children. *Body Image, 3,* 113–120.

James, P. T. (2004). Obesity: The worldwide epidemic. *Clinics in Dermatology, 22,* 276–280.

Jolliffe, D. (2004). Extent of overweight among US children and adolescents from 1971 to 2000. *International Journal of Obesity and Related Metabolic Disorders, 28,* 4–9.

Kirkpatrick, S. W., & Sanders, D. M. (1978). Body image stereotypes: A developmental comparison. *Journal of Genetic Psychology, 132,* 87–95.

Klaczynski, P. A., Goold, K. W., & Mudry, J. J. (2004). Culture, obesity stereotypes, self-esteem, and the "thin ideal": A social identity perspective. *Journal of Youth and Adolescence, 33,* 307–317.

Kraig, K. A., & Keel, P. K. (2001). Weight-based stigmatization in children. *International Journal of Obesity, 25,* 1661–1666.

Kumanyika, S., Jeffrey, R. W., Morabia, A., Ritenbaugh, C., & Antipatis, V. J. (2002). Obesity prevention: The case for action. *International Journal of Obesity, 26,* 425–436.

Latner, J. D., Rosewall, J. K., & Simmonds, M. B. (2007). Childhood obesity stigma: Association with television, videogame, and magazine exposure. *Body Image, 4,* 147–155.

Latner, J. D., Simmonds, M., Rosewall, J. K., & Stunkard, A. J. (2007). Assessment of obesity stigmatization in children and adolescents: Modernizing a standard measure. *Obesity Research, 15,* 3078–3085.

Latner, J. D., & Stunkard., A. J. (2003). Getting worse: The stigmatization of obese children. *Obesity Research, 11,* 452–456.

Latner, J. D., Stunkard, A. J., & Wilson, G. T. (2005). Stigmatized students: Age, sex, and ethnicity effects in the stigmatization of obesity. *Obesity Research, 13,* 1226–1231.

Lemm, K. M. (2006). Positive associations among interpersonal contact, motivation, and implicit and explicit attitudes towards gay men. *Journal of Homosexuality, 51,* 79–99.

Lemm, K. M., Lane, K. A., Sattler, D. N., Khan, S. R., & Nosek, B. A. (2008). Assessing implicit cognitions with a paper-format Implicit Association Test. In M. A. Morrison & T. G. Morrison (Eds.), *Psychology of modern prejudice* (pp. 123–146). Hauppauge, NY: Nova Science Publishers.

Lerner, R. M., & Korn, S. J. (1972). The development of body build stereotypes in males. *Child Development, 43,* 908–920.

Lewis, R. J., Cash, T. F., Jacobi, L., & Bubb-Lewis, C. (1997). Prejudice toward fat people: The development and validation of the Anti-fat Attitudes Test. *Obesity Research, 5,* 297–307.

Lobstein, T., & Frelut, M. L. (2003). Prevalence of overweight among children in Europe. *Obesity Reviews, 4,* 195–200.

McArthur, L. H. (1995). Nutrition and non-nutrition majors have more favorable attitudes toward overweight people than personal overweight. *Journal of the American Dietetic Association, 95,* 593–596.

McArthur, L. H., & Ross, J. K. (1997). Attitudes of registered dietitians toward personal overweight and overweight clients. *Journal of the American Dietetic Association, 97,* 63–66.

Meyer, D. E., & Schvaneveldt, R. W. (1971). Facilitation in recognizing pairs of words: Evidence of a dependence between retrieval operations. *Journal of Experimental Psychology, 90,* 227–234.

Meyer, I. H. (2003). Prejudice as stress: Conceptual and measurement problems. *American Journal of Public Health, 93,* 262–265.

Morgan, S. B., Bieberich, A., Walker, M., & Schwerdtfeger, H. (1998). Children's willingness to participate in activities with a handicapped peer: Am I more willing than my classmates? *Journal of Pediatric Psychology, 22,* 367–375.

Morrison, T. G., Morrison, M. A., Hopkins, C., & Rowan, E. T. (2004). Muscle mania: Development of a new scale examining the drive for muscularity in Canadian males. *Psychology of Men and Masculinity, 5,* 30–39.

Morrison, T. G., & O'Connor, W. E. (1999). Psychometric properties of a scale measuring negative attitudes toward overweight individuals. *Journal of Social Psychology, 139,* 436–445.

Musher-Eizenman, D. R., Holub, S. C., Barnhart Miller, A., Goldstein, S. E., & Edwards-Leeper, L. (2004). Body size stigmatization in preschool children: The role of control attributions. *Journal of Pediatric Psychology, 29,* 613–620.

Myers, A., & Rosen, J. C. (1999). Obesity stigmatization and coping: Relation to mental health symptoms, body image, and self-esteem. *International Journal of Obesity, 23,* 221–230.

Nosek, B. A., Greenwald, A. G., & Banaji, J. R. (2007). The Implicit Association Test at age 7: A methodological and conceptual review. In J. A. Bargh (Ed.), *Automatic processes in social thinking and behaviour* (pp. 265–292). Hove, UK: Psychology Press.

Oberrieder, H., Walker, R., Monroe, D., & Adeyanju, M. (1995). Attitude of dietetics students and registered dietitians toward obesity. *Journal of the American Dietetic Association, 95,* 914–916.

O'Brien, K. S., Hunter, J. A., & Banks, M. (2007). Implicit anti-fat bias in physical educators: Physical attributes, ideology and socialization. *International Journal of Obesity, 31,* 308–314.

O'Bryan, M., Fishbein, H. D, & Ritchey, P. N. (2004). Intergenerational transmission of prejudice, sex role stereotyping and intolerance. *Adolescence, 39,* 407–426.

Ogden, J., & Sidhu, S. (2006). Adherence, behavior change, and visualization: A qualitative study of the experiences of taking an obesity medication. *Journal of Psychosomatic Research, 61,* 545–552.

Ojerholm, A. J., & Rothblum, E. D. (1999). The relationships of body image, feminism, and sexual orientation in college women. *Feminism & Psychology, 9,* 431–448.

Penny, H., & Haddock, G. (2007). Anti-fat prejudice among children: The 'mere proximity effect' in 5–10 year olds. *Journal of Experimental Social Psychology, 43,* 678–683.

Perez-Lopez, M. S., Lewis, R. J., & Cash, T. F. (2001). The relationship of anti-fat attitudes to other prejudicial and gender-related attitudes. *Journal of Applied Social Psychology, 31,* 683–697.

Polinko, N. K., & Popovich, P. M. (2001). Evil thoughts but angelic actions: Responses to overweight job applicants. *Journal of Applied Social Psychology, 31,* 905–924.

Popkin, B. M., & Doak, C. M. (1998). The obesity epidemic is a worldwide phenomenon. *Nutrition Reviews, 56,* 106–114.

Puhl, R. M., & Brownell, K. D. (2001). Obesity, bias, and discrimination. *Obesity Research, 8,* 788–805.

Puhl, R. M., & Brownell, K. D. (2003). Psychosocial origins of obesity stigma: Toward changing a powerful and pervasive bias. *Obesity Review, 4,* 213–227.

Puhl, R. M., & Brownell, K. D. (2006). Confronting and coping with weight stigma: An investigation of overweight and obese adults. *Obesity, 14,* 1802–1815.

Puhl, R. M., Moss-Racusin, C. A., & Schwartz, M. B. (2007). Internalization of weight bias: Implications for binge eating and emotional well-being. *Obesity, 15,* 19–23.

Puhl, R. M., Schwartz, M. B., & Brownell, K. D. (2005). Impact of perceived consensus on stereotypes about obese people: A new approach for reducing bias. *Health Psychology, 24,* 517–525.

Quinn, D. M., & Crocker, J. (1999). When ideology hurts: Effects of belief in the Protestant ethic and feeling overweight on the psychological well-being of women. *Journal of Personality and Social Psychology, 77,* 402–414.

Regan, P. C. (1996). Sexual outcasts: The perceived impact of body weight and gender on sexuality. *Journal of Applied Social Psychology, 26,* 1803–1815.

Richardson, S. A., Goodman, N., Hastorf, A. H., & Dornbusch, S. M. (1961). Cultural uniformity in reaction to physical disabilities. *American Sociological Review, 26,* 241–247.

Richardson, S. A., & Royce, J. (1968). Race and physical handicap in children's preferences for other children. *Child Development, 39,* 467–480.

Robinson, B. E., Bacon, J. G., & O'Reilly, J. (1993). Fat phobia: Measuring, understanding and changing anti-fat attitudes. *International Journal of Eating Disorders, 14,* 467–480.

Rudman, L. A., Feinberg, J., & Fairchild, K. (2002). Minority members' implicit attitudes: Automatic ingroup bias as a function of group status. *Social Cognition, 20,* 294–320.

Schwartz, M. B, Chambliss, H. O., Brownell, K. D., Blair, S. N., & Billington, C. (2003). Weight bias among health professionals specializing in obesity. *Obesity Research, 11,* 1033–1039.

Schwartz, M. B., Vartanian, L. R., Nosek, B. A., & Brownell, K. D. (2006). The influence of one's own body weight on implicit and explicit anti-fat bias. *Obesity, 14,* 440–447.

Sigelman, C. K. (1991). The effect of causal information on peer perceptions of children with physical problems. *Journal of Applied Developmental Psychology, 12,* 237–253.

Siperstein, G. N. (1980). *Development of the Adjective Checklist: An instrument for measuring children's attitudes towards the handicapped.* Unpublished manuscript, University of Massachusetts, Boston.

Siperstein, G. N., & Bak, J. (1977). *Instruments to measure children's attitudes towards the handicapped: Adjective Checklist and Activity Preference List.* Unpublished manuscript, University of Massachusetts, Boston.

Smith, C. A., Schmoll, K., Konik, J., & Oberlander, S. (2007). Carrying weight for the world: Influence of weight descriptors on judgments of large-sized women. *Journal of Applied Social Psychology, 37,* 989–1006.

Springer, D. W., Abell, N., & Hudson, W. W. (2002). Creating and validating rapid assessment instruments for practice and research: Part 1. *Research on Social Work Practice, 12,* 408–439.

Staffieri, J. R. (1967). A study of social stereotype of body image in children. *Journal of Personality & Social Psychology, 7,* 101–104.

Staffieri, J. R. (1972). Body build and behavioral expectations in young females. *Developmental Psychology, 6,* 125–127.

Stager, S. F., & Burke, P. J. (1982). A re-examination of body build stereotypes. *Journal of Research in Personality, 16,* 435–446.

Streiner, D. L. (2003). Being inconsistent about consistency: When coefficient alpha does and doesn't matter. *Journal of Personality Assessment, 80,* 217–222.

Swami, V., & Tovée, M. J. (2005). Female physical attractiveness in Britain and Malaysia: A cross-cultural study. *Body Image, 2,* 115–128.

Teachman, B. A., & Brownell, K. D. (2001). Implicit anti-fat bias among health professionals: Is anyone immune? *International Journal of Obesity, 25,* 1525–1531.

Teachman, B. A., Gapinski, K. D., Brownell, K. D., Rawlins, M., & Jeyaram, S. (2003). Demonstrations of implicit anti-fat bias. *Health Psychology, 22,* 68–78.

Thompson, S. H., & Sargent, R. G. (2000). Black and White women's weight-related attitudes and parental criticism of their childhood appearance. *Women & Health, 30,* 77–92.

Tiggemann, M., & Anesbury, T. (2000). Negative stereotyping of obesity in children: The role of controllability beliefs. *Journal of Applied Social Psychology, 30,* 1977–1993.

Tiggemann, M., & Rothblum, E. D. (1988). Gender differences in social consequences of perceived overweight in the United States and Australia. *Sex Roles, 18,* 75–86.

Tiggemann, M., & Wilson-Barrett, E. (1998). Children's figure ratings: Relationship to self-esteem and negative stereotyping. *International Journal of Eating Disorders, 23,* 83–88.

Tovée, M. J., Reinhardt, S., Emery, J., & Cornelissen, P. (1998). Optimum body-mass index and maximum sexual attractiveness. *The Lancet, 352,* 548.

Trafimow, D., & Sheeran, P. (1998). Some tests of the distinction between cognitive and affective beliefs. *Journal of Experimental Social Psychology, 34,* 378–397.

Tropp, L. R., & Pettigrew, T. F. (2005). Differential relationships between intergroup contact and affective and cognitive dimensions of prejudice. *Personality and Social Psychology Bulletin, 31,* 1145–1158.

Turnbull, J. D., Heaslip, S., & McLeod, H. A. (2000). Pre-school children's attitudes to fat and normal male and female stimulus figures. *International Journal of Obesity, 24,* 1705–1706.

Vartanian, L. R., Herman, C. P., & Polivy, J. (2005). Implicit and explicit attitudes towards fatness and thinness: The role of the internalization of societal standards. *Body Image, 2,* 373–381.

Wade, T. J., Fuller, L., Bresnan, J., Schaefer, S., & Mlynarski, L. (2007). Weight halo effects: Individual differences in personality evaluations and perceived life success of men as a function of weight? *Personality and Individual Differences, 42,* 317–324.

Wade, T. J., Loyden, J., Renninger, L., & Tobey, L. (2003). Weight halo effects: Individual differences in personality evaluations as a function of weight? *Personality and Individual Differences, 34,* 263–268.

Wang, S. S., Brownell, K. D., & Wadden, T. A. (2004). The influence of the stigma of obesity on overweight individuals. *International Journal of Obesity, 28,* 1333–1337.

Weng, L.-J. (2004). Impact of the number of response categories and anchor labels on coefficient alpha and test re-test reliability. *Educational and Psychological Measurement, 64,* 956–972.

Wilson, T. D., Lindsey, S., & Schooler, T. Y. (2000). A model of dual attitudes. *Psychological Review, 107,* 101–126.

Wittenbrink, B., Judd, C. M., & Park, B. (1997). Evidence for racial prejudice at the implicit level and its relationship with questionnaire measures. *Journal of Personality & Social Psychology, 72,* 262–274.

World Health Organization (WHO). (1997). *Obesity: Preventing and managing the global epidemic* (Report of the WHO consultation of obesity). Geneva, Switzerland: Author.

World Health Organization (WHO). (2000). *Obesity: Preventing and managing the global epidemic* (WHO Obesity Technical Report Series No. 894). Geneva, Switzerland: Author.

Yuker, H. E., Allison, D. B., & Faith, M. S. (1995). Methods for measuring attitudes and beliefs about obese people. In D. B. Allison (Ed.), *Handbook of assessment methods for eating behaviors and weight-related problems* (pp. 81–118). Thousand Oaks, CA: Sage.

CHAPTER 4

Assessment of Body Image

Hemal P. Shroff, Rachel M. Calogero, and J. Kevin Thompson

T he field of body image has experienced a phenomenal growth in recent years. In 2004, a new journal, *Body Image: An International Journal of Research,* was launched by Elsevier to provide a forum for publishing papers in this area. The field of body image was once closely linked to that of eating disorders, but the construct is now often studied in a variety of fields, including, oncology, dentistry, surgery, sociology, nutrition, and obesity (Cash & Pruzinsky, 2002). In addition, measurement of body image in younger samples and men has received a great deal of attention in recent years (Cafri & Thompson, 2007; Yanover & Thompson, 2009). The expansion of the field in general has been paralleled by a dramatic increase in the number of measures developed to assess some dimension of "body image."

In this chapter, we aim to briefly cover the broad categories of measures, discuss recent innovations, and outline important methodological issues. It is not possible for us to discuss all the measures in detail; therefore, we will focus our discussion on those measures that have been widely used and received rather extensive psychometric evaluation. We provide information regarding many of the available measures in Table 4.1. Within the text and in the table, we categorize measures using standard

terminology into the following dimensions of body image: subjective and affective, cognitive, and behavioral. We also include a subsection on new and widely used measures that examine sociocultural and interpersonal influences on body image because of their relevance for assessing associated features of body image disturbance that may have treatment indications. It should be noted that we do not discuss perceptual measures in this chapter because they are seldom used in clinical practice, and there is an ongoing debate regarding whether these measures provide a distinct index of perceptual body image (J. K. Thompson & Gardner, 2002). Also, at the end of this chapter, we offer some detailed guidelines for choosing a measure based on gender, age, and ethnicity.

It is important to keep in mind that in selecting a measure, one should always give careful consideration to the psychometric qualities of the instrument and the validation sample for the specific scale. For instance, scales developed with an adult eating disordered clinical sample may not necessarily be appropriate for use with a community sample of adolescents. In Table 4.1, we provide reliability data for the measures that are reviewed. The standard requirement for a scale to have acceptable reliability is a reliability coefficient of

(Text continues on page 126)

Table 4.1 Categorical Listing of Body Image Measures With Psychometric and Descriptive Information

Subjective and Affective Measures

Measure	Author(s)	Reliability	Description
Body Dysmorphic Disorder Diagnostic Module	Phillips (1996)	Kappa: .96	Interview for BDD based on *DSM* criteria.
Body Dysmorphic Disorder Examination	Rosen and Reiter (1994)	IC: .81–.93; R: .87–.94 TR: .87–.94	Interview that assesses multiple components of BDD.
Body Esteem Scale-Children	Mendelson and White (1985); Cecil and Stanley (1997)	IC: (split half) = .85	Measures children's agreement with statements about one's body.
Body Esteem Scale–Adolescents and Adults	Mendelson, Mendelson, and White (2001)	IC: .81–.94	Twenty-three items assess three factors in adults and adolescents: appearance, attribution, and weight.
Body Image Assessment	Williamson, Gleaves, Watkins, and Schlundt (1993)	TR: current: .90, ideal: .71	Select current and ideal body shape from nine female figures that range from underweight to overweight.
Body Image Assessment–Children	Veron-Guidry and Williamson (1996)	TR (immediate): current = .94, ideal = .93; (1 week): current = .79, current/ideal = .67	Select current and ideal body shape from nine body figures that range from underweight to overweight.
Body Image Assessment–Revised	Beebe, Holmbeck, and Grzeskiewicz (1999)	TR: 2 weeks, cognitive = .74, affective = .79, desired = .70, cognitive-desired discrepancy = .67, affective-desired discrepancy = .79, affective-desired discrepancy = .63	Select cognitive and affective body estimates and desired body size from nine female figures that range from underweight to overweight. Normed with college females.

Measure	Author(s)	Reliability	Description
Body Image Coping Strategies Inventory	Cash, Santos, and Williams (2004); Cash and Grasso (2006)	Multiple studies: IC > .70	Twenty-nine items assess how individuals cope with various situations that threaten their body image on a 3-point Likert-type scale; three subscales (Avoidance, Appearance Fixing, Positive-Rational Acceptance).
Body Image Disturbance Questionnaire	Cash, Phillips, Santos, and Hrabosky (2004)	IC: .89	Items assess broad array of aspects of body image disturbance.
Body Image and Eating Questionnaire	Thelen, Powell, Lawrence, and Kuhnert (1992)	IC: all values ≥ .68	Fourteen items focus on overweight concerns, dieting, and restraint; for use with younger children.
Body Image Quality of Life Inventory	Cash and Fleming (2002)	IC = .95 TR: 2–3 weeks = .79	Assesses the impact of one's body image on 19 life domains using a 7-point Likert-type scale ranging from *very negatively* (−3) to *very positively* (+3).
Body Image Questionnaire	Huddy, Nieman, and Johnson (1993)	TR: 6 weeks: .97	Twenty items on a 3-point Likert scale from *agree* (1) to *disagree* (3).
Body Image States Scale	Cash, Fleming, and Alindogan (2002)	IC: females = .77 (neutral), .90 (negative), .88 (negative), .81 (positive), .80 (positive) IC: males = .62 (neutral), .66 (negative), .78 (negative), .83 (positive), .84 (positive) TR: females = .77, males = .72	Measures body image across five different contexts: neutral, negative (day at the beach and magazine models), and positive (party compliments and ideal weight).

(Continued)

Table 4.1 (Continued)

Measure	Author(s)	Reliability	Description
Body Mass Index Silhouette Matching Test	Peterson, Ellenberg, and Crossan (2003)	TR: males' current = .79, females' current = .85; males' ideal = .83, females' ideal = .82	Interval scale of 27 items along with four gender-specific figures to anchor for older children.
Body Parts Satisfaction Scale–Revised	Petrie, Tripp, and Harvey (2002)	IC: Study 1, body = .89, face = .76 IC: Study 2, body = .89, face = .74	Fourteen items assess satisfaction with various body sites on a 6-point Likert-type scale in adult women and men; two factors—body and face.
Body Satisfaction Scale	Siegel, Yancey, Aneshensel, and Schuler (1999)	IC: .73–.80	Rate satisfaction with four aspects of pubertal development; for males and females.
Body Shape Questionnaire	Cooper, Taylor, Cooper, and Fairburn (1987); Rosen, Jones, Ramirez, and Waxman (1996)	TR: .88	Thirty-four items assess adult men and women's concern with body shape and size.
Body Uneasiness Test (BUT)	Cuzzolaro, Vetrone, Marano, and Garfinkel (2006)	IC: BUT-A = .79–.90; BUT-B = .69–.90 TR: 1 week = BUT-A = .71–.91 (nonclinical); .80–.94 (clinical): BUT-B = .78–.94 (nonclinical); .68–.92 (clinical)	Thirty-four items assess body shape and/or weight dissatisfaction, behaviors, and feelings, and 37 items assess concern about specific body parts or functions; for males and females.
Breast/Chest Rating Scale	J. K. Thompson and Tantleff (1992)	TR: current = .85; ideal breast = .81, ideal chest = .69	Select current and ideal breast/chest ratings from five male and five female schematic figures, ranging from small to large upper torso.

Measure	Author(s)	Reliability	Description
Color-A-Person Dissatisfaction Test	Wooley and Roll (1991)	IC: .74–.85 TR: 2 weeks = .72–.84, 4 weeks = .75–.89	Uses five colors to indicate level of satisfaction with body sites by masking on a schematic figure for both men and women.
Contour Drawing Rating Scale	M. A. Thompson and Gray (1995); Wertheim, Paxton, and Tilgner (2004)	TR: 1 week, self = .79 TR: .65–.87	Select ideal and current self from nine male and nine female schematic figures, ranging from underweight to overweight. (Wertheim sample: adolescents).
Drive for Bulk	Furnham and Calnan (1998)	IC: .70	Rate desire to be bigger and to gain weight; for males between ages 16 and 18 years.
Drive for Muscularity Scale (DMS)	McCreary and Sasse (2000); McCreary, Sasse, Saucier, and Dorsch (2004)	IC: Full DMS-Males = .85, MBI-Males = .88; MB-Men = .81; Full DMS-Females = .82	Fourteen items assess drive for muscularity: Muscle-Oriented Body Image (MBI; seven items), Muscle-Oriented Behavior (MB; seven items).
Drive for Muscularity–Body Image subscale	(1) McCreary and Sasse (2000) (2) Cafri, van den Berg, and Thompson (2006)	(1) IC = .84 (whole scale) (2) IC = .90 (subscale)	Seven items assess satisfaction with appearance (specifically muscular physique); adolescents and young adults.
Eating Disorder Inventory-2 Body Dissatisfaction subscale	Garner (1991)	IC >.70 for multiple samples, including individuals with eating disorders and non-eating-disordered controls	Nine items assess dissatisfaction with specific body parts.

(Continued)

Table 4.1 (Continued)

Measure	Author(s)	Reliability	Description
Feelings of Fatness Questionnaire	Roth and Armstrong (1993)	IC: Troubles = .96, Satisfaction = .98	Measures the extent to which females feel thin or fat across 61 situations; two subscales: Troubles (38 items) and Satisfaction (23 items).
Figure Rating Scale	Stunkard, Sorenson, and Schulsinger (1983); J. K. Thompson and Altabe (1991)	TR: 2 weeks: ideal; males = .82, females = .71, Self-think: males = .89, females = .92, females = .81; Self-feel; males = .81; females = .83	Select ideal and current self from nine male and female figures that vary from underweight to overweight. Normed with college males and females.
Goldfarb Fear of Fat Scale	Goldfarb, Dykens, and Gerrard (1985)	IC: .70; TR = .88	Ten items assess overconcern with fatness and body size.
Kid's Eating Disorder Survey	Childress, Brewerton, Hodges, and Jarrell (1993)	TR (4 months): .83 for entire survey; not given for figures only	Choose ideal and current self from eight male and eight female figure drawings: for preadolescent childres, Grades 5 to 8. Items relate to weight control behaviors.
Male Body Attitudes Test	Tylka, Bergeron, and Schwartz (2005)	IC: .80–.94; TR: .81–.94	Twenty-four items assess body image related to muscularity, body fat, body shape, and height.

Measure	Author(s)	Reliability	Description
McKnight Risk Factor Survey (MFRS-III)	Shisslak et al. (1999)	IC: elementary = .82; middle school = .86; high school = .87 TR: elementary = .79; middle school = .84; high school = .90	Five items assess concern with weight and shape; elementary, middle and high school children.
Multidimensional Body-Self Relations Questionnaire–Appearance Evaluation subscale	Cash (body-images.com); Brown, Cash, and Mikulka (1990)	IC > .70 for multiple samples, including men and women	Seven items assess overall appearance satisfaction.
Muscle Appearance Satisfaction Scale	Mayville, Williamson, White, Netemeyer, and Drab (2002)	IC: .74–.79 (subscales); TR: .76–.89 (subscales)	Nineteen items assess excessive concern with muscularity in males; five subscales (bodybuilding dependence, muscle checking, substance use, injury, and muscle satisfaction).
Muscle Dysmorphic Disorder Inventory	Hildebrandt, Langenbucher, and Schlundt (2004)	IC: .77–.85; TR: .81–.87	Thirteen items; three subscales (Desire for Size, Appearance Intolerance, Functional Impairment) in males using a 5-point Likert-type scale.
Physical Appearance State and Trait Anxiety Scale (PASTAS)	Reed, Thompson, Brannick, and Sacco (1991)	IC: trait = .82–88, state = .82–92 TR: 2 weeks = .87	Assesses trait or state anxiety associated with 16 body sites (8 weight related, 8 non-weight related).
Self-Image Questionnaire for Young Adolescents–Body Image subscale	Petersen, Schulenberg, Abramowitz, Offer, and Jarcho (1984)	IC: boys = .81, girls =.77 TR: 1 year = .60; 2 years = .44	Eleven items assess positive feelings toward the body in 10- to 15-year-old boys and girls.

(Continued)

Table 4.1 (Continued)

Measure	Author(s)	Reliability	Description
Situational Inventory of Body Image Dysphoria (SIBID)–Short Form	Cash (2002)	IC: females = .94–.96; males = .93–.94 TR: 1 month, females = .87; males = .81	Twenty items; short form of SIBID. Men and women rate how often they experience negative body image emotions in various situations.
Somatomorphic Matrix	(1) Gruber, Pope, Borowiecki, and Cohane (1999) (2) Cafri, Roehrig, and Thompson (2004)	(1) Not available (2) TR: females = .35–.75; males = .45–.80	Assesses current and ideal muscularity and body fat dimensions in men and women; available in (1) computer and (2) paper-and-pencil forms.

Cognitive Measures

Measure	Author(s)	Reliability	Description
Appearance Schemas Inventory–Revised	Cash, Melnyk, and Hrabosky (2004)	IC = total-women = .88; total-men = .90; self-eval-women = .82; self-eval-men = .84; motivational-women = .90, motivational-men = .91	Twenty items assess beliefs and assumptions about the importance and influence of appearance in one's life on a 5-point Likert-type scale; two subscales (Self-Evaluative Saliance [12 items], Motivational Saliance [8 items]); for males and females.
Assessment of Body Image Cognitions	Jakatdar, Cash, and Engle (2006)	IC > .70	Thirty-seven items assess eight types of distorted thinking about own physical appearance.
Beliefs About Appearance Scale	Spangler and Stice (2001)	IC: .94, .95, .96 (three samples, respectively) TR: 3 weeks = .83 (Sample 3); 10 months = .73 (Sample 2)	Twenty items assess one's beliefs about consequences of appearance for relationships, achievement, self-view, and feelings on a 5-point Likert-type scale.

Measure	Author(s)	Reliability	Description
Body Attitude Test (BAT)–Japanese version	Kashima, Yamashita, and Okamoto (2003)	IC: .90	Twenty items measure body dissatisfaction.
Body Image Automatic Thoughts Questionnaire	Cash, Lewis, and Keeton (1987)	IC: .90	Measures frequency of 37 negative and 15 positive body image cognitions in women.
Body Image Ideals Questionnaire	Cash and Szymanski (1995)	IC: discrepancy = .75; importance = .82	Ratings of ideal and actual self on 10 attributes related to weight/appearance and strength/importance of attribute.
Body Image Ideals Questionnaire–Expanded	Szymanski and Cash (1995)	IC: .81–.95	Ratings of one's specific attributes from own viewpoint and that of romantic partner based on "ideal" and "actual."
Bulimia Cognitive Distortions Scale–Physical Appearance subscale	Schulman, Kinder, Powers, Prange, and Gleghorn (1986)	IC: .97 (entire scale)	Measures agreement with 25 statements related to physical appearance–related cognitions.
Drive for Muscularity Attitudes Questionnaire	Morrison, Morrison, Hopkins, and Rowan (2004)	IC: .84 (Study 1), .82 (Study 2); .79 (protein supplement), .72 (weight training), .45 (cardio exercise)	Eight items assess attitudes toward muscularity in males.
Eating Disorder Belief Questionnaire–Self Acceptance & Acceptance by Others subscales	Rose, Cooper, and Turner (2006)	IC: .85 (self-acceptance), .94 (acceptance by others)	Six items assess how attractive one will feel if one is slim (self-acceptance); nine items assess how others will feel if body is slim/toned (acceptance by others).
Swansea Muscularity Attitudes Questionnaire	Edwards and Launder (2000);	IC: .86–.92; .58–.70 (for 2-item subscale)	Nineteen items assess intention to become more muscular (eight items), positive attributes of muscularity (nine items), and muscle-building activities (two items).

(Continued)

Table 4.1 (Continued)

Behavioral Measures

Measure	Author(s)	Reliability	Description
Body Checking Questionnaire	Reas, Whisenhunt, and Netemetyer (2002)	IC: .88 (overall appearance), .92 (specific body parts), .83 (idiosyncratic checking) TR: 2 weeks = .94	Twenty-three items assess body-checking behaviors related to overall appearance, specific body parts, and idiosyncratic checking behaviors in adult females.
Body Image Avoidance Questionnaire	Rosen, Srebnik, Saltzberg, and Wendt (1991)	IC: .89; TR: 2 weeks = .87	Frequency of body image avoidance behaviors.

Sociocultural and Interpersonal Influences

Measure	Author(s)	Reliability	Description
Body Comparison Scale	Fisher and Thompson (1998)	IC: .95	Assesses tendency to compare specific body sites with others.
Fear of Negative Appearance Evaluation Scale	Lundgren, Anderson, and Thompson (2004)	IC = .94	Measures affective reaction to perceived negative evaluation by others. The original measure consisted of eight items. In the second study, it was reduced it to 6 items.
Feedback on Physical Appearance Scale	Tantleff-Dunn, Thompson, and Dunn (1995)	IC: .84 TR: 2 weeks = .82	Twenty-six items assess verbal and nonverbal appearance-related commentary on a 5-point Likert-type scale; adults.
Ideal Body Internalization Scale– Revised	Stice, Shaw, and Nemeroff (1998)	IC: .88 TR: 1 year = .59	Ten items assess agreement with cultural ideal for female body.

Measure	Author(s)	Reliability	Description
Objectified Body Consciousness Scale	McKinley and Hyde (1996); Lindberg, Hyde and McKinley (2006)	IC: body surveillance: .79–.89; body shame = .75	Sixteen items assess body surveillance (eight items) and body shame (eight items); modified version used with preadolescents and adolescents.
Perception of Teasing Scale	J. K. Thompson, Cattarin, Fowler, and Fisher (1995)	IC: general weight = .94, competency = .78	Twelve items assess frequency and emotional response to general weight teasing and competency teasing.
Physical Appearance Comparison Scale	J. K. Thompson, Heinberg, and Tantleff (1991)	IC = .78; TR = .72	Assesses tendency to compare own appearance with others.
Self-Objectification Questionnaire	Noll and Fredrickson (1998)	NA	Rank order of 10 attributes (5 appearance-based, 5 non–appearance based) based on how important the attribute is to the physical self-concept.
Sociocultural Attitudes Towards Appearance Scale–3	J. K. Thompson, van den Berg, Roehrig, Guarda, and Heinberg, (2004)	IC: .93	Thirty items measure multiple aspects of societal influence on appearance and consists of four distinct subscales: Pressures, Information, Internalization-General, Internalization-Athlete.
Sociocultural Internalization of Appearance Questionnaire–Adolescents	Keery, Shroff, Thompson, Wertheim, and Smolak (2004)	IC: .83–.92 (U.S. and international samples)	Five items measure thin-ideal internalization in adolescent girls.

NOTE: BDD = body dysmorphic disorder; IC = internal consistency; TR = test-retest reliability; NA = not available.

around .70 (J. K. Thompson, 2004). When a measure is considered for clinical or research purposes, it is important to select a measure that has acceptable reliability and validity and has been evaluated on a sample that is similar to the one under consideration. Some measures have received limited validity work, but others have received extensive validation (such as the Eating Disorders Inventory–Body Dissatisfaction scale and the Multidimensional Body Self-Relations Questionnaire; see Cash, 2000; Garner, 2004). In the sections that follow, we discuss measures that fit into widely accepted categorical dimensions of body image, with an intent of providing a broad overview of the possible measures that might be included in an assessment battery. Again, this is a highly selective review, and the reader is also encouraged to examine the broader range of potential measures that are available in Table 4.1.

Measurement Categories

Subjective and Affective Measures

Subjective and affective measures tap into a dimension of body image that is usually labeled *satisfaction* (J. K. Thompson, Heinberg, Altabe, & Tantleff-Dunn, 1999). The satisfaction may be site specific (e.g., waist, hips) or may involve a more global self-evaluation of overall appearance. There are two primary methods for assessing the subjective and affective component. One method consists of using figural stimuli consisting of a range of images (usually schematic line drawings or silhouettes) that differ in body size and/or shape. The stimuli are presented to the participants, who are asked to select the image that represents their ideal self and their real (current) self. The discrepancy between their current and ideal selves is used as the index of dissatisfaction. The second category consists of questionnaire measures that typically ask respondents to complete a variety of items designed to assess body satisfaction or an affective dimension of body image. Examples of these two types of measurement strategies (figural

rating scales, questionnaire measures) are provided below.

A variety of figural stimuli measures have been created in the past two decades (Table 4.1). A measure that has been developed specifically for children is the Body Image Assessment–Children (Veron-Guidry & Williamson, 1996). This scale is particularly useful as it has separate figures for children and for adolescents, so that the participants make their ratings using figures similar to themselves in body composition and pubertal status. A figural scale that has been used with adult women is the Contour Drawing Rating Scale (J. K. Thompson et al., 1999; M. A. Thompson & Gray, 1995). Two widely used figural scales allow for the assessment of dissatisfaction related to overall weight and muscularity. The Somatomorphic Matrix is a two-dimensional computerized body image test that can be used to assess self and ideal body image in relation to muscularity and body fat (Gruber, Pope, Borowiecki, & Cohane, 1999). The test is available for both genders and consists of 100 images arranged in a 10×10 matrix, representing 10 degrees of adiposity and 10 degrees of muscularity. The Somatomorphic Matrix Modification is a paper-and-pencil modification of the original somatomorphic matrix (Cafri & Thompson, 2004c). The Bodybuilder Image Grid (Hildebrandt, Langenbucher, & Schlundt, 2004) is a paper-and-pencil measure that has figures arranged in a 6×5 matrix with body fat and muscularity varying on two separate dimensions (i.e., six degrees of body fat and five degrees of muscularity).

With regard to questionnaire measures, there is also a wide variety available to assess the subjective and/or affective component of body image. Some of these measures are global or generic in nature and provide an overall estimate of body dissatisfaction or focus on specific sites. The Self Image Questionnaire for Young Adults (Petersen, Schulenberg, Abramowitz, Offer, & Jarcho, 1984) includes a subscale that provides a global measure of body satisfaction for adolescents. The Appearance Evaluation subscale of the Multidimensional Body Self-Relations Questionnaire (Cash, 2000) is a measure that has been used in numerous studies, with adult men and women of different ethnicities (see www.body-images.com). A sample item from this scale is "I like my looks just the way they are." The Body Shape Questionnaire (Cooper, Taylor, Cooper, & Fairburn, 1987) assesses the experience of "feeling fat" with items such as, "Have you worried about your flesh not being firm enough?"

Other measures offer site-specific information regarding satisfaction or body image affect, such as the Body Uneasiness Test (Cuzzolaro, Vetrone, Marano, & Garfinkel, 2006), created for adolescents and adults, which has items that assess concern about specific body parts. Likewise, the Body Dissatisfaction subscale of the Eating Disorder Inventory–3 (Garner, 2004) asks participants to rate satisfaction with nine weight-relevant body sites, including the stomach, hips, thighs, and so forth. This scale has also been widely used with adults and adolescents and has a wealth of normative information for use with individuals with eating disorders. The Body Parts Satisfaction Scale (Petrie, Tripp, & Harvey, 2002) also assesses satisfaction with various body sites in adult men and women.

Some scales assess a more specific affective component of body image. For instance, the Physical Appearance State and Trait Anxiety Scale (Reed, Thompson, Brannick, & Sacco, 1991) provides for an assessment of anxiety regarding weight and non-weight-related (hair, eyes, face) body aspects. Cash's (1994, 2002) Situational Inventory of Body Image Dysphoria scale taps into negative body image–related emotions that accompany exposure to various situations.

Cognitive Measures

Scales assessing cognitive components of body image include those that evaluate thoughts or beliefs about one's appearance. For example, Cash, Melnyk, and Hrabosky's (2004) Appearance Schema Inventory–Revised assesses beliefs about appearance that may reflect a rather ingrained aspect of body image schema. The Body Image Automatic Thoughts Questionnaire (Cash, Lewis,

& Keeton, 1987) has subscales that assess Positive and Negative body-related cognitions. A relatively new and somewhat unique measure is the Eating Disorder Belief Questionnaire, which contains the Self-Acceptance subscale and the Acceptance by Others subscale (Rose, Cooper, & Turner, 2006). The subscales assess how an individual will feel if her or his body is toned and how others will feel if her or his body is toned. Within this category are a variety of measures related to appearance ideals and self-schema (e.g., Stein & Hedger, 1997; Szymanski & Cash, 1995).

Behavioral Assessment

Behavioral measures attempt to document the specific observational manifestation of body image disturbance, such as avoidance or body checking. One of the first measures of this type was a self-report measure developed by Rosen, Srebnik, Saltzberg, and Wendt (1991), the Body Image Avoidance Questionnaire. The Body Checking Questionnaire (Reas, Whisenhunt, & Netemeyer, 2002) is one of the more recent innovations in this area; a 23-item scale that indexes a variety of body-checking behaviors. Although only a few questionnaire measures specifically focus on behavioral issues, some of the measures of body dysmorphic disorder (see Table 4.1) provide an assessment of the behavioral component. Interestingly, most of the measures in this category provide a self-report of one's behaviors—there remains a need for further development of objective measures of behavioral avoidance.

Interview Scales

In addition to the above-mentioned methods of assessment, interview strategies have been used with children, adolescents, and adults. The Eating Disorder Examination (EDE; Fairburn & Cooper, 1993) is a semi-structured interview of eating pathology currently in its 12th edition. The interview has subscales related to body image (shape and weight concerns). Two interviewers provide symptom ratings in this assessment tool. The interview was originally designed for adults, but Bryant-Waugh, Cooper, Taylor, and Lask (1996) modified the EDE and administered it to children and found that the measure works well with children. The Structured Interview for Anorexia and Bulimic Disorders (SIAB) also has a body image scale as one of its six factors (Fichter, Herpertz, Quadflieg, & Herpertz-Dahlmann, 1998). The Interview for Diagnosis of Eating Disorders–IV (Kutlesic, Williamson, Gleaves, Barbin, & Murphy-Eberenz, 1998) includes symptom ratings for body image disturbance, as well as the other *DSM* criteria for eating disorders (anorexia nervosa, bulimia nervosa, binge eating disorder, and eating disorder not otherwise specified).

Body Dysmorphic Disorder

Body dysmorphic disorder (BDD) is an extreme form of body image disturbance wherein the disparagement of a particular aspect of appearance may be very severe, even delusional. In recent years, a variety of measures have been developed to assess this disorder. For adolescents, the Body Image Rating Scale (BIRS) has been designed to assess the presence and severity of BDD and its associated features (Mayville, Katz, Gipson, & Cabral, 1999). The scale consists of 15 items in a Likert-type format that focuses on cognitive, affective, and behavioral features of BDD. The most widely used interview measure of BDD is the Body Dysmorphic Disorder Examination (BDDE; Rosen & Reiter, 1996), which has 34 items that index symptoms of BDD. The content of the interview includes preoccupation/negative evaluation of appearance, self-consciousness, excessive importance given to appearance in self-evaluation, avoidance of social situations or activities, camouflaging appearance, and body-checking behavior.

The Body Dysmorphic Disorder Diagnostic Module (BDDDM) is an interview based on *DSM-IV* diagnostic criteria that is designed similar to other Structured Clinical Interview for DSM

Disorders (SCID) modules to determine whether a diagnosis of body dysmorphic disorder is appropriate (Phillips, 1996). The BDD modification of the Yale-Brown Obsessive-Compulsive Scale (Y-BOCS) is a 12-item interview that assesses severity of BDD symptoms (Phillips, 1996). These items assess BDD-related thoughts, behaviors, insight, and avoidance.

Within the field of BDD, Pope and colleagues have identified a clinical disorder that corresponds to a pathological preoccupation with the pursuit of a muscular ideal, referred to as *muscle dysmorphia* (Pope, Katz, & Hudson, 1993; Pope, Gruber, Choi, Olivardia, & Phillips, 1997). In muscle dysmorphia, a person is described as experiencing cognitive symptoms, including extreme body dissatisfaction and repeated thoughts of not being sufficiently muscular, along with behavioral symptoms such as substance abuse (e.g., use of anabolic steroids), strict dieting, compulsive weight lifting, and mirror checking (Olivardia, 2004). Some of the measures included in Table 4.1 that assess a muscularity component of body image (Drive for Muscularity, Muscle Areas Satisfaction Scale, etc.) are also useful in providing information related to diagnosing muscle dysmorphia.

Recent Advances

One of the recent trends in body image assessment work is the development of a variety of measures designed to index constructs that are closely related to body image and/or that might be considered risk factors for the development of body image disturbance. For instance, the Body Image Coping Strategies Inventory (Cash, Santos, & Williams, 2004) looks at how individuals cope with situations that threaten their body image. The Body Image Quality of Life Inventory (Cash & Fleming, 2002) asks respondents about the effect of their body image on a variety of life domains (home, work, etc.).

A variety of sociocultural and interpersonal factors, such as media influences and psychosocial pressures (e.g., teasing), have been associated with body image disturbance. Utilization of these measures may be useful not only for understanding factors that are connected to an individual's body image but also assist in identifying variables that may be linked to disturbed eating patterns (Levine & Harrison, 2004; J. K. Thompson, van den Berg, Roehrig, Guarda, & Heinberg, 2004). One of the most commonly used measures in this category is the Sociocultural Attitudes Towards Appearance Questionnaire–Third Revision (J. K. Thompson et al., 2004), which measures multiple aspects of societal influence on appearance, including four subscales: Pressures, Information, Internalization-General, Internalization-Athlete. This scale has also been validated for use with clinical eating disorders populations (Calogero, Davis, & Thompson, 2004).

Internalization measures that examine the extent to which the "thin ideal" present in the media is internalized by an individual are also in this category of measures (e.g., Sociocultural Internalization of Appearance Questionnaire–Adolescents [Keery, Shroff, Thompson, Wertheim, & Smolak, 2004]; Ideal Body Internalization Questionnaire [Stice, Shaw, & Nemeroff, 1998]). Appearance comparison scales (e.g., the Physical Appearance Comparison Scale [J. K. Thompson, Heinberg, & Tantleff, 1991]) assess the degree to which an individual compares himself or herself with peers, models, and others. Research with these types of measures are frequently used in studies evaluating risk for body image and eating disturbances (e.g., Shroff & Thompson, 2006a, 2006b).

Recently developed measures of body objectification are also relevant to the measurement of body image. One commonly used measure in this category is the Objectified Body Consciousness Scale (OBC; McKinley & Hyde, 1996), which includes two subscales related to how individuals respond to cultural pressures to meet appearance ideals. The Body Surveillance subscale assesses the degree to which an individual engages in habitual monitoring of their external appearance. The Body Shame subscale assesses the degree to which an individual feels like a bad person if not meeting societal appearance ideals. The OBC scale has been modified recently to provide a validated measure of objectified body consciousness in preadolescents and adolescents (Lindberg, Hyde, & McKinley, 2006). The Self-Objectification Questionnaire (Noll & Fredrickson, 1998) provides a short rank-order scale that is used to measure the extent to which an individual values observable appearance-based attributes over nonobservable competence-based attributes as most important to their physical self-concept. Research with these measures has frequently used them to assess the extent to which individuals view their bodies as objects to be looked at and evaluated by others, which, in turn, has been linked to an increased risk for body image and eating disturbances (Calogero, Davis, & Thompson, 2005; Tiggemann & Lynch, 2001; Tiggemann & Slater, 2001).

Researchers are also beginning to realize the value of cross-cultural studies of body image. To that end, several studies have examined the relevance and applicability of translating measures created in English into other languages. For example, Kashima, Yamashita, and Okamoto (2003) have translated the Body Attitude Test into Japanese, and Thurfjell, Edlund, Arinell, Hagglof, and Engstrom (2003) have created a Swedish translation of the Body Dissatisfaction subscale of the Eating Disorders Inventory for Children. Both of these scales show good internal consistency in the samples in which they were studied. Rousseau, Knotter, Barbe, Raich, and Chabrol (2005) have used a French version of the Body Shape Questionnaire with university female students. In addition, Lau, Lum, Chronister, and Forrest (2006) have translated the Body Parts Satisfaction Scale and the Body Comparison Scale (Fisher & Thompson, 1998) into Chinese. Yamamiya, Shroff, and Thompson (2008) translated a variety of measures into Japanese. These new measures will allow researchers to assess the same construct across cultures and to perform comparative studies. Such studies may shed some light on factors leading to body image disturbance in various cultures around the world.

Methodological Issues

An important consideration about body image scales is whether the clinician or researcher is attempting to assess a state or trait dimension. In most cases, measures assess traits; however, a few state measures have been developed. Primarily, these measures have been used in experimental studies designed to investigate the impact of specific variables (e.g., exposure to media images) on body image (J. K. Thompson, 2004). These scales could potentially be used in a clinical setting as a gauge of the immediate, within-session improvement in body image. One such measure is the state subscale of the Physical Appearance State and Trait Anxiety Scale (Reed et al., 1991). Cash, Fleming, and Alindogan (2002) have also created the Body Image States scale, which offers the advantage of being rather short (six items) so that it can be used efficiently for multiple ratings.

Another methodological issue, touched on early in this chapter, is that some of the measures created for the assessment of some component of body image were standardized on relatively small samples and may have limited evidence of reliability and validity. In addition, the samples are not always clinical in nature (i.e., individuals with a diagnosis of an eating disorder or body dysmorphic disorder). As mentioned earlier, they may have limited generalizability due to limited work with a variety of ages and/or ethnicities. A further limitation of body image measures is that no reliable measures for very young children (i.e., younger than 6 years) have been developed.

The ethnicity of the standardization sample should be taken into account. For example, using a figural rating scale, a sample of Moroccan Sahraoui women rated their ideal body size as significantly *larger* than their rating of an average body size (Rguibi & Belahsen, 2006), which is in contrast to the typical findings among White, European American samples of women. In this sample, greater body dissatisfaction predicted attempts to gain weight as opposed to lose weight. Ethnic differences in response to body image measures have also been observed based on the degree of assimilation and/or acculturation into other cultural contexts. For example, again using figural rating scales, research has indicated that Latina women born in the United

States endorse an even thinner ideal body size than European American women, whereas Latina women who immigrated to the United States endorsed a larger body ideal (Lopez, Blix, & Blix, 1995). Although limited work has assessed levels of different body image dimensions with a variety of ethnic groups, it is important to consider ethnic differences when interpreting individual responses to body image measures and to seek out this information when it is available.

The gender and sexual orientation of the standardization sample should also be taken into account. For example, the body objectification measures have been primarily developed for and tested in samples of heterosexual women; however, recent research has provided more information about men's body surveillance and body shame (Hebl, King, & Lin, 2004), as well as gay men (Martins, Tiggemann, & Kirkbride, 2007) and lesbian women (Kozee & Tylka, 2006), indicating different levels and patterns of relations among body objectification and body image disturbances across these populations.

Conclusions and Practical Considerations

We now offer some specific guidelines for selecting a measure. One of the strategies that has guided our decision over the past several years (e.g., J. K. Thompson et al., 1999) is to include a variety of measures that tap into different dimensions of body image disturbance, especially when involved in clinical work. (The decision for research purposes may be more specific and targeted, depending on the research question.) For instance, we generally include at least one measure that assesses a more abstract aspect of appearance (e.g., not weight related or specific to a certain body site). One widely used measure of this aspect of body image is the Multidimensional Body Self-Relations Questionnaire–Appearance Evaluation subscale (MBSRQ-AE; Brown, Cash, & Mikulka, 1990). We also typically include a measure of weight-specific body image, such as the Eating Disorder

Inventory–Body Dissatisfaction subscale. Another measure that might be included is a measure that assesses a variety of different sites, such as the MBSRQ–Body Areas Satisfaction Scale. A nice addition to questionnaire measures is a figural rating scale, such as the Contour Drawing Rating scale (M. A. Thompson & Gray, 1995).

The above measures generally index the affective and subjective nature of body image; therefore, it may also be useful to add a measure or two that involves cognitive disturbances (see Table 4.1). These types of measures are very helpful for providing evidence of disturbed thinking patterns that might be addressed in a clinical intervention for body image or related disturbances (e.g., eating disorders). For instance, the Appearance Schemas Inventory–Revised (Cash, Melnyk, & Hrabosky, 2004) and the Assessment of Body Image Cognitions (Jakatdar, Cash, & Engle, 2006) are two measures that appear to have excellent psychometric properties.

Especially when dealing with boys or men or an athletic sample, it might be important to include a measure that allows for the specific assessment of muscularity dissatisfaction. As Table 4.1 shows, many of these measures have been developed in recent years, including the Drive for Muscularity Scale (McCreary, Sasse, Saucier, & Dorsch, 2004), Drive for Muscularity Attitudes Questionnaire (Morrison, Morrison, Hopkins, & Rowan, 2004), and others (for a review, see Cafri & Thompson, 2007).

If an initial assessment suggests the possible presence of body dysmorphic disorder, it would be important to include a measure that assesses this more severe form of disturbance such as the Body Dysmorphic Disorder Examination (Rosen & Reiter, 1996) or the Body Dysmorphic Disorder Diagnostic Module (Phillips, 1996).

There are a few sources that someone interested in the assessment of body image can return to periodically for updates on measures and assessment issues. First, the journal *Body Image* (Elsevier.com) frequently has articles that include development and validation of new measures. Second, Tom Cash's Web site (body-images.com)

contains detailed advice on his measures of body image, which are quite numerous. Third, our Web site (bodyimagedisturbance.org) contains information on the measures that we have developed that assess body image and/or related constructs (such as social and interpersonal influences on body image). Fourth, it is very important to stay current with the scientific literature because new measures appear with regularity and old measures are reexamined. For instance, Pook, Tuschen-Caffier, and Brähler (2008) recently evaluated eight different versions of the Body Shape Questionnaire. Measures are also often modified and evaluated for use with samples cross-culturally; for instance, Yamamiya et al. (2008) recently evaluated several measures on a Japanese sample. Therefore, when considering a measure that has been available for several years, it is often useful to conduct a literature review to see if the measure has been modified and/or whether the measure has received new evaluation with a sample that it may not have been tested upon previously.

In conclusion, this chapter has provided a fairly selective review of measures commonly used in the assessment of body image. The clinician or researcher has a rather daunting task when faced with the variety and plethora of measures available for selection. We hope this chapter offers a few guidelines that reduce the complexity involved in the evaluation of body image disturbance.

References

Beebe, D. W., Holmbeck, G. N., & Grzeskiewicz, C. (1999). Normative and psychometric data on the Body Image Assessment–Revised. *Journal of Personality Assessment, 73,* 374–394.

Brown, T. A., Cash, T. F., & Mikulka, P. J. (1990). Attitudinal body-image assessment: Factor analysis of the Body Self Relations Questionnaire. *Journal of Personality Assessment, 55,* 135–144.

Bryant-Waugh, R. J., Cooper, P. J., Taylor, C. L., & Lask, B. D. (1996). The use of the Eating Disorder Examination with children: A pilot study. *International Journal of Eating Disorders, 19,* 391–397.

Cafri, G., Roehrig, M., & Thompson, J. K. (2004). Reliability assessment of the somatomorphic matrix. *International Journal of Eating Disorders, 35,* 597–600.

Cafri, G., & Thompson, J. K. (2004a). *Development of a modified version of the somatomorphic matrix.* Unpublished measure.

Cafri, G., & Thompson, J. K. (2004b). Evaluating the convergence of muscle appearance attitude measures. *Assessment, 11,* 224–229.

Cafri, G., & Thompson, J. K. (2004c). Measuring male body image: A review of the current methodology. *Psychology of Men & Masculinity, 5,* 18–29.

Cafri, G., & Thompson, J. K. (2007). Measurement of the muscular ideal. In J. K. Thompson & G. Cafri (Eds.), *The muscular ideal.* Washington, DC: American Psychological Association.

Cafri, G., van den Berg, P., & Thompson, J. K. (2006). Pursuit of muscularity in adolescent boys: Relations among biopsychosocial variables and clinical outcomes. *Journal of Clinical Child and Adolescent Psychology, 35,* 283–291.

Calogero, R. M., Davis, W. N., & Thompson, J. K. (2004). The Sociocultural Attitudes Toward Appearance Scale (SATAQ-3): Reliability and normative data for eating disorder patients. *Body Image: An International Journal of Research, 1,* 193–198.

Calogero, R. M., Davis, W., N., & Thompson, J. K. (2005). The role of self-objectification in the experience of women with eating disorders. *Sex Roles, 52,* 43–50.

Cash, T. F. (1994). The Situational Inventory of Body-Image Dysphoria: Contextual assessment of a negative body image. *The Behavior Therapist, 17,* 133–134.

Cash, T. F. (2000). *The users' manuals for the Multidimensional Body-Self Relations Questionnaire, Situational Inventory.* Retrieved September 2007 from Body-images.com

Cash, T. F. (2002). The Situational Inventory of Body-Image Dysphoria: Psychometric evidence and development of a short form. *International Journal of Eating Disorders, 32,* 362–366.

Cash, T. F., & Fleming, E. C. (2002). The impact of body image experiences: Development of the Body Image Quality of Life Inventory. *International Journal of Eating Disorders, 31,* 455–460.

Cash, T. F., Fleming, E. C., & Alindogan, J. (2002). Beyond body image as a trait: The development and validation of the Body Image States Scale. *Eating Disorders: The Journal of Treatment and Prevention, 10,* 103–113.

Cash, T. F., & Grasso, K. (2005). The norms and stability of new measures of the multidimensional body image construct. *Body Image, 2,* 199–203.

Cash, T. F., & LeBarge, A. S. (1996). Development of the Appearance Schemas Inventory: A new cognitive body image assessment. *Cognitive Therapy and Research, 20,* 37–50.

Cash, T. F., Lewis, R. J., & Keeton, P. (1987, March). *Development and validation of the Body-Image Automatic Thoughts Questionnaire: A measure of body-related cognitions.* Paper presented at the meeting of the Southeastern Psychological Association, Atlanta, GA.

Cash, T. F., Melnyk, S. E., & Hrabosky, J. I. (2004). The assessment of body image investment: An extensive revision of the Appearance Schemas Inventory. *International Journal of Eating Disorders, 35,* 305–316.

Cash, T. F., Phillips, K. A., Santos, M. T., & Hrabosky, J. I. (2004). Measuring "negative body image": Validation of the Body Image Disturbance Questionnaire in a nonclinical population. *Body Image, 1,* 363–372.

Cash, T. F., & Pruzinsky, T. (2002). Future challenges for body image theory, research, and clinical, practice. In T. F. Cash & T. Pruzinsky (Eds.), *Body images: A handbook of theory, research, and clinical practice* (pp. 509–516). New York: Guilford.

Cash, T. F., Santos, M., & Williams, E. (2004). *Coping with body-image threats and challenges: Validation of the Body Image Coping Strategies Inventory.* Unpublished manuscript.

Cash, T. F., & Szymanski, M. L. (1995). The development and validation of the Body-Image Ideals Questionnaire. *Journal of Personality Assessment, 64,* 466–477.

Cecil, H., & Stanley, M. A. (1997). Reliability and validity of adolescents' scores on the Body Esteem Scale. *Educational and Psychological Measurement, 57,* 340–356.

Childress, A. C., Brewerton, T. D., Hodges, E. L., & Jarrell, M. P. (1993). The Kids' Eating Disorders Survey (KEDS): A study of middle school students. *Journal of the American Academy of Child and Adolescent Psychiatry, 32,* 843–850.

Cooper, P. J., Taylor, M. J., Cooper, Z., & Fairburn, C. G. (1987). The development and validation of the Body Shape Questionnaire. *International Journal of Eating Disorders, 6,* 485–494.

Cuzzolaro, M., Vetrone, G., Marano, G., & Garfinkel, P. E. (2006). The Body Uneasiness Test (BUT): Development and validation of a new body image assessment scale. *Eating and Weight Disorders, 11,* 1–13.

Edwards, S., & Launder, C. (2000). Investigating muscularity concerns in male body image: Development of the Swansea Muscularity Attitudes Questionnaire. *International Journal of Eating Disorders, 28,* 120–124.

Fairburn, C. G., & Cooper, Z. (1993). The Eating Disorder Examination (12th ed.). In C. G. Fairburn & G. T. Wilson (Eds.), *Binge eating: Nature, assessment, and treatment* (pp. 317–360). New York: Guilford.

Fichter, M. M., Herpertz, S., Quadflieg, N., & Herpertz-Dahlmann, B. (1998). Structured interview for anorexic and bulimic disorders for DSM-IV and ICD-10: Updated (third) revision. *International Journal of Eating Disorders, 24,* 227–249.

Fisher, E., & Thompson, J. K. (1998). *Social comparison and body image: An investigation of body comparison processes using multidimensional scaling.* Unpublished manuscript.

Furnham, A., & Calnan, A. (1998). Eating disturbance, self-esteem, reasons for exercising and body weight dissatisfaction in adolescent males. *European Eating Disorders Review, 6,* 58–72.

Garner, D. (1991). *Eating Disorder Inventory–2: Professional manual.* Odessa, FL: Psychological Assessment Resources.

Garner, D. (2004). *Manual for the Eating Disorders Inventory–3 (EDI-3).* Odessa, FL: Psychological Assessment Resources.

Goldfarb, L. A., Dykens, E. M., & Gerrard, M. (1985). The Goldfarb Fear of Fat Scale. *Journal of Personality Assessment, 49,* 329–332.

Gruber, A. J., Pope, H. G., Borowiecki, J., & Cohane, G. (1999). The development of the somatomorphic matrix: A bi-axial instrument for measuring body image in men and women. In T. S. Olds, J. Dollman, & K. I. Norton (Eds.), *Kinanthropometry VI* (pp. 217–231). Sydney, Australia: International Society for the Advancement of Kinanthropometry.

Hebl, M. R., King, E. B., & Lin, J. (2004). The swimsuit becomes us all: Ethnicity, gender, and vulnerability to self-objectification. *Personality and Social Psychology Bulletin, 30,* 1322–1331.

Hildebrandt, T., Langenbucher, J., & Schlundt, D. G. (2004). Muscularity concerns among men:

Development of attitudinal and perceptual measures. *Body Image, 1,* 169–181.

Huddy, D. C., Nieman, D. C., & Johnson, R. L. (1993). Relationship between body image and percent body fat among college male varsity athletes and nonathletes. *Perceptual and Motor Skills, 77,* 851–857.

Jakatdar, T. A., Cash, T. F., & Engle, E. K. (2006). Body-image thought processes: The development and initial validation of the Assessment of Body-Image Cognitive Distortions. *Body Image, 3,* 325–333.

Kashima, A., Yamashita, T., & Okamoto, A. (2003). Japanese version of the Body Attitude Test: Its reliability and validity. *Psychiatry and Clinical Neurosciences, 57,* 511–516.

Keery, H., Shroff, H., Thompson, J. K., Wertheim, E., & Smolak, L. (2004). The Sociocultural Internalization of Appearance Scale–Adolescent version. *Eating and Weight Disorders: Studies on Anorexia, Bulimia and Obesity, 9,* 56–61.

Kozee, H. B., & Tylka, T. L. (2006). A test of objectification theory with lesbian women. *Psychology of Women Quarterly, 30,* 348–357.

Kutlesic, V., Williamson, D. A., Gleaves, D. H., Barbin, J. M., & Murphy-Eberenz, K. P. (1998). The Interview for the Diagnosis of Eating Disorders IV: Application to DSM-IV diagnostic criteria. *Psychological Assessment, 10,* 41–48.

Lau, A. S., Lum, S. K., Chronister, K. M., & Forrest, L. (2006). Asian American college women's body image: A pilot study. *Cultural Ethnicity and Minority Psychology, 12,* 259–274.

Levine, M. P., & Harrison, K. (2004). Media's role in the perpetuation and prevention of negative body image and disordered eating. In J. K. Thompson (Ed.), *Handbook of eating disorders* (pp. 695–717). New York: John Wiley.

Lindberg, S. M., Hyde, J. S., & McKinley, N. M. (2006). A measure of objectified body consciousness for preadolescent and adolescent youth. *Psychology of Women Quarterly, 30,* 65–76.

Lopez, E., Blix, G. G., & Blix, A. G. (1995). Body image of Latinas compared to body image of non-Latina White women. *Health Values: The Journal of Health, Behavior, Education, and Promotion, 19,* 3–10.

Lundgren, J., Anderson, D. A., & Thompson, J. K. (2004). Fear of negative appearance evaluation: Development and evaluation of a new construct for risk factor work in the field of eating disorders. *Eating Behaviors, 5,* 75–84.

Martins, Y., Tiggemann, M., & Kirkbride, A. (2007). Those Speedos become them: The role of self-objectification in gay and heterosexual men's body image. *Personality and Social Psychology Bulletin, 33,* 634–647.

Mayville, S., Katz, R. C., Gipson, M. T., & Cabral, K. (1999). Assessing the prevalence of body dysmorphic disorder in an ethnically diverse group of adolescents. *Journal of Child and Family Studies, 8,* 357–362.

Mayville, S. B., Williamson, D. A., White, M. A., Netemeyer, R., & Drab, D. L. (2002). Development of the muscle appearance satisfaction scale: A self-report measure for the assessment of muscle dysmorphia symptoms. *Assessment, 9,* 351–360.

McCreary, D. R., & Sasse, D. K. (2000). An exploration of the drive for muscularity in adolescent boys and girls. *Journal of American College Health, 48,* 297–304.

McCreary, D. R., Sasse, D. K., Saucier, D. M., & Dorsch, K. D. (2004). Measuring the drive for muscularity: Factorial validity of the drive for muscularity scale in men and women. *Psychology of Men & Masculinity, 5,* 49–58.

McKinley, N. M., & Hyde, J. S. (1996). The Objectified Body Consciousness Scale: Development and validation. *Psychology of Women Quarterly, 20,* 181–215.

Mendelson, B. K., Mendelson, M. J., & White, D. R. (2001). Body Esteem Scale for adolescents and adults. *Journal of Personality Assessment, 76,* 90–106.

Mendelson, B. K., & White, D. R. (1985). Development of self-body-esteem in overweight youngsters. *Developmental Psychology, 21,* 90–96.

Morrison, T. G., Morrison, M. A., Hopkins, C., & Rowan, E. T. (2004). Muscle mania: Development of a new scale examining the drive for muscularity in Canadian Males. *Psychology of Men and Masculinity, 5,* 30–39.

Noll, S. M., & Fredrickson, B. L. (1998). A mediational model linking self-objectification, body shame, and disordered eating. *Psychology of Women Quarterly, 22,* 623–636.

Olivardia, R. (2004). Body dysmorphic disorder. In J. K. Thompson (Ed.), *Handbook of eating disorders and obesity* (pp. 542–561). Hoboken, NJ: John Wiley.

Petersen, A. C., Schulenberg, J. E., Abramowitz, R. H., Offer, D., & Jarcho, H. D. (1984). A Self-Image Questionnaire for Young Adolescents (SIQYA): Reliability and validity studies. *Journal of Youth and Adolescence, 13,* 93–111.

Peterson, M., Ellenberg, D., & Crossan, S. (2003). Body-image perceptions: Reliability of a BMI-based silhouette matching test. *American Journal of Health Behavior, 27,* 355–363.

Petrie, T. A., Tripp, M. M., & Harvey, P. (2002). Factorial and construct validity of the Body Parts Satisfaction Scale–Revised: An examination of minority and non-minority women. *Psychology of Women Quarterly, 26,* 213–221.

Phillips, K. A. (1996). *The broken mirror.* New York: Oxford University Press.

Pook, M., Tuschen-Caffier, B., & Brähler, E. (2008). Evaluation and comparison of different versions of the Body Shape Questionnaire. *Psychiatry Research, 158,* 67–73.

Pope, H., Gruber, A., Choi, P., Olivardia, R., & Phillips, K. (1997). An underrecognized form of body dysmorphic disorder. *Psychosomatics, 38,* 548–557.

Pope, H., Katz, D., & Hudson, J. (1993). Anorexia nervosa and "reverse anorexia" among 108 male bodybuilders. *Comprehensive Psychiatry, 34,* 406–409.

Reas, D. L., Whisenhunt, B. L., & Netemeyer, R. (2002). Development of the Body Checking Questionnaire: A self-report measure of body checking behaviors. *International Journal of Eating Disorders, 31,* 324–333.

Reed, D. L., Thompson, J. K., Brannick, M. T., & Sacco, W. P. (1991). Development and validation of the Physical Appearance State and Trait Anxiety Scale (PASTAS). *Journal of Anxiety Disorders, 5,* 323–332.

Rguibi, M., & Belahsen, R. (2006). Body size preferences and sociocultural influences on attitudes towards obesity among Moroccan Sahraoui women. *Body Image, 3,* 395–400.

Rose, K. S., Cooper, M. J., & Turner, H. (2006). The eating disorder belief questionnaire: Psychometric properties in an adolescent sample. *Eating Behaviors, 7,* 410–418.

Rosen, J. C., & Reiter, J. (1996). Development of the Body Dysmorphic Disorder Examination. *Behaviour Research and Therapy, 34,* 755–766.

Rosen, J. C., Jones, A., Ramirez, E., & Waxman, S. (1996). Body shape questionnaire: Studies of validity and reliability. *International Journal of Eating Disorders, 20,* 315–319.

Rosen, J. C., Srebnik, D., Saltzberg, E., & Wendt, S. (1991). Development of a body image avoidance questionnaire. *Psychological Assessment, 3,* 32–37.

Roth, D., & Armstrong, J. (1993). Feelings of Fatness Questionnaire: A measure of the cross-situational variability of body experience. *International Journal of Eating Disorders, 14,* 349–358.

Rousseau, A., Knotter, A., Barbe, P., Raich, R., & Chabrol, H. (2005). Validation of the French version of the Body Shape Questionnaire. *Encephale, 31,* 162–173.

Schulman, R. G., Kinder, B. N., Powers, P. S., Prange, M., & Gleghorn, A. A. (1986). The development of a scale to measure cognitive distortions in bulimia. *Journal of Personality Assessment, 50,* 630–639.

Shisslak, C. M., Renger, R., Sharpe, T., Crago, M., McKnight, K. M., Gray, N., et al. (1999). Development and evaluation of the McKnight Risk Factor Survey for assessing potential risk factor and protective factors for disordered eating in preadolescent and adolescent girls. *International Journal of Eating Disorders, 25,* 195–214.

Shroff, H., & Thompson, J. K. (2006a). Multiple aspects of influence for body image among adolescents: A test of the tripartite influence model. *Body Image, 3,* 17–23.

Shroff, H., & Thompson, J. K. (2006b). Peer influences, body image dissatisfaction, eating dysfunction and self-esteem in adolescent girls. *Journal of Health Psychology, 11,* 533–551.

Siegel, J. M., Yancey, A. K., Aneshensel, C. S., & Schuler, R. (1999). Body image, perceived pubertal timing, and adolescent mental health. *Journal of Adolescent Health, 25,* 155–165.

Spangler, D. L., & Stice, E. (2001). Validation of the Beliefs About Appearance Scale. *Cognitive Therapy and Research, 25,* 813–827.

Stein, K. E., & Hedger, K. M. (1997). Body weight and shape self-cognitions, emotional distress, and disordered eating in middle adolescent girls. *Archives of Psychiatric Nursing, 11,* 264–275.

Stice, E., Shaw, H., & Nemeroff, C. (1998). Dual pathway model of bulimia nervosa: Longitudinal support for dietary restraint and affect-regulation mechanisms. *Journal of Social and Clinical Psychology, 17,* 129–149.

Stunkard, A. J., Sorenson, T. I., & Schulsinger, F. (1983). Use of the Dutch Adoption Register for the study of obesity and thinness. In S. Kety, L. P. Rowland, R. L. Sidman, & S. W. Matthysse (Eds.), *The genetics of neurological and psychiatric disorders* (pp. 115–120). New York: Raven.

Szymanski, M. L., & Cash, T. F. (1995). Body-image disturbances and self-discrepancy theory: Expansion of the Body-Image Ideals Questionnaire. *Journal of Social and Clinical Psychology, 14,* 134–146.

Tantleff-Dunn, S., Thompson, J. K., & Dunn, M. E. (1995). The Feedback on Physical Appearance Scale (FOPAS): Questionnaire development and psychometric evaluation. *Eating Disorders: The Journal of Treatment and Prevention, 3,* 332–341.

Thelen, M. H., Powell, A. L., Lawrence, C., & Kuhnert, M. E. (1992). Eating and body image concern among children. *Journal of Clinical Child & Adolescent Psychology, 21,* 41–46.

Thompson, J. K. (2004). The (mis)measurement of body image: Ten strategies for improving assessment for clinical and research purposes. *Body Image: An International Journal of Research, 1,* 7–14.

Thompson, J. K., & Altabe, M. N. (1991). Psychometric qualities of the Figure Rating Scale. *International Journal of Eating Disorders, 10,* 615–619.

Thompson, J. K., Cattarin, J., Fowler, B., & Fisher, E. (1995). The Perception of Teasing Scale (POTS): A revision and extension of the Physical Appearance Related Teasing Scale (PARTS). *Journal of Personality Assessment, 65,* 146–157.

Thompson, J. K., & Gardner, R. (2002). Measuring perceptual body image among adolescents and adults. In T. F. Cash & T. Pruzinsky (Eds.), *Body image: A handbook of theory, research and clinical practice* (pp. 135–141). New York: Guilford.

Thompson, J. K., Heinberg, L. J., Altabe, M. N., & Tantleff-Dunn, S. (1999). *Exacting beauty: Theory, assessment and treatment of body image disturbance.* Washington, DC: American Psychological Association.

Thompson, J. K., Heinberg, L. J., & Tantleff, S. (1991). The Physical Appearance Comparison Scale. *The Behavior Therapist, 14,* 174.

Thompson, J. K., & Tantleff, S. T. (1992). Female and male ratings of upper torso: Actual, ideal, and stereotypical conceptions. *Journal of Social Behavior and Personality, 7,* 345–354.

Thompson, J. K., van den Berg, P., Roehrig, M., Guarda, A. S., & Heinberg, L. J. (2004). The Sociocultural Attitudes Towards Appearance Questionnaire-3 (SATAQ-3): Development and validation. *International Journal of Eating Disorders, 35,* 293–304.

Thompson, M. A., & Gray, J. J. (1995). Development and validation of a new body-image assessment tool. *Journal of Personality Assessment, 64,* 258–269.

Thurfjell, B., Edlund, B., Arinell, H., Hagglof, B., & Engstrom, I. (2003). Psychometric properties of Eating Disorder Inventory for Children (EDI-C) in Swedish girls with and without a known eating disorder. *Eating and Weight Disorders, 8,* 296–303.

Tiggeman, M., & Lynch, J. (2001). Body image across the life span in adult women: The role of self-objectification. *Developmental Psychology, 37,* 243–253.

Tiggemann, M., & Slater, A. (2001). A test of objectification theory in former dancers and non-dancers. *Psychology of Women Quarterly, 25,* 57–64.

Tylka, T. L., Bergeron, D., & Schwartz, J. P. (2005). Development and psychometric evaluation of the Male Body Attitudes Scale (MBAS). *Body Image, 2,* 161–175.

Veron-Guidry, S., & Williamson, D. A. (1996). Development of a body image assessment procedure for children and preadolescents. *International Journal of Eating Disorders, 20,* 287–293.

Wertheim, E. H., Paxton, S. J., & Tilgner, L. (2004). Test-retest reliability and construct validity of Contour Drawing Rating Scale scores in a sample of early adolescent girls. *Body Image, 1,* 199–205.

Williamson, D. A., Gleaves, D. H., Watkins, P. C., & Schlundt, D. G. (1993). Validation of the self-ideal body size discrepancy as a measure of body dissatisfaction. *Journal of Psychopathology and Behavioral Assessment, 15,* 57–68.

Wooley, O. W., & Roll, S. (1991). The Color-a-Person Body Dissatisfaction Test: Stability, internal consistency, validity, and factor structure. *Journal of Personality Assessment, 56,* 395–413.

Yamamiya, Y., Shroff, H., & Thompson, J. K. (2008). The tripartite influence model of body image and eating disturbance: A replication with a Japanese sample. *International Journal of Eating Disorders, 41,* 88–91.

Yanover, T., & Thompson, J. K. (2009) Assessment of body image in children and adolescents. In L. Smolak & J. K. Thompson (Eds.), *Body image, eating disorders and obesity in youth* (2nd ed., pp. 177–192). Washington, DC: American Psychological Association.

CHAPTER 5

Measures of Restrained Eating

Conceptual Evolution and Psychometric Update

Michael R. Lowe and J. Graham Thomas

R esearch on restrained eating was first published more than 30 years ago. During this period, much has been learned about the psychometric properties of the three primary measures of restrained eating. One purpose of the present chapter is to supplement and update the thorough review of restraint measures provided by Allison and Gorman in the first edition of this book. We have retained the psychometric information from their chapter and updated it with data published since 1995.

Since the first studies on restrained eating were published in 1975 (Herman & Mack, 1975; Herman & Polivy, 1975), another major development has been an evolution—some might say a revolution—in the very meaning of *restrained eating*. That is, at a conceptual level, it has become clearer what these measures are—and are not— measuring, and these newer findings are often inconsistent with the way in which the measures were originally conceptualized. Because the psychometric properties of a measure only become meaningful when some consensus exists on the concept or domain assessed by that measure, it is critical to review research that can help specify what *restrained eating* means and what restrained eating measures are assessing.

We first provide a brief historical overview of the three main measures of restrained eating and the rationale for their development. This is followed by a consideration of studies, most of which have been published since the first edition of this book, that have raised questions about what these scales are measuring. The final section provides an update on the psychometric properties of restraint scales, again focusing primarily on the three most widely used measures of restraint.

A Brief History of Measures of Restrained Eating

The first measure of restrained eating, the Restraint Scale (RS), was developed by Herman and Polivy (1975) with the final, 10-item revised version published in 1978 (see Herman & Polivy, 1980). The rationale for the development of the RS grew out of the work of Schachter and Rodin (1974) and Nisbett (1972) on factors controlling food intake in the obese. Herman and Polivy (1975) and Herman and Mack (1975) reasoned that normal-weight individuals who were constantly dieting and holding their weight below its biological set point would demonstrate anomalies in eating behavior that resembled those shown by obese individuals in prior research. This reasoning directly followed from Nisbett's (1972) hypothesis that differences in eating behavior between normal-weight and overweight individuals were due to the overweight individuals keeping their body weight suppressed below its biologically appropriate level to conform to social norms. The RS was used to identify normal-weight individuals whose body weight was kept suppressed by constant dieting. Subsequent research has indeed found that the RS identifies normal-weight individuals who differ from unrestrained individuals on a wide variety of behavioral, cognitive, and physiological measures (Herman & Polivy, 1984; Lowe, 1993; Lowe & Kral, 2006).

Nonetheless, Stunkard and Messick (1985) noted several serious problems with the RS. First, they reviewed evidence showing that restrained, overweight individuals—unlike normal-weight restrained eaters—did not overeat following consumption of a preload. This contradicted Herman and Polivy's (1975) assumption that previously observed differences in eating behavior between normal-weight and obese individuals were due to greater dieting in the obese. If this were true, then restrained obese individuals should be at least as susceptible to preload-induced overeating as normal-weight restrained eaters. Second, they noted that the RS measured not only dietary restraint but also weight fluctuations. Weight fluctuation is often higher in obese individuals for reasons having nothing to do with dieting behavior (e.g., if the degree of weight fluctuation that individuals experience is a constant fraction of their body mass, obese individuals will experience larger fluctuations

in absolute terms; see Drewnowski, Riskey, & Desor, 1982). Furthermore, Drewnowski et al. (1982) showed that two weight fluctuation items account for 70% of the variance in total RS scores and also found that obese persons actually scored lower on the dietary concern factor of the RS. These problems led Stunkard and Messick to develop a new measure of restraint—the restrained eating scale—which is one of three factors in their Three-Factor Eating Questionnaire (TFEQ; now called the Eating Inventory [EI]). The TFEQ-R scale represented a major improvement in the assessment of restrained eating because it eliminated two confounds—between dieting and overeating and between restrained eating and overweight—that characterize the RS. Investigators studying restrained eating broadly agree that the TFEQ-R, relative to the RS, represents a "purer" measure of restraint that is more likely to reflect actual efforts to restrict dietary intake (Stunkard & Messick, 1985; van Strien, 1999).

van Strien, Frijters, Bergers, and DeFares (1986) noted many of the same problems with the RS that Stunkard and Messick (1985) described. To address these limitations, they developed the Dutch Eating Behavior Questionnaire (DEBQ) that included a restrained eating scale. Their restraint scale is quite similar to Stunkard and Messick's TFEQ-R measure, in part because both groups used items from a measure developed by Pudel, Metzdorff, and Oetting (1975) to construct their scales. Pudel et al.'s scale assessed "latent obesity" or the tendency of some normal-weight individuals to exhibit eating patterns previously associated with obesity. A major advantage of both the TFEQ-R and DEBQ-R scales is that they (unlike the RS) reflect "pure" dietary restraint, permitting the dissociation of restrained eating from its opposite—overconsumption. Interestingly, the TFEQ-R and DEBQ-R scales have weak or nonexistent relationships with the other subscales of the Eating Inventory and DEBQ that tap different types of excessive eating (stemming from disinhibition, hunger, negative emotions, and external food stimuli).

Developments in the Definition and Conceptualization of Restrained Eating

The majority of early theorizing about restrained eating and its possible psychobiological effects was produced by Herman, Polivy, and their colleagues (Herman & Polivy, 1984). However, during the past 30 or so years, there have been a variety of research findings that have (a) raised questions about the meaning and definition of restrained eating and (b) shed new light on what measures of restrained eating are—and are not—assessing. In the next several sections, we review this literature because it suggests that traditional theorizing about restrained eating and its putative effects is in need of major revision.

The Meaning of Restrained Eating

Most researchers have defined restrained eating in a manner similar to the following: Restrained eating refers to conscious efforts to restrict food intake for the purpose of weight control. Over the years, Herman and Polivy have defined the term in different ways, including the suppression of body weight below one's body weight set point (Herman & Polivy, 1975), the imposition of a cognitively defined "diet boundary" to limit food intake (Herman & Polivy, 1984), and a history of repeatedly going on and off diets, referred to as "unsuccessful dieting" (Heatherton, Herman, Polivy, King, & McGree, 1988).

From one perspective, it is certainly possible that a restrained eater on the RS would have all three characteristics implied by these definitions: that her weight would be well below her highest weight ever (and perhaps therefore well below her body weight "set point"), that she would impose a diet boundary on her eating to establish permissible caloric intake, and that she had been on and off diets repeatedly in the past. However, as Lowe (1993) pointed out, these are characteristics that could also be used to differentiate three different *types* of restrained eaters: those who

(a) are well below their highest weights ever by virtue of intentional weight loss (weight suppressors), (b) are currently on a diet to lose weight (current dieters), or (c) have engaged in repeated cycles of dieting and overeating in the past (frequent dieters and overeaters). Importantly, even though most restrained eaters will be characterized by one or more of these designations, these three types of dieting are theoretically independent: Knowing a person's status on any one of these three dieting types does not necessarily tell you anything about his or her standing on the others. Furthermore, because these different dieting patterns are associated with different appetitive and behavioral responses, Lowe pointed out that measuring a single construct of "restraint" could conceal important differences between these dieting subtypes. For instance, Lowe, Whitlow, and Bellwoar (1991) found that restrained eaters who were not currently dieting ate somewhat more with than without a preload, whereas current dieters ate much less with than without a preload. Another example comes from Lowe, Thomas, Safer, and Butryn (2007), who recently reported that weight suppression was positively associated with binge-eating frequency among individuals diagnosed with bulimia nervosa (which is consistent with Russell's [1979] original theorizing about the role of significant weight losses in bulimia), whereas scores on the Eating Disorders Examination–Restrained Eating subscale were negatively associated with binge-eating frequency (which is inconsistent with the cognitive-behavioral model of bulimia).

Another major development regarding the meaning of restraint involves the motivation underlying restrained eating. At different times, Herman and Polivy have viewed restrained eating as a way of examining the effects of dieting to avoid weight gain (Herman & Polivy, 1975), as a factor contributing to weight gain and obesity (Polivy & Herman, 1983), and as a major cause of eating disorders (Polivy & Herman, 1985). Despite these wide variations in the purported significance of restrained eating, the same scale (the RS) has been used to measure restraint, and essentially the same theory (that dieting behavior sows the seeds of its own destruction) has been used to account for these varied functions of restrained eating. However, when particular subtypes of dieting are examined in relation to outcomes traditionally studied in the restraint literature, the need to go beyond the use of a single, monolithic measure of restraint emerges again. For example, weight suppressors, who, according to the set point model (Herman & Polivy, 1975), should be hyperresponsive to appetitive stimuli, instead show rigorous eating control following a preload (Lowe & Kleifield, 1988) and reduced sweetness preferences (Kleifield & Lowe, 1991). When applied to those with bulimia nervosa, restraint theory predicts that bulimic individuals who are currently dieting should binge more than bulimic nondieters; instead, the opposite relationship has been found in two studies (Lowe, Gleaves, & Murphy-Eberenz, 1998; Lowe et al., 2007).

These findings indicate that the advisability of using the RS to study restrained eating depends on the investigator's research objectives. If the objective is to study "restrained eating" as operationalized by the RS (which involves the simultaneous measurement of several constructs—dieting, overeating, weight fluctuations, overweight), then the RS could be appropriate to use—and has the advantage of being characterized by a large corpus of previously published findings. (Alternatively, investigators are increasingly using a combination of the TFEQ-R and disinhibition scales from the EI [e.g., Westenhoefer, Broeckmann, Munch, & Pudel, 1994; Williamson et al., 1995]—based on the reasonable assumption that those who score high on both resemble restrained eaters measured by the RS—because this approach permits them to study both the independent and interactional relationship of restrained eating and predisposition toward overeating on outcomes of interest.) If the objective of a study is to examine particular types of dieting, on the other hand, then an alternative to the RS should be considered—for example, by measuring one of the three types of dieting behavior outlined by Lowe (1993) or by putting

people on short-term weight loss diets (Presnell & Stice, 2003).

What Are Restraint Scales Measuring?

As noted above, Herman and Polivy (1975) originally conceived of restrained eaters as individuals who were "constantly dieting and concerned with not gaining weight, and who presumably would gain substantial weight if they were to 'let themselves go'" (p. 667). Although these authors subsequently de-emphasized this characterization of restrained eaters in favor of a more cognitively focused perspective (Herman & Polivy, 1984) that emphasized drive for thinness (Polivy & Herman, 1987), it appears—as we shall see shortly—that this original viewpoint may actually best capture the nature of restrained eaters' vulnerability to aberrations in their appetitive and consummatory responses.

Twenty-five years ago, when no one realized that developed countries were entering the early stages of explosive growth in the prevalence of obesity, dieting in normal-weight individuals (and normal-weight women in particular) was assumed to reflect an unhealthy need to achieve a slim body to conform with societal norms of attractiveness (Striegel-Moore, Silberstein, & Rodin, 1986). As Polivy and Herman put it in 1987, "Nowadays, women are induced to strive toward a condition of ruddy-cheeked emaciation" (p. 635). This emphasis on attaining the "thin ideal" has been widely accepted as the primary driver of restrained eating among individuals in the normal weight range. Thus, restraint theory has gone 180 degrees from its original belief that restrained eating is motivated by an effort to prevent weight gain (Herman & Polivy, 1975) to the belief that it is motivated by the yearning for an unrealistically thin body (Polivy & Herman, 1987).

These seemingly contradictory possibilities might be clarified by drawing two distinctions regarding restrained eaters' motivation for weight control. The first distinction involves restrained eaters' goals for weight change. Restrained eaters have elevated levels of body dissatisfaction (Ruderman & Grace, 1988) and both desire a thinner body (Polivy & Herman, 1987) and fear weight gain (Vartanian, Herman, & Polivy, 2005). Presumably, most restrained eaters would like to consume fewer calories than they expend and lose some weight, thereby moving closer to their desired goal and further away from the feared outcome of weight gain. However, Polivy and Herman's assumption that restrained eaters are driven to reach unhealthy levels of body weight conflates restrained eaters' desire to be *thinner* (e.g., to lose a few pounds) with their desire to be objectively *thin* (e.g., to achieve a body weight far below their medically appropriate weight for their height). A recent study (Chernyak & Lowe, 2007) compared unrestrained and restrained eaters on drive for thinness, fear of fatness, and drive to be objectively thin (defined as being 15% below their medically appropriate weight for height). Restrained eaters scored significantly higher than unrestrained eaters on the first two measures but did not differ from unrestrained eaters on the third measure. These findings suggest that while restrained eaters would like to avoid weight gain or to lose a small amount of weight, they do not have an unhealthy drive to become pathologically thin. Therefore, it appears that restrained eaters are not as strongly motivated to lose weight as has often been assumed. The fact that most restrained eaters are not currently dieting to lose weight (Lowe, 1993) is consistent with this conclusion.

The second distinction involves the extent to which restrained eaters, whatever their weight control goals, are actually reducing their caloric intake. Restrained eaters assessed with the RS are assumed to vacillate between periods of caloric restriction and overindulgence without losing weight in absolute terms (Heatherton, Polivy, & Herman, 1991). Restrained eaters on the other two restraint measures are generally assumed to be more successful at caloric restriction, especially since these measures are viewed as purer measures of the actual cognitions and behaviors involved in dieting (Stunkard & Messick, 1985; van Strien,

1999). However, although past lab studies sometimes found that restrained eaters consume less food than unrestrained eaters, recent evidence indicates that restrained eaters, no matter how they are identified, do not eat less in the natural environment than unrestrained eaters (Stice, Cooper, Schoeller, Tappe, & Lowe, 2007).

Stice, Fisher, and Lowe (2004) examined five dietary restraint scales that were developed to assess intentional dietary restriction for the purposes of weight control. These scales showed weak and generally nonsignificant correlations with objectively measured caloric intake during unobtrusively observed eating episodes across four studies (mean $r = -.07$; range: $-.34$ to $.20$; Stice et al., 2004). For example, the average correlation between three dietary restraint scales and observed caloric intake of students consuming meals in a cafeteria was $-.09$.

In response to these validity findings, van Strien, Engels, van Staveren, and Herman (2006) noted that short-term caloric intake may not be representative of long-term caloric intake and suggested that researchers test whether dietary restraint scales show inverse correlations with objective measures of longer term caloric intake. Four previous studies (reviewed in Stice et al., 2007) that examined this question found no relationship between caloric intake and several measures of restrained eating. In a recent follow-up study, Stice et al. (in 2007) reported on three additional studies that found that the TFEQ-R scale was not correlated with doubly labeled water-estimated energy intake over 2-week periods or with observationally measured caloric intake over 3 months. Taken together, the foregoing findings suggest that dietary restraint scales may not be valid measures of naturalistic dietary restriction and imply the need to reinterpret findings from studies that have used dietary restraint scales. As Lowe and Levine (2005), Lowe and Butryn (2007), and Stice et al. (2007) have recently suggested, part of this reinterpretation should be based on the idea that measures of restrained eating reflect *relative* dietary restriction (i.e., relative to the positive energy balance that would result if a restrained eater no longer practiced restraint) rather than *absolute* dietary restriction (i.e., relative to energy balance or to the intake of unrestrained eaters).

Two other teams of researchers have come to similar conclusions. First, Gorman, Allison, and Primavera (1993) and Allison, Kalinsky, and Gorman (1992) conducted a factor analysis of the TFEQ-R scale and found that it contained two factors that they called cognitive restraint and behavior restraint. They analyzed their data using nonlinear techniques that take into account situations where items differ substantially in their endorsement rates. Their results suggested that the TFEQ-R items form a continuum that begins with relatively common thoughts of reducing eating and ends with overt, deliberate, but relatively rare actions to reduce eating. These results indicate that even measures that ostensibly reflect "successful" restraint do not identify individuals who eat less than unrestrained eaters.

Second, Larsen, van Strien, Eisinga, Herman, and Engels (2007) recently factor analyzed the DEBQ-R among a large sample of weight-concerned individuals and found that a two-factor solution fit the data well. The two factors differentiated between restrained eating intentions and restrained eating behavior. In line with Allison et al.'s (1992) work, they found that participants scored higher on dieting intentions than dieting behavior. They also found that that more restrained eating behavior was related to "*less* external and emotional eating, whereas more restrained intentions (without restrained behavior) were related to *more* external and emotional eating" (p. 106). These results are reminiscent of the distinction Lowe et al. (1991) made between restrained eaters who are and are not currently dieting to lose weight, with the former group showing a counterregulatory eating pattern and the latter group showing eating regulation.

We should also note that the same questions about the relationships between food restriction, overeating, and weight control have been raised in research in children. Birch, Fisher, and Davison (2003) found that 5-year-old girls whose mothers

reported using restrictive feeding practices were more likely to exhibit eating in the absence of hunger at 9 years of age. This was especially true of girls who were already overweight at the age of 5. These results are suggestive of a gene-by-environment interaction in which overweight girls are genetically predisposed to be highly sensitive to environmental influences over eating. There is no way of knowing from these data whether mothers' restrictive eating practices are causally related to later vulnerability to eating in the absence of hunger, if they reflect mothers' concerns about concurrent weight gain in their children and have no causal influence, or if this relationship is due to some as yet unidentified variable.

All the research reviewed in this section suggests that, despite their *desire* to be thinner, in functional terms, most restrained eaters are at best employing restraint to avoid weight gain, not to lose weight. This conclusion is supported by research showing that measures of restrained eating prospectively predict weight gain rather than weight loss (French, Jeffery, & Wing, 1994; Klesges, Isbell, & Klesges, 1992; Stice, Presnell, Shaw, & Rohde, 2005). It appears that, just as most obese individuals who lose weight via dieting eventually regain it (Sarwer & Wadden, 1999), restrained eating may forestall but usually does not prevent weight gain. One additional reason to suggest that much of restrained eaters' motivation for weight control stems from concerns about gaining weight is that restrained eaters show levels of certain hormones (e.g., reduced leptin, increased cephalic phase insulin) that makes them metabolically predisposed toward weight gain (Lowe & Kral, 2006). Although these findings theoretically could be due to metabolic adaptations to weight loss dieting, the evidence reviewed above indicates that restrained eaters are not in negative energy balance. In sum, it appears that our understanding of the nature of the motivation that has fueled the tremendous increase in dieting behavior in the past few decades has come full circle. Herman and Polivy (1975) started out believing that restrained eating was driven by the desire to avoid weight gain secondary to being below one's biologically determined body weight set point value. If one replaces the notion that a body weight set point is "pulling" weight upward from within (e.g., via the hypothalamus [Nisbett, 1972]) with the idea that an obesogenic environment is "pulling" weight upward from without (Lowe & Butryn, 2007; Lowe & Levine, 2005) then Herman and Polivy's original theorizing appears to be closest to the truth. That is, normal-weight restrained eaters and dieters appear to have a predisposition toward weight gain in an obesogenic environment (e.g., Lowe et al., 2006), but this characteristic would presumably remain latent in environments where food was difficult to come by. From this perspective, the fact that the first research on restrained eating was conducted around the same time that the obesity epidemic began is probably no coincidence.

One caveat is needed before bringing this section of the chapter to a close. The fact that measures of restrained eating generally do not reflect caloric restriction or weight loss dieting should not be taken to mean that diet-induced weight loss is not a risk factor for the development of eating disorders. On one hand, it does appear that the multiple findings in the literature showing that measures of restrained eating or dieting prospectively predict increased bulimic symptoms are not due to low-calorie dieting (Stice et al., 2007). On the other hand, there is good evidence that extreme dieting that produces rapid, extensive weight loss may indeed help cause bulimia nervosa (Butryn & Wadden, 2005; Garner & Fairburn, 1988; Keys, Brozek, Henschel, Mickelsen, & Taylor, 1950; Russell, 1979). These findings are a further indication that it behooves researchers to think carefully about precisely what construct they are interested in investigating when studying "restrained eating" and to tailor their measures of that construct accordingly.

Herman and Polivy's Restraint Scale

Description

Herman and Mack (1975) originally developed the Restraint Scale (RS) to identify normal-weight individuals who attempt to limit their food intake in an effort to resist biological pressures toward weight gain. The original scale consisted of 5 items measuring chronic dieting. The items were rationally derived and selected for face validity. The scale was tested on a sample of 45 women, which produced a Cronbach's alpha coefficient of 0.65. Herman and Polivy (1975) revised the instrument to include 11 items, with 6 items forming a Diet and Weight History subscale (alpha coefficient 0.62) and the remaining 5 items forming a Concern With Dieting subscale (alpha coefficient 0.68). The subscales correlated at 0.48, and the alpha coefficient for the whole scale was 0.75. The final iteration of the RS (Herman & Polivy, 1980) consists of 10 items. Polivy, Herman, and Howard (1988) describe the RS as "a 10-item self report questionnaire assessing weight fluctuations, degree of chronic dieting, and related attitudes toward weight and eating" (p. 377). The preponderance of published research using the RS has used this 10-item version.

Herman and Polivy (1975) subdivided the RS into two subscales. The Weight Fluctuation (WF) subscale (Items 2, 3, 4, and 10) measures both instability in weight and a history of overweight. The Concern for Dieting (CD) subscale (Items 1, 5, 6, 7, 8, and 9) assess preoccupation with food, overconcern about eating, and overeating tendencies. Thus, an individual who scores highly on both subscales is likely to be characterized by a history of overweight, a desire to weigh less, and unstable body weight. Notably, the RS should not be considered a measure of actual hypocaloric dieting or energy deficit (Polivy et al., 1988). High scores on the RS are prospectively associated with greater fluctuations in body weight (Heatherton, Polivy, & Herman, 1991; Tiggemann, 1994). Some (Heatherton et al., 1988) have cited the link between restraint scores and weight fluctuation as support for the idea that the concept of restraint should include efforts to restrict eating to control one's weight *and* the periodic failure of restraint resulting in episodes of overeating (i.e., disinhibited eating). The RS is consistent with this formulation of restraint and the associated theory that dieting is a major cause of overeating and eating disorders (Polivy & Herman, 1985). As noted previously, this theory has undergone increased scrutiny (e.g., Lowe & Kral, 2006; Stice et al., 2007).

Sample

The RS was initially tested on samples of 42 (Herman & Mack, 1975) and 45 (Herman & Polivy, 1975) female college students. The great majority of psychometric studies using the RS have been done with normal-weight and overweight female college students. It is occasionally used with eating-disordered individuals but rarely with clinical populations of overweight individuals.

Norms

Studies that incorporate the RS as a measure of primary interest tend to use the RS in one of two ways: either as a continuous measure of restrained eating or as a tool to dichotomize a sample into restrained and unrestrained eaters. In the former case, the RS is typically analyzed with regression methods to investigate constructs that may be associated with restraint. This analytic strategy is desirable because it preserves the full variability of the RS. In the latter case, after participants have been classified as restrained eaters or unrestrained eaters, the two groups are compared on some measure(s), often in an analysis of variance (ANOVA). Historically, the latter approach was more common than the former. Typically, a median split was used to create groups of restrained and unrestrained eaters of approximately equal size. However, medians varied across samples, which resulted in different cutoffs for identifying restrained eaters. Concern over the failure to consistently identify a homogeneous set of restrained eaters across studies led some researchers to adopt the most frequently observed RS median (a score 15) as the standard cutoff for use in studies of restrained eating. This approach has the strength of standardization of the definition of restrained eaters but also the weakness of using dissimilar strategies of defining restrained eating in earlier and later studies of this construct. Furthermore, there is some evidence that medians on the RS are decreasing over time (e.g., medians were in the 15–17 range in the 1970s but are most often in the 12–14 range more recently), which casts doubt on the utility of a preselected cutoff to identify restrained eaters.

Table 5.1 presents sample sizes, means, and standard deviations for the RS, as well as its subscales, for a variety of samples. The average score for normal-weight women (mostly from samples of college students) is about 13. The corresponding value for men is 10. These values are useful for determining whether a particular sample is unusually high or low on restraint. It is important to keep in mind that RS scores may differ by nationality, weight status, eating disorder status, or other personal characteristics.

Table 5.1   Mean Restraint Scale Scores Reported in the Literature

Scale and Participants	Author	n	Mean	SD
Whole scale				

American adults
  Female
  Male
	French, Jeffery, and Wing (1994)	
		103
		99
			
			14.6
			11.0
				
				5.5
				5.0

American adult women	Timmerman and Gregg (2003)	120	20.5	4.6
American overweight adults	Williamson et al. (2007)	46	13.4	6.0

American college students
  Female
  Male
	Allison, Kalinsky, and Gorman (1992)	901
		617
		282
			15.1
			16.4
			12.3
				7.0
				6.9
				6.4

American college students
  Female
  Male
	Boerner, Spillane, Anderson, and Smith (2004)	
		215
		214
			
			13.0
			8.9
				
				6.1
				5.5

American college students
  Female
  Male
	Klem, Klesges, Bene, and Mellon (1990)	497
		346
		151
			12.6
			13.4
			10.8
				5.9
				5.8
				5.8

American female college students	Urland and Ito (2005)	82	13.8	6.6
Australian female college students	Griffiths et al. (2000)	82	12.1	6.0
British adolescent women	Cole and Edelmann (1987)	184	10.6	5.9
British women	Wardle and Beales (1987)	102	13.5	5.4
British men	Wardle and Beales (1987)	45	8.5	5.8

Canadian college students
  Female
  Male
	Oates-Johnson and DeCourville (1999)	220
		159
		61
			11.6
			12.8
			8.5
				6.6
				6.5
				5.7

Canadian college students
  Female
  Male
	Rotenberg and Flood (2000)	
		159
		61
			
			12.8
			8.5
				
				6.5
				5.7

Dutch obese women	Westerterp-Plantenga, Kempen, and Saris (1998)	57	20	3.5
Portuguese female college students	Scagliusi et al. (2005)	62	11.3	5.0

(Continued)

Table 5.1 (Continued)

Scale and Participants	Author	n	Mean	SD
Portuguese women				
With anorexia nervosa	Scagliusi et al. (2005)	15	17.3	9
With bulimia nervosa	Scagliusi et al. (2005)	24	28.1	13.0
Weight fluctuation scale				
Overweight American adults	Williamson et al. (2007)	46	6.9	3.2
American college students	Allison et al. (1992)	901	5.8	3.3
Female		617	5.9	3.3
Male		282	5.3	3.5
American college students	Boerner et al. (2004)			
Female		215	5.3	2.9
Male		214	4.8	3.3
American college students	Klem, Klesges, Bene, et al. (1990)			
Female		346	5.0	
Male		151	4.8	
British adolescent women	Cole and Edelmann (1987)	184	4.1	2.8
British women	Wardle and Beales (1987)	102	4.9	2.8
British men	Wardle and Beales (1987)	45	3.1	3.1
Concern with dieting scale				
American adults	Williamson et al. (2007)	46	6.4	4.7
American college students	Allison et al. (1992)	901	9.3	4.7
Female		617	10.4	4.6
Male		282	6.9	3.9
American college students	Boerner et al. (2004)			
Female		215	7.7	3.9
Male		214	4.0	3.2
American college students	Klem, Klesges, Bene, et al. (1990)			
Female		346	8.4	4.0
Male		151	5.9	3.4
British adolescent women	Cole and Edelmann (1987)	184	6.2	3.5
British women	Wardle and Beales (1987)	102	7.8	3.7
British men	Wardle and Beales (1987)	45	4.7	3.0

It appears that the practice of dichotomizing individuals into restrained and unrestrained eaters as the primary method of analysis should be discontinued. Stein (1988) demonstrated that an ANOVA design in which participants are dichotomized into groups based on RS score may have less predictive power in a preload study than a regression model in which RS scores are treated as continuous. Maxwell and Delaney (1993) confirmed that using median splits to form factors in a grouped design reduces statistical power. The authors also reported that dichotomizing participants based on a median split may produce erroneous conclusions about interactions among factors. This is especially relevant, as interactions between restraint status and various disinhibiting stimuli form the basis of many studies on restrained eating. Allison, Gorman, and Primavera (1993) discussed the disadvantages of dichotomization in general. Given these findings, the use of full RS scores in regression models is encouraged over the dichotomization of participants into restraint groups based on a median split. An exception may be made in situations where a strong theoretical or empirical basis exists for identifying specific groups of participants based on their RS score. Furthermore, though treating restraint scores continuously is preferable, because the majority of studies have treated restraint as a dichotomy, it is a good idea for researchers to analyze their results both ways so the categorical results can more easily be compared with past studies. A final reason to analyze results dichotomously in secondary analyses is that certain outcomes showing a nonlinear distribution may produce significant results using a median split but not with using continuous scores.

Age

There are a dearth of studies examining the relationship between the RS and age. Two studies including college students ranging from ages 17 to 57 years failed to find a relationship between RS and age (Allison et al., 1992; Klem, Klesges, Bene, & Mellon, 1990). However, little can be concluded from these studies because the most participants were between the ages of 18 and 22 years. The point in the human life span when dietary restraint typically asserts itself is unknown. A study by Cole and Edelmann (1987) observed a typical distribution of restraint scores in a sample of adolescent women with a mean age of 15 years old (see Table 5.1).

Gender

Boerner, Spillane, Anderson, and Smith (2004) observed higher RS total scores and CD subscale scores, but not WF subscale scores, among college women as compared with men. This pattern was also found by Allison et al. (1992). Klem, Klesges, Bene, and Mellon (1990) found that college women scored higher than men on the CD subscale but not the WF subscale or total RS. Oates-Johnson and DeCourville (1999) reported that college women scored significantly higher than men on the RS. This pattern was also observed by Rotenberg and Flood (2000). French et al. (1994) found that women scored higher on the RS than men in a sample of 202 adults, about a quarter of whom reported that they were actively dieting to lose or maintain weight. In a sample of adults, Klesges et al. (1992) reported higher restraint score in women than men. Thus, women appear to report systematically greater restraint on the RS than men. Concern for dieting seems to be more responsible for this difference than a history of weight fluctuation.

Reliability

Internal Consistency

The RS has been shown to have good internal consistency (Cronbach's alpha greater than .75) when used with normal-weight, non-eating-disordered samples. Table 5.2 illustrates the lower alpha levels that are observed in overweight and eating-disordered groups. This difference in alphas is likely attributable to restricted range within the overweight and eating-disordered subgroups. Crocker and Algina (1986) point out that Pearson product-moment correlations are lower when the variance of one or more variables in the analysis is restricted. As alpha depends on both the number of items and the correlation between items, subgroups of participants who respond in a systematically similar manner will produce lower alphas than more diverse subgroups that show greater variability in their scores. Drewnowski et al. (1982) were the first to point out that overweight and obese individuals are likely to score highly on the RS, and specifically the WF subscale, as a result of large weight fluctuations due, at least in part, to their increased adipose tissue rather than to restrained eating or concern about their weight. This potential measurement artifact may be a further source of homogeneity and subsequent lower internal consistency among overweight samples.

The CD and WF subscales show predictably lower alpha levels than the full RS score, presumably due to their smaller number of items. The alphas range from .66 to .71 for the CD subscale and from .70 to .80 for the WF subscale (Allison et al., 1992; Herman & Polivy, 1975; Klem, Klesges, Bene, & Mellon, 1990). van Strien, Breteler, and Ouwens (2002) and van Strien, Herman, Engels, Larsen, and van Leeuwe (2007) examined the internal consistency of the CD and WF subscales after removing Item 6 because of possible criterion confounding (Stice, Ozer, & Kees, 1997) and Item 10 because of inconsistent subscale factor loadings (Blanchard & Frost, 1983; Lowe, 1984; Overduin & Jansen, 1996). The resulting alphas for a group of 209 Dutch female college students were .77 for the five CD items and .70 for the three WF items (van Strien et al., 2002). van Strien et al. (2007) replicated the analysis with 349 normal-weight Dutch female college students and 409 overweight Dutch women and found alphas of .81 and .68 for the altered CD and WF scales for the normal-weight students and alphas of .65 and .72 for the altered CD and WF scales for the overweight women. Boerner et al. (2004) found that alphas for the total RS and its subscales are slightly higher for women than men. Klem, Klesges, Bene, et and Mellon (1990) determined that alphas for the RS and its subscales are equivalent for men and women, as well as for Blacks and Whites.

Test-Retest Reliability

RS scores appear to be stable over time (see Table 5.3). A somewhat lower coefficient was obtained with the Scagliusi et al. (2005) Portuguese translation of the RS.

Validity

There are a multitude of studies linking the RS to various aspects of eating behaviors, psychopathology, personality factors, and other constructs. It is beyond the scope of this chapter to review all of these reports; furthermore, most of them were not designed to test the validity of the RS. Rather, studies have been included that were (a) designed explicitly to test the

Table 5.2   Reliability of Dietary Restraint Scales: Internal Consistency

Reference	n	Coefficient alpha	Sample Characteristics
RS			
Allison, Kalinsky, and Gorman (1992)	823	.83	Normal-weight college students
Allison et al. (1992)	78	.72	Obese college students
Allison et al. (1992)	901	.82	Above two samples combined
Boerner, Spillane, Anderson, and Smith. (2004)	214	.76	Male college students
Boerner et al. (2004)	215	.82	Female college students
Laessle, Tuschl, Kotthaus, and Pirke (1989)	60	.78	Normal-weight women 18 to 30 years old; mostly college students
Rudderman (1983)	89	.86	Normal-weight female college students
Rudderman (1983)	58	.51	Obese female college students
W. G. Johnson, Lake, and Mahan (1983)	51	.79	Normal weight
W. G. Johnson et al. (1983)	58	.50	Obese nondieters
W. G. Johnson et al. (1983)	27	.83	Obese dieters
W. G. Johnson et al. (1983)	26	.57	Bulimic women 13 to 41 years old
Klem, Klesges, Bene, and Mellon (1990)	497	.78	College students (151 men; 346 women)
Klem, Klesges, Bene, et al. (1990)	124	.68	Obese college students
Klem, Klesges, Bene, et al. (1990)	373	.78	Normal weight college students
Oates-Johnson and DeCourville (1999)	220	.84	College students (61 men; 159 women)
Ouwens, van Strien, van der Staak (2003)	209	.83	Female college students
Rotenberg and Flood (1999)	58	.78	Female college students
Rotenberg and Flood (2000)	319	.77	College students (112 men; 207 women)
Urland and Ito (2005)	82	.85	Normal-weight female college students
van Strien, Cleven, and Schippers (2000)	200	.73	Female college students
van Strien, Herman, Engels, Larsen, and van Leeuwe (2007)	349	.84	Normal-weight female college students
van Strien et al. (2007)	409	.73	Overweight, nonobese women

(Continued)

Table 5.2 (Continued)

Reference	n	Coefficient alpha	Sample Characteristics
TFEQ-R			
Allison et al. (1992)	823	.91	Normal-weight college students
Allison et al. (1992)	78	.88	Obese college students
Allison et al. (1992)	901	.90	Above two samples combined
Boerner et al. (2004)	214	.89	Male college students
Boerner et al. (2004)	215	.90	Female college students
Laessle et al. (1989)	60	.80	Normal-weight women 18 to 30 years old; mostly college students
Ouwens et al. (2003)	209	.88	Female college students
Ricciardelli, Tate, and Williams (1997)	171	.91	Female college students
Simmons, Smith, and Hill (2002)	392	.87	American female 7th graders
Simmons et al. (2002)	300	.88	American female 10th graders
Stunkard and Messick (1988)	45	.92	Unrestrained eaters
Stunkard and Messick (1988)	53	.79	Restrained eaters
Stunkard and Messick (1988)	98	.93	Above two samples combined
van Strien et al. (2000)	200	.80	Female college students
DEBQ-R			
Allison et al. (1992)	823	.95	Normal-weight college students
Allison et al. (1992)	78	.91	Obese college students
Allison et al. (1992)	901	.95	Above two samples combined
Banasiak et al. (2001)	393	.94	Grade 9 female adolescents
Laessle et al. (1989)	60	.89	Normal-weight women 18 to 30 years old; mostly college students
Ouwens et al. (2003)	209	.94	Female college students
van Strien, Frijters, Bergers, and Defares (1986)	114	.94	Obese adults (71 men; 73 women)
van Strien, Frijters, et al. (1986)	996	.95	Normal-weight adults (427 men; 569 women)
van Strien, Frijters, et al. (1986)	1169	.95	Above two samples combined
van Strien et al. (2000)	200	.94	Female college students
van Strien et al. (2007)	349	.93	Normal-weight female college students
van Strien et al. (2007)	409	.89	Overweight, nonobese women

NOTE: DEBQ-R = Dutch Eating Behavior Questionnaire–Restraint subscale; RS = Restraint Scale; TFEQ-R = Three-Factor Eating Questionnaire–Restraint scale.

Table 5.3   Reliability of Dietary Restraint Scales: Test-Retest Reliability

Reference	n	Coefficient	Interval	Sample Characteristics
RS				
Allison, Kalinsky, and Gorman (1992)	34	.95	2 weeks	College students
Hibscher and Herman (1997)	86	.92	"A few weeks"	Male college students
Polivy, Herman, and Howard (1988)	514	.93	1 week	College students (166 men; 348 women)
Kickham and Gayton (1977)	44	.93	4 weeks	Normal-weight college students (16 men; 28 women)
Klesges, Klem, Epkins, and Klesges (1991)	305	.74	2½ years	98 men, 207 women
Scagliusi et al. (2005)	50	.64	1 month	Female college students
TFEQ-R				
Allison et al. (1992)	34	.91	2 weeks	College students
Bond, McDowell, and Wilkinson (2001)	64	.81	1 year	College students
Stunkard and Messick (1988)	17	.93	4 weeks	College students
DEBQ-R				
Allison et al. (1992)	34	.92	2 weeks	College students
Banasiak et al. (2001)	165	.85	4 to 5 weeks	High school students

NOTE: DEBQ-R = Dutch Eating Behavior Questionnaire–Restraint subscale; RS = Restraint Scale; TFEQ-R = Three-Factor Eating Questionnaire–Restraint scale.

validity of the RS or (b) report results that may be interpreted after the fact as support for, or evidence against, the theoretical assumptions that serve as a foundation for the development and continued use of the RS.

Content Validity

The RS was originally designed to be used with normal-weight individuals. Furthermore, factor-analytic studies of the Restraint Scale often obtain different factor solutions as a function of the number of overweight participants in the sample. Thus, studies including a large proportion of overweight participants are covered in their own section below.

Factorial Composition in Primarily Normal-Weight Samples

The two-factor model of the RS, including the CD and WF subscales that Herman and Polivy (1975) identified during the original development of the RS, is the most widely validated and frequently used conceptualization of the measure. This model has been supported by a variety of studies, including primarily normal-weight participants (Allison et al., 1992; Blanchard & Frost, 1983; Cole & Edelmann, 1987; Drewnowski et al., 1982; Heatherton et al., 1988; Lowe, 1984; Polivy et al., 1988; Ruderman, 1983). In most cases, Items 1, 5, 6, 7, 8, and 9 load on the CD factor, and Items 2, 3, 4, and 10 load on the WF factor (Blanchard & Frost, 1983; Drewnowski et al., 1982; Ruderman, 1983). Two factors often account for 50% to 60% of the variance. Herman and Polivy (1975) originally found the correlation among the two factors to be .48, while the more recent studies found subscale correlations ranging from .17 to .62.

Further evidence for the usual two-factor model was found by Allison et al. (1992), who performed orthogonal and oblique confirmatory factor analyses. The CD and WF factors accounted for 39% and 15% of the total variance, respectively. The original CD and WF scales correlated at .50.

Boerner et al. (2004) used structure equation modeling to conduct a confirmatory factor analysis on the RS. To facilitate the analysis, they combined items into parcels for factors with four or more items. The sample included 215 female and 214 male college students. The results indicated that the standard two-factor structure was a less than optimal fit using the comparative fit index (CFI = .85) but a fair fit using the root mean square error of approximation (RMSEA = .08). Similarly, in a series of factor analyses by Klem, Klesges, and Shadish (1990) on a sample of 229 college students (117 men, 112 women), the traditional two-factor model was only a fair fit with the data.

Occasionally, studies find more than two factors in the RS. Often, the results are attributed to the poor performance of certain specific items. van Strien et al. (2002) point out that there is generally poor consensus on the factorial assignment of Items 6 (splurging), 7 (thoughts about food), and 10 (history of overweight). The authors used maximum likelihood factor analysis to examine the RS responses from a sample of 209 female college students. The initial results suggested that a three-factor model fit the data the best, c^2 (35) = 13.65, p = .75. After oblique rotation, most items had high loadings on the first factor (36% of the variance), but the items from the WF subscale (2, 3, 4, 10) had the highest loadings on this factor. The five items from the CD subscale (1, 5, 7, 8, 9) and one item from the WF subscale (10) loaded highly on the second factor (9% of the variance). All items loaded negatively on the third factor (only 3% of the variance). Item 6 loaded highly on the first and third factors. When a two-factor solution was examined, Items 1, 6, and 10 were observed to load highly on both factors. The authors repeated their analysis after eliminating Items 6 and 10 due to their failure to load reliably on a single factor. Item 1 was kept because it was "considered central to the concept of dietary concern." The best-fit model included two factors, c^2 (13) = 12.55, with Items 2, 3, and 4 loading on the first factor (WF; 33% of the variance) and Items 1, 5, 7, 8, and 9 loading on the second factor (CD; 14% of the variance).

In a sample of 110 college students, Williams, Spencer, and Edelmann (1987) used principal components analysis to identify three factors with an eigenvalue greater than 1.4. The first factor included items primarily from the WF (1, 2 3, 4, 10) subscale, the second included items primarily from the CD subscale (5, 6, 8), and the third factor, labeled *attention to food intake,* included Items 2, 7, and 9. In this case, Item 2 loaded on the second and third factors. The three factors accounted for 27.7%, 21.4%, and 13.8% of the variance, respectively.

The findings of van Strien et al. (2002) and Williams et al. (1987) serve as a reminder that Herman and Polivy's conceptualization of restraint, as measured by the RS, includes several aspects of eating and attitudes, behaviors, and personal history that are related, but not perfectly so. Researchers who intended to measure the construct of restrain as conceptualized by Herman and Polivy need to recognize that the heterogeneity of constructs being assessed may be problematic. Those who desire a more "pure" (i.e., unidimensional) measure restraint are encouraged to use the restraint subscale from the Three Factor Eating Questionnaire or the Dutch Eating Behavior Questionnaire.

The developers of the RS intended it to be used as a single-factor measure (Polivy et al., 1988), and in most situations involving normal-weight samples, it should be used that way in primary analyses. Use of the total RS score will allow comparison with the majority of studies that have been conducted using the RS. However, the accumulated psychometric evidence suggests that the RS is multifactorial. van Strien et al. (2002) state that "use of total RS scores should be strongly discouraged" because the CD and WF subscales appear to measure qualitatively different constructs that may relate to outcomes such as disinhibited eating in different directions. Furthermore, the CD and WF subscales may interact in unpredictable ways. As such, it may often prove instructive to conduct secondary analyses that reanalyze data using the separate CD and WF subscales. If results replicate with one factor but not the other, it may provide valuable information about the source of the findings with the full scale.

Factorial Composition in Samples With a Significant Proportion of Overweight Participants

The two-factor model of the RS does not appear to be as reliable in samples composed primarily of overweight or eating-disordered participants. Most often, these studies report three or more factors (W. G. Johnson, Corrigan, Crusco, & Schlundt, 1986; W. G. Johnson, Lake, & Mahan, 1983; Lowe, 1984; Ruderman, 1983). Oblique factor rotation on samples including large numbers of obese participants often finds that Items 6 and 7 load on a third factor, possibly related to overeating. For example, Ruderman (1983) identified a four-four factor solution in a sample of 58 obese college students with a principal components factor analysis with orthogonal rotation. The factors consisted of a Weight Fluctuation dimension (25% of the variance), a Binge dimension (17% of the variance), a Tendency to Diet dimension (15% of the variance), and an Overconcern With Dieting dimension (12% of the variance). In addition, Lowe's (1984) exploratory principal components analysis found three factors with eigenvalues > 1.0. After oblique rotation, Items 1, 5, 8, 9, and 10 loaded on the first factor (29.3% of the variance), dubbed *dietary concern and weight history.* The second factor (28.3% of the variance), *weight fluctuation,* consisted of Items 2 to 4. Items 6 and 7 loaded on a third factor (17.6% of the variance).

The greater the proportion of overweight people in a sample, the more factors emerge (Ruderman, 1986). This factor instability may be a sign of differential validity or the result of restricted variance due to homogeneity of the sample. When a sample is homogeneous, the correlation coefficients among items are reduced, leading to an increased likelihood of the identification of additional factors in a factor-analytic study.

Factor Stability

A few studies have been conducted to test the factor stability of the RS. Blanchard and Frost (1983) found the factor structure of the RS to be stable across two samples of female college students. Tucker's (1951) congruence coefficient (CC) was above .99 for both factors, indicating excellent factor stability. Allison et al. (1992) found that the CC for the RS factors for males and females was over .95. For random splits of the sample, the CC was over .99. A comparison of obese and nonobese subjects produced a CC of .96 for the CD factor and .92 for the WF factor. Boerner et al. (2004) used the guidelines described by Hoyle and Smith (1994) to test the factor stability of the RS for a sample of college men ($n = 214$) and women ($n = 215$). The authors conclude that the RS is invariant across gender.

Construct Validity: Convergent and Discriminant Validity

As opposed to other restraint scales that appear to measure actual dieting behaviors associated with caloric restriction (e.g., TFEQ, DEBQ), the RS appears to measure failed attempts at dieting (Heatherton et al., 1988). Researchers frequently consider the construct of restraint, *as measured by the RS,* to encompass both efforts at restricting food intake *and* episodes of overeating (van Strien, 1997). This conceptualization of restraint, as measured by the RS, was supported in analyses by van Strien et al. (2007), who used confirmatory factor analysis to examine the RS in relation to other measures of dieting, overeating, and body dissatisfaction in a sample of normal-weight ($n = 349$) and overweight ($n = 409$) females. A three-factor model was posited. The first factor, labeled *overeating,* consisted of the TFEQ disinhibition scale, the DEBQ emotional eating scale, DEBQ external eating scale, the Eating Disorder Inventory Revised (EDI-II) bulimic eating scale, and the question, "Have you ever had an eating binge, i.e., you ate an amount of food others would consider unusually large?" The second factor, labeled *dieting,* consisted of the DEBQ restraint scale, the TFEQ restraint scale, and the question, "Are you currently dieting?" The third factor, labeled *body dissatisfaction,* consisted of the EDI-II drive for thinness and body dissatisfaction scales. The confirmatory factor analyses were conducted at the level of scale scores rather than individual items. A model in which the RS loaded on all three factors was a better fit of the data than a model in which the RS loaded only on the dieting factor. The association of the RS with the overeating factor supports the conceptualization of the RS as a measure of unsuccessful dieting.

Further support for the RS as a measure of unsuccessful dieting comes from a study by K. K. J. Ferguson, Brink, Wood, and Koop (1992), who studied the individual RS item responses of a group of overweight participants in a dieting program. A group of 41 female and 41 male successful dieters was identified, who lost at least 5% of their body weight and maintained the loss for a year with no more than 5 lbs. regain. Unsuccessful dieters, including 32 women and 28 men, failed to meet these benchmarks. Unsuccessful dieters were more likely than successful dieters to endorse items related to overeating and food obsession, such as, "Do you eat sensibly in front of others and splurge alone?" and "Do you give too much time and thought to food?" On the other hand, unsuccessful dieters were less likely to endorse items related to restriction of food intake, such as, "How conscious are you of what you are eating?" This study is partly consistent and partly inconsistent with what Herman and Polivy's restraint theory would predict: Unsuccessful dieters were higher on disinhibiton items but *lower* on restriction items. According to Herman and Polivy, unsuccessful dieters should be higher on both because the continuing attempts to restrict presumably should be fueling the overeating.

Weight and Obesity Status

Given that the RS is associated with both efforts at caloric restriction *and* a propensity toward overeating, it is not surprising that researchers have found a variety of relationships with weight and obesity status. Researchers have studied the relationship between the RS and weight primarily by correlating RS scores with body weight and body mass index (BMI), comparing the weight and BMI of restrained and unrestrained eaters, and comparing RS scores among normal-weight and overweight participants. Drewnowski et al. (1982) found a relationship between only the WF subscale and percentage overweight. Drewnowski et al. also found that overweight participants scored higher than normal-weight participants on the total RS and the WF subscale but not the CD subscale. Because greater weight fluctuations in overweight individuals could stem from biological characteristics of adipose tissue per se (rather than from repeated periods of weight loss dieting and disinhibition-induced weight regain), Drewnowski et al. suggested that the RS may not be an appropriate measure of restrained eating in overweight individuals. However, Lowe (1984) found that CD ($r = .41$) but not WF ($r = -.01$) was related to overweight status in a sample of 217 college students (96 men, 118 women, 3 unknown). The discrepancy between the Lowe and Drewnowski et al. findings is likely the result of a greater proportion of overweight participants in the Drewnoswki sample. This interpretation is supported by Allison et al. (1992), who found that obese participants ($n = 78$) obtained significantly higher scores on the RS and the WF subscale but not CD.

In two studies, Ruderman (1983, 1985) found correlations of .37 and .38 between RS scores and percentage overweight. In a study comparing overweight and nonoverweight participants, Klem, Klesges, Bene, and Mellon (1990) found that overweight participants obtained significantly higher scores on the CD and WF subscales, as well as on the total RS. In a sample of 358 adults (201 men and 157 women), de Castro (1995) found that higher RS scores were associated with higher body weights. Similarly, a Portuguese translation of the RS was significantly correlated with BMI in a sample of patients suffering from anorexia nervosa or bulimia nervosa ($r = .38$) and non-eating-disordered controls ($r = .43$; Scagliusi et al., 2005). Lowe (1984) found that restrained eaters had greater relative weights than unrestrained eaters, even though all participants were within the normal weight range.

The RS failed to prospectively predict changes in body weight in three studies involving college students (Klesges, Klem, Epkins, & Klesges, 1991; Lowe et al., 2006; Tiggemann, 1994). However, Klesges et al. (1992) found that RS scores predicted weight gain among adult women but not men over a 1-year period when the relationship was analyzed in a multiple linear regression, including other physiological, demographic, and activity variables. Williamson et al. (2007) reported that RS scores increased during a weight loss intervention, but changes in RS were not correlated with relative energy balance during the diet.

There appears to be a relationship between the RS and body weight. However, the relationship is not consistent across samples and may be artificially inflated among overweight and obese individuals. Given that nearly all literature on the RS has involved primarily normal-weight individuals, that overweight restrained eaters and dieters do not behave like those of normal weight (Lowe et al., 1991; Ruderman, 1986), and that the RS has weaker psychometric properties in overweight individuals, the RS is not well suited as a measure of restrained eating in overweight samples.

Naturalistic Food Consumption

Several authors have attempted to find a relationship between the RS and measures of naturalistic food consumption. However, most of these studies rely on self-reported dietary intake via food diaries, which have poor validity in general (Bandini, Schoeller, Dyr, & Dietz, 1990; Lichtman et al., 1992; Livingstone, Prentice, & Strain, 1990; Prentice et al., 1986), but especially among overweight samples (Lichtman et al., 1992; Prentice et al., 1986) and restrained eaters (for a review, see Maurer et al., 2006). Both of these groups tend to underreport food intake to a significantly greater degree than unrestrained normal-weight individuals.

Laessle, Tuschl, Kotthaus, and Pirke (1989) failed to find a correlation between RS ($r = -.04$) and mean caloric intake over a 7-day period in a sample of 60 normal-weight women. Similarly, de Castro (1995) found no relationship between total caloric intake and RS over a 7-day period in a sample of 201 male and 157 female adult participants. In a study by French et al. (1994), RS score was not related to caloric intake over a 6-month period, as measured by the Block Food Frequency Questionnaire (FFQ; Block et al., 1986). All three of these studies relied on self-reported intake. The fact that restrained eaters are more likely to underreport their actual food intake could be masking a tendency toward greater intake in restrained eaters. Consistent with this speculation are findings indicating that measures of restrained eating prospectively predict weight gain rather than weight loss (Stice et al., 2004).

Eating Disorders and Psychopathology

The creators of the RS have suggested that dietary restraint and eating-disordered attitudes and behaviors are inherently related and have gone so far as to say that the type of dieting that is measured by the RS can lead to the development of eating disorders (Heatherton & Polivy, 1992; Polivy & Herman, 1985). A variety of cross-sectional studies support this claim. Ruderman and Grace (1987) found that the RS was correlated with the BULIT (Smith & Thelen, 1984), a measure of bulimia, in a sample of 108 women. The partial correlation between the BULIT and the CD subscale of the RS was still statistically significant when WF subscale scores were controlled. However, the relationship between WF and the BULIT was nonsignificant when the CD scores were controlled. In a sample of college students (Boerner et al., 2004), the RS total score was significantly correlated with the BULIT-R (Thelen, Farmer, Wonderlich, & Smith, 1991) among both men ($r = .56$, $n = 214$) and women ($r = .69$, $n = 215$). In addition, scores for both men ($r = .46$) and women ($r = .64$) were correlated with a measure of anorexic symptomatology, the Eating Attitudes Test (EAT; Garner & Garfinkel, 1979). Using a Portuguese translation of the RS, Scagliusi et al. (2005) found that bulimics ($n = 24$) scored significantly higher on the RS than anorexics ($n = 15$), who obtained significantly greater scores than non-eating-disordered college students ($n = 57$). Prussin and Harvey (1991) compared a subsample of 38 individuals meeting *DSM-III-R* criteria for bulimia to 136 non-eating-disordered participants in a sample of normal-weight female runners. Bulimic participants had significantly higher RS scores. Bourne, Bryant, Griffiths, Touyz, and Beaumont (1998) found that the RS and its subscales were significantly correlated with greater frequency and intensity of disordered eating behaviors, as measured with the Eating Behavior Rating Scale (Wilson, Touyz, Dunn, & Beumont, 1989), during a video-recorded test meal. Griffiths et al. (2000) found significant relationships between the RS and abnormal eating attitudes and general dissatisfaction with one's life in a sample of 82 college students.

Prospective studies have confirmed that elevated RS scores predict the future onset of binge eating (Stice, Killen, Hayward, & Taylor, 1998) and bulimic pathology (Killen, Taylor, Hayward, & Wilson, 1994; Killen et al., 1996). In a sample of 967 adolescent girls who were followed over a 4-year period, Killen, Hayward, Wilson, and Taylor (1994) found that girls who developed bulimic symptoms had greater scores on both the CD and WF subscales of the RS at baseline compared to girls who remained asymptomatic. In a similar study of 543 female high school students, Stice et al. (1998) reported that RS scores at baseline predicted onset of objective binge eating, subjective binge eating, and purging. Two items referring to binge eating were removed from the RS for this analysis because of concerns regarding criterion confounding, which are discussed below.

Scores on the RS are clearly associated with measures of eating-disordered attitudes and behaviors. This is not surprising since dieting is a cardinal feature of both anorexia and bulimia nervosa, and overeating is a cardinal feature of bulimia nervosa. In addition, there is some evidence that RS scores are associated with depression and general dissatisfaction with life. However, Stice et al. (1997) suggest that the relationships observed between the RS and measures of eating-disordered symptomatology are the result of criterion confounding of the RS, which includes items related to disinhibited eating, a close relation of binge eating. When these items were removed (Items 6 and 8), the relationship between the RS and measures of disordered eating were significantly reduced among a sample of 117 female college students. The relationships were further weakened when items pertaining to weight fluctuation (which may create an artificial relationship between the RS and measures of eating-disordered symptomatology) were removed. The authors' argument for criterion confounding of the RS is strengthened by the fact that the DEBQ-R, which does not included items related to weight fluctuation or disinhibited eating, did not show equivalent relationships with measures of disordered eating.

Because the RS and other measures of restrained eating have been linked to the development of unhealthy eating behaviors, it is now widely accepted that "dieting" plays a causal role in the onset of eating disorders (e.g., Hawkins & Clement, 1984; Heatherton & Polivy, 1992; Polivy & Herman, 1985). In rare cases involving radical dieting and extensive weight loss to subnormal levels, there is reason to believe that such a connection exists (e.g., Butryn & Wadden, 2005). However, experimental evidence suggests that prescribed diets involving gradual weight loss reduce binge eating in normal-weight and overweight individuals (for a review, see Stice et al., 2004). This evidence, combined with studies indicating that restraint scales do not reflect hypocaloric dieting (Stice et al., 2007), seriously questions the prevalent assumption that garden-variety dieting helps cause eating disorders.

Susceptibility to Response Sets

Historically, restrained eaters were thought to be motivated by a desire to attain a thin body to conform to socially defined standards for attractiveness (Polivy & Herman, 1987). Furthermore, some items on the RS, especially those related to overeating, may be embarrassing to endorse. Thus, it seems plausible that the RS may be influenced by social desirability bias, which is the inclination to present oneself in a manner that will be viewed favorably by others. Several researchers have tested this theory by correlating the RS with measures of social desirability responding. Most measures of social desirability responding present participants with a list of behaviors that are either socially desirable but infrequently practiced or frequently practiced but socially undesirable. Attempts to "fake good" are indicated by endorsement of the former type of behavior and denial of the latter type. The Minnesota Multiphasic Personality Inventory (MMPI) L, or "lie" scale, is possibly the most well-known measure of social desirability responding. The items comprising the Edwards Social Desirability Scale (Edwards, 1957), and some items from the Marlowe-Crowne Social Desirability Scale (MCSD; Crowne & Marlowe, 1964) were taken from the MMPI.

W. G. Johnson et al. (1983, 1986) found small and nonsignificant correlations between the RS, the MMPI Lie scale, and the MCSD for bulimics, obese nondieters, and "normals." However, the relationship between the RS and the MMPI Lie scale ($r = -.33$), as well as the RS and MCSD ($r = -.51$), was moderate and negative for a sample of 27 obese dieters (W. G. Johnson et al., 1983). Ruderman (1983) found the opposite; the relationship between the RS and the Eysenck Lie Scale was stronger for nonobese participants ($r = -.70$) than obese participants ($r = -.13$). Other studies have found small and nonsignificant correlations between the RS and the Edwards Social Desirability Scale (Kickham & Gayton, 1977) and the RS and MCSD among normal-weight participants (Corrigan & Ekstrand, 1988; Ruderman, 1983) and obese participants (Ruderman, 1983). In a subset of participants ($n = 73$), Allison et al. (1992) found that the RS correlated with the MCSD ($r = -.27$) and the Edwards Social Desirability Scale ($r = -.05$). The authors also found that RS items that were rated as more desirable were endorsed more frequently. In the same study, when participants were instructed to "create the most favorable impression you can," scores on the RS were low (mean = 8.75). When instructed to "create the worst possible impression," the mean score was very high (mean = 30.65).

Generally, the relationship between the RS and social desirability scales is negative, meaning that high scores on the RS are associated with relatively elevated endorsement of socially undesirable behavior. These findings present an interesting contrast to restraint theory, which suggests that restrained eaters' behavior is motivated by a desire to attain a more socially desirable appearance. Regardless, the RS is transparent and can easily be "faked" good or bad. Finally, McCrae and Costa (1983a, 1983b) point out that correlations between a psychometric instrument and measures of social desirability responding should not necessarily be taken as a sign of invalidity of the instrument. It is generally undesirable to have a measure correlate with socially desirable motives, unless such a relationship can be argued to be part of the construct the measure is supposed to assess. In the case of the RS, the creators of the scale explicitly state that individuals who score highly on the measure are presumed to be highly influenced by socially dictated standards for appearance (Polivy & Herman, 1987).

Predictions of Laboratory Behavior

The RS is well known for its ability to predict disinhibited eating in laboratory studies using the preload paradigm (Herman & Polivy, 1984; Lowe, 1993). In these studies, participants are typically designated as restrained or unrestrained eaters based on the median score of the RS. Half of each group will be assigned to consume a high-calorie preload, such as a milkshake, before they participate in a "taste test" of palatable food, such as ice cream. The outcome measure is the amount of food consumed during the taste test, which is surreptitiously monitored by the experimenter. Unrestrained eaters typically compensate for a preload by consuming fewer calories in the preload than in the no-preload condition. Restrained eaters show the opposite trend: They will show evidence of disinhibited eating and consume somewhat *more* after than in the absence of a preload. This pattern of findings is typically observed only when dietary restraint is measured with the RS but not other measures such as the TFEQ or DEBQ (Lowe, 1993).

Notably, a caloric preload is not the only stimulus that will lead to disinhibited eating. Emotional distress (Herman & Polivy, 1980), threat of electric shock (Herman & Polivy, 1975), and increased cognitive load (Ward & Mann, 2000) also result in disinhibition. Furthermore, restrained eaters will exhibit disinhibited eating when they are led to believe that they have consumed a high-calorie preload when in fact the preload they consumed was low in calories (e.g., Heatherton, Polivy, & Herman, 1989). Thus, disinhibited eating seems to occur when restrained eaters believe that their efforts at caloric restriction have been "blown" or when they are distracted from their efforts at restraint by an engrossing or distressing stimulus.

The trend toward disregulation of food intake by restrained eaters was also observed in a study by Westerterp-Plantenga, Wouters, and ten Hoor (1991) in which 6 obese and 18 normal-weight women were served a four-course meal. Participants were allowed to eat as much as they wished during the second course, but the amount of food served during the other three courses was fixed. Eating behavior was observed, and the amount of food eaten was surreptitiously measured by a scale under the participant's plate. Participants who were low on the RS scale showed a decreased rate of intake following the first course. Restrained women showed a pattern of progressive linear intake across the meal. This result may reflect the same process (lack of response to eating what is normally a satiating amount of food) as observed in preload studies, even though the indicator was different (rate of eating over the meal).

The relationship between the RS and eating behavior observed in the laboratory is complex (Lowe, 1993). A sizable minority of studies have failed to find evidence of disinhibited eating in restrained eaters (e.g., Ouwens, van Strien, & van der Staak, 2003; van Strien, Cleven, & Schippers, 2000), while some have found that the effect of disinhibition is better accounted for by other constructs such as attributional style (Rotenberg & Flood, 2000). In addition, van Strien et al. (2002) found that the WF and CD subscales interacted with the preload in opposite directions in the prediction of food intake during the taste test, suggesting that the component parts of Herman and Polivy's Restraint Scale may be differentially related to behavioral outcomes. Finally, as with other aspects of restrained eating, the outcome of laboratory studies seems partly dependent on the participants' weights. van Strien et al. (2007) note that the disinhibition effect has never been observed in overweight restrained eaters. This observation reinforces the recommendation that the RS not be used in overweight samples.

While some of the laboratory studies cited here seem to suggest that restrained eaters eat less than unrestrained eaters in the absence of a disinhibiting stimulus (Herman & Polivy, 1984), a series of studies by Stice and colleagues (Stice et al., 2004, 2007) strongly suggest that such laboratory-based findings of reduced eating by restrained eaters in the laboratory do not generalize to their food intake outside the laboratory.

Readability

The reading level of the RS has been estimated to be between the fourth and ninth grades (Allison & Franklin, 1993).

Stunkard and Messick's TFEQ-R Scale

Description

The Three Factor Eating Questionnaire (TFEQ), also known as the Eating Inventory (Stunkard & Messick, 1988), was created by Stunkard and Messick (1985) in response to a developing awareness of the limitations of the RS. The authors expressed concerns with regard to the content of the RS and its construct validity. In regards to the content of the RS, the authors point out that, while the RS was not designed to measure the behavior of over-weight and obese persons, its creators had suggested that the RS measured the construct of dieting as *separate* from the construct of overweight. Furthermore, they indicated that the cause of many behaviors associated with obesity was a history of dieting per se (Hibscher & Herman, 1977). However, it became increasingly apparent that the RS was indeed influenced by obesity. Some studies reported that overweight restrained eaters did not show evidence of disinhibited eating as did normal-weight restrained eaters. Furthermore, the RS contains items related to weight fluctuation that may artificially inflate the scale scores of persons suf-fering from overweight and obesity. Finally, the relationships that researchers reported for the RS and various outcome measures such as food consumption varied in strength and even direction, and the relationships seemed to vary by obesity status. Herman and Polivy's hypothesis that restraint accounted for the eating behavior of obese individuals was not sup-ported by reports that restrained obese individuals did not demonstrate counterregulatory eating (Ruderman, 1986).

In response to these concerns, as well as the desire for a measure that would be more reli-ably related to food intake in normal-weight and obese persons, Stunkard (1981) and later Stunkard and Messick (1985) developed the restraint scale of the TFEQ (TFEQ-R). The first ver-sion of the TFEQ borrowed several items from the RS and Pudel et al.'s (1975) Latent Obesity Questionnaire, and 17 original items were also included. The variety of questions included in the scale reflects Stunkard and Messick's intention to capture several facets of eating behavior, including but not limited to dietary restraint.

The original 67-item scale was administered to a sample of 220 participants, including both genders and persons of both obese and normal weight. An exploratory factor analysis includ-ing all participants suggested three factors, representing behavioral restraint, lability in behav-ior and weight, and hunger. The results were essentially equivalent when separate factor analyses were conducted for men and women, as well as three groups of participants who were ostensibly low, medium, and high on restraint.

On the basis of these preliminary results, the authors modified some items and added oth-ers in an effort to capture more accurately the constructs measured by each of the newly iden-tified factors and to heighten the distinctiveness of each factor. A new sample, consisting of 53 (7 men and 46 women) participants in the same intensive weight loss program and 45 (5 men, 13 women, and 27 of indeterminate gender) completed a questionnaire comprising 93 items, including those that were unchanged, modified, and newly written. Of those, 58 items were selected for inclusion in the final version of the TFEQ. The items in the final measure were selected because of significant partial correlations with their provisional factors, while holding the other two subscales constant. Finally, the subscales were given new names: Cognitive Control of Eating (Factor I), Disinhibition (Factor II), and Susceptibility to Hunger (Factor III). Cronbach's alpha was .92, .91, and .85 for Factors I, III, and III, respectively. A cor-relation of −.43 was found for Factors I and II, −.03 for Factors I and III, and .42 for Factors II and III. Although the scale was originally published as the Three-Factor Eating Questionnaire (Stunkard & Messick, 1985), it is now published by the Psychological Corporation as the *Eating Inventory* (Stunkard & Messick, 1988). For the purposes of the present chapter, we shall confine our discussion mainly to the Restraint Factor scale and shall refer to the restraint scale of the TFEQ as the TFEQ-R.

Sample

As described in the previous section, a preliminary set of items was tested on a sample of 97 men and 123 women. The sample consisted of 78 "dieters" who were members of an intensive weight loss group, 62 nonobese "free eaters" who were selected by the dieters, and 80 persons who were chosen by the dieters for geographic proximity. The ages of the participants ranged from 17 to 77 years with a mean of 44.

A second sample of 53 dieters (7 men and 46 women) and 45 free eaters (5 men, 13 women, and 27 of indeterminate gender) was used to refine the instrument. As before, the free eaters were nominated by the dieters, who were recruited from an intensive weight loss program. This second sample was used to identify the norms in the next section.

Norms

Means, sample sizes, and standard deviations for participant groups on the TFEQ-R are presented in Table 5.4. As with other measures of restraint, studies often report lower TFEQ-R scores for men than women (e.g., Bellisle et al., 2004; de Castro, 1995). Stunkard and Messick (1988) suggest tentative TFEQ-R guidelines of 0 to 10 as "low average," 11 to 13 as "high," and 14 or more as "clinical range." Care should be taken when attempting to classify persons into high- or low-restraint groups, as TFEQ-R scores differ by gender and nationality. Furthermore, scores should be interpreted in the context of the other characteristics of the responder. For example, a low TFEQ-R score in an obese person with obesity-related health problems may be a cause for concern, whereas a high restraint score in a thin woman could be problematic.

It should also be noted that researchers sometimes change the dichotomized response format of the true/false items in the TFEQ-R to a 4-point response scale. This practice seems especially common in twin studies of the genetic component of eating behaviors (e.g., Neale, Mazzeo, & Bulik, 2003; Tholin, Rasmussen, Tynelius, & Karlson, 2005). While this practice may facilitate studies of heredity, the TFEQ-R scores reported in these studies are not directly comparable to studies using the standard scoring rubric.

Reliability

Internal Consistency

As can been seen in Table 5.2, Cronbach's alpha for the TFEQ-R is routinely reported to be at or greater than .80. Unlike the RS, the TFEQ appears to be equally reliable for normal-weight and obese persons.

Test-Retest

Stunkard and Messick (1985) cited an unpublished manuscript by Ganley that reported a test-retest correlation over a 1-month interval to be .93. Allison et al. (1992) found test-retest

Table 5.4   Mean Three-Factor Eating Questionnaire–Restraint Scale (TFEQ-R) Scores Reported in the Literature

Participants	Author	n	Mean	SD
Unrestrained eaters	Stunkard and Messick (1985)	62	6.0	5.5
Swedish control group	Bjorvell et al. (1986)[a]	58	9.8	4.2
Chilean university students	Lolas (1987)[a]	88	7.7	5.1
U.S. control sample	Ganley (1986)[a]	30	11.0	5.3
American adult men	French, Jeffery, and Wing (1994)	99	5.9	4.2
American adult women	French et al. (1994)	103	9.1	4.2
Postmenopausal American women At baseline At 4-year follow-up	Hays, Bathalon, Robenoff, McCrory, and Roberts (2006)	 36 36	 10.6 9.0	 6.9 5.5
American adults	Williamson et al. (2007)	46	7.8	4.1
Japanese high school girls	Nogami (1986)[a]	243	5.6	3.7
Female White American college students	Atlas, Smith, Hohlstein, McCarthy, and Kroll (2002)	300	10.4	5.4
Female African American college students		200	8.9	5.3

American college students
    Females only
    Males only
	Allison et al. (1992)	901
		617
		282
			9.0
			10.26
			6.1
				5.8
				5.6
				5.1

American male college students	Boerner, Spillane, Anderson, and Smith (2004)	214	4.7	4.7
American female college students	Boerner et al. (2004)	215	8.2	5.7
Australian female college students	Ricciardelli, Tate, and Williams (1997)	172	15.9	8.4
Japanese nursing students	Nogami (1986)[a]	270	6.3	3.6
German women	Laessle, Tuschl, Kotthaus, and Pirke (1989)	62	6.5	4.7
German women in a weight reduction program	Westenhoefer (1991)	46,132	13.1	4.3
German men in a weight reduction program	Westenhoefer (1991)	8,393	10.6	4.7

a. Reported in Stunkard and Messick (1988).

reliability to be .91 over a 2-week span. Bond, McDowell, and Wilkinson (2001) reported a test-retest coefficient of .81 over 1 year.

Validity

Content Validity

Factorial Composition. While the focus of this chapter is measures of restraint, findings involving the other two TFEQ subscales are reviewed below because they can help shed light on the domain assessed by the TFEQ-R. Factor analyses of the full TFEQ, including items from all three subscales, typically find that a three-factor solution fits the data well. Stunkard and Messick (1985) conducted several factor analyses during development of the measure, with the express intention of creating distinct subscales. Little variation in the factor structure was found between dieters in a weight loss program who were ostensibly restrained eaters and neighbors of the dieters who were ostensibly moderately restrained. However, the factor structure for a group of "free eaters" was slightly less simple, possibly because of infrequent endorsement of items related to restraint and disinhibition. Regardless, the restraint factor (Factor I) was robust across all groups. Highly similar results were obtained by Hyland, Irvine, Thacker, and Dan (1989) and Ganley (1988).

Boerner et al. (2004) used structural equation modeling to conduct a confirmatory factor analysis of several measures of eating attitudes and behaviors simultaneously. Items from the subscales of each measure were combined into item parcels to facilitate analysis. The authors found that the typical three-factor model fit the TFEQ very well. Similar results were obtained by Atlas, Smith, Hohlstein, McCarthy, and Kroll (2002). In contrast, Mazzeo, Aggen, Anderson, Tozzi, and Bulik (2003) tested three models of the TFEQ using two types of confirmatory factor analysis and found that none of the models produced an acceptable fit of the data. However, the authors used a modified TFEQ that excluded 15 items and altered the response option for some other items. It is unclear to what degree the results reported in this study may have been affected by Mazzeo et al.'s manipulation of the TFEQ.

Of greater relevance to the study of restrained eating are studies that focus more specifically on the 21 items of the TFEQ-R. Ricciardelli and Williams (1997) examined the factor structure of the TFEQ-R. The sample consisted of 144 female college students. A principal components analysis with varimax rotation identified three factors. The first factor, accounting for 33.5% of the variance, included six items and was labeled *emotional/cognitive concerns for dieting*. The second factor contained seven items, accounted for 7.8% of the variance, and was labeled *calorie knowledge*. The third factor was made up of five items, accounting for 6.6% of the variance, and was labeled *behavioral dieting control*. Three items failed to load on any of the factors. Ricciardelli and Williams suggested that Factors I and III are similar to the constructs of cognitive restraint and behavioral restraint that have been identified in the literature on problem drinking. They conclude that Factor III may be a better measure of successful dieting than the total TFEQ-R, as Factor III was negatively correlated with BMI.

Westenhoefer (1991) identified two highly correlated sources of variance in the TFEQ-R using a variant of discriminant analysis. In a sample of 46,132 female and 8,393 male Germans in a weight loss program, factors were identified representing "Flexible" control and "Rigid" control over eating. Persons scoring highly on the rigid control scale were characterized by a dichotomized, "all-or-nothing" approach to eating. They reported dieting frequently but did not seem to follow any specific plan. On the other hand, individuals scoring highly on flexible control reported eating more slowly, taking smaller helpings, and controlling their eating by using situation-specific guidelines rather than inflexible rules. Rigid control was associated with high disinhibition, whereas flexible control was linked to low disinhibition.

Allison et al. (1992) conducted a principal components factor analysis on the TFEQ-R responses of 901 college students. While the Minimum Average Partial (MAP) test (Zwick & Velicer, 1986) suggested a one-factor solution, and goodness-of-fit indices were good to fair for this model, a two-factor solution similar to that found by Westenhoefer (1991) was eventually retained. Catell's scree test and the Guttman-Kaiser eigenvalues > 1 rule each suggested a two-factor solution. Varimax rotation was attempted but later abandoned when an oblique rotation yielded a simpler factor pattern. The two factors seemed to represent a cognitive dimension (35% of the variance) and a behavioral dimension (6% of the variance) of restraint. However, the correlation between the factors was high ($r = .56$). The authors concluded that the TFEQ-R contains two highly correlated primary factors that can be considered nested within a broader secondary factor.

Gorman et al. (1993) conducted a further analysis of the findings reported in Allison et al. (1992). The high correlation between the two factors and the substantially greater endorsement of items in the cognitive restraint factor as compared to the behavior restraint factor led the authors to consider alternative methods of analyzing the data. Psychometric research has shown that conventional linear factor analysis techniques will often produce spurious factors when items differ considerably in their endorsement rates (G. A. Ferguson, 1941; Gibson, 1967; Horst, 1965; McDonald & Ahlawat, 1974). Thus, Gorman et al. reanalyzed the data using nonlinear techniques, including multidimensional scaling and Rasch model scaling (Hambleton, Swaminathan, & Rogers, 1991), that alleviate the biases of traditional methods. The results suggested that the TFEQ-R items form a continuum that begins with relatively common thoughts of reducing eating and ends with overt, deliberate, but relatively rare actions to reduce eating.

Taken together, these findings suggest that the TFEQ-R performs well as a unidimensional measure of restrained eating but that it can also be further bifurcated into a cognitive and a behavioral component. There is evidence that these two components may form a continuum ranging from typical thoughts of reducing intake to actual behaviors at limiting consumption that are rarely followed through with. While further research involving nonlinear analytic techniques is needed to strengthen this conceptualization of the TFEQ-R, it appears that these results dovetail nicely with recent data suggesting that restrained eaters on the TFEQ-R do not actually reduce their food intake below their energy needs, even though they may wish they could do so (Stice et al., 2004, 2007).

Factor Stability

Allison et al. (1992) found that Tucker's CC was high for random splits of the subject sample (CC > .97) but only modest (CC < .90) when comparing obese and normal-weight participants and low when comparing across gender (CC < .90). However, Boerner et al. (2004) found that the TFEQ-R was invariant across gender using the steps described by Hoyle and Smith (1994) for testing measurement invariance. Atlas et al. (2002) found that the TFEQ-R performed equally well for African Americans as Whites. More research is needed to compare the performance of the TFEQ-R in obese and normal-weight participants.

Construct Validity: Convergent and Divergent Validity

Relationships Among the TFEQ Subscales

Stunkard and Messick intended for the subscales of the TFEQ to be conceptually and empirically distinct. For the most part, this goal seems to have been accomplished, although there is notable overlap between the TFEQ-R and the other subscales, in some reports. For example, Atlas et al. (2002) found a moderately strong correlation between the TFEQ-R and the TFEQ Hunger subscale for both White ($r = .74$) and African American ($r = .77$) women. However, the correlation between the TFEQ-R and the TFEQ Disinhibition subscale was substantially stronger for White ($r = .47$) than African American ($r = .05$) women. Despite the correlations that have been observed in such studies, the TFEQ subscales were never intended to be combined into a single "total" score, and there is no evidence that such an amalgam has any theoretical or empirical utility.

The TFEQ subscales appear to relate to each other differently for obese and normal-weight individuals but similarly across gender. Bellisle et al. (2004) studied these relationships in a sample of 2,509 adults of both genders and varying weights. While correlations between the TFEQ-R and the Disinhibition and Hunger subscales were positive in the lowest BMI groups (i.e., BMI < 27), the relationship became increasingly more negative as BMI increased. In persons with BMI greater than 45, TFEQ-R was moderately negatively correlated with the Disinhibition subscale in women and men. In the same BMI category, the relationship between TFEQ-R and Hunger was $r = -.30$ for women and $r = -.12$ for men. Similar results were found by Foster et al. (1998), who reported moderately negative correlations between TFEQ-R and Disinhibition, as well as between TFEQ-R and Hunger, among overweight women seeking behavioral treatment for weight loss. In a sample of U.S. college students, Boerner et al. (2004) found that the TFEQ-R and Disinhibition subscale was moderately positively correlated among men and women. The correlation between TFEQ-R and Hunger was very weak for men and women. Similarly, in two samples of Dutch female college students, TFEQ-R was correlated with Disinhibition at $r = .36$ and $r = .42$ (Ouwens et al., 2003; van Strien et al., 2000, respectively). In a study by van Strien et al. (2007), a significant difference was observed in the correlation between TFEQ-R and Disinhibition for normal-weight ($r = .41$) and overweight ($r = .07$) subsamples. For people in the normal weight range, it may be that people with low Disinhibition or Hunger scores have very low risk for weight gain (they may be "naturally thin"), whereas those with higher scores may attempt to counter their chronic vulnerability to overeating and weight gain by being more restrained. Among those already obese, most may already be frequently overeating relative to their normal-weight peers, but those who are currently restraining their eating are (at least temporarily) reducing their vulnerability to this overeating.

Weight and Obesity Status

During the measure development process, Stunkard and Messick (1985) found a correlation of .20 between restraint and weight. Since then, a variety of relationships have been reported. Allison et al. (1992) found no significant differences between obese and nonobese participants on the TFEQ-R. Ricciardelli and Williams (1997) reported that the TFEQ-R correlated with BMI ($r = .25$), previous dieting ($r = .64$), and current dieting ($r = .65$) in a sample of female college students. Beiseigel and Nickols-Richardson (2004) found that a subgroup of normal-weight college women with high scores on the TFEQ-R possessed more fat mass (as measured by dual-energy X-ray absorptiometry) and had a higher body fat percentage than a subgroup of women with low restraint scores.

When a French translation of the TFEQ-R was administered to 1,554 participants, 955 of whom were in the obese range, the TFEQ-R scale was positively associated with BMI in men but not in women (Bellisle et al., 2004). Obese and nononbese women did not differ significantly on the TFEQ-R. Furthermore, being obese as a child and/or adolescent was generally associated with more intense restraint, disinhibition, and hunger in adults, whether or not the subject was still obese at the time of the test. The authors conclude that some level of restraint may allow some children to grow out of obesity. This study was conducted with obese persons and their first-degree relatives, so the results may not be generalizable to persons with no family history of obesity.

De Lauzon-Guillain et al. (2006) studied the relationship between eating behavior and weight gain in a community sample of 466 adults and 271 adolescents over a 2-year period in France. At baseline, a French translation of the TFEQ-R was positively associated with BMI in normal-weight participants but not overweight adults. While TFEQ-R scores did not predict changes in adiposity, a higher initial BMI was associated with a larger increase in TFEQ-R. Similarly, Hays, Bathalon, Roubenoff, McCrory, and Roberts (2006) examined predictors of weight change in a sample of 36 nonobese postmenopausal women in a 4-year longitudinal study. Hunger was the only TFEQ subscale that predicted weight gain.

While the previous studies found either a positive relationship or no relationship between TFEQ-R and body size, Westenhoefer, Stunkard, and Pudel (1999) found that the TFEQ-R was negatively associated with BMI in both male and female Germans in a computer-assisted weight loss program. TFEQ-R was also positively associated with successful weight loss. Although not discussed by the authors, there were also apparently significant interactions between TFEQ-R and Disinhibition, such that the antiobesity effects of restraint were stronger at higher levels of disinhibition. This pattern of results was also observed by Williamson et al. (1995). These results are consistent with the previously mentioned argument that dietary restraint may be a desirable characteristic in already overweight individuals.

Westenhoefer et al. (1999) further parsed their results by the flexible and rigid control subscales developed by Westenhoefer (1991). These analyses revealed that rigid control is associated with increased Disinhibition and higher BMI, whereas flexible control is associated with lower Disinhibition and lower BMI. Furthermore, successful weight losers had more flexible control at the beginning of the program and increased their flexible control scores during the program, whereas less successful participants had lower scores at the beginning and did not increase them during the program. Differences for rigid control, while statistically significant, were considerably smaller. The authors conclude that flexible control, but not rigid control, is associated with successful weight reduction. However, just as the potential causal association between restraint and overeating is open to debate (e.g., overeating may increase restraint, not vice versa), so is the causal status of rigid and flexible dieting. It is possible that flexible dieters are able to be flexible because their overeating tendencies are not as severe, whereas rigid dieters have learned that they can only control their eating by employing more definitive dieting rules.

Generally, the TFEQ-R seems to be linked with successful weight loss. In addition to the studies described previously, Foster et al. (1998) found that weight loss treatment was associated with significant increases in restraint and decreases in disinhibition and hunger. Before treatment, higher restraint scores were associated with lower body weights, and greater increases in restraint were correlated with greater weight losses. In a study of 46 adults (26 men and 20 women) seeking weight loss treatment, TFEQ-R scores increased significantly in treatment groups but not the control group (Williamson et al., 2007). Notably, of several measures of dietary restraint, the TFEQ-R was the only measure to be correlated with energy balance (as measured by a combination of doubly labeled water and change in body composition). However, it was the *change* in TFEQ-R, not its absolute value, that was associated with energy balance. Increases in TFEQ-R were associated with an energy deficit. Very little or no change in TFEQ-R was associated with energy excess. TFEQ-R is also related to weight maintenance. Westerterp-Plantenga, Kempen, and Saris (1998) found that participants who successfully maintained weight loss following a very low-calorie diet experienced greater increases in TFEQ-R during the diet, as compared to participants with poorer weight maintenance, who did not experience as great an increase in TFEQ-R while dieting.

TFEQ-R scales have also been linked to the construct of weight suppression (i.e., the difference between current and highest ever weight). de Castro (1995) reported an interaction between TFEQ-R and gender in the prediction of weight suppression in a sample of 201 male and 157 female adults. When participants were trichotomized based on their TFEQ-R scores, the current weights of high-restraint men were 10.5% below their highest weights, whereas the current weights of the moderate- and low-restraint groups were closer to their highest weights (5.2% and 6.6% below their highest weights, respectively). This pattern was not observed for women, who were 6.9% below their highest ever weight in all three restraint groups.

Naturalistic Food Consumption

de Castro (1995) reported that highly restrained eaters had significantly lower self-reported caloric intake than dieters with low restraint. The differences resulted from significantly lower intakes of fat and carbohydrate in restrained eaters (although the usual cautions about under-reporting in restrained eaters apply). In addition, overall daily intakes were less variable with higher levels of restraint. Participants high in restraint had lower deprivation ratios but not satiety ratios. This suggests that highly restrained participants ate significantly less than unrestrained eaters relative to their period of premeal deprivation than did the less restrained subjects, but there was no differential effect of meal size on time to next meal.

In a study of food intake and physical activity, French et al. (1994) found that women who scored highly on the TFEQ-R reported significantly lower caloric intake, lower percent calories from sweets, and less frequent sweets consumption than women with low TFEQ-R scores. Men with high TFEQ-R scores reported a significantly greater percentage of calorie intake from protein and carbohydrate and less frequent consumption of beef, pork, whole milk, and sweets.

Lahteenmaki and Tuorila (1995) studied the relationship between the TFEQ-R and the desired use and liking of a variety of foods in a sample of 253 women and 11 men attending Weight Watchers in Finland. The TFEQ-R was negatively related to the reported use of some food groups such as fruit-based sweet foods, butter, margarine, and regular-fat cheese but not to their desired use or liking. Beiseigel and Nickols-Richardson (2004) found that college women who score highly on the TFEQ-R consumed more servings of fruits and vegetables per day compared to women in a low-restraint group.

Care must be taken when drawing inferences from studies linking the TFEQ-R to lower caloric intake and/or healthier intake (e.g., fewer fats/sweets, more fruits and vegetables) as restrained eaters are known to underestimate their caloric intake to a greater degree than restrained eaters (for a review, see Maurer et al., 2006). Furthermore, the source of the underreporting seems to be disproportionately accounted for by the unhealthiest foods (Maurer et al., 2006).

Eating Disorders and Psychopathology

A plethora of studies report cross-sectional correlations for the TFEQ-R and measures of eating disorders. For example, Boerner et al. (2004) found a correlation of .43 for men and .52 for women between the TFEQ-R and the Bulimia Test–Revised (BULIT-R; Thelen et al., 1991). Similarly, the correlation between the TFEQ-R and the EAT (Garner & Garfinkel, 1979) was .45 for men and .64 for women. Atlas et al. (2002) found that the TFEQ-R correlated with the BULIT-R at .47 for White and .69 for African American college women. Ricciardelli, Tate, and Williams (1997) found evidence that body dissatisfaction may mediate the relationship between the TFEQ-R and the BULIT-R. However, their conclusions are limited by the cross-sectional nature of their research design. Rigid and flexible (Westenhoefer, 1991) control over eating appears to be differentially related to measures of eating disorders. In a field survey of 1,838 West Germans, rigid control was associated with more frequent and more severe binge episodes, whereas flexible control was associated with the opposite (Westenhoefer et al., 1999). The TFEQ-R as a whole was not related to binge frequency or severity. High scores on the TFEQ-R were associated with greater risk for using purging behaviors such as diuretics, laxatives, appetite suppressants, vomiting, physical exercise, and bodybuilding. Higher rigid control was associated with a higher risk of using all of these purging techniques except physical exercise and bodybuilding. Higher flexible control was associated with a lower risk of using diuretics or appetite suppressants and a higher likelihood of using physical exercise or bodybuilding as methods of weight control. Despite the correlations between the TFEQ-R and measures of eating-disordered attitudes and behaviors, Safer, Agras, Lowe, and Bryson (2004) reported that TFEQ-R scores did not decrease significantly during cognitive-behavioral therapy for bulimia in a sample of 134 women.

Correlations between the TFEQ-R and measures of eating-disordered symptomatology should not be interpreted as supporting a causal link between this measure of dieting and eating disorders. For one, the studies finding such a relationship were all done with nonclinical populations, and only a very small percentage was likely to suffer from an eating disorder. Also, if there were a causal link, then those bulimic individuals who are actually dieting to try to lose weight should show particularly high levels of binge eating. Instead, strict dieting is associated with reduced, rather than enhanced, binge-eating frequency (Lowe et al., 1998, 2007). Finally, the observation that TFEQ-R scores do not decrease during treatment (Safer et al., 2004) for bulimia seems to suggest that the construct of dieing tapped by the TFEQ-R is not an important factor in the maintenance of this eating disorder. Prospective studies are needed to determine what, if any, role this type of dieting may play in the development and maintenance of disordered eating.

Susceptibility to Response Sets

Allison et al. (1992) found weak correlations between the TFEQ-R and the Edwards and Marlowe-Crowne Social Desirability Scales ($r = .05$ and $-.21$, respectively). Furthermore, ratings of the social desirability of each item did not correlate with the frequency with which they were endorsed. Finally, instructions to "fake good" and "fake bad" did not result in significantly different means on the TFEQ-R. On the basis of these results, the authors conclude that the TFEQ-R is not unduly influenced by socially desirable responding.

Predictions of Laboratory Behavior

One of the most well-known qualities of Herman and Polivy's Restraint Scale is its ability to predict disinhibited eating in the laboratory setting. In contrast, the TFEQ-R is not typically linked to disinhibited eating in preload/taste test studies (Lowe & Maycock, 1988; Rogers & Hill, 1989; Tuschl, Laessle, Platte, & Pirke, 1990; Westerterp, Nicolson, Boots, Mordant, & Westerterp, 1988; Westerterp-Plantenga et al., 1991). It is more common to find that a tendency toward disinhibited eating, as measured by the Disinhibition subscale of the TFEQ, for example, is a better predictor of overeating (e.g., Ouwens et al., 2003; van Strien et al., 2000). The discrepancy between the RS and the TFEQ-R in the prediction of disinhibited eating often has been explained by the assertion that the TFEQ-R tends to select a broad range of dieters, including those who are successful and unsuccessful, whereas the RS tends to select primarily failed dieters who have a tendency toward overeating (for a review, see van Strien, 1999). Thus, van Strien (1999) recommended that the TFEQ-R be used in conjunction with the TFEQ Disinhibition subscale to independently study the individual and combined associations of these constructs with eating behavior.

Readability

The reading level of the TFEQ-R has been estimated to be between the sixth and ninth grades (Allison & Franklin, 1993).

Availability

The TFEQ can be purchased from Harcourt Assessment (harcourtassessment.com).

Dutch Eating Behavior Questionnaire

Description

van Strien, Frijters, Bergers, et al. (1986) created the Dutch Eating Behavior Questionnaire (DEBQ) to facilitate research on the development and maintenance of human obesity. The measure was created partly in response to psychosomatic theory, externality theory, and Herman and Polivy's restraint theory, all of which suggest that obesity is attributable to overeating.

The DEBQ was created in response to the same criticisms of the RS that led Stunkard and Messick to develop the TFEQ. While the TFEQ was published before the DEBQ, the two measures were under development at about the same time. In fact, both scales borrowed items from Pudel's et al.'s (1975) Latent Obesity Questionnaire, which may partially explain any correlation observed between the DEBQ and TFEQ restraint scales. In addition to a restraint subscale that was intended to be distinct from measures of overeating and independent of obesity status, the DEBQ includes subscales for emotional eating and external eating. The restraint subscale includes items pertaining to deliberate, planned weight control. The emotional eating subscale prompts individuals to indicate how often they experience a desire to eat as a result of unpleasant emotions such as anxiety, sadness, and boredom. The external eating subscale has items that refer to increased consumption or desire for food in the presence of food-related stimuli.

During the initial measure development process of the DEBQ, a pool of 100 items taken from previous measures, including the Eating Patterns Questionnaire and the Eating Behavior Inventory (O'Neil et al., 1979), were administered to a sample of 140 participants, including normal-weight and obese individuals. A series of factor analyses and item analyses were used to identify items that appeared factorially simple (i.e., tended to load only on one factor). In addition, some items were revised, and new items created, to increase the distinctiveness of the subscales.

The final scale consisted of 33 items divided among three subscales. The response options for each item are on a Likert-type scale with the following categories: *never* (1), *seldom* (2), *sometimes* (3), *often* (4), and *very often* (5). The subscales of the DEBQ are typically scored by calculating the average response for all items in each scale. Although the developers' intention was to create a measure with three distinct factors, a fourth factor was identified during the final analyses that represented emotional eating while bored. This fourth factor was not included as a formal subscale, as it contained items that loaded highly on other subscales, and was not of specific theoretical interest. For our purposes, all further discussion will be limited to the restraint subscale (DEBQ-R) of the DEBQ.

Sample

The final form of the DEBQ was tested on a sample of 517 male and 653 female participants, 114 of whom were obese.

Norms

Table 5.5 presents norms for the DEBQ restraint scale. Women appear to score higher on the DEBQ-R than men, and obese individuals seem to have higher scores than persons of normal weight. Care should be taken when classifying individuals as restrained and unrestrained as no empirically validated cutoff exists, and the distribution of scores varies by nationality. Although sample medians are often used to create two restraint groups, it is generally preferable to treat the DEBQ-R score (or any restraint score) as continuous when possible.

Reliability

Internal Consistency

The rigorous development process of the DEBQ resulted in a restraint factor with high internal consistency. As can be seen in Table 5.2, Cronbach's alpha is generally greater than .90. Furthermore, the scale appears to be equally reliable in normal-weight and obese individuals.

Table 5.5 Mean Dutch Eating Behavior Questionnaire–Restraint Subscale (DEBQ-R) Scores Reported in the Literature

Participants	Author	n	Mean	SD
Dutch adults	van Strien, Frijters, Bergers, and Defares (1986)	1169	2.2	0.9
Men only		498	1.8	0.8
Obese men only		71	2.3	0.8
Nonobese men only		427	1.8	0.7
Women only		642	2.5	0.9
Obese women only		73	3.0	0.8
Nonobese women only		569	2.4	0.9
Dutch college students	Ouwens, van Strien, and van der Staak (2003)	209	2.6	0.9
Dutch college students	van Strien, Cleven, and Schippers (2000)	200	2.6	0.8
Normal-weight female Dutch college students	van Strien, Herman, Engels, Larsen, and van Leeuwe (2007)	349	2.6	0.8
Overweight, nonobese Dutch women	van Strien et al. (2007)	409	3.2	0.7
American college students	Allison, Kalinsky, and Gorman (1992)	901	2.9	1.0
Men only		281	2.3	0.9
Obese men only		7	3.1	0.8
Nonobese men only		274	2.3	0.0
Women only		607	3.1	1.0
Obese women only		23	3.2	0.8
Nonobese women only		584	3.1	1.0
Australian Grade 9 female adolescents	Banasiak, Wertheim, Koerner, and Voudouris (2001)	393	2.7	0.8
English men	Wardle (1986)	45	1.9	0.8
English women	Wardle (1986)	102	2.7	0.0
German women	Laessle, Tuschl, Kotthaus, and Pirke (1989)	60	2.4	0.6

Test-Retest

In a sample of 165 adolescent girls, Banasiak, Wertheim, Koerner, and Voudouris (2001) found the test-retest reliability of the DEBQ-R to be .85 after a delay of 4 to 5 weeks. The retest coefficient for a 2-week span was .92.

Validity

Factorial Composition

Few published studies have tested the factor structure of the DEBQ. Of those that have, the majority found that a simple three-factor solution including all 33 items fits the data quite well, with a restraint factor that is clearly separate from the factors representing emotional eating and external eating (van Strien, Frijters, Bergers, et al.,1986; Wardle, 1987). van Strien, Frijters, Bergers, et al. (1986) also found the factor structure to be invariant for both genders and persons of obese and normal weight.

Two other studies investigated the factor structure of the 10-item DEBQ restraint scale. After completing both exploratory and confirmatory factor analyses, Allison et al. (1992) concluded that the DEBQ-R was best described by a unifactorial solution accounting for 68% of the variance. However, Ogden (1993) observed that the DEBQ-R contains two potentially confounded aspects of dietary restraint: attempts at food restriction and actual restrictive behavior. To examine this possibility, she conducted an exploratory factor analysis of a modified DEBQ-R in which extra items were added to questions, including the word *try,* that specifically distinguished between intended restraint and successful restraint. In addition, two new items were added: "Do you attempt to diet in order to lose weight?" and "Do you regard yourself as a successful dieter?" All items but Item 4 loaded on a single factor containing the two additional items, which suggests that individuals do not distinguish between attempts at restraint and actual restraint behaviors. However, the possibility remains that restrained eating varies on a single continuum ranging from intentions to diet to actual restrictive behaviors, as was found in studies of the TFEQ-R by Gorman et al. (1993) and Allison et al. (1992).

Factor Stability

During the measure development process, van Strien, Frijters, Bergers, et al. (1986) noted that the pattern of item-total scale correlations was similar for obese and normal-weight participants. Allison et al. (1992) conducted separate factor analyses of the DEBQ-R for obese and normal-weight participants, for men and women, and for random splits of the sample. They found that Tucker's congruence coefficients were at least .990 in each split. Based on these data, the factor stability of the DEBQ-R seems excellent.

Construct Validity: Convergent and Discriminant Validity

Preliminary evidence suggests that the restraint subscale of the DEBQ is minimally related to the other two DEBQ subscales. van Strien, Frijters, Bergers, et al. (1986) report that the DEBQ restraint scale correlated at .37 with the DEBQ emotional eating scale and .16 with the DEBQ external eating subscale in a mixed sample of normal-weight and obese individuals.

Weight and Obesity Status

The mean DEBQ-R scores of 76 friendship cliques consisting of 523 adolescent girls were correlated with mean clique BMI ($r = .38$; Paxton, Schutz, Wertheim, & Muir, 1999). In a randomized controlled trial of behavioral weight loss interventions, DEBQ-R scores increased significantly in the three treatment conditions but not in a control condition (Williamson et al., 2007). The sample consisted of 46 overweight ($25 < BMI < 30$ kg/m^2) individuals.

Ogden (1993) studied a sample of "successful," "reasonable," and "failed" dieters, who were categorized based on whether they rated their success at dieting as higher, equivalent, or lower than their attempts at dieting, respectively. DEBQ-R scores were highest among the failed dieters, lowest among the successful dieters, and intermediate among the reasonable dieters. While this finding suggests that the DEBQ-R is related to unsuccessful attempts at dieting, care must be taken when interpreting the results, as there is no assessment of the reliability or validity of the self-reported measures of dieting frequency or success used in this study.

Naturalistic Food Consumption

Several studies have reported moderate negative correlations between caloric intake and the DEBQ-R. In a sample of 50 female undergraduates and university staff, Wardle and Beales (1987) found a correlation of −.28 between the DEBQ-R and caloric intake over a 1-day period, as assessed by interviewers trained in conducting 24-hour food recalls. Similarly, in a sample of 110 Dutch women, van Strien, Frijters, Staveren, Defares, and Deurenberg (1986) reported a correlation of −.47 between the DEBQ-R and a measure of deviation from required energy intake, which was computed by subtracting the mean caloric intake across three 24-hour food recalls from an estimate of the number of calories needed for weight maintenance. This finding suggests that individuals who score high on the DEBQ-R consume fewer calories than what is needed to sustain their current body weight. Some of this difference may be the result of ingesting fewer high-calorie foods, as the DEBQ-R also correlated at −.28 with fat intake and −.38 with sugar intake. Laessle et al. (1989) also found that the DEBQ-R correlated at −.49 with a measure of caloric intake based on computer-assisted analysis of 7-day food diaries that were completed by 60 normal-weight women. Collectively, these studies seem to indicate that the DEBQ-R identifies individuals with comparatively lower food intake, which may result in negative energy balance. However, this conclusion is qualified by previously mentioned research that finds restrained eaters systematically underreport their food intake to a greater degree than unrestrained eaters and that the source of the underreporting is disproportionately accounted for by the unhealthiest foods (Stice et al., 2004, 2007).

Prediction of Laboratory Behavior

Unlike the Restraint Scale, higher scores on the DEBQ-R are not typically associated with disinhibited eating behavior in preload studies. Of the studies that failed to detect disinhibited eating following a preload, two studies found a small but significant positive relationship between the DEBQ-R and food consumption during the "taste test" (van Strien et al., 2000; Wardle & Beales, 1987), while one other did not (Ouwens et al., 2003). Despite the lack of a disinhibition effect, participants scoring high on the DEBQ-R have been known to exhibit increased food consumption following a cognitive task (Lattimore & Caswell, 2004; Wallis & Hetherington, 2004) and a task involving ego threat (Wallis & Hetherington, 2004). In addition, female restrained eaters (as identified by a median split of DEBQ-R scores) tended to consume more calories than unrestrained eaters, when given ad libitum access to large amounts of palatable food (Jansen, 1996). Notably, unrestrained eaters were able to estimate their caloric intake quite well, while restrained eaters underestimated their intake.

Disordered Eating and Psychopathology

Like other measures of dietary restraint, the DEBQ-R is often correlated with eating-disordered attitudes and behaviors, as well as general measures of psychopathology. In a sample of 123 young adults, DEBQ-R was significantly associated with a measure of anxiety, but only for women (Jeffery & French, 1999). DEBQ-R was not associated with depression in either gender. Paxton et al. (1999) studied restraint and disordered eating in 79 friendship cliques consisting of 523 adolescent girls. The DEBQ-R was significantly correlated with mean clique scores for body image concerns and extreme weight loss behavior but not depression, self-esteem, or anxiety. Stice et al. (1997) reported correlations of .62, .53, and .69 between the DEBQ-R and the BULIT-R total score, the BULIT-R binge control subscale, and the bulimia factor of the EAT, respectively, among 117 female college students. However, some of the relationship between the DEBQ-R and measures of psychopathology may be explained by other variables. For example, in a study of 1,177 adolescent girls over a 1-year period, F. Johnson and Wardle (2005) found that the cross-sectional and prospective relationships between the DEBQ-R and symptoms of bulimia, low self-esteem, and depression were better accounted for by body dissatisfaction. The presence and later development of abnormal eating attitudes was the only outcome with which restraint was independently associated.

Susceptibility to Response Sets

The DEBQ-R does not appear to be unduly influenced by social desirability responding or dissimulation. The correlation between the DEBQ-R and social desirability scales such as the Marlowe-Crowne Social Desirability Scale ($r = -.08$) and the Edwards Social Desirability Scale ($r = -.24$) appears to be weak and statistically nonsignificant (correlation coefficients from Allison et al., 1992; also see Corrigan & Ekstrand, 1988; van Strien, Frijters, Roosen, Knuiman-Hijl, & Defares, 1985). When each item of the DEBQ-R was rated for its social desirability, Allison et al. (1992) found that the social desirability ratings correlated with item endorsement at .67, indicating that the more desirable items were endorsed more frequently. When participants were instructed to "fake good" or "fake bad," the resulting mean DEBQ-R scores were not significantly lower or higher than when such instructions were not given. These findings indicate that the DEBQ-R scale has good discriminant validity.

Readability

The reading level of the TFEQ-R has been estimated to be between the fifth and eighth grades (Allison & Franklin, 1993).

Availability

The DEBQ-R was originally printed in van Strien, Frijters, Bergers, et al. (1986).

Other Scales

The RS, TFEQ-R, and DEBQ-R are typically the measures of choice when studying restrained eating. However, there are a few other scales worth mentioning, although most of the following lack much psychometric evidence to support their reliability or validity. One exception is the restraint scale of the Eating Disorders Examination, which is available in questionnaire (EDE-Q; Fairburn & Beglin, 1994) and interview (EDE; Fairburn & Cooper, 1993) forms. The EDE is primarily a diagnostic tool for anorexia and bulimia nervosa, for which its reliability and validity have been well demonstrated. However, the EDE is intended for use only in eating-disordered samples. As such, the restraint subscale is not appropriate for use with nonclinical samples.

A restraint interview was created by Rand and Kuldau (1991) for use with nonclinical samples that may have certain advantages, including the potential for phone-based assessment and no requirement of reading skills on the part of the subject. Also, there is some thought that interviews may be less susceptible to dissimulation, given a skilled interviewer. Child versions of the RS and TFEQ were developed by Hill et al. (Hill, Rogers, & Blundell, 1989; Hill, Weaver, & Blundell, 1990). Other instruments that purport to measure restraint have been developed by Coker and Roger (1990) and Smead (1990).

Relationships Among the Restraint Scales

Intercorrelations among the RS, TFEQ-R, and DEBQ-R are illustrated in Table 5.6. The TFEQ-R borrowed items from the RS, and the TFEQ-R and DEBQ-R both contain items from Pudel et al.'s (1975) Latent Obesity Scale. Thus, high correlations among the three restraint measures are not surprising. The correlations among measures appear to be similar for men and women. In contrast, correlations among scales appear to be lower for overweight than normal-weight individuals, especially for correlations between the RS and the other two scales. van Strien et al. (2007) report that the correlations between the RS (including the total score and both subscales) and the DEBQ-R and TFEQ-R are significantly lower for overweight women than normal-weight women. As discussed previously, the RS was not designed for use with overweight individuals and has questionable validity when used with this population. The lower correlations among restraint scales for overweight individuals are further evidence that the restraint constructs applied to normal-weight individuals do not translate perfectly to overweight samples.

Wardle (1986) reported greater correlations between the DEBQ-R and the RS CD subscale ($r = .75$ for women and $r = .76$ for men) than the RS WF subscale ($r = .24$ for women and $r = .37$ for men). A similar pattern of results was reported by Boerner et al. (2004) for the relationship between the TFEQ-R and RS subscales, as well as by van Strien et al. (2007) for the RS subscales and both the TFEQ-R and DEBQ-R. These findings suggest that the three scales share common variance related to cognitive restraint but that the RS WF subscale measures a dimension that the other two scales do not address.

The relationships among the three restraint measures have also been tested by conducting factor analyses on the scale scores for the restraint scales and sometimes other measures of eating behavior and weight concerns. For example, Allison et al. (1992) took the factors identified in factor analyses of each individual restraint scale and performed a second-order principal components factor analysis on these factors to look for overlap among the scales. The result was a three-factor solution. The first factor represented cognitive restraint and had high loadings from

Table 5.6   Intercorrelations Among Restraint Scales

Reference	n	Coefficient alpha	Sample Characteristics
RS and TFEQ-R			
Allison, Kalinsky, and Gorman (1992)	901	.74	Obese and normal-weight college students
Boerner, Spillane, Anderson, and Smith (2004)	214	.63	Male college students
Boerner et al. (2004)	215	.68	Female college students
Laessle, Tuschl, Kotthaus, and Pirke (1989)	60	.35	Normal-weight women
Ouwens, van Strien, and van der Staak (2003)	209	.73	Female college students
van Strien, Cleven, and Schippers (2000)	200	.57	Female college students
Williamson et al. (2007)	46	.51	Overweight men and women
van Strien, Herman, Engels, Larsen, and van Leeuwe (2007)	349	.74	Normal-weight female college students
van Strien et al. (2007)	409	.35	Overweight, nonobese women
RS and DEBQ-R			
Allison et al. (1992)	901	.80	Obese and normal-weight college students
Laessle et al. (1989)	60	.59	Normal-weight women
Ouwens et at. (2003)	209	.69	Female college students
Stice, Ozer, and Kees (1997)	117	.83	Female college students
van Strien et al. (2000)	200	.55	Female college students
Williamson et al. (2007)	46	.55	Overweight men and women
van Strien et al. (2007)	349	.71	Normal-weight female college students
van Strien et al. (2007)	409	.36	Overweight, nonobese women
Wardle (1986)	147	.72	Female college students
Wardle (1986)	147	.75	Male college students
TFEQ and DEBQ-R			
Allison et al. (1992)	901	.89	Obese and normal-weight college students
Laessle et al. (1989)	60	.66	Normal-weight women
Ouwens et at. (2003)	209	.85	Female college students
van Strien et al. (2000)	200	.75	Female college students
Williamson et al. (2007)	46	.69	Overweight men and women
van Strien et al. (2007)	349	.86	Normal-weight female college students
van Strien et al. (2007)	409	.66	Overweight, nonobese women

NOTE: DEBQ-R = Dutch Eating Behavior Questionnaire–Restraint subscale; RS = Restraint Scale; TFEQ-R = Three-Factor Eating Questionnaire–Restraint scale.

the RS Concern With Dieting subscale, the DEBQ-R, and the TFEQ-R Factor I (cognitive restraint). The second factor consisted of Factor I (cognitive restraint) and Factor II (behavioral restraint) from the TFEQ-R and was therefore determined to be representative of a general restraint factor specific to the TFEQ-R. The third factor included only the RS Weight Fluctuation subscale. The authors concluded that the three scales share some common variance but that the TFEQ-R is the only scale that measures behavioral restraint, and the RS WF subscale is the only measure of weight fluctuation.

Laessle et al. (1989) conducted a factor-analytic investigation that included the RS, the DEBQ-R, and the TFEQ restraint and disinhibition scales, as well as measures of weight history, self-reported mean daily caloric intake, disordered eating, and body figure consciousness. The first factor had high loadings from the RS, scales representing counterregulatory or disinhibited eating (the Eating Disorder Inventory Bulimia subscale and the TFEQ Disinhibition subscale), and measures representing body concern (Eating Disorder Inventory Body Dissatisfaction and Drive for Thinness subscales and the Body Shape Questionnaire). The second factor had high loadings from the RS and weight-related measures (BMI, maximum BMI, and a BMI fluctuation index). The third factor had high loadings from the TFEQ-R and the DEBQ-R, as well as a negative loading on mean caloric intake.

van Strien et al. (2007), noting the three-factor solution obtained by Laessle et al. (1989), conducted a series of confirmatory factor analyses to determine how the three measures of restraint would load on three factors representing overeating, dieting, and body dissatisfaction. The overeating factor included the Eating Disorder Inventor Bulimia subscale, the DEBQ Emotional Eating and External Eating subscales, and the question, "Have you ever had an eating binge, i.e., you ate an amount of food others would consider unusually large?" The dieting factor included the question, "Are you currently dieting?" The body dissatisfaction factor included the Eating Disorder Inventory Drive for Thinness and Body Dissatisfaction subscales. The best-fit models for the TFEQ-R and DEBQ-R were the ones in which these scales loaded only on the dieting factor but not the overeating or body dissatisfaction factors. This was true for normal-weight and overweight subsamples. In contrast, the best-fit model for the RS was the one in which it loaded on all three factors, rather than just the dieting factor. There was an association between dieting and overeating in the normal-weight sample that was absent in the overweight sample.

The results of Laessle et al. (1989) and van Strien et al. (2007) seem to confirm that the TFEQ-R and DEBQ-R are "purer" measures of restraint, whereas the RS taps constructs related to unsuccessful dieting such as overeating and weight fluctuation. Furthermore, the findings of van Strien et al. may explain why overweight individuals do not show disinhibited eating in preload studies; they lack the association between restraint and overeating that is present among normal-weight individuals.

Future Research Directions

One priority for future research is improving our understanding of what the different restraint scales are actually measuring. Our review makes it clear that the RS reflects both the tendency to lose control over eating and the effort to resist that tendency. The fact that the RS taps both tendencies simultaneously might be advantageous for some research questions, but the field's understanding of factors that promote and inhibit overeating would be better served by research designs that analytically separate these two factors. Research that has categorized participants on both the TFEQ disinhibition scale and the TFEQ restraint scale (e.g., Westenhoefer et al., 1994) represents one way of doing this.

For the TFEQ-R and the DEBQ-R, it is becoming apparent that these scales do not identify individuals who are in negative energy balance or who are restricting their energy intake relative to unrestrained eaters (Stice et al., 2004, 2007). However, they may be restricting their intake relative to what they would *like* to eat (Lowe & Butryn, 2007). Although forced preloads do not elicit counterregulatory eating in restrained eaters identified by these scales, it is possible that such individuals would nonetheless show poorer eating regulation in situations in which multiple disinhibiting influences are operating simultaneously (e.g., a social gathering where alcohol and a variety of palatable foods are being consumed). It is possible that simply providing ice cream following a milkshake preload simply does not constitute a disinhibiting context powerful enough to overcome these restrained eaters' efforts to avoid overconsumption (e.g., Jansen, 1996).

Another major implication of the evidence reviewed in this chapter is that none of the measures of restrained eating reflects *dieting* as that term is usually understood—that is, losing weight by eating less than needed. Indeed, as Lowe (1993) suggested, "dieting to lose weight" and "restrained eating" appear to be two different constructs that are associated with different and sometimes opposing effects on behavior. Although measures of restrained eating have been shown to be related to a variety of domains (affective, cognitive, behavioral, physiological, and genetic), it cannot be assumed that these associations are due to hypocaloric dieting. Thus, future research is needed to study the effects of "restrained eating" separately from dieting (both in terms of self-labeled current dieting and documented weight loss dieting). Furthermore, if Lowe and Levine (2005) are correct that most restrained eating research should be interpreted in terms of the consequences of eating less than desired rather than eating less

than needed, then new explanations may be needed for many of the findings documented in the restraint literature.

Finally, it is very important to keep in mind that the vast majority of research on restrained eating has been correlational in nature. This, of course, leaves open the question of whether restraint plays the causal role it is assumed to play in eating disregulation and eating disorders. Indeed, when dieting status has been experimentally manipulated, its effects are often opposite (e.g., Foster, Wadden, Kendall, Stunkard, & Vogt, 1996; Presnell & Stice, 2003) to those predicted by the original restraint model (Herman & Polivy, 1975, 1984). This suggests that restrained eating per se may not be responsible for the effects that are often associated with it. Alternatively, since most normal-weight restrained eaters are prone toward weight gain, it may be that restraint acts to moderate a predisposition toward weight gain such that restraint slows but usually does not prevent eventual weight gain. Also, it is important to keep in mind that, to the extent that restrained eating does have causal effects on behavior, they may be quite different depending on why a person is attempting to exercise dietary restraint. For example, an anorexic restrictor, a normal-weight person who is struggling to avoid weight gain, and an obese binge eater may all be "restrained eaters," but the form and consequences of such restraint may be quite different in each.

References

Allison, D. B., & Franklin, R. D. (1993). The readability of three measures of dietary restraint. *Psychotherapy in Private Practice, 12*(3), 53–57.

Allison, D. B., Gorman, B. S., & Primavera, L. H. (1993). Some of the most common questions asked of statistical consultants: Our favorite responses and recommended readings. *Genetic, Social, and General Psychology Monographs, 119*, 153–185.

Allison, D. B., Kalinsky, L. B., & Gorman, B. S. (1992). A comparison of the psychometric properties of three measures of dietary restraint. *Psychological Assessment, 4*, 391–398.

Atlas, J., Smith, G., Hohlstein, L., McCarthy, D., & Kroll, L. (2002). Similarities and differences between Caucasian and African American college women on eating and dieting expectancies, bulimic symptoms, dietary restraint, and disinhibition. *International Journal of Eating Disorders, 32*, 326–334.

Banasiak, S., Wertheim, E., Koerner, J., & Voudouris, N. (2001). Test-retest reliability and internal consistency of a variety of measures of dietary restraint and body concerns in a sample of adolescent girls. *International Journal of Eating Disorders, 29*, 85–89.

Bandini, L. G., Schoeller, D. A., Dyr, H. N., & Dietz, W. H. (1990). Validity of reported energy intake in obese and nonobese adolescents. *American Journal of Clinical Nutrition, 52*, 421–425.

Beiseigel, J., & Nickols-Richardson, S. (2004). Cognitive eating restraint scores are associated with body fatness but not with other measures of dieting in women. *Appetite, 43*, 47–53.

Bellisle, F., Clement, K., LeBarzic, M., LeGall, A., GuyGrand, B., & Basdevant, A. (2004). The eating inventory and body adiposity from leanness to massive obesity: A study of 2509 adults. *Obesity Research, 12*, 2023–2030.

Birch, L. L., Fisher, J. O., & Davison, K. K. (2003). Learning to overeat: Maternal use of restrictive practices promotes girls' eating in the absence of hunger. *American Journal of Clinical Nutrition, 78*, 215–220.

Blanchard, F. A., & Frost, R. O. (1983). Two factors of restraint: Concern for dieting and weight fluctuation. *Behaviour Research and Therapy, 21*, 259–267.

Block, G., Hartman, A. M., Dresser, C. M., Carroll, M. D., Gannon, J., & Gardner, L. (1986). A data-based approach to diet questionnaire design and testing. *American Journal of Epidemiology, 124*, 453–469.

Boerner, L. M., Spillane, N. S., Anderson, K. G., & Smith, G. T. (2004). Similarities and differences between women and men on eating disorder risk factors and symptom measures. *Eating Behaviors, 5*, 209–222.

Bond, M. J., McDowell, A. J., & Wilkinson, J. Y. (2001). The measurement of dietary restraint, disinhibition and hunger: An examination of the factor structure of the three factor eating questionnaire (TFEQ). *International Journal of Obesity & Related Metabolic Disorders: Journal of the International Association for the Study of Obesity, 25*, 900–906.

Bourne, S. K., Bryant, R. A., Griffiths, R. A., Touyz, S. W., & Beumont, P. J. V. (1998). Bulimia nervosa, restrained, and unrestrained eaters: A comparison of non-binge eating behavior. *International Journal of Eating Disorders, 24*, 185–192.

Butryn, M. L., & Wadden, T. A. (2005). Treatment of overweight in children and adolescents: Does dieting increase the risk of eating disorders? *International Journal of Eating Disorders, 37*, 285–293.

Chernyak, Y., & Lowe, M. R. (2007, October). *Differentiating drive for thinness and drive to be thin: Restrained eaters and bulimic individuals have different motives for dieting.* Poster session presented at the annual meeting of the Eating Disorders Research Society, Pittsburg, PA.

Coker, S., & Roger, D. (1990). The construction and preliminary validation of a scale for measuring eating disorders. *Journal of Psychosomatic Research, 34*, 223–231.

Cole, S., & Edelmann, R. (1987). Restraint, eating disorders and need to achieve in state and public school subjects. *Personality and Individual Differences, 8*, 475–482.

Corrigan, S. A., & Ekstrand, M. L. (1988). An investigation of the construct validity of the Dutch Restrained Eating Scale. *Addictive Behaviors, 13*, 303–306.

Crocker, L., & Algina, J. (1986). *Introduction to classical and modern test theory.* New York: Holt, Rinehart & Wilson.

Crowne, D. P., & Marlowe, D. (1964). *The approval motive: Studies in evaluative dependence.* New York: John Wiley.

de Castro, J. (1995). The relationship of cognitive restraint to the spontaneous food and fluid intake of free-living humans. *Physiology & Behavior, 57*, 287–295.

De Lauzon-Guillain, B., Basdevant, A., Romon, M., Karlsson, J., Borys, J. M., Charles, M. A., et al. (2006). Is restrained eating a risk factor for weight gain in a general population? *American Journal of Clinical Nutrition, 83*, 132–138.

Drewnowski, A., Riskey, D., & Desor, J. A. (1982). Feeling fat yet unconcerned: Self-reported overweight and the restraint scale. *Appetite, 3*, 273–279.

Edwards, A. L. (1957). *The social desirability variable in personality assessment and research.* New York: Dryden.

Fairburn, C. G., & Beglin, S. J. (1994). Assessment of eating disorders: Interview or self-report questionnaire? *International Journal of Eating Disorders, 16,* 363–370.

Fairburn, C. G., & Cooper, Z. C. (1993). The eating disorder examination (12th edition). In C. G. Fairburn & G. T. Wilson (Eds.), *Binge eating: Nature, assessment, and treatment* (pp. 317–360). New York: Guilford.

Ferguson, G. A. (1941). The factorial interpretation of test difficulty. *Psychometrika, 6,* 323–329.

Ferguson, K. J., Brink, P. J., Wood, M., & Koop, P. M. (1992). Characteristics of successful dieters as measured by guided interview responses and restraint scale scores. *Journal of the American Dietetic Association, 92,* 1119–1121.

Foster, G. D., Wadden, T. A., Kendall, P. C., Stunkard, A. J., & Vogt, R. A. (1996) Psychological effects of weight loss and regain: A prospective evaluation. *Journal of Consulting and Clinical Psychology, 64,* 752–757.

Foster, G. D., Wadden, T. A., Swain, R. M., Stunkard, A. J., Platte, P., & Vogt, R. A. (1998). The eating inventory in obese women: Clinical correlates and relationship to weight loss. *International Journal of Obesity & Related Metabolic Disorders: Journal of the International Association for the Study of Obesity, 22,* 778–785.

French, S. A., Jeffery, R. W., & Wing, R. R. (1994). Food intake and physical activity: A comparison of three measures of dieting. *Addictive Behaviors, 19,* 401–409.

Ganley, R. M. (1988). Emotional eating and how it relates to dietary restraint, disinhibition, and perceived hunger. *International Journal of Eating Disorders, 7,* 635–647.

Garner, D. M., & Fairburn, C. G. (1988). Relationship between anorexia nervosa and bulimia nervosa: Diagnostic implications. In D. M. Garner & P. E. Garfinkel (Eds.), *Diagnostic issues in anorexia nervosa and bulimia nervosa* (p. 56). New York: Brunner/Mazel.

Garner, D. M., & Garfinkel, P. E. (1979). The eating attitudes test: An index of the symptoms of anorexia nervosa. *Psychological Medicine, 9,* 273–279.

Gibson, W. A. (1967). A latent structure for the simplex. *Psychometrika, 32,* 33–46.

Gorman, B. S., Allison, D. B., & Primavera, L. H. (1993). *The scalability of items of the three-factor eating questionnaire restraint scale: When is a per-*

sonality scale a "scale"? Arlington, VA: Eastern Physiological Association Convention.

Griffiths, R. A., MalliaBlanco, R., Boesenberg, E., Ellis, C., Fischer, K., Taylor, M., et al. (2000). Restrained eating and sociocultural attitudes to appearance and general dissatisfaction. *European Eating Disorders Review, 8,* 394–402.

Hambleton, R. K., Swaminathan, H., & Rogers, H. J. (1991). *Fundamentals of item response theory.* Newbury Park, CA: Sage.

Hawkins, R. C. I., & Clement, P. F. (1984). Binge eating: Measurement problems and a conceptual model. In R. C. Hawkins, W. J. Fremouw, & P. F. Clement (Eds.), *The binge purge syndrome: Diagnosis, treatment, and research* (pp. 229–253). New York: Springer.

Hays, N., Bathalon, G., Roubenoff, R., McCrory, M., & Roberts, S. (2006). Eating behavior and weight change in healthy postmenopausal women: Results of a 4-year longitudinal study. *Journals of Gerontology: Series A: Biological Sciences and Medical Sciences, 61A,* 608–615.

Heatherton, T. F., Herman, C. P., & Polivy, J. (1991). Effects of physical threat and ego threat on eating behavior. *Journal of Personality and Social Psychology, 60,* 138–143.

Heatherton, T. F., Herman, C. P., Polivy, J., King, G. A., & McGree, S. T. (1988). The (mis)measurement of restraint: An analysis of conceptual and psychometric issues. *Journal of Abnormal Psychology, 97,* 19–28.

Heatherton, T. F., & Polivy, J. (1992). *Chronic dieting and eating disorders: A spiral model.* In C. H. Janis, D. L. Tennenbaum, S. E. Hobfoll, & M. A. P. Stephens (Eds.), *The etiology of bulimia nervosa: The individual and familial context* (pp. 133–155). Washington, DC: Hemisphere Publishing Corporation.

Heatherton, T. F., Polivy, J., & Herman, C. P. (1989). Restraint and internal responsiveness: Effects of placebo manipulations of hunger state on eating. *Journal of Abnormal Psychology, 98,* 89–92.

Heatherton, T. F., Polivy, J., & Herman, C. P. (1991). Restraint, weight loss, and variability of body weight. *Journal of Abnormal Psychology, 100,* 78–83.

Herman, C. P., & Mack, D. (1975). Restrained and unrestrained eating. *Journal of Personality, 43,* 647–660.

Herman, C. P., & Polivy, J. (1975). Anxiety, restraint, and eating behavior. *Journal of Abnormal Psychology, 84,* 666–672.

Herman, C. P., & Polivy, J. (1980). *Obesity.* Philadelphia: Saunders.

Herman, C. P., & Polivy, J. (1984). A boundary model for the regulation of eating. In A. J. Stunkard & E. Stellar (Eds.), *Eating and its disorders* (pp. 141–156). New York: Raven.

Hibscher, J. A., & Herman, C. P. (1977). Obesity, dieting, and the expression of "obese" characteristics. *Journal of Comprehensive Physiological Psychology, 91,* 374–380.

Hill, A. J., Rogers, P. J., & Blundell, J. E. (1989). Dietary restraint in young adolescent girls: A functional analysis. *British Journal of Clinical Psychology, 28,* 165–176.

Hill, A. J., Weaver, C., & Blundell, J. E. (1990). Dieting concerns of 10-year-old girls and their mothers. *British Journal of Clinical Psychology, 29,* 346–348.

Horst, P. (1965). *Factor analysis of data matrices.* New York: Holt, Rinehart and Winston.

Hoyle, R. H., & Smith, G. T. (1994). Formulating clinical research hypotheses as structural equation models: A conceptual overview. *Journal of Consulting and Clinical Psychology, 62,* 429–440.

Hyland, M. E., Irvine, S. H., Thacker, C., & Dan, P. L. (1989). Psychometric analysis of the Stunkard-Messick Eating Questionnaire (SMEQ) and comparison with the Dutch Eating Behavior Questionnaire (DEBQ). *Current Psychology: Research & Reviews, 8,* 228–233.

Jansen, A. (1996). How restrained eaters perceive the amount they eat. *British Journal of Clinical Psychology, 35,* 381–392.

Jeffery, R. W., & French, S. A. (1999). Preventing weight gain in adults: The pound of prevention study. *American Journal of Public Health, 89,* 747–751.

Johnson, F., & Wardle, J. (2005). Dietary restraint, body dissatisfaction, and psychological distress: A prospective analysis. *Journal of Abnormal Psychology, 114,* 119–125.

Johnson, W. G., Corrigan, S. A., Crusco, A. H., & Schlundt, D. G. (1986). Restraint among bulimic women. *Addictive Behaviors, 11,* 351–354.

Johnson, W. G., Lake, L., & Mahan, J. M. (1983). Restrained eating: Measuring an elusive construct. *Addictive Behaviors, 8,* 413–418.

Keys, A., Brozek, K., Henschel, A., Mickelsen, O., & Taylor, H. L. (1950). *The biology of human starvation.* Minneapolis: University of Minnesota Press.

Kickham, K., & Gayton, W. F. (1977). Social desirability and the restraint scale. *Psychological Reports, 40,* 550.

Killen, J. D., Hayward, C., Wilson, D. M., & Taylor, C. B. (1994). Factors associated with eating disorder symptoms in a community sample of 6th and 7th grade girls. *International Journal of Eating Disorders, 15,* 357–367.

Killen, J. D., Taylor, C. B., Hayward, C., Haydel, K. F., Wilson, D. M., Hammer, L., et al. (1996). Weight concerns influence the development of eating disorders: A 4-year prospective study. *Journal of Consulting and Clinical Psychology, 64,* 936–940.

Killen, J. D., Taylor, C. B., Hayward, C., & Wilson, D. M. (1994). Pursuit of thinness and onset of eating disorder symptoms in a community sample of adolescent girls: A three-year prospective analysis. *International Journal of Eating Disorders, 16,* 227–238.

Kleifield, E., & Lowe, M. R. (1991). Weight loss and sweetness preferences: The effects of recent versus past weight loss. *Physiology and Behavior, 49,* 1037–1042.

Klem, M. L., Klesges, R. C., Bene, C. R., & Mellon, M. W. (1990). A psychometric study of restraint: The impact of race, gender, weight and marital status. *Addictive Behaviors, 15,* 147–152.

Klem, M. L., Klesges, R. C., & Shadish, W. (1990, November). *Application of confirmatory factor analysis to the dietary restraint scale.* Paper presented to the Association for the Advancement of Behavior Therapy, San Francisco.

Klesges, R. C., Isbell, T. R., & Klesges, L. M. (1992). Relationship between dietary restraint, energy intake, physical activity, and body weight: A prospective analysis. *Journal of Abnormal Psychology, 101,* 668–674.

Klesges, R. C., Klem, M. L., Epkins, C. C., & Klesges, L. M. (1991). A longitudinal evaluation of dietary restraint and its relationship to changes in body weight. *Addictive Behaviors, 16,* 363–368.

Laessle, R. G., Tuschl, R. J., Kotthaus, B. C., & Pirke, K. M. (1989). A comparison of the validity of three scales for the assessment of dietary restraint. *Journal of Abnormal Psychology, 98,* 504–507.

Lahteenmaki, L., & Tuorila, H. (1995). Three-factor eating questionnaire and the use and liking of sweet and fat among dieters. *Physiology & Behavior, 57,* 81–88.

Larsen, J. K., van Strien, T., Eisinga, R., Herman, C. P., & Engels, R. C. M. E. (2007). Dietary restraint: Intention versus behavior to restrict food intake. *Appetite, 49,* 100–108.

Lattimore, P., & Caswell, N. (2004). Differential effects of active and passive stress on food intake in restrained and unrestrained eaters. *Appetite, 42,* 167–173.

Lichtman, S. W., Pisarska, K., Berman, E., Pestone, M., Dowling, H., Offenbacher, E., et al. (1992). Discrepancy between self-reported and actual caloric intake and exercise in obese subjects. *New England Journal of Medicine, 327,* 1893–1898.

Livingstone, M. B., Prentice, A. M., & Strain, J. J. (1990). Accuracy of weighed dietary records in studies of diet and health. *British Medical Journal, 300,* 708–712.

Lowe, M. R. (1984). Dietary concern, weight fluctuations and weight status: Further explorations of the restraint scale. *Behaviour Research and Therapy, 22,* 243–248.

Lowe, M. R. (1993). The effects of dieting on eating behavior: A three-factor model. *Psychological Bulletin, 114,* 100–121.

Lowe, M. R., Annunziato, R. A., Markowitz, J. T., Didie, E., Bellace, D. L., Riddell, L., et al. (2006). Multiple types of dieting prospectively predict weight gain during the freshman year of college. *Appetite, 47,* 83–90.

Lowe, M. R., & Butryn, M. (2007). Hedonic hunger: A new dimension of appetite? *Physiology & Behavior, 91,* 432–439.

Lowe, M. R., Gleaves, D. H., & Murphy-Eberenz, K. P. (1998). On the relation of dieting and bingeing in bulimia nervosa. *Journal of Abnormal Psychology, 107,* 263–271.

Lowe, M. R., & Kleifield, E. (1988). Cognitive restraint, weight suppression, and the regulation of eating. *Appetite, 10,* 159–168.

Lowe, M. R., & Kral, T. V. E. (2006). Stress-induced eating in restrained eaters may not be caused by stress or restraint. *Appetite, 46,* 16–21.

Lowe, M. R., & Levine, A. S. (2005). Eating motives and the controversy over dieting: Eating less than needed versus less than wanted. *Obesity Research, 13,* 797–805.

Lowe, M. R., & Maycock, B. (1988). Restraint, disinhibition, hunger and negative affect eating. *Addictive Behaviors, 13,* 369–377.

Lowe, M. R., Thomas, J. G., Safer, D. L., & Butryn, M. L. (2007). The relationship of weight suppression and dietary restraint to binge eating in bulimia nervosa. *International Journal of Eating Disorders, 40,* 640–644.

Lowe, M. R., Whitlow, J. W., & Bellwoar, V. (1991). Eating regulation: The role of restraint, dieting, and weight. *International Journal of Eating Disorders, 10,* 461–471.

Maurer, J., Taren, D. L., Teixeira, P. J., Thomson, C. A., Lohman, T. G., Going, S. B., et al. (2006). The psychosocial and behavioral characteristics related to energy misreporting. *Nutrition Reviews, 64*(Pt. 1), 53–66.

Maxwell, S. E., & Delaney, H. D. (1993). Bivariate median splits and spurious statistical significance. *Psychological Bulletin, 113,* 181–190.

Mazzeo, S., Aggen, S., Anderson, C., Tozzi, F., & Bulik, C. (2003). Investigating the structure of the eating inventory (three-factor eating questionnaire): A confirmatory approach. *International Journal of Eating Disorders, 34,* 255–264.

McCrae, R. R., & Costa, P. T. (1983a). Joint factors in self-reports and ratings: Neuroticism, extraversion and openness to experience. *Personality and Individual Differences, 4,* 245–255.

McCrae, R. R., & Costa, P. T. (1983b). Social desirability scales: More substance than style. *Journal of Consulting and Clinical Psychology, 51,* 882–888.

McDonald, R. P., & Ahlawat, K. S. (1974). Difficulty factors in binary data. *British Journal of Mathematical and Statistical Psychology, 27,* 82–99.

Neale, B., Mazzeo, S., & Bulik, C. (2003). A twin study of dietary restraint, disinhibition and hunger: An examination of the eating inventory (three factor eating questionnaire). *Twin Research, 6,* 471–478.

Nisbett, R. E. (1972). Hunger, obesity, and the ventromedial hypothalamus. *Psychological Review, 79,* 433–453.

Oates-Johnson, T., & DeCourville, N. (1999). Weight preoccupation, personality, and depression in university students: An interactionist perspective. *Journal of Clinical Psychology, 55,* 1157–1166.

Ogden, J. (1993). The measurement of restraint: Confounding success and failure? *International Journal of Eating Disorders, 13,* 69–76.

O'Neil, P. M., Currey, H. S., Hirsch, A. A., Malcom, R. J., Sexauer, J. D., Riddle, F. E., et al. (1979). Development and validation of the eating behavior inventory. *Journal of Psychopathology and Behavioral Assessment, 1,* 123–132.

Ouwens, M., van Strien, T., & van der Staak, C. F. (2003). Tendency toward overeating and restraint as predictors of food consumption. *Appetite, 40,* 291–298.

Overduin, J., & Jansen, A. (1996). A new scale for use in non-clinical research into disinhibitive eating.

Personality and Individual Differences, 20, 669–677.

Paxton, S. J., Schutz, H. K., Wertheim, E. H., & Muir, S. L. (1999). Friendship clique and peer influences on body image concerns, dietary restraint, extreme weight-loss behaviors, and binge eating in adolescent girls. *Journal of Abnormal Psychology, 108,* 255–266.

Polivy, J., & Herman, C. P. (1983). *Breaking the diet habit: The natural weight alternative.* New York: Basic Books.

Polivy, J., & Herman, C. P. (1985). Dieting and binging: A causal analysis. *American Psychologist, 40,* 193–201.

Polivy, J., & Herman, C. P. (1987). Diagnosis and treatment of normal eating. *Journal of Consulting and Clinical Psychology, 55,* 635–644.

Polivy, J., Herman, C. P., & Howard, K. (1988). The restraint scale: Assessment of dieting. In M. Hersen & A. S. Bellack (Eds.), *Dictionary of behavioral assessment techniques* (p. 377). New York: Pergamon.

Prentice, A. M., Black, A. E., Coward, W. A., Davies, H. L., Goldberg, G. L., & Murgatroyd, P. (1986). High levels of energy expenditure in obese women. *British Medical Journal, 292,* 983–987.

Presnell, K., & Stice, E. (2003). An experimental test of the effect of weight-loss dieting on bulimic pathology: Tipping the scales in a different direction. *Journal of Abnormal Psychology, 112,* 166–170.

Prussin, R. A., & Harvey, P. D. (1991). Depression, dietary restraint, and binge eating in female runners. *Addictive Behaviors, 16,* 295–301.

Pudel, V., Metzdorff, M., & Oetting, M. (1975). Zur personlichkeit adiposer in psychologischen tests unter berucksichtigung latent fettsuchtiger [The personality of obese persons in psychological tests with special consideration on latent obesity]. *Zeitschrift fur Psychosomatische Medizin und Psychoanalyse, 21,* 345–361.

Rand, C. S., & Kuldau, J. M. (1991). Restrained eating (weight concerns) in the general population and among students. *International Journal of Eating Disorders, 10,* 699–708.

Ricciardelli, L., Tate, D., & Williams, R. (1997). Body dissatisfaction as a mediator of the relationship between dietary restraint and bulimic eating patterns. *Appetite, 29,* 43–54.

Ricciardelli, L., & Williams, R. (1997). A two-factor model of dietary restraint. *Journal of clinical psychology, 53,* 123–131.

Rogers, P. J., & Hill, A. J. (1989). Breakdown of dietary restraint following mere exposure to food stimuli: Interrelationships between restraint, hunger, salivation, and food intake. *Addictive Behavior, 14,* 387–397.

Rotenberg, K. J., & Flood, D. (1999). Loneliness, dysphoria, dietary restraint and eating behavior. *International Journal of Eating Disorders, 25,* 55–64.

Rotenberg, K. J., & Flood, D. (2000). Dietary restraint, attributional styles for eating, and preloading effects. *Eating Behaviors, 1,* 63–78.

Ruderman, A. J. (1983). The restraint scale: A psychometric investigation. *Behaviour Research and Therapy, 21,* 253–258.

Ruderman, A. J. (1985). Restraint, obesity and bulimia. *Behaviour Research and Therapy, 23,* 151–156.

Ruderman, A. J. (1986). Dietary restraint: A theoretical and empirical review. *Psychological Bulletin, 99,* 247–262.

Ruderman, A. J., & Grace, P. S. (1987). Restraint, bulimia, and psychopathology. *Addictive Behaviors, 12,* 249–255.

Ruderman, A. J., & Grace, P. S. (1988). Bulimics and restrained eaters: A personality comparison. *Addictive Behaviors, 13,* 359–368.

Russell, G. (1979). Bulimia nervosa: An ominous variant of anorexia nervosa. *Psychological Medicine, 9,* 429–448.

Safer, D., Agras, W. S., Lowe, M., & Bryson, S. (2004). Comparing two measures of eating restraint in bulimic women treated with cognitive-behavioral therapy. *International Journal of Eating Disorders, 36,* 83–88.

Sarwer, D. B., & Wadden, T. A. (1999). The treatment of obesity: What's new, what's recommended. *Journal of Women's Health and Gender-Based Medicine, 8,* 483–493.

Scagliusi, F. B., Polacow, V. O., Cordas, T. A., Coelho, D., Alvarenga, M., Philippi, S. T., et al. (2005). Test-retest reliability and discriminant validity of the restraint scale translated into Portuguese. *Eating Behaviors, 6,* 85–93.

Schachter, S., & Rodin, J. (1974). *Obese humans and rats.* Washington, DC: Erbaum/Halsted.

Simmons, J. R., Smith, G. T., & Hill, K. K. (2002). Validation of eating and dieting expectancy measures in two adolescent samples. *International Journal of Eating Disorders, 31,* 461–473.

Smead, V. S. (1990). A psychometric investigation of the rigorous eating scale. *Psychological Reports, 67,* 555–561.

Smith, M. C., & Thelen, M. H. (1984). Development and validation of a test for bulimia. *Journal of Consulting and Clinical Psychology, 52,* 863–872.

Stein, D. M. (1988). The scaling of restraint and the prediction of eating. *International Journal of Eating Disorders, 7,* 713–717.

Stice, E., Cooper, J., Schoeller, D., Tappe, K., & Lowe, M. (2007). Are dietary restraint scales valid measures of moderate-to long-term dietary restriction? Objective biological and behavioral data suggest not. *Psychological Assessment, 19,* 449–458.

Stice, E., Fisher, M., & Lowe, M. R. (2004). Are dietary restraint scales valid measures of dietary restriction? Unobtrusive observational data suggest not. *Psychological Assessment, 16,* 51–59.

Stice, E., Killen, J. D., Hayward, C., & Taylor, C. B. (1998). Age of onset for binge eating and purging during late adolescence: A 4-year survival analysis. *Journal of Abnormal Psychology, 107,* 671–675.

Stice, E., Ozer, S., & Kees, M. (1997). Relation of dietary restraint to bulimic symptomatology: The effects of the criterion confounding of the restraint scale. *Behaviour Research and Therapy, 35,* 145–152.

Stice, E., Presnell, K., Shaw, H., & Rohde, P. (2005). Psychological and behavioral risk factors for obesity onset in adolescent girls: A prospective study. *Journal of Consulting and Clinical Psychology, 73,* 195–202.

Striegel-Moore, R. H., Silberstein, L. R., & Rodin, J. (1986). Toward an understanding of risk factors for bulimia. *American Psychologist, 41,* 246–263.

Stunkard, A. J. (1981). *The body weight regulatory system: Normal and distributed mechanisms.* New York: Raven.

Stunkard, A. J., & Messick, S. (1985). The three-factor eating questionnaire to measure dietary restraint, disinhibition and hunger. *Journal of Psychosomatic Research, 29,* 71–83.

Stunkard, A. J., & Messick, S. (1988). *The eating inventory.* San Antonio, TX: Psychological Corporation.

Thelen, M. H., Farmer, J., Wonderlich, S., & Smith, M. (1991). A revision of the bulimia test: The BULIT-R. *Psychological Assessment, 3,* 119–124.

Tholin, S., Rasmussen, F., Tynelius, P., & Karlsson, J. (2005). Genetic and environmental influences on eating behavior: The Swedish young male twins study. *American Journal of Clinical Nutrition, 81,* 564–569.

Tiggemann, M. (1994). Dietary restraint as a predictor of reported weight loss and affect. *Psychological Reports, 75*(Pt. 2), 1679–1682.

Timmerman, G. M., & Gregg, E. K. (2003). Dieting, perceived deprivation, and preoccupation with food. *Western Journal of Nursing Research, 25,* 405–418.

Tucker, L. R. (1951). *Personnel research report* (No. 984, Contract DA-49–083, Department of the Army). Princeton, NJ: ETS.

Tuschl, R. J., Laessle, R. G., Platte, P., & Pirke, K. (1990). Differences in food-choice frequencies between restrained and unrestrained eaters. *Appetite, 14,* 9–13.

Urland, G. R., & Ito, T. A. (2005). Have your cake and hate it, too: Ambivalent food attitudes are associated with dietary restraint. *Basic and Applied Social Psychology, 27,* 353–360.

van Strien, T. (1997). The concurrent validity of a classification of dieters with low versus high susceptibility toward failure of restraint. *Addictive Behaviors, 22,* 587–597.

van Strien, T. (1999). Success and failure in the measurement of restraint: Notes and data. *International Journal of Eating Disorders, 25,* 441–449.

van Strien, T., Breteler, M. H. M., & Ouwens, M. A. (2002). Restraint scale, its sub-scales concern for dieting and weight fluctuation. *Personality and Individual Differences, 33,* 791–802.

van Strien, T., Cleven, A., & Schippers, G. (2000). Restraint, tendency toward overeating and ice cream consumption. *International Journal of Eating Disorders, 28,* 333–338.

van Strien, T., Engels, R. C. M. E., van Staveren, W., & Herman, C. P. (2006). The validity of dietary restraint scales: Comment on Stice et al. (2004). *Psychological Assessment, 18,* 89–94.

van Strien, T., Frijters, J. E., Bergers, G. P. A., & Defares, P. B. (1986). Dutch Eating Behaviour Questionnaire for assessment of restrained, emotional and external eating behaviour. *International Journal of Eating Disorders, 5,* 295–315.

van Strien, T., Frijters, J. E. R., Roosen, R. G. F. M., Knuiman-Hijl, W. F. H., & Defares, P. B. (1985). Eating behavior, personality traits and body mass in women. *Addictive Behaviors, 10,* 333–343.

van Strien, T., Frijters, J. E. R., Staveren, W. A., Defares, P. B., & Deurenberg, P. (1986). The predictive validity of the Dutch restrained eating questionnaire. *International Journal of Eating Disorders, 5,* 747–755.

van Strien, T., Herman, C. P., Engels, R. C. M. E., Larsen, J. K., & van Leeuwe, J. F. J. (2007). Construct validation of the restraint scale in normal-weight and overweight females. *Appetite, 49,* 109–121.

Vartanian, L. R., Herman, C. P., & Polivy, J. (2005). Implicit and explicit attitudes toward fatness and thinness: The role of the internalization of societal standard. *Body Image, 2,* 373–381.

Wallis, D. J., & Hetherington, M. M. (2004). Stress and eating: The effects of ego-threat and cognitive demand on food intake in restrained and emotional eaters. *Appetite, 43,* 39–46.

Ward, A., & Mann, T. (2000). Don't mind if I do: Disinhibited eating under cognitive load. *Journal of Personality and Social Psychology, 78,* 753–763.

Wardle, J. (1986). The assessment of restrained eating. *Behaviour Research and Therapy, 24,* 213–215.

Wardle, J. (1987). Eating style: A validation study of the Dutch Eating Behaviour Questionnaire in normal subjects and women with eating disorders. *Journal of Psychosomatic Research, 31,* 161–169.

Wardle, J., & Beales, S. (1987). Restraint and food intake: An experimental study of eating patterns in the laboratory and in normal life. *Behaviour Research and Therapy, 25,* 179–185.

Westenhoefer, J. (1991). Dietary restraint and disinhibition: Is restraint a homogeneous construct? *Appetite, 16,* 45–55.

Westenhoefer, J., Broeckmann, P., Munch, A. K., & Pudel, V. (1994). Cognitive control of eating behaviour and the disinhibition effect. *Appetite, 23,* 27–41.

Westenhoefer, J., Stunkard, A., & Pudel, V. (1999). Validation of the flexible and rigid control dimensions of dietary restraint. *International Journal of Eating Disorders, 26,* 53–64.

Westerterp, K. R., Nicolson, N. A., Boots, J. M., Mordant, A., & Westerterp, M. S. (1988). Obesity, restrained eating and the cumulative intake curve. *Appetite, 11,* 119–128.

Westerterp-Plantenga, M. S., Kempen, K. P., & Saris, W. H. (1998). Determinants of weight maintenance in women after diet-induced weight reduction. *International Journal of Obesity & Related Metabolic Disorders: Journal of the International Association for the Study of Obesity, 22,* 1–6.

Westerterp-Plantenga, M. S., Wouters, L., & ten Hoor, F. (1991). Restrained eating, obesity, and cumulative food intake curves during four-course meals. *Appetite, 16,* 149–158.

Williams, A., Spencer, C. P., & Edelmann, R. J. (1987). Restraint theory, locus of control and the situational analysis of binge eating. *Personality and Individual Differences, 8,* 67–74.

Williamson, D. A., Lawson, O. J., Brooks, E. R., Wozniak, P. J., Ryan, D. H., Bray, G. A., et al. (1995). Association of body mass with dietary restraint and disinhibition. *Appetite, 25,* 31–41.

Williamson, D. A., Martin, C. K., York-Crowe, E., Anton, S. D., Redman, L. M., Han, H., et al. (2007). Measurement of dietary restraint: Validity tests of four questionnaires. *Appetite, 48,* 183–192.

Wilson, A. J., Touyz, S. W., Dunn, S. M., & Beumont, P. (1989). The Eating Behavior Rating Scale (EBRS): A measure of eating pathology in anorexia nervosa. *International Journal of Eating Disorders, 8,* 583–592.

Zwick, W. R., & Velicer, W. F. (1986). Comparison of five rules for determining the number of components to retain. *Psychological Bulletin, 99,* 432–442.

CHAPTER 6

Measures of Physical Activity and Exercise

Donna Spruijt-Metz, David Berrigan, Louise A. Kelly,
Rob McConnell, Donna Dueker, Greg Lindsey, Audie
A. Atienza, Selena Nguyen-Rodriguez, Melinda L. Irwin,
Jennifer Wolch, Michael Jerrett, Zaria Tatalovich, and Susan Redline

Introduction

Why Measure Physical Activity?

Physical activity has many health benefits, including reduced obesity (Goran, Reynolds, & Lindquist, 1999; Bergman, Ader, Huecking, & Van Citters, 2002); reduced risk for cardiovascular disease (McTiernan, Ulrich, Slate, & Potter, 1998), osteoporosis (Stallings, 1997; Lysen & Walker, 1997), and type 2 diabetes (Diabetes Prevention Program Research Group, 2002); the reduction of breast cancer risk by as much as 40% (McTiernan et al., 2003; A. Patel & Bernstein, 2006; Thune, Brenn, Lund, & Gaard,

1997; Verloop, Rookus, van der Kooy, & van Leeuwen, 2000); reduction of risk for many other cancers, including colon (Slattery et al., 1997; Wu, Paganini-Hill, Ross, & Henderson, 1987) and endometrial cancer (Friedenreich & Orenstein, 2002; Sturgeon et al., 1993); and improved mental health and well-being (Suitor & Kraak, 2007). Measurement of physical activity levels can thus inform medical decisions, decisions pertaining to an individual's exercise needs, competing programmatic interventions, and the management of public facilities. Therefore, accurate measures of physical activity and inactivity are essential to assess physical activity levels and to determine the effectiveness of interventions to

AUTHORS' NOTE: This work was supported by the NCI Centers for Transdisciplinary Research on Energetics and Cancer (TREC) (U54CA116847, U54CA116848, U54CA116849, U54CA116867, U01CA116850). All authors except Dr. Lindsey are members of the Physical Activity, Sleep and Environmental Measures Working Group, funded by NCI as part of the TREC initiative. We are grateful to Capt. Richard Troiano for his expert comments on an earlier draft on this chapter. The opinions or assertions contained herein are the private ones of the authors and are not considered as official or reflecting the views of the National Institutes of Health.

increase physical activity and decrease sedentary behaviors (Sirard & Pate, 2001).

What Is Physical Activity?

Physical activity is conceived of as bodily movement that is produced by the contraction of muscle and increases energy expenditure (U.S. Department of Health and Human Services [DHHS], 1996). In this conceptualization, some form of physical activity takes place during daily chores, leisure activities, organized sports, workouts, and sleep.

Exercise (exercise training) is defined separately as planned structured and repetitive bodily movement done to promote or maintain one or more components of physical fitness (Institute of Medicine, 2002). Although physical activity and exercise are defined differently, they are often captured together in measures of overall levels of physical activity. Depending on the hypotheses of a particular study and the measures chosen, it may or may not be important to tease these apart.

Sedentary behavior (sometimes labeled *inactivity*) and sleep have tended to be conceptualized as the absence of movement, living on a continuum from movement (activity) to sedentary behaviors (inactivity) to sleep, and not necessarily requiring separate measures. However, to understand the full spectrum of human activity/movement, researchers in the field of physical activity research are beginning to develop a comprehensive battery of distinct measures for all aspects of activity/movement, including sedentary behaviors and sleep.

As the field expands, many researchers agree that to fully understand physical activity, they must measure the entire spectrum of bodily movement in context. Important advances are being made in the conceptualization and measurement of environmental aspects of physical activity, including technological advances in geographical information and placement systems.

Overview of This Chapter

This chapter is a product of a collaboration of the members of the Physical Activity, Sleep and Environmental Measures Working Group, which is part of the Centers for Transdisciplinary Research on Energetics and Cancer, an initiative of the National Cancer Institute. In it, we explore the complex task of measurement of physical activity. The chapter begins with a primer on how to select physical activity measures for research and evaluation purposes. Then, the more "traditional" genres of physical activity measures are reviewed, moving from objective (observation, accelerometers, and pedometers) through subjective measures (such as self-report by questionnaire). Next, the measurement of sleep and movement in sleep are discussed. This is followed by a discussion of the measurement of physical activity in the environment. An introduction to emerging technologies for the measurement of physical activity and some of the challenges that this wealth of measures poses to the researcher close the chapter.

Some further aspects of our choices in preparing this review are worth highlighting. This review is not intended to provide specific recommendations concerning a single measure of physical activity (PA) appropriate for a given study. Our primary aims are to highlight some of the main considerations associated with selecting a set of PA measurement tools and to showcase new developments in measurement of energy expenditure that are worth considering when designing studies concerning physical activity. These developments include a growing interest in sleep as an element of the activity and energy balance equation, an intense recent focus on the potential influence of the built environment on physical activity, and the potential for new technologies to enhance our ability to capture the nature, context, and, to some extent, the consequences of physical activity.

Measures of physical activity are frequently validated against "gold standards" or criterion measures. These include energy expenditure (doubly labeled water), heart rate (by monitor), and cardiorespiratory fitness (indirect calorimetry or heart rate). However, it must be noted that energy expenditure, fitness, and heart rate can be construed—at least to some extent—as *outcomes* of physical activity. All three constructs are distinct from physical activity, and this may limit their functionality as criterion measures for validation of physical activity measures. For this reason, direct observation of movement has been put forward as the most appropriate standard for physical activity assessment, certainly for children (Sirard & Pate, 2001). As this chapter will illustrate, the task of measuring physical activity is complex. Therefore, we have restricted this chapter to a discussion of the ever-widening array of direct measures of physical activity and movement. Indirect measures of physical activity, including energy expenditure (doubly labeled water) and heart rate (by monitor), are not included in this chapter. Other chapters in this volume, particularly Chapter 16, examine indirect measures of physical activity.

A Brief Word on Measures of Physical Fitness

The complexities of measuring physical fitness are as subtle as those of measuring physical activity. Furthermore, physical fitness is often considered an *outcome* of physical activity rather than a *component* thereof. Therefore, we have chosen not to review the many measures of physical fitness in this chapter. However, because fitness is closely tied to physical activity, we will give a brief overview of fitness measurement here and then refer the interested reader to the considerable literature on fitness assessment. Components of physical fitness include cardiorespiratory endurance, flexibility, muscular strength, and endurance (Baranowski et al., 1992; Casperson, Powell, & Christenson, 1985; Pate, 1988). Other components often tested include balance, agility, flexibility, and coordination (U.S. DHHS, 1996). Body composition is considered by some as a component of physical fitness (Heyward, 2006), but it is more often construed as an outcome of physical fitness (M. S. Johnson et al., 2000). VO_{2max}—maximal oxygen uptake (also called *aerobic power* or *directly measured maximal aerobic power*)—is the gold standard for measuring cardiorespiratory fitness. VO_{2max} is assessed by

walking, running, and cycling and is measured using expired air composition and respiratory volume during maximal exertion, usually in a laboratory situation because of equipment requirements. Field measures of fitness often involve running, jogging, or walking a specified distance or time and are converted to an estimate of VO_{2max}. Submaximal cycle ergometer tests with measured heart rate are also common cardiovascular fitness measures (Sallis, 1993). Tests of muscular strength and endurance include pull-ups, palms-forward pull-ups and palms-facing chin-ups, modified pull-up tests, bench press, bent-arm hangs, and several measures of flexibility (such as the sit-and-reach test; U.S. DHHS, 1996). Two of the most widely used field measures for physical fitness testing in healthy populations include AAHPERD's Physical Best battery (McSwegin, 1989) and the Cooper Institute's Fitnessgram (Welk, Morrow, & Falls, 2002). All of these measures are extremely age and health status sensitive and are not safe, valid, or accurate for all populations. Specific protocols must be used to accommodate the participants being tested. For a scholarly review of fitness assessment, there are several excellent books available, including Hayward's (2006) volume.

Learning Objectives

We hope that this chapter will serve as an entrée to diverse topics in the measurement of PA and guide creative thinking about measurement of PA in diverse research and applied activities. The chapter is intended to help people consider what they should measure to address the specific goals of their task. Further review, collaboration, and expert consultation will be required to select the optimal tools available in this rapidly evolving aspect of energy balance–related research.

Modalities for Measuring Physical Activity

Increasing our understanding of physical activity and exercise behavior involves acquisition of information about people's patterns of activity and exercise. These behaviors can be studied through direct observation, measurement of activity using devices such as pedometers or accelerometers, use of indirect measures such as heart rate or capacity for oxygen exchange, analyses of self-reports of activity on questionnaires, or measurement and analysis of sleep patterns and other periods of activity, inactivity, and sedentariness. Physical activity is subject to Counting (people who are active in a recreational area or steps on a pedometer), Looking (direct observation), Asking (surveys and questionnaires, interviews, diaries, logs), Inference (through indirect measures such as calorimetry and doubly labeled water), and objective Measurement (accelerometry). We developed the acronym for all these modalities, CLAIM, to represent the breadth and depth of choices that must be made when measuring physical activity.

Every measurement approach to PA has its caveats. The very act of recording or (self-)observation may influence a participant's behavior (reactivity; Welk, 2002). Because no single approach to the study of physical activity provides complete information, multiple approaches generally are preferred because their use enables complementary insights that enrich interpretations and understanding.

Domains of Measurement

Regardless of measurement modality, physical activity is usually captured in one of five domains of measurement: (1) *intensity,* which is the ratio of working metabolic rate to resting metabolic rate (METs), where one MET, or metabolic equivalent, represents the metabolic rate of an individual at rest and is estimated at 3.5 mL of oxygen consumed per kilogram of body mass per minute, or 1 kcal/kg/h; (2) *energy expenditure* in kilocalories (kcal) or kilocalories per kilogram of body weight; (3) time spent (*duration*) and/or (4) *type* of specific activity (e.g., leisure, occupational, household, organized sports; Ainsworth,

Haskell, et al., 1993); and (5) *frequency* with which a particular activity is undertaken—how often in a day, week, month, or year—depending on the nature of the research question. Some questionnaires are designed to measure intensity, duration, and frequency of very specific activities only, such as questionnaires that only measure walking. Depending on the measurement modalities employed, these domains can be combined in many ways—for instance, in order to capture time spent at a particular level of intensity in a specific type of activity.

Choosing Measures of Physical Activity: The Six Constraints

Research and evaluation projects may require very specific instruments designed to assess particular kinds of physical activity in one or more settings. Thus, there is no prescription for objective versus subjective measurement or for one specific survey tool. Instead, for any given study, the investigators must determine what they want to measure and what tool they can best use in the face of temporal, budgetary, and population constraints. Major constraints include the following:

1. *The research hypothesis and physical activity domains of interest.* The choice of measures must be closely matched to the research hypotheses. For instance, to understand dose response in an intervention to lower stress by physical activity, researchers might be interested in frequency, intensity, and duration of bouts of physical activity. This might be accomplished by using an accelerometer. An intervention to increase certain kinds of physical activity, such as walking, might aim to specifically measure the targeted activity, and it might not always be important to measure physical activity in other domains. This might be accomplished by using a questionnaire. The energetic effects of unintentional activity, such as fidgeting, might be of interest to understand the effects of movement on metabolism. This might require direct observation, doubly

labeled water, or calorimetry. To understand the effects of new urban trail landscaping on recreational trail use at a population level, researchers might use a combination of infrared sensors and geographic information systems (GIS).

2. The target population. Choice of measures and data analyses should furthermore be closely matched to the targeted population. Language and reading level must be taken into account for questionnaires or interviews. In particular, the age of subjects must be taken into consideration. Questionnaires that have been validated in adults will not necessarily be valid in children. In fact, surveys that have been validated in 14- to 16-year-olds are more than likely invalid in 10- to 12-year-olds. Accelerometers produce data that are translated (usually to time spent in light, moderate, and vigorous activity) prior to data analysis using count cut points to define boundaries between METs. Cut points must be chosen that are appropriate for the age group being studied and for the specific accelerometer being used (Freedson, Pober, & Janz, 2005).

3. Special populations. Finally, working with special populations may inform or dictate the choice of measures. For instance, when working with cancer patients and survivors, assessment methods need to be particularly sensitive to measure change in physical activity duration and intensity, as well as types of physical activity. For some cancer survivors who are receiving treatment, certain activities of daily living become difficult to do (e.g., grocery shopping). Questionnaires that assess only recreational physical activity will not be sensitive enough to measure activities of daily living. Very young children or people suffering from cognitive impairment may be unable to answer questions about their daily activities, and parents or caretakers may be asked to provide proxy information.

4. Budgetary considerations. Data collection is expensive, and the availability of resources for its acquisition generally is limited. For instance, even if objective measurement of physical activity is desired, accelerometers that costs upwards of $300 a piece may be beyond a study budget. For any study, the most complete and complex data are always desirable. However, these come at ever-increasing costs, and there is a tipping point, or a point of diminishing returns, where the cost (in money or person-hours) can no longer be justified in the context of the study, the sample size cannot carry the variable load, or data collection at ever-increasing costs incurs proportionally reduced returns. Hence, analysts must specify research questions carefully and consider the trade-offs among methods for acquiring information to ensure that the methods chosen will provide the requisite data within the financial and time constraints governing the investigation.

5. Recommendations. U.S. physical activity recommendations currently emphasize achieving 30 minutes or more of moderate-intensity physical activity 5 or more days per week (U.S. DHHS, 1996), and for healthy adults, it has been argued that such activities should occur in bouts of 10+ minutes (Pate et al., 1995). However, more recent reviews have suggested that 60+ minutes of moderate to vigorous PA 5 or more days per week may be required for weight loss or to maintain weight loss (U.S. Department of Agriculture, 2005). Furthermore, few studies explicitly contrast the health benefits of different patterns of physical activity such as 10-minute bouts versus activity that occurs in shorter time intervals (Macfarlane, Taylor, & Cuddihy, 2006). Further use of devices such as accelerometers could help address this gap in the literature (Troiano, 2008). Guidelines for physical activity levels will continue to evolve as we learn more about associations between PA and health for specific populations and specific outcomes. Notwithstanding debates (on recommendations concerning physical activity levels and health benefits of various bout lengths) and measurement shortcomings (many self-report instruments do not allow the assessment of the number of days in which PA occurred), there is often a strong interest in assessing adherence to current PA recommendations, particularly in evaluation and public health–oriented studies. This interest may constrain the choice of measurement tools or require incorporations of multiple tools in a given study.

6. *Time constraints.* Complete assessments of physical activity in multiple domains may require the employment of lengthy instruments. In studies where physical activity is a primary manipulation or outcome, lengthy measures may be warranted and may not overburden participants. However, participant burden and complex studies that involve multiple psychosocial and environmental mediators and moderators of a physical activity may dictate feasibility of various measures. It is thus important to remember that such long instruments cannot always be included in telephone surveys or in the context of studies measuring many different constructs.

Choosing Multiple Measures of Physical Activity

As research in the field progresses, many studies have moved to incorporate more than one measurement modality to capture physical activity. Table 6.1 shows how multiple measures of physical activity were matched to population and research questions (as reflected in the title of the projects) across three centers and 12 studies that comprise the Transdisciplinary Centers for Energetics and Cancer. Table 6.1 includes measures of physical activity and sleep for each study. Many of the studies have also incorporated several measures of the built environment, such as street connectivity and availability of parks and trails, not depicted in Table 6.1.

Measuring Physical Activity by Direct Observation

Observation of Physical Activity and Exercise Using Instruments

Direct observation of physical activity, which can be accomplished through field observation or with instrumentation, is one of the most basic approaches to the acquisition of information about behaviors. Direct observation provides information about how people exercise and play, how environments shape their activities, and how people use specific facilities such as parks, sidewalks, or trails. Direct observation of behaviors thus can inform decisions that include medical decisions about an individual's exercise needs, public health decisions about competing programmatic interventions to encourage physical activity, and public works decisions about the management of public facilities. In general, direct observation by field observers can provide richer information than direct observation by instrumentation but at higher costs, mainly because of the costs of labor. Approaches involving observation through instrumentation generally are difficult to implement over large areas and typically provide less information about the personal characteristics of individuals such as age, gender, race, or ethnicity that are important in understanding behavior. The trade-offs among approaches are clear if one compares the types of data obtained through use of various tools. One such comparison example would be the use of SOFIT and SOPLAY by observers in the field (see below) with the data obtained from infrared monitors that will be illustrated here.

Direct observation of physical activity and exercise has been undertaken in management of public works, especially in recreation and transportation, for many years, primarily for purposes such as determining priorities for expansion or maintenance of facilities. For example, public works managers historically have installed pneumatic tubes on bikeways and paths to obtain counts of users to inform decisions that require information about level of use. In the field of recreation, general guidelines for planning park and greenway facilities published by the National Recreation and Park Association (Mertes & Hall, 1996) require information about use relative to facility capacity. Researchers have summarized data related to the use of particular facilities such as bike paths (Hunter & Huang, 1995) and sidewalks (Davis, King, & Robertson, 1998), although

(Text continues on page 197)

Table 6.1 Projects, Populations, and Physical Activity/Sleep Measures Across the four NCI Centers for Transdisciplinary Research in Energetics and Cancer (University of Southern California: PI Michael Goran, Case Western Reserve University: PI Nathan Berger, Fred Hutchinson Cancer Research Center: PI Anne McTiernan, University of Minnesota: PI Robert Jeffries)

Project Title	Population: Age, Gender, Ethnicity	Study Design	Subjective PA Measures	Objective PA Measures	Subjective Sleep Measures	Objective Sleep Measures
Insulin Resistance Syndrome Pathway Factors and Colon Polyps (L. Li)	21–80 years Male and female	Prospective case control study	AAFQ (C. L. Craig et al., 2003)	None	None	None
Determinants of Obesity and Metabolic Dysfunction in Adolescents (S. Redline)	16–19 years Male and female	Longitudinal cohort	3DPAR (Kriska et al., 1990; Kriska & Bennett, 1992) PA items from Nurses' Health Survey	Accelerometry: uniaxial CSA, WAM 6471 Epochs: 1 minute 5–7 days	Sleep-wake inference via 5- to 7-day sleep diary (Kump et al., 1994) Snoring and sleep habits via Cleveland Sleep & Health Questionnaire (Wolfson et al., 2003), Sleep Habits (Pate, Ross, Dowda, Trost, & Sirard, 2003), and Epworth Sleepiness Scale (Aaron et al., 1995)	Sleep times via wrist actigraphy for 5–7 days Overnight polysomnography
Etiology of Adolescent Obesity (L. Lytle)	15–18 years One adult caregiver Male and female	Cohort study	3DPAR (Pate et al., 2003) IPAQ (Godin & Shepard, 1985) MAQ-A (C. L. Craig et al., 2003)	Accelerometry: MTI Actigraph (Model #7164) Epochs: 30 seconds 7 days	Sleep items adapted from NEDS (Night Eating)	None

(Continued)

Table 6.1 (Continued)

Project Title	Population: Age, Gender, Ethnicity	Study Design	Subjective PA Measures	Objective PA Measures	Subjective Sleep Measures	Objective Sleep Measures
Household Environmental Weight Gain Prevention (S. French)	Birth to adults (all ages) Male and female	Group randomized trial	3DPAR (Staten et al., 2001) IPAQ (Backhaus, Junghanns, Broocks, Riemann, & Hohagen, 2002; Buysse, Reynolds, Monk, Berman, & Kupfer, 1989; Carpenter & Andrykowski, 1998)	None	None	None
Women, Oxidative Stress, Estrogens and Exercise (WISER) (M. Kurzer)	18–30 years Female	Randomized control trial	Adapted MAQ (Kriska et al., 1990; Kriska & Bennett, 1992)	None	Snoring and sleep habits via leveland Sleep & Health Questionnaire (Levine, Kaplan, et al., 2003; Levine, Lewis, et al., 2003) and Sleep Habits (Pate et al., 2003)	None
Obesity-Related Metabolic Risk for Cancer: Ethnicity and Response to Exercise in Minority Youth Goran, M)	9th - 12th grade Male & Female African-American & Latino	Randomized control trial	3DPAR (Johns, 1992)	Accelerometry: Actigraph Epochs: 15sec 7 days	None	None
Insulin Resistance and Declining	8–11 years Female African	Longitudinal observation study	PA items from YRBS High School Survey MAQ-A (Spilsbury et al.,	Accelerometry: Actigraph Epochs: 15	None	None

Project Title	Population: Age, Gender, Ethnicity	Study Design	Subjective PA Measures	Objective PA Measures	Subjective Sleep Measures	Objective Sleep Measures
Levels in African Americans and Latina Girls (D. Spruijt-Metz)	and Latino		3DPAR (Puhl, Greaves, Hoyt, & Barnowski, 1990)			
Influence of Built Environments on the Development of Obesity During Childhood (M. Jerrett)	9–11 years Male and female Multiethnic	Longitudinal cohort	Items developed to assess PA and time outdoors in 5- to 7-year-olds (no validated measure available for this age group) Parent completed survey	Pedometry: Yamax SW-701 Collected at 6–7 years 3 days	None	None
Preventing Obesity in Worksites (S. Beresford)	18–65 years Male and female	Randomized control trial	Abbreviated GLTEQ (Rowe, van der Mars, Schuldheisz, & Fox, 2004) Abbreviated IPAQ (Pope, Coleman, Gonzalez, Barron, & Heath, 2002)	Pedometry: New Lifestyles (NL)-2000 piezoelectric 4–7 days Subsample NL-800 7 days	None	None
Glycemic Load & Obesity Effects on	18–45 years Male and female	Randomized control crossover feeding trial	AAFQ (McKenzie, Sallis, Nader, Patterson, et al., 1991)	None	Sleep quality via PSQI (Heath, Coleman, Lensegrav, & Fallon, 2006)	None

(Continued)

Table 6.1 (Continued)

Project Title	Population: Age, Gender, Ethnicity	Study Design	Subjective PA Measures	Objective PA Measures	Subjective Sleep Measures	Objective Sleep Measures
Cancer Biomarkers (J. Lampe and M. Neuhouser)			Daily activity recorded on daily food intake record			
Exercise and Diet: Biomarkers and Mechanisms in Humans (A. McTiernan and N. Ulrich)	Postmenopausal Female	Randomized control trial	Adapted MAQ (McKenzie, Sallis, Nader, Patterson, et al., 1991)	Pedometry: Accusplit 7 days	Insomnia via WHIIRS (McKenzie, Marshall, Sallis, & Conway, 2000)	None
Fitness, Fatness and Cancer: Biomarkers in Overweight Adolescent Girls (G. Duncan)	14–18 years Female	Pilot study: cross-sectional and prospective arms	3DPAR		Sleepiness via modified Epworth Sleepiness Scale Sleep habits via Adolescent Sleep-Wake Scale	None

NOTE:3DPAR = 3-Day Physical Activity Recall; AAFQ = Arizona Activity Frequency Questionnaire; GLTEQ = Godin Leisure-Time Exercise Questionnaire; IPAQ = International Physical Activity Questionnaire; MAQ-A = Modifiable Activity Questionnaire for Adolescents; PA = physical activity; PSQI = Pittsburg Sleep Quality Index; WHIIRS = Women's Health Initiative Insomnia Rating Scale; YRBS = Youth Risk Behavior Surveillance Survey.

the quality of information available about the "number of bicyclists and pedestrians by facility or geographic area" is "poor," and the "priority for better data" remains "high" (U.S. Department of Transportation, 2000, p. 45). With increased interest in the public health benefits of physical activity and exercise, interest in direct observation of use of facilities has increased, demand for more detailed information has grown, and new technologies for observation have been developed.

Instruments available for monitoring physical activity and exercise include pneumatic tubes for counting bicyclists; infrared sensors for counting path, trail, or sidewalk users; and digital video cameras for observing numbers, patterns, and characteristics of park or facility users. These instruments can be purchased from different manufacturers that provide varying levels of support for operations. New devices that combine features of existing instruments are becoming available (e.g., infrared sensors with magnets to detect cyclists and provide separate counts of pedestrians and cyclists).

Table 6.2 is a general overview of the types of information that can be obtained with different instruments. Table 6.2 also summarizes some considerations in the use of these different technologies. Criteria for choosing among instruments include type of information desired, accuracy, durability, reliability, ease of operation, and cost. For example, pneumatic tubes may be an efficient way to obtain information about cyclists' use of multiuse trails, but if information about use by both cyclists and pedestrians is required, then infrared sensors may be needed. If more information than simple traffic counts is needed (e.g., direction of travel or characteristics of users), then infrared sensors will be insufficient, and analysts will need to consider video technology or supplementing instrumentation with field observations, recognizing that, in either case, the costs will be higher. With any of the instruments, similar considerations must be given to site selection, mounting and installation of equipment, strategies to deter vandalism, and protocols for maintenance, data collection, and analytic procedures. The types

of trade-offs inherent in choices made concerning measurement modalities can be illustrated through the following example.

Monitoring Trail Traffic in Indiana

In 2000, the Indiana Departments of Natural Resources and Transportation initiated the Indiana Trail Study, a project to count and interview users on six trails across the state (Eppley Institute for Parks and Public Lands, 2001). The primary aims of the project were to obtain counts of users on separate, multiuse trails and information about user patterns and preferences for trail use. Results of the study have been used to inform trail planning and investment decisions in the state. In 2005, with support from the Active Living Research (ALR) program sponsored by the Robert Wood Johnson Foundation, the Indianapolis trail monitoring network was expanded from 6 to 30 locations, creating the most comprehensive, longest running monitoring system in the United States (Lindsey, Han, Wilson, & Yang, 2006; Lindsey, Wilson, Rubchinskaya, Yang, & Han, 2007). The primary aims of the ALR project were to identify environmental correlates of trail traffic, explain variation in trail traffic, develop a model for forecasting trail traffic, and measure elasticity of trail traffic in response to policy variables. Obtaining objective measures of trail use (i.e., traffic) was thus integral to both studies.

Choice of Observation Methods

Because documenting levels of trail use or trail traffic—not mode of use—was a principal objective of each study, researchers chose to use infrared monitors supplemented with direct observation of trail users in the field as the principal means of observation. Pneumatic tubes were not used to count users because they would have provided information only about use by cyclists, and video monitoring was not used because it was too expensive to install and would have required labor-intensive coding and analysis of the video imagery.

Table 6.2 General Overview of Instruments for Observing Physical Activity and Exercise

Instruments/ Devices	Examples of Information Provided	Considerations in Use

Turn-styles	Counts of users of controlled-access play areas or pedestrian pathways	Limited applicability (specific areas/facilities) and type of information (counts)
		 Durable and generally reliable
		 Sources of error:
		     Children carried may not be counted (undercount)
		     Users may spin turn-style (overcount)

Pneumatic tubes or pressure pads	Tubes: counts of bicyclists on street bikeways, trails, or paths
	 Pads: counts of traffic
		Limited applicability (linear facilities) and type of information (counts)
		 Tubes durable and generally reliable
		 Pads must be buried outdoors and do not work where ground freezes
		 Pads can be used indoors
		 Sources of error:
		     Pedestrians stepping on tubes
		     Potential malfunctioning or vandalism
		     Multiple steps on pads

Infrared counters	Counts of pedestrians or cyclists on paths, trails, or sidewalks	Limited applicability (linear facilities) and type of information (counts both cyclists and pedestrians but does not differentiate mode of use)
		 Durable and generally reliable
		 Requires power source and frequent downloading of information (1–2 times/week to once per 4–6 weeks depending on level of use and capacity of counter)
		 Sources of error:
		     Users passing simultaneously
		     Human error in downloading information
		     Potential malfunctioning due to weather or insect infestation or vandalism

Video cameras	Counts, patterns, and characteristics of users of park spaces or facilities or trails and paths	Potential broad applicability for variety of parks, spaces, and facilities, but problems of site selection and installation are complex
		 Technology proven for security but few applications for physical activity known
		 Requires power source, periodic data collection (remote transmittal of data is expensive), and time-consuming reanalysis of data to extract relevant information
		 Sources of error:
		     Potential malfunctioning or vandalism
		     Poor image quality may hinder interpretation
		     Human error in downloading and coding

The battery-operated infrared monitors include a transmitter, which emits a beam of infrared pulses, and a receiver that records an event whenever the beam is broken. The length of time the beam must be interrupted (i.e., the number of pulses that must be missed) before an event is recorded can be varied to permit monitoring of different types of use. Experimentation with the infrared monitors to determine proper settings revealed that sensors systematically undercount users because only single events are recorded when multiple users pass the monitor simultaneously. Field observations of trail use then were completed to determine magnitudes of error and to provide general information about mode of use (i.e., cycling, walking, running, skating, wheelchairs, or strollers) and user characteristics (e.g., gender, race, and individual or group use). Analyses revealed that the error rate was a function of traffic flow, with more errors occurring with higher flow rates. Because hourly counts are the building block for most other analyses (i.e., estimates of daily or seasonal use) and are important for determining periods of peak demand used in traffic safety analyses, observed use was regressed on trail monitor counts for each hour of field observation to develop an hourly correction equation (Lindsey et al., 2006). The correction equation then was applied to each hour of monitoring data prior to aggregation into daily, monthly, or annual totals.

Operational Logistics, Problems, and Challenges

Development of the monitoring system required a set of decisions regarding site selection, monitor installation, and data collection that were partially dependent on the chosen technology. A project goal was to obtain counts for trail segments representative of the entire trail network at an affordable cost. The process of site selection involved trade-offs between scope of coverage and costs of instrumentation, data collection, and system maintenance. The decision eventually was made to install counters for trail segments approximately one mile long, with deviations to account for natural or manmade break points along each trail. This approach ensured coverage for the entire 33-mile trail network on segments that were considered short enough to capture major changes in traffic flow with relative geographic specificity.

The monitoring units were installed on respective sides of a trail right-of-way approximately 36 to 42 inches above the ground on treated timber posts. The units were housed in custom-built aluminum boxes to protect them from the weather and to minimize potential for vandalism. Operational problems included vandalism, infestation by insects, and loss of power supply.

Data collection required trips to the monitor, downloading of traffic counts using a data collector, and uploading data into a computer for analyses. The monitoring units had the capacity to record either 8,000 or 16,000 events, which, depending on the trail segment and season, was sufficient to last anywhere from 2 or 3 days to 2 or 3 months. The frequency for collecting data from each monitor was a function of both monitor capacity and the need to ensure operations and prevent loss of data. Heavily used sites were visited as needed (e.g., twice per week) to prevent loss of information associated with the monitor reaching capacity. Monitors on segments with lower use were visited at least every 2 weeks to ensure they were operating and had not been vandalized even though they had capacity and power to operate for longer periods of time without downloading.

The monitors record the time of day when the infrared beam is interrupted. Data analyses involve exporting data (i.e., the list of times the beam was broken) from the monitor database into generally available spreadsheets and statistical databases for data cleaning, aggregation, and analyses. Data cleaning involves inspection and identification of anomalies such as extremely large counts for short periods of time that seem unlikely given patterns of use for the particular segment. Analytic choices include retaining the data, censoring the data from the database and using fewer observations in the analysis, or censoring the data or imputing a replacement value from other data believed to be valid. The choice among alternatives depends on a number of factors, including the total number of observations available.

Challenges in Technologically Based Observation of Physical Activity and Exercise Behavior

This overview with an example illustrates the trade-offs and challenges inherent in measuring physical activity and exercise behaviors using instruments. Lessons learned include the following:

- The research question should guide the choice of technology. Although increasingly sophisticated devices for observation are becoming available, their applicability depends on the research question of interest. More complex technologies potentially can provide more information and answer more questions but at higher cost along with greater potential for complications.

- All technologies have limitations. Systematic bias associated with use of a technology does not preclude use of the technology if the bias is known and can be taken into account in subsequent analyses. Identification of limitations or systematic error in any instrumentation therefore is essential prior to deployment.

- Different types of instrumentation require different commitments of resources to data collection, cleaning, and management. The costs of resources for these activities must be considered during the original choice of methods.

- Measures of use of facilities (i.e., user counts) that historically have been collected by public works managers to inform investment and maintenance decisions for recreational or transportation facilities may not include sufficient information about users and their characteristics to target public health interventions. Direct field observations and other techniques such as surveys and questionnaires often will be required to obtain the information needed to inform most programmatic and policy decisions related to physical activity and exercise behavior.

Direct Observational Techniques for Assessing Physical Activity

Direct observational (DO) techniques for assessing physical activity offer a variety of reliable approaches to collecting contextually rich information on physical activity. DO involves an observer recording observations while watching the subject or subjects of interest (Fairweather, Reilly, Grant, Whittaker, & Paton, 1999; Finn & Specker, 2000; Kelly, Reilly, Grant, & Paton, 2004; Reilly et al., 2003; Sirard & Pate, 2001; Welk, Corbin, & Dale, 2000). While considerable time and effort are required to conduct DO studies, the detail provided makes it a highly useful method for characterizing the different dimensions of an individual's physical activity. DO allows investigators to describe the mode, intensity, and duration of subjects' activities, as well as the interactions they have with the environment and other individuals.

This technique has been used most frequently in research for the study of preschool and school-aged children when other methods were not feasible (Montoye, Kemper, Saris, & Washburn, 1996). DO is particularly appropriate when determining physical activity in children who historically have poor self-report data. DO also lends itself well as one of the best criterion measures to validate other assessment tools (Welk, Corbin, & Dale, 2000), including accelerometers, heart rate monitors, calorimetry, and other quantitative physical activity or energy expenditure measures.

The two most popular direct observation methods for quantifying physical activity in children are the Children's Physical Activity Form (CPAF; O'Hara, 1989) and the Children's Activity Rating Scale (CARS; Puhl, Greaves, Hoyt, & Baranowski, 1990). Other common tools include the System for Observing Fitness Instruction Time (SOFIT) and the System for Observing Play and Leisure Activity in Youth

(SOPLAY). SOFIT is an adaptation of the SOPLAY system used to assess physical activity in children and adults using public parks in a variety of surrounding neighborhoods.

Children's Physical Activity Form

The CPAF was originally developed to evaluate a fitness-oriented physical U.S. education curriculum (Baranowski, Dworkin, & Cieslik, 1984). In this observational technique, physical activities are categorized into four *distinct* categories, representing different levels of intensity of movement by direct observation. The categories are as follows:

1. Stationary, no limb movement (e.g., sitting, lying, standing still)

2. Stationary, with limb movement (e.g., bouncing a ball, painting, completing a jigsaw)

3. Slow trunk movement (e.g., walking, twisting)

4. Rapid trunk movement (e.g., running, skipping)

The trained observer records the amount of activity that is occurring in each minute interval and records this by marking a number on a CPAF recording form. If the child is carrying out a particular type of movement or is inactive for *greater* then 15 seconds, a mark is placed in the according activity level box. Since the type and intensity of movement can change several times in 1 minute, observers are instructed to reflect this by checking all categories of the child's activity occurring in that minute. Therefore, each 1-minute interval may have several different categories, although no one category can be checked twice within the same minute (O'Hara, 1989).

Scoring of the CPAF. An intensity of activity point score is calculated for every minute of activity by a trained observer. For each minute, the proportion of the minute (in seconds) is allocated to an activity level depending on whether that level has been checked for that minute. Activity points, which are ordinal in value, are assigned to each of the ordinal levels of movement. That is, each 15 seconds of stationary, no movement (SNM) receives 1 activity point; stationary limb movement (SLM) receives 2 points, slow trunk movement (STM) receives 3 points, and rapid trunk movement (RTM) receives 4 points (O'Hara, 1989).

For example, if a minute had checks in three boxes, it would be scored as follows: 60 seconds/3 checks = 20 seconds per category checked. If in the above minute, the observer had checked the three activity points in the SNM, STM, and RTM boxes, the activity point for that 1 minute would be calculated as follows:

$$SNM = 1 \text{ activity point} * 20 \text{ seconds} = 20 \text{ activity points.}$$

$$STM = 2 \text{ activity points} * 20 \text{ seconds} = 60 \text{ activity points.}$$

$$RTM = 4 \text{ activity points} * 20 \text{ seconds} = 80 \text{ activity points.}$$

$$TOTAL = 160 \text{ activity points.}$$

Therefore, the child would have scored as having expended 160 activity points for this minute. Such calculations were conducted for each minute of activity. The minimal numbers of activity points per minute are 60; the maximum activity points are 240.

Children's Activity Rating Scale

CARS is a rating scale that was developed to provide an activity score representative of physical activity in young children (Puhl et al., 1990). It has been used successfully to measure physical activity in young children (ages 3–5 years) from different ethnic groups (Finn & Specker, 2000). Common activities by preschool children can be classified into five levels according to this rating system (Puhl et al., 1990). Level 1 activities are sedentary. Level 2 activities are sedentary but include movement of the limbs or torso. Activities in Levels 3 to 5 require translocation (moving the body from one location to another). The speed or intensity of the activities determines the level. By using the coding rules by Puhl et al. (1990), a level of physical activity observed for a 3-second duration or repeated in brief duration (< 3 seconds) at least three times within 15 seconds is recorded using a standard score sheet. Only one activity at each level is recorded, with up to five scores being recorded within each minute. All levels within the minute are then averaged and the mean minute CARS score recorded (Puhl et al., 1990).

System for Observing Fitness Instruction Time

SOFIT is a direct observational tool originally developed for assessment of physical education classes in elementary schools (McKenzie, Sallis, & Nader, 1991). SOFIT measures three aspects of the subject's activities:

1. The activity level of the subject (laying, sitting, standing, walking, and vigorous activity)

2. The context of the physical education (PE) lesson being taught (general content, general knowledge, fitness knowledge, fitness practice, skill practice, game play, other)

3. The degree of involvement of the PE teacher (promotes fitness, demonstrates fitness, general instruction, management, observation, other)

Trained observers watch a subject for 10 seconds and, at a prerecorded signal, spend 10 seconds scoring the subject's behavior, the context of the class lesson being taught, and the involvement of the physical education teacher. Observe-record intervals are combined to form 20-second time periods. Time periods are summed to give a total estimate of time spent at each activity level with three periods comprising 1 minute of activity (McKenzie, Sallis, & Nader, 1991). During data analysis, the time spent at the "walking" and

"vigorous activity" intensity levels is often combined to give an estimate of time spent in moderate to vigorous physical activity (MVPA), allowing for comparison with national fitness recommendations (Pope, Coleman, Gonzalez, Barron, & Heath, 2002; U.S. DHHS, 1996).

SOFIT has been employed in the assessment of PE classes in numerous settings(Nader, 2003; Scruggs, Beveridge, Watson, & Clocksin, 2005) and has been validated using heart rate monitors and accelerometers for use with children in PE classes ranging from the 3rd to 12th grades (McKenzie, Sallis, & Armstrong, 1994; McKenzie, Sallis, Nader, Patterson, et al., 1991; Pope et al., 2002; Rowe, Schuldheisz, & van der Mars, 1997; Rowe, van der Mars, Schuldheisz, & Fox, 2004). Various adaptations of the SOFIT tool have been developed, including a six-category activity variable and a continuous observation method (SOFIT-CO). The SOFIT-6 differentiates the walking and vigorously active categories into "light," "moderate," and "vigorous" physical activity (Pope et al., 2002). SOFIT-6 showed significant correlation with heart rate monitoring but suffered from low interrater reliability when compared to the original SOFIT measure. In a modification to the SOFIT tool allowing for continuous observation (SOFIT-CO), variations in nonexercise activity thermogenesis (NEAT; J. A. Levine, Schleusner, & Jensen, 2000), or fidgeting, were implemented recently. SOFIT-CO shows a high degree of interrater agreement and is currently being validated against the original SOFIT.

Relative to other direct observation tools, SOFIT benefits from a relatively low observer training time and high interrater reliability (McKenzie, Sallis, & Nader, 1991; Pope et al., 2002). One limitation of the SOFIT tool is its reliance on momentary time sampling, in which observations are based on the subject's actions at the *end* of each observation period and do not necessarily account for activities performed at the beginning or during the observation period (Heath, Coleman, Lensegrav, & Fallon, 2006; McKenzie, Sallis, & Nader, 1991).

System for Observing Play and Leisure Activity in Youth and System for Observing Play and Recreation in Communities

SOPLAY and the System for Observing Play and Recreation in Communities (SOPARC) are two tools used to measure the activity of groups of individuals in unsupervised settings (i.e., outside PE classes). SOPLAY has been specifically employed to measure the free-play energy expenditure of children in outdoor settings, typically on school playgrounds (McKenzie, Marshall, Sallis, & Conway, 2000), and has been most widely used to record activities in children before and after school, as well as during recess and lunch periods in middle schools. SOPARC differs from SOPLAY in that it has been adapted for use with adults and children in parks and other public recreational facilities (McKenzie, Cohen, Sehgal, Williamson, & Golinelli, 2006). Furthermore, SOPARC is also employed to assess utilization of park spaces and improvements and to date has been used only in urban parks in the L.A. area.

Both SOPARC and SOPLAY are based on a time sampling method with variable observe/record intervals. The area to be observed is selected beforehand and scored based on several characteristics, including accessibility, supervision, and physical improvements (play equipment, basketball hoops, etc.) that make the area suitable for group activities (Sallis et al., 2001). Four 1-hour sessions are selected throughout the day in a sequential order. Once the observation period begins, trained observers sweep the play area from left to right, recording the number of individuals at each activity level, as well as the primary sport or activity they are engaged in. Each sweep focuses on a different set of subjects, usually determined by gender, race, or other readily visible characteristics (McKenzie et al., 2000).

In both the SOPARC and SOPLAY tools, physical activity is measured as one of three categories, including "sedentary," "walking," and "very active" levels. These categories have been validated in children using heart rate monitors and accelerometers (McKenzie, Sallis, Nader, Patterson, et al., 1991). Average activity (or energy expenditure) for an entire play area is estimated for different periods of the day. In SOPLAY, these time periods are typically defined as before school, after school, and during recess, whereas in SOPARC, they are chosen based on morning, afternoon, and evening and according to the seasons. Energy expenditure can be estimated by combining the number of people engaging in each activity and their intensity of activity (McKenzie et al., 2006).

Like all measures, both SOPARC and SOPLAY have their advantages and disadvantages and must be chosen based on study design and the variables that need to be measured. Both measures may underestimate activity time (and energy expenditure) due to the fact that people who leave the target area before the specified recording period are not included as having been in the target area. Both measures may also overestimate activity time by counting people twice as they move from target area to target area. Furthermore, the measures may provide inaccurate estimates of activity levels because subjects are scored at the time the observer sees them, and other behaviors are missed. The primary advantages of SOPARC and SOPLAY are that they provide tools to systematically measure activity in outdoor and unstructured activity settings. The measures can provide contextually rich data that can be used in conjunction with more objective physical activity measures (i.e., accelerometry).

Validation of the Direct Observation Method for Assessing Physical Activity

DO is probably the most appropriate criterion measure of physical activity and patterns of physical activity for young children (Sirard & Pate, 2001). The direct observation technique is ideal when behavior is the main focus of concern. It can allow for several different dimensions of activity (e.g., type, intensity, and duration) to be simultaneously recorded (Melanson & Freedson, 1996; O'Hara, 1989).

For the most accurate recording, the sampling interval should be sensitive to brief periods of activity and not exclude short bursts of activity. This is a major concern when measuring children, in whom activity patterns are believed to be constantly changing (L. M. Klesges & Klesges, 1987). Welk et al. (2000) noted that as a method for assessing physical activity, DO was highly suited for studies involving children. However, because it is highly labor intensive, its greatest value probably lies in the validation of other methods of physical activity assessments, such as accelerometry.

The observational method would also appear to be appropriate when the observation period is short, such as during a physical activity class (O'Hara, 1989). The observational method is not limited by recall or self-reporting biases that can occur in questionnaires or activity diaries. Validity of direct observational methods based on comparison to heart rate is high with correlations ranging from $r = 0.61$ to 0.91 (O'Hara, 1989), and heart rate and oxygen consumption are significantly different among the observed physical activity levels categorized by the various direct observation methods (Bailey et al., 1995; Puhl et al., 1990).

Limitations of the Direct Observation Method for Assessing Physical Activity

DO as a method for assessing physical activity has a number of limitations. The system can be costly to implement due to its labor intensiveness. Observers are expensive to recruit and train, and multiple observers are needed to assess a number of people reliably (O'Hara, 1989). However, possibly the greatest limitation is the effect of the observer. If the observed subject is aware of the observer, his or her behavior may be modified. Fortunately, available studies have demonstrated that most observed children ignore the observers after a few minutes (Puhl et al., 1990). This may not always hold in adolescents and adults. Because observation is time-consuming and expensive, it is really suited only for relatively small groups. Also, observations are confined to relatively short periods and may not,

therefore, reflect habitual physical activity accurately. Video recording of sessions can provide material that can be used to improve training as well as check the reliability and reproducibility of the activity assessments (Montoye et al., 1996).

Direct Objective Measures

Overview

Consistent with the definition that physical activity is bodily movement that produces energy expenditure above basal level, motion sensors (i.e., pedometers and accelerometers) can be used to detect body movement and hence provide an estimate of physical activity. Advancements in technology have increased the sophistication, sensitivity, and accuracy of these instruments.

Pedometers

Invention of the pedometer has been credited to Leonardo DaVinci (Tudor-Locke, 2002). The modern pedometer, an improvement over the gear-driven device with a pendulum arm, was developed in Japan in the 1960s. Dr. Yoshiro Hatano advocated the use of the pedometer and encouraged people to take 10,000 steps a day, approximately equivalent to a 5-mile walk. This amount of walking approximates current recommendations for adults to be moderately active for 30 minutes daily and has been shown to be associated with improvements in health indicators such as blood pressure, body mass, and glucose tolerance (Iwane et al., 2000; Swartz, Strath, et al., 2003; Tudor-Locke & Bassett, 2004). Pedometers have been promoted as a motivational tool in public health campaigns to achieve the goal of 10,000 steps daily.

Internal Mechanisms and Other Pedometer Features

There are currently three types of mechanisms found in pedometers. Spring-loaded pedometers

Table 6.3   Validation of Observational Methods

Instrument	Technique	Participants	Reliability	Criterion Measure	Validity	Reference
CPAF	Four categories of behavior in PE class; 1-minute time sampling interval	8- to 10-year-olds	96%–98% interobserver agreement	Heart rate monitors	$R = 0.61-0.72$	O'Hara, Baranowski, Simons-Morton, Wilson, and Parcel (1989)
CARS	Five categories of behavior averaged in 1-minute intervals	3- to 5-year-olds	84% ± 10% in 3- to 4-year-olds	VO_2 Heart rate monitor	Heart rates and VO_2 levels were significantly different at all five activity categories ($p < .05$)	Puhl, Greaves, Hoyt, and Baranowski (1990)
SOFIT	Five categories of behavior in PE class; 10-second momentary time-sampling interval	Grades 9–12	Lying: $r = 0.997$ Sitting: $r = 0.998$ Standing: $r = 0.997$ Walking: $r = 0.997$ Jogging: $r = 0.995$	VO_2 Heart rate monitor	Heart rates were significantly different for all categories except for lying and sitting levels ($p < .05$). VO_2 was significantly different between standing and walking ($p < .05$).	Rowe, van der Mars, Schuldheisz, and Fox (2004)
		Grades 3–5	Interrater $r = 0.98$	TriTrac accelerometer	TriTrac cutpoints and SOFIT categories $r = 0.60$ (95% CI: 0.43–0.73)	Pope, Coleman, Gonzalez, Barron, and Heath (2002)

(Continued)

Table 6.3 (Continued)

Instrument	Technique	Participants	Reliability	Criterion Measure	Validity	Reference
SOPARC	Three energy categories in parks; sweep designated play area for 1-hour interval twice per day		Target areas interrater r > 0.97 Number of participants interrater r > 0.84 Participant characteristics interrater r > 0.88	Heart rate monitors	Activity categories have been previously validated (McKenzie, Sallis, Nader, Patterson, et al., 1991)	McKenzie, Cohen, Sehgal, Williamson, and Golinelli (2006)
SOPLAY	Three energy categories and 14 activity categories; sweep designated playground three times per day	Grades 6–8	Sedentary interrater r = 0.98 Walking interrater r = 0.94–0.98 Very active interrater r = 0.76–0.97	Heart rate monitors	Activity categories have been previously validated (McKenzie, Sallis, Nader, Patterson, et al., 1991)	McKenzie, Marshall, Sallis, and Conway (2000)

NOTE: CARS = Children's Activity Rating Scale; CI = confidence interval; CPAF = Children's Physical Activity Form; PE = physical education; SOFIT = System for Observing Fitness Instruction Time; SOPLAY = System for Observing Play and Leisure Activity in Youth; SOPARC = System for Observing Play and Recreation in Communities.

have a horizontal lever that moves up and down with the hip's vertical movements. When a step is taken, the hip moves vertically, which causes the lever to move. The movement of the lever opens and closes an electrical circuit, and the lever arm makes an electrical contact and a step is counted (Schneider, Crouter, & Bassett, 2004). Magnetic reed proximity switch pedometers also have a spring-suspended horizontal lever arm. There is a magnet attached to the lever arm, and the magnet moves up and down when the hip moves. The magnetic field triggers a switch that causes the step to be counted. Piezoelectric pedometers use an accelerometer-type mechanism (described elsewhere in this chapter).

In addition to the type of mechanism, pedometer models vary in other features. Some models use algorithms to estimate distance walked and calories expended. Crouter, Schneider, Karabulut, and Bassett (2003) found that pedometers were less accurate for assessing distance than for estimating step counts and even less accurate for assessing caloric expenditure. Most pedometers display cumulative step counts until the count is cleared. Some newer models log and store step counts daily and have computer downloading options (Crouter et al., 2003). One new pedometer, the Sportbrain™, records step counts in 60-second epochs, which are stored for later downloading. This device could potentially be used to identify periods during which the instrument was not worn, based on long periods with zero steps, and periods of moderate and vigorous physical activity based on a threshold of steps per minute. To our knowledge, there has been no published validation of the accuracy of this instrument.

Step Count as an Indicator of Physical Activity

There are a multitude of pedometers on the market. Choice of pedometers for research depends on (1) hypotheses (step counts vs. energy expenditure or other outcomes of interest), (2) population (some pedometers are validated in adults but not children, for instance), (3) available funds (costs vary widely), (4) research setting (lab or free living, for instance), and probably most important, (5) validity of the model as relates to 1, 2, and 4 above. Numerous studies have evaluated the validity of pedometer counts as a measurement of physical activity in various populations in comparison with direct observation, accelerometry, and energy expenditure. A review of that literature is beyond the scope of this chapter. However, Tudor-Locke, Williams, Reis, and Pluto (2002) reviewed 25 studies and found a strong correlation of pedometer counts with accelerometer output (median of reported correlations $r = 0.86$) and with directly observed activity time (median $r = 0.82$). These correlations varied depending on the accelerometer used, the type of activity, and the population under study. Correlation between pedometers and energy expenditure varied widely (median $r = 0.68$).

Accuracy of pedometers depends on the model used and on walking speed in treadmill and track studies and in free-living conditions studies. Crouter et al. (2003) compared several pedometers at five different speeds on a treadmill. Most models underestimated steps at 54 m/min (a slow walk), compared to direct observation, and accuracy varied between models. Other studies also showed that accuracy was lower at a slow pace (< 3 miles per hour; Tudor-Locke, Williams, et al., 2002). Different models were also found to vary in accuracy in adult subjects walking 400 meters around a track (Schneider, Crouter, Lukajic, & Bassett, 2003). Because models change frequently, any recommendation for a specific pedometer model is likely to be outdated quickly. Japanese industrial standards require that pedometers have less than 3% margin of error, and Japanese Yamax™ brand pedometers consistently have been found to be accurate in a variety of settings and have been widely used in research studies (Crouter et al., 2003; Le Masurier, Lee, & Tudor-Locke, 2004; Schneider et al., 2003). In a free-living validation study, for example, Schneider et al. (2003) compared step values of 13 different models of pedometers to a Yamax™ criterion pedometer in adult subjects. Five pedometer models underestimated steps, and three overestimated steps. However, the best pedometer may depend on the conditions under study. For example, piezoelectric pedometers may be less likely to undercount steps at slower walking speed than spring-levered pedometers (Melanson et al., 2004), but the piezoelectric mechanism theoretically may be more sensitive to nonstep movement such as fidgeting, twisting, bending, or mechanical vibration such as riding in a car (Beets, Patton, & Edwards, 2005; Tudor-Locke, Ainsworth, Thompson, & Matthews, 2002). The trade-off in sensitivity against false-positive counts depends in part on the acceleration threshold and may be a function of the spring tension in spring-loaded pedometers (Beets et al., 2005; Schneider et al., 2004).

Pedometer Applications in Field Studies

Pedometers provide an objective measurement of physical activity at low cost. Thus, for large observational or intervention studies, they are an attractive alternative to self-report of physical activity, which is limited by recall bias, compliance, and accuracy, and to accelerometry, which is expensive to conduct in large populations (Tudor-Locke, Ham, et al., 2004). Pedometers have been shown to assess physical activity accurately in populations of schoolchildren, a group for which self-report may be even less reliable than in adults (Scruggs et al., 2003; Tudor-Locke, Lee, Morgan, Beighle, & Pangrazi, 2006). Pedometers have been used to assess physical activity in observational studies in adult populations (Strycker, Duncan, Chaumeton, Duncan, & Toobert, 2007; Tudor-Locke et al., 2002; Tudor-Locke, Ham, et al., 2004). Pedometers have also been used extensively as a motivational tool providing a record of physical activity to participants in intervention studies to increase activity in diabetics, elderly subjects with osteoarthritis, and other diverse populations (Araiza, Hewes, Gashetewa, Vella, & Burge, 2006; Merom et al., 2007; Talbot, Gaines, Huynh, & Metter, 2003; Tudor-Locke, Bell, et al., 2004). For observational studies in which large numbers of pedometers are to be used, intramodel variability is potentially an issue (Beets et al., 2005). Schneider et al. (2003) evaluated intramodel variability between pedometers worn on the left and right hips. Only 1 of 10 pedometers evaluated had poor intramodel reliability (Cronbach's alpha < 0.80), but only a limited number of instruments were evaluated. A shake test has been suggested as a crude way of conducting quality control of a large number of instruments in the field setting (Vincent & Sidman, 2003).

There are some limitations to pedometers as indicators of physical activity beyond the accuracy of the measurement discussed above. As with accelerometers, activity may be poorly estimated if someone besides a study participant wears it, and steps will be falsely counted if the pedometer is shaken. Cumulative step counts over periods long enough to estimate usual physical activity, at least 3 days in adults and 7 days in children (Trost, Pate, Freedson, Sallis, & Taylor, 2000; Tudor-Locke et al., 2005), will not identify periods or duration of low, moderate, and vigorous physical activity. For example, a subject taking 10,000 steps daily could accumulate the steps over the course of the day through walking or by taking a single 5-mile run. In addition, pedometers measure only ambulatory activity; therefore, physical activities such as bicycling and swimming go unrecorded. Compliance can be an issue, and self-report is the only way to distinguish a low step count due to not wearing the pedometer from a low count due to inactivity. People may also increase their activity in response to wearing the pedometer ("reactivity"), leading to an overestimation of typical activity levels (Strycker et al., 2007; Tudor-Locke et al., 2006).

Pedometer Applications in Overweight and Obese Populations

Pedometers have been used to motivate physical activity in intervention studies of overweight and obese groups (Araiza et al., 2006; Clarke et al., 2007). Obese adults take less steps per day than normal-weight adults (Chan, Spangler, Valcour, &

Tudor-Locke, 2003), and people taking less than 5,000 steps/day were more likely to be overweight (Tudor-Locke et al., 2001). However, this association with obesity may be at least in part an artifact of underestimated step counts by pedometers, which has been found in some (Crouter, Schneider, & Bassett, 2005; Melanson et al., 2004) but not all (Swartz, Bassett, Moore, Thompson, & Strath, 2003) studies of overweight and obese adults. This may be due to the known pedometer undercount of steps at a slow walking pace, especially with spring-loaded pedometers. Spring-loaded pedometers may underestimate step counts in overweight individuals because the device must be in a vertical plane for steps to be recorded accurately. In obese individuals, the pedometer may tip forward out of the vertical plane. In a study of the effects of body mass index (BMI), waist circumference, and pedometer tilt on the accuracy of spring-loaded and piezoelectric pedometers, Crouter et al. (2005) found pedometer tilt influenced accuracy of the spring-loaded pedometer more than waist circumference or BMI. The piezoelectric pedometer's accuracy was not affected by these factors.

Pedometer Applications in the Elderly

Because the elderly and infirm often walk slowly or with a shuffling gait, pedometers may have reduced accuracy in these groups. Cyarto, Myers, and Tudor-Locke (2004) found that steps were underestimated in an elderly group at slower walking speeds. They also found that gait disorders also reduced pedometer accuracy.

Pedometer Applications in Children

Children may walk at a slow pace that results in underestimates in step counts, and some pedometer models may not be sensitive enough to detect a child's steps, especially in younger children. Beets et al. (2005) tested the accuracy of pedometer steps during both treadmill walking and self-paced walking in children. At speeds less than 54 m/min, there was poor agreement between pedometer counts and observer counts for the two models of pedometers they tested. However, there was good agreement between pedometer counts and observer counts for both models during the self-paced walking test.

When establishing steps/day goals, 10,000 steps may be too low for children. The 2001–2002 President's Challenge Physical Activity and Fitness Awards Program recommended 11,000 steps for girls and 13,000 steps for boys (Tudor-Locke, Pangrazi, et al., 2004). These values were based on norm-referenced standards. Tudor-Locke, Pangrazi, et al. (2004) used BMI-referenced standards and recommended 12,000 steps/day for girls 6 to 12 years old and 15,000 steps/day for boys 6 to 12 years old.

Pedometer: Conclusions and Recommendations

Pedometers provide a useful tool for motivating physical activity and a low-cost alternative to accelerometry for assessment of physical activity in large field studies. In general, pedometer data should be reported as steps, rather than relying on manufacturer algorithms for estimating energy expenditure or distance (Schneider et al., 2003).When choosing a pedometer model, it is important to consider the population under study. For the elderly and obese subjects, pedometers may underestimate step counts (but piezoelectric models may be less subject to error, especially at low speed, other factors being equal). In adults, 3 days of pedometer monitoring typically predict average weekly physical activity, and 7 days are needed to estimate typical physical activity levels in children.

In field studies, individual pedometers can be crudely validated by shaking each a specific number of times and the number recorded by the pedometer compared to the number of shakes. Validation can also be done by wearing the pedometer for a short distance and comparing the pedometer counts to an observer recorded count (Melanson et al., 2004).

Accelerometers

Activity monitors were developed in part as a response to the sometimes dubious reliability of self-report measures and the complexity of heart rate monitoring. Accelerometers measure accelerations caused by bodily movement in one (uniaxial), two (biaxial), or three (triaxial) planes of motion. A number of accelerometers, varying in size, cost, and weight, are commercially available such as the Caltrac, Actigraph (uniaxial), Actiwatch and Actical (biaxial), and Tritrac and RT3 (triaxial).

Accelerometers are more sophisticated electronic devices than the previously mentioned pedometers. In contrast to the spring mechanisms of pedometers, accelerometers use piezoelectric transducers and microprocessing that converts recorded accelerations from an analog signal to a quantifiable digital signal referred to as counts. Recent advances in integrated circuitry and memory capacity have produced sensitive, unobtrusive accelerometers that measure the intensity, frequency, and duration of movement for extended periods (Sirard & Pate, 2001).

Uniaxial Accelerometers

The Caltrac was one of the first commercially available accelerometers. It is also one of the largest commercially available accelerometers ($14 \times 8 \times 4$ cm). The Caltrac provides information on activity counts and energy expenditure. The latter can be calculated by summing the predicted resting metabolic rate (RMR), but because the RMR is based on equations for adults, using this function for children is not recommended (Sallis, Buono, Roby, Carlson, & Nelson, 1990). The unique feature of the Caltrac is that it has a special entry for activities such as cycling, weight lifting, and stair climbing.

The Actigraph (Actigraph, LLC, Pensacola, Florida) is one of the most widely used accelerometers for physical activity research. The Actigraph (WAM-7164 and GT1M models) uses an internal piezoelectric cantilever beam that creates a charge proportional to the magnitude of the movement. The Actigraph accurately and consistently measures

and records time-varying accelerations in magnitude from approximately 0.05 to 2 Gs. The acceleration signal is sampled and digitized by a 12-bit analog to digital converter at a sampling rate of 30 times per second (30 Hz). Once digitized, the signal passes through a digital filter, and this filter limits the accelerations to a frequency range of 0.25 to 2.5 Hz. This frequency range best reflects human motion and rejects motion from other sources such as traveling in a car. The filter produces an output that responds linearly to changing accelerations within a defined range. Each sample is summed and stored over a user-specified time period (i.e., epoch). Epochs range from 1 second to several minutes; for example, using a 1-minute epoch, the Actigraph can record 356 consecutive days of data. The Actigraph can be preprogrammed to begin recording on a specific date and time. The Actigraph is small and unobtrusive ($3.8 \times 3.7 \times 1.8$ cm), making it an attractive method for collecting physical activity data, which makes it particularly suitable for use with young children. Various models can record activity data and pedometer data, energy expenditure, skin temperature, or ambient light level. The newer GT1M models have the added advantage of being water resistant and have rechargeable batteries. However, battery charge intervals can be an issue in longer duration studies since the storage capacity of the devices exceeds the battery life. Therefore, care must be taken in study design to match data collection protocols and charge intervals.

Biaxial Accelerometers

The Actiwatch (Mini Mitter Co., Inc., Bend, Oregon) is one of the most widely used *biaxial* accelerometers (i.e., measures activity in two planes). The Actiwatch is a small ($2.8 \times 2.5 \times 1.0$ cm), lightweight (18 g), and waterproof (1 m) motion sensor. The Actiwatch can be worn at the wrist, ankle, or waist and contains a sensor capable of detecting acceleration in all directions.

The Actiwatch is sensitive to movements in the 0.05- to 7-Hz frequency range. The Actiwatch sensor integrates the degree and speed of motion and produces an electrical current (voltage) that varies in magnitude. An increased degree of speed and motion causes an increased voltage in the sensor. The voltage corresponds to a number of activity counts, which the monitor stores. The maximum sampling frequency is 32 Hz. The Actiwatch has been programmed with a calibration coefficient to normalize data between watches. This removes most if not all variation between units due to sensors. However, to date, there are few published data on the reliability and reproducibility of the Actiwatch.

A computer clock sets the Actiwatch. The unit marks elapsed time, as it contains a crystal that oscillates 32 times per second. When a sampling epoch is chosen, the Actiwatch is then instructed to wait a specific number of oscillations before storing the number of activity counts. This also applies to delayed starting times. The Actiwatch communicates with the computer via a reader/interface unit, which plugs into the RS-232 serial port of the computer; therefore, it requires no external power supply. The watch has a short-range telemetric link established between the watch and the reader. Communicating with the watch occurs when it is placed on the reader in the proper position (i.e., when the ready LED is lit). Once the watch is placed, reading and writing to the watch can occur. A single lithium coin cell watch battery powers the Actiwatch. If the battery runs out while the watch is logging, all the data taken up to that point will be stored. The projected battery life is 180 days, but this will vary depending on the number of times the watch is read or written to. The standard watch can log 8,000 data points (each one is an 8-bit type). If the epochs are set for 1 minute, the monitor will run consecutively for 5.5 days. However, an Actiwatch with 32K memory can run for 32,000 data points and, with a 1-minute epoch, can run for 22 days consecutively.

Triaxial Accelerometers

The Actical (Mini Mitter Co., Inc., Bend, Oregon) is one of the newest multidirectional accelerometers to come onto the market. The Actical uses a multidirectional, piezoelectric accelerometer

to create a charge proportional to the magnitude of the movement and is sensitive to movements in the 0.5- to 3-Hz range. Similar to the Actiwatch, the Actical is a small (2.9 × 3.7 × 1.1 cm), lightweight (18 g), waterproof (1 m) motion sensor and can be worn at the wrist, ankle, or waist. Physical activity data are stored over a user-specified time period (i.e., epoch) ranging from 15 seconds to several minutes and can be preprogrammed to turn itself on, on a specific date and time. Unlike the Actiwatch, the Actical has been designed to measure whole-body physical activity. Actical can provide calculated energy expenditure values for active energy expenditure (AEE) in kilocalories and total energy expenditure in METs in kcal/kg/min.

The RT3 (Stayhealthy, Inc., Monrovia, California) measures activity in three dimensions and has recently replaced the Tritrac R3D. The RT3 uses an integrated triaxial accelerometer that integrates measurement of the three vectors into a single chip. With the RT3 worn on the hip, the vectors are as follows: vertical (x), anteroposterior (y), and mediolateral (z). The RT3 is the largest of the motion sensors with a size and mass (including the battery) of 7.1 × 5.6 × 2.8 cm and weighs 65.2 g. The RT3 provides triaxial vector data in activity units, METs, or kilocalories. The RT3 is not able to accurately calculate metabolic calorie burn in children younger than age 10, but it can be used as an activity monitor.

The Tracmor2 (Philips Research, Eindhoven, Netherlands) consists of three one-dimensional accelerometers. It calculates the sum of the amplified and bandpass-filtered acceleration curves from anterior-posterior, vertical, and mediolateral movements of the trunk. The Tracmor2 is a smaller version of the Tracmor with a size and mass of 7 × 2 × 0.8 cm and weight of 30 g. While studies using the Tracmor2 accelerometer have been published, this accelerometer is not commercially available at this time.

Accelerometers: Reproducibility

It is a well-established principle of science that reliability is an essential prerequisite for validity.

Despite this principle, there is a paucity of research on the reliability of accelerometers. Most manufacturing companies perform calibration checks as part of a quality assurance check before shipping, to ensure that the devices are each measuring and summarizing raw accelerometer data in a similar way. However, researchers began to conduct separate calibration studies to check reliability. The most common design has been to use high-precision shaker devices to examine technical reliability over multiple trials (Brage, Brage, Wedderkopp, & Froberg, 2003; Fairweather et al., 1999; Metcalf, Curnow, Evans, Voss, & Wilkin, 2002; S. M. Powell, Jones, & Rowlands, 2003).

Studies with the Actigraph (WAM-7164) have demonstrated good intra- and interinstrument coefficient of variation. Brage, Brage, et al. (2003) noted a mean intrainstrument coefficient of variability (CV) for all units of 4.4%, but large variations were noted at very low and very high accelerations. With respect to interinstrument reliability, the intraclass correlation coefficients (ICCs) were 0.96 to 0.99. Metcalf et al. (2002) evaluated the reliability of the older model of the ActiGraph monitor (CSA) using a turntable device. They reported low intrainstrument coefficients of variation (1.83%) and slightly higher interinstrument coefficients of variation of 5%. Fairweather et al. (1999), using a high-precision shaker device, found a CV of 3% and correlations between pairs of accelerometers of $r = 0.98$–0.99. Studies with the Tritrac-R3D have demonstrated good interinstrument reliability (ICC of $r = 0.97$; Kochersberger, McConnell, Kuchibhatla, & Pieper, 1996) and acceptably small coefficients of variation of 1.8% (Nichols, Morgan, Sarkin, Sallis, & Calfas, 1999).

An alternative design for reliability research has been to compare outputs from two units on opposite sides of the hips. Using a treadmill protocol with varying speeds, Trost et al. (2000) found an intraclass reliability coefficient of $r = 0.87$ for two accelerometers worn on the left and right hips. A study on the Tritrac-R3D (Nichols et al., 1999) reported ICC values ranging from $R^2 = 0.73$ to $R^2 = 0.87$ for two different Tritrac-R3D

monitors worn during free-living activity. A study on the RT3 (S. M. Powell et al., 2003) employed a contralateral hip lab-based study design to evaluate the interinstrument reliability. Interinstrument CV for the vector sum during the locomotor activities was less than 6%; however, relatively high variations were evident during the sit-to-stand task (8%–25%). No significant between-unit differences for activity counts were recorded during the rest.

Accelerometers: Validity

Several studies have investigated the validity of the Caltrac using a number of measurement techniques, with conflicting results. In an adult study, Montoye et al. (1983) reported a strong linear relationship between activity counts and oxygen consumption ($r = -0.74$) across a wide range of activity levels (e.g., slow walking and running) but also reported a moderate amount of individual variation in this relationship (nearly 2 METs). These results suggest that the Caltrac had the ability to differentiate between dynamic activities of lower and higher intensities but was not able to differentiate between low- and moderate-intensity activities (i.e., 2 vs. 4 METs), particularly for activities involving complex movement patterns. Data from children have shown that AEE derived from the doubly labeled water technique was not correlated with Caltrac activity counts ($r = -0.09$) or with Caltrac AEE ($r = 0.22$; R. K. Johnson, Russ, & Goran, 1998). Using direct observation, the mean correlation between 1 hour of direct observation and Caltrac activity counts was $r = 0.35$ but increased when the observation period was extended to 1 day ($r = 0.54$; R. C. Klesges, Klesges, Swenson, & Pheley, 1985). Correlations between calorimeter values and Caltrac activity counts were poor in one study ($r = 0.11$–0.14; Bray, Wong, Morrow, Butte, & Pivarnik, 1994) but high in another ($r = 0.82$; Sallis et al., 1990). Heart rate and Caltrac activity counts were moderately correlated in one study ($r_{d1} = 0.54$, $r_{d2} = 0.42$; Sallis et al., 1990), but correlations were lower in another study (Allor & Pivarnik, 2001). Caltrac activity counts and Caltrac energy expenditure were moderately to highly correlated with self-reported energy expenditure in two studies ($r_{d1} = 0.49$, $r_{d2} = 0.39$ [Sallis et al., 1990]; $r = 0.76$ [Allor & Pivarnik, 2001]).

Pediatric studies on the validity of the Actiwatch are also conflicting. One study compared direct observation scores using the CARS with Actiwatch activity counts in preschool children (Finn & Specker, 2000). The within-child correlation ranged from $r = 0.03$ to $r = 0.92$, with a median of $r = 0.74$. Another study, using direct observation (CPAF) in preschool children, found a mean correlation of 0.16 (Kelly et al., 2004). The validity of the Actiwatch, as measured with direct calorimetry, a Doppler microwave sensor, heart rate telemetry, and the CSA, was high in a study with older children with correlations ranging from $r = 0.66$ to $r = 0.89$ (Puyau, Adolph, Vohra, & Butte, 2002).

The validity of the ActiGraph was examined in a number of studies using a variety of techniques from criterion to subjective. Melanson and Freedson (1995) demonstrated the Actigraph (WAM-7164) monitor to be a valid measure of treadmill walking and running in 15 adult men and 13 adult women (ages 12.0 ± 1.0 years and 21.0 ± 1.1 years, respectively) using energy expenditure assessed via indirect calorimetry as the criterion measure (Melanson & Freedson, 1995). Sirard, Melanson, Li, and Freedson (2000) evaluated the Actigraph (WAM-7164) monitor while quantifying physical activity in 19 free-living subjects (means age 25 ± 3.6 years) using an activity diary as the comparative measure. King, Torres, Potter, Brooks, and Coleman (2004) evaluated the validity of the Actigraph (WAM-7164) and four other accelerometers against indirect calorimetry in 22 adults (mean age 24.7 ± 5.4 years for women and 25.2 ± 4.5 years for men). The researchers concluded that Actigraph (WAM-7164) monitoring might be useful in field situations where total physical activity and patterns of physical activity are the desired outcome.

In pediatric studies, activity counts were moderately correlated with all measures of energy expenditure derived from the doubly labeled water technique ($r = 0.39–0.58$; Ekelund et al., 2001). Observed activity was correlated with Actigraph activity counts in preschool children ($r = 0.72$, $p < .001$ [Kelly et al., 2004]; $r = 0.87$, $p < .001$ [Fairweather et al., 1999]). Using indirect calorimetry, Trost et al. (1998) found that activity counts from Actigraph (MTI/CSA) monitors were strongly correlated with energy expenditure ($r = 0.86$, 0.87; $p < .001$), oxygen consumption ($r = 0.86$, 0.87; $p < .001$), heart rate ($r = 0.77$; $p < .001$), and treadmill speed ($r = 0.90$, 0.89; $p < .001$). Energy expenditure estimated from a regression equation based on counts was highly correlated with actual energy expenditure ($r = 0.62–0.85$; $p < .01$). Janz (1994) assessed the validity of an older version of the MTI/CSA model, the WAM 7164 monitor, as a field measure of physical activity in 31 children ages 7 to 15 who wore the belt for 12 hours per day for 3 consecutive days using heart rate telemetry as the comparative measure. Correlation coefficients between MTI/CSA counts pre minute (cpm) and various indices of heart rate, including average net heart rate and number of minutes with heart rate greater than or equal to 150 beats×min^{-1}, were statistically significant and ranged from 0.50 to 0.74 ($p < .05$). Table 6.4 summarizes available studies of the validity of the various models of accelerometers in children, and Table 6.5 summarizes some of the key studies of the validity of various models of accelerometers in adults.

Monitor Placement

The positioning of a motion sensor on the body is another important consideration for investigators, particularity when working with children. Studies comparing different placement options indicate that accelerometers work best when placed on the hip or on the lower back or as close as possible to the subject's center of mass (Fairweather et al., 1999; Nilsson, Ekelund, Yngve, & Sjöström, 2002; Welk, Blair, Wood, Jones, & Thompson, 2000). It makes little difference whether the monitor is worn on the right or

Table 6.4 Validity of Accelerometers in Children

Monitor	Variables	Participants	Criterion	Validity	Reference
Caltrac	Activity counts	17 boys, 14 girls; 8 ± 2.0 years	DLW	$r = -0.09$	Johnson, Russ, and Goran (1998)
Caltrac	Total counts·h free-play^{-1}	18 boys, 12 girls; 2–6 years	FATS DO	$r = 0.35-0.54$	R. C. Klesges, Klesges, Swenson, and Pheley (1985)
Caltrac	Total counts·h^{-1}	17 boys, 13 girls; 2–4 years	FATS DO	Spearman $r = 0.54$	L. M. Klesges and Klesges (1987)
Caltrac	24 hours; counts; TEE; SEE; WEE	40 girls; 10–16 years	Whole-room calorimeter (24 hours, TEE, SEE, and WEE)	$r = 0.80$ w/TEE $r = 0.84$ w/SEE $r = 0.85$ w/WEE	Bray, Wong, Morrow, Butte, and Pivarnik (1994)
Caltrac	Total counts·h^{-1}	20 boys, 15 girls; 10.8 years	HR	$r = 0.54$	Sallis, Buono, Roby, Carlson, and Nelson (1990)
Caltrac	kcal×h^{-1}	46 girls; 12 ± 0.6 years	HR	$r = 0.28$	Allor and Pivarnik (2001)
Actiwatch	Mean counts·min^{-1}	40 children; 3–4 years	CARS DO		Finn and Specker (2000)
Actiwatch	Mean counts·min^{-1}	30 boys, 48 girls; 3–4 years	CPAF DO	$r = 0.16$	Kelly, Reilly, Grant, and Paton (2004)
Actiwatch	AEE, PA	26 children; 6–16 years	Whole-room calorimeter, Doppler microwave, heart rate	$r = 0.66-0.89$	Puyau, Adolph, Vohra, and Butte (2002)
Actigraph	Mean counts·min^{-1}	15 boys, 11 girls; 9.1 ± 0.3 years	DLW	$r = 0.39-0.58$	Ekelund et al. (2001)
Actigraph	Mean counts·min^{-1}	30 boys, 48 girls; 3–4 years	CPAF DO	$r = 0.72$	Kelly et al. (2004)
Actigraph	Mean counts·min^{-1}	11 children; 4 ± 0.4 years	CPAF DO	$r = 0.87$	Fairweather, Reilly, Grant, Whittaker, and Payton (1999)
Actigraph	Mean counts·min^{-1}	19 boys, 11 girls; 10–14 years	Indirect calorimeter	$r = 0.77-0.87$	Trost (2001)
Actigraph	Mean counts·min^{-1}	31 children; 7–15 years	HR	$r = 0.50-0.74$	Janz (1994)

NOTE: AEE = active energy expenditure; CARS = Children's Activity Rating Scale; CPAF = Children's Physical Activity Form; DLW = doubly labeled water; DO = direct observation; FATS = Fargo activity time sampling survey; HR = heart rate; PA = physical activity; TEE = total energy expenditure; SEE = sedentary energy expenditure; WEE = waking energy expenditure.

Table 6.5 Validity of Accelerometers in Adults

Monitor	Variables	Participants	Criterion	Validity	Reference
Caltrac	Activity counts	21 adults	VO$_2$	$r = 0.63$	Montoye, Kemper, Saris, and Washburn (1996)
Actigraph	Mean counts·min^{-1}	28 adults	EE	EE ($r = 0.66$–0.82) Relative VO$_2$ ($r = 0.77$–0.89) Heart rate ($r = 0.66$–0.80) Treadmill speed ($r = 0.82$–0.92)	Melanson and Freedson (1996)
Actigraph	Total counts per day	19 adults	Diary	$r = 0.51$	Sirard, Melanson, Li, and Freedson (2000)
Actigraph	Mean counts·min^{-1}	21 adults	EE	$r = 0.58$–0.73	King, Torres, Potter, Brooks, and Coleman (2004)
RT3	Mean counts·min	21 adults	EE	$r = 0.34$–0.61	King et al. (2004)
Bio-Trainer	Mean counts·min	21 adults	EE	$r = 0.39$–0.69	King et al. (2004)

NOTE: VO$_2$ = oxygen consumption; EE = energy expenditure.

left hip, but the need for a standard protocol would suggest that one side be used consistently. The right hip has become the most common placement for monitors (Kelly et al., 2004; Penpraze, Reilly, Grant, Paton, & Aitchison, 2006; Penpraze et al., in press; Reilly et al., 2004; Trost, 2001; Trost et al., 2000).

Accelerometers: Number of Days

Currently, there is limited evidence on how many (number of days and hours per day) and which days (consecutive/nonconsecutive and weekdays/weekends) accelerometry monitoring should be carried out to be confident of obtaining a representative measurement of PA in children. At present, there is limited evidence documenting recommended measurement periods in free-living environments. In the literature, examples of monitoring periods include as few as 2 days, 3 or 4 days (including 1 weekend day), 7 days, and up to 2 weeks (Casperson et al., 1985; Diabetes Prevention Program Research Group, 2002; McTiernan et al., 1998; McTiernan et al., 2003; Thune et al., 1997). There appears little theoretical or empirical evidence base for the duration of monitoring. However, it is not clear from the published work if any of these monitoring periods can provide a reliable measurement of young children's physical activity. A recent publication by Penpraze and colleagues (2006) suggested that a monitoring period of 7 days and

10 hours per day produces the highest level of reliability, but surprisingly, short monitoring periods may provide adequate levels of reliability. These shorter monitoring durations can be on nonconsecutive days and need not include a weekend day. The wide-ranging differences in the approach to PA monitoring highlight the need for evidence that supports the measurement periods. In addition, consistency of measurement periods across all studies will allow meaningful comparisons to be made between studies.

Cutoff Points

In physical activity/sedentary behavior, epidemiology researchers are often interested in minutes of time or percentage of time spent in selected physical activity intensity categories that are operationally defined as sedentary, light, moderate, and vigorous physical activity. Subsequently, to convert the accelerometer output to measures of behavior, age-appropriate cutoff points that define activities of different intensity have to be applied. To date, there are a number of published pediatric cutoffs to define physical activity (Freedson et al., 2005; Puyau et al., 2002; Schmidt, Freedson, & Chasan-Taber, 2003; Sirard, Trost, Pfeiffer, Dowda, & Pate, 2005; Trost, 2001; Trost et al., 1998) and sedentary behavior (Reilly et al., 2003). However, levels of sedentary behavior and MVPA are highly sensitive to the cutoff points chosen (Penpraze et al., in press). Using the same data but applying different cutoff points can dramatically alter the assessment of how inactive or active respondents are.

This methodological problem is important and requires urgent attention. To address this problem, investigators are advised to use age-appropriate published cutoffs that have been established using criterion measures of physical activity (i.e., doubly labeled water, direct observation, and calorimeters). However, appropriate choice of cut points may depend on the distribution of activities in the respondent population, and if there is heterogeneity in these activities, it may prove difficult to select a set of cut points

that allows unbiased translation of activity scores into METS.

Epoch Length

In conjunction with deciding what motion sensor to use, how many days to monitor, and which cutoffs to use, investigators must also decide how frequently the data will be collected. Measuring physical activity and sedentary behavior by accelerometers employs a rapid sampling of accelerometer counts over a predetermined and preset time sampling period commonly known as an *epoch*. Early studies typically used 1-minute epochs, mainly due to limited memory storage capacities. However, newer models have increased their memory capacity, making data collection with very small epochs (i.e., 1 second) feasible. Much of the pediatric research has used cutoffs based on 1-minute epochs. While this might have minimum impact on physical activity assessment in adults, it has been suggested that the use of the 1-minute epoch may be problematic in children, especially young children, as it may obscure the very short bursts of moderate to vigorous activity, which are believed to be frequent in nature (Trost, 2001; Welk et al., 2000). The results of one empirical study suggest that the use of the 1-minute epoch may be inappropriate and may result in underestimation of moderate to vigorous physical activity (Nilsson et al., 2002).

Analysis of Accelerometry Data: Best Practices

Defining a Day. One of the most challenging aspects of accelerometers is managing and understanding the large amount of data collected. This is made amplified when data are collected using shorter epochs (i.e., 15 seconds). Some of the challenging decisions an investigator faces even before data collection begins include how to define a day, how to clean the data, and how to collapse and analyze the data. Defining a day is probably the most important decision an investigator is faced with. Defining a day is difficult, in the current literature; days have been defined as "waking hours" (i.e., the participant wears the monitor from the moment he or she gets up until he or she goes to bed, excluding all hours spent sleeping). Other investigators have decided to standardize the collection time to a predetermined time period such as 8 a.m. to 9 p.m. for all study participants. The most important task is ensuring that sufficient data have been collected to get a representative sample of the participants' habitual physical activity. It is also important to remember that the definition of a day will vary with different age groups. Very young children such as preschoolers and the elderly have typically shorter "waking hours" than teenagers, so care must be taken to make sure that the age of the participant is taken into consideration when defining a day.

Identification of Wearing Period. Identifying when a participant is truly wearing the accelerometer from when he or she is not can be difficult due to bouts of inactivity. Distinguishing between the two can be somewhat difficult as continuous zero readings can occur for a number of reasons: The participant (1) took the accelerometer off during these periods for a reason, (2) removed it to bathe or went swimming, (3) removed it for a sporting event, (4) removed the accelerometer as it was causing discomfort or was embarrassed to wear it, or (5) was inactive during this period (e.g., watching TV, playing computer games, or napping). Therefore, algorithms are often used to analyze these data. However, different algorithms can effect identification of physical activity behaviors significantly. For example, stringent algorithms may result in significantly lower wearing time, the lowest activity counts per minute per day, and fewer minutes of moderate to vigorous physical activity per day. To date, there is no consensus of what algorithm is the most accurate. Current literature has reported the use of algorithms ranging from 10 minutes to 60minutes (Brage et al., 2004; Brage, Wedderkopp, Franks, Andersen, & Froberg, 2003; Cradock et al., 2004; Ekelund, Yngve, Brage, Westerterp, & Sjöström, 2004;

Goran & Reynolds, 2005; Masse et al., 2005; Riddoch et al., 2004; Schmidt et al., 2003). Assuming that adults remain still for longer periods of time than children (especially young children), it may be more appropriate to use longer bouts of zero counts with adults. To date, we do not have any empirical data to support this suggestion; further studies are urgently needed to address this question. Researchers, however, should clearly specify in all their manuscripts the decision rules that they used to identify periods of accelerometer inactivity and periods when the accelerometer was presumably not worn. Ideally, all accelerometer data might be processed by one person only to reduce this decision-making bias.

Making Sense of Accelerometry Data. Once all of the above-mentioned decisions have been made (including choice of accelerometer, epochs, cutoffs, placement, number of days, valid days, and how to decide if an accelerometer was really worn) and once the data have been collected, there remains the enormous task of cleaning, collapsing, and analyzing an immense amount of data. Although these important topics are beyond the scope of the current chapter, we refer the interested reader to the 2005 *Medicine & Science in Sports & Exercise* special issue on accelerometry (Troiano, 2005).

Self-Report

Self-report of physical activity is one of the least costly, simplest to implement, and therefore most frequently used modalities for collecting information on an individual's patterns of physical activity, particularly in large epidemiological studies. Self-report measures come in a number of formats that will yield very different information. Table 6.6 gives an overview of self-report modalities.

Self-report offers deeply contextual, often qualitative data and reflects different aspects of people's lives. The tools for measuring physical activity discussed up to this point can deliver

Table 6.6 Self-Report Modalities and Data Yielded

Modality of Report	Examples of Questions Asked	Reporter	Data Yielded	Levels of Analysis (Depending on Specific Instrument)
A. Screener	Do you walk on a particular trail, or do you participate in an after-school sport?	Individual or by proxy (i.e., parent, teacher, caretaker)	Usually binary yes or no	Type of activity Frequency
B. Standardized surveys	Considering [time period X], how many times on the average do you do [activity X] for more than [X] minutes?	Individual or by proxy (i.e., parent, teacher, caretaker)	Time spent in specific activities kcal over time in specific activities METs over time in specific activities Types of activities preferred Frequency, duration, and intensity of physical activity	Type of activity intensity Duration Frequency
C. Interviews	Same as A and B but can also include what, when, where, and why questions about time use that are less amenable to questionnaire form	Same as A and B	Same as A and B but can also yield rich qualitative and contextual data	
D. Diaries and logs	Usually set up to be filled in per day or per hour/half-hour period	Same as A and B	Same as A and C	

data on several health-related dimensions of physical activity, including caloric expenditure and aerobic intensity. However, short of continual direct observation, data from questionnaires, surveys, diaries, and other forms of self-report are the only data that tell us which kind of physical activity is being undertaken. Only through self-report can an informed picture of all aspects of human daily physical activity be developed. The import of this endeavor cannot be underestimated. All forms of caloric expenditure are not equal to all people. Exploration of the differential impact of different forms of energy expenditure on health outcomes and disease risk has driven research and treatment programs. For instance, 100 calories expended in weight-bearing exercise might be important to prevent osteoporosis, while 100 calories expended in swimming or biking might be more effective to promote cardiovascular health. Understanding the types of physical activity that people undertake in their leisure time has informed many aspects of public policy and is beginning to inform urban design. This understanding can be obtained only from self-report.

When actigraphy and other forms of direct objective measures of physical activity became affordable and user-friendly enough to be used in research, the possibility of finding a definitive measure of physical activity seemed close at hand. However, Figures 6.1 and 6.2 illustrate the fact that objective measures are not yet a panacea. These figures also demonstrate the importance of self-report data. Figure 6.1 illustrates one day of actigraph data from a middle-aged man. From the figure, it would appear that he is fairly sedentary, with the exception of a peak in the evening between 8 and 9 p.m. We don't know what kind of activity he undertook at that time. It looks like he might not have been wearing the actigraph between 12 a.m. and 7:30 p.m. and again from approximately 1 to 2 p.m. He does not appear to meet any of the various guidelines for daily physical activity. However, Figure 6.2, which incorporates data from a carefully kept diary, not only shows us what kind of activity he undertook in

the evening but also reveals that he took a swim from 1 to 2 p.m. This added qualitative information changes our interpretation of the amount of physical activity that he accrued in that day. If the swimming was lap swimming and not, for instance, playing in a pool with small children, then this man would easily meet the current Institute of Medicine physical activity recommendations of 60 minutes a day for this particular day (Institute of Medicine, 2002).

It is beyond the scope of this chapter to develop a comprehensive list and review of self-report measures of physical activity. Literally hundreds of self-report measures explore different aspects/domains of physical activity in different populations, many of them available on the Web. For instance, James Sallis offers many of the questionnaires that he used in his extensive work on physical activity on his Web site at www-rohan.sdsu.edu/faculty/sallis/measures.html. The IPAQ (International Physical Activity Questionnaire) and accompanying documentation is available online at www.ipaq.ki.se. Active Living Research, supported by the Robert Wood Johnson Foundation, also has a battery of measures and tools available at www.activelivingresearch.org/resourcesearch/toolsandmeasures. An excellent, but not comprehensive, compendium review of 32 physical activity questionnaires was published in a special issue of the journal *Medicine & Science in Sports & Exercise* in 1997 (Volume 29, number 6, June 1997 supplement), and several chapters have appeared detailing measures in specific populations, such as Sirard and Pate's (2001) publication on measuring physical activity in children.

A Case Study in Self-Report Measurement: Walking and Bicycling

The preceding section of this chapter highlighted challenges in selecting self-report instruments for physical activity, largely associated with recreation, sport, and leisure activities. In recent years, there has been an intense interest in

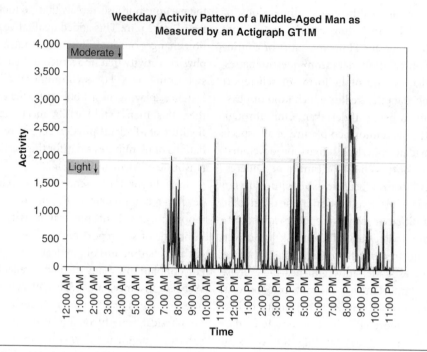

Figure 6.1   Weekday Activity Pattern of a Middle-Aged Man as Measured by an Actigraph GT1M

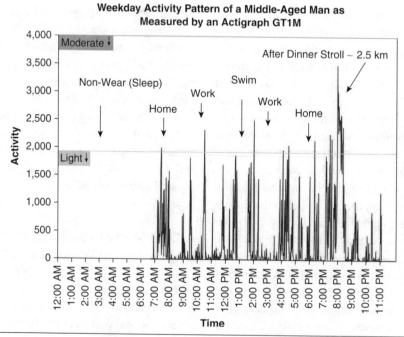

Figure 6.2   Weekday Activity Pattern of a Middle-Aged Man as Measured by an Actigraph GT1M Including Self-Report Data

walking (both for transportation and leisure) as a component of physical activity that could contribute to health (Haskell et al., 2007). Here we illustrate the depth of this literature by describing questionnaires that attempt to elicit self-report levels of walking over multiple time scales and for diverse purposes. We also reference diverse papers reporting efforts to validate these surveys. This discussion highlights the importance of selecting a physical activity self-report instrument that serves the specific purpose of your study and the weaknesses of self-report as the sole quantitative measure of physical activity in any domain.

Relevant surveys were identified through a combination of PubMed searches for keywords, snowball techniques, and consultation with experts to identify relevant surveys by name. Such surveys may appear in diverse national and international government surveys (such as the BRFSS, NHIS, ADD HEALTH, YRBS, NHANES, CHIS, IPAQ, etc.) or in the peer-reviewed literature (Aadahl & Jorgensen, 2003; Ainsworth, Bassett, et al., 2000; Ainsworth, Jacobs, Leon, Richardson, & Montoye, 1993; Ainsworth, Leon, Richardson, Jacobs, & Paffenbarger, 1993; Ainsworth, Richardson, Jacobs, Leon, & Sternfeld, 1999; Ainsworth, Sternfeld, Richardson, & Jackson, 2000; Albanes, Conway, Taylor, Moe, & Judd, 1990; Bassett, Cureton, & Ainsworth, 2000; Bonnefoy et al., 2001; Brownbill, Lindsey, Crncevic-Orlic, & Ilich, 2003; Chasan-Taber, Erickson, Nasca, Chasan-Taber, & Freedson, 2002; Conway, Irwin, & Ainsworth, 2002; C. L. Craig et al., 2003; C. L. Craig, Russell, & Cameron, 2002; De Abajo, Larriba, & Marquez, 2001; Dipietro, Caspersen, Ostfeld, & Nadel, 1993; Elley, Kerse, Swinburn, Arroll, & Robinson, 2003; Elosua et al., 2000; George, 1996; Gregg et al., 1999; Harada, Chiu, King, & Stewart, 2001; Hovell, Hofstetter, Sallis, Rauh, & Barrington, 1992; Jacobs, Ainsworth, Hartman, & Leon, 1993). We then used a combination of bibliographic tools and author contacts to find validation studies. This compilation was not based on a formal meta-analytic review; it was intended to be a robust

sample of major instruments. Complete details and a searchable data base are available at http://appliedresearch.cancer.gov/tools/paq. A total of 71 Physical Activity Questionnaires (PAQs; http://appliedresearch.cancer.gov/tools/paq/reflist.html) were identified from surveys, cohort studies, and diverse epidemiological studies. They included walking and biking questions from physical activity questionnaires.

In addition, a total of 35 validation studies, described in 70 peer-reviewed publications documenting these PAQs, was compiled with information on author, date of survey, methods, sampling, and summary results (see cites above and the following: Kohl, Blair, Paffenbarger, Macera, & Kronenfeld, 1988; Konradi & Lyon, 2000; Kriska et al., 1990; Kriska et al., 1988; Kruskall, Campbell, & Evans, 2004; LaPorte et al., 1983; Leon, Jacobs, DeBacker, & Taylor, 1981; Littman et al., 2004; Miller, Freedson, & Kline, 1994; A. Norman, Bellocco, Bergstrom, & Wolk, 2001; Oliveria, Kohl, Trichopoulos, & Blair, 1996; Philippaerts & Lefevre, 1998; Philippaerts, Westerterp, & Lefevre, 1999; Pols et al., 1995; Pols, Peeters, Kemper, & Collette, 1996; Pols, Peeters, Ocke, Bueno-de-Mesquita, et al., 1997; Pols, Peeters, Ocke, Slimani, et al., 1997; Rauh, Hovell, Hofstetter, Sallis, & Gleghorn, 1992; Resnicow et al., 2003; Richardson, Ainsworth, Wu, Jacobs, & Leon, 1995; Richardson, Leon, Jacob, Ainsworth, & Serfass, 1994; Roeykens et al., 1998; Schuler, Richardson, Ochoa, & Wang, 2001; Siconolfi, Lasater, Snow, & Carleton, 1985; Singh, Fraser, Knutsen, Lindsted, & Bennett, 2001; Singh, Tonstad, Abbey, & Fraser, 1996; Starling, Matthews, Ades, & Poehlman, 1999; Staten et al., 2001; Stel et al., 2004; Stewart et al., 2001; Suleiman & Nelson, 1997; Tuero, De Paz, & Marquez, 2001; Voorrips, Ravelli, Dongelmans, Deurenberg, & Van Staveren, 1991; Walsh, Hunter, Sirikul, & Gower, 2004; Wareham et al., 2002; Wareham et al., 2003; Washburn & Ficker, 1999; Washburn, Goldfield, Smith, & McKinlay, 1990; Washburn, McAuley, Katula, Mihalko, & Boileau, 1999; Washburn, Smith, Jette, & Janney, 1993; Weiss et al., 1990; Wendel-Vos, Schuit, Saris, & Kromhout, 2003; Westerterp et al., 1992; Wilbur, Holm, & Dan, 1993;

Wolf et al., 1994; Yore, Ham, Kohl, Ainsworth, & LaMonte, 2004; Young, Jee, & Appel, 2001; see also http://appliedresearch.cancer.gov/tools/paq/valida tion.html).

Analysis of these diverse survey instruments, all aimed at a rather small subset of all kinds of PA— namely, walking and bicycling alone—highlights some points to consider when selecting a self-report instrument in addition to some of the general survey response characteristics relevant to any study incorporating self-report (Tourangeau, Rips, & Rasinski, 2000). First, walking and/or bicycling surveys use various time intervals for activity, including day, week, month, year, most recent/last occasion, and others. Second, surveys may query walking and bicycling separately or in combination. Third, walking or bicycling might be studied for exercise, leisure, transportation, occupation, combined, or other functions. Fourth, transportation walking surveys were sometimes organized by destination such as work, work or school, activities, work or activities, or all of these destinations. Finally, it is also possible to cross-tabulate temporal domains by duration and interval. For example, a survey question might ask about bicycling in minutes in the past year.

These five categories are tabulated in the Web site above, which allows searching for a specified set of characteristics. It is not obvious that reliability and validity are correlated with the temporal and functional domains listed; therefore, readers must consider selecting a survey that matches the goals of their study. We suspect that similar considerations apply to self-report standardized surveys concerning general levels of physical activity or specific leisure time activities. However, we do recognize that the cognitive challenges of asking about structured activities such as tennis in the past week may be reduced compared to the problem of aggregating a behavior such as walking that occurs for multiple purposes over diverse time scales.

Reliability and validity studies do not seem to provide a very clear guide to the selection of an optimal standardized survey for measurement of walking and bicycling (http://appliedresearch

.cancer.gov/tools/paq/validation.html). Such studies use diverse methods to measure validity, multiple studies give different results, and studies often address energy expenditure overall, without determining if the survey instrument is measuring a specific behavior with any degree of validity and/or reliability.

In sum, this case study of a detailed review of survey instruments aimed at measuring walking and bicycling suggests that investigators should focus first on measurement of the salient duration, interval, function, and destinations of interest. Then efforts to review validity and reliability of the instruments are appropriate. Of course, these considerations apply most directly to measures of specific kinds of physical activity. If the aim is to measure energy expenditure, then the focus must generally be extended to include various kinds of physical activity, although great care should obviously be taken to determine exactly what kinds of physical activity might yield a valid measure of energy expenditure and are therefore of interest in the study. Finally, reliability and validity are usually studied in rather restricted demographic samples, and it is doubtful that rankings in such measures of survey performance will be consistent across age, race, socioeconomic status, or health-related classes.

Choosing Self-Report Measures

To close this section on self-report, it is clear that the array of possible self-report measures is large. Although many criteria can be relevant to any given study of physical activity, we suggest that two major considerations should guide the choice of appropriate measures for any study. These are the following:

1. *Match self-report instrument to research hypotheses.* Because different self-report instruments provide largely different information, the outcome of interest is the first consideration. Self-report measures should be chosen so that

the data yielded (frequency, intensity, duration, and/or type of activity) will be appropriate to address hypotheses.

2. Ensure that the instrument is reliable and valid in the targeted population. Validity and reliability of a questionnaire is important, and the questionnaire of choice should preferably be validated in the target group to be studied. Questionnaires developed to understand physical activity in outback Australian 15- to 18-year-olds will most likely not be valid in a sample of urban Los Angeles 10- to 12-year-olds. Examples of important differences between these two populations that could interfere with questionnaire validity might include reading level, language use, and difference in available activities.

Sleep

Historical Background

The study of movement during sleep has been increasingly incorporated into the field of research on energy expenditure and health. The modern age of sleep medicine began with the discovery in 1953 of rapid eye movement (REM) sleep periods by Aserinsky and Kleitman, followed later by the description of periodic sleep cycles by Dement and Kleitman (1957). These seminal observations resulted from the astute application of overnight recording of electroencephalography (EEG, measuring brain cortical activity) and electrooculography (EOG, measuring eye movements) and other physiological signals, an approach termed *polysomnography* (PSG). These pioneering studies established that indices of autonomic activity covaried with levels of cortical activity and eye movements in nonrandom patterns, suggesting the occurrence of dreaming as well as distinct states of consciousness. Over the subsequent 60 years, sleep physiology continued to be studied with the use of PSG, as well as with other physiological monitors, questionnaires, and imaging techniques, leading

to remarkable advances in the understanding of the neurophysiological basis of sleep as well as the role of sleep in the pathogenesis of numerous health conditions. Over the past 10 years, much attention has been directed at the role of sleep disruptions, sleep disorders, and sleep duration in the pathoetiology of health conditions. There are accumulating data indicating broad adverse health effects attributable to insufficient sleep. It is clear that sleep deprivation has adverse effects on mood, neurocognitive function, and quality of life (Gottlieb et al., 2005). In addition, large epidemiological studies have demonstrated significant associations between short sleep duration with diabetes, cardiovascular disease, hypertension and mortality, and, as described below, obesity. In particular, a 10% to 60% increased odds of glucose intolerance or diabetes has been observed in adults reporting < 6 or 7 hours of sleep per night (Ayas et al., 2003), with risk as high as 250% for those getting < 5 hours of sleep (S. R. Patel et al., 2004; Wingard & Berkman, 1983). Reduced sleep time has also been associated with an approximately 30% increased odds of coronary heart disease (Spiegel, Leproult, Tasali, Penev, & Van Cauter, 2003; Van Cauter, Plat, & Copinschi, 1998) and mortality (Spiegel, Tasali, Penev, & Van Cauter, 2004).

Measuring Sleep as an Element of Activity: Relevance to Energetics Research

It has been only recently that a link between sleep duration, and possibly sleep quality, and energy balance has been established. This handbook perhaps contains the first section dealing with sleep measurement embedded in a chapter that addresses measurement of physical activity— a domain more traditionally associated with energy balance. However, as described below, the epidemiological and experimental data linking short sleep duration to weight and weight gain are both compelling and continue to grow.

Insufficient Sleep and Hormonal Dysregulation

Insufficient sleep likely increases the risk of obesity through effects on hormonal dysregulation, with specific effects on the hypothalamic-pituitary axis and sympathetic overactivity (Locard et al., 1992). Abnormalities in insulin, cortisol, and growth hormone secretion have been observed following experimental sleep restriction. In addition, sleep deprivation causes morning leptin (an appetite-suppressing hormone) levels to drop by approximately 20% and ghrelin (an appetite-stimulating hormone) to increase by 18% (Sekine et al., 2002). Subjective ratings of appetite and hunger increase following moderate degrees of experimental sleep deprivation and are also associated with cravings for high-carbohydrate, high-fat containing foods (von Kries, Toschke, Wurmser, Sauerwald, & Koletzko, 2002). Thus, a range of hormonal responses to sleep deprivation likely occurs that predispose people to altered energetics.

Insufficient Sleep and Obesity Risk

Numerous epidemiological studies of children, adults, and the elderly have demonstrated a 40% to 400% increased odds of obesity for individuals with short sleep duration (Seicean et al., 2007). In adults, risk of obesity or weight gain generally has been associated with average self-reported sleep durations of < 5 or 6 hours per night. In children, who require more sleep than adults, short sleep has been defined using age-specific thresholds (Iglowstein, Jenni, Molinari, & Largo, 2003). In several pediatric studies, short sleep duration, defined using age-specific values, was similarly or more strongly associated with obesity as were traditional risk factors. Among more than 1,000 French children, of all environmental risk factors examined, short sleep duration was the strongest predictor of obesity at age 5 years (i.e., relative risk for short sleep was 4.9 vs. 1.3 and 2.1 for snacks and TV watching, respectively; National Sleep Foundation, 2000). In more

than 8,000 Japanese children ages 6 to 7 years, a significant dose-response relationship was demonstrated between late bedtime or short sleeping hours and childhood obesity. Even after considering effects of age, sex, parental obesity, and other lifestyle factors, young children sleeping < 8 hours/night were almost threefold more likely to be obese compared to children sleeping > 10 hours/night (Carskadon, Wolfson, Acebo, Tzischinsky, & Seifer, 1998). Similar findings were reported from a German study of 5- to 6-year-olds, reporting obesity in 5.4% as compared to 2.1% of children sleeping < 10 hours/night and > 11.5 hours, respectively, with significant associations persisting after adjusting for parental education, BMI of the parent, birth weight, TV watching, and snacking behavior (Spilsbury et al., 2004). Recent data from a middle-class U.S. high school survey of almost 500 students showed that self-reported sleep of < 5 hours was associated with an eight-fold increase in overweight compared to sleep of > 8 hours (Dahl, 1996). Longitudinal data from the Zurich Cohort Study as well as the Nurses' Health Study also show that shorter sleep time predicts incident weight gain in adults (Rechtschaffen & Kales, 1968), with the latter study of almost 70,000 nurses followed over 16 years showing that the relative risk of a 15-kg weight gain to be 1.32 (95% confidence interval [CI]: 1.19, 1.47) for those sleeping < 5 hours per night. Preliminary data from two large cohorts of older men and women (Study of Osteroporetic Fractures), using actigraphy performed over several nights to provide objective estimates of sleep duration, have shown sleep durations of < 5 hours per night as well as low sleep efficiency to be associated with higher BMI, even after adjusting for multiple confounders.

Declines in Sleep

The importance of these observations relative to the current obesity epidemic is underscored by the progressive decrease in sleep duration in the community. Between 1959 and 2002, median sleep time decreased from 8 to 7 hours, with the percentage of adults usually getting < 7 hours of sleep rising from 15% to 39% (ASDA Report, 1992). Much of the reduction in sleep time reflects changes in behavior, including late-night TV viewing or Internet use (reported by 43% of adults) or keeping late hours to attend to work needs (reported by 45%). Sleep deprivation has also increased in preadolescents and adolescents, with > 33% of teens getting less than the recommended 9 hours of sleep (Whitney, Lind, & Wahl, 1998). Insufficient sleep in adolescents likely reflects the influences of social/school pressures, along with biological changes in circadian rhythm and sleep architecture that occur in this developmental stage. Certain ethnic groups may be particularly at risk for insufficient sleep. For example, Black boys are almost five times more likely to have delayed bedtimes compared to White children (Iber et al., 2004).

Sleep and Other Obesity Risk Factors

The need to consider sleep in obesity research is also underscored by the potential interactions between insufficient sleep and other obesity risk factors. Reduced sleep has been implicated in mood swings and irritability, which may alter food consumption, as well as fatigue, which may negatively affect physical activity (Ancoli-Israel et al., 2003). However, to date, little research has comprehensively used transdisciplinary methods to consider traditional and novel risk factors, such as sleep patterns, for understanding energy balance. As described below, there are multiple methods for measuring sleep in experimental, clinical, and epidemiological research that may significantly complement the information gathered on traditional obesity risk factors.

Methods in Sleep Assessment

The following sections review the key methods for assessing sleep, particularly sleep duration. These include PSG, wrist actigraphy, and questionnaires.

Measuring Sleep Using Polysomnography. As the introduction to this section alluded to, the gold standard for assessing sleep is PSG, which is a method for collecting multiple channels of data to measure neurophysiological indicators of sleep state. By combining data on EEG, EOG, and chin EMG and using well-standardized approaches for assessing patterns of these signals across the night, sleep can be precisely staged in 30-second epochs as wake or Stage 1, 2, 3, 4, or REM sleep, with each stage characterized by different EEG frequencies and amplitude patterns, corresponding to distinct states associated with different degrees of arousability and autonomic activation (Acebo et al., 1999). In addition to identifying sleep stages, abrupt discrete changes in background EEG are identified and scored as "arousals" (Morgenthaler et al., 2007). These data are summarized to provide indices of total sleep time, percentage of the sleep period asleep (sleep efficiency), time awake after sleep onset (WASO), duration and percentage of sleep period in each sleep stage, and total arousals per sleep hour. Thus, a comprehensive assessment of sleep duration (i.e., total sleep time) and sleep quality (sleep efficiency, WASO, arousal index, number of shifts in sleep state, and percentage of time in deeper [Stages 3, 4 and REM] vs. lighter [Stage 1 and 2 sleep) is possible. When scored by trained polysomnologists, these data can be highly reliable, with excellent epoch-by-epoch levels of agreement (kappa statistics > 0.80; Ancoli-Israel et al., 2003). Laboratory-based PSG, however, has a known "first night effect" due to poor sleep occurring during an initial recording night in an unfamiliar environment. New technology, however, permits these measurements, traditionally made in highly controlled laboratory settings, to be made in more natural home environments. When performed in the home, there is moderate to high levels of night-to-night reproducibility for percentage of slow-wave sleep and the arousal index but less agreement for total sleep time, sleep efficiency, and REM sleep (Tikotzky & Sadeh, 2001). The relative cost and complexity of these procedures has limited the widespread use of such measurements in large-scale studies, with monitoring usually limited to only one or two nights. However, given the detailed physiological data attainable with PSG, its use in at least selected subgroups participating in studies of sleep and obesity may importantly enhance the interpretation of data derived from other sources, such as actigraphy and questionnaire.

Measuring Sleep Using Actigraphy. Over the past 25 years, as both interest in making objective measures of sleep outside of a laboratory setting and technological advances in monitoring equipment have grown, there has been a progressive increased use of actigraphy for making inferences on sleep and wake activity. The use of wrist actigraphy as a method of estimating sleep time and sleep patterns has the benefits of (1) providing more objective data than sleep diaries or questionnaires and (2) being less intrusive and expensive than PSG, with the ability to collect data over multiple nights in the participant's normal sleep setting with minimal intrusion. Actigraphs detect and digitally store movement (or acceleration) counts. When worn on the trunk, this technology has been used to estimate overall activity and make inferences on energy consumption. However, when worn on a limb (typically a non-dominant wrist), with data processed using specific software, such activity counts provide estimates of sleep and wake bouts, including several measures analogous to those made with PSG, such as total sleep time, sleep efficiency, WASO, sleep onset and offset times, and daytime measurements of napping behavior. Several commercially available actigraphs and various models with differing computer algorithms and signal collection approaches are available. Most actigraphs use a piezoelectric sensor that generates a signal based on movement. The analog signal is digitized and for each 30-second or 1-minute epoch, an activity count is calculated and stored. There are currently three data modes available in wrist actigraphs: Proportional integration mode calculates the area under the curve for each epoch, time above threshold (TAT)

counts the amount of time per epoch that the signal is above a set threshold, and zero-crossing mode (ZCM) counts the number of times per epoch that the signal crosses a threshold (set very close to zero; Ancoli-Israel et al., 2003). Among sources of variability that may influence the derived data are the sensitivity of accelerometers, filters applied to reduce detection of fast movements unlikely to represent purposeful (wake) behaviors, duration of epochs used for analyses, and the processing and scoring algorithms used to translate activity to sleep-wake estimates.

Studies have shown that more than two nights of monitoring are needed to provide reliable estimates of sleep patterns (Gupta, Mueller, Chan, & Meininger, 2002). In children and adolescents, data loss of up to 28% has been reported, and 7 days of monitoring, including one weekday and weekend night, is recommended. Sleep logs, requiring participants or their caregivers to record sleep and wake times, times when the monitor is removed, and so on, are generally recommended to collect concurrent complementary information and help ascertain when monitors are removed or situations of increased movement occur (e.g., riding in a vehicle), which may create wake activity patterns that do not represent state changes.

Recommendations for the role of these devices in clinical practice have been published (Sadeh, Sharkey, & Carskadon, 1994), as have a comprehensive review of both research and clinical issues in using actigraphy (Morgenthaler et al., 2007). Normative data are available for most age groups other than young adults. Predictive accuracy has been established for actigraphy using a variety of approaches. In aggregate, studies have shown that actigraphic measures of sleep patterns predict daytime levels of sleepiness and developmental changes in children (Kushida et al., 2001), sleep symptoms (N. J. Johnson et al., 2007), responsiveness to sleep interventions (N. J. Johnson et al., 2007), and BMI levels (Buysse, Reynolds, Monk, Berman, & Kupfer, 1989). Sleep-wake inference by actigraphy has been shown to be moderately accurate in comparison to PSG in adult and infant populations (D. W. Levine, Lewis, et al.,

2003) and in a mixed sample of healthy adults and adolescents (Quan et al., 1997). Some data indicate that sleep periods are more accurately identified than wake periods, although overall validity of each measurement varies with the sensitivities used to classify given epochs as sleep or wake. A review of 108 studies showed that the overall correlations between total sleep time obtained by actigraphy and PSG was on average 0.71 but with a range of 0.15 to 0.92 (Johns, 1992). Any factor that may influence movement patterns in wakefulness or sleep may be anticipated to alter the validity of actigraphy. These include age, gender, physical and psychiatric disorders, and sleep disorders. In general, the highest levels of agreement have been reported for individuals with no known sleep or serious health problems. Situations where movements during sleep may be increased, such as sleep apnea or periodic limb movements, may tend to underestimate sleep. In contrast, conditions where individuals spend long periods resting quietly while awake (including depression and older age) may result in overestimation of sleep duration. The overall accuracy of actigraphy degrades with shorter sleep duration and more fragmented sleep or lower sleep efficiency (Devine, Hakim, & Green, 2005). A study of adults referred to a sleep laboratory showed that actigraphy overestimated sleep duration by an average of 20 minutes (up to 1.8 hours) and overestimated sleep efficiency by 4.4% (up to 29%; Monk et al., 2003). In contrast, actigraphy tended to underestimate sleep time in a group of 181 adolescents (Wolfson et al., 2003). This study also showed that lower levels of reliability for sleep duration were found in boys compared to girls and in those with sleep apnea compared to those without sleep apnea (Wiggs, Montgomery, & Stores, 2005). Thus, in the settings of sleep or health disorders, actigraphy may provide reliable estimates of within-subject changes (e.g., provide information on responsiveness to an intervention) but may be less useful for characterizing between-subject differences in sleep time. Actigraphy and questionnaires also may be used as complementary sources of information, identifying where there are consistencies and inconsistencies in other objective or subjective information.

Sleep Questionnaires

A large number of sleep questionnaires have been developed that variably attempt to characterize sleep adequacy (including sleep duration, timing, and restorative functions), sleep maintenance (or the converse, sleep fragmentation or interruptions), sleep behaviors and attitudes, daytime consequences (e.g., hypersomnolence), and sleep disorders (sleep apnea, periodic limb movements, insomnia). Instruments with the strongest levels of validation and most widespread use include the Pittsburgh Sleep Quality Index (a 19-item instrument with a global score and subscales that include sleep quality, latency, duration, sleep efficiency, disturbances, hypnotic use, and daytime dysfunction; Hauri & Wisbey, 1992), the Women's Health Study Insomnia Severity Scale (a 5-item instrument that assesses sleep duration and sleep quality; Spilsbury et al., 2004), the Sleep Heart Health Study Sleep Habits Questionnaire (with special emphasis on sleep apnea symptoms; Monk et al., 1994), and the Epworth Sleepiness Scale (an 8-item questionnaire designed to assess subjective sleepiness; Knutson & Lauderdale, 2007). A recent systematic review of 22 sleep questionnaires provides detailed information on the psychometric properties of many commonly used instruments (D. L. Craig, 1981; Mueller et al., 1986; Saris, Snel, Baecke, van Waesberghe, & Binkhorst, 1977). Since the strongest epidemiological associations between sleep parameters and obesity are for sleep duration, the remaining section focuses on approaches to assessing usual sleep duration and timing of sleep.

Most commonly, sleep duration is assessed with use of a sleep survey instrument or a sleep diary (completed over several days). Sleep questionnaires vary in whether they ask participants to record their usual sleep duration or record their usual bed and wake times. Since the former approach is simpler (i.e., requiring only one question and avoiding data coding of clock times), it has been used most often when sleep assessment has been added to ongoing health surveys. However, it is likely that many people, even when correctly identifying their bed and wake times, fail to accurately calculate the interval between these times and/or will tend to report what they believe is a "normal" sleep duration. This question also does not address the timing of sleep, which may be shifted in certain groups. Some but not all questionnaires ask participants to report separately for weekend versus weekday (or work/school or other days)—distinctions that are important in understanding cumulative sleep debt. One major problem in asking participants to record their usual sleep and wake times is the ambiguity of wording used to identify times when subjects actually fell asleep and woke up and got out of bed, as contrasted with "going to bed" and "waking up." To address this, one instrument, the Sleep Timing Questionnaire, specifically defined "Good Night Time" and "Good Morning Time." With this approach, within-subject reliability over an average test-retest period of 108 days for self-reported bed and wake times was 0.71 and .83, respectively, and the correlation of each with actigraphic measures of bed and wake times was .59 and .77, thus showing promise as a useful tool for identifying sleep timing and duration.

A study of U.S. high school students using the Sleep Habits Survey (asking participants to "figure out their usual sleep time on a school night") showed that self-reported sleep duration was correlated with sleep duration measured by both actigraphy ($r = .53$) and a sleep diary ($r = .64$; Bassett, 2000; Chen & Bassett, 2005; Tudor-Locke & Myers, 2001). However, in other studies, compared to PSG, sleep duration estimated by self-report was underestimated and sleep latency overestimated. In certain subgroups, differences may be more pronounced. For example, sleep duration reported by parents of children with attention-deficit hyperactivity disorder shows no correlation with actigraphy, and patients with

insomnia may be particularly subject to underreporting sleep duration and overestimating sleep latency (Prochaska, Zabinski, Calfas, Sallis, & Patrick, 2000). Nonetheless, despite these limitations, most of the epidemiological studies linking obesity and short sleep used questionnaire data, with most employing a simple question on sleep duration, providing evidence for predictive validity.

Sleep diaries, which have been in use for more than 30 years, ask the participant to record, on a daily basis, the time he or she went to bed and awoke each day over a several-day period. The advantages of diaries include the potentially enhanced reliability achieved by averaging over several nights and the added accuracy achieved with direct recording as compared to recall. However, staff and participant burden is also increased, and data often are missing.

Various diaries differ in whether information is entered only in the morning upon awakening or also require the subject to complete it in the evening, how much other information relevant to sleep (or obesity) is collected (e.g., beverage and caffeine consumption, naps, illness, medications, activities), and the duration of recording. One would anticipate that, similar to actigraphy, greater reliability would be achieved as the number of recording days is increased. As described for questionnaires, each diary differs in the specific words used to identify sleep and bed times, with some instruments also asking participants to record both the times they went to bed ("lights out") and then how long it took to fall asleep. Versions for pediatric populations have been developed, with parent or joint parent-child completion of the diaries, with normative data available (Evers & Carol, 2007).

Two studies in pediatric and adolescent samples from Japan have shown high levels of agreement between sleep times estimated by 7-day diaries with 7-day actigraphy (correlations of > .95; Atienza, Oliveira, Fogg, & King, 2006), with only a reported 8-minute average difference in sleep duration measurement using the two techniques. Using the Pittsburgh Sleep Diary in 234 adults, high correlations were observed between sleep duration assessment by the diary and actigraphy ($ps < .006$; Stone, Shiffman, Atienza, & Nebeling, 2007). In contrast, a low correlation was reported between self-reported sleep duration as assessed with a single item to data obtained from a 2-day diary ($r = .27$), with sleep diary data showing an average 48-minute longer weekday sleep duration than self-report (G. J. Norman et al., 2007).

Measuring Sleep: Summary and Conclusions

Emerging data indicate that sleep duration and perhaps sleep quality operate as novel risk factors for obesity. The tools for measuring sleep vary from intensive neurophysiological assessments made with PSG to objective measures made with actigraphy to subjective assessments by questionnaires. Similar to physical activity measurement, there likely is complementary information available through the use of both questionnaires and actigraphy. There are several approaches to quantifying sleep duration. However, when possible, ascertainment of bed/sleep and wake times is likely to be most useful because this provides information on both sleep duration and timing of the sleep period. Given the informativeness of sleep diary information, many of the activity logs used for recording physical activity in energetics studies may be expanded to include sleep data, providing an efficient approach for obtaining daily self-reported activity information for both physical activity and sleep. PSG, although not easily performed in large numbers of individuals, can provide important detail on sleep architecture not otherwise available through other instrumentation. As a "gold-standard" tool for sleep measurements, it may also be useful for providing corroborative data in subgroups studied with less intensive means or for characterizing specific sleep disorders.

Measuring Inactivity or Sedentariness

Interest in measuring physical inactivity, or sedentary behavior that is not sleep, is relatively new and likely stems from the repeated finding that time spent in front of the television is securely tied to obesity in children (Robinson, 1999) as well as adults (Kronenberg et al., 2000). By definition, sedentary behaviors are low-intensity/low–energy expenditure activities (Hardy, Bass, & Booth, 2007; Must & Tybor, 2005). Several attempts have been made to narrowly quantify sedentariness either by intensity or time, including accelerometer cutoff points (less than 1,100 cpm in 3- to 4-year-old children; Reilly et al., 2003), less than 10 minutes of continuous physical activity weekly (overweight African American adults; Brown, Miller, & Miller, 2003; Yancey et al., 2004), and activities that expend less than 1.5 METs (adolescent girls; Hardy et al., 2007).

A relative newcomer to the realm of sedentary behavior is the study of nonexercise activity thermogenesis (NEAT). Some but not all components of NEAT fall into the category of sedentary behavior. According to J. A. Levine (2004), NEAT is "the energy expended for everything that is not sleeping, eating, or sports-like exercise. It includes the energy expended walking to work, typing, performing yard work, undertaking agricultural tasks, and fidgeting" (p. E675). Sedentary aspects of NEAT, conceptualized as aspects of posture (sitting and lying), have been measured by inclinometers (Lanningham-Foster et al., 2005).

We have yet to converge on an agreed-upon, well-defined spectrum of "sedentariness." While the need to understand sedentariness as an important health behavior, distinct from physical activity, has become increasingly clear, the study of sedentary behavior most frequently focuses on media-based behaviors (television, computer, and video games; Spanier, Marshall, & Faulkner, 2006), and few measures have been dedicated exclusively to understanding the complexities of sedentary behaviors (Hardy et al., 2007). Sedentariness is often gleaned by using measures originally intended to capture physical activity, such as accelerometry (Hardy et al., 2007) or items from existing surveys, such as the short form of the International Physical Activity Questionnaire (IPAQ) in adults (Brown, Trost, Bauman, Mummery, & Owen, 2004) or various physical activity recall instruments in children (Jago, Anderson, Baranowski, & Watson, 2005). However, these measures do not cover the range of sedentary behaviors. Sedentary behaviors change over the life span and cover a huge range of behaviors, including stroller time, classroom time, homework, small screen time (SSR—computer and video games), hanging out with friends, talking on the phone, motorized transportation, time spent sitting at a desk, reading, and wheelchair time. Furthermore, understanding the nature of behaviors that we commonly consider sedentary is complex. On one hand, with the advent of computer games such as *Dance Dance Revolution* and Wii, playing computer games can no longer be categorized as "sedentary" across the board. On the other hand, behaviors that once demanded a moderate amount of energy expenditure, such as some daily domestic tasks, require significantly less energy expenditure when performed with the aid of machines or equipment (Lanningham-Foster, Nysse, & Levine, 2003).

Where Physical Activity Happens: Conceptualizing and Measuring the Built Environment

Evidence continues to mount that sedentary lifestyles and associated health problems, such as obesity, diabetes, and heart disease (Anderson et al., 2005; Calle & Kaaks, 2004; Deckelbaum & Williams, 2001), are more prevalent in urban areas characterized by lack of parks and open space and by sprawl, where the arrangement of land uses and specific features of urban form discourage walking and other types of physical activity (Frank, Andresen, & Schmid, 2004; Lopez, 2004; Lopez-Zetina, Lee, & Friis, 2006;

Vandegrift & Yoked, 2004). Experts in public health, transportation, recreation, and urban planning increasingly seek a more comprehensive understanding of the mechanisms by which urban form shapes human activity patterns. These efforts are part of larger initiatives to promote active living and contribute to overall public health and quality of life in urban settings.

A number of studies point out that human activity patterns and associated health status are together influenced in part by the nature of the built environment, as well as individual factors and the larger social environment (Figure 6.3). For example, specific land use characteristics, such as residential density, connectivity, the mix of land uses, and the presence/accessibility of parks, recreational facilities, golf courses, and so on, together establish the types and amounts of movement possible in the urban environment (Bedimo-Rung, Mowen, & Cohen, 2005; Ewing, Schmid, Killingsworth, Zlot, & Raudenbush, 2003; Frank et al., 2004; Handy, Boarnet, Ewing, & Killingsworth, 2002; Jackson & Kochtitzky, 2001; Janz, Burns, & Levy, 2005; Lopez, 2004; Lopez-Zetina et al., 2006; K. E. Powell, 2005; Sallis et al., 2006; Zimring, Joseph, Nicoll, & Tsepas, 2005). The growing interest in the effects of urban form on physical activity has thus focused attention on conceptualizing the urban built environment and measuring relevant aspects of the cityspace that may either promote or hinder physical activity.

Conceptualizing the Built Environment

There are many approaches to conceptualizing the built environment of cities and deriving associated measures. Urban form can be considered in terms of the broad spatial organization of activity centers, for example, whether the metropolis has a single downtown or many subcenters of employment and housing. Another angle is to characterize the distribution of demographic subgroups of the population, focusing

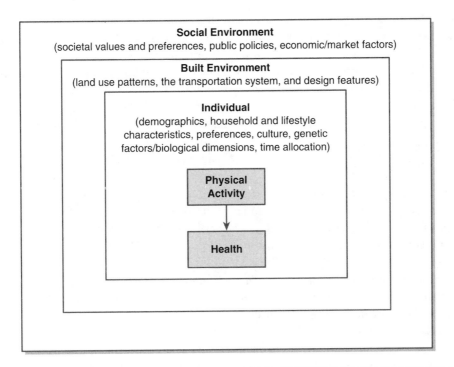

Figure 6.3   How the Built Environment Influences Physical Activity

SOURCE: National Research Council (2005, p. 4).

on the extent of segregation or the presence of barrios, ghettos, or suburban ethnic enclaves. A third avenue of considering urban form emphasizes density and land use mix and hence whether the city's built environment encourages automobile use or walking.

For purposes of relating aspects of the built environment to physical activity, however, it is vital to employ a framework centered on perception. The use of the built environment by residents is largely driven by their perceptions of place and access to various destinations of importance to everyday life, such as job centers, schools, or parks.

One framework, developed by the urban theorist Kevin Lynch (1960), is particularly useful in the present context. His approach specifically identifies those elements of urban form that shape the ways in which residents perceive the city's landscape—perceptions that in turn influence their decisions about how they navigate or wayfind, their mode of transportation, and their daily activity patterns.

Lynch's (1960) lexicon of urban form elements, which together shape what he termed "the image of the city," includes *districts, edges, paths, nodes,* and *landmarks.*

- *Districts* form distinct neighborhoods or easily recognized zones that are internally homogeneous.

- *Paths* connect people and land uses within and between districts.

- *Nodes* are destinations and places where people gather.

- *Edges* are the boundaries and barriers between districts.

- *Landmarks* serve to guide people through their neighborhoods.

Lynch (1960) analyzed the problems that arise when key elements of the built environment are not "legible." Here we use Los Angeles as an example to illustrate the structure of a section of the city and why it might be difficult to imagine or navigate (Figure 6.4).

Measuring Districts, Paths, Nodes, Edges, and Landmarks

Characteristics of Lynch's (1960) lexicon of the urban built environment can be captured in two ways: as a result of perception studies (e.g., through the creation of cognitive maps based on interviews) or on the basis of objective data collected from a wide variety of sources and compiled within a geographic information system (GIS) model. There are no validated, widely used instruments for the capture of perceptions of the urban built environment, and thus any specific study of physical activity and the built environment involving perception will include study-specific instruments that capture how individual subjects imagine the city. GIS models are basically geo-referenced data sets that can be conceived of as layers of spatial information, which together constitute a series of overlay maps. Increasingly, researchers can access a wide variety of secondary data sources that provide objective measures of the built environment and can be stored, analyzed, and displayed via GIS. Figure 6.5 shows an example of a 500-meter buffer around schools in Santa Monica, California. The buffers intersect with all fast-food outlets, which can be tabulated as a means of characterizing the foodscape near the schools.

There are a number of ways to characterize elements of urban form, at various spatial scales, using spatially referenced GIS attributes from many sources. Some data can be derived from national public- and private-sector sources; the precise nature and format of other data, available only locally, will necessarily be more variable.

For example, *districts* can be characterized using Business Analyst for ArcGIS (ESRI, Redlands, California). Business Analyst offers a large number of data sets on population and housing units, as well as their characteristics, street density, percent of district land area, park density, number of schools, density of businesses and jobs, landmarks, and other features of districts. Demographic data are drawn from the 1990 and 2000 U.S. census data (STF 1 and STF 3 tables), both using 2000 geography, plus 2003 estimates and 2008 projections, all of which are available at various spatial scales, such as county, ZIP code, census tract, and block group. Economic indicators are also included from federal sources on a small area basis. Traffic data are available as part of the data set (Dynamap/Transportation v.6.0) compiled by Geographic Data Technology (GDT). Commercial data are compiled, including an infoUSA database of more than 12 million businesses documenting industry, sales volume, employees, geography, and so on.

Nodes are destinations and places within districts where people gather. Again using ESRI Business Analyst data, specific types of nodes can be identified, and access to such nodes can be calculated. Nodes of note include parks, pay and free recreational facilities, shopping centers, and entertainment uses. With a particular district, access measures can be calculated, such as distance (or time-distance or road-network distance) to parks, other recreational and entertainment facilities, shopping, fast-food outlets, or school, to assess the impact of nodal density and proximity on physical activity (see Figure 6.6).

More detailed measures can also be developed, such as ratios of fast-food outlets (e.g., convenience stores and fast-food outlets) to full-service food outlets (e.g., grocery stores), using ESRI Business Analyst data. In addition, data on shopping centers from the National Research Board are included in Business Analyst for centers with more than 100,000 square feet of gross leaseable area.

For *paths*, which are primarily streets and roadways, the objective is to characterize their scale and volume of traffic. Public transport network data, often available from cities and counties, typically include frequency of buses (from

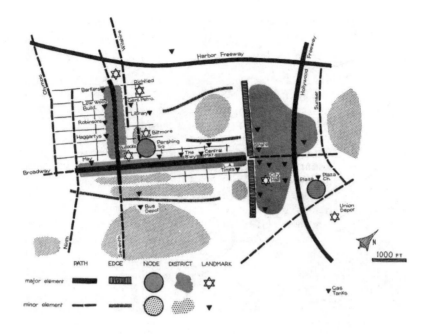

Figure 6.4   Problems "Reading" Districts, Paths, Edges, Nodes, and Landmarks in Los Angeles

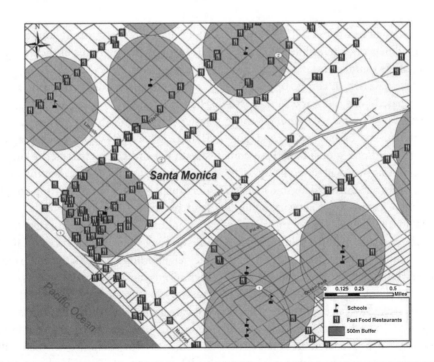

Figure 6.5   Fast-Food Outlets Within 500 Meters of Schools in Santa Monica, California

SOURCE: ESRI Business Analyst, 2004.

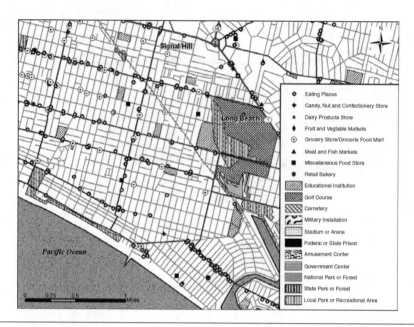

Figure 6.6   Map of Business Destinations, Road Networks, and Land Use in Long Beach, California

SOURCE: ESRI Business Analyst, 2004.

bus timetables) and bus routes. ESRI Streetmaps USA offers road network data, while Tele Atlas, a private firm, offers traffic count data at the road link level. These data, which consist of position-accurate GIS-based road networks and corresponding link-based traffic volume and vehicle fraction data, can be connected to and augmented by state and/or regional data. Path connectivity can be measured in several ways. The structure of a district can be determined from the length of streets and street network patterns as captured in the digital road network files, while various modeling methods can be used to calculate the routes linking specific origins and destinations. These include Arc 9 routing algorithms (e.g., to school); the gamma index, which assesses connectivity by calculating the ratio of the number of links to the maximum number of possible links given a specified number of nodes; the ratio of the number of circuits (routes) in a system to the maximum number of possible circuits, which is computed; the number of intersections with

more than three legs throughout a district; and road types based on ratios of the length of major to minor roads.

Edges may serve as barriers to connectivity. High-resolution (10-meter) topography data in raster format USGS Digital Elevation Model (DEM), as well as National Hydrography data on stream networks, can characterize the terrain of the built environment and identify physical barriers such as rivers or cliffs or topography, while land use data (described above) can highlight large industrial land uses that can constitute barriers to movement. Major roads slicing through the neighborhood with high traffic volumes and high speeds can also form edges that may impede travel by foot or bicycle. These traffic and road data are available through transportation data as described above and can also be used to measure the sinuosity (or curvature) of roads, block size, and T intersections. Neighborhoods with better interconnectivity are expected to promote more travel on foot.

Beyond Lynch: Urban Fabric and Sprawl

There remain key aspects of the urban built environment that are important to understanding physical activity but are not fully captured by Lynch's (1960) framework. Although the framework is scalable (in other words, applicable to the analysis of both small areas within the city as well as entire metropolitan areas), it is most useful for studies with a relatively small-scale orientation, such as the neighborhood or community, because it does not address the influence of larger parameters of urban spatial organization on residents' physical activity, particularly their decisions to walk, bike, or drive.

For instance, at the meso-urban scale, which might capture a major subarea of the metropolis such as the central city or suburban ring, the nature of the *urban fabric* could be vital. The character of the urban fabric—its density and land use mix—can determine the extent to which residents may have easy access to and thus be inclined to walk or bicycle to potential destinations such as work, shopping and other services, or recreation. Although the urban fabric of smaller scale areas ("districts") is also important, the nature and variation of the urban fabric at the meso-urban scale can profoundly shape daily activity patterns, including the decision to engage in physical activity. For example, a cluster of high-density, mix-use districts creates an urban fabric that encourages a lifestyle based on walking or biking to work, shopping, or leisure; where large subareas of a metropolis are low density and homogeneous with regard to land use (e.g., a cluster of bedroom suburbs designed on a cul-de-sac model), the necessity of driving to most destinations may systematically undermine habits of walking to work, to see friends, or to use common services or amenities.

To measure urban fabric, researchers can use basic parameters such as population density (which can be measured in several ways) from the U.S. census. Most urban regions maintain high-resolution land use classification data that can be used to characterize land use mix. A variety of land use segregation measures can then be used to portray the extent of heterogeneity of the urban fabric. Such measures include indices of segregation (concentration, dissimilarity, isolation, clustering, etc.), as well as measures derived from landscape ecology that capture fragmentation of land use distributions. Frank et al. (2006) have reviewed various measures of "walkability" that may promote utilitarian travel by foot. These measures include net residential density, density of intersections per square kilometer (as a proxy for street connectivity), area of retail floor space around the home, and land use mix. The latter measures the relative diversity of land use in an area around the residence or school of a study subject. In this regard, ESRI's Arc 9.2 includes spatial analysis tools (FRAGSTATS) that provide a wide range of segregation and landscape fragmentation measures that allow additional analysis, such as the impacts of edge effects (that can create barriers between land use "patches") on physical activity. Satellite data also are becoming more widely used to characterize land use in urban regions. For example, a green cover network can be developed using the Normalized Difference Vegetation Index (NDVI) classification system. The NDVI is based on Landsat satellite images and is useful for understanding the interaction between physical activity and the presence of nature in the city (see Figure 6.7).

In addition, the macro-urban scale of an entire metropolitan area can be characterized by extent of *urban sprawl*, measured by such parameters as the region-wide segregation of populations and land uses, density and/or discontinuous (or leap-frog) development, and average commute distances. Although evidence is mixed, some research suggests that higher levels of physical activity are linked to metropolitan regions that are compact and conserve open space. Conversely, a more sprawling urban form, in which residences and workplaces are far apart and where access to services is low and requires automobile trips, may reduce discretionary time, establish driving as the dominant travel mode, and thus discourage physical activity.

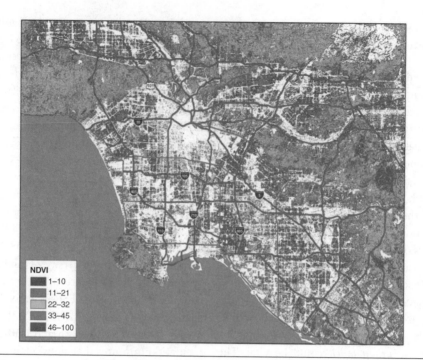

Figure 6.7   Normalized Difference Vegetation Index Across the Los Angeles Metropolitan Area

SOURCE: Landsat images captured on February 3, 2003.

NOTE: Areas shown in white have no green cover, while the darkest areas have the highest levels of green cover in the region.

Sprawl Indices

A variety of "sprawl indices" have been developed to characterize the extent of urban sprawl. For example, Galster et al. (2001) defined sprawl as a pattern of land use in urban area that exhibits low levels of some combination of eight distinct dimensions of land use: (1) density, (2) mixed use, (3) proximity, (4) continuity, (5) concentration, (6) centrality, (7) nuclearity, and (8) clustering. Each dimension reflects spatial relationships among units of analysis that were established by assigning housing units from 1990 census blocks to 1- and ½ -mile square grids. Low scores on each dimension were indicative of sprawl. In contrast, Ewing, Pendall, and Chen (2002) used 22 variables that were collected at a variety of scales to describe different aspects of urban dynamics and developmental patterns at the metropolitan level. These indicators were grouped into four dimensions of sprawl: residential density; neighborhood mix of homes, jobs, and services; strength of activity centers and downtowns; and accessibility of the street network. These factors were combined to produce the overall sprawl index for assessment of the impact of sprawl on certain aspects of daily life, including walking.

Measuring Physical Activity in the Built Environment: Future Directions

Although built environment characterization has improved over the past 10 years, there is still relatively little understanding or cross-validation of whether environments hypothesized to promote activity are associated with objective measures. Recent advances in GPS technologies and new wearable technologies capable of sensing activity levels and a wide range of heart and lung functions appear likely to be gaining wider use in research linking physical activity assessments to the built environment. Continuous, lightweight, and accurate GPS units are now available and can be deployed in larger population studies. These recently have been combined with accelerometers to assess the likely location of physical activity. Rodriguez, Brown, and Troped (2005) performed a pilot study and found that about two thirds of the times, moderate to vigorous physical activity could be successfully located using a GPS.

In parallel with these developments, wearable ambulatory technologies have emerged, allowing for real-time monitoring of cardiovascular, respiratory, and physical activity. For example, "life shirts" by Vivometrics (Grossman, 2004), which weigh only 8 ounces, can be used to collect continuous, time-stamped measurements of activity with accelerometers and pulmonary function. The possibility of merging these technologies with ambient and personal activity modeling using GPS will expand knowledge on understanding and integrate social-spatial patterns into assessment of which specific environments are most likely to promote physical activity. These data will be important for understanding the relative locations that promote activity and inactivity in children (e.g., points of high physical activity may occur in and around neighborhood park space but not near busy roads), which in turn can be used to refine future built environment measures and potentially to target intervention studies.

Innovative Technologies and Methodologies for Physical Activity Research

Since the late 1970s and early 1980s, researchers have used computer technology to monitor and assess exercise behavior among patients and individuals in the general population (Kroeze, Werkman, & Brug, 2006). Since then, the processing speed and complexity of the technology have increased exponentially, while the size of portable computers and computer processors has become a fraction of the size of the initial technology (and getting smaller). The emergence of powerful microprocessors has provided researchers (and practitioners) with ways to collect data on specific aspects of physical activity, particularly in two areas: activity assessment and behavioral modification of activity (i.e., intervention). This section discusses technological advances and innovations in both physical activity assessment and intervention, as well as the opportunities and challenges that arise from using ever more powerful computer technology to assess and modify physical activity.

Technological Innovations in Physical Activity Assessment

The electronic assessment of physical activity behavior has advanced substantially since pioneering research in the area of cardiovascular research that used computer technology to record an immediate physiologic response to physical activity behavior—namely, changes in heart rate. The development of electronic pedometers and accelerometers afforded opportunities to directly assess certain physical activity behaviors (e.g., walking, running); frequency, duration, and intensity can be on several devices, and newer devices can connect to desktop computers and the Internet (e.g., Sport Brain; G. J. Norman et al., 2007). The methodological and conceptual issues related to pedometers and accelerometers have been discussed by others (Hurling et al., 2007; Nawyn, Intille, & Larson, 2006; Patrick, Intille, & Zabinski, 2005).

Further innovation in tools to objectively assess physical activity behavior include (1) the use of GPS to assess location and movement among individuals, either as stand-alone portable units (Hurling et al., 2007; Oliveira, Morton, Atienza, Gardner, & King, 2005) or integrated into mobile phone technology (Atienza et al., 2007); (2) the further miniaturization of mobile wireless sensors (e.g., accelerometers) that either stand alone or are integrated into mobile phone technology; and (3) the development of devices that assess multiple objective aspects of physical activity (e.g., BodyMedia assesses motion, galvanic skin response, and temperature). With advances in technology, it is currently possible to assess concurrently physical activity behavior and related physiologic processes 24 hours a day, 7 days a week (for extended periods of time depending on battery life of the sensors). However, electronic tools traditionally used by researchers to objectively assess physical activity currently provide little information about the specific types of activity being performed (walking upstairs vs. walking on a flat path) and cannot yet assess certain types of activities (e.g., swimming, strength training). Future innovations in pattern recognition of data and technology development may remedy these current weaknesses in the objective assessment of physical activity.

Self-reported assessment of physical activity behavior has also seen rapid advances due to the use and proliferation of increasingly more powerful computer technology. Paper-and-pencil measures of behavior have been created in computerized format, allowing for faster analysis and interpretation of the information provided (Collins, Murphy, & Strecher, 2007). The proliferation of the Internet has also provided researchers with an alternative way to efficiently gather and store self-reported physical activity information electronically (Staten et al., 2001). More recently, mobile electronic devices (e.g., PDAs, mobile phones) have been used to assess self-reported physical activity information, as well as related psychosocial and contextual factors, in real time and in the real world (Stone et al., 2007). Advantages to assessing physical activity behavior electronically include the ability to date and time stamp the assessment (which is particularly useful when examining assessment adherence), the ability to gather data in the real world in closer temporal proximity to when activities actually occur, and the capability of immediately analyzing the information gathered

through electronic means. Still, several of the methodological limitations of paper-and-pencil physical activity measures (e.g., self-report bias, social desirability) remain with self-reported physical activity assessed electronically.

The integration of self-reported and multiple objective measures of physical activity gathered electronically may help to offset the weaknesses inherent in objective and self-reported activity measures. However, the optimal integration of electronically assessed objective and self-reported activity, collected either concurrently or in an asynchronous manner, remains a key challenge facing researchers. It is possible that information from the various measures may provide contradictory information. Managing the time-intensive large data sets that can be produced with the electronic capture of physical activity information, particularly data collected in real time, can also pose a daunting challenge to researchers. Furthermore, the ability to concurrently assess psychological, social, environmental, and other contextual variables that relate physical activity behavior may require that researchers employ complex statistical methods (e.g., hierarchical linear modeling, structural equation modeling, etc.) to analyze the complex data collected (Spilsbury et al., 2004).

Technological Innovations in Physical Activity Interventions

The use of computer technology to modify and improve physical activity behavior has proceeded in several research phases (Kump et al., 1994). The first generation of studies used technology (primarily desktop computers) to create computerized tailored information (e.g., pamphlets, newsletters, and reports) in efforts to increase physical activity behavior. However, there was little evidence of overall effectiveness for these first-generation intervention studies (see review by Kroeze et al., 2006). In second-generation physical activity intervention studies using technology, individuals actually interacted with the technology in efforts to increase physical activity behavior. Technology used in these second-generation intervention studies has included Web sites, e-mail, a computer automated telephone system, and CD-ROMs (see review by G. J. Norman et al., 2007). In their systematic review, G. J. Norman and colleagues (2007) found the effectiveness of these second-generation physical intervention studies to be mixed.

A third generation of intervention studies has arisen where researchers are employing mobile technology (e.g., PDAs, mobile phones) to provide real-time or just-in-time feedback to individuals as they go about their daily lives (Pate, Ross, Dowda, Trost, & Sirard, 2003). These mobile devices can operate independently or in connection with other technology (e.g., Internet, desktop computer, accelerometers, etc.). Initial results in studies using randomized controlled research designs have found that the use of mobile devices for intervention purposes can increase physical activity levels among adults (C. L. Craig et al., 2002). Although promising, these third-generation intervention studies are in their infancy, and firm conclusions cannot be drawn.

One key challenge in the area of technology and physical activity interventions is that research methodologies have not kept pace with the rapid evolution and proliferation of technology, and the traditional research designs are not optimal for maximizing and tailoring behavioral interventions, given the richness of the electronic data collected (Aaron et al., 1995). Novel research methods for behavioral interventions using technology have been developed to capitalize on extensive data that can be collected (e.g., the multiphase optimization strategy; Collins et al., 2007), but physical activity intervention researchers have yet to adopt these novel methods.

The electronics industry has been developing increasingly more powerful and precise electronic tools for physical activity. Electronic tools exist to assess multiple activities, such as biking, running, and hiking (Polar). Electronic sensors are now being imbedded into clothes and shoes with wireless connection to mobile devices, such as iPods (Nike + iPod) and electronic wrist watches (Polar + Adidas). With the increasing power of smaller and smaller processors, the ubiquity of mobile technology (e.g., mobile phones), and the ability to provide real-time or just-in-time motivational feedback to individuals based on personalized data collected in the real world, physical activity researchers will have a greater range of tools at their disposal.

Conclusions

Physical activity plays a key role in mental and physical health through direct effects on risks of adverse health outcomes and through indirect effects on energy balance, obesity, cognitive status, mood, and social function. In the first edition of this handbook, the authors of a comparable chapter lucidly and concisely reviewed a relatively small set of valid and reliable instruments, which were largely aimed at measuring self-reported levels of leisure time physical activity. This longer chapter highlights the enormous growth in the field of physical activity assessment in three main areas. First, there has been a tremendous growth in the notion that physical activity can be measured via diverse methods, including observation, self-report, and objective measurement via a variety of gadgets. This chapter has tried to describe some of the promise and some of the pitfalls of the objective measurement approach. One of the conclusions of our review and thinking has been that while objective measurement represents a huge advance in the study of physical activity, it is not a panacea and may complement but cannot replace self-report.

The second main point of this chapter is to highlight the fact that there are literally hundreds of different self-report instruments to assess PA in multiple domains. These instruments are relatively easily available because of improved dissemination via the Internet, and it is no longer possible (if it ever was) to state that there is a single best instrument. We believe that each investigator must carefully delineate the goal of his or her research, evaluation, or surveillance study and consider the optimal tool or tools for measuring physical activity in that context. These efforts must be guided by consideration of some major constraints that can influence any kind of study, and we list a few of these in the chapter.

Third, measurement of physical activity occurs in diverse populations. Diversity in public health studies almost always encompasses age, gender, race/ethnicity, socioeconomic status, and often a myriad of other factors. There has been substantial growth in the past decade in the assessment of physical activity in children and disabled populations. It is not yet clear if new tools are needed to measure physical activity in other demographic groups, although questionnaires developed specifically for different racial groups have been validated. Fourth, there is a growing realization that it is worth thinking about physical activity in multiple domains, including work, routine activities, transportation, and, of course, leisure. Furthermore, sleep and sedentary behaviors are now recognized as important elements in the energy balance equation. Fifth, physical activity occurs in diverse contexts, and measurement of physical activity may be incomplete without measurement of the social and physical environments in which it occurs. Finally, technology matters, and we include a section on technological developments that are likely to guide the future of research and practice in the measurement of physical activity in multiple domains and diverse populations. So the future is exciting yet challenging. On one hand, there has been an exponential growth in the tools available for measuring physical activity. On the other hand, great care is required to select the tool that matches a study question, target population, and project budget.

References

Aadahl, M., & Jorgensen, T. (2003). Validation of a new self-report instrument for measuring physical activity. *Medicine & Science in Sports & Exercise, 35,* 1196–1202.

Aaron, D. J., Kriska, A. M., Dearwater, S. R., Cauley, J. A., Metz, K. F., & LaPorte, R. E. (1995). Reproducibility and validity of an epidemiologic questionnaire to assess past year physical activity in adolescents. *American Journal of Epidemiology, 142,* 191–201.

Acebo, C., Sadeh, A., Seifer, R., Tzischinsky, O., Wolfson, A. R., Hafer, A., et al. (1999). Estimating sleep patterns with activity monitoring in children and adolescents: How many nights are necessary for reliable measures? *Sleep, 22,* 95–103. (Erratum appears in *Sleep,* 1999, *22,* 143.)

Ainsworth, B. E., Bassett, D. R., Jr., Strath, S. J., Swartz, A. M., O'Brien, W. L., Thompson, R. W., et al. (2000). Comparison of three methods for measuring the time spent in physical activity. *Medicine & Science in Sports & Exercise, 32,* S457–S464.

Ainsworth, B. E., Haskell, W. L., Leon, A. S., Jacobs, D. R., Montoye, H. J., Sallis, J. F., et al. (1993). Compendium of physical activities: Classification of energy costs of human physical activities. *Medicine & Science in Sports & Exercise, 25,* 71–80.

Ainsworth, B. E., Jacobs, D. R., Jr., Leon, A. S., Richardson, M. T., & Montoye, H. J. (1993). Assessment of the accuracy of physical activity questionnaire occupational data. *Journal of Occupational Medicine, 35,* 1017–1027.

Ainsworth, B. E., Leon, A. S., Richardson, M. T., Jacobs, D. R., & Paffenbarger, R. S, Jr. (1993). Accuracy of the College Alumnus Physical Activity Questionnaire. *Journal of Clinical Epidemiology, 46,* 1403–1411.

Ainsworth, B. E., Richardson, M. T., Jacobs, D. R., Jr., Leon, A. S., & Sternfeld, B. (1999). Accuracy of recall of occupational physical activity by questionnaire. *Journal of Clinical Epidemiology, 52,* 219–227.

Ainsworth, B. E., Sternfeld, B., Richardson, M. T., & Jackson, K. (2000). Evaluation of the Kaiser physical activity survey in women. *Medicine & Science in Sports & Exercise, 32,* 1327–1338.

Albanes, D., Conway, J. M., Taylor, P. R., Moe, P. W., & Judd, J. (1990). Validation and comparison of eight physical activity questionnaires. *Epidemiology, 1,* 65–71.

Allor, K. M., & Pivarnik, J. M. (2001). Stability and convergent validity of three physical activity assessments. *Medicine & Science in Sports & Exercise, 33,* 671–676.

Ancoli-Israel, S., Cole, R., Alessi, C., Chambers, M., Moorcroft, W., & Pollak, C. P. (2003). The role of actigraphy in the study of sleep and circadian rhythms. *Sleep, 26,* 342–392.

Anderson, L. H., Martinson, B. C., Crain, A. L., Pronk, N. P., Whitebird, R. R., O'Connor, P. J., et al. (2005). Health care charges associated with physical inactivity, overweight, and obesity. *Preventing Chronic Disease, 2,* A09.

Araiza, P., Hewes, H., Gashetewa, C., Vella, C. A., & Burge, M. R. (2006). Efficacy of a pedometer-based physical activity program on parameters of diabetes control in type 2 diabetes mellitus. *Metabolism, 55,* 1382–1387.

ASDA Report. (1992). EEG arousals: Scoring rules and examples. *Sleep, 15,* 173–184.

Aserinsky, E., & Kleitman, N. (1953). Regularly occurring periods of eye motility, and concomitant phenomena, during sleep. *Science, 118,* 273–274.

Atienza, A. A., Hesse, B. W., Baker, T. B., Abrams, D. B., Rimer, B. K., Croyle, R. T., et al. (2007). Critical issues in eHealth research. *American Journal of Preventive Medicine, 32,* S71–S74.

Atienza, A. A., Oliveira, B., Fogg, B. J., & King, A. C. (2006). Using electronic diaries to examine physical activity and other health behaviors of adults age 50+. *Journal of Aging and Physical Activity, 14,* 192–202.

Ayas, N. T., White, D. P., Manson, J. E., Stampfer, M. J., Speizer, F. E., Malhotra, A., et al. (2003). A prospective study of sleep duration and coronary heart disease in women. *Archives of Internal Medicine, 163,* 205–209.

Backhaus, J., Junghanns, K., Broocks, A., Riemann, D., & Hohagen, F. (2002). Test-retest reliability and validity of the Pittsburgh Sleep Quality Index in primary insomnia. *Journal of Psychosomatic Research, 53,* 737–740.

Bailey, R., Olson, J., Pepper, S., Proszasz, J., Barstow, T., & Cooper, D. (1995). The level and tempo of children's physical activities: An observational study. *Medicine & Science in Sports & Exercise, 27,* 1033–1041.

Baranowski, T., Bouchard, C., Bar-Or, O., Bricker, T., Heath, G., Kimm, S. Y., et al. (1992). Assessment, prevalence, and cardiovascular benefits of physical activity and fitness in youth. *Medicine & Science in Sports & Exercise, 24,* S237–S247.

Barnowski, T., Dworkin, R. J., & Cieslik, C. J. (1984). Reliability and validity of self-report for aerobic activity: Family health project. *Research Quarterly for Exercise and Sport, 55,* 309–317.

Bassett, D. R, Jr.. (2000). Validity and reliability issues in objective monitoring of physical activity. *Research Quarterly for Exercise & Sport, 71,* S30–S36.

Bassett, D. R., Jr., Cureton, A. L., & Ainsworth, B. E. (2000). Measurement of daily walking distance-questionnaire versus pedometer. *Medicine & Science in Sports & Exercise, 32,* 1018–1023.

Bedimo-Rung, A. L., Mowen, A. J., & Cohen, D. A. (2005). The significance of parks to physical activity and public health: A conceptual model. *American Journal of Preventive Medicine, 28,* 159–168.

Beets, M. W., Patton, M. M., & Edwards, S. (2005). The accuracy of pedometer steps and time during walking in children. *Medicine & Science in Sports & Exercise, 37,* 513–520.

Bergman, R. N., Ader, M., Huecking, K., & Van Citters, G. (2002). Accurate assessment of beta-cell function: The hyperbolic correction. *Diabetes, 51*(Suppl. 1), S212–S220.

Bonnefoy, M., Normand, S., Pachiaudi, C., Lacour, J. R., Laville, M., & Kostka, T. (2001). Simultaneous validation of ten physical activity questionnaires in older men: A doubly labeled water study. *Journal of the American Geriatrics Society, 49,* 28–35.

Brage, S., Brage, N., Wedderkopp, N., & Froberg, K. (2003). Reliability and validity of the computer science and applications accelerometer in a mechanical setting. *Measurement in Physical Education and Exercise Science, 7,* 101–119.

Brage, S., Wedderkopp, N., Ekelund, U., Franks, P. W., Wareham, N. J., Andersen, L. B, et al. (2004). Objectively measured physical activity correlates with indices of insulin resistance in Danish children. *International Journal of Obesity, 28,* 1503–1508.

Brage, S., Wedderkopp, N., Franks, P. W., Andersen, L. B., & Froberg, K. (2003). Reexamination of validity and reliability of the CSA monitor in walking and running. *Medicine & Science in Sports & Exercise, 35,* 1447–1454.

Bray, M. S., Wong, W. W., Morrow, J. R., Jr., Butte, N. F., & Pivarnik, J. M. (1994). Caltrac versus calorimeter determination of 24-h energy expenditure in female children and adolescents. *Medicine & Science in Sports & Exercise, 26,* 1524–1530.

Brown, W. J., Miller, Y. D., & Miller, R. (2003). Sitting time and work patterns as indicators of overweight and obesity in Australian adults. *International Journal of Obesity & Related Metabolic Disorders, 27,* 1340–1346.

Brown, W. J., Trost, S. G., Bauman, A., Mummery, K., & Owen, N. (2004). Test-retest reliability of four physical activity measures used in population surveys. *Journal of Science & Medicine in Sport, 7,* 205–215.

Brownbill, R. A., Lindsey, C., Crncevic-Orlic, Z., & Ilich, J. Z. (2003). Dual hip bone mineral density in postmenopausal women: Geometry and effect of physical activity. *Calcified Tissue International, 73,* 217–224.

Buysse, D. J., Reynolds, C. F., III, Monk, T. H., Berman, S. R., & Kupfer, D. J. (1989). The Pittsburgh sleep quality index: A new instrument for psychiatric practice and research. *Psychiatry Research, 28,* 193–213.

Calle, E. E., & Kaaks, R. (2004). Overweight, obesity and cancer: Epidemiological evidence and proposed mechanisms. *Nature Reviews Cancer, 4,* 579–591.

Carpenter, J. S., & Andrykowski, M. A. (1998). Psychometric evaluation of the Pittsburgh Sleep Quality Index. *Journal of Psychosomatic Research, 45,* 5–13.

Carskadon, M. A., Wolfson, A. R., Acebo, C., Tzischinsky, O., & Seifer, R. (1998). Adolescent sleep patterns, circadian timing, and sleepiness at a transition to early school days. *Sleep, 21,* 871–881.

Casperson, C. J., Powell, K. E., & Christenson, G. M. (1985). Physical activity, exercise, and physical fitness: Definitions and distinctions for health-related research. *Public Health Reports, 100,* 126–131.

Chan, C. B., Spangler, E., Valcour, J., & Tudor-Locke, C. (2003). Cross-sectional relationship of pedometer-determined ambulatory activity to indicators of health. *Obesity Research, 11,* 1563–1570.

Chasan-Taber, L., Erickson, J. B., Nasca, P. C., Chasan-Taber, S., & Freedson, P. S. (2002). Validity and reproducibility of a physical activity questionnaire in women. *Medicine & Science in Sports & Exercise, 34,* 987–992.

Chen, K. Y., & Bassett, D. R., Jr.. (2005). The technology of accelerometry-based activity monitors: Current and future. *Medicine & Science in Sports & Exercise, 37,* S490–S500.

Clarke, K. K., Freeland-Graves, J., Klohe-Lehman, D. M., Milani, T. J., Nuss, H. J., & Laffrey, S. (2007). Promotion of physical activity in low-income mothers using pedometers. *Journal of the American Dietetic Association, 107,* 962–967.

Collins, L. M., Murphy, S. A., & Strecher, V. (2007). The multiphase optimization strategy (MOST) and the sequential multiple assignment randomized trial (SMART): New methods for more potent eHealth interventions. *American Journal of Preventive Medicine, 32,* S112–S118.

Conway, J. M., Irwin, M. L., & Ainsworth, B. E. (2002). Estimating energy expenditure from the Minnesota Leisure Time Physical Activity and Tecumseh Occupational Activity questionnaires: A doubly labeled water validation. *Journal of Clinical Epidemiology, 55,* 392–399.

Cradock, A. L., Wiecha, J. L., Peterson, K. E., Sobol, A. M., Colditz, G. A., & Gortmaker, S. L. (2004). Youth recall and Tritrac accelerometer estimates of physical activity levels. *Medicine & Science in Sports & Exercise, 36,* 525–532.

Craig, C. L., Marshall, A. L., Sjöström, M., Bauman, A. E., Booth, M. L., Ainsworth, B. E., et al. (2003). International physical activity questionnaire: 12-country reliability and validity [see comment]. *Medicine & Science in Sports & Exercise, 35,* 1381–1395.

Craig, C. L., Russell, S. J., & Cameron, C. (2002). Reliability and validity of Canada's Physical Activity Monitor for assessing trends. *Medicine & Science in Sports & Exercise, 34,* 1462–1467.

Craig, D. L. (1981). Microprocessor heart rate histogram recorder for ambulatory monitoring of daily physical activity. *Medical & Biological Engineering & Computing, 19,* 367–369.

Crouter, S. E., Schneider, P. L., & Bassett, D. R., Jr.. (2005). Spring-levered versus piezo-electric pedometer accuracy in overweight and obese adults. *Medicine & Science in Sports & Exercise, 37,* 1673–1679.

Crouter, S. E., Schneider, P. L., Karabulut, M., & Bassett, D. R, Jr.. (2003). Validity of 10 electronic pedometers for measuring steps, distance, and energy cost. *Medicine & Science in Sports & Exercise, 35,* 1455–1460.

Cyarto, E. V., Myers, A. M., & Tudor-Locke, C. (2004). Pedometer accuracy in nursing home and community-dwelling older adults. *Medicine & Science in Sports & Exercise, 36,* 205–209.

Dahl, R. E. (1996). The regulation of sleep and arousal: Development and psychopathology. *Development and Psychopathology, 8,* 3–27.

Davis, S. E., King, L. E., & Robertson, H. D. (1998). Predicting pedestrian crosswalk volumes. *Transportation Research Record, 1168,* 25–29.

De Abajo, S., Larriba, R., & Marquez, S. (2001). Validity and reliability of the Yale Physical Activity Survey in Spanish elderly. *Journal of Sports Medicine & Physical Fitness, 41,* 479–485.

Deckelbaum, R. J., & Williams, C. L. (2001). Childhood obesity: The health issue. *Obesity Research, 9,* s239–s243.

Dement, W., & Kleitman, N. (1957). Cyclic variations in EEG during sleep and their relation to eye movements, body motility, and dreaming. *Electroencephalography and Clinical Neurophysiology, 9,* 673–690.

Devine, E. B., Hakim, Z., & Green, J. (2005). A systematic review of patient-reported outcome instruments measuring sleep dysfunction in adults. *Pharmacoeconomics, 23,* 889–912.

Diabetes Prevention Program Research Group. (2002). Reduction in the incidence of type 2 diabetes with lifestyle intervention or metformin. *New England Journal of Medicine, 346,* 393–403.

Dipietro, L., Caspersen, C. J., Ostfeld, A. M., & Nadel, E. R. (1993). A survey for assessing physical activity among older adults. *Medicine & Science in Sports & Exercise, 25,* 628–642.

Ekelund, U., Sjöström, M., Yngve, A., Poortvliet, E., Nilsson, A., Froberg, K., et al. (2001). Physical activity assessed by activity monitor and doubly labeled water in children. *Medicine & Science in Sports & Exercise, 33,* 275–281.

Ekelund, U., Yngve, A., Brage, S., Westerterp, K., & Sjöström, M. (2004). Body movement and physical activity energy expenditure in children and adolescents: How to adjust for differences in body size and age. *American Journal of Clinical Nutrition, 79,* 851–856.

Elley, C. R., Kerse, N. M., Swinburn, B., Arroll, B., & Robinson, E. (2003). Measuring physical activity in primary health care research: Validity and reliability of two questionnaires. *New Zealand Family Physician, 30,* 171–180.

Elosua, R., Garcia, M., Aguilar, A., Molina, L., Covas, M. I., & Marrugat, J. (2000). Validation of the Minnesota Leisure Time Physical Activity Questionnaire in Spanish women. Investigators of the MARATDON Group. *Medicine & Science in Sports & Exercise, 32,* 1431–1437.

Eppley Institute for Parks and Public Lands. (2001). *Summary report: Indiana Trails Study, a study of trails in six Indiana cities.* Bloomington: Indiana University, Eppley Institute for Parks and Public Lands.

Evers, W., & Carol, B. (2007). An Internet-based assessment tool for food choices and physical activity

behaviors. *Journal of Nutrition Education & Behavior, 39,* 105–106.

Ewing, R., Pendall, R., & Chen, D. D. T. (2002). *Measuring sprawl and its impact.* Smart Growth America. http://www.smartgrowthamerica.org/sprawlindex/sprawlindex.html

Ewing, R., Schmid, T., Killingsworth, R., Zlot, A., & Raudenbush, S. (2003). Relationship between urban sprawl and physical activity, obesity, and morbidity. *American Journal of Health Promotion, 18,* 47–57.

Fairweather, S. C., Reilly, J. J., Grant, S., Whittaker, A., & Payton, J. Y. (1999). Using the Computer Science and Applications (CSA) activity monitor in preschool children. *Pediatric Exercise Science, 11,* 413–420.

Finn, K. J., & Specker, B. (2000). Comparison of Actiwatch activity monitor and Children's Activity Rating Scale in children. *Medicine Science Sports & Exercise, 32,* 1794–1797.

Frank, L. D, Andresen, M., & Schmid, T. (2004). Obesity relationships with community design, physical activity and time spent in cars. *American Journal of Preventive Medicine, 27,* 87–96.

Frank, L. D., Sallis, J. F., Conway, T. L., Chapman, J., Saelens, B., & Bachman, W. (2006). Multiple pathways from land use to health: Walkability associations with active transportation, body mass index, and air quality. *Journal of the American Planning Association, 72,* 75–87.

Freedson, P., Pober, D., & Janz, K. F. (2005). Calibration of accelerometer output for children. *Medicine & Science in Sports & Exercise, 37,* S523–S530.

Friedenreich, C. M., & Orenstein, M. R. (2002). Physical activity and cancer prevention: Etiologic evidence and biological mechanisms. *Journal of Nutrition, 132,* 3456S–3464S.

Galster, G., Hanson, R., Ratcliffe, M. R., Wolman, H., Coleman, S., & Freihage, J. (2001). Wrestling sprawl to the ground: Defining and measuring an elusive concept. *Housing Policy Debate, 12,* 681–717.

George, J. D. (1996). Alternative approach to maximal exercise testing and VO_2 max prediction in college students. *Research Quarterly for Exercise & Sport, 67,* 452–457.

Godin, G., & Shephard, R. J. (1985). A simple method to assess exercise behavior in the community. *Canadian Journal of Applied Sport Sciences, 10,* 141–146.

Goran, M. I., & Reynolds, K. (2005). Interactive Multimedia for Promoting Physical Activity (IMPACT) in children. *Obesity Research, 13,* 762–771.

Goran, M. I., Reynolds, K. D., & Lindquist, C. H. (1999). Role of physical activity in the prevention of obesity in children. *International Journal of Obesity & Related Metabolic Disorders, 23,* S18–S33.

Gottlieb, D. G., Punjabi, N. M., Newman, A. B., Resnick, H. E., Redline, S., Baldwin, C. M., et al. (2005). Short sleep time is associated with diabetes mellitus and impaired glucose tolerance. *Archives of Internal Medicine, 165,* 863–867.

Gregg, E. W., Kriska, A. M., Salamone, L. M., Wolf, R. L., Roberts, M. M., Ferrell, R. E., et al. (1999). Correlates of quantitative ultrasound in the Women's Healthy Lifestyle Project. *Osteoporosis International, 10,* 416–424.

Grossman, P. (2004). The LifeShirt: A multi-function ambulatory system monitoring health, disease, and medical intervention in the real world. *Studies in Health Technology and Informatics, 108,* 133–141.

Gupta, N. K., Mueller, W., Chan, H., & Meininger, J. C. (2002). Is obesity associated with poor sleep quality in adolescents? *American Journal of Human Biology, 14,* 762–768.

Handy, S. L., Boarnet, M. G., Ewing, R., & Killingsworth, R. E. (2002). How the built environment affects physical activity: Views from urban planning. *American Journal of Preventive Medicine, 23,* 64–73.

Harada, N. D., Chiu, V., King, A. C., & Stewart, A. L. (2001). An evaluation of three self-report physical activity instruments for older adults. *Medicine & Science in Sports & Exercise, 33,* 962–970.

Hardy, L. L., Bass, S. L., & Booth, M. L. (2007). Changes in sedentary behavior among adolescent girls: A 2.5-year prospective cohort study. *Journal of Adolescent Health, 40,* 158–165.

Haskell, W. L., Lee, I.-M., Pate, R. R., Powell, K. E., Blair, S. N., Franklin, B. A., et al. (2007). Physical activity and public health: Updated recommendation for adults from the American College of Sports Medicine and the American Heart Association. *Circulation, 116,* 1081–1093.

Hauri, P. J., & Wisbey, J. (1992). Wrist actigraphy in insomnia. *Sleep, 15,* 293–301.

Heath, E. M., Coleman, K. J., Lensegrav, T. L., & Fallon, J. A. (2006). Using momentary time sampling to estimate minutes of physical activity in physical education: Validation of scores for the system for observing fitness instruction time. *Research Quarterly for Exercise and Sport, 77,* 142–146.

Heyward, V. H. (2006). *Advanced fitness assessment and exercise prescription.* Champaign, IL: Human Kinetics.

Hovell, M. F., Hofstetter, C. R., Sallis, J. F., Rauh, M. J., & Barrington, E. (1992). Correlates of change in walking for exercise: an exploratory analysis. *Research Quarterly for Exercise & Sport, 63,* 425–434.

Hunter, W., & Huang, H. (1995). User counts on bicycle lanes and multiuse trails in the United States. *Transportation Research Record, 1502,* 45–47.

Hurling, R., Catt, M., Boni, M. D., Fairley, B. W., Hurst, T., Murray, P., et al. (2007). Using Internet and mobile phone technology to deliver an automated physical activity program: Randomized controlled trial. *Journal of Medical Internet Research, 9,* e7.

Iber, C., Redline, S., Gilpin, A., Quan, S., Zhang, L., Gottlieb, D., et al. (2004). Polysomnography performed in the unattended home vs. the attended laboratory setting: Sleep Heart Health Study methodology. *Sleep, 27,* 536–540.

Iglowstein, I., Jenni, O. G., Molinari, L., & Largo, R. H. (2003). Sleep duration from infancy to adolescence: Reference values and generational trends. *Pediatrics, 111,* 302–307.

Institute of Medicine. (2002). *Dietary reference intakes for energy, carbohydrates, fiber, fat, protein and amino acids (macronutrients).* Washington, DC: National Academies Press.

Iwane, M., Arita, M., Tomimoto, S., Satani, O., Matsumoto, M., Miyashita, K., et al. (2000). Walking 10,000 steps/day or more reduces blood pressure and sympathetic nerve activity in mild essential hypertension. *Hypertension Research, 23,* 573–580

Jackson, R. J., & Kochtitzky, C. (2001). *Creating a healthy environment: The impact of the built environment on public health.* Washington, DC: Sprawl Watch Clearinghouse.

Jacobs, D. R., Jr., Ainsworth, B. E., Hartman, T. J., & Leon, A. S. (1993). A simultaneous evaluation of 10 commonly used physical activity questionnaires. *Medicine & Science in Sports & Exercise, 25,* 81–91.

Jago, R., Anderson, C. B., Baranowski, T., & Watson, K. (2005). Adolescent patterns of physical activity differences by gender, day, and time of day.

American Journal of Preventive Medicine, 28, 447–452.

Janz, K. F. (1994). Validation of the CSA accelerometer for assessing children's physical activity. *Medicine & Science in Sports & Exercise, 26,* 369–375.

Janz, K. F., Burns, T. L., & Levy, S. M. (2005). Tracking of activity and sedentary behaviors in childhood: The Iowa Bone Development Study. *American Journal of Preventive Medicine, 29,* 171–178.

Johns, M. W. (1992). Reliability and factor analysis of the Epworth Sleepiness Scale. *Sleep, 15,* 376–381.

Johnson, M. S., Figueroa-Colon, R., Herd, S. L., Fields, D. A., Sun, M., Hunter, G. R., et al. (2000). Aerobic fitness, not energy expenditure, influences subsequent increase in adiposity in Black and White children. *Pediatrics, 106,* e50.

Johnson, N. J., Kirchner, H. L., Storfer-Isser, A., Cartar, L., Ancoli-Israel, S., Emancipator, J. L., et al. (2007). Sleep estimation using wrist actigraphy in adolescents with and without sleep disordered breathing: A comparison of three data modes. *Sleep, 30,* 899–905.

Johnson, R. K., Russ, J., & Goran, M. I. (1998). Physical activity related energy expenditure in children by doubly labeled water as compared with the Caltrac accelerometer. *International Journal of Obesity & Related Metabolic Disorders, 22,* 1046–1052.

Kelly, L. A., Reilly, J. J., Grant, S., & Paton, J. Y. (2004). Comparison of two accelerometers for assessment of physical activity in pre-school children. *Pediatric Exercise Science, 16,* 324–333.

King, G. A., Torres, N., Potter, C., Brooks, T. J., & Coleman, K. J. (2004). Comparison of activity monitors to estimate energy cost of treadmill exercise. *Medicine & Science in Sports & Exercise, 36,* 1244–1251.

Klesges, L. M., & Klesges, R. C. (1987). The assessment of children's physical activity: A comparison of methods. *Medicine & Science in Sports & Exercise, 19,* 511–551.

Klesges, R. C., Klesges, L. M., Swenson, A. M., & Pheley, A. M. (1985). A validation of two motion sensors in the prediction of child and adult physical activity levels. *American Journal of Epidemiology, 122,* 400–410.

Knutson, K. L., & Lauderdale, D. S. (2007). Sleep duration and overweight in adolescents: Self-reported sleep hours versus time diaries. *Pediatrics, 119,* e1056–1062.

Kochersberger, G., McConnell, E., Kuchibhatla, M. N., & Pieper, C. (1996). The reliability, validity, and stability of a measure of physical activity in the elderly. *Archives of Physical Medicine and Rehabilitation, 77,* 793–795.

Kohl, H. W., Blair, S. N., Paffenbarger, R. S., Jr., Macera, C. A., & Kronenfeld, J. J. (1988). A mail survey of physical activity habits as related to measured physical fitness. *American Journal of Epidemiology, 127,* 1228–1239.

Konradi, D. B., & Lyon, B. L. (2000). Measuring adherence to a self-care fitness walking routine. *Journal of Community Health Nursing, 17,* 159–169.

Kriska, A. M., & Bennett, P. H. (1992). An epidemiological perspective of the relationship between physical activity and NIDDM: From activity assessment to intervention. *Diabetes-Metabolism Reviews 8,* 355–372.

Kriska, A. M., Knowler, W. C., LaPorte, R. E., Drash, A. L., Wing, R. R., Blair, S. N., et al. (1990). Development of questionnaire to examine relationship of physical activity and diabetes in Pima Indians. *Diabetes Care, 13,* 401–411.

Kriska, A. M., Sandler, R. B., Cauley, J. A., LaPorte, R. E., Hom, D. L., & Pambianco, G. (1988). The assessment of historical physical activity and its relation to adult bone parameters. *American Journal of Epidemiology, 127,* 1053–1063.

Kroeze, W., Werkman, A., & Brug, J. (2006). A systematic review of randomized trials on the effectiveness of computer-tailored education on physical activity and dietary behaviors. *Annals of Behavioral Medicine, 31,* 205–223.

Kronenberg, F., Pereira, M. A., Schmitz, M. K., Arnett, D. K., Evenson, K. R., Crapo, R. O., et al. (2000). Influence of leisure time physical activity and television watching on atherosclerosis risk factors in the NHLBI Family Heart Study. *Atherosclerosis, 153,* 433–443.

Kruskall, L. J., Campbell, W. W., & Evans, W. J. (2004). The Yale Physical Activity Survey for older adults: predictions in the energy expenditure due to physical activity. *Journal of the American Dietetic Association, 104,* 1251–1257.

Kump, K., Whalen, C., Tishler, P. V., Browner, I., Ferrette, V., Strohl, K. P., et al. (1994). Assessment of the validity and utility of a sleep-symptom questionnaire. *American Journal of Respiratory & Critical Care Medicine, 150,* 735–741.

Kushida, C. A., Chang, A., Gadkary, C., Guilleminault, C., Carrillo, O., & Dement, W. C. (2001). Comparison of actigraphic, polysomnographic, and subjective assessment of sleep parameters in sleep-disordered patients. *Sleep Medicine, 2,* 389–396.

Lanningham-Foster, L. M., Jensen, T. B., McCrady, S. K., Nysse, L. J., Foster, R. C., & Levine, J. A. (2005). Laboratory measurement of posture allocation and physical activity in children. *Medicine & Science in Sports & Exercise, 37,* 1800–1805.

Lanningham-Foster. L., Nysse, L. J., & Levine, J. A. (2003). Labor saved, calories lost: The energetic impact of domestic labor-saving devices. *Obesity Research, 11,* 1178–1181.

LaPorte, R. E., Black-Sandler, R., Cauley, J. A., Link, M., Bayles, C., & Marks, B. (1983). The assessment of physical activity in older women: Analysis of the interrelationship and reliability of activity monitoring, activity surveys, and caloric intake. *Journal of Gerontology, 38,* 394–397.

Le Masurier, G. C., Lee, S. M., & Tudor-Locke, C. (2004). Motion sensor accuracy under controlled and free-living conditions. *Medicine & Science in Sports & Exercise, 36,* 905–910.

Leon, A. S., Jacobs, D. R., Jr., DeBacker, G., & Taylor, H. L. (1981). Relationship of physical characteristics and life habits to treadmill exercise capacity. *American Journal of Epidemiology, 113,* 653–660.

Levine, D. W., Kaplan, R. M., Kripke, D. F., Bowen, D. J., Naughton, M. J., & Shumaker, S. A. (2003). Factor structure and measurement invariance of the Women's Health Initiative Insomnia Rating Scale. *Psychological Assessment, 15,* 123–136.

Levine, D. W., Lewis, M. A., Bowen, D. J., Kripke, D. F., Kaplan, R. M., Naughton, M. J., et al. (2003). Reliability and validity of the Women's Health Initiative Insomnia Rating Scale. *Psychological Assessment, 15,* 137–148.

Levine, J. A. (2004). Nonexercise activity thermogenesis (NEAT): Environment and biology. *American Journal of Physiology and Endocrinology Metabolism, 286,* E675–E685.

Levine, J. A., Schleusner, S. J., & Jensen, M. D. (2000). Energy expenditure of nonexercise activity. *American Journal of Clinical Nutrition, 72,* 1451–1454.

Lindsey, G., Han, Y., Wilson, J., & Yang, J. (2006). Neighborhood correlates of urban trail traffic. *Physical Activity and Health, 1,* S134–S152.

Lindsey, G., Wilson, J., Rubchinskaya, E., Yang, J., & Han, Y. (2007). Estimating urban trail traffic: Methods for existing and proposed trails. *Landscape and Urban Planning, 81,* 299–315.

Littman, A. J., White, E., Kristal, A. R., Patterson, R. E., Satia-Abouta, J., & Potter, J. D. (2004). Assessment of a one-page questionnaire on long-term recreational physical activity. *Epidemiology, 15,* 105–113.

Locard, E., Mamelle, N., Billette, A., Miginiac, M., Munoz, F., & Rey, S. (1992). Risk factors of obesity in a five year old population. Parental versus environmental factors. *International Journal of Obesity and Related Metabolic Disorders, 16,* 721–729.

Lopez, R. (2004). Urban sprawl and risk for being overweight or obese. *American Journal of Public Health, 94,* 1574–1579.

Lopez-Zetina, J., Lee, H., & Friis, R. (2006). The link between obesity and the built environment: Evidence from an ecological analysis of obesity and vehicle miles of travel in California. *Health Place, 12,* 656–664.

Lynch, K. (1960). *Image of the city.* Cambridge: MIT Press.

Lysen, V. C., & Walker, R (1997). Osteoporosis risk factors in eighth grade students. *Journal of School Health, 67,* 317–321.

Macfarlane, D. J., Taylor, L. H., & Cuddihy, T. F. (2006). Very short intermittent vs continuous bouts of activity in sedentary adults. *Preventive Medicine, 43,* 332–336.

Masse, L. C., Fuemmeler, B. F., Anderson, C., Matthews, C. E., Trost, S. G., Catellier, D. J., et al. (2005). Accelerometer data reduction: A comparison of four reduction algorithms on select outcome variables. *Medicine & Science in Sports & Exercise, 37,* S544–S554.

McKenzie, T. L., Cohen, D. A., Sehgal, A., Williamson, S., & Golinelli, D. (2006). System of Observing Play and Recreation in Communities (SOPARC): Reliability and feasibility measures. *Journal of Physical Activity and Health, 3,* S208–S222.

McKenzie, T. L., Marshall, S. J., Sallis, J. F., & Conway, T. L. (2000). Leisure-time physical activity in school environments: An observational study using SOPLAY. *Preventive Medicine, 30,* 70–77.

McKenzie, T. L., Sallis, J. F., & Armstrong, C. A. (1994). Association between direct observation and accelerometer measures of children's physical activity during physical education and recess. *Medicine & Science in Sports & Exercise, 26,* 143.

McKenzie, T. L., Sallis, J. F., & Nader, P. R. (1991). SOFIT: System for Observing Fitness Instruction Time. *Journal of Teaching in Physical Education, 11,* 195–205.

McKenzie, T. L., Sallis, J. F., Nader, P. R., Patterson, T. L., Elder, J. P., Berry, C. C., et al. (1991). BEACHES: An observational system for assessing children's eating and physical activity behaviors and associated events. *Journal of Applied Behavior Analysis, 24,* 141–151.

McSwegin, P. (1989). *Physical best: The AAHPERD guide to physical fitness education and assessment.* Reston, VA: American Alliance for Health, Physical Education, Recreation, and Dance.

McTiernan, A., Kooperberg, C., White, E., Wilcox, S., Coates, R., Adams-Campbell, L. L., et al. (2003). Recreational physical activity and the risk of breast cancer in postmenopausal women: The Women's Health Initiative Cohort Study [see comment]. *Journal of the American Medical Association, 290,* 1331–1336.

McTiernan, A., Ulrich, C., Slate, S., & Potter, J. (1998). Physical activity and cancer etiology: Associations and mechanisms. *Cancer Causes & Control 9,* 487–509.

Melanson, E. L., & Freedson, P. S. (1995). Validity of the Computer Science and Applications, Inc. (CSA) activity monitor. *Medicine & Science in Sports & Exercise, 27,* 934–940.

Melanson, E. L., & Freedson, P. S. (1996). Physical activity assessment: A review of methods. *Critical Reviews in Food Science and Nutrition, 36,* 385–396.

Melanson, E. L., Knoll, J. R., Bell, M. L., Donahoo, W. T., Hill, J. O., Nysse, L. J., et al. (2004). Commercially available pedometers: Considerations for accurate step counting. *Preventive Medicine, 39,* 361–368.

Merom, D., Rissel, C., Phongsavan, P., Smith, B. J., Van Kemenade, C., Brown, W. J., et al. (2007). Promoting walking with pedometers in the community: The step-by-step trial. *American Journal of Preventive Medicine, 32,* 290–297.

Mertes, J. D., & Hall, J. R. H. (1996). *Park, recreation, open space, and greenway guidelines.* Ashburn, VA: National Recreation and Park Association.

Metcalf, B. S., Curnow, J. S., Evans, C., Voss, L. D., & Wilkin, T. J. (2002). Technical reliability of the CSA activity monitor: The EarlyBird Study. *Medicine & Science in Sports & Exercise, 34,* 1533–1537.

Miller, D. J., Freedson, P. S., & Kline, G. M. (1994). Comparison of activity levels using the Caltrac accelerometer and five questionnaires. *Medicine & Science in Sports & Exercise, 26,* 376–382.

Monk, T. H., Buysse, D. J., Kennedy, K. S., Pods, J. M., DeGrazia, J. M., & Miewald, J. M. (2003). Measuring sleep habits without using a diary: The sleep timing questionnaire. *Sleep, 26,* 208–212.

Monk, T. H., Reynolds, C. F., Kupfer, D. J., Buysse, D. J., Coble, P. A., Hayes, A. J., et al. (1994). The Pittsburgh Sleep Diary. *Journal of Sleep Research, 3,* 111–120.

Montoye, H. J., Kemper, H. C., Saris, W. H., & Washburn, R. A. (1996). *Measuring physical activity and energy expenditure.* Champaign, IL: Human Kinetics.

Montoye, H. J., Washburn, R., Servais, S., Ertl, A., Webster, J. G., & Nagle, F. J. (1983). Estimation of energy expenditure by a portable monitor. *Medicine & Science in Sports & Exercise, 15,* 403–407.

Morgenthaler, T., Alessi, C., Friedman, L., Owens, J., Kapur, V., Boehlecke, B., et al. (2007). Practice parameters for the use of actigraphy in the assessment of sleep and sleep disorders: An update for 2007. *Sleep, 30,* 519–529.

Mueller, J. K., Gossard, D., Adams, F. R., Taylor, C. B., Haskell, W. L., Kraemer, H. C., et al. (1986). Assessment of prescribed increases in physical activity: application of a new method for microprocessor analysis of heart rate. *American Journal of Cardiology, 57,* 441–445.

Must, A., & Tybor, D. J. (2005). Physical activity and sedentary behavior: A review of longitudinal studies of weight and adiposity in youth. *International Journal of Obesity and Related Metabolic Disorders, 29,* S84–S96.

Nader, P. R. (2003) Frequency and intensity of activity of third-grade children in physical education. *Archives of Pediatrics & Adolescent Medicine, 157,* 185–190.

National Research Council. (2005). *Does the built environment influence physical activity? Examining the evidence.* Washington, DC: Transportation Research Board.

National Sleep Foundation. (2000). *Omnibus Sleep in America Poll.* Washington, DC: Author.

Nawyn, J., Intille, S. S., & Larson, K. (2006, September). *Embedding behavior modification strategies into consumer electronic devices.* Paper presented at the 8th international conference of UbiComp 2006, Orange County, CA.

Nichols, J. F., Morgan, C. G., Sarkin, J. A., Sallis, J. F., & Calfas, K. J. (1999). Validity, reliability, and calibration of the Tritrac accelerometer as a measure of physical activity. *Medicine & Science in Sports & Exercise, 31,* 908–912.

Nilsson, A., Ekelund, U., Yngve, A., & Sjöström M. (2002). Assessing physical activity among children with accelerometers using different time sampling intervals and placements. *Pediatric Exercise Science, 14,* 87–96.

Norman, A., Bellocco, R., Bergstrom, A., & Wolk, A. (2001). Validity and reproducibility of self-reported total physical activity: Differences by relative weight. *International Journal of Obesity & Related Metabolic Disorders, 25,* 682–688.

Norman, G. J., Zabinski, M. F., Adams, M. A., Rosenberg, D. E., Yaroch, A. L., & Atienza, A. A. (2007). A review of e-Health interventions for physical activity and dietary behavior change. *American Journal of Preventive Medicine, 33,* 336–345.

O'Hara, N. (1989). Validity of the observation of children's physical activity. *Research Quarterly for Exercise and Sport, 60,* 42–47.

O'Hara, N. M., Baranowski, T., Simons-Morton, B. G., Wilson, B. S., & Parcel, G. (1989). Validity of the observation of children's physical activity. *Research Quarterly for Exercise & Sport, 60,* 42–47.

Oliveira, B., Morton, J., Atienza, A. A., Gardner, C., & King, A. C. (2005, April). *Randomized controlled pilot study of a handheld computer delivered intervention to promote brisk walking in sedentary middle-aged and older adults.* Paper presented at the 26th Annual Meeting & Scientific Sessions of the Society of Behavioral Medicine, Boston.

Oliveria, S. A., Kohl, H. W., III, Trichopoulos, D., & Blair, S. N. (1996). The association between cardiorespiratory fitness and prostate cancer. *Medicine & Science in Sports & Exercise, 28,* 97–104.

Pate, R. R. (1988). The evolving definition of physical fitness. *Quest, 40,* 174–179.

Pate, R. R., Pratt, M., Blair, S. N., Haskell, W. L., Macera, C. A., Bouchard, C., et al.. (1995). Physical activity and public health: A recommendation from the Centers for Disease Control and Prevention and the American College of Sports Medicine. *Journal of the American Medical Association, 273,* 402–407.

Pate, R. R., Ross, R., Dowda, M., Trost, S., & Sirard, J. (2003). Validation of a 3-day physical activity recall instrument in female youth. *Pediatric Exercise Science, 15,* 257–265.

Patel, A., & Bernstein, L. (2006). Physical activity and cancer incidence: Breast cancer. In A. McTiernan (Ed.), *Physical activity, energy balance, and cancer: Etiology and prognosis.* New York: Marcel Dekker.

Patel, S. R., Ayas, N. T., Malhotra, M. R., White, D. P., Schernhammer, E. S., Speizer, F. E., et al. (2004). A prospective study of sleep duration and mortality risk in women. *Sleep, 27,* 440–444.

Patrick, K., Intille, S. S., & Zabinski, M. F. (2005). An ecological framework for cancer communication: Implications for research. *Journal of Medical Internet Research, 7,* e23.

Penpraze, V., Kelly, L. A., Montgomery, C., Jackson, D., Paton, J., Aitchison, T., et al. (In press). Effect of Actigraph cut-point on level of physical activity and sedentary behavior in young children. *International Journal of Obesity.*

Penpraze, V., Reilly, J. J., Grant, S., Paton, J. Y., & Aitchison, T. A. (2006). Monitoring of physical activity in young children: How much is enough? *Pediatric Exercise Science, 18,* 483–491.

Philippaerts, R. M., & Lefevre, J. (1998). Reliability and validity of three physical activity questionnaires in Flemish males. *American Journal of Epidemiology, 147,* 982–990.

Philippaerts, R. M., Westerterp, K. R., & Lefevre, J. (1999). Doubly labelled water validation of three physical activity questionnaires. *International Journal of Sports Medicine, 20,* 284–289.

Pols, M. A., Peeters, P. H., Bueno-De-Mesquita, H. B., Ocke, M. C., Wentink, C. A., Kemper, H. C., et al. (1995). Validity and repeatability of a modified Baecke questionnaire on physical activity. *International Journal of Epidemiology, 24,* 381–388.

Pols, M. A., Peeters, P. H., Kemper, H. C., & Collette, H. J. (1996). Repeatability and relative validity of two physical activity questionnaires in elderly women. *Medicine & Science in Sports & Exercise, 28,* 1020–1025.

Pols, M. A., Peeters, P. H., Ocke, M. C., Bueno-de-Mesquita, H. B., Slimani, N., Kemper, H. C., et al. (1997). Relative validity and repeatability of a new questionnaire on physical activity. *Preventive Medicine, 26,* 37–43.

Pols, M. A., Peeters, P. H., Ocke, M. C., Slimani, N., Bueno-de-Mesquita, H. B., & Collette, H. J. (1997). Estimation of reproducibility and relative validity of the questions included in the EPIC Physical Activity Questionnaire. *International Journal of Epidemiology, 26*(Suppl. 1), S181–S189.

Pope, R. P., Coleman, K. J., Gonzalez, E. C., Barron, F., & Heath, E. M. (2002). Validity of a revised System for Observing Fitness Instruction Time (SOFIT). *Pediatric Exercise Science, 14,* 135–146.

Powell, K. E. (2005). Land use, the built environment, and physical activity: A public health mixture; a public health solution. *American Journal of Preventive Medicine, 28,* 216–217.

Powell, S. M., Jones, D. I , & Rowlands, A. V. (2003). Technical variability of the RT3 accelerometer. *Medicine & Science in Sports & Exercise, 35,* 1773–1778.

Prochaska, J. J., Zabinski, M. F., Calfas, K. J., Sallis, J. F., & Patrick, K. (2000). PACE+: Interactive communication technology for behavior change in clinical settings. *American Journal of Preventive Medicine, 19,* 127–131.

Puhl, J., Greaves, K., Hoyt, M., & Barnowski, T. (1990). Children's Activity Rating Scale (CARS): Description and evaluation. *Research Quarterly for Exercise and Sport, 61,* 26–36.

Puyau, M. R., Adolph, A. L., Vohra, F. A., & Butte, N. F. (2002). Validation and calibration of physical activity monitors in children. *Obesity Research, 10,* 150–157.

Quan, S. F., Howard, B. V., Iber, C., Kiley, J. P., Nieto, F. J., O'Connor, G. T., et al. (1997). The Sleep Heart Health Study: Design, rationale, and methods. *Sleep, 20,* 1077–1085.

Rauh, M. J., Hovell, M. F., Hofstetter, C. R., Sallis, J. F., & Gleghorn, A. (1992). Reliability and validity of self-reported physical activity in Latinos. *International Journal of Epidemiology, 21,* 966–971.

Rechtschaffen, A., & Kales, A. (1968). *A manual of standardized techniques and scoring system for sleep stages of human subjects* (NIH Pub. No. 204). Washington, DC: Government Printing Office.

Reilly, J. J., Coyle, J., Kelly, L. A., Burke, G., Grant, S., & Paton, J. Y. (2003). An objective method for measurement of sedentary behavior in young children. *Obesity Research, 11,* 1155–1158.

Reilly, J. J., Jackson, D. M., Montgomery, C., Kelly, L. A., Slater, C., Grant, S., et al. (2004). Total energy expenditure and physical activity in young Scottish children: Mixed longitudinal study. *Lancet, 363,* 211–212.

Resnicow, K., McCarty, F., Blissett, D., Wang, T., Heitzler, C., & Lee, R. E. (2003). Validity of a modified CHAMPS physical activity questionnaire among African-Americans. *Medicine & Science in Sports & Exercise, 35,* 1537–1545.

Richardson, M. T., Ainsworth, B. E., Wu, H. C., Jacobs, D. R., Jr., & Leon, A. S. (1995). Ability of the Atherosclerosis Risk in Communities (ARIC)/Baecke Questionnaire to assess leisure-time physical activity. *International Journal of Epidemiology, 24,* 685–693.

Richardson, M. T., Leon, A. S., Jacobs, D. R., Jr., Ainsworth, B. E., & Serfass, R. (1994). Comprehensive evaluation of the Minnesota Leisure Time Physical Activity Questionnaire. *Journal of Clinical Epidemiology, 47,* 271–281.

Riddoch, C. J., Bo Andersen, L., Wedderkopp, N., Harro, M., Klasson-Heggebo, L., Sardinha, L. B., et al. (2004). Physical activity levels and patterns of 9-and 15-yr-old European children. *Medicine & Science in Sports & Exercise, 36,* 86–92.

Robinson, T. N. (1999). Reducing children's television viewing to prevent obesity: A randomized controlled trial. *Journal of the American Medical Association, 282,* 1561–1567.

Rodriguez, D. A., Brown, A. L., & Troped, P. J. (2005). Portable global positioning units to complement accelerometry-based physical activity monitors. *Medicine & Science in Sports & Exercise, 37,* S572–S581.

Roeykens, J., Rogers, R., Meeusen, R., Magnus, L., Borms, J., & de Meirleir, K. (1998). Validity and reliability in a Flemish population of the WHO-MONICA Optional Study of Physical Activity Questionnaire. *Medicine & Science in Sports & Exercise, 30,* 1071–1075.

Rowe, P., Schuldheisz, J. M., & van der Mars, H. (1997). Measuring physical activity in physical education: Validation of the SOFIT direct observation instrument for use with first to eighth grade students. *Pediatric Exercise Science 9,* 136–149.

Rowe, P., van der Mars, H., Schuldheisz, J., & Fox, S. (2004). Measuring students' physical activity levels: Validating SOFIT for use with high-school students. *Journal of Teaching in Physical Education, 23,* 235–251.

Sadeh, A., Sharkey, K. M., & Carskadon, M. A. (1994). Activity-based sleep-wake identification: An empirical test of methodological issues. *Sleep, 17,* 201–207.

Sallis, J. F. (1993). Epidemiology of physical activity and fitness in children and adolescents. *Critical Reviews in Food Science & Nutrition, 33,* 403–408.

Sallis, J. F., Buono, M. J., Roby, J. J., Carlson, D., & Nelson, J. A. (1990). The Caltrac accelerometer as a physical activity monitor for school-age children. *Medicine & Science in Sports & Exercise, 22,* 698–703.

Sallis, J. F., Cervero, R., Ascher, W., Henderson, K., Kraft, M. K., & Kerr, J. (2006). An ecological approach to creating active living communities. *Annual Review of Public Health, 27,* 297–322.

Sallis, J. F., Conway, T. L., Prochaska, J. J., McKenzie, T. L., Marshall, S. J., & Brown, M. (2001). The association of school environments with youth physical activity. *American Journal of Public Health, 91,* 618–620.

Saris, W. H., Snel, P., Baecke, J., van Waesberghe, F., & Binkhorst, R. A. (1977). A portable miniature solid-state heart rate recorder for monitoring daily physical activity. *Biotelemetry, 4,* 131–140.

Schmidt, M. D., Freedson, P. S., & Chasan-Taber, L. (2003). Estimating physical activity using the CSA accelerometer and a physical activity log. *Medicine & Science in Sports & Exercise, 35,* 1605–1611.

Schneider, P. L., Crouter, S. E., & Bassett, D. R. (2004). Pedometer measures of free-living physical activity: Comparison of 13 models. *Medicine & Science in Sports & Exercise, 36,* 331–335.

Schneider, P. L., Crouter, S. E., Lukajic, O., & Bassett, D. R., Jr.. (2003). Accuracy and reliability of 10 pedometers for measuring steps over a 400-m walk. *Medicine & Science in Sports & Exercise, 35,* 1779–1784.

Schuler, P. B., Richardson, M. T., Ochoa, P., & Wang, M. Q. (2001). Accuracy and repeatability of the Yale physical activity survey in assessing physical activity of older adults. *Perceptual & Motor Skills, 93,* 163–177.

Scruggs, P. W., Beveridge, S. K., Eisenman, P. A., Watson, D. L., Shultz, B. B., et al. (2003). Quantifying physical activity via pedometry in elementary physical education. *Medicine & Science in Sports & Exercise, 35,* 1065–1071.

Scruggs, P. W., Beveridge, S. K., Watson, D. L., & Clocksin, B. D. (2005). Quantifying physical activity in first-through fourth-grade physical education via pedometry. *Research Quarterly for Exercise & Sport, 76,* 166–175.

Seicean, A., Redline, S., Seicean, S., Kirchner, H. L., Gao, Y., Sekine, M., et al. (2007). Association between short sleeping hours and overweight in adolescents: Results from a US suburban high school survey. *Sleep Breath, 11,* 285–293.

Sekine, M., Yamagami, T., Handa, K., Saito, T., Nanri, S., Kawaminami, K., et al. (2002). A dose-response relationship between short sleeping hours and childhood obesity: Results of the Toyama Birth Cohort Study. *Child Care Health Development, 28,* 163–170.

Siconolfi, S. F., Lasater, T. M., Snow, R. C., & Carleton, R. A. (1985). Self-reported physical activity compared with maximal oxygen uptake. *American Journal of Epidemiology, 122,* 101–105.

Singh, P. N., Fraser, G. E., Knutsen, S. F., Lindsted, K. D., & Bennett, H. W. (2001). Validity of a physical activity questionnaire among African-American Seventh-day Adventists. *Medicine & Science in Sports & Exercise, 33,* 468–475.

Singh, P. N., Tonstad, S., Abbey, D. E., & Fraser, G. E. (1996). Validity of selected physical activity questions in white Seventh-day Adventists and non-Adventists. *Medicine & Science in Sports & Exercise, 28,* 1026–1037.

Sirard, J. R., Melanson, E. L., Li, L., & Freedson, P. S. (2000). Field evaluation of the Computer Science and Applications, Inc. physical activity monitor. *Medicine & Science in Sports & Exercise, 32,* 695–700.

Sirard, J. R., & Pate, R. R. (2001). Physical activity assessment in children and adolescents. *Sports Medicine, 31,* 439–454.

Sirard, J. R., Trost, S. G., Pfeiffer, K. A., Dowda, M., & Pate, R. R. (2005). Calibration and evaluation of an objective measure of physical activity in preschool children. *Journal of Physical Activity and Health, 2,* 345–357.

Slattery, M. L., Potter, J., Caan, B., Edwards, S., Coates, A., Ma, K. N., et al. (1997). Energy balance and colon cancer—beyond physical activity. *Cancer Research, 57,* 75–80.

Spanier, P. A., Marshall, S. J., & Faulkner, G. E. (2006). Tackling the obesity pandemic: A call for sedentary behaviour research. *Canadian Journal of Public Health, 97,* 255–257.

Spiegel, K., Leproult, R., Tasali, E., Penev, P., & Van Cauter, E. (2003). Sleep curtailment results in decreased leptin levels and increased hunger and appetite. *Sleep, 26,* A174.

Spiegel, K., Tasali, E., Penev, P., & Van Cauter, E. (2004). Brief communication: Sleep curtailment in healthy young men is associated with decreased leptin levels, elevated ghrelin levels, and increased hunger and appetite. *Annals of Internal Medicine, 141,* 846–850.

Spilsbury, J. C., Storfer-Isser, A., Drotar, D., Rosen, C. L., Kirchner, L. H., Benham, H., et al. (2004). Sleep behavior in an urban US sample of school-aged children. *Archives of Pediatrics & Adolescent Medicine, 158,* 988–994.

Stallings, V. A (1997). Calcium and bone health in children: A review. *American Journal of Therapeutics 4,* 259–273.

Starling, R. D., Matthews, D. E., Ades, P. A., & Poehlman, E. T. (1999). Assessment of physical activity in older individuals: A doubly labeled water study. *Journal of Applied Physiology, 86,* 2090–2096. (Erratum appears in *Journal of Applied Physiology,* 2001, *90*(5), following table of contents.)

Staten, L. K., Taren, D. L., Howell, W. H., Tobar, M., Poehlman, E. T., et al. (2001). Validation of the Arizona Activity Frequency Questionnaire using doubly labeled water [see comment]. *Medicine & Science in Sports & Exercise, 33,* 1959–1967.

Stel, V. S., Smit, J. H., Pluijm, S. M. F., Visser, M., Deeg, D. J. H., & Lips, P. (2004). Comparison of the LASA Physical Activity Questionnaire with a 7-day diary and pedometer. *Journal of Clinical Epidemiology, 57,* 252–258.

Stewart, A. L., Mills, K. M., King, A. C., Haskell, W. L., Gillis, D., & Ritter, P. L. (2001). CHAMPS physical activity questionnaire for older adults: Outcomes for interventions. *Medicine & Science in Sports & Exercise, 33,* 1126–1141.

Stone, A., Shiffman, S., Atienza, A. A., & Nebeling, L. (2007). *The science of real-time data capture: Self-reports in health research.* New York: Oxford University Press.

Strycker, L. A., Duncan, S. C., Chaumeton, N. R., Duncan, T. E., & Toobert, D. J. (2007). Reliability of pedometer data in samples of youth and older women. *International Journal of Behavioral Nutrition and Physical Activity, 4,* 4.

Sturgeon, S. R., Brinton, L. A., Berman, M. L., Mortel, R., Twiggs, L. B., Barrett, R. J., et al. (1993). Past and present physical activity and endometrial cancer risk. *British Journal of Cancer, 68,* 584–589.

Suitor, C. W., & Kraak, V. I. (2007). *Adequacy of evidence for physical activity guidelines development.* Washington, DC: National Academies Press.

Suleiman, S., & Nelson, M. (1997). Validation in London of a physical activity questionnaire for use in a study of postmenopausal osteopaenia. *Journal of Epidemiology & Community Health, 51,* 365–372.

Swartz, A. M., Bassett, D. R., Jr., Moore, J. B., Thompson, D. L., & Strath, S. J. (2003). Effects of body mass index on the accuracy of an electronic pedometer. *International Journal of Sports Medicine, 24,* 588–592.

Swartz, A. M., Strath, S. J., Bassett, D. R., Moore, J. B., Redwine, B. A., Groer, M., et al. (2003). Increasing daily walking improves glucose tolerance in overweight women. *Preventive Medicine, 37,* 356–362.

Talbot, L. A., Gaines, J. M., Huynh, T. N., & Metter, E. J. (2003). A home-based pedometer-driven walking program to increase physical activity in older adults with osteoarthritis of the knee: A preliminary study. *Journal of the American Geriatric Society, 51,* 387–392.

Thune, I., Brenn, T., Lund, E., & Gaard, M. (1997). Physical activity and the risk of breast cancer. *New England Journal of Medicine, 336,* 1269–1275.

Tikotzky, L., & Sadeh, A. (2001). Sleep patterns and sleep disruptions in kindergarten children. *Journal of Clinical Child Psychology, 30,* 581–591.

Tourangeau, R., Rips, L. J., & Rasinski, K. A. (2000). *The psychology of survey response.* Cambridge, UK: Cambridge University Press.

Troiano, R. P. (2005). A timely meeting: Objective measurement of physical activity. *Medicine & Science in Sports & Exercise, 37,* S487–S489.

Troiano, R. P., Berrigan, D., Dodd, K. W., Mâsse, L. C., Tilert, T., & McDowell, M. A. (2008). Physical activity in the United States measured by accelerometer. *Medicine & Science in Sports & Exercise, 40,* 181–188.

Trost, S. G. (2001). Objective measurement of physical activity in youth: Current issues, future directions. *Exercise and Sport Science Reviews, 29,* 32–36.

Trost, S. G., Pate, R. R., Freedson, P. S., Sallis, J. F., & Taylor, W. C. (2000). Using objective physical activity measures with youth: How many days of monitoring are needed? *Medicine & Science in Sports & Exercise, 32,* 426–431.

Trost, S. G., Ward, D. S., Moorehead, S. M., Watson, P. D., Riner, W., & Burke, J. R. (1998). Validity of the computer science and applications (CSA) activity monitor in children. *Medicine & Science in Sports & Exercise, 30,* 629–633.

Tudor-Locke, C. (2002). Taking steps toward increased physical activity: Using pedometers to measure and motivate. *Research Digest, 3,* 1–8.

Tudor-Locke, C., Ainsworth, B. E., Thompson, R. W., & Matthews, C. E. (2002). Comparison of pedometer and accelerometer measures of free-living physical activity. *Medicine & Science in Sports & Exercise, 34,* 2045–2051.

Tudor-Locke, C., Ainsworth, B. E., Whitt, M. C., Thompson, R. W., Addy, C. L., & Jones, D. A. (2001). The relationship between pedometer-determined ambulatory activity and body composition variables. *International Journal of Obesity and Related Metabolic Disorders, 25,* 1571–1578.

Tudor-Locke, C., & Bassett, D. R., Jr.. (2004). How many steps/day are enough? Preliminary pedometer indices for public health. *Sports Medicine, 34,* 1–8.

Tudor-Locke, C., Bell, R. C., Myers, A. M., Harris, S. B., Ecclestone, N. A., Lauzon, N., et al. (2004). Controlled outcome evaluation of the First Step Program: A daily physical activity intervention for individuals with type II diabetes. *International Journal of Obesity and Related Metabolic Disorders, 28,* 113–119.

Tudor-Locke, C., Bell, R. C., Myers, A. M., Harris, S. B., Lauzon, N., & Rodger, N. W. (2002). Pedometer-determined ambulatory activity in individuals with type 2 diabetes. *Diabetes Research and Clinical Practice, 55,* 191–199.

Tudor-Locke, C., Burkett, L., Reis, J. P., Ainsworth, B. E., Macera, C. A., & Wilson, D. K. (2005). How many days of pedometer monitoring predict weekly physical activity in adults? *Preventive Medicine, 40,* 293–298.

Tudor-Locke, C., Ham, S. A., Macera, C. A., Ainsworth, B. E., Kirtland, K. A., Reis, J. P., et al. (2004). Descriptive epidemiology of pedometer-determined physical activity. *Medicine & Science in Sports & Exercise, 36,* 1567–1573.

Tudor-Locke, C., Lee, S. M., Morgan, C. F., Beighle, A., & Pangrazi, R. P. (2006). Children's pedometer-determined physical activity during the segmented school day. *Medicine & Science in Sports & Exercise, 38,* 1732–1738.

Tudor-Locke, C., & Myers, A. M. (2001). Challenges and opportunities for measuring physical activity in sedentary adults. *Sports Medicine, 31,* 91–100.

Tudor-Locke, C., Pangrazi, R. P., Corbin, C. B., Rutherford, W. J., Vincent, S. D., Raustorp, A., et al. (2004). BMI-referenced standards for recommended pedometer-determined steps/day in children. *Preventive Medicine, 38,* 857–864.

Tudor-Locke, C., Williams, J. E., Reis, J. P., & Pluto, D. (2002). Utility of pedometers for assessing physical activity: Convergent validity. *Sports Medicine, 32,* 795–808.

Tuero, C., De Paz, J. A., & Marquez, S. (2001). Relationship of measures of leisure time physical activity to physical fitness indicators in Spanish adults. *Journal of Sports Medicine & Physical Fitness, 41,* 62–67.

U.S. Department of Agriculture, U.S. Department of Health and Human Services. (2005). *Dietary guidelines for Americans* (6th ed.). Washington, DC: Author.

U.S. Department of Health and Human Services. (1996). *Physical activity and health: A report of the Surgeon General.* Atlanta, GA: U.S. Department of Health and Human Services, Centers for Disease Control and Prevention, National Center for Chronic Disease Prevention and Health Promotion.

U.S. Department of Transportation, Bureau of Transportation. (2000). *Bicycle and pedestrian data: Sources, needs, and gaps.* Washington, DC: Author.

Van Cauter, E., Plat, L., & Copinschi, G. (1998). Interrelations between sleep and the somatotropic axis. *Sleep, 21,* 553–566.

Vandegrift, D., & Yoked, T. (2004). Obesity rates, income, and suburban sprawl: An analysis of US states. *Health Place, 10,* 221–229.

Verloop, J., Rookus, M. A., van der Kooy, K., & van Leeuwen, F. E. (2000). Physical activity and breast cancer risk in women aged 20–54 years. *Journal of the National Cancer Institute, 92,* 128–135.

Vincent, S. D., & Sidman, C. L. (2003). Determining measurement error in digital pedometers. *Measurement in Physical Education and Exercise Science, 7,* 19–24.

von Kries, R., Toschke, A. M., Wurmser, H., Sauerwald, T., & Koletzko, B. (2002). Reduced risk for overweight and obesity in 5- and 6-y-old children by duration of sleep: A cross-sectional study. *International Journal of Obesity and Related Metabolic Disorders, 26,* 710–716.

Voorrips, L. E., Ravelli, A. C., Dongelmans, P. C., Deurenberg, P., & van Staveren, W. A. (1991). A physical activity questionnaire for the elderly. *Medicine & Science in Sports & Exercise, 23,* 974–979.

Walsh, M. C., Hunter, G. R., Sirikul, B., & Gower, B. A. (2004). Comparison of self-reported with objectively assessed energy expenditure in Black and White women before and after weight loss. *American Journal of Clinical Nutrition, 79,* 1013–1019.

Wareham, N. J., Jakes, R. W., Rennie, K. L., Mitchell, J., Hennings, S., & Day, N. E. (2002). Validity and repeatability of the EPIC-Norfolk Physical Activity Questionnaire. *International Journal of Epidemiology, 31,* 168–174.

Wareham, N. J., Jakes, R. W., Rennie, K. L., Schuit, J., Mitchell, J., Hennings, S., et al. (2003). Validity and repeatability of a simple index derived from the short physical activity questionnaire used in the European Prospective Investigation into Cancer and Nutrition (EPIC) study. *Public Health Nutrition, 6*, 407–413.

Washburn, R. A., & Ficker, J. L. (1999). Physical Activity Scale for the Elderly (PASE): The relationship with activity measured by a portable accelerometer. *Journal of Sports Medicine & Physical Fitness, 39*, 336–340.

Washburn, R. A., Goldfield, S. R., Smith, K. W., & McKinlay, J. B. (1990). The validity of self-reported exercise-induced sweating as a measure of physical activity. *American Journal of Epidemiology, 132*, 107–113.

Washburn, R. A., McAuley, E., Katula, J., Mihalko, S. L., & Boileau, R. A. (1999). The physical activity scale for the elderly (PASE): Evidence for validity. *Journal of Clinical Epidemiology, 52*, 643–651.

Washburn, R. A., Smith, K. W., Jette, A. M., & Janney, C. A. (1993). The Physical Activity Scale for the Elderly (PASE): Development and evaluation. *Journal of Clinical Epidemiology, 46*, 153–162.

Weiss, T. W., Slater, C. H., Green, L. W., Kennedy, V. C., Albright, D. L., & Wun, C. C. (1990). The validity of single-item, self-assessment questions as measures of adult physical activity. *Journal of Clinical Epidemiology, 43*, 1123–1129.

Welk, G. (2002). *Physical activity assessments for health-related research.* Champaign, IL: Human Kinetics.

Welk, G. J., Blair, S. N., Wood, K., Jones, S., & Thompson, R. W. (2000). A comparative evaluation of three accelerometry-based physical activity monitors. *Medicine & Science in Sports & Exercise, 32*, S489–S497.

Welk, G. J., Corbin, C. B., & Dale, D. (2000). Measurement issues in the assessment of physical activity in children. *Research Quarterly for Exercise and Sport, 71*, 59–73

Welk, G. J., Morrow, J. R. J., & Falls, H. B. (2002). *Fitnessgram reference guide.* Dallas, TX: Cooper Institute.

Wendel-Vos, G. C. W., Schuit, A. J., Saris, W. H. M., & Kromhout, D. (2003). Reproducibility and relative validity of the short questionnaire to assess health-enhancing physical activity. *Journal of Clinical Epidemiology, 56*, 1163–1169.

Westerterp, K. R., Saris, W. H. M., Bloemberg, B. P. M., Kempen, K., Caspersen, C. J., & Kromhout, D.

(1992). Validation of the Zutphen Physical Activity Questionnaire for the Elderly with doubly labeled water. *Medicine & Science in Sports & Exercise, 24*, S68.

Whitney, C. W., Lind, B. K., & Wahl, P. W. (1998). Quality assurance and quality control in longitudinal studies. *Epidemiology Review, 20*, 71–80.

Wiggs, L., Montgomery, P., & Stores, G. (2005). Actigraphic and parent reports of sleep patterns and sleep disorders in children with subtypes of attention-deficit hyperactivity disorder. *Sleep, 28*, 1437–1445.

Wilbur, J., Holm, K., & Dan, A. (1993). A quantitative survey to measure energy expenditure in midlife women. *Journal of Nursing Measurement, 1*, 29–40.

Wingard, D. L., & Berkman, L. F. (1983). Mortality risk associated with sleeping patterns among adults. *Sleep, 6*, 102–107.

Wolf, A. M., Hunter, D. J., Colditz, G. A., Manson, J. E., Stampfer, M. J., Corsano, K. A., et al. (1994). Reproducibility and validity of a self-administered physical activity questionnaire. *International Journal of Epidemiology, 23*, 991–999.

Wolfson, A. R., Carskadon, M. A., Acebo, C., Seifer, R., Fallone, G., Labyak, S. E., et al. (2003). Evidence for the validity of a sleep habits survey for adolescents. *Sleep, 26*, 213–216.

Wu, A. H., Paganini-Hill, A., Ross, R. K., & Henderson, B. E. (1987). Alcohol, physical activity and other risk factors for colorectal cancer: A prospective study. *British Journal of Cancer, 55*, 687–694.

Yancey, A. K., Wold, C. M., McCarthy, W. J., Weber, M. D., Lee, B., Simon, P. A., et al. (2004). Physical inactivity and overweight among Los Angeles County adults [see comment]. *American Journal of Preventive Medicine, 27*, 146–152.

Yore, M. M., Ham, S. A., Kohl, I. H. W., Ainsworth, B. E. F., & LaMonte, M. (2004). Reliability and validity of BRFSS Walking Questions. *Medicine & Science in Sports & Exercise, 36*, S111.

Young, D. R., Jee, S. H., & Appel, L. J. (2001). A comparison of the Yale Physical Activity Survey with other physical activity measures. *Medicine & Science in Sports & Exercise, 33*, 955–961.

Zimring, C., Joseph, A., Nicoll, G. L., & Tsepas, S. (2005). Influences of building design and site design on physical activity: Research and intervention opportunities. *American Journal of Preventive Medicine, 28*, 186–193.

CHAPTER 7

Measuring Food Intake in Free-Living Populations

Focus on Obesity

Lauren Lissner and Nancy Potischman

The purpose of this chapter is to review current knowledge of methods for studying food intake in observational studies of free-living populations, with special focus on obese and overweight groups, as well as other difficult-to-measure populations. Examples will be given from several studies that have focused specifically on dietary methodology evaluation issues in obesity, including questionnaire development, documentation of errors, and analytical considerations.

Accurate assessment of dietary intake in obese individuals is of special concern in population-based nutrition research, in view of dramatically increased prevalence rates of obesity together with the growing list of obesity-related comorbidities and health consequences. This issue is also of obvious relevance within clinical settings in which dietary intake is being monitored. Yet, surprisingly little is known on how to obtain accurate measures of dietary intake in the obese, and this issue is widely viewed as one of the weak links in nutritional epidemiology. Thus, dietary instrumentation in obese individuals is a topic that urgently requires attention by researchers in nutrition.

Underreporting Bias and Obesity

Measurement of habitual food intake is known to include varying levels of measurement error depending on the type of dietary assessment method used and the bias of respondents. In particular, measuring dietary intakes of free-living obese subjects is problematic because they may be more prone to underreporting bias compared to their normal-weight counterparts. In

AUTHORS' NOTE: We thank Drs. Fran Thompson, Rachel Ballard-Barbash, Susan Krebs-Smith, Amy Subar, June Stevens, and Berit Heitmann for their helpful comments.

addition to generalized under- or overreporting, there are other forms of misreporting of intake, including omissions and insertions of specific types of foods. It has been proposed that these biases are related to social desirability factors (Hebert, Clemow, Pbert, Ockene, & Ockene, 1995) and may involve a combination of conscious and unconscious errors (Hise, Sullivan, Jacobsen, Johnson, & Donnelly, 2002; Muhlheim, Allison, Heshka, & Heymsfield, 1998; Roth, Snyder, & Pace, 1986). It follows that inadequate measures of usual diet in obese individuals may lead to misleading or inaccurate observed associations between diet and obesity-related health outcomes.

The specific existence of obesity-related underreporting was rather controversial until the advent of doubly labeled water (DLW) gave support to previously anecdotal evidence of such a bias (Prentice et al., 1986; Schoeller, 1999). Briefly, DLW is a "recovery" biomarker (Kaaks, Ferrari, Ciampi, Plummer, & Riboli, 2002), one with quantitative retrieval and directly related to intake. It is now widely used to estimate energy intake in free-living, weight-stable subjects and is believed to be unbiased with respect to obesity. The DLW method has been shown to be accurate to 1%, and the within-subject variation in total daily energy expenditure for those with stable weight and activity is approximately 9% (Black, Coward, Cole, & Prentice, 1996). Because the isotopic materials are costly, particularly O^{18}, which has fluctuating costs, and analysis requires specialized, expensive equipment, this method cannot be considered routine. However, it is now possible to apply the DLW method to studies involving hundreds of participants rather than the samples sizes of 5 to 20 that characterized earlier applications (Schoeller, 1999). This method has demonstrated clearly that obese subjects consume more energy while tending to report less than their normal-weight counterparts. Use of this technique has revealed that in some obese subjects, presence of an observer to record intake or belief that investigators know true intake can affect the quality of reported energy intakes (Hise et al., 2002; Muhlheim et al., 1998).

Selective Underreporting

Investigators have attempted to evaluate disproportionate misreporting of macronutrient and other specific aspects of the diet. Studies involving urinary nitrogen as a biomarker for total protein intake (Johansson, Bingham, & Wahter, 1999) have been consistent with the conclusion that obese individuals consume more protein than they report (Heitmann & Lissner, 1995; Hultén, Bengtsson, & Isaksson, 1990). Disproportionate misreporting of the nonprotein fraction of the diet has also been examined, using estimated energy expenditure and urinary nitrogen to demonstrate increasing underreporting error with increasing levels of body mass index (BMI) (Heitmann & Lissner, 1995). In contrast, a few studies specifically examining biases in reported percentage of energy as protein, as opposed to total protein intake, suggested relative overreporting of the protein fraction of the diet (Heitmann & Lissner, 1995; Heitmann, Lissner, & Osler, 2000; Lissner, Heitmann, & Lindroos, 1998; Lissner, Lindroos, & Sjöström, 1998; Lissner et al., 2007). Selective underreporting of socially undesirable food types has been documented using a number of other approaches, ranging from direct covert observation (Poppitt, Swann, Black, & Prentice, 1998) to more indirect assessments of dietary characteristics of "underreporters" (Tooze et al., 2004). Limitations in the science of dietary biomarkers constrain our understanding of how this type of selective underreporting can affect observations in nutritional epidemiology.

Other Aspects of Underreporting

Overweight per se is one of many factors that are associated with underreporting and misreporting (Maurer et al., 2006; Tooze et al., 2004). Other factors believed to be equally or more important are dietary restraint (see also Chapter 5, this volume) and social desirability (Hebert et al., 1995), while preliminary evidence exists that dietary disinhibition, body image, depression, anxiety, and fear of negative evaluation may also be related to underreporting and other errors (Maurer et al., 2006). In addition, there may be marked shifts in caloric intake in obese individuals due to intermittent energy restriction and the probability of dieting during the assessment period (Ballard-Barbash, Graubard, Krebs-Smith, Schatzkin, & Thompson, 1996). Thus, it may be difficult to assess "usual" intake when studies can only sample subjects once or a limited number of times. The relative importance of these different factors is difficult to compare across studies but appears to vary widely in magnitude. Because many such traits are likely to be associated with obesity, a better understanding of these complex relationships is probably needed to improve the accuracy of dietary reporting in contemporary population studies.

As the prevalence of obesity increases in most populations studied, both total and selective reporting biases are likely to influence reporting accuracy in an increasing proportion of the population. In addition, underreporting of total intake and/or socially undesirable foods has implications in the management of obesity in both treatment and primary preventive contexts. The extent to which obese individuals underreport certain types of food is difficult to document under survey conditions, and there is evidence that similar biases exist in nonoverweight groups (Asbeck et al., 2002), although the magnitude of underreporting may be smaller. In the next section, we give a brief overview of selected dietary assessment instruments that are currently used for dietary assessment of free-living populations. Some but not all of these methodologies have been specifically assessed with respect to obesity-related reporting errors and biases.

Overview of Dietary Assessment Methods

Numerous chapters, journal supplements, and even textbooks have covered the topic of dietary assessment methods (Gibson, 2005; Thompson & Byers, 1994; Thompson & Subar, 2001; Willett,

1998). In this section, we briefly overview currently used methods (Table 7.1) and direct readers interested in more detailed information about dietary methods to the references provided in this chapter. In addition, Chapter 12 of the present volume offers an overview of dietary methodologies with a focus on applications in children.

Food Frequency Questionnaires

A variety of dietary methods can be used in studies of free-living populations, but some are more amenable to very large studies (more than 100,000 subjects) due to ease of administration and associated costs. The food frequency questionnaire (FFQ) is considered the method of choice in very large studies. Commonly used FFQs in the United States include the Block FFQ (http://www .nutritionquest.com/products/questionnaires_scree ners.htm), the National Cancer Institute (NCI) Diet History Questionnaire (DHQ) (http://riskfactor .cancer.gov/DHQ/index.html), and the Harvard-Willett Questionnaire. These instruments are publicly available, either for a fee or free, and have support for converting the frequency data into nutrient and food data. The validity of these instruments has been found to be generally comparable, especially after adjustment for energy intake. In one comparative study (Subar et al., 2001), subjects completed either the NCI DHQ and the Block FFQ or the NCI DHQ and the Harvard-Willett FFQ, and 26 nutrients were compared between FFQs and with four 24-hour recalls. Although the DHQ and Block instruments had higher correlations with the 24-hour recalls for many nutrients, all three were comparable after energy adjustment and suitable for studying diet and disease relationships.

The FFQ is most often self-administered and can be mailed or given to subjects to complete at their leisure. It is a retrospective method asking respondents to report their usual frequency of consumption of each item from a list of foods, for a specific period (several months or a year). Food lists vary according to the purpose of the study and study population. Frequency of consumption

Table 7.1 Advantages and Disadvantages of Dietary Assessment Instruments

Instrument	Advantages	Disadvantages	Selected Studies With an Obesity Focus
Food frequency questionnaire	Usual individual intake asked Aims to capture whole diet Low investigator cost Does not affect eating behavior	Intake often misreported Not quantifiably precise Difficult cognitive task for respondent	Subar et al. (2003) Tooze et al. (2004) Lindroos, Lissner, and Sjöström (1993, 1999) Lissner et al. (2007)
Diet history	Usual individual intake asked Aims to capture whole diet Information often available on foods consumed by meal Does not affect eating behavior	Intake often misreported Not quantifiably precise Difficult cognitive task for respondent Can have high investigator burden	Heitmann and Lissner (1995) Heitmann, Lissner, and Osler (2000) Rothenberg, Bosaeus, Lernfelt, Landahl, and Steen (1998) Martin, Tapsell, Denmeade, and Batterham (2003)
Food record	Intake quantified Describes total diet Could enhance self-monitoring for weight control	Affects eating behavior Intake often underreported Reports of intake decrease with time May lead to substantial sample bias High investigator cost High respondent burden Extensive respondent training and motivation required Many days needed to capture individual's usual intake	Lindroos et al. (1993) Lafay et al. (1997) Martin, Tapsell, Batterham, and Russell (2002)

Instrument	Advantages	Disadvantages	Selected Studies With an Obesity Focus
24-hour dietary recall	Intake quantified Describes total diet Appropriate for most populations: low sample bias Relatively low respondent burden	Intake often underreported High investigator cost Many days needed to capture individual's usual intake	Johansson, Wikman, Ahrén, Hallmans, and Johansson (2001) Ferrari et al. (2002) Subar et al. (2003) Tooze et al. (2004) Lissner et al. (2007)
Brief instruments	Usual individual intake often asked Low investigator cost Low respondent burden Does not affect eating behavior	Intake often misreported Not quantifiably precise Assessment limited to small number of nutrients/foods	Obesity issues have not been assessed

SOURCE: Adapted with permission from Thompson, F. E., & Subar, A. F. (in press). Dietary assessment methodology. In A. M. Coulson & C. J. Boushey (Eds.), *Nutrition in the prevention and treatment of disease* (2nd ed.). New York: Academic Press.

categories also varies by questionnaire but usually includes categories of per day, week, month, or year. There are two main types of FFQ that differ in the information obtained about portion size. The semi-quantitative FFQ specifies some or all of the portion sizes, and the respondent chooses among the range of portions or reports frequency of consumption of a particular portion. The non-quantitative FFQ does not include portion size information which would seem to be a potential limitation in obese populations. Some FFQs may also inquire about whether the subject has changed consumption patterns recently or is on a weight reduction or other special diet. The nutrient estimates from these instruments generally rank individuals adequately but cannot capture true absolute intakes of most nutrients (Willett, 1998). Differentiating low and high consumers of the dietary components is usually adequate for epidemiologic studies, but combining the frequency information with other markers of nutritional intake or nutritional status can aid in classifying individuals (Potischman, 2003) or describing usual intakes in a population (Dodd et al., 2006, Freedman et al., 2004). Shortened versions of FFQs have been developed (e.g., Block, Hartman, & Naughton, 1990), which seem appropriate for some circumstances in that they can perform similarly to the longer versions (Potischman et al., 1999). Questionnaires asking frequency information related to very short lists of foods have also been developed with a focus on a specific aspect of diet, such as a particular nutrient of interest (see screeners below).

Diet History

The Diet History (DH) questionnaire is another common method used in epidemiologic studies (e.g., Eiben et al., 2004; Heitmann & Lissner, 1995;

Liu, et al., 1994; Rothenberg, Bosaeus, Lernfelt, Landahl, & Steen, 1998). The DH is a retrospective assessment method ascertaining a respondent's typical food intake by collecting descriptive detail and amount information about each food. The major limitation of DH questionnaires is the fact that the method is not as straightforward as other self-administered instruments and therefore typically requires a trained interviewer to administer the DH in person or by telephone. DHs may include questions on meal patterns, lists of common foods, and groups of generic food (Kohlmeier, 1994; Kohlmeier, Mendez, McDuffie, & Miller, 1997). This diet method estimates usual intake of various foods and nutrients to rank subjects but, similar to the FFQ, may not capture absolute intake of a particular nutrient of interest as not all foods consumed are queried. With special reference to energy, this method is similar to others in that it has been shown to underestimate energy intake in obese individuals, when compared to DLW or to energy requirement estimated by body composition (Heitmann & Lissner, 1995; Rothenberg et al., 1998).

Food Records

Food records are a form of diary wherein the subjects record food intake at the time of consumption, over a number of days, usually 4 to 7, not necessarily sequential ones. Most studies ask respondents to enter the information on hard-copy form, although tape-recording and electronic weighing also have been used to collect descriptive and quantity information. The food record method requires the subject to document the portion consumed either through estimating portion size with household measures or portion size props ("estimated FR") or by weighing all foods before and after consumption ("weighed FR"). The recorded information is also reviewed by a nutritionist with queries to the subjects regarding missing details; one study on this topic found large differences after review (Cantwell et al., 2006) while another found less dramatic differences (Kolar et al., 2005), and neither reported

on differences by body weight status of the subjects. After receiving the diaries, the information is coded and entered into computer programs to derive average daily intake estimates for the whole period. These data are thought to reflect absolute intake, although more than 4 to 7 days of intake may be required to describe usual intake over a specific time period, such as "in the past year" or "usual," which may take several weeks for estimates of usual amounts of calories. A major limitation of this methodology is that the act of recording intake often results in modified intakes and may result in biased reporting. It is well established that self-monitoring or recording daily intakes via food record is a useful tool in weight loss programs (Boutelle & Kirshenbaum, 1998; Streit, Stevens, Stevens, & Rossner, 1991). Because obese subjects are likely to have experience with this, it has been speculated that obesity-related underestimation of usual intake may be particularly problematic with this method, due to changing consumption patterns while recording intake.

Food records are currently not appropriate in large population studies but have been used in smaller studies or in representative subgroups of larger studies with the results extrapolated or inferred for the whole group. A newer application of this approach, aimed at reducing costs for this methodology, is completion of food records by all subjects included in a large study, with later nested sampling of cases and controls to code and use in the analysis (Bingham et al., 2003; Freedman et al., 2006).

Twenty-Four-Hour Recalls

The 24-hour recall (24HR) is another method that may be applied to large studies but requires multiple administrations and some spontaneity of administration to avert planned eating or reporting. The 24HR is a retrospective assessment method in which an interviewer prompts a respondent to recall and describe all foods and beverages consumed in the preceding 24 hours or the preceding day. The interview may be conducted in person or by telephone and may be paper and pencil or computer-assisted. Portion size estimating aids assist the respondent to recall amounts consumed. It is important to keep in mind when planning studies that data from weekends should be represented, although they may be particularly difficult to collect. The methodology for conducting the 24HR has evolved during the past two decades. Among the methods reported are the three-pass method, the U.S. Department of Agriculture's five-pass method, University of Minnesota's protocol for the Nutrition Data System, the Bogalusa Heart Study protocol, and others (Dennis, Ernst, Hjortland, Tillotson, & Grambsch, 1980; Frank, Berenson, Schilling, & Moore, 1977; Guenther, DeMaio, Ingwersen, & Berlin, 1996; Moshfegh, Borrud, Perloff, & LaComb, 1999; U.S. Department of Agriculture [USDA], 1997). The 24HR will result in average daily intake of a variety of nutrients and is considered the gold standard for estimating population distributions of intakes (USDA) and absolute intakes for a given day.

The number of recalls needed depends on the research or public health focus, variability in the population, and the nutrients of interest. For studies evaluating diet and disease outcomes, multiple days of intake may be required (e.g., 7–14 days depending on the nutrient; Hartman et al., 1990). It has been observed that, for research purposes, two to four 24HRs may be necessary to attain reasonable validity with DLW and urinary nitrogen (Schatzkin et al., 2003). Usual intake of the population can be modeled by a variety of methods (Dodd et al., 2006) and requires two 24HRs. Preliminary research has indicated that 24HR data can be refined with information from a food frequency questionnaire without portion size information, called a food propensity questionnaire (FPQ), to obtain improved distributions of usual intake (Carriquiry, 2003; Subar et al., 2006; Tooze et al., 2006).

Considering different methods, data from the 24HR are considered the most valid, particularly for population distributions, but this comes at a cost. The major limitation of this method is the requirement of being interviewer administered, although several groups are currently developing self-administered versions (Subar et al., 2007; Vereecken, Covents, Matthys, & Maes, 2005). Another limitation is that the 24HR be administered spontaneously so that subjects do not modify intake for the day of recall. This is particularly difficult to achieve in large studies where investigators must coordinate administration of many unannounced 24HRs on any given day. Currently, administration of unplanned telephone 24HRs is difficult because many individuals use only cellular phones with no telephone listing, and others use answering machines or caller identification to screen incoming phone calls. Finally, time constraints related to a possibly 30- to 40-minute interview may decrease compliance. Administration in a clinical setting can be spontaneous for one or possibly two administrations, but subjects may come to expect such interviews and thereby alter intake the day prior to the visit in anticipation of the recall. These issues may be more complex for obese subjects if they are cognizant of food issues and experienced with altering intakes or reporting. This method is sensitive to problems of memory, and obesity-related underreporting is often documented with this instrument.

Finally, 24HR can be useful in developing and validating new frequency-based methods, adjusting for attenuation of risk estimates, and calibrating instruments used in international studies (Slimani et al., 2002). The problem of harmonizing dietary data across different countries (e.g., within Europe) has underscored the importance of the 24HR due to its inherent flexibility and open-ended structure.

Screeners and Checklists

Screening instruments typically include 7 to 30 questions, usually in food frequency format describing how often the foods are consumed. These simplified screeners have been developed to assess specific intakes such as percent calories from fat, fruit and vegetable servings, dairy products, fiber, added sugar, calcium and vitamin D, folic acid, and soy intakes (http://riskfactor.cancer.gov/diet/screeners/;http://www.nutritionquest.com/products/questionnaires_screeners.htm). Figure 7.1 shows an example of a fat screener developed from 24HR recalls in older U.S. subjects (Thompson et al., 2007), which is now being evaluated in intervention studies (Thompson, Midthune, et al., 2008). Some screeners have been calibrated against longer instruments or 24HRs and have been designed to accomplish crude divisions of the population on a particular nutrient or food (e.g., consuming five servings of fruit and vegetables per day; Thompson, Subar, Smith, et al., 2002). These instruments have been found useful for surveillance of intakes in population groups (e.g., National Health Interview Survey; Thompson et al., 2005), but given their focus on select dietary constituents, they may have limited utility for most epidemiologic purposes. Whether these instruments might be more or less useful in overweight individuals has not been investigated specifically.

A related methodology of interest is the Checklist or Daily Food List, which includes a short list of foods; the subjects check those that were consumed on a given day and complete this task every day for 3 to 30 days. The subject should complete the checklist over the course of the day, with a check or mark each time a particular food is eaten (see Figure 7.2; Thompson et al., 2006). These data share qualities with diet records in that the subject completes the intake information on the day it is consumed for some given number of days. These data can be used to estimate usual intake for that period of time or in conjunction with other data (Thompson et al., 2006) to decrease the measurement error in other instruments, such as the FFQ. Due to the limited number of foods and the grouping of foods in a one-page list, the instrument has some limitations, but new work is being conducted to incorporate it in the arsenal of instruments to be administered in research settings. The current checklists have not been evaluated with respect to validity in overweight or obese populations;

however, one evaluation of 30 consecutive days did indicate that the recording did not alter intakes that were being assessed (Thompson, Subar, Brown, et al., 2002). Although this study did not evaluate reactivity by BMI status, this method holds promise as longer recording instruments have been shown to result in modified intakes, especially among obese individuals.

Food Balance Data

Food supply data on an aggregate (usually national) level can be used in ecological studies of diet and health outcomes. For instance, this approach has been employed in attempts to relate dietary factors to obesity in populations, both at the country level and in describing trends in a given country over time (Gross, Ford, & Liu, 2004; Heini & Weinsier, 1997; Lissner & Heitmann, 1995). This, like all ecological research, is subject to the "ecological fallacy" if associations are confounded or do not match individual-based results. While use of food supply data has a number of important sources of error (e.g., wastage, nonhuman consumption, food from home gardens, and other sources outside of commercial exchange), this approach may have some value when studying items that are liable to be underestimated due to social desirability related factors. For instance, a study of alcohol usage on an isolated Norwegian island community indicated far lower consumption by self-reports compared to direct inventory of alcohol consumption on the island (Høyer, Nilssen, Brenn, & Schirmer, 1995). Although ecological studies have limitations, these studies have utility in providing evidence, generating hypotheses, and sparking further individual-level studies.

Other Novel Approaches

Many new methodologies are currently being developed and tested for use in free-living populations. One such method is a self-administered

NATIONAL CANCER INSTITUTE
QUICK FOOD SCAN

| ID # Place Label Here |

1. Think about your eating habits over the past 12 months. About how often did you eat or drink each of the following foods? Remember breakfast, lunch, dinner, snacks, and eating out. Blacken in only one bubble for each food.

TYPE OF FOOD	Never	Less Than Once Per Month	1-3 Times Per Month	1-2 Times Per Week	3-4 Times Per Week	5-6 Times Per Week	1 Time Per Day	2 or More Times Per Day
Cold cereal	O	O	O	O	O	O	O	O
Skim milk, on cereal or to drink	O	O	O	O	O	O	O	O
Eggs, fried or scrambled in margarine, butter, or oil	O	O	O	O	O	O	O	O
Sausage or bacon, regular-fat	O	O	O	O	O	O	O	O
Margarine or butter on bread, rolls, pancakes	O	O	O	O	O	O	O	O
Orange juice or grapefruit juice	O	O	O	O	O	O	O	O
Fruit (not juices)	O	O	O	O	O	O	O	O
Beef or pork hot dogs, regular-fat	O	O	O	O	O	O	O	O
Cheese or cheese spread, regular-fat	O	O	O	O	O	O	O	O
French fries, home fries, or hash brown potatoes	O	O	O	O	O	O	O	O
Margarine or butter on vegetables, including potatoes	O	O	O	O	O	O	O	O
Mayonnaise, regular-fat	O	O	O	O	O	O	O	O
Salad dressings, regular-fat	O	O	O	O	O	O	O	O
Rice	O	O	O	O	O	O	O	O
Margarine, butter, or oil on rice or pasta	O	O	O	O	O	O	O	O

2. Over the past 12 months, when you prepared foods with margarine or ate margarine, how often did you use a reduced-fat margarine?

O	O	O	O	O	O
DIDN'T USE MARGARINE	Almost never	About ¼ of the time	About ½ of the time	About ¾ of the time	Almost always or always

3. Overall, when you think about the foods you ate over the past 12 months, would you say your diet was high, medium, or low in fat?

O	O	O
High	Medium	Low

Figure 7.1   Sixteen-Item Percent Energy From Fat Screener Developed From 24-Hour Recall Data in Older U.S. Adults

1. What day is today?

☐ Sunday   ☐ Monday   ☐ Tuesday   ☐ Wednesday   ☐ Thursday   ☐ Friday   ☐ Saturday

2. How to Record Foods

- **Check (✓) a box for every food you eat at a different meal or snack.**

  Example: I ate 1 roll at lunch and 1 roll at dinner.

  ☑☑☐☐☐ Rolls, English muffins, bagels

- Do NOT count the number of pieces or servings of the **same** food you eat at a meal or snack.

  Example: I ate two rolls at dinner.

  ☑☐☐☐☐ Rolls, English muffins, bagels

- **Record mixtures** (sandwiches, casseroles, salads, pasta, and stir-fry dishes) by checking each food in the mixture.

  Example: I ate a turkey sandwich (2 slices of bread) lettuce and mustard.

  ☑☐☐☐☐ All other bread (NOT in pizza)

  ☑☐☐☐☐ Chicken, turkey, duck alone or in mixtures (but NOT in the foods in Box A)

  ☑☐☐☐☐ Lettuce in other mixtures, such as sandwiches

- For additional examples, see back cover.

3. Now fill in the foods you eat today in Boxes A–G.

A. Chili, Mexican Food, Pizza, Soup

Do NOT count ingredients in these foods anywhere else.

☐☐☐☐☐ Chili (All kinds)

☐☐☐☐☐ Mexican food mixtures, such as tacos, tostados, burritos, fajitas, enchiladas

☐☐☐☐☐ Pizza (All kinds)

☐☐☐☐☐ Soup (All kinds)

B. Meat, Poultry, Fish

☐☐☐☐☐ Beef, pork, ham, bacon, sausage alone or in mixtures (but NOT in the foods in Box A)

☐☐☐☐☐ Chicken, turkey, duck alone or in mixtures (but NOT in the foods in Box A)

☐☐☐☐☐ Fish, seafood alone or in mixtures (but NOT in the foods in Box A)

C. Dairy, Eggs

☐☐☐☐☐ Cheese (All kinds)

☐☐☐☐☐ Yogurt (All kinds)

☐☐☐☐☐ Eggs (All kinds)

D. Fruits, Vegetables

☐☐☐☐☐ Fruit cocktail, fruit salad

☐☐☐☐☐ All other fruits (NOT juice)

If different fruits are eaten at the same time, check a box for each fruit.

☐☐☐☐☐ Potatoes alone or in mixtures (All kinds, but NOT chips and NOT in soup)

☐☐☐☐☐ Cooked dried beans, such as pinto, lima, lentils (but NOT in the foods in Box A)

☐☐☐☐☐ Salad greens, such as lettuce and spinach

☐☐☐☐☐ Lettuce in other mixtures, such as sandwiches

☐☐☐☐☐ All other vegetables alone or in mixtures, such as salads (but NOT in the foods in Box A)

If different vegetables are eaten at the same time, check a box for each vegetable.

☐☐☐☐☐ Tomato sauce, such as in spaghetti and lasagna (but NOT in the foods in Box A)

E. Snack Foods, Desserts

☐☐☐☐☐ Candy (All kinds)

☐☐☐☐☐ Cookies, pie, cake, brownies

☐☐☐☐☐ Ice cream, sorbet, frozen yogurt

☐☐☐☐☐ Popcorn, crackers, chips, pretzels

F. Cereals, Breads, Grains

☐☐☐☐☐ Cereal, hot or cold (All kinds)

☐☐☐☐☐ Rolls, English muffins, bagels

☐☐☐☐☐ All other bread (NOT in pizza)

☐☐☐☐☐ Tortillas (NOT in mixtures)

☐☐☐☐☐ Doughnuts, Danish, sweet rolls, muffins, dessert breads, pop-tarts

☐☐☐☐☐ Pancakes, waffles, French toast

☐☐☐☐☐ Rice alone or in mixtures (but NOT in the foods in Box A)

☐☐☐☐☐ Pasta, spaghetti, noodles alone or in mixtures (but NOT in chili or soup)

G. Spreads, Dressings

Do NOT count the items below if only used in cooking.

☐☐☐☐☐ Butter or margarine added to each different food

☐☐☐☐☐ Mayonnaise or salad dressing, including low-fat, added to each different food

Comments

Did you have any difficulty understanding how to fill out the form today? If so, please explain.

_____

_____

_____

4. Please review. Do you remember anything else?

Figure 7.2   Daily Checklist to Be Completed as Foods Are Consumed Over the Course of a Day for Multiple Consecutive Days

24HR is Web based and freely available to researchers and clinicians (http://riskfactor .cancer.gov/tools/instruments/asa24.html). This new 24HR is based on the American standard of the USDA multiple-pass methodology used in National Health and Nutrition Examination Survey (NHANES) and has audio components and a guide to assist completion by subjects unfamiliar with computers and low-literacy groups. Work is under way to establish a Spanish version of this instrument and possibly versions for other countries. A similar computer-assisted 24HR system, the Young Adolescent's Nutrition Assessment on Computer (YANA-C), is being used in the Healthy Lifestyle by Nutrition in Adolescence (HELENA) study in Europe (Vereecken et al., 2005; Vereecken et al., 2008). It should be noted, however, that the instrument may require some supervision. Other Web-based nutrition analysis programs are available, such as Formula for Life (www.formulaforlife.com), Fit Day (www.fitday.com), USDA My Pyramid (www.mypyramidtracker.gov), NutriWatch (www .nutrawatch.com), and Nutrition Analysis Tools and System (www.nat.uiuc.edu). Although these are self-administered systems for respondents that can provide feedback on daily intakes, these systems are not necessarily for researchers due to lack of detail questions about each food. All of the 24HR-based systems have the limitation of requiring administration on a specified day while also requiring spontaneity to avoid changes in behavior and furthermore have documented underreporting errors among overweight respondents.

Other new technologies include use of photographs from digital cameras and cellular phones for 24HRs (see Glanz & Murphy, 2007, for review). Nutrax (http://nutraxcorp.com/research .html) incorporates use of digital photographs that can be loaded onto a computer and then merged with other data entered by hand to derive nutrient information. These methods are not yet ready for researchers and need to be tested in small studies. Portion size estimation from photographs is a challenge, and standardization across individuals may be difficult in some population groups. Documentation of cafeteria food choices for specific individuals has been achieved through use of "smart cards" (Lambert et al., 2005). Such systems can be useful for collecting data limited to one meal but hold promise for other applications in the future.

Use of barcodes on food items has been of interest to nutritionists for some years (Anderson et al., 1999), but their usage is not yet feasible in surveys or epidemiologic research. Although a database is available on the Internet (http://www.glondon .com/) linking the barcodes to food identification and nutrients, a pilot study (Bryant, Ward, & Stevens, 2006) found this database far too limited and not feasible for research purposes. Work is under way to create a larger database, but currently there is no publicly available system to link the barcodes to foods, nutrients, and food groups. In addition, there is concern about the rapid appearance of new foods on the markets and that the nutrient content of products with the same barcode may change rapidly over time. A system will need to be established to maintain such a database in a standardized manner.

Recording of intake on a personal digital assistant (PDA) is another technology that is currently evolving. A recent workshop delineated the issues related to electronic real-time data capture wherein the dietary component was addressed along with other health behaviors (http://dccps.cancer.gov/ hprb/real-time/ index.html). PDAs have been used in clinical settings and in weight loss programs. Evaluation of the electronic technology shows it to be similar to traditional methods of recording food intake (Beasley, Riley, & Jean-Mary, 2005; Yon, Johnson, Harvey-Berino, Gold, & Howard, 2007), and one study reported better compliance with dietary goals during the observation period (Glanz, Murphy, Moylan, Evensen, & Curb, 2006). For observational studies, this method would share limitations similar to food records (Yon, Johnson, Harvey-Berino, & Gold, 2006) as subjects are requested to document intake at every eating occasion. The field is rapidly advancing, and testing of these new technologies will emerge in the next few years.

Examples of Three Studies Documenting Obesity-Related Bias in Free-Living Populations

In this section, we focus on three dietary surveys in free-living populations that specifically addressed the issue of obesity-related reporting bias, using various traditional instruments.

Swedish Obese Subjects

The first set of studies described here was designed with the overall aim to measure dietary intake in severely obese adults who were potential participants in a controlled surgical intervention study. The instrument was a semi-quantitative food frequency questionnaire designed to capture intake patterns and dietary problem areas for obese Swedes (Lissner, Lindroos, & Sjöström, 1998; questionnaire reproduced in Lindroos, Lissner, & Sjöström, 1999). For instance there was special probing on frequency and composition of sandwiches, size of candy and usual portions included on a plate model of main meals. This method performed well in initial validation studies, in fact capturing much more of obese subjects' usual intakes than a 4-day food record (Lindroos et al., 1999). This comparative success of the FFQ, relative to the food diary, drew attention to episodic undereating as a potential explanation for low intakes during food recording periods, a phenomenon that has subsequently been demonstrated by other researchers (Goris, Westerterp-Plantenga, & Westerterp, 2000). Although subsequent validation results for the Swedish Obese Subjects (SOS) method were suggestive of some energy underreporting even by FFQ, compared to 24-hour indirect calorimetry (Lindroos, Lissner, & Sjöström, 1999). This method is fairly unique in having captured realistic intakes in highly cooperative and motivated subjects, intakes that were significantly higher than those of population-based controls (Lindroos et al., 1997), giving an early indication that an FFQ-based approach might produce a lesser degree of obesity-specific underreporting than food records. In a supplementary methodological development in this same study, it was observed that obese women, compared to population controls, reported more eating occasions and that these occurred later in the day, in addition to consuming more total energy by the FFQ method described previously (Bertéus Forslund, Lindroos, Sjöström, & Lissner, 2002).

MONICA-Denmark

The next studies to be addressed here are the MONICA-Denmark energy and protein validation studies (Heitmann & Lissner, 1995; Heitmann et al., 2000). These were population-based surveys that collected information on usual intake by diet history and included in the examination protocol PABA-validated urinary nitrogen, body composition by bioelectric impedance, and reports of usual levels of physical activity. These measures made it possible to derive a minimally biased estimate of protein underreporting relative to energy underreporting. These studies demonstrated that protein is underreported but to a lesser extent than other parts of the diet and that this may be particularly true in obese subjects. The logical implication of this observation is that fat, carbohydrate, and/or alcohol must be disproportionately underreported. A similar finding was also made in the SOS study described above (Lissner, Lindroos, & Sjöström, 1998). The observation that certain parts of the diet are reported better than others is not surprising and is also consistent with direct observation of subjects in a laboratory setting. In one such study, where subjects underreported certain types of foods and beverages (e.g., snacks, alcohol) more than others, obese and nonobese subjects showed similar underreporting patterns (Poppitt et al., 1998). This underscores the idea noted previously (Muhlheim et al., 1998) that underreporting in free-living obese populations may exceed that occurring under controlled conditions when the subject is aware of being observed.

Observing Protein and Energy Nutrition: The OPEN Study

The final examples are from the OPEN study, which used two recovery biomarkers (doubly labeled water and PABA-validated urinary nitrogen) to document underreporting of energy and protein intake in a U.S. population, with two different dietary instruments: 24HR (Raper, Perloff, Ingwersen, Steinfeldt, & Anand, 2004) and a food frequency questionnaire (Subar et al., 2001). In the initial reports from OPEN, body mass index and a number of other psychosocial variables were examined as explanatory factors for underreporting (Subar et al., 2003; Tooze et al., 2004). Because BMI was confirmed to be the strongest determinant of underreporting, more detailed analyses followed the initial work, with a particular focus on obesity (Lissner et al., 2007). One methodological observation in OPEN was that both obese and nonobese groups reported lower mean intakes by FFQ than by a five-pass 24HR, although biomarker-based information indicated significant underreporting with both of the dietary instruments. The distributions of true energy intake and that reported by both dietary methods are shown in Figures 7.3 and 7.4, stratified according to whether or not subjects were obese. Interestingly, there seemed to be a gender difference in obesity-specific underreporting by the two instruments. Among women, the "true" energy requirement (from DLW) was 378 kcal greater in obese than in nonobese groups; the FFQ was able to detect a statistically significant portion of this "true" extra energy consumption, while the 24HR did not. Among men, the DLW-based energy requirement was 485 kcal greater in the obese group; however, neither FFQ nor 24HR detected a difference in energy consumption. Combining protein and energy estimates, obese men significantly overreported the proportion of energy from protein using the 24HR but not with the FFQ. At the individual level, correlations between energy expenditure and reported energy intake tended to be weaker in obese than

in nonobese groups, particularly with the 24HR. This work added to existing evidence that neither of these commonly used dietary reporting methods adequately measures energy or protein intake in obese groups. The 24HR, while capturing more realistic energy *distributions* for usual intake, appeared to be particularly problematic in the obese.

In summary, the OPEN study is unique in having examined two different dietary methods with attention to obesity-related biases detected by two biomarkers. Combining individual- and group-level information from this study, it appears that the method that best captured total energy intakes of the study population may be more biased with respect to obesity. For instance, although total underreporting was most pronounced with the FFQ, among women, this method was not associated with significant obesity-related energy underreporting. Using definitions from previous OPEN studies (Subar et al., 2003), the percentage of women who could be classified as "underreporters" on the FFQ was 46% in both obese and nonobese groups. The 24HR also yielded lower individual correlations between intakes and biomarkers in obese compared to nonobese men and women. These observations suggest certain advantages of the FFQ despite its generalized underestimation of total intake.

Analytical Issues Relevant in Obesity

Energy Adjustment: Does It Reduce Underreporting Bias?

It has been suggested that various procedures to adjust nutrient intake for total energy intake may reduce the problem of obesity-related underreporting. This suggestion assumes that underreporting of a given nutrient is proportional to underreporting of total energy, an assumption that can be challenged on the basis of much existing evidence on the selectivity of under- and overreporting different

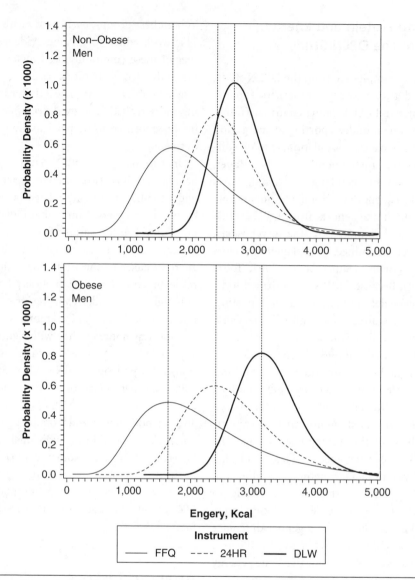

Figure 7.3 Smoothed Distributions of Usual Total Energy Intake in Obese and Nonobese Men, Estimated From the DLW Energy Expenditure and the Two Dietary Assessment Methods

NOTE: The mode of each distribution is indicated by a dotted line to facilitate comparison of instruments across subgroups. Adapted from Lissner et al. (2007).

parts of the diet. However, assuming that part of the obesity-related underreporting (e.g., portion sizes) occurs across the whole diet, it may be that energy adjustment corrects for part of the bias. In the OPEN study described above (Lissner et al., 2007), it was of interest to observe that protein per energy correlations (i.e., biomarker-based protein-energy percent vs. dietary protein-energy percent) were generally stronger than correlations based on absolute protein levels, suggesting that energy adjustment may correct somewhat for measurement error and may improve ranking of individuals with respect to protein. This was the case in obese as well as nonobese groups described

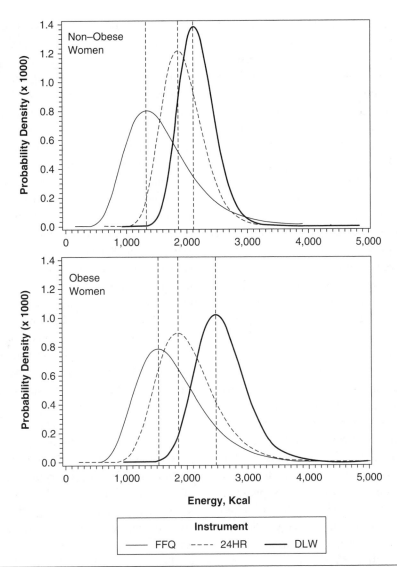

Figure 7.4   Smoothed Distributions of Usual Total Energy Intake in Obese and Nonobese Women, Estimated From the DLW Energy Expenditure and the Two Dietary Assessment Methods

NOTE: The mode of each distribution is indicated by a dotted line to facilitate comparison of instruments across subgroups. Adapted from Lissner et al. (2007).

there, providing some support for energy adjustment procedures when obesity is a main focus. Also, in the Whitehall study of socioeconomic status (SES) as a possible source of bias (Stallone, Brunner, Bingham, & Marmot, 1997), the energy adjustment method is identified as an approach that reduced bias without exclusion of low-energy reporters. The authors concluded that energy adjustment may be the preferred method for correcting for systematic underreporting. The authors speculate that false associations may be seen before such adjustment (i.e., higher SES associated with higher fat intake). This is in contrast to the widely accepted approach of excluding implausible energy reporters (Goldberg et al., 1991). There is always a danger, when excluding implausibly low values, that these represent some of the same individuals who are truly in the ranks of low consumers, albeit not as low as reported. Historically, the handling of outliers has been a subjective decision left to the investigator, with some standards recommended for handling outliers and influential points based on energy (Willett, 1998) or for each nutrient of interest (Thompson, Kipnis, et al., 2008). However, outliers may be particularly problematic with misreporting among obese and need careful consideration and testing.

A separate but related area involves the dietary energy density per se, or energy per volume consumed. Energy adjustment procedures (i.e., adjustment of dietary fat for total energy intake) may be accomplishing much more than adjusting for generalized dietary underreporting. Positive associations frequently reported between energy-adjusted dietary fat and obesity (Lissner & Heitmann, 1995) may also reflect to a large extent associations between high energy density and obesity. The idea that energy density is an underlying cause of overeating on a high-fat diet has been confirmed by a number of studies (Rolls et al., 1999, reviewed in Levitsky, 2001). It is important for future studies of diet in free-living populations to collect data on energy density in studies of dietary risk factors for obesity while also recognizing that energy adjustment can profoundly affect the associations with the nutrients being studied.

Portion Size Issues

Dietary methodologists have long debated the potential gain in accuracy to be expected from allowing subjects to choose their usual portion sizes for included items in a FFQ. Some investigators report improved performance of FFQs, compared with reference instruments, when respondents are asked to specify their portion size (Block et al., 1986; Cummings, Block, McHenry, & Baron, 1987). When this choice is not available, standard portion sizes are assumed,

often gender and/or age specific. The assumption of standard portion sizes is supported by work that showed a dominance of within-person (rather than between-person) variance in portion sizes, potentially making it difficult for subjects to specify their usual portion sizes (Hunter et al., 1988). The authors suggested that specification of a standard portion size may not introduce a large error in the estimation of food and nutrient intake. This assumption is likely to be questioned by obesity researchers who are interested in the etiologic role of portion size on the epidemic. For instance, Lindroos et al. (1993, 1997) found that variability in portion size of components of the plate model explained a significant portion of the surfeit in reported energy intake by obese women, suggesting that portion sizes picked up relevant information in addition to frequency of items consumed... Similarly, in an intervention among high-risk women (Eiben & Lissner, 2006), use of the same depicted portion sizes explained a significant part of the observed 1-year weight changes (not published). Finally, the InterGene Study (Berg et al., 2005) has used a single series of four portion sizes and asked subjects to make a generalized estimate of their usual portion size, for all meal components depicted on the plate (Figure 7.5). In this study, it was found that portion size was significantly larger in obese compared to nonobese subjects, although no obesity-related differences were observed for total energy calculated from the FFQ part of the questionnaire (Berg et al., 2009). These studies highlight the potential importance of documenting portion size in studies of obesity and obesity-related comorbidities.

Photographs have been tested against observed intake or plates of food in front of subjects and have suggested that sets of three and eight photographs of portions (Turconi et al., 2005; Nelson, Atkinson, & Darbyshire, 1994, respectively) are useful for respondents and may be superior to average portion size assumptions. In one study, use of photographs resulted in minimal bias related to BMI (Turconi et al., 2005). Although research on this methodology continues, it seems

26. How large portions do you eat?

Describe you own portion size relative to the pictures below. Choose the one that best matches your portions.

Like half of portion A.......... ☐

Like portion A.......... ☐

Right between portion A and B.......... ☐

Like portion B.......... ☐

Right between portion B and C.......... ☐

Like portion C.......... ☐

Right between portion C and D.......... ☐

Like portion D.......... ☐

Larger than portion D.......... ☐

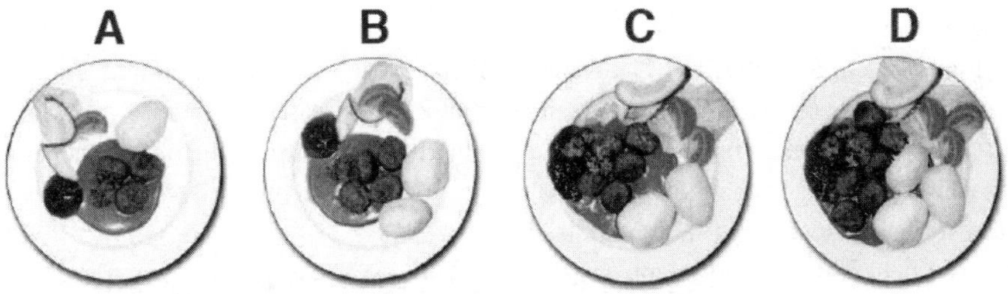

Figure 7.5 Photograph of Four Portion Size Pictures (A–D) Used in the InterGene Dietary Survey

reasonable to assume that photographs associated with food on standard plates may be easier for respondents than estimating intakes from words describing standard measures or units (e.g., one sandwich). Prior to conducting a large prospective study of diet and disease in Europe, investigators tested photographs for an FFQ and found some overestimation by those who consumed small portions and the reverse for those who consumed large portions (Faggiano et al., 1992). This flattened-slope phenomenon has been observed previously in many settings and now is being observed when photographs are used as portion size aids (Faggiano et al., 1992; Nelson & Atkinson, 1996). Nonetheless, there may be less bias with photographs than with other portion size methods (Nelson, Atkinson, & Darbyshire, 1996), and therefore using photographs as a cognitive recall aid may prove to be useful in future studies.

Analysis of Foods and Eating Patterns

An alternative approach to characterizing diet by calculating nutrient intakes, eating patterns (also referred to as food or dietary patterns) are often defined by grouping foods and nutrients according to some criteria of nutritional health (Newby & Tucker, 2004). A typical example is a healthy index score developed on a priori assumptions of diet quality. For example, a refined version of the Healthy Eating Index, based on compliance to the Dietary Guidelines for Americans, was shown to be highly predictive of chronic disease, particularly cardiovascular disease, in two U.S. cohorts (McCullough & Willett, 2006). Alternatively, empirically defined eating patterns can be derived statistically and evaluated a posteriori. Factor and cluster analyses are the most commonly used approaches. Both a priori and a posteriori food pattern definitions have been used to test obesity-related dietary characteristics. It has been hypothesized that data derived from food patterns analyses may be less vulnerable to obesity-related biases than estimates of nutrient intake. A systematic review of the literature by Togo and coworkers (2001) indeed found that obese study populations have demonstrably different patterns of intake compared to normal-weight populations, particularly when assessed via healthy eating indices, but not consistently so. A follow-up of this review, using prospective research design, tested the predictive value of food patterns identified by factor analysis, in relation to subsequent weight gain, and did not succeed in identifying high-risk dietary patterns (Togo, Osler, Sørensen, & Heitmann, 2004). In contrast, a recent paper by Newby and coworkers (2006) found that a change in food pattern was predictive of weight change, particularly in the obese. It may be speculated that analysis of food patterns often fails to identify obesogenic dietary traits because data collected are susceptible to the same reporting biases that are apparent with conventional nutrient analysis. However, examination of food-based patterns may give results that are relevant to types of foods chosen and in the best case may be amenable to food-based recommendations to prevent weight gain.

Other Special Populations

Biases in Case-Control Studies

Within observational epidemiology, study design plays an obvious and influential role in the validity of dietary data. Case series within case-control studies provide a well-recognized example of special circumstances that may bias conclusions about dietary risk factors. In particular, the case-control design, based on comparing exposure rates in defined case groups compared to controls without that disease, may be subject to a variety of differential errors related to the fact that the cases are aware that they have a medical condition while controls are not. As illustrated by Giovannucci and coworkers (1993a, 1993b), there is evidence that alcohol, total fat intake, and saturated fat intake may be differentially recalled in individuals before and after their diagnoses, in this case, of breast cancer. This bias has not always been observed, however (Friedenreich, Howe, & Miller, 1991; Holmberg et al., 1996). Psychological reasons for bias among cases have been speculated to range from finding an explanation for one's disease to denial of a potentially causal factor. While these findings may not constitute sufficient evidence to discontinue the case-control design in nutritional epidemiology, they serve to reinforce the importance of design and recall factors when studying populations with a wide variety of health problems beyond obesity. It should be remembered that many diseases are themselves associated with obesity, which may further compound dietary reporting errors in a case-control study.

Children and Adolescents

Methods for assessing diet in children, either directly or by parental proxy, are covered in depth in Kral et al. (2008). In brief, the average age at which children develop the cognitive skills relevant to self-reporting of diet intake differs cross-culturally and between individuals, and the minimum age at which children gain the ability to conceptualize the time frames used in dietary instruments (i.e., 24 hours, 1 week, 1 month) is not well established. The ability of children younger than 10 years to give valid responses to food frequency questionnaires covering periods greater than 1 day is questionable because of their inability to conceptualize frequency and averaging. The need for adult assistance in dietary reporting is also driven by the limited scope of the child's experience and knowledge of food preparation and detail (e.g., fat content of milk). It is generally recognized that adults reporting their young children's intakes are also likely to be affected by social desirability biases reflecting the desire to report that their children consume healthy diets (USDA, 2005).

Adolescents, on the other hand, are frequently asked to report their own diets. Some of the challenges of assessing diet in adolescents include rapidly changing eating habits due to growth, unstructured eating of many snacks and skipping meals, eating away from home much of the time, and the high prevalence of restrained eating, particularly among girls. In addition, similar to adults, overweight and obesity in adolescents may lead to underreporting of intake; up to 40% of energy may not be reported in obese adolescents (Bandini, Schoeller, Cyr, & Dietz, 1990). Energy underreporting also increases with age across adolescence, as evidenced with DLW studies by Livingstone and Robson (2000). Obesity-related underreporting by food record (also compared to DLW) has been documented in Swedish children (Bratteby, Sandhagen, Fan, Enghardt, & Samuelson, 1998).

FFQs have been developed for adolescents (Rockett et al., 1997) and in the near future, electronic and Web-based tools will have increasing appeal within this age group. Research in school settings has many advantages and has been administered successfully in HELENA (Vereecken et al., 2005, 2008). There are difficulties, however, including increasing time pressures on school curriculum, limited time for recruitment, and adequate explanation of study forms and procedures. Alternative approaches and settings that appeal to young people are needed (Coufopoulos, Maggs, & Hackett, 2001; Frank, 1994). It is unclear which methods may avoid or minimize some of the biased reporting related to overweight and restrained eating that are known to exist in this age group.

International Studies: Is Underreporting Universal?

While numerous population studies have documented general and obesity-related reporting errors, it has been pointed out by Harrison et al. (2000) that a relative dearth of data on this problem exists from developing countries and those in economic transition. To address this issue, a dietary survey was conducted among Egyptian women in 1993–1994, using the 24HR method, which in fact revealed a much lesser degree of underreporting than that typically observed among U.S. and European surveys (Harrison, et al., 2000). Only 10% of Egyptian women reported implausibly low intakes, compared to one third of American women surveyed in the 1994–1996 Continuing Survey of Food Intakes of Individuals. However, significant obesity-related underreporting was observed, even in the Egyptian sample. Other work, in Indonesian women measured across pregnancies, found somewhat higher levels of underreporting (16%–18% after first trimester), and this study was able to confirm that both obesity and low education were factors associated with underreporting, similar to findings in other regions (Winkvist, Persson, & Hartini, 2002). A final example, from Jamaica (Mendez, Wynter, Wilks, & Forrester, 2004), indicated relatively more underreporting of energy in women than in men and more overreporting in younger adults, along with the usual obesity-related bias. Moreover, they confirmed reports of a more socially desirable diet in low energy reporters and illustrated that inclusion of implausible reporters may yield less credible associations.

Populations Studied During Pregnancy

Assessment of dietary intake in pregnant women is a special challenge in nutritional epidemiology due to numerous potential reporting biases, many of which are common to both pregnant and nonpregnant populations. As mentioned previously, obesity-related underreporting has been documented in pregnant women. Other likely sources of error that may affect validity of dietary data in pregnancy include changes related to nausea (e.g., low intakes, vomiting, and rapid changes in diet related to heartburn) constipation, cravings, and specific food cultures. In addition, it must be acknowledged that pregnant women may be particularly susceptible to the bias of reporting a good diet, given the recognized health implications of poor nutrition on the developing fetus. In view of the emphasis on healthy eating and recommended weight gain across the pregnancy, as well as monitoring these factors in the clinical setting, there is great potential for misreporting of intakes. Obese women may be more sensitive to these lifestyle recommendations, especially if low weight gains have been recommended. It is considered important to specifically validate existing methodologies if they are to be used in a population of pregnant women and, if these are not acceptable, to develop new methods. Examples of validated methodologies include those specially developed for the Danish National Birth Cohort (Olsen, Melbye, Olsen, Sørensen, & Aaby, 2001; http://www.ssi.dk/sw9314.asp) and the Norwegian Mother and Child Study (Brantsaeter et al., 2007). Since both of these studies are large (~100,000 each), an FFQ approach was chosen. These methods provide information on usual diet, and additional questions can be added to identify specific aspects of diet (e.g., omega-3 fatty acid intake) (Mikkelsen, Osler, & Olsen, 2006) or dietary change that may be of interest. Another example, the Avon Longitudinal Study of Pregnancy and Childhood (ALSPAC), included 12,000 women who completed an FFQ with 43 food group items as well as detailed questions on type and amount of fat, alcohol, bread, and milk consumption (Rogers & Emmett, 1998). Finally, it should be kept in mind that validation by biomarkers may be problematic in pregnant women due to the variability in plasma volume expansion (Faupel-Badger, Hsieh, Troisi, Lagiou, & Potischman, 2007). Not only is it important to obtain blood specimens at the same gestational age, but also the variability in plasma volume expansion across women of differing body sizes and ethnicities should be considered.

Populations Undergoing an Intervention

Just as knowledge of being observed is likely to change dietary behavior in obese and other weight-conscious population groups, such biases are also likely to occur in association with any experimental manipulation or quasi-experimental intervention. This type of bias may be relevant in interpreting dietary information collected by health trials in free-living populations. For instance, the Women's Health Initiative documented decreases in reported dietary fat intake in the intervention group that exceeded changes reported by the control group. It was encouraging to note that changes in fat intake significantly predicted simultaneous weight changes in both groups, consistent with an etiologic role of a high-fat diet in development of overweight (Howard, Manson, et al., 2006). However, no corresponding differences in cardiovascular or cancer outcomes were observed between the intervention and control groups (Howard, Van Horn, et al., 2006; R. L. Prentice et al., 2006), and one explanation for this is that the intervention group may have been "talking a good diet" more so than the control group. Preliminary evidence from a DLW validation substudy within this trial is consistent with such an interpretation (Neuhouser et al., 2008).

Conclusions on Measuring Intakes in Obese Populations

While a general underreporting bias exists in free-living populations reporting their diets, regardless of weight status, all evidence points to this problem being magnified in the obese. Data from affluent and transitional countries suggest that this tendency may be universal, at least in regions of relative nutritional adequacy. However, existing data suggest that it is possible to obtain valid intake data on sufficiently motivated obese subjects, that underreporting occurs disproportionately for different fractions of the diet, and that the choice between diet recall versus frequency-based methods is not obvious since the former method may capture more realistic intakes while the latter may be less biased with respect to obesity. Obesity-related underreporting biases have been reported for most of the commonly used dietary assessment instruments, but relatively little focus has been placed on how to solve this problem.

A major concern surrounding obesity-related reporting bias is its potential impact on epidemiologic studies evaluating diet and disease outcomes. Differentially greater underreporting with higher BMI could attenuate relative risk estimates for dietary factors that are truly associated with the outcome, although the reverse may also occur (Heitmann & Lissner, 2005; Lissner, Heitmann, & Lindroos, 1998; Lissner, Lindroos, & Sjöström, 1998). Procedures have been employed to correct for effects of reporting errors in FFQs (Rosner, Willett, & Spiegelman, 1989). However, there is evidence that similar BMI-related underreporting and other systematic and person-specific biases occur with calibration instruments, such as 24HRs, thereby diminishing the effectiveness of this correction method (Kipnis et al., 2003; Subar et al., 2003).

Available results from OPEN and other studies involving reporting error have implications for the design of future studies in nutritional epidemiology. In OPEN, the higher performance of the five-pass 24HRs method in capturing mean intakes, relative to FFQ, must be weighed against the observation that the FFQ performed better or at least as well in a number of obesity-related comparisons. In this context, a possible future strategy could be to develop methodologies that combine the recall, checklist and FFQ methodologies. Moreover, continued efforts to develop our knowledge of the role of dietary patterns in obesity are likely to be important since this type of analysis may capture aspects of the obesogenic diet that are not obtained in traditional nutrient analyses. Finally, continued work on psychological and behavioral characteristics associated with underreporting is needed to move forward in developing dietary methodologies suitable for contemporary populations. Given the known importance of obesity vis-à-vis a number of chronic disease endpoints, it is critical to develop instruments that can rank and

differentiate obese and nonobese individuals with respect to dietary intakes.

References

Anderson, A. S., Maher, L., Ha, T. K., Cooney, J., Eley, S., Martin, M., et al. (1999). Evaluation of a barcode system for nutrient analysis in dietary surveys. *Public Health Nutrition, 2,* 579–586.

Asbeck, I., Mast, M., Beirwag, A., Westenhofer, J., Acheson, K. J., & Muller, M. J. (2002). Severe underreporting of energy intake in normal weight subjects: Use of an appropriate standard and relation to restrained eating. *Public Health Nutrition, 5,* 683–690.

Ballard-Barbash, R., Graubard, I., Krebs-Smith, S. M., Schatzkin, A., & Thompson, F. E. (1996). Contribution of dieting to the inverse association between energy intake and body mass index. *European Journal of Clinical Nutrition, 50,* 98–106.

Bandini, L. G., Schoeller, D. A., Cyr, H. N., & Dietz, W. H. (1990). Validity of reported energy intake in obese and nonobese adolescents. *American Journal of Clinical Nutrition, 52,* 421–425.

Beasley, J., Riley, W. T., & Jean-Mary, J. (2005). Accuracy of a PDA-based dietary assessment program. *Nutrition, 21,* 672–677.

Berg, C., Lappas, G., Wolk, A., Strandhagen, E., Toren, K., Rosengren, A., et al. (2009). Eating patterns and portion size associated with obesity in a Swedish population. *Appetite, 52,* 21–26.

Berg, C., Rosengren, A., Aires, N., Lappas, G., Toren, K., Thelle, D., et al. (2005). Trends in overweight and obesity from 1985–2002 in Göteborg, West Sweden. *International Journal of Obesity, 29,* 916–924.

Bertéus Forslund, H., Lindroos, A. K., Sjöström, L., & Lissner, L. (2002). Meal patterns and obesity in Swedish women: A simple instrument describing usual meal types, frequency and temporal distribution. *European Journal of Clinical Nutrition, 56,* 740–747.

Bingham, S., Luben, R., Welch, A., Wareham, N., Khaw, K.-T., & Day, N. (2003). Are imprecise methods obscuring a relation between fat and breast cancer? *Lancet, 362,* 212–214.

Black, A. E., Coward, W. A., Cole, T. J., & Prentice, A. M. (1996). Human expenditure in affluent societies: An analysis of 574 doubly-labeled water measurements. *European Journal of Clinical Nutrition, 50,* 70–92.

Block, G., Hartman, A. M., Dresser, C. M., Carroll, M. D., Gannon, J., & Gardner, L. (1986). A data-based approach to diet questionnaire design and testing. *American Journal of Epidemiology, 124,* 453–469.

Block, G., Hartman, A. M., & Naughton, D. (1990). A reduced dietary questionnaire: Development and validation. *Epidemiology, 1,* 58–64.

Boutelle, K. N., & Kirshenbaum, D. S. (1998). Further support for consistent self-monitoring as a vital component of successful weight control. *Obesity Research, 5,* 219–224.

Brantsaeter, A. L., Haugen, M., Rasmussen, S. E., Alexander, J., Samuelsen, S. O., & Meltzer, H. M. (2007). Urine flavonoids and plasma carotenoids in the validation of fruit, vegetable and tea intake during pregnancy in the Norwegian Mother and Child Cohort Study (MoBa). *Public Health Nutrition, 10,* 838–847.

Bratteby, L. E., Sandhagen, B., Fan, H., Enghardt, H., & Samuelson, G. (1998). Total energy expenditure and physical activity as assessed by the doubly labeled water method in Swedish adolescents in whom energy intake was underestimated by 7-d diet records. *American Journal of Clinical Nutrition, 67,* 905–911.

Bryant, M., Ward, D., & Stevens, J. (2006). Feasibility of measuring food availability in the home using handheld scanners. *FASEB Journal,* abstract 379.3.

Cantwell, M. M., Millen, A. E., Carroll, R., Mittl, B. L., Hermansen, S., Brinton, L. A., et al. (2006). Assessment of dietary intake: Does a debriefing session with a nutritionist improve dietary assessment using food diaries? *Journal of Nutrition, 136,* 440–445.

Carriquiry, A.L. (2003). Estimation of usual intake distributions of nutrients and foods. *Journal of Nutrition, 133,* 601S–608S.

Coufopoulos, A. M., Maggs, C., & Hackett, A. (2001). Doing dietary research with adolescents: The problems of data collection in the school setting. *International Journal of Health Promotion and Education, 39,* 100–105.

Cummings, S. R., Block, G., McHenry, K., & Baron, R. B. (1987). Evaluation of two food frequency methods of measuring dietary calcium intake. *American Journal of Epidemiology, 126,* 796–802.

Dennis, B., Ernst, N., Hjortland, M., Tillotson, J., & Grambsch, V. (1980). The NHLBI nutrition data system. *Journal of the American Dietetic Association, 77,* 641–647.

Dodd, K. W., Guenther, P. M., Freedman, L. S., Subar, A. F., Kipnis, V., Midthune, D., et al. (2006). Statistical methods for estimating usual intake of nutrients and foods: A review of the theory. *Journal of the American Dietetic Association, 106,* 1640–1650.

Eiben, G., Andersson, C. S., Rothenberg, E., Sundh, V., Steen, B., & Lissner, L. (2004). Secular trends in diet among elderly Swedes: Cohort comparisons over three decades. *Public Health Nutrition, 7,* 637–644.

Eiben, G., & Lissner, L. (2006). Health Hunters: An intervention to prevent overweight and obesity in young high-risk women. *International Journal of Obesity (London), 30,* 691–696.

Faggiano, F., Vineis, P., Cravanzola, D., Pisani, P., Xompero, G., Riboli, E., et al. (1992). Validation of a method for the estimation of food portion size. *Epidemiology, 3,* 379–382.

Faupel-Badger, J. M., Hsieh, C.-C., Troisi, R., Lagiou, P., & Potischman, N. (2007). Plasma volume expansion in pregnancy: Implications for biomarkers in population studies. *Cancer Epidemiology Biomarkers & Prevention, 16,* 1720–1723.

Ferrari, P., Slimani, N., Ciampi, A., Trichopoulou, A., Naska, A., et al. (2002). Evaluation of under- and overreporting of energy intake in the 24-hour diet recalls in the European Prospective Investigation into Cancer and Nutrition (EPIC). *Public Health Nutrition, 5,* 1329–1345.

Frank, G. C. (1994). Environmental influences on methods used to collect dietary data from children. *American Journal of Clinical Nutrition, 59,* 207S–211S.

Frank, G. C., Berenson, G. S., Schilling, P. E., & Moore, M. C. (1977). Adapting the 24-hr. recall for epidemiologic studies of school children. *Journal of the American Dietetic Association, 71,* 26–31.

Freedman, L. S., Midthune, D., Carrol, R. J., Krebs-Smith, S., Subar, A. F., Troiano, R. P., et al. (2004). Adjustments to improve the estimation of usual dietary intake distributions in the population. *Journal of Nutrition, 134,* 1836–1843.

Freedman, L. S., Potischman, N., Kipnis, V., Midthune, D., Schatzkin, A., Thompson, F. E., et al. (2006). A comparison of two dietary instruments for evaluating the fat-breast cancer relationship. *International Journal of Epidemiology, 35,* 1011–1021.

Friedenreich, C. M., Howe, G. R., & Miller, A. B. (1991). An investigation of recall bias in the reporting of past food intake among breast cancer cases and controls. *Annals of Epidemiology, 1,* 439–453.

Gibson, R. S. (2005). *Principles of nutritional assessment* (2nd ed.). New York: Oxford University Press.

Giovannucci, E., Stampfer, M. J., Colditz, G. A., Manson, J. E., Rosner, B. A., Longnecker, M. P., et al. (1993a). Recall and selection bias in reporting past alcohol consumption among breast cancer cases. *Cancer Causes & Control, 4,* 441–448.

Giovannucci, E., Stampfer, M. J., Colditz, G. A., Manson, J. E., Rosner, B. A., Longnecker, M., et al. (1993b). A comparison of prospective and retrospective assessments of diet in the study of breast cancer. *American Journal of Epidemiology, 137,* 502–511.

Glanz, K., & Murphy, S. (2007). Dietary assessment and monitoring in real time. In A. A. Stone, S. Schiffman, A. A. Atienza, & L. Nebeling (Eds.), *The science of real-time data capture: Self-reports in health research* (pp. 151–168). New York: Oxford University Press.

Glanz, K., Murphy, S., Moylan, J., Evensen, D., & Curb, J. D. (2006). Improving dietary self-monitoring and adherence with hand-held computers: A pilot study. *American Journal of Health Promotion, 20,* 165–170.

Goldberg, G. R., Black, A. E., Jebb, S. A., Cole, T. J., Murgatroyd, P. R., Coward, W. A., et al. (1991). Critical evaluation of energy intake data using fundamental principles of energy physiology: 1. Derivation of cut-off limits to identify under-recording. *European Journal of Clinical Nutrition, 45,* 569–581.

Goris, A. H. C., Westerterp-Plantenga, M. S., & Westerterp, K. R. (2000). Undereating and under-recording of habitual food intake in obese men: Selective underreporting of fat intake. *American Journal of Clinical Nutrition, 71,* 130–134.

Gross, L. S., Li, L., Ford, E. S., & Liu, S. (2004). Increased consumption of refined carbohydrates and the epidemic of type 2 diabetes in the United States: An ecologic assessment. *American Journal of Clinical Nutrition, 79,* 774–779.

Guenther, P. M., DeMaio, T. J., Ingwersen, L. A., & Berlin, M. (1996). The multiple-pass approach for the 24-h recall in the continuing survey of food intakes by individuals, 1994–96. *FASEB Journal, 10,* a198.

Harrison, G. G., Galal, O. M., Ibrahim, N., Khorshid, A., Stormer, A., Leslie, J., et al. (2000).

Underreporting of food intake by dietary recall is not universal: A comparison of data from Egyptian and American women. *Journal of Nutrition, 130,* 2049–2054.

Hartman, A. M., Brown, C. C., Palmgren, J., Pietinen, P., Verkasalo, M., Myer, D., et al. (1990). Variability in nutrient and food intakes among older middle-aged men: Implications for design of epidemiologic and validation studies using food recording. *American Journal of Epidemiology, 132,* 999–1012.

Hebert, J., Clemow, L., Pbert, L., Ockene, I. S., & Ockene, J. K. (1995). Social desirability bias in dietary self-report may compromise the validity of dietary intake measures. *International Journal of Epidemiology, 24,* 389–398.

Heini, A. F., & Weinsier, R. L. (1997). Divergent trends in obesity and fat intake patterns: The American paradox. *American Journal of Medicine, 102,* 259–264.

Heitmann, B., & Lissner, L. (1995). Dietary underreporting by obese individuals: Is it specific or nonspecific? *British Medical Journal, 311,* 986–989.

Heitmann, B. L., & Lissner, L. (2005). Can adverse effects of dietary fat intake be overestimated as a consequence of dietary fat underreporting. *Public Health Nutrition, 8,* 1332–1337.

Heitmann, B. L., Lissner, L., & Osler, M. (2000). Do we eat less fat, or just report so? *International Journal of Obesity and Related Metabolic Disorders, 24,* 435–442.

Hise, M. E., Sullivan, D. K., Jacobsen, D. J., Johnson, S. L., & Donnelly, J. E. (2002). Validation of energy intake measurements determined from observer-recorded food records and recall methods compared with doubly labeled water method in overweight and obese individuals. *American Journal of Clinical Nutrition, 75,* 263–267.

Holmberg, L., Ohlander, E. M., Byers, T., Zack, M., Wolk, A., Bruce, A., et al. (1996). A search for recall bias in a case-control study of diet and breast cancer. *International Journal of Epidemiology, 25,* 235–244.

Howard, B. V., Manson, J. E., Stefanick, M. L., Beresford, S. A., Frank, G., Jones, B., et al. (2006). Low-fat dietary pattern and weight change over 7 years: The Women's Health Initiative Dietary Modification Trial. *Journal of the American Medical Association, 295,* 39–49.

Howard, B. V., Van Horn, L., Hsia, J., Manson, J. E., Stefanick, M. L., Wassertheil-Smoller, S., et al. (2006). Low-fat dietary pattern and risk of cardiovascular disease: The Women's Health

Initiative Randomized Controlled Dietary Modification Trial. *Journal of the American Medical Association, 295,* 655–666.

Høyer, G., Nilssen, O., Brenn, T., & Schirmer, H. (1995). The Svalbard study 1988–89: A unique setting for validation of self-reported alcohol consumption. *Addiction, 90,* 539–544.

Hultén, B., Bengtsson, C., & Isaksson, B. (1990). Some errors in a longitudinal dietary survey revealed by the urine nitrogen test. *European Journal of Clinical Nutrition, 44,* 169–174.

Hunter, D. J., Sampson, L., Stampfer, M. J., Colditz, G. A., Rosner, B., & Willett, W. C. (1988). Variability in portion sizes of commonly consumed foods among a population of women in the United States. *American Journal of Epidemiology, 127,* 1240–1249.

Johansson, G., Bingham, S., & Wahter, M. (1999). A method to compensate for incomplete 24 h urine collections in nutritional epidemiology studies. *Public Health Nutrition, 2,* 587–591.

Johansson, G., Wikman, A., Ahrén, A. M., Hallmans, G., & Johansson, I. (2001). Underreporting of energy intake in repeated 24-hour recalls related to gender, age, weight status, day of interview, educational level, reported food intake, smoking habits and area of living. *Public Health Nutrition, 4,* 919–927.

Kaaks, R., Ferrari, P., Ciampi, A., Plummer, M., & Riboli, E. (2002). Uses and limitations of statistical accounting for random error correlations in the validity of dietary questionnaire assessments. *Public Health Nutrition, 5,* 969–976.

Kipnis, V., Subar, A. F., Midthune, D., Freedman, L. S., Ballard-Barbash, R., Troiano, R. P., et al. (2003). Structure of dietary measurement error: Results of the OPEN Biomarker Study. *American Journal of Epidemiology, 158,* 14–21.

Kohlmeier, L. (1994). Gaps in dietary assessment methodology: Meal vs list-based methods. *American Journal of Clinical Nutrition, 59,* 175s–179s.

Kohlmeier, L., Mendez, M., McDuffie, J., & Miller, M. (1997). Computer-assisted self-interviewing: a multimedia approach to dietary assessment. *American Journal of Clinical Nutrition, 65,* 1275S–1278S.

Kolar, A. S., Patterson, R. E., White, E., Neuhouser, M. L., Frank, L. L., Standley, J., et al. (2005). A practical method for collecting 3-day food records in a large cohort. *Epidemiology, 16,* 579–583.

Lafay, L., Basdevant, A., Charles, M. A., Vray, M., Balkau, B., Borys, J. M., et al. (1997). Determinants and nature of dietary underreporting in a free-living population: The Fleurbaix Laventie Ville Sante (FLVS) Study. *International Journal of Obesity and Related Metabolic Disorders, 21,* 567–573.

Lambert, N., Plumb, J., Looise, B., Johnson, I. T., Harvey, I., Wheeler, C., et al. (2005). Using smart card technology to monitor the eating habits of children in a school cafeteria: 1. Developing and validating the methodology. *Journal of Human Nutrition and Dietetics, 18,* 243–254.

Levitsky, L. (2001). Macronutrient intake and the control of body weight. In A. M. Coulson, C. L. Rock, & E. R. Monsen (EDs.), *Nutrition in the prevention and treatment of disease* (pp. 499–516). New York: Academic Press.

Lindroos, A. K., Lissner, L., Mathiassen, M. E., Karlsson, J., Sullivan, M., Bengtsson, C., et al. (1997). Dietary intake in relation to restrained eating, disinhibition, and hunger in obese and nonobese Swedish women. *Obesity Research, 5*(3), 175–182.

Lindroos, A. K., Lissner, L., & Sjöström L. (1993). Validity and reproducibility of a self-administered dietary questionnaire in obese and non-obese subjects. *European Journal of Clinical Nutrition, 47,* 461–481.

Lindroos, A. K., Lissner, L., & Sjöström, L. (1999). Does degree of obesity influence the validity of reported energy and protein intake? Results from the SOS Dietary Questionnaire. Swedish Obese Subjects. *European Journal of Clinical Nutrition, 53,* 375–378.

Lissner, L., & Heitmann, B. (1995). Dietary fat and obesity: Evidence from epidemiology. *European Journal of Clinical Nutrition, 49*(2), 79–90

Lissner, L., Heitmann, B., & Lindroos, A. K. (1998). Measuring intake in free-living humans: A question of bias. *Proceedings of the Nutrition Society, 57,* 333–339.

Lissner, L., Lindroos, A. K., & Sjöström, L. (1998). Swedish Obese Subjects (SOS): An obesity intervention study with a nutritional perspective. *European Journal of Clinical Nutrition, 52,* 316–322.

Lissner, L., Troiano, R. P., Midthune, D., Heitmann, B. L., Kipnis, V., Subar, A. F., et al. (2007). OPEN about obesity: Recovery biomarkers, dietary reporting errors and BMI. *International Journal of Obesity (London), 31,* 956–961.

Liu, K., Slattery, M., Jacobs, D. R., Jr., Cutter, G., McDonald, A., Van Horn, L., et al. (1994). A study of the reliability and comparative validity of the CARDIA dietary history. *Ethnicity & Disease, 4,* 15–27.

Livingstone, M. B., & Robson, P. J. (2000). Measurement of dietary intake in children. *Proceedings of the Nutrition Society, 59,* 279–293.

Martin, G. S., Tapsell, L. C., Batterham, M. J., & Russell, K. G. (2002). Relative bias in diet history measurements: A quality control technique for dietary intervention trials. *Public Health Nutrition, 5,* 537–545.

Martin, G. S., Tapsell, L. C., Denmeade, S., & Batterham, M. J. (2003). Relative validity of a diet history interview in an intervention trial manipulating dietary fat in the management of Type II diabetes mellitus. *Preventive Medicine, 36,* 420–428.

Maurer, J., Taren, D. L., Teixeira, P. J., Thomson, C. A., Lohman, T. G., Going, S. B., et al. (2006). The psychosocial and behavioral characteristics related to energy misreporting. *Nutrition Review, 64,* 53–66.

McCullough, M. L., & Willett, W. C. (2006). Evaluating adherence to recommended diets in adults: The Alternate Healthy Eating Index. *Public Health Nutrition, 9,* 152–157.

Mendez, M. A., Wynter, S., Wilks, R., & Forrester, T. (2004). Under- and overreporting of energy is related to obesity, lifestyle factors and food group intakes in Jamaican adults. *Public Health Nutrition, 7,* 9–19.

Mikkelsen, T. B., Osler, M., & Olsen, S. F. (2006). Validity of protein, retinol, folic acid and n-3 fatty acid intakes estimated from the food-frequency questionnaire used in the Danish National Birth Cohort. *Public Health Nutrition, 9,* 771–778.

Moshfegh, A. M., Borrud, L. G., Perloff, P., & LaComb, R. (1999). Improved method for the 24-hour dietary recall for use in national surveys. *FASEB Journal, 13,* A603.

Muhlheim, L. S., Allison, D. R., Heshka, S., & Heymsfield, S. B. (1998). Do unsuccessful dieters intentionally underreport food intake? *International Journal of Eating Disorders, 24,* 259–266.

Nelson, M., Atkinson, M., & Darbyshire, S. (1994). Food photography. I: The perception of food portion size from photographs. *British Journal of Nutrition, 72,* 649–663.

Nelson, M., Atkinson, M., & Darbyshire, S. (1996). Food photography II: Use of food photographs for estimating portion size and the nutrient content of meals. *British Journal of Nutrition, 76,* 31–49.

Neuhouser, M., Tinker, L., Shaw, P. A., Schoeller, D., Bingham, S. A., Horn, L. V., et al. (2008). Use of recovery biomarkers to calibrate nutrient consumption self-reports in the Women's Health Initiative. *American Journal of Epidemiology, 167,* 1247–1259.

Newby, P. K., & Tucker, K. L. (2004). Empirically derived eating patterns using factor or cluster analysis: A review. *Nutrition Review, 62,* 177–203.

Newby, P. K., Weismayer, C., Akesson, A., Tucker, K. L., & Wolk, A. (2006). Longitudinal changes in food patterns predict changes in weight and body mass index and the effects are greatest in obese women. *Journal of Nutrition, 136,* 2580–2587.

Olsen, J., Melbye, M., Olsen, S. F., Sørensen, T. I., & Aaby, P. (2001). The Danish National Birth Cohort: Its background, structure and aim. *Scandinavian Journal of Public Health, 29,* 300–307.

Poppitt, S., Swann, D., Black, A. E., & Prentice A. M. (1998). Assessment of selective under-reporting of food intake by both obese and non-obese women in a metabolic facility. *International Journal of Obesity, 22,* 303–311.

Potischman, N. (1993). Biological and methodologic issues for Nutritional Biomarkers. *J. Nutr, 133,* 875S–880S.

Potischman, N., Carroll, R. J., Iturria, S. J., Mittl, S., Curtin, J., Thompson, F. E., et al. (1999). Comparison of the 60- and 100-item NCI-Block questionnaires with validation data. *Nutrition and Cancer, 34,* 70–75.

Potischman, N., & Freudenheim, J. (2003). Biomarkers of nutritional exposure and nutritional status: An overview. *Journal of Nutrition, 133,* 873S–874S.

Prentice, A. M., Black, A. E., Coward, W. A., Davies, H. L., Goldberg, G. R., Murgatroyd, P. R., et al. (1986). High levels of energy expenditure in obese women. *British Medical Journal, 292,* 983–987.

Prentice, R. L., Caan, B., Chlebowski, R. T., Patterson, R., Kuller, L. H., Ockene, J. K., et al (2006). Low-fat dietary pattern and risk of invasive breast cancer: The Women's Health Initiative Randomized Controlled Dietary Modification Trial. *Journal of the American Medical Association, 295,* 629–642.

Raper, N., Perloff, B., Ingwersen, L., Steinfeldt, L., Anand, J., et al. (2004). An overview of USDA's dietary intake data system. *Journal of Food Composition and Analysis, 17,* 545–555.

Rockett, H. R., Breitenbach, M., Frazier, A. L., Witschi, J., Wolf, A. M., Field, A. E., et al. (1997). Validation of a youth/adolescent food frequency question-naire. *Preventive Medicine, 26,* 808–816.

Rogers, I., & Emmett, P. (1998). Diet during pregnancy in a population of pregnant women in South West England. ALSPAC Study Team. Avon Longitudinal Study of Pregnancy and Childhood. *European Journal of Clinical Nutrition, 52,* 246–250.

Rolls, B. J., Bell, E. A., Castellanos, V., Chow, M., Peklman, C. L., & Thorwart, M. L. (1999). Energy density but not fat content of foods affected energy intake in lean and obese women. *American Journal of Clinical Nutrition, 69,* 863–871.

Rosner, B., Willett, W. C., & Spiegelman, D. (1989). Correction of logistic regression relative risk esti-mates and confidence intervals for systematic within-person measurement error. *Statistics in Medicine, 8,* 1051–1069.

Roth, D. L., Snyder, C. R., & Pace, L. M. (1986). Dimensions of favourable self-presentation. *Journal of Personality and Social Psychology, 51,* 867–874.

Rothenberg, E., Bosaeus, I., Lernfelt, B., Landahl, S., & Steen, B. (1998). Energy intake and expenditure: Validation of a diet history by heart rate monitor-ing, activity diary and doubly labeled water. *European Journal of Clinical Nutrition, 52,* 832–838.

Schatzkin, A., Kipnis, V., Carroll, R. J., Midthune, D., Subar, A. F., Bingham, S., et al. (2003). A comparison of a food frequency questionnaire with a 24-hour recall for use in an epidemiological cohort study: Results from the biomarker-based Observing Protein and Energy Nutrition (OPEN) study. *International Journal of Epidemiology, 32,* 1054–1062.

Schoeller, D. A. (1999). Recent advances from applica-tion of doubly labeled water to measurement of human energy expenditure. *Journal of Nutrition, 129,* 1765–1768.

Slimani, N., Kaaks, R., Ferreari, P., Casagrande, C., Clavel-Chapelon, F., Lotze, G., et al. (2002). European Prospective Investigation into Cancer and Nutrition (EPIC) calibration study: Rationale, design and population characteristics. *Public Health Nutrition, 5,* 1125–1145.

Stallone, D. D., Brunner, E. J., Bingham, S. A., & Marmot, M. G. (1997). Dietary assessment in Whitehall II: The influence of reporting bias on apparent socioeconomic variation in nutrient intakes. *European Journal of Clinical Nutrition, 51,* 815–825.

Streit, K. J., Stevens, N. H., Stevens, V. J., & Rossner, J. (1991). Food records: A predictor and modifier of weight change in a long-term weight loss program. *Journal of the American Dietetic Association, 91,* 213–216.

Subar, A. F., Dodd, K. W., Guenther, P. M., Kipnis, V., Midthune, D., McDowell, M., et al. (2006). The food propensity questionnaire: Concept develop-ment, and validation for use as a covariate in a model to estimate usual food intake. *Journal of the American Dietetic Association, 106,* 1556–1563.

Subar, A. F., Kipnis, V., Troiano, R., Midthune, D., Schoeller, D. A., Bingham, S., et al. (2003). Using intake biomarkers to evaluate the extent of dietary misreporting in a large sample of adults: The OPEN Study. *American Journal of Epidemiology, 158,* 1–13.

Subar, A. F., Thompson, F. E., Kipnis, V., Midthune, D., Hurwitz, P., McNutt, S., et al. (2001). Com-parative validation of the Block, Willett and National Cancer Institute Food Frequency Questionnaires: The Eating at America's Table Study (EATS). *American Journal of Epidemiology, 154,* 1089–1099.

Subar, A. F., Thompson, F. E., Potischman, N., Forsyth, B. H., Buday, R., Richards, D., et al. (2007). Formative research of a quick list for an automated self-administered 24-hour dietary recall. *Journal of the American Dietetic Association, 107,* 1002–1007.

Thompson, F. E., & Byers, T. (1994) Dietary Assessment Resource Manual. *Journal of Nutrition, 124*(Suppl. 11S), 2245S–2317S.

Thompson, F. E., Kipnis, V., Midthune, D., Freedman, L. S., Carroll, R. J., Subar, A. F., et al. (2008). Performance of a food frequency questionnaire in the U.S. National Institutes of Health–AARP Diet and Health Study. *Public Health Nutrition, 11,* 183–195.

Thompson, F. E., Midthune, D., Subar, A. F., Kipnis, V., Kahle, L. L., & Schatzkin, A. (2007). Development and evaluation of a short instrument to estimate usual dietary intake of percentage energy from fat. *Journal of the American Dietetic Association, 107,* 760–767.

Thompson, F. E., Midthune, D., Subar, A. F., McNeel, T., Berrigan, D., & Kipnis, V. (2005). Dietary intake estimates in the National Health Interview Survey, 2000: Methodology, results, and interpre-tation. *Journal of the American Dietetic Association, 105,* 352–363.

Thompson, F. E., Midthune, D., Williams, G., Yaroch, A. L., Hurley, T. G., Resnicow, K., et al. (2008).

Evaluation of a short dietary assessment instrument for percent energy from fat in an intervention study. *Journal of Nutrition, 138*, 193S–199S.

Thompson, F. E., & Subar, A. F. (2001). Dietary assessment methodology. In A. M. Coulson, C. L. Rock, & E. R. Monsen (Eds.), *Nutrition in the prevention and treatment of disease* (pp. 3–30). New York: Academic Press.

Thompson, F. E., Subar, A. F., Brown, C. C., Smith, A. F., Sharbaugh, C. O., Jobe, J. B., et al. (2002). Cognitive research enhances accuracy of food frequency questionnaire reports: Results of an experimental validation study. *Journal of the American Dietetic Association, 102*, 212–225.

Thompson, F. E., Subar, A., Potischman, N., Midthune, D., Kipnis, V., Troiano, R. P., et al. (2006). *A checklist-adjusted food frequency method for assessing dietary intake*. Paper presented at the Sixth International Conference on Dietary Assessment Methods: Complementary Advances in Diet and Physical Activity Assessment Methodologies, Copenhagen, Denmark.

Thompson, F. E., Subar, A. F., Smith, A. F., Midthune, D., Radimer, K. L., Kahle, L. L., et al. (2002). Fruit and vegetable assessment: Performance of 2 new short instruments and a food frequency questionnaire. *Journal of the American Dietetic Association, 102*, 1764–1772.

Togo, P., Osler, M., Sørensen, T. I., & Heitmann, B. L. (2001). Food intake patterns and body mass index in observational studies. *International Journal of Obesity and Related Metabolic Disorders, 25*, 1741–1751.

Togo, P., Osler, M., Sørensen, T. I., & Heitmann, B. L. (2004). A longitudinal study of food intake patterns and obesity in adult Danish men and women. *International Journal of Obesity and Related Metabolic Disorders, 28*, 583–593.

Tooze, J. A., Midthune, D., Dodd, K. W., Freedman, L. S., Krebs-Smith, S. M., Subar, A. F., et al. (2006). A new statistical method for estimating the usual intake of episodically consumed foods with application to their distribution. *Journal of the American Dietetic Association, 106*, 1575–1587.

Tooze, J. A., Subar, A. F., Thompson, F. E., Troiano, R., Schatzkin, A., & Kipnis, V, (2004). Psychosocial predictors of energy underreporting in a large

doubly labelled water study. *American Journal of Clinical Nutrition, 79*, 795–804.

Turconi, G., Guarcello, M., Berzolari, F. G., Carolei, A., Bazzano, R., & Roggi, C. (2005). An evaluation of a colour food photography atlas as a tool for quantifying food portion size in epidemiological dietary surveys. *European Journal of Clinical Nutrition, 59*, 923–931.

U.S. Department of Agriculture (USDA), Agricultural Research Service. (1997). *Design and operation: The continuing survey of food intakes by individuals and the diet and health knowledge survey, 1994–96*. Hyattsville, MD: Author.

U.S. Department of Agriculture (USDA), ORC/Macro. (2005). *Food Assistance and Nutrition Research Program: Developing effective wording and format options for a children's nutrition behavior questionnaire for mothers of children in kindergarten* (USDA Contractor and Cooperator Report No. 10). Hyattsville, MD: Author.

Vereecken, C. A., Covents, M., Matthys, C., & Maes, L. (2005). Young adolescents' nutrition assessment on computer (YANA-C). *European Journal of Clinical Nutrition, 59*, 658–667.

Vereecken, C. A., Covents, M., Sichert-Hellert, W., Alvira, J. M., Le Donne, C., De Henauw, S., et al. (2008). Development and evaluation of a self-administered computerized 24-h dietary recall method for adolescents in Europe. *International Journal of Obesity, 32*(Suppl. 5), S26–S34.

Willett, W. (1998). *Nutritional epidemiology.* New York: Oxford University Press.

Winkvist, A., Persson, V., & Hartini, T. N. (2002). Underreporting of energy intake is less common among pregnant women in Indonesia. *Public Health Nutrition, 5*, 523–529.

Yon, B. A., Johnson, R. K., Harvey-Berino, J., & Gold, B. C. (2006). The use of a personal digital assistant for dietary self-monitoring does not improve the validity of self-reports of energy intake. *Journal of the American Dietetic Association, 106*, 1256–1259.

Yon, B. A., Johnson, R. K., Harvey-Berino, J., Gold, B. C., & Howard, A. B. (2007). Personal digital assistants are comparable to traditional diaries for dietary self-monitoring during a weight loss program. *Journal of Behavioral Medicine, 30*, 165–175.

CHAPTER 8

Measuring Food Intake, Hunger, Satiety, and Satiation in the Laboratory

John Blundell, Kees de Graaf, Graham Finlayson, Jason C. G. Halford,
Marion Hetherington, Neil King, and James Stubbs

Why Study Appetite in the Laboratory?

Over the years, the phenomenon of human appetite has become a significant force in advocating healthy living and promoting optimal functioning in people. An appropriate control over appetite—including the selection of foods and their consumption in appropriate amounts—is a factor in the regulation of body weight and in its dysregulation in obesity and eating disorders, as well as in a range of metabolic and psychological diseases (Blundell, 1995). Accordingly, it has become increasingly necessary to be able to accurately and reliably measure appetite under a variety of conditions in diverse environments.

The laboratory is one particular environment that provides the possibility of assessing various aspects of appetite under controlled circumstances free from the turbulence of a natural social environment. It should be made clear at the outset that the purpose of measuring appetite in the laboratory is not to attempt to replicate the quality of the natural free-living world with its profusion of distractors and interfering variables. The purpose of laboratory research is to study appetite free from the social chaos in which it is normally expressed and, through appropriate control procedures, to isolate specific factors and to study their effects on the expression of appetite uncontaminated by extraneous input.

The essence of measuring food intake in the laboratory is set out in Figure 8.1, which illustrates in brief schematic form the structure of the locations and circumstances under which eating can be measured.

The major contrast is between a strict laboratory environment (embodying a strong control over the surroundings and the experimental events) and the free-living situation (in which minimal control is applied). Clearly, different methods are required to gather data in such different circumstances, and there are differences in the nature and status of the data collected. The main

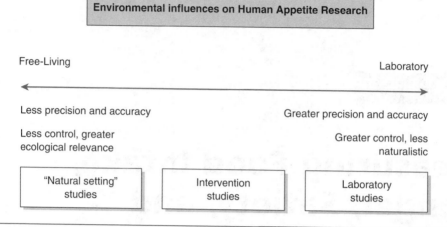

Figure 8.1   Conceptual Description of the Relationship Between Laboratory and Free-Living Research

distinction is between precision and accuracy, at one end of the spectrum, and naturalness at the other. Eating data gathered under laboratory conditions are usually precisely and accurately related to the behavior through which they were emitted, but the circumstances are not natural (because people do not normally eat alone in a cubicle or small room isolated from social stimuli). On the other hand, eating under free-living conditions can be considered natural, but it is often not precisely or accurately related to the behavior that forms the target of interest. The dimension of precision-naturalness can be considered as a gradient. Even in the laboratory, the score for naturalness need not be zero since participants normally (but not always) put food into the mouth using hands, eating implements, and so on. In most experimental situations, there is a trade-off between precision and naturalness, and the researcher has to make a decision about the value of modulating one in favor of the other. The decision depends, of course, on the research question itself; a laboratory study of food intake will only be relevant for certain types of research inquiries.

The laboratory study of appetite has been used for decades to investigate causal mechanisms believed to be responsible for eating. This enterprise is normally referred to as a study of the "control of eating" within the framework of

"regulation of body weight." This exercise continues to be important for the development and elucidation of theoretical principles underlying human appetite. However, there is also a need for controlled studies of appetite for more practical reasons—for example, in the development of functional foods for appetite control (Dye & Blundell, 2002) and the investigation of the mode of action of antiobesity drugs—at least those believed to work via a reduction in food intake (e.g., Blundell et al., 2006; B. J. Rolls, Shide, Thorwart, & Ulbrecht, 1998; S. Smith et al., 2007). In both of these circumstances, an accurate assessment of appetite (food intake, food selection, hunger sensations, etc.) is essential to define the efficacy of the food (or food ingredient) or drug. It is therefore important that the laboratory study of appetite should be able to describe a *methodological platform,* with a specific set of tools, that can be used consistently and reliably in different locations to provide comparable results.

Principles and Concepts

Most researchers carry in their "mind's eye" a conceptual framework that is used to organize the research approach. This framework will, of course, incorporate the key variables believed to be responsible for influencing food intake, hunger, and food choice. In recent years, one major question that has framed research inquiries includes the contrast between homeostatic and hedonic influences over eating. In addition, many researchers have based a research approach on the energy balance model in which energy intake is understood in relation to the various forms of energy expenditure (behavioral and metabolic) and changes in body composition.

Considering the short-term control of food intake, it is readily recognized that food intake is an episodic activity that is expressed as a pattern of eating episodes. An experimental approach has developed based on the measurement of the size of an eating episode (or repeated episodes). The episode is normally called a meal (or test meal) and is at the center of the laboratory measurement of food intake. Consequently, processes of importance for study include those that determine eating within the meal itself and those that precede or follow the meal. The terms *prepran-dial*, *prandial*, and *postprandial* are often used. The various processes, attributes of foods, and related psychological and behavioral states are often contained within the concept of the "satiety cascade" proposed about 20 years ago (Blundell, Rogers, & Hill, 1987).

Figure 8.2a contains the simplest description of the satiety cascade and illustrates the separation of the processes of satiation and satiety. Satiation is used to describe the processes that bring an episode of eating to an end; it therefore incorporates all of those events that operate during the course of the meal itself. Satiety is defined as the inhibition of further eating together with the (usual) suppression of hunger (and increase in fullness) that occurs once eating has ceased. Broadly speaking, satiation controls the size of meals, whereas satiety may be said to influence the intermeal interval (though this is rarely measured). Both satiation and satiety can vary in duration and intensity, and the expression of each depends on the strength and speed of the onset of physiological signals (generated by the action of food) and by the nature of the food itself. Because of the separate identities of satiation and satiety, different experimental procedures are required to measure each of these sets of processes. At this stage, it can be mentioned that satiation is especially influenced by a number of aspects of food, including the amount offered (portion size), energy density, and sensory features, including taste, texture, diversity (variety), and palatability. Satiety is influenced by the total energy consumed (sometimes briefly by weight and volume), macronutrient composition, presence and type of fiber (nondigestible polysaccharides, resistant starch, viscous or non-viscous, etc.), and specific components designed to affect physiological satiety signaling systems. It follows, of course, that if satiation is modulated by food properties that lead to a change in meal size, then the food in that meal will modulate satiety in the subsequent postprandial period. Even though satiation and satiety are integrated in the overall control of the eating pattern, it is important to recognize their theoretical independence and to have experimental procedures to measure each separately. In addition, there are likely to be interindividual differences in the rates at which satiety develops as well as intraindividual differences in satiety development according to food properties (e.g., satiety quotient).

Figure 8.2b illustrates in pictorial form some of the macro-attributes of food that can influence satiation and, in turn, satiety. One strength of laboratory-based research is that it can be used to accurately control one set of attributes (e.g., sensory–taste, textural–qualities of food) to allow the measurement of the impact of other attributes such as palatability, energy density, macronutrient composition, and so forth. Although in theory, such control could be exerted across the entire diet and for long periods, in practice this is difficult and inconvenient. Therefore, a short-term study of one or two meals under laboratory conditions can be used as a behavioral assay to understand the effect of adjusting particular parameters.

Figure 8.2c further extends the graphical representation of the satiety cascade to indicate the classes of physiological signals that contribute to satiation and to the time course of satiety. More detailed descriptions of the physiological components of the system can be found elsewhere (e.g., Badman & Flier, 2005; Berthoud, 2006; Schwartz & Morton, 2002). Carefully monitored studies in the laboratory environment have become mandatory for defining the actions of physiological processes associated with eating and, in particular, for identifying the strength and timing of signaling mechanisms for satiation and satiety. Under these circumstances, the satiety cascade can serve as a guide to indicate how a particular experimental design can be used to investigate specific processes underlying the control of food intake.

Quality Control in the Laboratory Environment

Conducting valid research in a laboratory environment obviously requires an appropriate experimental design incorporating the control and isolation of variables, together with sufficient power to test the hypothesis under scrutiny. However, the outcome of a study can only be as good as the quality of the data collected. It is

therefore essential that procedures are put in place to govern the conduct of the experimenters at every stage of the data collection process. This is known as good laboratory practice (GLP). Strictly speaking, there is no official code of practice for behavioral studies in contrast to those for pharmaceutical research, for example. However, there are standards that should be met to ensure that experimental procedures are enacted in a uniform and consistent manner on every occasion and with every subject. The maintenance of a consistent experimental procedure is best ensured through the use of standard operating procedures (SOPs). These are clearly written statements that carry instructions for every task that an experimenter will undertake during the course of a study. There should be, for example, an SOP for the interaction between an experimenter and the subject/participant that dictates the information and contact that will be delivered. Similar rules apply for the preparation of all test foods, including the accurate weighing of food—usually to the nearest 0.1 g—before and after consumption. Since food intake is often the major parameter of interest—either as a dependent or independent variable—SOPs are essential to control these procedures in the laboratory

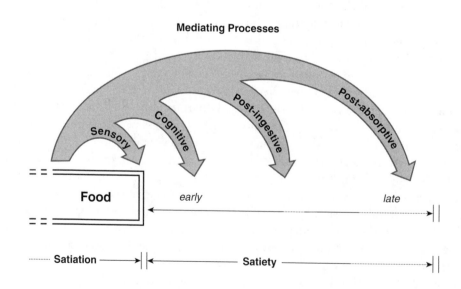

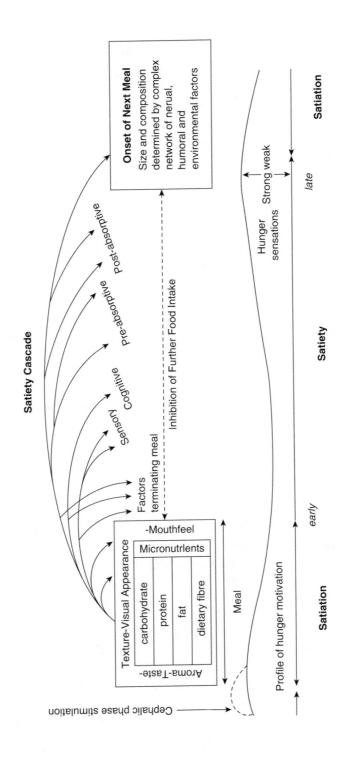

b

287

c

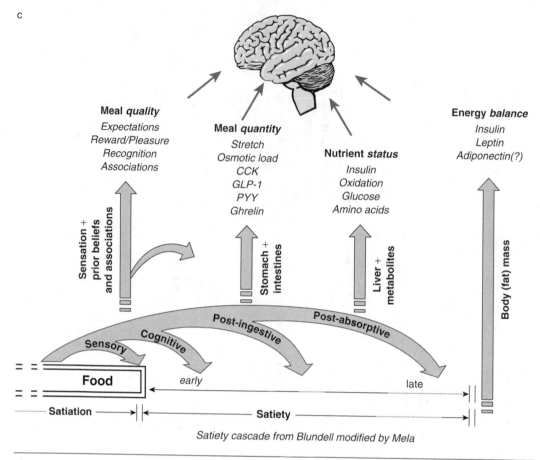

Satiety cascade from Blundell modified by Mela

Figure 8.2   Three Versions of the Satiety Cascade Illustrating the Difference Between (a) Satiation and Satiety, (b) Influence of Contextual Factors on These Processes, (c) and Some of the Physiological Mechanisms Involved

kitchen. SOPs should also be in place for recording data (adding or subtracting weights of food, for example) and for transferring written data to electronic files. Since errors in computation and transcription are a fundamental feature of data collection (the human error), it is essential that every item of data collected and written down (or typed in) should be checked independently by a coexperimenter. It can be assumed, with high certainty, that experimenters make errors in the recording of data, so every effort should be made to minimize these effects. Again, this can best be achieved through the use of clearly stated SOPs that incorporate data checking (and often double checking). This can be particularly important, for example, if paper-and-pencil-type visual analog scales are used that require the manual measurement of marks on hundreds of lines.

It is the precision and accuracy of every item of data collection (including every item of food) that forms the basis of GLP and that can safeguard the validity of laboratory investigations of food intake. Conversely, it is extremely easy to undermine the value of experimental control by a casual and informal approach to the basics of food intake measurement. A turbulent and unprofessional laboratory environment is the behavioral equivalent of "dirty test tubes."

A final aspect of GLP for laboratory feeding studies is the security of the data collected. This is paramount in some commercially sponsored studies in which the data could subsequently be used in judicial proceedings. Although most of the time researchers will be concerned with their data as evidence in arguments in scientific journals, the same principles of security should apply. Once data have been collected, checked, and entered into files, they should be protected from subsequent amendment, except under special cases described in the protocol. The fundamental data comprising the data output of an investigation should be preserved for a minimum number of years (usually 5 to 7). Sometimes the stage of formally securing the data is called the database lock. This is a good practice for researchers to adopt. It is in the area of data security where university researchers can learn from commercially sponsored research in which future interrogation of data is a possibility. Most researchers using their data output to publish findings in scientific journals will never have their data files inspected; nevertheless, it is good practice to operate as if this could be the case.

What Is a Food Intake Laboratory?

Strictly defined, a laboratory will be a purpose-built facility specifically designed to carry out measurements on food intake and associated variables. A basic facility normally includes a laboratory kitchen for the accurate and safe preparation of foods together with a suite of small rooms, cubicles, or shielded spaces where subjects can be presented with test foods in a quiet, calm, and controlled environment free from distractors. The laboratory should have the capacity for subjects to eat alone with no social contact with other participants and no distraction from the environment. However, since some designs may require social contact, the laboratory may also provide a communal dining area for group eating. A laboratory also often includes a reception area where subjects can be met, check in for studies, fill in screening questionnaires, and receive information and instructions relevant to the study. Some laboratories may be extended into a clinical research

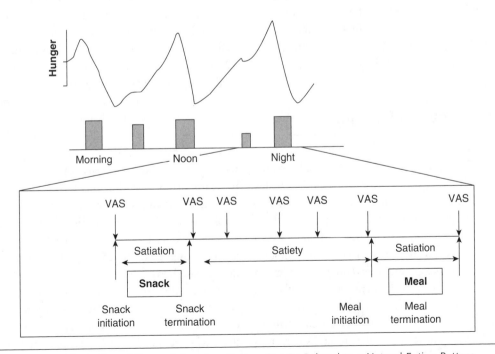

Figure 8.3   Illustration of How a Laboratory Design Can Be Related to a Natural Eating Pattern

facility with rooms set aside for the measurement of anthropometric and physiological variables and for blood taking. Other laboratories incorporate rooms specialized for energy balance measurements with indirect calorimetry equipment, body composition analyzers, and physical activity equipment. A few laboratories have rooms set up with special techniques such as Universal Eating Monitors (UEMs). Consequently, a food intake laboratory can range from a simple structural arrangement for the measurement of eating under controlled conditions to an extended research facility capable of measuring food intake in relation to energy balance and body composition and physiological parameters.

However, although a laboratory can be defined as a physical structure, there is also the conceptual recognition of a "laboratory." This implies the carrying out of research under controlled and systematic environmental conditions that characterize a laboratory. This laboratory approach can be enacted in various establishments, including clinics, institutes, departments where the clear intention is to obtain accurate measures of food consumption and related variables. As long as the procedural and methodological requirements are met, then a "laboratory" investigation need not involve a specific structure labeled with that title.

Experimental Designs

In laboratory research, no single experimental design can provide a resolution for all research questions. Using the scheme set out in Figure 8.3, two basic approaches emerge that are designed to measure the influence of a manipulation upon either satiation or satiety. The question of which design to use will depend on the research question and the nature of the intervention. A design to measure satiation will focus on manipulations that produce intrameal effects, including the amount of food offered, energy density, sensory qualities, liquid versus solid state, and so on. This approach is designed to measure within-meal

effects, or effects occurring during the eating process. The second approach is designed to measure effects following (not during) the ingestion of food (postprandial) and takes the form of a preload–test meal design or a meal-to-meal arrangement (Kissileff, 1984). Although the preload–test meal strategy has been particularly attractive in laboratory-based research, it is now common to find the preload (independent variable) presented as a meal rather than as a small amount of food prior to a meal (Burns et al., 2000; Cani, Joly, Horsemans, & Delzenne, 2006; King, Craig, Pepper, & Blundell, 2005). The principle of the satiety design remains, however, to prescribe an eating episode in which the parameters of the food are strictly fixed (weight, volume, energy density, percent macronutrients, etc.) with only the variable under investigation allowed to vary.

Procedures for Assessing Satiation

As defined earlier, satiation is the process that brings a meal to an end. Satiation determines the size of an eating occasion. Verbal reports on the processes that bring a meal to an end indicate that "fullness" and "boredom with taste" are two major reasons to stop eating (Hetherington, 1995; Mook & Votaw, 1992; Tuomisto, Tuomisto, Hetherington, & Lappalainen, 1998). These reasons may differ depending on whether we deal with the consumption of a single food or a composite meal. With a single food, it is more likely that boredom of taste becomes involved, whereas with composite dishes/meals, fullness may be more important in ending the meal.

Satiation is important because it determines meal size. Within the perspective of energy balance and obesity, it is instructive to note that there is no strong relationship between eating frequency and body weight (e.g., Bellisle, McDevitt, & Prentice, 1997; Whybrow, Mayer, Kirk, Mazlan, & Stubbs, 2007). As obese people ingest more energy than nonobese people, one might infer that meal size may be the key factor in the overconsumption of energy in obese people. However, the possible contribution of meals and snacks to overeating is still a highly debated issue, which is outside the scope of this chapter.

Before focusing on the methodology of measuring satiation, it should be realized that in real life, most meals/snacks/eating occasions are terminated through environmental factors/cues such as portion size. In most cases, people consume most (or all) of the food on the plate. In a field study with U.S. soldiers on the consumption of about 5,700 main meals and 8,800 snacks, it was observed that soldiers ate 100% of their portion in 80% to 90% of the cases. Even if foods were neither liked nor disliked (a 5 on the 9-point hedonic scale), people ate on average 87% of their meal (C. de Graaf et al., 2005).

Satiation is measured through the measurement of ad libitum food consumption of particular experimental foods under standardized conditions. The ad libitum consumption of foods varies to a large extent. For example, in a study on sensory-specific satiation, Weenen, Stafleu, and de Graaf (2005) observed that people ate on average 70 to 80 g from savory cheese biscuits, whereas they ate about five times as much of pears in light-sugared syrup. This was not due to differences in liking as the pears and biscuits were about equally liked. Studies such as this indicate that people do not automatically eat the same weight/volume of foods presented, and experimenters should be prepared to deal with this situation.

The proper methodology of the measurement of satiation takes into consideration the properties of food and the environmental/contextual factors that may be involved in meal termination. In view of the processes of the satiety cascade (see Figure 8.2), it is clear that sensory factors play a major role in satiation. Many studies showed that palatability has a strong effect on ad libitum food intake, both from controlled experimental studies (e.g., C. de Graaf, de Jong, & Lambers, 1999) as well as from more real-life studies (e.g., C. de Graaf et al., 2005). So, when studying the effect of particular food properties on satiation, it is important that the experimental foods are similarly liked.

The satiety cascade also shows that cognitive factors may play an important role in meal termination. On the basis of the consumption of thousands and thousands of foods through our lifetime, we gradually learn to estimate the satiating effects of many foods. We "know" that we need to consume two slices of bread and cheese for breakfast to prevent the irritating occurrence of hunger during the morning. These learning mechanisms determine our expectations about the satiating properties of foods and probably also determine how much we put on our plate (e.g., Brunstrom, 2007). This also affects how much we eat ad libitum from particular food in experimental situations.

A crucial role in this learned response (expectations) about satiation is the energy density of the product. In the example above where subjects consumed five times the amount in grams (weight) of pears compared to cheese biscuits, the energy density of the savory cheese biscuits (2268 kJ/100 g) was about eight times higher than the energy density of the pears (272 kJ/100 g). At first sight, it seems that regular portion sizes of low-energy density foods (e.g., many liquids) are much higher than regular portion sizes of high-energy density foods (e.g., chocolate, cheese, peanuts, etc.). However, there are no systematic data in scientific papers comparing portions sizes of low-energy density foods to portion sizes of high-energy density foods. Nevertheless, this observation implies that it is crucial to match foods for energy density when investigating the effect of food properties on satiation.

Experimental data on the effect of varying energy density on ad libitum food intake (with matched sensory properties) suggest that people are slow to respond to (covert) changes in energy density (e.g., Blundell, Lawton, Cotton, & Macdiarmid, 1996; Kendall, Levitsky, Strupp, & Lissner, 1991; Lissner, Levitsky, Strupp, Kalkwarf, & Roe, 1987). This may be especially the case for liquid foods and fast foods, which do not lead to strong sensory cues (DiMeglio & Mattes, 2000; Raben, Vasilaras, Moller, & Astrup, 2002). Fast foods are foods that are easy to ingest without much chewing effort. The absence of clear sensory cues may prevent people from learning to associate the oral sensory cues during eating with the postingestive metabolic consequences.

The texture of foods is also important in satiation. People consume more ad libitum from more liquid foods than they consume of more solid foods. This is related to the rate of eating, which is higher in liquids than in (semi)solids (Zijlstra, Mars, de Wijk, Westerterp-Plantenga, & de Graaf, 2008). The higher eating rate may be caused by the bite/swallow size, which is probably higher in liquids compared to (semi)solids. Eating 500 g of apples takes about 17 minutes; drinking the equivalent amount of apple juice can be done in 1.5 minutes (Haber, Heaton, & Murphy, 1977). These observations imply that controlling for texture may be an important prerequisite when investigating the effects of food properties on meal termination.

Another cognitive factor that plays a role in meal termination is knowledge about the time until the next meal. In a study of C. de Graaf et al. (1999), subjects consumed more from an ad libitum test meal when they knew they had no access to food the next 2 hours compared to a situation where the next meal was 20 minutes ahead. So, people anticipated with their consumption on the future availability of foods. It is clear that the amount that people eat is also determined by the motivational state of subjects; people eat more when they are hungry compared to when they are satiated. Therefore, it is important that people have a similar state of satiety before presenting them with an ad libitum meal.

People will have certain ideas about the satiating effect of particular foods. These learned responses are mostly in concurrence with other sensory/environmental cues. When emptying a bottle of soft drinks, the weight of the bottle is a clear cue of how much has been drunk. In an innovative study, the importance of concurrent (visual) cues in meal satiation was studied by Wansink, Painter, and North (2005). He showed that the ad libitum consumption of soup was strongly influenced by the visual cues with respect to the emptiness of the bowl of soup from which the soup was eaten. In one condition, people were (unconsciously) deceived, as the soup was refilled partially through an invisible tube. In the tube condition, people ate about 73% more, while the perceived consumption was about equal. This study illustrates that people use many environmental (and not internal cues) to decide whether they should continue to eat.

In summary, the amount that we eat from a particular product is influenced by a variety of factors related to the properties of food and the context in which the food is consumed. In general, ad libitum consumption of foods is a learned response based on associations between the sensory properties of foods and its metabolic consequences after ingestion. When studying the effect of properties on meal termination from a scientific point of view, it is necessary to vary one factor while holding other important factors constant. This implies that when studying satiation, we need to take into consideration the palatability, energy density, and texture of foods; the motivational state (hungry vs. satiated) of subjects; potential important environmental cues (e.g., visual cues, plate size, effort to eat); and cognitive factors. All of these factors can influence the effects of similar caloric loads on satiation. A further important issue is the interindividual variation in the rate of satiation for comparable caloric loads.

Procedures for Assessing Satiety: The Preload Type Design

With the exception of observational approaches, the most basic form of experimental design used to measure food and energy intake (EI) in the laboratory is the "preload test meal" paradigm, which has been used to assess the short-term effect of a wide range of manipulations on subjective motivation to eat and often intake at a subsequent test meal (Hulshof & de Graff, 1993; Kissileff, 1984; B. Rolls et al., 1991; B. Rolls et al., 1994; Spitzer & Rodin, 1981). These experiments are most profitably conducted using a within-subject repeated-measures design, in which subjects serve as their own controls. This is important since there is considerable interindividual variability in food intake behavior, which can reduce the power of between-subjects designs.

It is apparent from Figure 8.2 that a number of aspects of an eating episode could influence the postprandial consequences (usually measured by the amount eaten at the subsequent [test] meal). These aspects include cognitive beliefs and expectations, sensory factors (taste and texture), total energy, proportion of macronutrients, and the presence of components likely to affect postingestive physiological processing. Consequently, one primary requirement of laboratory research is to be able to hold constant all of these variables except the one whose influence is being investigated. Often, it requires considerable skill and effort to be able to match preloads or preload meals so that subjects cannot detect any apparent differences. Experimental control over the parameters of the preload is a paramount consideration in laboratory research.

What is a preload? It is debatable when the term *preload* was first used, but the term has come to be recognized as an eating episode (smaller than a meal and often about 1 MJ in energy value) that is given at a particular interval (often 30 to 90 minutes) before the presentation of a test meal (usually at a usual mealtime). The outcome of a preload–test meal design will therefore depend critically on the parameters of the preload, the duration of the preload test meal interval, and the nature of the test meal. The key to using this design appropriately is plausibility. The design should provide a fair test of the hypothesis. This means that the manipulated variable should be sufficiently large to be detectable. Some preload manipulations are too small to exert any meaningful impact over the postingestive period (and therefore over the test meal itself). The interval between the preload and the test meal also should be realistic and appropriate to the anticipated action of the active variable in the preload. Clearly, if the preload–test meal interval (the postingestive

window; Cotton, Westrate, & Blundell, 1996) is too small, then the effect will not be detected. It follows that a preload test meal interval can be too long (action of the preload has decayed before the test meal is presented) or too short (action of the preload occurs after the test meal is finished). Two common causes of a failure to detect an effect in this type of design are the minimal size of the preload manipulation (or the active variable) and a test meal presented at an inappropriate time. A cynic might add that this may sometimes be the unwritten objective behind the study, and given the strong commercial interest in the effects of foods on satiety, it is necessary to be watchful for choice of implausible parameters. The injudicious choice of experimental parameters can easily lead to a null outcome in preload research.

Because of the arbitrary nature of the choice of parameters in the preload test meal design, many experimenters have opted for a meal-to-meal strategy in which Meal 1 is fixed and incorporates the independent variable and Meal 2 is ad libitum and is the dependent variable. Of course, some of the same considerations apply about the size and detectability of the independent variable, but the interval is normally based on realistic eating habits and is therefore plausible. Because of the interest attached to snacking, a variation of the preload and meal-to-meal approach is the manipulated snack. It is important to note that the participant's eating and drinking behavior should be monitored between preload (or snack) and test meal. This is easy if the interval is short but can become more difficult for longer intervals. In addition to the importance of the preload and the interval until measurement, the nature of the test meal itself can also affect the outcome, and the choice of the structure of the meal can be critical.

For example, varying the palatability of foods in the test meal influences the degree of compensation generated by preloads that vary in size (e.g., Robinson, Gray, Yeomans, & French, 2005). A large homogeneous meal in contrast to a buffet meal containing a variety of foods can also affect the measured outcome (Raynor & Epstein, 2000).

Of course, it should be kept in mind that the impact of a preload or a preload meal can be monitored sensitively by subjective sensations using visual analog scales; these scales can sometimes detect the effect of a preload that has no measured impact on food ingestion itself (test meal). Consequently, a strong design will normally incorporate the measurement of subjective sensations and objective food intake.

The use of subjective rating scales to track the temporal profile of postingestive effects draws attention to the "time course" of satiety. Postingestive effects of food consumption vary in intensity and duration, and under sensitive conditions, both of these can be detected. It follows that the influence of postingestive events will be reflected in the "time" elapsed until the return of the desire to eat (next request for food) or in the amount eaten in a meal presented at a predetermined time. Theoretically, the duration of the postmeal interval could be used as a measure of satiety. However, it should be borne in mind that the timing of meals is highly conditioned in most humans (de Castro, 1987; de Castro & Elmore, 1988). The second strategy is the most commonly used—mainly because of the convenience for the experimenter—but it should not be overlooked that the strength of satiety can be measured along a temporal dimension. Satiety can therefore be quantified by time (until next eating episode) or amount (of food consumed).

Modifications of the Basic Design

Lawton, Burley, Wales, and Blundell (1993) have extended the preload–test meal design by altering the composition of possible test meals available. This means the test meal is an outcome variable in relation to the preload, and the preload plus test meal together become the input manipulation, whose effects on subsequent intake can be assessed. While subject to some of the constraints of the preload design, this adaptation enhances the ecological validity of the experiment by producing a feeding sequence similar to that

encountered in everyday life and measures feeding over the course of a day, which appears to be the minimal shortest time window that can be used to make any statements about the possible effects of a given manipulation on energy balance (EB). A further adaptation to the preload design has been used by Foltin et al. (Foltin, Fischman, Emurian, & Rachlinski, 1988; Foltin, Fischman, Moran, Rolls, & Kelly, 1990; Foltin et al., 1992), who provided subjects in the laboratory setting with a variety of familiar food items and covertly manipulated one mandatory meal, usually lunch. This again has the advantage of enhancing the ecological validity of the experimental design and enables the experiment to be conducted over more than one day. More recently, a multiple-preload design has been used to assess the effect of snack composition on the food and EI of an otherwise ad libitum diet of fixed composition over 7 days per treatment). Thus, while the original preload-testmeal paradigm has certain limitations, this basic experimental design can be extended to study feeding behavior and its likely effects on EB.

Manipulating the Whole Diet (Not Just a Single Meal)

As interest has focused on the effect of dietary parameters (e.g., nutrient composition, energy density, sensory characteristics) on EI and EB, the use of manipulated diets in laboratory studies of feeding has become common (e.g., Kendall et al., 1991; Lawton et al., 1993; Lissner et al., 1987; O'Reilly, Stubbs, Johnstone, Mara, & Robertson, 1997; Stubbs & Harbron, 1996; Stubbs, Harbron, Murgatroyd, & Prentice, 1995; Tremblay et al., 1991). Under these conditions, the diet can represent aspects of both the manipulated input and the measured outcome variable in an experiment. The degree of manipulation can vary from highly precise systematic manipulation of the nutrient ratios and/or energy density of all foods on the diet to partial manipulations of the whole diet (O'Reilly et al., 1997; Stubbs & Harbron, 1996; Stubbs et al., 1995). For example, manipulations that use foods with a food quotient of [FQ = (EI as protein/total EI × RQ protein) + (EI as lipid/total EI × RQ lipid) + (EI as carbohydrate/total EI × RQ carbohydrate)] classify high- or low-fat foods as above or below 0.85 (Tremblay et al., 1991). It is important in such studies for the experimenter to describe meticulously the nature of the manipulation, including, for instance, whether energy density also altered with the nutrient ratio of the diet. What was the range of variation in the composition of foods with an FQ above 0.85? Whenever a study uses a manipulated diet, the design of that diet places certain constraints on the behavior of the subject. In real life, subjects are able to vary the energy density, composition, amount, and solid food-to-fluid ratio of the foods they select and ingest. Very few laboratory designs enable this degree of behavioral flexibility and often view variations in more than one dietary parameter as a contamination of the cause-effect relationship under scrutiny. Herein lies a further dilemma to the investigator, because allowing an increased range of the subject's behavioral response decreases the signal-to-noise ratio in the manipulation and so may weaken the detection of the cause-effect relationship under investigation. On the other hand, the more controlled the dietary manipulation, the more constrained the subject is in his or her behavioral response. It is important to emphasize, rather than to understate or rationalize, the limitations of the experimental design in research reports. This allows the influence of the experimental context on experimental outcomes to be assessed. For example, comparing studies that use overt and covertly manipulated diets confirms that cognition and/or learning play important roles in mechanisms of caloric compensation (Stubbs, 1995).

Role of Learning With Manipulated Diets

Considering the issue of learning in relation to the type of manipulated diet used, an interesting phenomenon has been observed in the growing number of studies that use covertly manipulated diets over periods ranging from a few days to a few weeks. These studies are characterized by a general tendency for subjects not to alter their food intake (FI) in response to the dietary manipulation, unless the manipulation produces a particularly large (physiological or orosensory) effect. Even then compensatory responses are somewhat blunted, and FI changes little. This means that a growing number of studies appear to suggest that maintaining a constant weight or volume of food intake appears to be a major outcome of subjects feeding in the laboratory. Why should weight and volume appear as important features that affect FI in some studies? (A liter of water would have weight and volume but would provide no energy or nutrients.) It has been argued that the ultimate function of satiety signals is to monitor the biological value of foods and to play a role in the processing of ingested nutrients. During the acquisition of learned feeding patterns, weight and volume of food will have become associated with (conditioned to) the important biological components of food—namely, energy value and nutrient composition. Following the ideas of Brunswik (1952), it has been argued that weight and volume become learned cues with high functional validity (proximal cues that correlate well with more distal cues such as hormone release, contact with gastrointestinal receptors, etc.). In other words, subjects learn to associate the weight and volume of specific, familiar foods that they habitually eat with the physiological consequences of ingesting those foods. However, in an experiment using manipulated foods, subjects are presented with foods that are not of a similar composition to those normally ingested, even if they look similar. Indeed, studies using covertly manipulated diets tend to strip learning cues out of the experiment by covertly altering food composition, dissociating the sensory and nutritional attributes of the foods, randomizing the order of experimental conditions to avoid learned order effects, and often using relatively unfamiliar foods. In the absence of familiar feeding cues, weight and volume of food may attain greater significance, under these experimental conditions. Furthermore, in studies where subjects feed ad libitum on covertly manipulated diets of a constant composition, they cannot alter the type, energy density, or composition of foods they eat to the extent that they can in real life (e.g., Kendall et al., 1991; Lissner et al., 1987; O'Reilly et al., 1997; Stubbs & Harbron, 1996; Stubbs et al., 1995). Hence, any compensatory feeding responses are likely to be more blunted under these experimental conditions relative to those encountered in real life. Because of these important constraints of the experimental design on feeding behavior, equal attention should be given to comparisons of overt and covert manipulations, as well as studies using familiar foods, to differentiate whether feeding responses were due to the overt/covert nature of the experiment or the nutritional nature of the dietary manipulation.

The Use of Familiar Foods

Ostensibly, it might appear that the use of familiar foods creates a microcosm of the real-life feeding situation and overcomes the constraints of using manipulated diets. However, the choice of foods provided in the laboratory is inevitably limited, and few reports give scientific explanations of why a certain range or selection of foods was made available to a group of subjects. Given that a number of dietary factors can influence food, energy, and nutrient intakes in laboratory studies, considerable attention should be paid to this aspect of dietary design. The use of familiar foods in the laboratory also decreases the precision of measurement since it is more difficult to quantify energy and nutrient intakes, especially if the foods are mixed as in real life. The use of familiar foods in discrete units affects the experimental context with as yet unquantified consequences. Other studies, particularly those of de Castro (1987; de Castro & Elmore, 1988), employ subjects to self-record intakes in the natural setting. While these studies are subject

to all of the errors associated with dietary surveys (especially misreporting of food intake; see above), they provide invaluable information regarding patterns of behavior in free-living subjects in their natural setting (see Figure 8.1). It is therefore valuable to attempt to compare more artificial manipulations in the laboratory (e.g., Kendall et al., 1991; Lissner et al., 1987; Lawton et al., 1993; O'Reilly et al., 1997; Stubbs & Harbron, 1996; Stubbs et al., 1995; Tremblay et al., 1991) with less precise but more naturalistic studies (de Castro, 1987; de Castro & Elmore, 1988).

Subjective Measures of Appetite

The visual analog scale (VAS) technique for measuring subjective appetite sensations is an important and useful contribution to appetite research by providing greater insights into eating than can be ascertained from voluntary food intake data alone. These additional features include revealing information that may not be readily inferred from food intake (Stratton et al., 1998), improve the interpretation of behavior, and allow measurement of the motivation to eat without contaminating the main behavioral outcome (Stubbs et al., 2000). VAS is a technique that provides a quantifiable objective measure translated from subjective sensations. As with other areas of psychology (e.g., pain research), VAS has now been accepted as the standard tool for assessing subjective appetite sensations.

VAS uses self-report methodology to assess the intensity of a variety of subjective states. The origin of VAS in appetite research dates back to Silverstone and Stunkard (1968). Since then, VAS has been employed as the standard methodology to measure the motivation to eat. Rogers and Blundell (1979) developed the original version of a portfolio of VAS questions that have since been adopted by many researchers.

Traditionally, VAS has been administered using the paper-and-pen (P&P) method. VAS typically takes the form of a 100-mm horizontal straight line that is unbroken and unmarked, with the two extreme states (minimum and maximum) anchored at either end by a question associated with a particular state (e.g., hunger). Variations in VAS do exist in the form of a 10-point Likert-type scale (e.g., Leathwood & Pollet, 1988), bipolar and unipolar scales (Merrill, Kramer, Cardello, & Schutz, 2002), a 150-mm horizontal line (Drapeau et al., 2007), and a 7-point scale with equally spaced qualitative labels (Holt, Brand-Miller, & Stitt, 2001). However, the 100-mm horizontal, unmarked line with anchored labels at the extreme (e.g., Figure 8.4) is the widely accepted form of VAS.

Procedure and Description

The original version of the VAS questionnaire (Rogers & Blundell, 1979) included six questions that relate to states of the motivation to eat. However, more recent questions include the following: How hungry do you feel now? How full do you feel now? How strong is your desire to eat now? and How much food do you think you could eat now? This last question is also known as prospective consumption. An advantage of the VAS technique is that the states (i.e., questions) and anchored labels can be modified to suit the manipulation and experimental design. Figure 8.4 shows the format for each of these questions and the appropriate anchored labels. The questions are designed to assess subjective states—that is, how the participant feels at the time of completion. Therefore, their subjective rating should reflect the intensity of that particular state at that time. The operative words in the anchored labels match the operative state that the particular question is assessing. It is accepted that each of the questions is assessing slightly different subjective appetite sensations—although they are all associated with the motivation to eat. The example questions in Figure 8.4 are designed to tap into different components of the motivation to eat. Therefore, a manipulation could affect each of the questions differentially. Participants will interpret the meaning of each question slightly differently. It is not usual practice to prescribe standardized definitions of each question.

VAS is completed by the participant at the required time of assessment. This is typically immediately before and after an eating episode and periodically (typically 1 hour) at intervals between eating episodes. The traditional P&P version

How hungry are you?

Not at all hungry _____ Extremely hungry

How full are you?

Not at all full _____ Extremely full

How strong is your desire to eat?

Not at all strong _____ Extremely strong

How much food do you think you could eat?

None at all _____ A large amount

Figure 8.4   Visual Analog Scales Widely Used in Food Intake Research

requires the participant to complete the VAS by placing a mark on a horizontal line at the intensity of his or her perceived feeling of that particular state. It is important to instruct participants that they should use the full range of the scale (100-mm line) and to bear in mind that the anchored labels (minimum and maximum) should be considered as extremes. For example, if the participant places the mark at the maximum end of the scale (i.e., very hungry), this is the hungriest state he or she has ever experienced. It is recommended to use an SOP in these instances, in which standard text is read verbatim to the participant. An SOP text for this is as follows:

Please place a vertical mark on the horizontal line depending on how you feel now. It is important that you rate how you actually feel now, and not how you might think you should feel, or how someone else might expect you to feel. Please consider the extreme labels—*not at all* and *extremely*—as the least hungry and the most hungry you have ever felt. When you complete the first question please proceed to the next and continue through the questions until you have completed them all.

It is only necessary to read this SOP text to the participant on the first occasion.

Recent Developments of VAS

The traditional paper-and-pencil VAS technique is still used in appetite studies, but it inherently involves some minor problems concerning validity and convenience. With the P&P method, it is possible that participants forget to complete question(s) during the test day. The implications of this are that participants either retrospectively complete the questions at the end of the day, which undermines the measurement of "state" sensations, or it inevitably leads to missing data. Equally important, it is possible that error is introduced into the method during the experimenter's

measurement of the location of the mark on the line and on entering the data from the paper version into a spreadsheet. In addition, this method of measuring, entering data, and quality control checking can be time-consuming and tedious. Sometimes these problems can be overcome by using machine-readable VAS, but even this procedure is not perfect and requires visual checking of the accuracy of the translation.

Recently, electronic versions of VAS known as the Electronic Appetite Rating System (EARS) have been developed that circumvent these problems (Delargy, Lawton, Smith, King, & Blundell, 1996; King, Lawton, Delargy, Smith, & Blundell, 1997; King, Lluch, Stubbs, & Blundell, 1997; Stubbs et al., 1997; Stubbs et al., 1999). The two most commonly used systems employ the Psion organizer (Delargy et al., 1996; King, Lawton, et al., 1997; King, Lluch, et al., 1997) and the Apple Newton Message Pad (Stubbs et al., 1997) to mimic the traditional P&P method of administering VAS. Some modifications and developments have occurred since the EARS procedure was first described (King, Lawton, et al., 1997; King, Lluch, et al., 1997). In essence, EARS is a technologically updated method of the P&P VAS method, which facilitates and enhances the quality of time-verified subjective appetite sensation data (see Figure 8.5). It makes use of a mobile, handheld personal computer and is based on original technology used in studies to track behavioral measures in shift workers (Totterdell & Folkard, 1992). A number of appetite laboratories have developed customized versions of the original EARS concept (King, Lawton, et al., 1997; King, Lluch, et al., 1997).

The personal handheld computer is small, light, and designed to be portable. The screen is of adequate size with a high-contrast, retardation film LCD. The EARS prompts the participant to complete a series of VAS that appears on the screen in sequence. The VAS appears on the screen in identical format to the P&P method (see Figure 8.2). The Psion EARS (Delargy et al., 1996; King, Lawton, et al., 1997; King, Lluch, et al., 1997) requires the participant to complete the

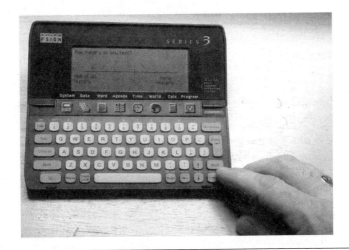

Figure 8.5   The Electronic Appetite Rating System (EARS) Developed for Ambulatory Recording of VAS

question by moving the cursor to the left or right across the horizontal line (using the appropriate cursor key) and then by pressing the "enter" key when the cursor has been correctly positioned. The Apple Newton (Stubbs et al., 1997; Stubbs et al., 2001) consists of a stylus-based graphical interface that allows the participant to use a stylus to place a vertical mark on the screen, which is more analogous to the P&P method.

The improved features of EARS include automatic verification of the date and time of completion of the VAS, identification of incomplete and/or incorrect entries, and preventing participants from retrospectively completing "missed" questions. It also provides an automatic measure of the intensity of the subjective rating. All these data are stored in the Psion or Apple Newton and automatically downloaded to a spreadsheet. The data are downloaded to a desktop or laptop via a cable and are transferred in a few seconds. The procedure will depend on the palmtop device used. Palmtop devices usually come with the appropriate software to transfer data to a desktop or laptop. Once the data are downloaded, they can be opened and viewed using Excel. Data are labeled by subject name, condition, date, time, question number (e.g., hunger, desire to eat), and the intensity of the subjective appetite sensation in millimeters.

Both the Apple Newton and Psion systems have been compared and validated against the traditional P&P method (Delargy et al., 1996; Stratton et al., 1998; Stubbs et al., 1997; Stubbs et al., 2000; Whybrow, Stephen, & Stubbs, 2006). These validation studies confirmed that the EARS produced similar findings to the P&P method and in general was a more preferred and acceptable method, as reported by the participants. It is important to note that two independent validation studies demonstrated that the EARS and P&P methods should not be used interchangeably in the same study (Stubbs et al., 2001; Whybrow et al., 2006). For a more detailed report of the validity and reliability of VAS and the EARS, the reader is referred to Stubbs et al. (2000) and Whybrow et al. (2006). It is often assumed that the EARS will reduce or prevent the frequency of missing data. However, validation work showed that the EARS produced more missing data because volunteers cannot retrospectively complete responses, unlike the paper-and-pen VAS.

Examples of Studies Using EARS

Since its development in the late 1990s, the EARS technique has been employed in a variety of intervention studies and clinical settings to provide a valid and improved method of data collection. These include using obese adults (Barkeling, King, Näslund, & Blundell, 2007; Näslund et al., 2004), renal patients (Oliver et al., 2004; Wright et al., 2001; Wright et al., 2003; Wright et al., 2004a, 2004b), obese children (Gately et al., 2007; King, Hester, & Gately, 2007), exercise interventions (Hubert, King, & Blundell, 1998; Hubert, Lluch, King, & Blundell, 2000; King, Appleton, Rogers, & Blundell, 1999; Lluch, King, & Blundell, 2000; Stubbs, Hughes, Johnstone, et al., 2004; Stubbs, Hughes, Ritz, et al., 2004; Stubbs, Sepp, Hughes, Johnstone, Horgan, et al., 2002; Stubbs, Sepp, Hughes, Johnstone, King, et al., 2002), and dietary manipulations (Blundell, Cooling, & King, 2002; King et al., 2005). In the renal studies by Wright et al., (2003), some of the patients were aged > 60 years. Therefore, EARS has been successfully used with participants differing in age, body weight, and gender and operating under a variety of experimental protocols.

The cost implications will vary depending on the type of palmtop or PDA device purchased. However, as with most other technological instruments, the cost per unit is decreasing. The EARS software developed for the Psion and Apple Newton is available from the authors, but programs can be commissioned to install VAS software on any mobile device. Indeed, there are examples of other electronic VAS systems (e.g., Yeomans, Gray, Mitchell, & True, 1997). More recently, an upgraded version of the EARS software has been applied using a Hewlett Packard PDA (HP6965). A number of pharmaceutical and nutrition companies have now developed in-house electronic data capture instruments based on the original concept of the EARS.

Validity, Sensitivity, and Reliability of VAS

A series of experimental studies has demonstrated that the VAS method of assessing subjective appetite sensations is sensitive to manipulations (for a review, see Stubbs et al., 2000). Sometimes subjective appetite sensations may be more sensitive to dietary manipulations than alterations in food intake (Johnstone, Stubbs, & Harbron, 1996).

In terms of reproducibility, when individuals are fed a diet to maintain energy balance via fixed meal and energy intake patterns, a consistent fluctuation in the diurnal profile of appetite sensations occurs. Other studies demonstrate the high reproducibility of VAS (Delargy et al., 1996; Stratton et al., 1998; Stubbs et al., 1997; Stubbs et al., 2001; Whybrow et al., 2006). A series of reviews and discussions has been dedicated to interrogating the validity and reliability of VAS (de Graaf, 1993; Flint, Raben, Blundell, & Astrup, 2000; Raben, Tagliabue, & Astrup, 1995; Reid, Johnstone, & Ryan, 1999). In addition, their ability to predict subsequent food intake has also been examined (Doucet, St-Pierre, & Almeras, 2003; Drapeau et al., 2005; Drapeau et al., 2007). The findings are mixed; some studies demonstrate that subjective appetite sensations are strong predictors of energy intake and others not. The reader is referred to the review by Stubbs et al. (2000) for a more detailed discussion of the predictive power of subjective appetite sensations. VAS is a reproducible method of assessing subjective appetite sensations—which is strengthened using a within-subjects design.

Quantifying Satiation and Satiety

When measured periodically during the test day, VAS provides diurnal profiles of subjective appetite sensations. This allows comparison of a range of manipulations and intervention trials. The VAS technique allows the continuous tracking of intrameal and intermeal changes in subjective appetite sensations. In turn, this provides a diurnal profile of subjective appetite sensations (see Figure 8.6). This example demonstrates the fluctuation in subjective appetite sensation induced by breakfast and snack meals.

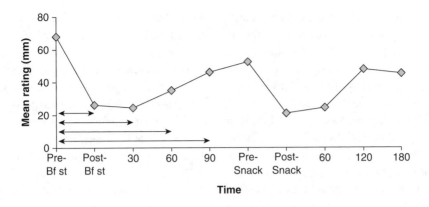

Figure 8.6   Procedure for Quantifying the Return of Hunger in Relation to the Energy Consumed in an Eating Episode

The two distinct phases of the satiety cascade described in an earlier section—satiation and satiety—can also be described as intra- and inter-meal satiety. In dietary manipulation studies, intrameal changes provide a comparison of the satiating power of the meals/diets. The following sections describe how these two phases can be used to calculate several indices of appetite.

Intra- and Intermeal Changes. By calculating the difference between the premeal and postmeal values, a delta VAS score is obtained (see Figure 8.6). Figure 8.6 is an example of intra- and inter-meal changes in hunger in a group of obese participants. The delta score is an indication of the acute power of the meal to suppress the motivation to eat (see Figure 8.4). This measure has been used to demonstrate changes in meal-induced satiation in obese children who experienced weight loss following a 6-week exercise and diet intervention (King et al., 2007).

Area Under the Curve. The area under the curve (AUC) provides an aggregate for each subjective appetite sensation. In essence, the AUC represents the area bounded by the hunger profile and is computed by the trapezoid measure or more readily as the mean of all the data points. The

AUC can be calculated for the whole of the measurement period or parts of the measurement period. It is usual to exclude baseline or fasting values when calculating the AUC. The rationale for doing this is to remove any bias or differences at baseline that might artificially alter the mean AUC and introduce more random variation into the measured response.

Recovery. The rate of return of hunger is an indication of the power of a food/meal to influence satiety. That is, the slower the return of hunger after a meal, the more powerful effect exerted on satiety. This is typically attained by calculating the difference between the postmeal value and the premeal value of the next eating episode (see Figure 8.6). An alternative approach is to calculate the time taken for subjective motivation to eat to return to 50% of its original (fasting or premeal) value.

Satiety Quotient. The original concept of developing an index to compare the satiating potency of foods was proposed by Kissileff (1984) and termed the *satiating efficiency.* One definition of the satiating efficiency of a food is "the effectiveness of a preload at suppressing test meal intake per unit of energy delivered." This concept was modified to include VAS ratings and was termed the *Satiety Quotient* (SQ; Green, Delargy, Joanes, & Blundell, 1997) and reflects a change in the rating score (mm) per unit (kcal) of energy consumed. Other similar concepts have been produced (e.g., Satiety Index—Holt, Miller, Petocz, & Farmakalidis, 1995), but the advantage of the SQ is that it provides a temporal measure of the satiating power of a meal or food. The SQ is an indicator of the power of a food, food component, or drug to suppress motivation to eat. The SQ provides an indication of the capacity of an individual's signaling system and is an interaction between the individual and the food. The SQ can therefore reveal features of the individual (who has eaten) or the food (that has been eaten).

In essence, the SQ is an expression of the change in motivation to eat as a function of energy consumed. Hence, SQ is calculated as follows:

$$SQ = \frac{\text{change in subjective appetite sensation (mm)}}{\text{Energy Intake (kcal or kJ)}}$$

The units of SQ are mm/kcal or mm/kJ and can be calculated temporally by subtracting the postingestive period value from the premeal (baseline) value (see Figure 8.6). The schematic diagram in Figure 8.6 describes how the SQ can be calculated for several time points to provide a temporal pattern of SQ. If the denominator (i.e., energy intake) is a constant, the SQ simply reflects the temporal change in subjective appetite sensation. The SQ provides added value when comparing foods or meals of varying energy intake. The SQ data presented in Figure 8.7 are an example of when this is useful. Therefore, deriving the SQ immediately after the meal and temporally afterwards provides valuable information about the immediate and delayed effect of foods or a meal. The SQ was used to compare the satiating power of three preloads varying in energy and macronutrient value: a high-energy, high-carbohydrate (CHO) meal (■); high-fat, high-energy meal (+); and a low-energy, high-CHO meal (*). Figure 8.7

shows that the low-energy, high-CHO meal suppressed hunger the most immediately after consumption per unit of energy, but by 17:00, the effect was reversed and the meal exerted the least reduction of hunger. This provides a good example of how the SQ can be used to demonstrate that the satiating efficiency of foods varies temporally. The SQ has been effectively used to assess the effect of a drug on appetite (Chapman et al., 2005) and the effect of food palatability (Yeomans, Mobini, Elliman, Walker, & Stevenson, 2006), as well as to characterize a low-satiety phenotype that can predict long-term changes in body weight (Drapeau et al., 2005; Drapeau et al., 2007). However, it should be noted that because of the nonlinear relationship between energy consumed and the consequent suppression of hunger, the SQ works optimally when used with a meal of fixed size.

Advantages and Wider Implications

In summary, the advantage of EARS is that it provides a high-quality and more efficient method of data collection and management. VAS is easy to administer and instruct for research participants to understand. The descriptors are provided, so participants do not need to generate their own descriptive terms, which produce a more standardized format that is less vulnerable to variability in interpretation. VAS is also flexible, in that the questions and anchored labels can be altered to suit the manipulation. VAS can also be administered to a large number of participants at a single time.

One of the key advantages of the EARS is that it can be used in the laboratory and free-living environment. In addition, it is more flexible by offering a wider range of applications. For example, with the improved technology and mobility of mobile devices, it will be possible to incorporate a self-report diary for food intake, physical activity, and adverse events. This could be very useful in clinical trials.

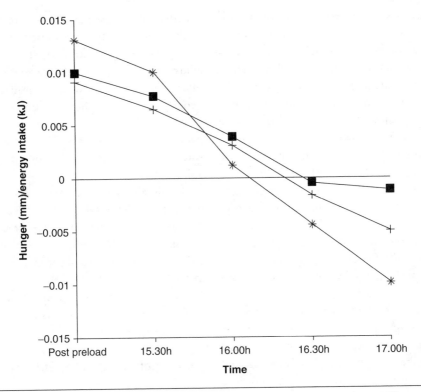

Figure 8.7   Changes in the Satiety Quotient (SQ) Over Time Following Three Different Isocaloric
Preload Manipulations

NOTE: The preload manipulation with the strongest action immediately after consumption (post preload) would have
the weakest action if measured at 17:00.

Sensory Aspects of Appetite Measurement

The measurement of sensory aspects of appetite as opposed to the psychophysical measurement of sensory characteristics (discrimination of tastes and odors, intensity ratings, etc.) has involved taste reactivity responses in a variety of species (including human infants; Steiner, Glaser, Hawilo, & Berridge, 2001), single-cell neuronal recording (E. T. Rolls, 2007), and self-report in humans (B. J. Rolls, Rolls, Rowe, & Sweeney, 1981). Hedonic responses to sensory features of food have been scrutinized using functional magnetic resonance imaging (fMRI) and other scanning technologies (Geliebter et al., 2006;

O'Doherty et al., 2000; Smeets & Westerterp-Plantenga, 2006).

Why is so much effort placed on the measurement of sensory aspects of appetite control? Since sensory characteristics of foods and drinks influence the hedonic judgment of the item, this, in turn, affects both food choice and intake. Food is a natural reward with three components: a "liking" or hedonic component, a motivational or "wanting" component, and a learned component (Berridge & Robinson, 2003).

Foods are chosen on the basis of their appearance, smell, texture, and taste, together with prior experience with those sensory attributes and their postingestive consequences. Humans are born with the ability to detect and respond to distinctive tastes. When exposed to a sweet stimulus, they indicate approach tendencies (positive affective responses such as smiling) but avoidance (negative affective responses such as gaping) to bitter tastes (Steiner, 1979). These gusto-facial responses are also observed in nonhuman primates (Steiner et al., 2001). The tendency to like sweet foods and to dislike bitter foods appears to be "hardwired." Therefore, infants must acquire preferences for a variety of complex foods beyond naturally sweet foods to meet complex nutritional needs. They do this by learning to associate particular sensory features of the food with their postingestive consequences (see Brunstrom, 2007, for a review). Sensory features of foods also influence how much is consumed once eating is initiated.

As soon as food is seen and smelled, preparation to eat is signaled by saliva secretion, cephalic phase hormone release, and indicators of arousal such as increased galvanic skin response and heart rate (Stroebele & de Castro, 2006). The sight and smell of foods with particular sensory properties (and prior learning histories) produce measurable anticipatory responses. For example, sham feeding a high-fat cake elicits greater levels of pancreatic polypeptide than sham feeding a low-fat cake (Crystal & Teff, 2006).

Sensory features of foods are detected and processed in the early stages of the satiety cascade (see Figure 8.2). Signals arising from the gut provide both orosensory-positive feedback and postingestive-negative feedback that control how much is consumed. Vagal efferent activity is stimulated by the presence of food in the gut, and this may induce further intake (Batterham & Bloom, 2003). Orosensory feedback stimulates eating while postingestive feedback inhibits eating (G. P. Smith, 2000). During the meal, positive orosensory stimulation eventually declines while negative feedback increases (Wiepkema, 1971). The meal ends when negative feedback exceeds or meets the strength of positive feedback (G. P. Smith, 1996).

Manipulating orosensory stimulation will enhance (or inhibit) the pleasantness of the food, and this influences intake. How are the effects of these manipulations measured in relation to appetite? A simple means of doing this is to adjust one aspect of the food, say sweetness, then offer both items (control and adjusted) simultaneously and measure how much of each is consumed. Indeed, this kind of forced-choice paradigm is routinely used in preference measurements (see Sclafani, 2004, for a review of the animal literature).

Simply altering the flavor of a food reliably increases the amount consumed (Bellisle, Lucas, Amrani, & Le Magnen, 1984; Henry et al., 2003; Yeomans et al., 1997). An increase of 10 mm on a 100-mm visual analog scale produces an increase in intake of around 100 g (Bobroff & Kissileff, 1986), and this has been confirmed elsewhere (Yeomans et al., 1997; Yeomans & Symes, 1999).

Fundamental Assessment Issues

Originally, in 1956, Le Magnen (see Le Magnen & Booth, 1999) set out to investigate the effects of manipulating sensory properties of food such as odor on amount consumed in the rat. He adapted rats over 32 days to a synthetic diet offered 2 hours in the morning and a standard diet 2 hours in the afternoon. The synthetic diets were presented with one of four different odors. After this period, the morning meal was changed to include presentation of each of the flavored diets for 30 minutes at a time. Simply changing the odor of the diet produced hyperphagia with 72% more consumed compared to the single-flavor condition. This experiment demonstrated the power of orosensory stimulation to disrupt appetite control. According to Le Magnen (Le Magnen & Booth, 1999), each of the four odors had "acquired a specific capacity to satiate the rat" but that providing the succession of four odors in the same meal "disturbed this adapted control and overeating was provoked" (Le Magnen & Booth, 1999).

The enhancing effect of variety has since been shown many times in humans (Hetherington,

Anderson, Norton, & Newson, 2006; B. J. Rolls, Rowe, et al., 1981). Thus, a simple measure of the impact of manipulating sensory aspects of food on appetite is to assess amount consumed. In an attempt to replicate Le Magnen's findings, Rolls and her colleagues also included ratings of the pleasantness of the taste of the foods offered (B. J. Rolls, Rolls, et al., 1981; B. J. Rolls, Rowe, et al., 1981). They found that self-reported pleasantness declined in response to the eaten food but not to other foods. This phenomenon, called *sensory-specific satiety*, demonstrated that the hedonic judgments of sensory and other characteristics of foods were not intrinsic to the food but changed as a function of intake. This methodology provided insight into the variety effect: that the hedonic response to the eaten food declines but remains positive to other uneaten foods. Offering different foods either simultaneously or in succession enhances intake within a meal.

Changes in response to a food stimulus as it is eaten to satiety can be measured using single-cell recording in the nonhuman primate brain (E. T. Rolls, Murzi, Yaxley, Thorpe, & Simpson, 1986). The firing rate of single cells in the hypothalamus declines in response to the presentation of cues associated with the eaten food. For example, presenting a model peanut to an alert macaque fed to satiety on real peanuts results in a decreased firing rate both to the real and the model peanut (E. T. Rolls et al., 1986). Clearly, this methodology cannot be applied easily to humans. Advances in neuroimaging techniques have provided a platform from which to investigate sensory aspects of appetite. For example, fMRI responsiveness to the odor of an eaten food declines relative to that for a different odor (O'Doherty et al., 2000), demonstrating sensory-specific satiety.

Description of the Methods

Investigating how sensory characteristics of foods influence intake involves both objective and subjective measures. Quantifying how much is consumed is achieved by weighing foods

before and after the meal. Investigators then translate weight (g) or number of units (portions) into energy and macronutrient composition. Subjective measures involve self-report of appetite (see section on VAS above) and the pleasantness of the foods offered.

To assess sensory-specific satiety, investigators screen participants (usually by telephone) to ensure that they like the foods in the study and that they have no allergies, medical conditions, or other contraindications (such as taking medications) that affect appetite. Those who are screened are then invited to the laboratory for a taste test to confirm liking for test foods. This highlights the difference between acceptance (a judgment made about the food as it is tasted) and preference (a judgment made about foods in relation to other foods from memory; Cardello & Maller, 1982). To be recruited into an experiment, participants should judge the food as more pleasant than neutral (say 50 mm on a 100-mm scale). The participant returns to the laboratory for the experimental session after the taste test with specific instructions about eating and activity before the test day. For example, for a lunchtime study, on the night before the session, participants are asked to avoid alcohol and to refrain from excessive exercise and then to eat and drink nothing after 10 p.m. They then attend the laboratory for a fixed breakfast or to consume their normal breakfast and, in both cases, to refrain from eating and drinking (except water) for at least 3 hours between breakfast and the lunch session. This is done to ensure that all participants are similarly food deprived for the experiment and in an equivalent state prior to each test session.

Upon arrival in the laboratory, participants record intake and activity during the previous evening to check compliance with instructions. If the participant has complied, then the experiment can begin. Typically, participants are asked to provide appetite ratings either on a fixed-point (Likert) or visual analog scale. They are then given a series of small containers with samples of foods to taste and rate. They are instructed to drink chilled water before and after each taste to clear the mouth. While the food is in the mouth, the participant is asked to rate how pleasant the appearance, smell, texture, and/or taste of the food is and how strong his or her desire to eat this food is at this moment. There may be as few as two foods (the target and one uneaten food) or as many as nine foods with the target embedded in the array. The order of foods tasted is maintained within and across sessions.

Participants rate the pleasantness of various sensory aspects of foods (appearance, smell, texture, and/or taste) on visual analog scales (100- to 500-mm lines). They are then offered a meal usually consisting of a large amount of the target food. The instruction given is to eat as much or as little as they wish to eat until they feel comfortably full. It is important to use a script for this instruction (as per SOPs discussed above) so that it does not vary (according to the SOP outlined earlier) and to encourage intake that is not a measure of capacity (how much can you eat?) but about satiety (how much do you wish to eat until you feel you have had enough?). When the meal is offered to the participant, a stopwatch or other timer is used. Time taken to consume the meal and time points beyond the meal for further ratings can be determined.

Since the dependent variable (amount consumed) can be influenced by the instruction, this must be carefully worded and delivered in the same way each time. Also, amount eaten can be influenced by portion size (B. J. Rolls, Roe, & Meengs, 2007). Therefore, the amount offered must be carefully controlled. This should be greater than a typical serving size to allow for individual differences in satiation but not too little to encourage "cleaning the plate." Meal size is generally piloted for participants to select an amount to be offered so that the lower and upper limits are known. If both men and women are involved in the study, then account must be taken of sex differences. Intake is influenced by the presence of others (Hetherington, Foster, Anderson, & Norton, 2006); therefore, most sensory-specific satiety experiments are conducted with participants eating alone with no distractions.

Participants must not read or listen to music during the test meal. Their attention should be focused on eating to facilitate satiation and for the experiment to be uncontaminated by extraneous variables.

Sensory-specific satiety is maximal immediately after eating, so a second set of ratings is generally administered 2 minutes after the meal has ended. Ratings can then be repeated at intervals following the meal for up to 2 or more hours (e.g., Hetherington, Rolls, & Burley, 1989). This method permits changes from baseline of the judged pleasantness of the food to be tracked before and after the meal and allows comparison of changes in pleasantness against amount eaten as well as changes in other subjective ratings, including appetite and mood.

The Universal Eating Monitor (UEM), first developed by Kissileff, Klingsberg, and Van Itallie (1980), permits ratings to be administered *during* the meal (e.g., Yeomans, 2000). Similarly, rate of eating, an important measure of appetitiveness, can be measured. However, interrupting participants to taste and rate foods during the meal may affect intake. Yeomans et al. (1997) reported that within-meal pauses after each 50 g of food eaten to rate appetite increased amount eaten. Investigators need to balance their interest in tracking changes in pleasantness and appetite during the meal against the impact this has on intake.

Modified sham feeding in humans involves chewing a meal but not swallowing. A meal that is sham fed for the time it would take to eat normally indicates that postingestive feedback is not necessary for the development of sensory-specific satiety (E. T. Rolls & Rolls, 1997; Smeets & Westerterp-Plantenga, 2006). Modified sham feeding involves chewing but not swallowing food and allows independent assessment of positive and negative feedback since orosensory stimulation is intact but gastric feedback is absent.

At the end of the test session, the investigator will have baseline ratings of appetite and pleasantness, the amount of food consumed, duration of eating (and rate if using the UEM), and ratings of appetite and pleasantness immediately after eating (during eating if using the UEM) and at intervals beyond the meal. Changes in subjective pleasantness and appetite can be tracked as a function of objectively measured intake. The participant may then return to the laboratory to undertake another session with independent variables manipulated such as food-related characteristics (sensory features, energy density, macronutrient composition, palatability) or group differences (age, weight, or clinical status).

Assessment of Sensory-Specific Effects in Different Groups

Sensory-specific satiety has been measured in children, adolescents, and young and older adults. Comparisons have been made between normal-weight, overweight, and obese individuals as well as patients with eating disorders, including anorexia nervosa, bulimia nervosa, and binge eating and other clinical conditions, including cancer (Davis, Walsh, Lagman, & Yavuszen, 2006). The primary reason is to compare "normal" satiation processes with a potentially aberrant expression of this. Thus, if obese individuals fail to show normal sensory-specific satiety, this may facilitate overeating. Snoek, Huntjens, Van Gemert, de Graaf, and Weenen (2004) compared sensory-specific satiety to high-fat foods between normal-weight and obese women. However, like others before them, no differences in sensory-specific satiety were found on the basis of weight status (Hetherington & Rolls, 1988, 1989).

Both age (B. J. Rolls & McDermott, 1991) and eating disorder diagnosis (Hetherington & Rolls, 1988, 1989) do produce differences in sensory-specific satiety. Older adults fail to show normal sensory-specific satiety (B. J. Rolls & McDermott, 1991) while children express sensory-specific satiety comparable with young adults (Birch & Deysher, 1986). This may reflect the true "anorexia" of aging in which appetite systems are impaired with aging (see Hetherington, 1998).

In contrast, patients with anorexia nervosa tend to express sensory-specific satiety very readily

and with relatively small amounts of food (Hetherington & Rolls, 1988), whereas patients with bulimia nervosa fail to show sensory-specific satiety alongside generally poor regulatory responses to preloads (Hetherington & Rolls, 1991). Failure to find differences between obese and normal-weight individuals is likely due to binge-eating status. For example, Mirch et al. (2006) found that overweight binge-eating children consumed more test meal and reported shorter satiety duration than overweight children with no previous history of binge eating. Therefore, normal sensory-specific satiety is expected across weight groups in the absence of binge eating, but binge eating weakens satiety mechanisms, including sensory-specific satiety.

Measuring Food Selection

Establishing a valid food selection methodology is fraught with pitfalls. This is one reason why the approach has not been developed extensively, and the area is ripe for innovation. The difficulty depends in large part on the degree of choice to be offered. Inviting participants to eat from a huge array of randomly assembled foods is not likely to lead to a clear understanding. For example, a free-selection buffet is a poor way of measuring preferences for particular macronutrients and will reveal very little about the determinants of food selection. A strong methodology will exert control over the significant nutritional and sensory aspects of each item so that the mechanisms underlying its selection can be identified. This can be achieved most readily when choices are restricted. The option facing experimenters is whether to use a two-choice model (e.g., protein vs. carbohydrate), a three-choice model (e.g., protein, carbohydrate, and fat), or a meal based on sensory-nutrient relationships (e.g., sweet or savory taste with high or low fat).

A common tool for assessing food selection in the laboratory is the simultaneous-choice model where the independent variable (e.g., macronutrient selection) is manipulated across multiple choices within one meal (e.g., high-protein vs. high-carbohydrate foods). Note that this model can be distinguished from the sequential-choice model where the independent variable is manipulated across two or more meals, consumed on separate days (Blundell, Burley, Cotton, & Lawton, et al., 1993).

The dependent variable is usually defined as the intake (energy or weight consumed) from each condition. The simultaneous-choice design is generally considered a reliable measure of spontaneous energy intake and food selection in the laboratory. In one within-subjects design, Arvaniti, Richard, and Tremblay (2000) used a three-choice model repeated over two sessions to test whether participants' selections were consistent. The authors reported high correlations between amount consumed in energy ($r = .97$), fat ($r = .97$), carbohydrate ($r = .92$), and protein ($r = .82$) between the experimental sessions when separated by at least 1 week.

The food (or food attributes) available in the environment is a major determining factor in food selection. Therefore, the food environment created in the laboratory situation will also largely determine the "free" selection of foods. For this reason, the choices offered should be carefully controlled, while the dimensions of interest to the research objectives are systematically manipulated. Food-specific attributes that influence food selection include branding and labeling, physical properties (liquid or solid), visual appearance, micronutrient content, energy density, texture and viscosity, temperature, familiarity, palatability, sensory properties, and macronutrient content. However, practical constraints usually dictate that test foods are selected or designed to vary as much as possible on the desired variable, while keeping variation in other confounding variables to an acceptable minimum.

In the past, very restricted designs that permit choices between two foods were frequently used to investigate the role of serotonin in carbohydrate selection (e.g., Wurtman & Wurtman, 1982–1983). However, the strength of such restricted procedures depends on the protein and carbohydrate choices being matched for fat

content, sweetness, palatability, and so on. With regard to the selection of dietary fat, a different model has used four choices where, rather than controlling for all sensory properties, the dimension of taste has been dichotomized into "sweet" and "savory" (see below).

Stubbs and colleagues developed an impressive but labor-intensive method of investigating macronutrient selection in the laboratory (Stubbs et al., 1997). They constructed a simultaneous-choice model consisting of three groups of food items rich in fat, carbohydrate, or protein (~60% by energy), with the remaining energy divided between the other macronutrients to counterbalance the conditions. Common, familiar foods were included to ensure participants had some experience with the postingestive consequences of each food option. The model controlled for differences in food preferences by involving a sizable range of foods in each condition (10 items) such that food selection would not be compromised by avoidance of one or two foods in a particular condition (see Table 8.1 for a list of foods used).

To test the paradigm, the authors employed a within-subjects design consisting of 4 treatment days. Participants received one of four breakfast plus snack preload conditions: high fat, high protein, high carbohydrate, or an equal mix of each macronutrient. These foods were closely matched for energy, volume, appearance, and density and varied in macronutrient content according to the proportions used in their simultaneous choice model. After consuming the breakfast and snack, participants were given ad libitum access to the lunch (as much or as little as they wanted). Lunchtime selection and intake were recorded in the laboratory by weighing foods before and after consumption. On examination of the lunchtime intake data, the authors found their method was sensitive to the macronutrient manipulation of the preloads. Administration of the high-fat preload (60% by energy) led to a selective decrease in fat and energy intake during the lunch. This indicates that the model is sensitive. Since its inception,

Table 8.1   Example 1: High-Protein, High-Carbohydrate, and High-Fat Foods Included in Simultaneous-Choice Model

High Protein	High Carbohydrate	High Fat	Salad
Shrimp sandwich	Lettuce and grape sandwich	Tuna and mayonnaise sandwich	Celery
Salmon sandwich	Banana sandwich	Egg and cheese sandwich	Cucumber
Tuna sandwich	Jam sandwich	Cheese sandwich	Lettuce
Corned beef sandwich	Honey sandwich	Salami sandwich	Sweet corn
Turkey breast	Savory rice	Pork pie	Cress
Chicken breast	Pot noodle	Sausage rolls	
Fromage frais	Pizza topping cracker	Philadelphia cheese and crispbread	
Crab sticks	Raisins	Pistachio nuts	
Crab pate cracker	Swiss roll	Nuts and raisins	
Cottage cheese cracker	Twiglets	Profiteroles and cream	

SOURCE: Stubbs et al. (1997).

this model of assessing food selection has not seen widespread use. However, this may be due more to the time and expense involved in preparation than to its methodological limitations or ecological validity.

Recently, a methodological platform has been developed using distinct real foods in conjunction with a computer procedure involving a parallel matrix of food photographs. Participants have the opportunity to make objective, real food choices (and eat the foods) and simulated selections via the computer (which they do not eat). This combined approach provides additional information on key determinants of food selection, based on the concept of liking versus wanting (Finlayson, King, & Blundell, 2007). Other indirect measures of wanting or motivation for food have also become available; for example, Epstein and colleagues have developed a food reinforcement task where participants "work" for food items on a progressive ratio schedule (e.g., Saelens & Epstein, 1996). Furthermore, some researchers are using food-based versions of the Stimulus-Response Compatibility Task often used in addiction research (e.g., Giesen,

Havermans, & Jansen, 2008). Further discussion will focus on the procedure described in Finlayson, King, and Blundell (2008) as it is especially relevant to experimental methodologies concerned with food selection.

A four-choice model was developed to assess food selection according to dimensions of fat content and taste properties. This 2×2 design (high or low fat with sweet or savory taste) allowed a variety of foods to be administered (thus enhancing ecological validity) while enabling a degree of counterbalancing of conditions. Foods were selected according to criteria of > 50% or < 25% fat by energy. Energy values and fat content were balanced across taste conditions, and taste properties were matched across fat conditions. In addition, acceptability and pleasantness of test foods were assessed using a taste panel. In this way, eight commercially available foods—two high-fat savory, two low-fat savory, two high-fat sweet, and two low-fat sweet items—were included (see Table 8.2).

The computer procedure was adapted from a tool used initially as a word list (Hill & Blundell, 1982–1983) and specifically developed to assess

Table 8.2   Example 2: High-Fat Savory, Low-Fat Savory, High-Fat Sweet, and Low-Fat Sweet Foods Included in Simultaneous-Choice Model

High-Fat Savory	Low-Fat Savory	High-Fat Sweet	Low-Fat Sweet
Ready-salted chips	Fresh garden salad	Milk chocolate	Fresh fruit salad
Cheddar cheese	Herb biscuits	Flapjack	Fruit biscuits

separate constructs of liking and wanting (Finlayson et al., 2008). The food stimuli presented in the procedure were selected based on dimensions of fat content and taste properties to match those used in the lunch model. The items were selected from a database of photographic stimuli by a panel of volunteers and sorted into conditions of high-fat savory, low-fat savory, high-fat sweet, and low-fat sweet foods. A total of 20 different photographs of household food items were included in the procedure (see Table 8.3).

The computer procedure incorporates measures of liking and wanting into a paradigm where relative preferences for each food condition are assessed. Separate tasks for each measure are used to prevent cross-contamination between measures. One task obtains introspective hedonic measures for each food item independently, using VAS. In addition, implicit wanting is measured indirectly by a behavioral forced-choice task. In this task, a food item from one of the four food conditions is paired with one item from the remaining conditions to form a series of 150 trials in which the goal is to select the food "you most want to eat now" (see Figure 8.8). By recording reaction time of selections made for stimuli in each food category, implicit changes in behavior related to the strength of motivation can be detected. Data from the forced-choice task together with VAS ratings of liking and wanting are recorded online.

This combined platform has been used in a study to investigate the effect of taste properties on food selection. Two preloads were designed to vary only in their sensory properties (savory or sweet taste). Participants attended the laboratory in a fasted state for two lunchtime visits. They

were required to complete the computer procedure before and after consumption of the savory or sweet preload (shown in Figure 8.9a). After a 30-minute rest, participants were given ad libitum access to the lunch (shown in Figure 8.9b). Acceptability of all foods was confirmed on a day prior to testing.

Results confirmed that the food selection model was sensitive to the preload manipulation. Intake of savory foods was lower in response to the savory preload. In contrast, the preload manipulation did not influence the selection of sweet foods. Findings from the computer procedure provided more information on the effects of the preloads. Consumption of the savory preload was associated with a number of sensory effects: A large decrease in ratings of liking and wanting for savory foods was revealed, while ratings for sweet foods were increased; conversely, implicit wanting increased for sweet foods, while no change was found for savory foods. In contrast, the sweet preload produced decreased ratings of liking and wanting for all foods and no effect on implicit wanting. Taken together, this combined model permitted a richer interpretation of food selection behavior. The preload manipulation was linked to changes in selection of savory foods in the lunch via effects brought about by the savory and not the sweet preload condition. Although combining real and photographic foods may enhance the assessment of food selection, there are also some limitations to this approach. It is unknown, for example, if visual representations of food are responded to in comparable ways to real foods. Furthermore, the photograph responses provide no information

Table 8.3   High-Fat Savory, Low-Fat Savory, High-Fat Sweet, and Low-Fat Sweet Food Stimuli Used in Food Preference Questionnaire

High-Fat Savory	Low-Fat Savory	High-Fat Sweet	Low-Fat Sweet
Ready-salted chips	Boiled new potatoes	Blueberry muffin	Fruit salad
Salted peanuts	Pilau rice	Cream cake	Marshmallows
Swiss cheese	Bread roll	Jam doughnut	Sugared popcorn
French fries	Spaghetti in sauce	Shortbread	Jelly babies
Mixed olives	Cheese biscuits	Milk chocolate	Strawberry Jell-O

SOURCE: Finlayson, King, and Blundell (2008).

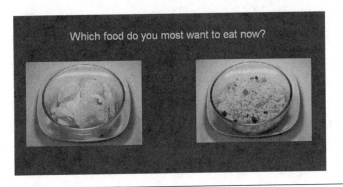

Figure 8.8   Monitor Display of Forced-Choice Components of the Food Preference Questionnaire

on the amount of food likely to be consumed, but they clearly indicate the direction and speed (implicit action) of the response.

Success of food selection methodologies rests on the clarity and lack of ambiguity in the choices offered so that there is transparency underlying the choices made. Ecological validity can be improved by increasing the number, familiarity, and acceptability of foods included in the model, which will also raise costs in terms of time and resources. Including fewer, carefully selected foods will allow greater manipulation of the independent variable, but this in turn must be sacrificed to some extent for sufficient control over confounding variables inherent to the available foods. Incorporating additional checks and measures of food selection can strengthen the interpretation of an effect, but interreliability of measures should be verified.

Automated Food Measuring Systems

While the macro-structural measures of eating behavior, such as total intake and intake of individual food items, potentially require little automation to record data, the measuring of minute-by-minute changes in human feeding behavior is far more methodologically challenging. It requires the constant monitoring of the research participant through direct observation, full automation, or a combination of both (Hill, Rogers, & Blundell, 1995).

a

b

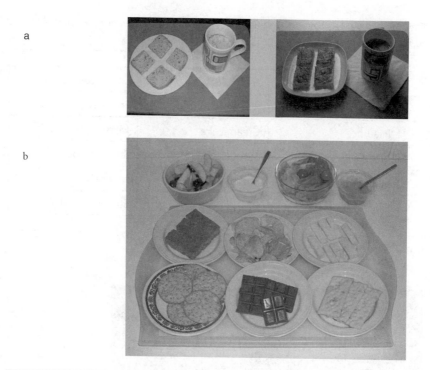

Figure 8.9   (a) Examples of Savory (Left) and Sweet (Right) Preloads Controlled for Energy, Volume, and Macronutrient Content and (b) Example of a Simultaneous-Choice Design Consisting of High-Fat Savory, Low-Fat Savory, High-Fat Sweet, and Low-Fat Sweet Foods

Why Measure Microstructure of Feeding Behavior?

The added value of an alternative technique is if it can reveal the effects of experimental manipulations or comparisons beyond the standard methodological approach. In the case of microstructural analysis, eating rate and changes in its trajectory (cumulative intake curves), both directly measured in micro-structural analysis, have been shown to be useful in detecting both the effects of experimental manipulations and individual differences in eating behavior. These changes in eating rate would be difficult, if not impossible, to identify using the macro-structural approach.

Examining within-meal eating rate has been useful in the study of drugs on eating behavior (Halford et al., 2007; Rogers & Blundell, 1979; Yeomans & Gray; 1997). Within-meal changes in

eating rate also have long history of use in defining an "obese eating style." Meyer and Pudel (1972) were among the first to observe decelerating cumulative intake curves associated with the normal biological development of satiety and the deviation from these characterizing the behavior of many obese (Stunkard, Coll, Lundquist, & Meyers, 1980; Stunkard & Kaplan, 1977). Failure to demonstrate a reduction in eating rate during a meal has been observed in obese children (Barkeling, Ekman, & Rössner, 1992; Laessle, Uhl, & Lindel, 2001; Laessle, Uhl, Lindel, & Müller, 2001), in syndromes characterized by severe obesity such as Prader-Willi (Lindgren et al., 2000), in the morbidly obese (Näslund, Gutniak, Skogar, Rössner, & Hellström, 1998), and sometimes (Halford et al., 2007) but not always in obese adults (Barkeling, Elfhag, Rooth, & Rössner, 2003; Westerterp-Plantenga, 2000).

Observation and Automation

To study eating rate, many researchers have visually coded eating behavior (Rogers & Blundell, 1979) while others developed automated means of assessing intake, such as the UEM (Guss & Kissileff, 2000). Coding of live or recorded behavior, like the automated measurement of behavior, has a long history in feeding research (Hill et al., 1995). Each provides advantages. By directly observing and coding behavior, experimenters can gain a rich variety of differing measures such as number of chews or swallows of food—and, consequently, chewing and swallowing rates as well as amount of chews per mouthful—but cannot estimate the amount consumed in each of these (Hill et al., 1995).

In contrast, those using automated procedures gain a more accurate measurement of the rate of consumption by continuously measuring what is removed from plate, glass, or bowl during the meal. Standard mechanistic approaches (see later) yield gram per minute intake, the most commonly analyzed automated behavioral measure, but also with finer resolution can determine amount per mouthful/spoonful and the intermouthful/spoonful interval. Moreover, the use of other novel automated techniques such as the BITE and the edogram (see below) could potentially yield most of the measures gained by behavioral monitoring. Therefore, automation can produce limitations on the type of data collected (although a combination of methodologies may remedy this), but the data yielded could be considered free from potential observer bias. Automation currently limits measurement of intake to one homogeneous liquid or semisolid set meals such as yogurts, soups, casseroles of various kinds, pasta meals, and Swedish hashes, preventing any study of food choice (Hill et al., 1995).

Development of Automation

Automated measurement of food intake in man can be traced to Jordan, Wieland, Zebley, Stellar, and Stunkard (1966) using a system of a straw and a hidden reservoir of liquid food. Meyer and Pudel (1972) used a similar dispenser to examine differences between overweight, normal-weight, and underweight participants. The authors characterized two types of intake patterns; the first type was a biological (negatively accelerating) satiation curve seen in most of the normal-weight participants, and the other was a linear intake trajectory that tended to be observed in the obese.

Other systems such as the BITE (Moon, 1979) and the edogram (Bellisle & Le Magnen, 1980; 1981; Bellisle et al., 1984) were subsequently developed to measure the intake of solid foods. The next major development came when Kissileff and colleagues developed the UEM, consisting of hidden scales connected to a computer (Guss & Kissileff, 2000; Kissileff & Guss, 2001; Kissileff et al., 1980; Kissileff, Thornton, & Becker, 1982). The electronic scales were hidden in a draw under the top of a standard wooden table, and on the scales a cutout panel of the table rested at the same height as the rest of the tabletop. The whole table was then covered in a table cloth (see Figure 8.10). The computer, connected to the scales located in a separate experimenter's room, measured the weight of the plate every 3 seconds, with the amount of the balance continually being subtracted at each time point from the initial amount. Experimenters could observe the participant's behavior though closed-circuit television monitors from the control room containing the UEM computer (Guss & Kissileff, 2000; Kissileff & Guss, 2001).

This basic design of the UEM has been replicated in systems such as the VIKTOR system, which has been used extensively in Sweden (e.g., Barkeling et al., 1992; Barkeling et al., 2003; Näslund et al., 1997; Näslund et al., 1998; Näslund et al., 1999), and derivations of the Sussex Meal Pattern Monitor (SMPM) used by laboratories in the United Kingdom (Halford et al., 2007; Yeomans, 2000). Modified versions of the UEM have also been developed in the Netherlands (Westerterp-Plantenga, 2000), Germany (Hubel, Laessle, Lehrke, & Jass, 2006; Laessle, Uhl, & Lindle; 2001; Laessle,

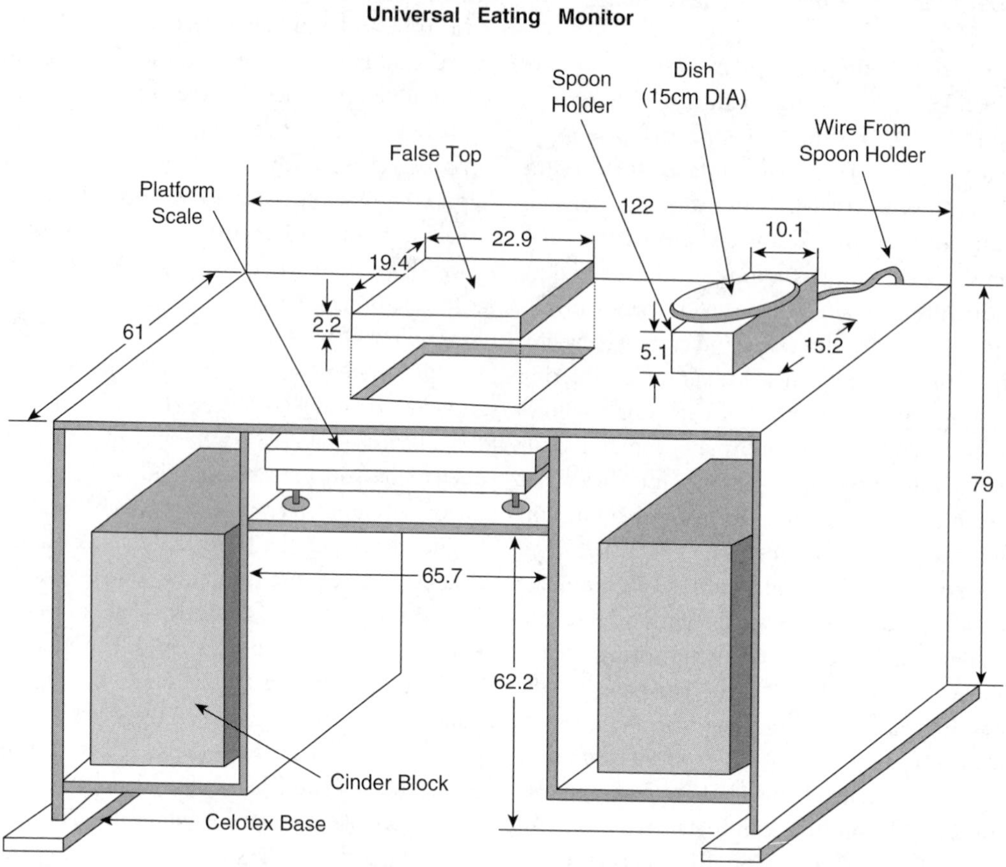

Universal Eating Monitor

Figure 8.10 The Universal Eating Monitor (UEM) Originally Designed by Kissileff, Klinsberg, and Van Itallie (1980)

Uhl, Lindel, & Müller, 2001), and the United States (Williamson et al., 2005; Williamson et al., 2006). These systems all generate eating curves (intake (g) against time (min)), which can be defined as decelerating or accelerating based on the coefficient of the slope of the curve.

However, beyond these eating rate measures, a number of researchers have focused on the relationship between changes in self-reported appetite (e.g., hunger and satiety) and cumulative intake within a meal. Such research has been useful in further characterizing satiety disturbances in bulimia nervosa (Kissileff et al., 1996) as well as the experimental effects of manipulations of volume, energy content, and palatability (Gray,

French, Robinson, & Yeomans, 2002, 2003; Robinson et al., 2005; Wentzlaff, Guss, & Kissileff, 1995; Yeomans, 1996, 2000; Yeomans et al., 1997; Yeomans, Lartamo, Proter, Lee, & Gray, 2001; Yeomans, Lee, Gray, & French, 2001). Different laboratories have collected these within-meal ratings in various ways using paper-and-pen methods with remote-controlled tape recordings (Guss & Kissileff, 2000; Wentzlaff et al., 1995) or a second computer for the participant to input the ratings (Westerterp-Plantenga, 2000). The SMPM allows the UEM computer to interrupt the participant to measure within-meal changes of appetite at either set time points or when specific amounts of food have been consumed (Yeomans, 2000).

The approach using serial interruptions of a meal to assess changes in appetite across the course of a meal was first used by Hill, Magson, and Blundell (1984; Wentzlaff et al., 1995), and this approach accounts for within- and between-participant differences in amount eaten in specific time periods, ensuring comparable ratings across and with subjects (Yeomans, 1996; Yeomans et al., 1997). However, researchers are mindful of the potential impact of interrupting participants while eating (Yeomans et al., 1997).

Validity and Reliability. Kissileff et al. (1982) demonstrated the relationship between UEM outcomes and self-reported real-world intakes (i.e., external validity). However, a true test of any measure of eating behavior is whether or not it varies in a way consistent with the expected nutritional, physiological, and psychological factors, including individual differences, associated with appetite expression. Various data sets show that UEM curves are influenced by gender and food deprivation, as well as by the composition and palatability of test meals, demonstrating that they are valid representations of the changes in appetite that occur within meals (for reviews, see Guss & Kissileff, 2000; Westerterp-Plantenga, 2000). With regard to manipulations in hunger, satiety, and palatability, measuring changes in within-meal appetite ratings may be particularly useful (Gray et al., 2002; Robinson et al., 2005; Yeomans, 2000).

UEM measurements such as cumulative intake curves have not always been able to discriminate the effects of administration of endogenous satiety factors such as glucagon-like peptide (GLP-1; Näslund et al., 1998; Näslund et al., 1999). Similarly, with the "satiety"-enhancing drug sibutramine, some researchers have failed to find any effect of drug on parameters of within-meal satiation such as eating rate or cumulative intake curves (Barkeling et al., 2003). Others have found significant effects on eating rate, reductions in within-meal hunger, increases in within-meal fullness, and a trend toward a great frequency of normal decelerating intake curves in the drug condition (Halford et al., 2007; see Figure 8.11), thus indicating that

within-meal satiation is produced by the drug. Therefore, measuring changes in appetite ratings during the meal may be particularly important in assessing the effects of hormones and drugs. These ratings can distinguish drugs such as naltrexone, known to effect palatability (ratings of how pleasant the food consumed is) rather than within-meal satiation (as measured by hunger and satiety ratings; Yeomans & Gray, 1997).

With regard to the reliability of these various micro-structural measures, many authors have commented on the consistency and stability of cumulative intake curves. In the early work of Jordan et al. (1966) and Meyer and Pudel (1972), consecutive trials showed that an individual's intake possessed large interindividual but small intraindividual variability. Modern UEM systems also possess good test-retest reliability for within-individual UEM curves (Hubel et al., 2006; Westerterp-Plantenga, 2000).

Overview and Future Developments

Justification

The presence of the obesity epidemic—with little prospect of a solution—increases the pressure on researchers to understand the processes controlling food intake. Central to this enterprise is the agreement on a strong scientific methodology that can provide reliable outcomes in different research environments and in the hands of different researchers. The methodology represents assays of behavior (and associated states) and should have the same scientific status as assays for measuring physiological variables, blood constituents, and so on. That is, the methods should give the same result independent of the research group and the testing environment. Among a number of exciting prospects, good measures of appetite control can act as biomarkers or predictors of likely weight gain and the development of obesity. This can be seen in the identification of the weak satiety phenotype

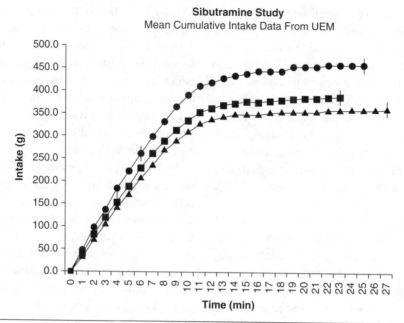

Figure 8.11   Cumulative Food Intake Curves From the UEM Showing Data for Placebo Condition (●) and Two Doses of Sibutramine (10 mg ■ & 15 mg ▲)

(Drapeau et al., 2007) and a weak compensatory index (Cecil et al., 2005).

Applications

Two applied areas where food intake methodology is becoming particularly important concern functional food research and antiobesity drug development. Both of these domains are growing in importance and intensity under pressure from the obesity epidemic. Food and nutrition companies are developing foods and food ingredients designed to exert specific effects on appetite control—and especially for the improvement of satiety. Eventually, claims will be made about the functions of such products. The substantiation of the claims, as well as their approval by appropriate legislative authorities, will depend on the presentation of scientific evidence from studies carried out under controlled conditions and conforming to guaranteed standards.

The pharmaceutical industry is also coming to rely on the strength of standardized measures of food intake and appetite motivation. At the present time, the degree of food intake suppression in Phase I clinical trials remains the best predictor of long-term weight loss in Phase III trials. In time, this will probably be replaced by more molecular (or genetic) biomarkers of subsequent weight loss. However, it is likely that pharmaceutical companies will continue to look for scientifically validated food intake studies carried out under controlled conditions and GLP standards.

Innovation

The capture of subjective sensations of appetite is often of equal importance to the measure of food intake itself. This is the case when the shape of the hunger or fullness profiles—or their dissociation one from the other—can throw light on the mechanisms underlying satiation or satiety. Such profiles can help to define the mechanisms and time course of a functional food or a drug. With this in mind, it is inevitable that automated electronic data capture devices will become much more sophisticated and more frequently used. In a short period of time, it is likely that they will replace paper-and-pencil scales. The advantages of an automated device are many, and instruments currently being developed can monitor other types of test information and a subject's personal data relevant to the food intake study.

Homeostasis and Hedonics

It is apparent that an ideological shift is taking place in the field of appetite control. After decades in which homeostatic principles have dominated thinking and theory, attention is being diverted to the role of hedonic processes controlling eating. For researchers focusing on the issue of overconsumption leading to obesity (a major current target of attention), it is being increasingly recognized—and admitted—that eating in the current obesigenic environment is stimulated by food hedonics rather than by signals of energy deficit. The term *hedonic hunger* has been coined to describe this phenomenon (Lowe & Butryn., 2007). This statement draws attention to the potency of sensory and hedonic factors of appetite control. Knowledge about the role of endocannabioids in appetite control, particularly about the function of a class of drugs known as CB1 receptor-inverse agonists, has further stimulated interest in the processes underlying food hedonics. Although it is apparent that these drugs influence homeostatic as well as hedonic mechanisms (Di Marzo & Mattias, 2005), their development has drawn attention to hedonics. It is therefore inevitable that the next few years will witness a rapid development in methodologies for the reliable measurement of hedonic processes, including liking and wanting, and the associated assessment of food selection and preference.

Quality Assurance

Food intake and associated sensations can be seen as scientific assays of the willingness to eat.

An assay must be reliable and valid. Therefore, a standardized methodology is an important step in the development of these laboratory procedures as measures of the operation of the appetite system. An agreed standard of working is important for theory development (so that researchers understand each other's ways of working) and for commercial applications (so that industrial partners can have faith in the outcomes of research). Alongside the tools and techniques themselves, we can describe a set of procedures to govern the conduct of researchers using the tools. This code of conduct represents GLP, the principles of which can be set down as part of the operating procedures for any laboratory. The standardized and accurate use of the tools together with principles for recording and storing data all add to the confidence in this field of appetite research.

References

Arvaniti, K., Richard, D., & Tremblay, A. (2000). Reproducibility of energy and macronutrient intake and related substrate oxidation rates in a buffet-type meal. *British Journal of Nutrition, 83,* 489–495.

Badman, M. K., & Flier, J. S. (2005). The gut and energy balance: Visceral allies in the obesity wars. *Science, 307,* 1907–1914.

Barkeling, B., Ekman, S., & Rössner, S. (1992). Eating behaviour in obese and normal weight 11-year-old children. *International Journal of Obesity, 16,* 335–360.

Barkeling, B., Elfhag, K., Rooth, P., & Rössner, S. (2003). Short-term effects of sibutramine (Reductil™) on appetite and eating behaviour and the long-term therapeutic outcome. *International Journal of Obesity, 27,* 693–700.

Barkeling, B., King, N., Näslund, E., & Blundell, J. E. (2007). Characterisation of obese people who claim to detect no relationship between their eating pattern and sensations of hunger and fullness. *International Journal of Obesity, 31,* 435–439.

Batterham, R. L., & Bloom, S. R. (2003). The gut hormone peptide YY regulates appetite. *Annals of the New York Academy of Science, 994,* 162–168.

Bellisle, F., & Le Magnen, J. (1980). The analysis of human feeding patterns: The edogram. *Appetite, 1,* 141–150.

Bellisle, F., & Le Magnen, J. (1981). The structure of meals in humans: Eating and drinking patterns in lean and obese subjects. *Physiology & Behavior, 27,* 649–658.

Bellisle, F., Lucas, F., Amrani, R., & Le Magnen, J. (1984). Deprivation, palatability and the microstructure of meals in human subjects. *Appetite, 5,* 85–94.

Bellisle, F., McDevitt, R., & Prentice, A. (1997). Meal frequency and energy balance. *British Journal of Nutrition, 77*(Suppl. 1), S71–S81.

Berridge, K. C., & Robinson, T. E. (2003). Parsing reward. *Trends in Neurosciences, 26,* 507–513.

Berthoud, H.-R. (2006). Homeostatic and non-homeostatic pathways involved in the control of food intake and energy balance. *Obesity, 14*(Suppl.), 197S–200S.

Birch, L. L., & Deysher, M (1986). Caloric compensation and sensory specific satiety: Evidence for self regulation of food intake by young children. *Appetite, 7,* 323–331.

Blundell, J. E. (1995). The psychobiological approach to appetite and weight control. In K. D. Brownell & C. G. Fairburn (Eds.), *Eating disorders and obesity: A comprehensive handbook.* New York: Guilford.

Blundell, J. E., Burley, V. J., Cotton, J. R., & Lawton, C. L. (1993). Dietary fat and the control of energy intake: Effects of fat on meal size and post-meal satiety. *American Journal of Clinical Nutrition, 57,* 772S–778S.

Blundell, J. E., Cooling, J., & King, N. A. (2002). Differences in postprandial responses to fat and carbohydrate loads in habitual high and low fat consumers (phenotypes). *British Journal of Nutrition, 88*(2), 125–132.

Blundell, J. E., Jebb, S., Stubbs, R. J., Wilding, J. R., Lawton, C. L., Browning, L., et al. (2006). Effect of rimonabant on energy intake, motivation to eat and body weight with and without hypocaloric diet: The REBA study. *Obesity Reviews, 7,* 104.

Blundell, J. E., Lawton, C. L., Cotton, J. R., & Macdiarmid, H. I. (1996). Control of human appetite: Implications for the intake of dietary fat. *Annual Review of Nutrition, 16,* 285–319.

Blundell, J. E., Rogers, P. J., & Hill, A. J. (1987). Evaluating the satiating power of foods: Implications for acceptance and consumption. In

J. Solms, D. A. Booth, R. M. Pangbourne, & O. Raunhardt (Eds.), *Food acceptance and nutrition* (pp. 205–219). London: Academic Press.

Bobroff, E. M., & Kissileff, H. R. (1986). Effects of changes in palatability on food intake and the cumulative food intake curve of man. *Appetite, 7,* 85–96.

Brunstrom, J. M. (2007). Associative learning and the control of human dietary behavior. *Appetite, 49,* 268–271.

Brunswik, E. (1952). *The conceptual framework of psychology: International encyclopedia of unified science.* Toronto: University of Toronto Press.

Burns, A. A., Livingstone, M. B. E., Welch, R. W., Dunne, A., Robson, P. J., Lindmark, L., et al. (2000). Short term effects of yoghurt containing a novel emulsion on energy and macronutrient intakes in non obese subjects. *International Journal of Obesity, 24,* 1419–1425.

Cani, P. D., Joly, E., Horsemans, Y., & Delzenne, N. M. (2006). Oligofructose promotes satiety in healthy human: A pilot study. *European Journal of Clinical Nutrition, 60,* 567–572.

Cardello, A. V., & Maller, O. (1982). Relationships between food preferences and food acceptance ratings. *Journal of Food Science, 47,* 1553–1557.

Cecil, J. E., Palmer, C. N. A., Wrieden, W., Murrie, I., Bolton-Smith, C., Watt, P., et al. (2005). Energy intakes after preloads: Adjustment not compensation. *American Journal of Clinical Nutrition, 82,* 302–308.

Chapman, I., Parker, B., Doran, S., Feinle-Bisset, C., Wishart, J., Strobel, S., et al. (2005). Effect of pramlintide on satiety and food intake in obese subjects and subjects with type 2 diabetes. *Diabetologia, 48,* 838–848.

Cotton, J. R., Westrate, J. A., & Blundell, J. E. (1996). Replacement of dietary fat with sucrose polyester: Effects on energy intake and appetite control in non-obese males. *American Journal of Clinical Nutrition, 63,* 891–896.

Crystal, S. R., & Teff, K. L. (2006). Tasting fat: Cephalic phase hormonal responses and food intake in restrained and unrestrained eaters. *Physiology & Behavior, 89,* 213–220.

Davis, M. P., Walsh, D., Lagman, R., & Yavuszen, T. (2006). Early satiety in cancer patients: A common and important but underrecognized symptom. *Supportive Care in Cancer, 14,* 693–698.

de Castro, J. (1987). Macronutrient relationships with meal patterns and mood in the spontaneous feeding behaviour of humans. *Physiology & Behavior, 39*, 561–569.

de Castro, J., & Elmore, D. (1988). Subjective hunger relationships with meal patterns in spontaneous feeding behaviour of humans: Evidence for a casual connection. *Physiology & Behavior, 43*, 159–165.

de Graaf, C., Cardello, A. V., Kramer, F. M., Lesher, L. L., Meiselman, H. L., & Schutz, H. G. (2005). Food acceptability in field studies with US Army men and women: Relationship with food intake and food choice after repeated expsoure. *Appetite, 44*, 23–31.

de Graaf, C., de Jong, L. S., & Lambers, A. C. (1999). Palatability affects satiation but not satiety. *Physiology & Behavior, 66*, 681–688.

de Graaf, K. (1993). The validity of appetite ratings. *Appetite, 21*, 156–160.

Delargy, H. J., Lawton, C. L., Smith, F. C., King, N. A., & Blundell, J. E. (1996). Electronic appetite rating system (EARS): Validation of continuous automated monitoring of motivation to eat. *International Journal of Obesity, 20*, 104.

Di Marzo, V., & Mattias, I. (2005). Endocannabinoid control of food intake and energy balance. *Nature Neuroscience, 8*, 585–589.

DiMeglio, D. P., & Mattes, R. D. (2000). Liquid versus solid carbohydrates: Effects on food intake and body weight. *International Journal of Obesity and Related Metabolic Disorders, 24*, 794–800.

Doucet, E., St-Pierre, S., & Almeras, N. (2003). Relation between appetite ratings before and after a standard meal and estimates of daily energy intake in obese and reduced obese individuals. *Appetite, 40*, 137–143.

Drapeau, V., Blundell, J., Therrien, F., Lawton, C., Richard, D., & Tremblay, A. (2005). Appetite sensations as a marker of overall intake. *British Journal of Nutrition, 93*, 273–280.

Drapeau, V., King, N., Hetherington, M., Doucet, E., Blundell, J., & Tremblay, A. (2007). Appetite sensations and satiety quotient: Predictors of energy intake and weight loss. *Appetite, 48*, 159–166.

Dye, L., & Blundell, J. E. (2002). Functional foods: Psychological and behavioural functions. *British Journal of Nutrition, 88*(Suppl. 2), S1–S28.

Finlayson, G. S., King, N. A., & Blundell, J. E. (2007). Liking vs. wanting food: Importance for human appetite control and weight regulation. *Neuroscience & Biobehavioral Reviews, 31*, 987–1002.

Finlayson, G. S., King, N. A., & Blundell, J. E. (2008). The role of implicit wanting in relation to explicit liking and wanting for food: Implications for appetite control. *Appetite, 50*, 120–127.

Flint, A., Raben, A., Blundell, J. E., & Astrup, A. (2000). Reproducibility, power and validity of visual analogue scales in assessment of appetite sensations in a single test meal studies. *International Journal of Obesity, 24*, 38–48.

Foltin, R., Fischman, M., Emurian, C., & Rachlinski, J. (1988). Compensation for caloric dilution in humans given unrestricted access to food in a residential laboratory. *Appetite, 10*, 13–24.

Foltin, R., Fischman, M., Moran, T., Rolls, B., & Kelly, T. (1990). Caloric compensation for lunches varying in fat and carbohydrate content by humans in a residential laboratory. *American Journal of Clinical Nutrition, 52*, 969–980.

Foltin, R., Rolls, B., Moran, T., Kelly, T., McNeilis, A., & Fischman, M. (1992). Caloric, but not macronutrient, compensation by humans for required-eating occasions with meals and snack varying in fat and carbohydrate. *American Journal of Clinical Nutrition, 55*, 331–342.

Gately, P. J., King, N., Greatwood, H., Humphrey, L. C., Radley, D., Cooke, C. B., et al. (2007). Does a high-protein diet improve weight loss in overweight and obese children attending a residential weight-loss camp? A controlled trial. *Obesity, 15*, 1527–1534.

Geliebter, A., Ladell, T., Logan, M., Schneider, T., Sharafi, M., & Hirsch, J. (2006). Responsivity to food stimuli in obese and lean binge eaters using functional MRI. *Appetite, 46*, 31–35.

Giesen, J. C. A. H., Havermans, R. C., & Jansen, A. (2008). Weight, gender and the reward value of food. *Appetite, 51*, 752.

Gray, R. W., French, S. J., Robinson, T. M., & Yeomans, M. R. (2002). Dissociation of the effects of preload volume and energy content on subjective appetite and food intake. *Physiology & Behavior, 76*, 57–64.

Gray, R. W., French, S. J., Robinson, T. M., & Yeomans, M. R. (2003). Increasing preload volume with water reduces rated appetite but not food intake in healthy men even with minimum delay between preload and test meal. *Nutritional Neuroscience, 6*, 29–37.

Green, S. M., Delargy, H. J., Joanes, D., & Blundell, J. E. (1997). A satiety quotient: A formulation to assess the satiating effect of food. *Appetite, 29*, 291–304.

Guss, J. L., & Kissileff, H. R. (2000). Microstructural analysis of human ingestive patterns: From description to mechanistic hypotheses. *Neuroscience & Biobehavioral Reviews, 24,* 261–268.

Haber, G. B., Heaton, K. W., & Murphy, D. (1977). Depletion and disruption of dietary fibre. *Lancet, 2,* 679–682.

Halford, J. C. G., Boyland, E., Dovey, T. M., Huda, M., Dourish, C. T., Dawson, G., et al. (2007). A double-blind, placebo-controlled crossover study to quantify the effects of sibutramine on energy intake and energy expenditure in obese subjects during a test meal using a Universal Eating Monitor (UEM) method. *International Journal of Obesity, 31*(Suppl. 1), s151.

Henry, C. J. K., Woo, J., Lightowler, H. J., Yip, R., Lee, R., Hui, E., et al. (2003). Use of natural food flavours to increase food and nutrient intakes in hospitalised elderly in Hong Kong. *International Journal of Food Sciences and Nutrition, 54,* 321–327.

Hetherington, M., & Rolls, B. J. (1988). Sensory specific satiety and food intake in eating disorders. In B. T. Walsh (Ed.), *Eating behavior in eating disorders* (pp. 141–160). Washington, DC: American Psychiatric Press.

Hetherington, M., & Rolls, B. J. (1989). Sensory-specific satiety in anorexia and bulimia nervosa. In L. Schneider, S. Cooper, & K. Halmi (Eds.), *Psychobiology of eating disorders: Pre-clinical and clinical perspectives* (pp. 257–264). New York: New York Academy of Sciences.

Hetherington, M., & Rolls, B. J. (1991). Eating behavior in eating disorders: Effects of preloads. *Physiology & Behavior, 50,* 101–108.

Hetherington, M., Rolls, B. J., & Burley, V. J. (1989). The time course of sensory-specific satiety. *Appetite, 12,* 57–68.

Hetherington, M. M. (1995). Sensory-specific-satiety and its importance in meal termination. *Neuroscience & Biobehavioral Reviews, 20,* 113–117.

Hetherington, M. M. (1998). Taste and appetite regulation in the elderly. *Proceedings of the Nutrition Society, 57,* 625–631.

Hetherington, M. M., Anderson, A. S., Norton, G. N. M., & Newson, L. (2006). Situational effects on meal intake: A comparison of eating alone and eating with others. *Physiology & Behavior, 88,* 498–505.

Hetherington, M. M., Foster, R., Anderson, A. S., & Norton, G. N. M. (2006). Understanding variety: Tasting different foods delays satiation. *Physiology & Behavior, 87,* 263–271.

Hill, A. J., & Blundell, J. E. (1982–1983). Nutrients and behaviour: Research strategies for the investigation of taste characteristics, food preferences, hunger sensations and eating patterns in man. *Journal of Psychiatric Research, 17,* 203–212.

Hill, A. J., Magson, L. D., & Blundell, J. E. (1984). Hunger and palatability: Tracking ratings of subjective experience before, during and after the consumption of preferred and un-preferred foods. *Appetite, 5,* 361–371.

Hill, A. J., Rogers, P. J., & Blundell, J. E. (1995). Techniques for the experimental measurement of human eating behaviour and food intake: A practical guide. *International Journal of Obesity, 19,* 361–375.

Holt, S. H., Brand-Miller, J. C., & Stitt, P. A. (2001). The effects of equal-energy portions of different breads on blood glucose levels, feelings of fullness and subsequent food intake. *Journal of the American Dietetic Association, 101,* 767–773.

Holt, S. H., Miller, J. C., Petocz, P., & Farmakalidis, E. (1995). A satiety index of common foods. *European Journal of Clinical Nutrition, 49,* 675–690.

Hubel, R., Laessle, R. G., Lehrke, S., & Jass, J. (2006). Laboratory measurement of cumulative food intake in humans: Results on the reliability. *Appetite, 6,* 57–62.

Hubert, P., King, N. A, & Blundell, J. E. (1998). Uncoupling the effects of energy expenditure and energy intake: Appetite response to short-term energy deficit induced by meal omission and physical activity. *Appetite, 31,* 9–19.

Hubert, P., Lluch, A., King, N. A., & Blundell, J. E. (2000). Selective effects of acute exercise and breakfast interventions on mood and motivation to eat. *Physiology & Behavior, 68,* 515–520.

Hulshof, T., & de Graff, C. (1993). The effects of preloads varying in physical state and fat content on satiety and energy intake. *Appetite, 21,* 273–286.

Johnstone, A. M., Stubbs, R. J., & Harbron, C. G. (1996). Effect of overfeeding macronutrients on day-to-day food intake in man. *European Journal of Clinical Nutrition, 50,* 418–430.

Jordan, H. A., Wieland, W. F., Zebley, S. P., Stellar, E., & Stunkard, A. J. (1966). Direct measurement of food intake in man: A method for objective study of eating behavior. *Psychosomatic Medicine, 28,* 836–842.

Kendall, A., Levitsky, D. A., Strupp, B. J., & Lissner, L. (1991). Weight-loss on a low fat diet: Consequence of the impression of the control of food intake in humans. *American Journal of Clinical Nutrition, 53*, 1124–1129.

King, N. A., Appleton, K., Rogers, P. J., & Blundell, J. E. (1999). Effects of sweetness and energy in drinks on food intake following exercise. *Physiology & Behavior, 6*, 375–379.

King, N. A., Craig, S. A., Pepper, T., & Blundell, J. E. (2005). Evaluation of the independent and combined effects of Xylitol and Litesse® polydextrose consumed as a snack on hunger and energy intake over 10 days. *British Journal of Nutrition, 93*, 911–955.

King, N. A., Hester, J., & Gately, P. J. (2007). The effect of a medium-term activity- and diet-induced energy deficit on subjective appetite sensations in obese children. *International Journal of Obesity, 31*, 334–339.

King, N. A., Lawton, C. L., Delargy, H. J., Smith, F. C., & Blundell, J. E. (1997). The electronic appetite rating system (EARS): A portable computerised method of continuous automated monitoring of motivation to eat and mood. In P. J. Wellman & B. G. Hoebel (Eds.), *Ingestive behavior protocols* (pp. 71–76). Northbrook, IL: Society for the Study of Ingestive Behavior.

King, N. A., Lluch, A., Stubbs, R. J., & Blundell, J. E. (1997). High dose exercise does not increase hunger or energy intake in free living males. *European Journal of Clinical Nutrition, 51*, 478–483.

Kissileff, H. (1984). Satiating efficiency and a strategy for conducting food loading experiments. *Neuroscience and Biobehavioral Reviews, 8*, 129–135.

Kissileff, H. R., & Guss, J. L. (2001). Microstructure of eating behaviour in humans. *Appetite, 36*, 70–78.

Kissileff, H. R., Klingsberg, G., & Van Itallie, T. B. (1980). Universal Eating Monitor for the continuous recording of solid or liquid consumption in man. *American Journal of Physiology, 238*, 14–22.

Kissileff, H. R., Thornton, J., & Becker, E. (1982). A quadratic equation adequately describes the cumulative food intake curve in man. *Appetite, 3*, 255–272.

Kissileff, H. R., Wentzlaff, T. H., Guss, J. L., Walsh, B. T., Devlin, M. J., & Thornton, J. C. (1996). A direct measure of satiety disturbance in patients with bulimia nervosa. *Physiology & Behavior, 60*, 1077–1085.

Laessle, R. G., Uhl, H., & Lindel, B. (2001). Parental influences on eating behaviour in obese and nonobese preadolescents. *International Journal of Eating Disorders, 30*, 447–453.

Laessle, R. G., Uhl, H., Lindel, B., & Müller, A. (2001). Parental influences on eating behaviour in obese and nonobese children. *International Journal of Obesity, 25*(Suppl. 1), s60–s62.

Lawton, C., Burley, V., Wales, J., & Blundell, E. (1993). Dietary fat and appetite control in obese subjects: Weak effects on satiation and satiety. *International Journal of Obesity, 17*, 1–8.

Le Magnen, J., & Booth, D. A. (1999). Appetite classics: The role of orosensory and postingestional effects of food in the control of intake: 1956–1963. *Appetite, 33*, 1.

Leathwood, P., & Pollet, P. (1988). Effects of slow release carbohydrates in the form of bean flakes on the evolution of hunger and satiety in man. *Appetite, 10*, 1–11.

Lindgren, A. C., Barkeling, B., Hägg, A., Ritzén, E. M., Marcus, C., & Rössner, S. (2000). Eating behaviour in Prader-Willi syndrome, normal weight and obese control groups. *Journal of Pediatrics, 137*, 50–55.

Lissner, L., Levitsky, D. A., Strupp, B. J., Kalkwarf, H. J., & Roe, D. A. (1987). Dietary fat and the regulation of energy intake in human subjects. *American Journal of Clinical Nutrition, 46*, 886–892.

Lluch, A., King, N. A., & Blundell, J. E. (2000). No energy compensation at the meal following exercise in dietary restrained and unrestrained women. *British Journal of Nutrition, 84*, 219–225.

Lowe, M. R., & Butryn, M. L. (2007). Hedonic hunger: A new dimension of appetite. *Physiology and Behavior, 91*, 432–439.

Mazlan, N., Horgan, G., Whybrow, S., & Stubbs, R. J. (2006). Effects of increasing increments of fat- and sugar-rich snacks in the diet on energy and macronutrient intake in lean and overweight men. *British Journal of Nutrition, 96*, 596–606.

Merrill, E. P., Kramer, F. M., Cardello, A., & Schutz, H. (2002). A comparison of satiety measures. *Appetite, 39*, 181–183.

Meyer, J.-E., & Pudel, V. (1972). Experimental studies on food-intake in obese and normal weight subjects. *Journal of Psychosomatic Research, 16*, 305–308.

Mirch, M. C., McDuffie, J. R., Yanovski, S. Z., Schollnberger, M., Tanofsky-Kraff, M., Theim, K. R., et al. (2006). Effects of binge eating on satiation, satiety, and energy intake of overweight children. *American Journal of Clinical Nutrition, 84*, 732–738.

Mook, D. G., & Votaw, M. C. (1992). How important is hedonism? Reasons given by college student for ending a meal. *Appetite, 18,* 69–75.

Moon, R. D. (1979). Monitoring human eating patterns during the ingestion of non-liquid foods. *International Journal of Obesity, 3,* 281–288.

Näslund, E., Barkeling, B., Gutniak, M., Blundell, J. E., Holst, J. J., Rössner, S., et al. (1999). Energy intake and appetite are suppressed by glucagon-like peptide (GLP)-1 in obese men. *International Journal of Obesity, 23,* 301–311.

Näslund, E., Gutniak, M., Skogar, S., Rössner, S., & Hellström, P. M. (1998). Glucagon-like peptide 1 increases the period of postprandial satiety and slows gastric emptying in obese men. *American Journal of Clinical Nutrition, 68,* 525–530.

Näslund, E., King, N., Mansten, S., Adner, N., Holst, J. J., Gutniak, M., et al. (2004). Prandial subcutaneous injections of GLP-1 cause weight loss in obese humans. *British Journal of Nutrition, 91,* 439–446.

Näslund, E., Melin, I., Grybäck, P., Hägg, A., Hellström, P. M., Jacobssson, H., et al. (1997). Reduced food intake after jejunoileal bypass: A possible association with prolonged gastric emptying and altered gut hormone patterns. *American Journal of Clinical. Nutrition, 65,* 26–32.

O'Doherty, J., Rolls, E. T., Francis, S., Bowtell, R., McGlone, F., Kobal, G., et al. (2000). Sensory-specific satiety-related olfactory activation of the human orbitofrontal cortex. *Neuroreport, 11,* 893–897.

Oliver, A., Wright, M., Matson, A., Woodrow, G., King, N., & Dye, L. (2004). Low sodium haemodialysis reduces interdialytic fluid consumption but paradoxically increases post-dialysis thirst. *Nephrology, Dialysis, Transplantation, 19,* 2883–2885.

O'Reilly, L. M., Stubbs, R. J., Johnstone, A. M., Mara, O., & Robertson, K. (1997). Covert manipulation of the energy density of mixed diets on ad libitum food intake in "free-living" humans. *Proceedings of the Nutrition Society, 56,* 127A.

Raben, A., Tagliabue, A., & Astrup, A. (1995). The reproducibility of subjective appetite sensations. *British Journal of Nutrition, 63,* 517–530.

Raben, A., Vasilaras, T. H., Moller, A. C., & Astrup, A. (2002). Sucrose compared with artificial sweeteners: Different effects on ad libitum food intake and body weight after 10 wk of supplementation on overweight subjects. *American Journal of Clinical Nutrition, 76,* 721–729.

Raynor, H. A., & Epstein, L. H. (2000). Effects of sensory stimulation and post-ingestive consequences on satiation. *Physiology & Behavior, 70,* 465–470.

Reid, C. A., Johnstone, A. M., & Ryan, L. M. (1999). What are psychometric assessments of appetite asking? A preliminary multivariate analysis. *International Journal of Obesity, 3,* 151A.

Robinson, T. M., Gray, R. W., Yeomans, M. R., & French, S. J. (2005). Test-meal palatability alters the effects of intra-gastric fat but not carbohydrate preloads on intake and related appetite in healthy volunteers. *Physiology & Behavior, 84,* 193–203.

Rogers, P. J., & Blundell, J. E. (1979). Effect of anorexic drugs on food intake and the micro-structure of eating in human subjects. *Psychopharmacology, 66,* 159–165.

Rolls, B., Kim, S., McNelis, A., Fischman, M., Foltin, R., & Moran, T. (1991). Time course of effects of preloads high in fat or carbohydrate on food intake and hunger ratings in humans. *American Journal of Physiology, 260,* R756–R763.

Rolls, B., Kim-Harris, S., Fischman, M. W., Foltin, R., Moran, T., & Stoner, S. (1994). Satiety after preloads with different amounts of fat and carbohydrate: Implications for obesity. *American Journal of Clinical Nutrition, 60,* 476–489.

Rolls, B. J., & McDermott, T. (1991). Effects of age on sensory-specific satiety. *American Journal of Clinical Nutrition, 54,* 988–996.

Rolls, B. J., Roe, L. S., & Meengs, J. S. (2007). The effect of large portion sizes on energy intake is sustained for 11 days. *Obesity, 15,* 1535–1543.

Rolls, B. J., Rolls, E. T., Rowe, E. A., & Sweeney, K. (1981). Sensory specific satiety in man. *Physiology & Behavior, 27,* 137–142.

Rolls, B. J., Rowe, E. A., Rolls, E. T., Kingston, B., Megson, A., & Gunnery, R. (1981). Variety in a meal enhances food intake in man. *Physiology & Behavior, 26,* 215–221.

Rolls, B. J., Shide, D. J., Thorwart, M. L., & Ulbrecht, J. S. (1998). Sibutramine reduces food intake in non-dieting women with obesity. *Obesity Research, 6,* 1–11.

Rolls, E. T. (2007). Sensory processing in the brain related to the control of food intake. *Proceedings of the Nutrition Society, 66,* 96–112.

Rolls, E. T., Murzi, E., Yaxley, S., Thorpe, S. J., & Simpson, S. J. (1986). Sensory-specific satiety: Food-specific reduction in responsiveness of ventral forebrain neurons after feeding in the monkey. *Brain Research, 12,* 79–86.

Rolls, E. T., & Rolls, J. H. (1997). Olfactory sensory-specific satiety in humans. *Physiology & Behavior, 61,* 461–473.

Saelens, B. E., & Epstein, L. H. (1996). Reinforcing value of food in obese and non-obese women. *Appetite, 27,* 41–50.

Schwartz, M. W., & Morton, G. J. (2002). Obesity: Keeping hunger at bay. *Nature, 418,* 595–597.

Sclafani, A. (2004). Oral and postoral determinants of food reward. *Physiology & Behavior, 81,* 773–779.

Silverstone, J. T., & Stunkard, A. J. (1968). The anorectic effect of dexamphetamine sulphate. *British Journal of Pharmacology and Chemotherapy, 33,* 513–522.

Smeets, A. J., & Westerterp-Plantenga, M. S. (2006). Oral exposure and sensory-specific satiety. *Physiology & Behavior, 89,* 281–286.

Smith, G. P. (1996). The direct and indirect controls of meal size. *Neuroscience & Biobehavioral Reviews, 20,* 41–46.

Smith, G. P. (2000). The controls of eating: A shift from nutritional homeostasis to behavioral neuroscience. *Nutrition, 16,* 814–820.

Smith, S., Blundell, J. E., Burns, C., Ellero, C., Schroeder, B., Kesty, N., et al. (2007). Pramlintide treatment reduces 24-hour caloric intake and meal sizes, and improves control of eating in obese subjects: A 6-week translational research study. *American Journal of Physiology (Endocrine and Metabolism), 293,* E620–E627.

Snoek, H. M., Huntjens, L., Van Gemert, L. J., de Graaf, C., & Weenen, H. (2004). Sensory-specific satiety in obese and normal-weight women. *American Journal of Clinical Nutrition, 80,* 823–831.

Spitzer, L., & Rodin, J. (1981). Human eating behaviour: A critical review of studies in normal weight and overweight individuals. *Appetite, 2,* 293–329.

Steiner, J. E. (1979). Human facial expressions in response to taste and smell stimulation. *Advances in Child Development and Behavior, 13,* 257–295.

Steiner, J. E., Glaser, D., Hawilo, M. E., & Berridge, K. C. (2001). Comparative expression of hedonic impact: Affective reactions to taste by human infants and other primates. *Neuroscience & Biobehavioral Reviews, 25,* 53–74.

Stratton, R. J., Stubbs, R. J., Hughes, D., King, N. A., Blundell, J. E., & Elia, M. (1998). Comparison of the traditional paper visual analogue scale questionnaire with an Apple Newton electronic appetite ratings system (EARS) in free living subjects feeding ad libitum. *European Journal of Clinical Nutrition, 52,* 737–741.

Stroebele, N., & de Castro, J. M. (2006). Influence of physiological and subjective arousal on food intake in humans. *Nutrition, 22,* 996–1004.

Stubbs, R. J. (1995). Macronutrient effects on appetite. *International Journal of Obesity, 19*(Suppl. 5), S11–S19.

Stubbs, R. J., & Harbron, C. G. (1996). Covert manipulation of the ratio of medium to long-chain triglycerides in isoenergetically dense diets: Effect on food intake in ad libitum feeding men. *International Journal of Obesity, 20,* 435–444.

Stubbs, R. J., Harbron, C., Murgatroyd, P., & Prentice, A. (1995). Covert manipulation of dietary fat and energy density: Effect substrate flux and food intake in men eating ad libitum. *American Journal of Clinical Nutrition, 62,* 1–14.

Stubbs, R. J., Hughes, D. A., Johnstone, A. M., Rowley, E., Ferris, S., Elia, M., et al. (2001). Description and evaluation of a Newton-based electronic appetite rating system for temporal tracking of appetite in human subjects. *Physiology & Behavior, 72,* 615–619.

Stubbs, R. J., Hughes, D. A., Johnstone, A. M., Rowley, E., Reid, C., Elia, M., et al. (2000). The use of visual analogue scales to assess motivation to eat in human subjects: A review of their reliability and validity with an evaluation of new hand-held computerized systems for temporal tracking of appetite ratings. *British Journal of Nutrition, 84,* 405–415.

Stubbs, R J., Hughes, D. A., Johnstone, A. M., Whybrow, S., Horgan, G. W., King, N., et al. (2004). Rate and extent of compensatory changes in energy intake and expenditure in response to altered exercise and diet composition in humans. *American Journal of Physiology, 286,* R350–R358.

Stubbs, R. J., Hughes, D. A., Ritz, P., Johnstone, A. M., Horgan, G. W., King, N., et al. (2004). A decrease in physical activity affects appetite, energy and nutrient balance in lean men feeding ad libitum. *American Journal of Clinical Nutrition, 79,* 62–69.

Stubbs, R. J., O'Reilly, L. M., Johnstone, A. M., Harrison, C. L., Clark, H., Franklin, M. F., et al. (1997). Description and evaluation of an experimental model to examine changes in selection between high protein, high carbohydrate and high fat foods in humans. *European Journal of Clinical Nutrition, 53,* 13–21.

Stubbs, R. J., Sepp, A., Hughes, D. A., Johnstone, A. M., Horgan, G. W., et al. (2002). The effect of graded levels of exercise on energy intake and balance in free-living men, consuming their normal diet. *European Journal of Clinical Nutrition, 56,* 129–140.

Stubbs, R. J., Sepp, A., Hughes, D. A., Johnstone, A. M., King, N., Horgan, G., et al. (2002). The effect of graded levels of exercise on energy intake and balance in free-living women. *International Journal of Obesity, 26,* 866–869.

Stunkard, A., Coll, M., Lundquist, S., & Meyers, A. (1980). Obesity and eating style. *Archives of General Psychiatry, 37,* 1127–1129.

Stunkard, A., & Kaplan, D. (1977). Eating in public places: A review of report of the direct observation of eating behaviour. *International Journal of Obesity, 1,* 89–101.

Totterdell, P., & Folkard, S. (1992). In situ repeated measures of affect and cognitive performance facilitated by use of a hand-held computer. *Behavior Research Methods, Instruments, and Computers, 24,* 545–553.

Tremblay, A., Lavallee, N., Almeras, N., Allard, L., Despres, J.-P., & Bouchard, C. (1991). Nutritional determinants of the increase in energy intake associated with a high-fat diet. *American Journal of Clinical Nutrition, 53,* 1134–1137.

Tuomisto, T., Tuomisto, M. T., Hetherington, M., & Lappalainen, R. (1998). Reasons for initiation and cessation of eating in obese men and women and the affective consequences of eating in everyday situations. *Appetite, 30,* 211–222.

Wansink, B., Painter, J. E., & North, J. (2005). Bottomless bowls: Why visual cues of portion size may influence intake. *Obesity Research, 13,* 93–100.

Weenen, H., Stafleu, A., & de Graaf, C. (2005). Dynamic aspects of liking: Post-prandial persistence of sensory specific satiety. *Food Quality and Preference, 16,* 528–535.

Wentzlaff, T. H., Guss, J. L., & Kissileff, H. R. (1995). Subjective ratings as a function of amount consumed: A preliminary report. *Physiology & Behavior, 57,* 1209–1214.

Westerterp-Plantenga, M. S. (2000). Eating behaviour in humans, characterized by cumulative food intake curves: A review. *Neuroscience & Biobehavioral Reviews, 24,* 239–248.

Whybrow, S., Mayer, C., Kirk, T. R., Mazlan, N., & Stubbs, R. J. (2007). Effects of two week's mandatory snack consumption on energy intake and energy balance. *Obesity, 15,* 673–685.

Whybrow, S., Stephen, J. R., & Stubbs, R. J. (2006). The evaluation of an electronic visual analogue scale system for appetite and mood. *European Journal of Clinical Nutrition, 60,* 558–560.

Wiepkema, P. R. (1971). Behavioural factors in the regulation of food intake. *Proceedings of the Nutrition Society, 30,* 142–149.

Williamson, D. A., Grislman, P. J., Lovejoy J., Greenway F., Volaufova, J., Main, C. K., et al. (2006). Effects of consuming mycoprotein, tofu or chicken upon subsequent eating behavior, hunger and satiety. *Appetite, 46,* 41–48.

Williamson, D. A., Ravussin, E., Wong, M. L., Wagner, A., Dipaoli, A., Caglayan, S., et al. (2005). Microanalysis of eating behavior of three leptin deficient adults treated with leptin therapy. *Appetite, 45,* 75–80.

Wright, M. J., Woodrow, G., O'Brien, S., Armstrong, E., King, N., Dye, L., et al. (2004a). Cholecystokonin and leptin: Their influence upon the eating behaviour and nutrient intake of dialysis patients. *Nephrology, Dialysis, Transplantation, 19,* 133–140.

Wright, M. J., Woodrow, G., O'Brien, S., Armstrong, E., King, N., Dye, L., et al. (2004b). Poldypisa: A feature of peritoneal dialysis. *Nephrology, Dialysis, Transplantation, 19,* 1–6.

Wright, M. J., Woodrow, G., O'Brien, S., King, N. A., Blundell, J. E., Brownjohn, A. M., et al. (2001). A novel technique to demonstrate disturbed appetite profiles in haemodialysis patients. *Nephrology, Dialysis, Transplantation, 16,* 1424–1429.

Wright, M. J., Woodrow, G., O'Brien, S., King, N., Dye, L., Blundell, J., et al. (2003). Disturbed appetite and nutrient intake in peritoneal dialysis patients. *Peritoneal Dialysis International, 23,* 550–556.

Wurtman, J. J., & Wurtman, R. J. (1982–1983). Studies on the appetite for carbohydrates in rats and humans. *Journal of Psychiatric Research, 17,* 213–221.

Yeomans, M. R. (1996). Palatability and the microstructure of feeding in humans: The appetizer effect. *Appetite, 27,* 119–133.

Yeomans, M. R. (2000). Rating changes over the course of meals: What do they tell us about motivation to eat? *Neuroscience & Biobehavioral Reviews, 24,* 249–259.

Yeomans, M. R., & Gray, R. W. (1997). Effects of naltrexone on food intake and changes in subjective appetite during eating: Evidence for opioid involvement in the appetizer effect. *Physiology & Behavior, 62,* 15–21

Yeomans, M. R., Gray, R. W., Mitchell, C. J., & True, S. (1997). Independent effects of palatability and within-meal pauses on intake and subjective appetite in human volunteers. *Appetite, 29,* 61–76.

Yeomans, M. R., Lartamo, S., Proter, E. L., Lee, M. D., & Gray, R. W. (2001). The actual, but not labelled, fat content of a soup preload alters short-term appetite in healthy men. *Physiology & Behavior, 73,* 533–540.

Yeomans, M. R., Lee, M. D., Gray, R. W., & French, S. J. (2001). Effects of test-meal palatability on compensatory eating following disguised fat and carbohydrate preloads. *International Journal of Obesity, 25,* 1215–1224.

Yeomans, M. R., Mobini, S., Elliman, T. D., Walker, H. C., & Stevenson, R. J. (2006). Hedonic and sensory characteristics of odors conditioned by pairing with tastants in humans. *Journal of Experimental Psychology: Animal Behavior Processes, 32,* 215–228.

Yeomans, M. R., & Symes, T. (1999). Individual differences in the use of pleasantness and palatability ratings. *Appetite, 32,* 383–394.

Zijlstra, N., Mars, M., de Wijk, R. A., Westerterp-Plantenga, M. S., & de Graaf, C. (2008). The effect of viscosity on ad-libitum food intake. *International Journal of Obesity, 34,* 676–683.

CHAPTER 9

Measuring Food Intake in Field Studies

Brian Wansink

"Cool Data"

When I was a PhD student, I heard two words that changed my research life.

At the time, a brilliant but underpublished assistant professor was given tenure at Stanford. He had published only three articles at the time. While this would be unheard of at most other research schools, the grapevine indicated that his tenure success was partially due to the overwhelming impact of these three articles. Shortly after his tenure announcement, I saw this professor at a campus running track. After a few laps of small talk, I asked him about his secret to research success. For the past 20 years, his two-word answer has influenced me more than anything I learned in my PhD program.

His secret to research success? "Cool data."

Cool data. That summarizes most of what many of us do *not* want to do. We tend to be experts at lab studies, complex modeling exercises, or short-term trials involving begrudging sophomores who need the extra credit. The last reason we joined academics was to run around in restaurants, movie theaters, bars, and dining rooms. Yet this is where some of this "cool data" hides. It is

data from real people in real situations, who are being observed, coded, measured, and dispassionately analyzed and reported (Schachter, 1971).

Cool data are hard to collect. They can be data collected in restaurants (Bell & Pliner, 2003), sports bars (Wansink & Cheney, 2005), household pantries (Terry & Beck, 1985), college cafeterias (Levitsky & Youn, 2004), food courts (Chandon & Wansink, 2007), elementary school lunchrooms (Kahn & Wansink, 2004), supermarkets (Iynegar & Lepper, 2000; Wansink, Kent, & Hoch, 1998), and movie theaters (Wansink & Park, 2001). They can also be data collected from unusual populations, such as preschoolers (Fisher, Rolls, & Birch, 2003) or amnesiacs (Rozin, Dow, Moscovitch, & Rajaram,1998), or which contrast data collected on the streets of Paris (Wansink, Payne, & Chandon, 2007) with that collected on the streets of Philadelphia (Rozin, Kabnick, Pete, Fischler, & Shields, 2003).

It is harder to get institutional review board (IRB) approval for cool data, they are harder to set up, they are harder to staff, and they are harder to analyze (Meiselman 1992). Yet what I have also learned is that cool data can capture imaginations; they can suddenly make science relevant to an unsuspecting segment, and they can almost always be published, eventually.

Over the years, I have struggled with many types of cool data. Some has been unpredictable, some has been costly, and some has ended up being influential (Bradburn, Sudman, & Wansink, 2004). In conducting over 200 studies, I have estimated this:

- Forty percent of the studies are disasters and need to be rethought because of a conceptual mistake or rerun because of a methodological mistake.

- Forty percent of the studies come out differently than hypothesized, leading to a new understanding, a new theory, and a new confirmatory study.

- Twenty percent of the studies come out perfectly predicted as hypothesized.

My favorite insights, and therefore my favorite studies, have almost always come from the second category. Part of this success has been because I have strived to set up studies in a way that generate diagnostic results. But that is only part of the key. Part of what distinguishes *great* papers from *no* paper is the ability to analyze field data to find the needle in the haystack. The purpose of this chapter is to provide some of these insights in how to set up cool data studies and how to analyze them to extract something that is true, insightful, and generalizable.

While the intent of using controlled field studies is to make our results powerful, impactful, and interesting, this does not always happen. What follows are some of the methods to try and mistakes to avoid.

The Emerging Importance of Field Studies

Until recently, intake research developed by borrowing constructs from parent disciplines (primarily economics and psychology) and modifying them to suit questions related to intake

behaviors. Recently, however, an emerging issue that is more uniquely central to intake—that of food intake volume and frequency—has become of increasing importance to consumers and public policy officials (Allison, Fontaine, Manson, Stevens, & VanItallie, 1999; French, Story, & Jeffery, 2001). Perhaps because there is a less established set of intake measurement procedures, methods, and analyses, the contributions in this area have been more sporadic and less consistent than in other areas. The objective of this chapter is to provide a framework that helps improve the probability of success and the consistency and synergy of intake-related field studies.

At this stage of development, there are many unexplained inconsistencies in intake studies. Some show that package shapes do not cause increases in intake (Raghubir & Krishna, 1999), while other studies do (Wansink, 2006). Some show intake to be driven by cognition (Berry, Beatty, & Klesges, 1985), while others show it driven by perceptions (Inman, 2001). Some show that attitude is related to intake, while others show it is not. We contend that many of these inconsistencies can be attributed to a wide variance in the methods, data analysis approaches, and reporting practices of intake studies. This chapter offers a framework for conducting intake studies, and it outlines methods and measures that would be most likely to lead to successful studies and accurate conclusions.

There is a basic distinction between "choosing" and "using" that makes research difficult to conduct without a framework. One way intake is distinct from choice is because it involves a behavior that can sometimes be more consequential than choice while also being less deliberate (Wansink & Sobal, 2007). Because intake has immediate implications for a person's gratification or even health, issues of intake frequency or volume are not always explained by rational economic models (Assunçao & Meyer, 1993). Importantly, there is also a motor component that distinguishes usage and intake studies from pencil-and-paper studies or even from those involving the selection and purchase of foods off of shelves (Schachter & Friedman, 1974).

A Framework for Defining, Measuring, and Analyzing Intake

The differences noted above can complicate the ability to investigate intake using standard models, methods, measures, or analyses. Such differences generate uncertainty as to whether weak effects in intake studies are due to noise introduced by the measure of the method or whether they are instead due to it being insignificant. A key objective here will be to increase effect size while decreasing systematic variation. There is a wide range of contexts in which this variation can occur. They can occur in studies of how the size, shape, variety, structure, or inventory level of a food influences intake. It can also occur in studies of how different advertising strategies influence intake frequency either in new situations or as substitutions for existing foods. They may also include situation variables such as how do social norms, the presence of others, or occasion-based usage influence intake differently (Clendenen, Herman, & Polivy, 1994; Fuenekes, de Graaf, & van Staveren, 1995).

There will be a number of benefits to a framework that improves the consistency in the way researchers use models, methods, and measures, as well as conduct analyses. First, such a framework will help researchers determine the most fruitful and sensitive way to study an intake-related variable without having the results obscured by unnecessary noise or inappropriate analysis. Second, it will help the area of consumer research grow in a more structured, synergistic manner by helping provide better structure to methods, measures, and analyses. Last, it will importantly encourage process models to be developed that can be useful in further understanding intake by helping examine it in an unconfounded, least invasive manner.

As shown in Figure 9.1, we first examine how intake can best be studied by increasing effect sizes and decreasing noise. Next, the timing of pre- and postintake measures is discussed. Last, analysis techniques that are somewhat unique to intake studies are investigated. This chapter examines intake primarily in the context of the usage volume and frequency of consumables.

Studying Intake

Intake can be examined by using lab experiments, field studies, surveys, or consumer panels, or it can be examined less directly by projecting intake from purchase data or by inferring intake from what is discarded. The specific research question dictates what method is most appropriate and can provide the strongest effects with the least interference.

The basic objective in developing a framework of intake measurement sensitivity is to increase relative effect sizes by reducing the systematic variation. One important way to accomplish this is to eliminate or control the potential sources of unwanted variation or noise associated with a study. Reducing systematic variance can be accomplished by developing intake models that help one articulate these differences. Developing a process model for intake experiments allows you to specify details and variables that your hypothesis involves (Baron & Kenny, 1986; Evans & Lepore, 1997). It allows for the examination of variables that could potentially obscure results or influence intake, and also considering alternate explanations, you can eliminate or add variables to decrease ambiguity and factors that could obscure hypothesized results.

For instance, consider the seemingly ubiquitous American phenomenon of cleaning one's plate. Research involving this tendency can simply show that it happens under different conditions and at different ages (Rolls, Engell, & Birch, 2000). These would be effect studies. Process studies would also try to explain why this happens. For instance, it might occur because the amount served to a person represents an implicit "consumption norm" (Wansink 2004) of how much is appropriate, typical, normal, and reasonable to consume. Therefore, one almost dutifully complies. By specifying this mediating variable ("the amount on my plate is the typical amount a person should eat"), one can begin to explain why an

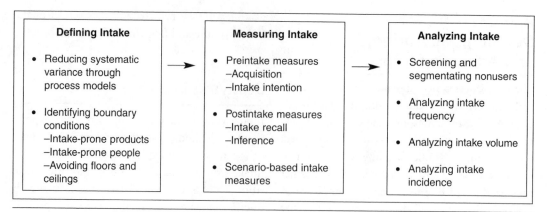

Figure 9.1   Different Forms of Intake-Related Variables

effect occurs. Effect studies explain "what," and process studies explain "why."

As will be explained in the next section, hypothesizing the different reasons why you think an independent variable might influence a dependent one can add a lot of precision to your field studies and to their analysis. One big reason for going to this extra effort is that it can help open up the "black box" of why people do what they do. A second reason is that it can help troubleshoot results that do not seem consistent with expectations or that seem too noisy to draw a conclusion.

In one study of Pacific combat veterans, we investigated how one's involvement in World War II influenced how much they would eat when they were introduced to a Chinese buffet dinner 55 years later (Wansink, 2006, pp. 154–156). The initial results were disappointing and showed no difference in comparison to a control group of the same age.

What we had not done is to fully articulate the reason why we thought they would eat less Chinese food (Wansink, van Ittersum, & Werle, in press). Our unarticulated reason was that we thought the negative feelings they had about their wartime experience in the Pacific would bias their long-term preference toward Asian food. Our implicit process model is outlined in Figure 9.2.

As noted, results of this study were disappointing. There was no difference between the veterans and a control group. Having a process

model enabled us to troubleshoot the data and determine whether the theory was wrong or whether there was another explanation. Of those veterans who enjoyed Chinese and Japanese food and still ate it with some frequency, there were no characteristics they had in common. Before the war, some had lived in big cities, some on farms. Some had graduated from college; others had never seen a ninth-grade classroom.

What did explain their behavior was the level of combat they had experienced as soldiers. When analyzing the profiles of those Pacific veterans who liked Chinese food, we did not find Marines who had been at Iwo Jima or infantry soldiers at Guadalcanal. What we found were mechanics, clerks, engineers, and truck drivers—enlisted men who did not experience the war from the front line. Although their wartime experience was a sacrifice, they did not come home with terrible associations that tainted the taste of food even 50 to 60 years later.

Having a process model enabled an analysis of the data that yielded insights other than what were expected. Even though our process model was wrong, it gave us a framework to analyze the data more completely. The subsequent insights were more on track with what is really true about the formation of long-term eating behaviors. This is one reason that developing a process model is an important way to start the planning of a field experiment.

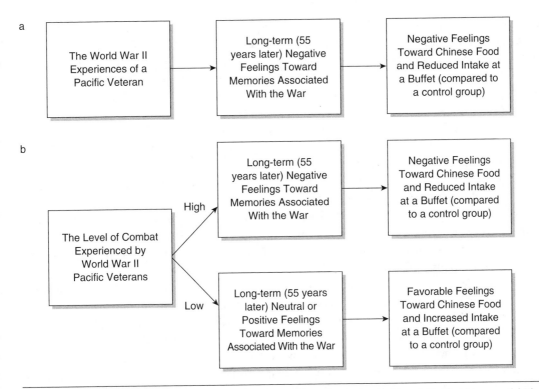

Figure 9.2   How World War II Was Believed to Influence the Eating Habits of Pacific Veterans: (a) The Original Incorrect Process Model and (b) Revised Process Model

Reducing Systematic Variance Through Intake Process Models

Increasing the relative effect size can be accomplished by using the appropriate method and by either controlling or eliminating those noise-related variations that may obscure hypothesized results. Many factors can influence intake and obscure the effects of a study. One way to determine those that would be most damaging to a study is to specifically articulate the process model that drives one's resulting hypotheses. This is important even for effect studies or calibration studies. Even though the focus of such studies may not be on the process leading to behavior (intake), per se, articulating such a model can help researchers to eliminate sources of unwanted variance (such as the time of day, the presence of others, the cost or availability of an item, etc.) or to control them.

For instance, suppose one is studying how lighting level influences how much a person eats. To estimate the most accurate influence of lighting, one should statistically eliminate the effects of other intervening variables, such as social facilitation (what others at the same table are doing). By measuring and accounting for the intake of other people at the table, a researcher can have a more pure examination of the influence of lighting (de Castro, 1994).

Regardless of whether one is studying the influence of variety, serving sizes, atmospherics, or structure on intake, it is important to hypothesize why intake should occur. Developing process models suggests not only the level at which to analyze data, as well as what potentially confounding variables should be measured, but it can also suggest which foods to use in the study (Rolls, Bell, & Waugh, 2000). Doing so will help control other variables or processes that might be seen as either confounds or as potentially explanatory causes. Even when these extraneous factors are not controllable, insights from a model can suggest measures that could serve as covariates or would enable post hoc tests to be conducted.

Explicitly articulating an intake model can help organize a study. Furthermore, doing so suggests important factors that must be controlled for and key measures that must be taken to best understand the process that is occurring. As an example, consider the process model illustrated in Figure 9.3. In this model, the relationship suggests a process model where two mediating factors—consumption norms and consumption monitoring—are suggested to explain why five common environmental cues have such an empirically robust influence on intake (Wansink, 2004).

The process of doing this enables researchers to articulate why hypothesized effects will occur, but it will also help them measure, control, or eliminate those factors that could mask or eliminate the hypothesized relationship. The impact of package size on intake, for instance, can be explained by scarcity research, by perceived differences in cost, or by a perceptual explanation (Wansink, 2006, p. 66). Articulating these alternatives can help a researcher design studies that either rule out or account for alternative explanations. It is important to show when an effect does work as well as when it does not. This helps other researchers to conduct more efficient follow-up studies, and it makes their efforts less derivative (Lawless, Bender, Oman, & Pelletier, 2003). As a result, researchers can investigate the fundamentals behind intake without having to conduct derivative or incremental research based on replications and slight extensions of existing studies.

Generating a process model also helps specify "boundary" conditions by knowing when and how effects will be found (Pliner, 1974). In this way, different antecedents will yield different results. One example of how an understanding of how boundary conditions influenced the analysis of many studies involves eating restraint. Understanding that there was a difference between restrained and unrestrained eaters disclosed many effects that were previously hidden (Polivy, Herman, Hackett, & Kuleshnyk, 1986; Polivy, Herman, Younger, & Erskine, 1979).

Increasing Effect Sizes by Identifying Boundary Conditions

By specifying a process model that relates how various factors influence intake, we can develop a better understanding of when an effect may or may not be observed. For example, in their study of pouring and intake behavior, Raghubir and Krishna (1999) found that less involved consumers were more influenced by the shape of packaging compared to more involved consumers. Given these conclusions, it is important that future studies related to package shape make certain their subjects are highly involved and are not distracted during the study. Not only do boundary conditions help develop stronger manipulations, but they also show conditions where the standard set of manipulations can be more effective than others.

Intake-Prone Foods

Some foods are more prone to intake acceleration or to variation in intake volume than others. Chandon and Wansink (2002), for instance, found that intake acceleration occurs with certain foods (such as yogurt) but not with others (such as ketchup). In this case, the intake of the more convenient and hedonic foods (yogurt) was more sensitive to stockpiling pressures than was ketchup (which less conveniently requires being eaten with a prepared food). Making these food-level distinctions is important because researchers can sometimes overrely on existing databases when testing intake-related hypotheses. If the existing categories on which there are data (e.g., coffee, ketchup, yogurt, etc.) are not categories that are prone to intake variation, however, researchers would be unfairly handicapping their hypotheses.

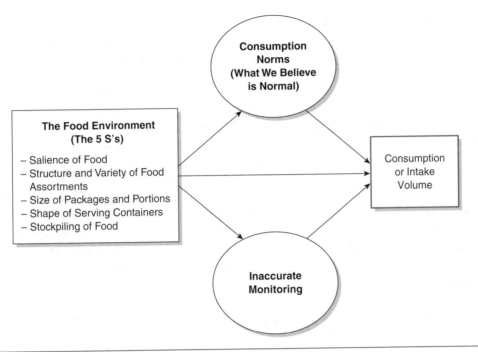

Figure 9.3   A Process Model of How the Food Environment Influences Consumption or Intake Volume

Recent studies have found that foods can be most acceptable to intake variations when they are hedonic and convenient to prepare and consume (Chandon & Wansink, 2002). Furthermore, it might also be that widely but irregularly consumed foods would be promising to examine as intake-prone categories. In contrast, foods that are widely enjoyed (such as coffee) but are consumed in reasonably regular patterns may not show the variation in intake that is necessary to provide an accurate examination of hypotheses.

Intake-Prone Populations

In attitude, perception, and cognition research, there is an understandable bias toward using the data from all participants who have been involved with a study. The rationale is that everyone has attitudes, perceptions, and cognitive processes that must be accounted for to accurately assess the influence of the different experimental treatments.

Measurement sensitivity in intake research, on the other hand, presupposes that users are different and potentially of more interest than nonusers. Since the key questions are focused on intake volume or frequency, it may not make sense to include participants who never have used (or who will never use) the food. For instance, a study using milk as a food stimulus can justly screen out participants who are lactose intolerant or otherwise allergic to milk. Similarly, it would also be acceptable to screen out nonusers of milk or people who simply do not drink it because they do not like its taste or texture. Studies that do not screen out nonusers are left with columns of zeros because regardless of the treatment condition, the consumer will not consume the food. While this may not be a problem if these nonusers are balanced across all cells of a design, this still generates unwanted variance that can be justly eliminated.

Yet just as nonusers add unwanted variance because they are qualitatively different than users, there may also be occasions when heavy users may be qualitatively different than light users. For instance, those with an alcohol dependency might behave qualitatively differently in a wine study than an occasional wine-with-dinner person, and Americans who have a "sweet tooth" behave qualitatively differently in a dessert study than most Asians, who have a stronger preference for less sweet, more savory snacks.

It is important to understand that screening heavy users is only justified when they are believed to qualitatively differ from lighter users. In general, it is still important to account for past usage when examining intake or usage behaviors. Past usage behavior can be used as a covariate for various analyses, or it can be used as a basis for categorizing heavier users from lighter users and analyzing each group separately.

Intake Floors and Ceiling

One difficulty with emerging fields of research lies not only in defining and measuring the *dependent* variables but also in determining the appropriate range of the *independent* variables that are examined. That is, to determine how different package sizes might influence one's intake volume, we must know the general range of sensitivity toward package size. If the small size package is such that most people empty the package on each intake occasion, it is a confounded test of the hypothesis because participants could not consume more even if they had wanted. It is therefore important to select packages that are large enough to not be fully consumed.

While the naive solution would be to increase the relative size of both packages to the point where there would be no ceiling effects, doing so would also result in diminishing effects. In his study of package sizes, Wansink (2006) showed that there becomes a point at which larger packages cease to have an effect on how much people consume. In effect, there is a point at which a person is just too full to eat (or drink) any more, regardless of how much stronger the manipulation becomes. If the manipulations are set outside this range of intake sensitivity, the resulting conclusions will be that the stimulus has no impact on intake. One solution to this involves calibration prestudies. Another involves collecting data

at three or more reasonably wide intervals of strength, knowing that only two may end up being of eventual interest because of either floor effects or ceiling (diminishing return) effects.

A related concern when examining quantities is the problem with satiation or flavor/category burnout. Inman (2001) identified that the burnout that is related to satiation can be delayed when a person switches between flavors within the same category. This can be one way in which to delay the effects of burnout in order to examine intake more extensively. Yet this underscores, more generally, the importance of understanding that satiation can cause a natural ceiling that we cannot easily observe. One solution for this is to be mindful of the time horizon under which a study is being conducted. The longer the time horizon, the less of a concern for burnout.

Selecting Intake Measures

Intake-related variables can be measured on various levels. This includes acquisition (such as purchase) and intended intake (which can be either short range or longer range), continues to actual intake, and can conclude with postintake reporting or residual analysis. Realizing that there are various levels on which intake can be examined becomes important in determining the most effective (and cost-efficient) way to study a research question. Figure 9.4 illustrates the different points at which intake can be measured. These can generally be characterized as preintake measures or postintake measures. If a research question does not necessitate the most involved measure (about intake, for example), it may be easier and less expensive to collect measures of intake intention instead.

It is important to distinguish between these different stages. It is often incorrectly assumed that one stage necessarily and accurately leads to another (Weingarten, 1984). For instance, it is often assumed that purchase will predictably lead to intake and that purchase data, therefore, are a surrogate for intake. While perhaps true under

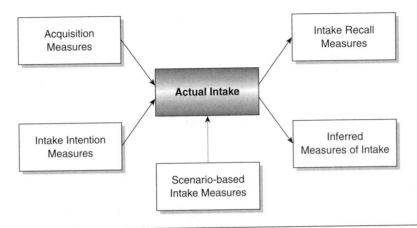

Figure 9.4   Different Forms of Intake-Related Measures

some conditions, there are still many foods that are thrown away or that sit unused and forgotten in the back of cupboards and pantries.

Preintake Measures

Acquisition Measures

As noted earlier, the intake rate of foods between purchase periods may be linear or consistent. While this may be true for some foods such as coffee or toothpaste, most other foods are less consistently consumed. Consider over-the-counter medicine, such as cold medicine or cough syrup. Such medicines are not consumed at a linear rate. Some consumers buy and consume this medicine immediately, while other consumers deplete it in tiered stages whenever they are sick. Still others stockpile the food for "insurance," while others purchase it and never use it because they either forgot about it or misplaced it. Scanner data do not tell us who in the household consumed the food, and they often assume a household size of one.

While the drawbacks of these have been noted earlier, there do seem to be conditions where they may be more justifiable. With frequently purchased goods, there is less likelihood that extraneous events (such as parties or guests) are causing untractable spikes in intake. With nonperishable items, there is less of a likelihood that things will be thrown away without being consumed. Last, when items are widely consumed around the household, it may be that they will be consumed at a more static rate than if there is only one person consuming the food.

Measuring Intake Intentions

The assumption of much marketing and sensory research is that if consumers rate a flavor as acceptable, they will consume it. Yet basic measures of attitude do not explain behavior and even less frequently relate to behavior (Garber, 2007). Because purchase and intake is a marketing-related objective in food development, intake intentions should be measured at the time of testing. Two ways of measuring one's intake intentions (for a particular time period, such as "within the next two weeks") are through likelihood measures or through estimates of one's future intake frequency. Likelihood measures can be directly obtained by asking an individual how likely (*highly unlikely* = 1 to *highly likely* = 9) it will be that he or she consumes the food within an upcoming time period. Intake intentions can also be measured by asking one to estimate how many times he or she might possibly consume the food within a similar time period (Wansink & Ray, 2000).

These two different measures of intake intent have different relative strengths. With infrequent users of a food, frequency estimates will be skewed toward 0 units (especially over a relatively short period of time). This is partially a drawback of numerical estimates that provide no gradation between 0 and 1 unit. In such cases, the frequency estimates provide less variance and less information than an estimate of intake likelihood. With light users, intake likelihood estimates will provide greater gradation in response and more sensitivity in detecting any potentially different effects that a particular set of sensory qualities would have on intake.

In contrast, with frequent or heavy users of a food, a frequency estimate is likely to be more accurate than a likelihood estimate. This is because the distribution of these frequency estimates is more likely to be normally distributed. As a result, a frequency estimate of one's intake intent is likely to provide more variance and more information about the intended intake of heavy users than is a likelihood measure, which would undoubtedly be at or near 1.0 (100% probable). With heavy users, frequency estimates would be a more accurate estimate of a heavy user's future intake frequency of a food.

When a sample consists of both heavy and light users, both likelihood and frequency measures should be used with both groups. However, in weighting the relative measures, frequency estimates should be weighted more heavily for consumers who are heavy users, and purchase likelihood measures should be weighted more heavily for consumers who are light users. Using both measures allows some degree of comparison, but weighting them allows more confidence in making segment-level conclusions.

In general, however, intake intention measures are most valid when they involve a readily accessible food that involves little or no preparation. The more intermediate steps that are involved (such as purchasing the food or preparing the food), the less accurate this measure becomes. In general, the direction of the bias for intake intention measures (frequency and likelihood) depends on the availability and convenience of the food.

When conditioning on past usage, it is important to check for differences across groups and foods. For frequently consumed foods, it may be that the difference between relatively heavy and relatively light consumers may not be important or diagnostic. Conversely, with very infrequently consumed foods, there may not be much of a difference between relatively heavy and light consumers because these differences might actually be caused by differences in consume volume per occasion and not by a wider number of occasions each.

The relation of intentions to usage is conditioned on many factors. It is critical to ask about intake in a specific situation. This is consistent with the view that attitudes are specific to a situation, and the key to linking attitude to behavior was to make sure that the attitude measure was carefully and specifically linked to behavior in an actual situation. The importance of linking attitude to specific situations is illustrated by the corresponding correlation increase. Estimates for general intake in three food categories had a correlation near .45; estimating the intake in specific situations increased the correlation to .77.

Postintake Measures

Measures of Intake Recall

It has long been recognized in social psychology that environmental factors can influence intake. One such confound involves those around us. There are social norms as to how much should or should not be consumed. These can involve social norms of underintake at an interview dinner or social norms of overintake at a New Year's party.

When studying unfamiliar foods, for instance, it is generally assumed that people have similar food experience backgrounds and that the treatments will have a general impact across all consumers. In contrast, with intake-related studies, one's past intake of the food and their liking of the food can easily create biases that need to be accounted for so they do not generate unwanted noise. For instance, with studies of how stockpiling influences intake, the treatment conditions may involve giving some participants high inventory levels of specific foods while giving others lower levels. In such circumstances, it is important to account for existing inventory levels and to account for any additional purchases that might occur during the test period.

On an immediate level, one's like or dislike of a food influences his or her intake. This is something that can be controlled by using past measures of attitude toward the food or toward the general category of foods it represents. Having people with a wide range of preferences for tuna fish or for chocolate can influence the results. Some of this would presumably be taken into account when screening or segmenting non-, light, and heavy users. In other cases, people do not have the opportunity to eat foods with the frequency they like (because of availability or diet restrictions). Yet their inherent preference for them would suggest they are different from light or nonusers who exhibit similar intake tendencies.

Estimated recall of intake can also be made and analyzed. While this is a reasonable surrogate for actual intake, it is influenced by factors such as the salience and the convenience of the food. Recent studies of chocolate intake have shown that people consume more chocolates when it is convenient and visible (on the desk) than when it is either inconvenient (2 meters from the desk) or convenient but not visible (in the desk). Yet their estimates of how much they eat were in the opposite direction. If the food was convenient, they overestimated how much they consumed, whereas if it was inconveniently located, they underestimated their intake of it (Painter, Wansink, & Hieggelke, 2002).

Residual and Inferential Measures of Intake

Just as preintake predictions about intake can be made forward from a purchase, postintake inferences can be made based on residual waste, including what a person does not eat or what a person throws away ("garbology").

Intake can be measured by how much people use, how much they do not use, or how much they remember using. Perhaps the easiest way to measure intake is by weighing or counting what is not eaten; this entails premeasuring portions and then weighing the food that was left uneaten.

One study, which measured the impact that container size and mood had on the intake of movie popcorn, gave people either large or extra-large containers of popcorn (Wansink & Kim, 2005). Prior to passing these out, each was weighed and the weight was written on the bottom of each container. Following the study, each container was collected, and the weight of the remaining popcorn was subtracted from the original weight to provide an estimate of intake. One danger of measuring residual intake is that it must be noted if people either spilled part of the container, whether they combined it with a friend, or whether they emptied the container and filled another container (or their pockets) with the food for later use. In all of these cases, the data from these people are eliminated from the study.

In general, when measuring usage, it is much more effective to weigh rather than count. This is true when giving foods to people and also when assessing the residual. Counting out exactly 300 jelly beans is much more time-consuming than making sure every container has the same number of grams of jelly beans. Following the study, determining the residual is much more easily done with a scale than with counting.

Scenario-Based Methods of Measuring Intake

One emerging method is that of scenario-based studies. Such studies present consumers with a scenario and ask them to predict what their intake would be under various manipulated circumstances. Scenario-based studies can be an effective means of investigating intake issues, particularly in the preliminary stages of a study or when beginning a program of research. While this is not as conclusive as having actual measures of intake (or of reported intake), it can be effective as a prestudy. This has even been used in early stages to determine how the size of containers would influence how much people poured. In these studies, consumers were given the stimuli (various-sized bottles of shampoo) and asked to indicate how much they would use by drawing a circle on one photograph of a hand. The area of the circle was then used as a surrogate for volume and used in the subsequent measures.

Intake studies conducted using scenario-based or hypothesized intake can be appropriate for academic research. Other times, however, it is also important to try and understand how such scenarios relate or map to actual intake so the size of the effect can be calibrated to determine whether it is worth intervention. This can be accomplished by re-creating the study in a field situation. As the number of these field replications grows, a more general estimate of the carryover of estimation and hypothesized intake measures can be made.

Analyzing Intake Studies

In analyzing intake studies, critically different methods used to analyze intake differ depending on whether it is volume, frequency, or incidence that is being studied. While each holds its own challenges, we will focus first on the practice of screening or segmenting nonusers and then address each in turn.

Screening and Segmenting Nonusers

Nonusers can create unwanted variance in intake-related studies through non-reporting or through reactivity. Screening nonusers out of an analysis can be critical in reducing variance that could otherwise obscure the effects through

non-reporting. This has frequently been done when studying volume, and it can also be justified when studying frequency.

Yet when studying incidence, screening out nonusers can be problematic. It would be easy to misclassify a person as a "nonuser" if too narrow of a time window or too restricted of a range of situations were investigated. There are many reasons why a person might choose to not consume a food. It may be occasion based (such as only eating cranberry sauce during holidays), or it might be joint decision based (such as being indifferent to anchovies but willing to eat them if ordered by a spouse or colleague). In either of these two cases, it is important to realize that there are differences between nonincidence that is caused by an absence of intake opportunity and nonincidence that is caused because one strongly dislikes a food and never consumes it.

Determining whether a participant should be screened out as a nonuser can present problems. Screening a person's food intake prior to a study can unintentionally foreshadow the purpose of the study and contaminate the results. One way to avoid this is to postscreen respondents instead of prescreen. This involves asking the screening questions (past usage frequency, most recent intake, etc.) following the collection of the measures for the primary dependent variables. At this point, reports of their past usage will not bias the primary measures, and consumers who simply do not use the food can be safely selected out of subsequent analyses. While nonuse of this food would result in data that would be thrown away, the screening can be done without fear of any contamination or demand effects.

There are times, however, when prescreening must be done for cost or efficiency reasons. In these cases, one less reactive way in which to prescreen consumers for a study is to ask them their past usage frequency of the food while also asking them about their frequency of a number of other related or unrelated foods that act as distracter items. Screening questions could be asked that do not directly investigate the target food but collect enough related data for an effective prescreen.

Separating consumers into different groups (such as non-, light, and heavy users) can be useful in determining the influence of marketing variables. Conditioning on past usage is particularly important when examining intake intentions and estimated intake.

Just as screening out nonusers can increase measurement sensitivity by reducing noise, sometimes focusing only on heavy users can increase sensitivity by magnifying the potential effects of certain treatments. One way to prescreen on this basis is by the absolute past frequency in which they have consumed a food.

In a study of how advertising variations influence intake, it was found that heavy users were more influenced by intake-oriented ads than light users but were more sensitive to treatment methods. As a result, differences that would be statistically insignificant for lighter users would be significant to heavy users.

Measuring Usage Frequency

Identify Broad Intake Intervals

It is important to not examine intake during potentially confounding time periods when the base rate of intake of the food is too low to be diagnostic (soup tests in the summer in Texas; cranberry sauce tests during the spring). It is critical that either diary panels or callbacks match the intake cycle interval. While some foods (such as coffee or toothpaste) are consumed at fairly standard rates, many others (particularly seasonal nonperishables) are not. Intake should be sampled across a long enough time frame to not be biased by accelerated intake that might occur during the early part of the purchase cycle or to be biased by the decelerated intake that might occur at later stages. The former bias would lead to a long-term overestimate of intake, and the latter would lead to a long-term underestimate.

It is also important to differentiate between intake driven by special occasions and intake that occurs in a more standard way during the typical passage of time. Chandon and Wansink (2007) show that it is important to differentiate between intake that is determined by salience and that driven by convenience.

Specifying Intake Situations and Usage Occasions

Although purchase intentions are often used as a dependent variable, intake intentions have a less developed history. Because of the differences between intake and purchase, there are legitimate concerns that intake intentions are not reliable surrogates for actual intake. Many of these concerns are valid when intake intention measures are incorrectly taken, but when carefully and correctly done, their reliability and validity improve.

As with attitude measures, intake measures should specify the time period and the intake situation. For instance, Wansink and Ray (2000) report that when people were asked to estimate their intake of a food in a specific situation (eating dinner within the next two weeks), they were more accurate than when estimating their total intake of soup over the same time period ($r = 0.77$ vs. $r = 0.58$).

One way to validate this relationship between intentions and intake is to conduct a split-half study. Such a study measures estimated and actual intake with one group (before and after being exposed to various stimuli) and measures only the actual intake of a second group (after being exposed to the same sets of stimuli). Comparing the two groups enables a researcher to assess potential demand effects. It also allows the researcher to determine how reliable intake intention estimates are in that situation by comparing intended and actual intake. Should they prove to be accurate and if they are not reactive (no demand effects), future studies of this type might be done more efficiently by simply using intake intentions.

Accounting for Usage Facilitators

Recall that certain foods might have different intake acceleration propensities than others because of physical characteristics such as

Table 9.1　Different Forms of Intake-Related Measures

Usage Level	Measures of Intake (Within Next 2 Weeks)	
	Likelihood Measure	Volume Measure
Light users		
Canned soup	.421	.151
Gelatin	.779	.580
Cranberry sauce	.490	.221
Average	.472	.161
Heavy users		
Canned soup	.190	.618
Gelatin	.233	.462
Cranberry sauce	.043	.207
Average	.197	.597

whether they are hedonic or utilitarian. It is also important to note that wide ranges of situations can influence intake and must also be accounted for. Recent studies indicate (Chandon & Wansink, 2002) that convenient-to-eat foods (such as ready-to-drink iced tea or premade pudding) have a much higher intake incidence than do foods that are less convenient to consume (such as ice tea mix or boxed pudding). Similarly, the basic convenience and salience of a food also influence how frequently it is eaten. A recent study showed that chocolate kisses that are more accessible and convenient (sitting on the desk) are eaten with greater frequency than those that are slightly less accessible and convenient (two meters from the desk; Painter et al., 2002).

The importance here is to try and account for environmental factors that can influence intake. This can be accomplished in either the design of a study or by controlling them by asking critical questions about convenience, salience, or accessibility. It seems that people feel a need to take a food's visibility and convenience into account when they try to estimate their prior intake of it

in such a way that a food that is inconvenient to consume may be eaten in larger amounts than are thought or recalled. Similarly, dietary researchers need to take into account the visibility and convenience of foods because not doing so might lead to biases in intake recall studies and diary panel estimates. One way to allow for such biases is to ask research participants to rate the visibility and convenience of the foods under investigation; these ratings can then be used either as covariates or as blocking or segmentation variables.

Comparative Versus Absolute Measures of Usage Frequency

Intake frequency is typically measured on an absolute level—units per week. It can also be measured, however, on a more comparative basis using either difference measures or an index. This would be akin to accounting for individual-level variation by accounting for within-subject effects. Such difference measures can involve the difference in intake between the test period and a pretest calibration period. They can also involve the differences in intake between the test period and one's usual or typical intake of the food over that same time interval. This can be expressed as a difference measure, but they have also been expressed as an index.

Another means of assessing intake is through the use of scaled comparison measures. Questions that address this typically ask a person to compare his or her intake with that of a typical intake period. They might then rate this on a 9-point scale (1 = I consumed less than is typical for me; 9 = I consumed more than is typical for me). While such comparative measures lack the appeal of an actual, tangible unit of measure, they appear highly sensitive to the treatments. They may be useful in prestudies as well as in final studies as a validation check or self-report in follow-up studies.

Measuring Intake Volume (Per Occasion)

Measuring intake volume is more straightforward than measuring intake frequency, yet still important. The issue of screening out nonusers is critical here as with intake frequency.

Actual Versus Inferred Intake

The two general methods for calculating intake are measuring actual intake volume or measuring residual intake, which is inferring intake based on the difference between the amount taken initially and the amount left after consumption.

A variation on these methods measures how much food is taken and assumes everything is consumed unless there is residual. A recent study of pouring behavior examined how glass sizes and shapes influenced pouring volume of juice at a summer camp. When people returned their dishes, the residual juice was subtracted from the amount originally poured. The difference was assumed to be what was consumed.

While this is a generally accepted measure, it needs to be underscored that it is inaccurate if a person spills or shares a food or if he or she saves it for a later time. To account for these, the person can be given an exit questionnaire that asks whether he or she spilled, shared, or saved the food in a pocket, purse, briefcase, or backpack. These people can then be eliminated from the study and reported as such. If it is critical that the study remain as unobtrusive as possible, unobtrusive video cameras can record intake behavior, and spilling, sharing, or saving can be coded and associated with the relevant person. This entails individual intake or assigned seating.

Counting Versus Weighing

Two different methods of determined intake volume are either to count or weigh the residual amount of the food that is left at the end of the intake episode. This can either be subtracted from what was originally taken by the consumer or by what was given to the consumer. In some instances, foods can be weighed, but in other instances, it is preferable from a design or a reporting standpoint to count the units consumed.

Weighing what is consumed is nearly always preferable to counting what is consumed. Indeed, with liquids and more continuous (mashed potatoes) or nonuniform consumables (such as French fries or meat), weighing can be the only option. Unfortunately, keeping track of what foods are taken and consumed based on weighing can be obtrusive and impractical for some studies. In these cases, it can be more advisable to discretely measure how much is taken either through unobtrusive observation or by recall questionnaires.

Certain foods lend themselves better to being counted (vs. weighed) than others. With more discrete or uniformly shaped foods, it may be preferable to measure or at least report them in terms of units. This is often true with candy (such as small candies or small candy bars), snacks (crackers, grapes, or cheese squares), or other small, pre-prepared foods. This has also been done successfully by asking the number cans of a soft drink or glasses of a beverage one has consumed during a time period. The importance of counting foods is that it can often be done less obtrusively than weighing. That is, people can be observed by confederates, they can be recorded by unobtrusive video cameras, or they can be questioned at the end of the episode.

Yet in other cases, it may be expedient to weigh a food in grams but report it in terms of units (or percentage of units). This can be done by weighing the food in the study and translating this measure to units. For instance, in studies of M&M and jelly bean intake, Kahn and Wansink (2004) used a residual weight measure in the methodologies but translated these weights into the number of M&Ms and number of jelly beans consumed for ease of reporting.

Accounting for Satiation

A key issue in examining intake was factoring in the effect that satiation from additional foods might have on the intake of the primary food being studied. For example, in one study of candy intake (Kahn & Wansink, 2004), consumers were given different varieties of candies that varied only in their color. The objective was to determine how variations in color influenced intake volume. Although carefully done across multiple locations with multiple groups, no differences were found. The methodology entailed bringing consumers in to a central mall location, giving them their choice of beverage, and assigning them to one of the candy conditions where they were given candy to eat as they watched television. In reviewing the methodology, it was later found that their selection of a beverage influenced how much candy they ate. Consumers who selected a sugared soft drink ate less candy than those who selected a diet soft drink, and both groups ate less than those selecting only water. When the study was rerun using only water, the expected differences in intake were consistent with what was hypothesized (Inman, 2001).

To make certain the effect sizes are as large as possible, one must determine how the presence of other foods influences intake. A recent field

study in which we investigated how the presence of others (manipulated through table size) influenced salty snack intake was conducted in a pub environment. We did not expect people to drink additional beverages than the ones we provided and carefully controlled. As a result, a good portion of the study was confounded because it did not also take into account the amount of beer that people drank. That is, while larger tables increased the amount that people eat, it also increased the amount they drank, and it is well established that the two variables are correlated.

It is also important in these studies of volume to take measures of critical covariates that can influence intake. Besides basic gender, age, height, and weight variables, it is also good to ask how many hours since their last meal, as well as a rating scale measuring the extent to which they are on a diet and watch what they eat. These measures should be used as covariates, and in the early stages of exploration, they can be assessed or analyzed separately to determine the strength of an effect. Not surprisingly, unless a ceiling is reached, the strongest differences between treatments are found among males in their early 20s who do not carefully monitor what or how much they eat.

Identifying the Appropriate Level of Analysis

One issue concerning intake is to not lose sight of the forest because of the trees. It is important that researchers consider a wide range of intake when analyzing how different factors influence intake. Consider a recent study that examined whether people consumed more olive oil or butter when eating bread dinner at a restaurant. While it was found that people ate many more calories of olive oil than butter on a piece of bread, they ate fewer pieces of bread. As a result, people do use more olive oil than butter when they eat a piece of bread, but they also eat fewer pieces of bread (Wansink & Linder, 2003). By broadening the field of focus, examining the amount of bread consumed, the results of the study became more conclusive.

When people were given olive oil in a restaurant, they consumed 26% more on each piece of bread than those given block butter, but they ended up consuming 23% less bread in total. This finding provides a novel look at a traditional dietary recommendation: When considering the health aspects in a diet, one needs to focus not only on fat calories but also on total calories. By eating less fat, one can unknowingly eat more carbohydrates—eating twice as many low-fat cookies trades off fat calories for an increased amount of carbohydrates. When focusing on the intake of a target food, it is critical to also analyze how that food influences the intake of related foods. A preoccupation with fat intake can distract health care professionals from understanding alternative effects that may bring their own set of health concerns.

Similarly, recent studies have investigated how the degree of heterogeneity in candy assortment influenced the intake of candy. In conducting the study, people were given one of the various assortments of candy, and the amount they ate was observed while they watched television. Because candy can make one thirsty, they were also given a selection of beverages. The data were inconclusive, and it was suspected that those who chose bottled soft drinks (instead of bottled water) might have varied how much candy they ate to keep their total sugar intake at a reasonable level. A subsequent study that provided only bottled water to people supported this conclusion, and the results were more in line with what was originally predicted.

Conclusion

"Cool data" are not easy data to collect. When it comes to field studies, the challenges of measuring intake for every procedure and set of measures have both advantages and disadvantages. As the need for precision and accuracy increases, increased confidence in intake methods and measures can be found by combining methods and triangulating on their conclusions (Sudman

& Wansink, 2002). For instance, combining a lab study with a field study can provide both the tight internal validity in the lab study with the external validity of the field study. Similarly, it can be useful to combine secondary data with recall surveys or to combine diary panels with laboratory experiments.

References

Allison, D. B., Fontaine, K., Manson, J. E., Stevens, J., & VanItallie, T. B. (1999). Annual deaths attributable to obesity in the United States. *Journal of the American Medical Association, 282,* 1530–1538.

Assunçao, J., & Meyer, R. J. (1993). The rational effect of price promotions on sales and consumption. *Management Science, 39,* 517–535.

Baron, R. M., & Kenny, D. A. (1986). The moderator-mediator variable distinction in social psychological research: Conceptual, strategic, and statistical consideration. *Journal of Personality and Social Psychology, 51,* 1173–1182.

Bell, R., & Pliner, P. L. (2003). Time to eat: The relationship between the number of people eating and meal duration in three lunch settings. *Appetite, 41,* 215–218.

Berry, S. L., Beatty, W. W., & Klesges, R. C. (1985). Sensory and social influences on ice-cream intake by males and females in a laboratory setting. *Appetite, 6,* 41–45.

Bradburn, N., Sudman, S., & Wansink, B. (2004). *Asking questions.* San Francisco: Jossey-Bass.

Chandon, P., & Wansink, B. (2002). When are stockpiled foods consumed faster? A convenience-salience framework of post-purchase intake incidence and quantity. *Journal of Marketing Research, 39,* 321–335.

Chandon, P., & Wansink, B. (2007). The biasing health halos of fast food restaurant health claims: Lower calorie estimates and higher side-dish consumption intentions. *Journal of Consumer Research, 34,* 301–314.

Clendenen, V., Herman, C. P., & Polivy, J. (1994). Social facilitation of eating among friends and strangers. *Appetite, 23,* 1–13.

de Castro, J. M. (1994). Family and friends produce greater social facilitation of food-Intake than other companions. *Physiology & Behavior, 56,* 445–455.

Evans, G. W., & Lepore, S. J. (1997). Moderating and mediating processing in environment-behavior research. In G. T. Moore & R. W. Marans (Eds.), *Advances in environment, behavior and design* (Vol. 4). New York: Plenum.

Fisher, J. O., Rolls, B. J., & Birch, L. L. (2003). Children's bite size and intake of an entree are greater with large portions than with age-appropriate or self - selected portions. *American Journal of Clinical Nutrition, 77*, 1164–1170.

French, S. A., Story, M., & Jeffery, R. W. (2001). Environmental influences on eating and physical activity. *Annual Review of Public Health, 22*, 309–325.

Fuenekes, G. I., de Graaf, C., & van Staveren, W. A. (1995). Social facilitation of food intake is mediated by meal duration. *Physiology & Behavior, 58*, 551–558.

Garber, L. (2007). Shape, size, and intake. *Journal of Marketing Research, 31*, 341–355.

Inman, J. J. (2001). The role of sensory specific satiety in attribute level variety seeking. *Journal of Consumer Research, 28*, 105–120.

Iynegar, S. S., & Lepper, M. R. (2000). When choice is demotivating: Can one desire too much of a good thing? *Journal of Personality and Social Psychology, 79*, 995–1006.

Kahn, B. E., & Wansink, B. (2004). The influence of assortment structure on perceived variety and intake quantities. *Journal of Consumer Research, 30*, 581–596.

Lawless, H. T., Bender, S., Oman, C., & Pelletier, C. (2003). Gender, age, vessel size, cup vs. straw sipping, and sequence effects on sip volume. *Dysphagia, 18*, 196–202.

Levitsky, D., & Youn, T. (2004). The more food young adults are served, the more they overeat. *Journal of Nutrition, 134*, 2546–2549.

Meiselman, H. L. (1992). Obstacles to studying real people eating real meals in real situations. *Appetite, 19*, 84–86.

Painter, J. E., Wansink, B., & Hieggelke, J. B. (2002). How visibility and convenience influence candy consumption. *Appetite, 38*, 237–238.

Pliner, P. (1974). On the generalizability of the externality hypothesis. In S. Schachter & J. Rodin (Eds.), *Obese humans and rats* (pp. 111–129). Potomac, MD: Lawrence Erlbaum.

Polivy, J., Herman, C. P., Hackett, R., & Kuleshnyk, I. (1986). The effects of self-attention and public attention on eating in restrained and unrestrained subjects. *Journal of Personality and Social Psychology, 50*, 1203–1024.

Polivy, J., Herman, C. P., Younger, J. C., & Erskine, B. (1979). Effects of a model on eating behavior: The induction of a restrained eating style. *Journal of Personality, 47*, 100–117.

Raghubir, P., & Krishna, A. (1999). Vital dimensions in volume perception: Can the eye fool the stomach? *Journal of Marketing Research, 36*, 313–326.

Rolls, B. J., Bell, E. A., & Waugh, B. A. (2000). Increasing the volume of a food by incorporating air affects satiety in men. *American Journal of Clinical Nutrition, 72*, 361–368.

Rolls, B. J., Engell, D., & Birch, L. L. (2000). Serving portion size influences 5-year-old but not 3-year-old children's food intakes. *Journal of the American Dietetic Association, 100*, 232–234.

Rozin, P., Dow, S., Moscovitch, M., & Rajaram, S. (1998). What causes humans to begin and end a meal? A role for memory for what has been eaten, as evidenced by a study of multiple meal eating in amnesic patients. *Psychological Science, 9*, 392–396.

Rozin, P., Kabnick, K., Pete, E., Fischler, C., & Shields, C. (2003). The ecology of eating: Smaller portion sizes in France than in the United States help explain the French paradox. *Psychological Science, 14*, 450–454.

Schachter, S. (1971). Some extraordinary facts about obese humans and rats. *American Psychologist, 26*, 129–144.

Schachter, S., & Friedman, L. N. (1974). The effects of work and cue prominence on eating behavior. In S. Schachter & J. Rodin (Eds.), *Obese humans and rats* (pp. 11–20). Potomac, MD: Lawrence Erlbaum.

Sudman, S., & Wansink, B. (2002). *Consumer panels* (2nd ed.). Chicago: American Marketing Association.

Terry, K., & Beck, S. (1985). Eating style and food storage habits in the home: Assessment of obese and nonobese families. *Behavior Modification, 9*, 242–261.

Wansink, B. (2004). Environmental factors that increase the food intake and intake volume of unknowing consumers. *Annual Review of Nutrition, 24*, 455–479.

Wansink, B. (2006). *Mindless eating: Why we eat more than we think*. New York: Bantam-Dell.

Wansink, B., & Cheney, M. M. (2005). Super bowls: Serving bowl size and food intake, *Journal of the American Medical Association, 293*, 1727–1728.

Wansink, B., Kent, R. J., & Hoch, S. J. (1998). An anchoring and adjustment model of purchase quantity decisions. *Journal of Marketing Research, 35*, 71–81.

Wansink, B., & Kim, J. (2005). Bad popcorn in big buckets: Portion size can influence intake as much as taste. *Journal of Nutrition Education and Behavior, 37*, 242–245.

Wansink, B., & Linder, L. W. (2003). Interactions between forms of fat consumption and restaurant bread consumption. *International Journal of Obesity, 27*, 866–868.

Wansink, B., & Park, S. (2001). At the movies: How external cues and perceived taste impact consumption volume. *Food Quality and Preference, 12*, 69–74.

Wansink, B., Payne, C. R., & Chandon, P. (2007). Internal and external cues of meal cessation: The French paradox redux? *Obesity, 15*, 2920–2924.

Wansink, B., & Ray, M. L. (2000). Estimating an advertisement's impact on one's consumption of a brand. *Journal of Advertising Research, 40*, 106–113.

Wansink, B., & Sobal, J. (2007). Mindless eating: The 200 daily food decisions we overlook. *Environment and Behavior, 39*, 106–123.

Wansink, B., van Ittersum, K., & Werle, C. (In press). How negative experiences shape long-term food preferences: Fifty years from the World War II combat front. *Appetite.*

Weingarten, H. P. (1984). Meal initiation controlled by learned cues: Basic behavioral properties. *Appetite, 5*, 147–158.

CHAPTER 10

Binge Eating and Purging

Giorgio A. Tasca, Valerie Krysanski,
Natasha Demidenko, and Hany Bissada

B inge eating and purging are key symptoms in eating disorders that have both diagnostic and prognostic significance. Binge eating is a central diagnostic criterion for bulimia nervosa (BN) and binge-eating disorder (BED; American Psychiatric Association [APA], 1994; Spitzer, Yanovski, Wadden, et al., 1993). It also occurs in approximately 40% to 50% of anorexia nervosa (AN) patients and is common in BN. Accordingly, the proper and accurate assessment of binge eating and purging is critical for the proper diagnosis and treatment planning of these disorders.

In this chapter, we define the parameters that must be addressed to reliably measure binge eating and purging. In doing so, we discuss some common difficulties encountered in attaining the desired uniformity in the definition of these parameters. Next, we review the methods available for assessing these behaviors. Assessment methods are organized into two categories: (1) self-report questionnaires and (2) structured clinical interviews. We discuss the most commonly used specific instruments, highlighting the psychometric properties, research evidence,

and relative advantages and disadvantages they offer the researcher and the clinician.

Definition of Binge Eating

The term *binge eating* is of recent origin in the clinical literature, and its emergence from the ancient diagnosis of bulimia is worth noting. The term *bulimia* comes from the Greek term *limos,* meaning hunger, and added to it is the prefix *bous,* which means ox; thus, when Hippocrates used the term *Boulimos,* he referred to a ravenous hunger similar to the hunger of an ox (Liddell & Scott, 1972).

It was in the context of anorexia nervosa that the modern notion of bulimia emerged as a medical term describing an abnormal craving for food that results in binge eating, followed by self-induced vomiting. This bulimic behavior has been known since the 1940s and was considered to be one possible presentation of anorexia nervosa. It was, however, in 1976 that Boskind-White described a group of patients who did not present with any significant weight loss and consequently could not be diagnosed with AN (Boskind-White & White, 1983). He used the term *bulimarexia* to describe this group of patients. Later in 1979, Palmer used the term *dietary chaos syndrome,* while in the same year, Russell (1979) coined the term *bulimia nervosa* to describe normal-weight bulimic patients. The term *binge eating* was introduced over 40 years ago by Stunkard (1959), who described recurrent overeating in a subgroup of obese patients who did not purge. Over the past two decades, the phenomenon of binge eating in the absence of the inappropriate compensatory behaviors has received increasing attention from researchers (Spitzer, Devlin, et al., 1992; Spitzer, Yanovski, Wadden, et al., 1993), until its eventual introduction in the fourth edition of the *Diagnostic and Statistical Manual of Mental Disorders* (*DSM-IV;* APA, 1994) as a specific example of an eating disorder not otherwise specified (EDNOS). It was included as a provisional diagnosis of "Binge Eating Disorder" in Appendix B of the *DSM-IV,* as a diagnostic category in need of further study.

Criteria for the Clinical Diagnosis of Binge Eating

According to the *DSM-IV* (APA, 1994), an episode of binge eating, in BN and BED, is characterized by both of the following: (1) eating, in a discrete period of time (e.g., within any 2-hour period), an amount of food that is definitely larger than most people would eat during a similar period of time and under similar circumstances and (2) a sense of lack of control over eating during the episode (e.g., a feeling that one cannot stop eating or control what or how much one is eating).

Parameters of Binge Eating

The Size of the Binge

DSM-IV criteria refer to the size of an objective binge as an amount of food that is definitely larger

than most people would eat during a similar period of time and under similar circumstances. When applying this criterion in practice, clinicians and researchers may have some difficulty distinguishing a true objective binge from overeating seen in many overweight people. Self-reports of binge eating frequently describe a sense of loss of control associated with a low caloric consumption, which would not qualify as a true objective binge-eating episode and have thus been referred to as "subjective binges." Beglin and Fairburn (1992) investigated the use of the word *binge* in a community sample of young women and found that young women placed a greater emphasis on loss of control when defining a binge and less on the quantity of food eaten (Beglin & Fairburn, 1992).

Some have argued that the reliability of quantifying a binge could be improved by using a cutoff of minimum caloric intake per binge. Fairburn (1987) recommended an average of 1,000 calories per binge to qualify as an objective binge. However, Rossiter and Agras (1990) found that nearly one third of binges in patients with BN consisted of less than 500 calories per binge. Although a cutoff of minimum caloric intake per binge would reduce the number of false positives, it may also result in an excessively high rate of false negatives. To avoid this drawback, we refer back to the *DSM-IV* criteria for binge eating, according to which, the clinician/researcher must consider the context in which an episode of binge eating occurred to determine if the amount of food consumed was large enough to qualify the episode as an objective binge.

The difficulty measuring objective binge episodes has led some to suggest that relying on self-report questionnaires (which accept participants' responses at face value) may generate less reliable results in distinguishing objective and subjective binge-eating episodes and overeating. More reliable results could be obtained using an investigator-based interview such as the Eating Disorder Examination (EDE; Fairburn & Cooper, 1993), in which a trained assessor classifies binges as objective or subjective according to specific guidelines, after obtaining a detailed account of the amount of food consumed by the subject during each binge-eating episode. The specifics of each instrument of measurement will be discussed later in this chapter.

The Frequency and Duration of Binge Eating

DSM-IV provided different parameters for BN and BED when addressing the frequency and the duration of binge eating. To qualify for the diagnosis of BN, *DSM-IV* stipulated that an individual must binge eat a minimum average of twice per week and for a minimum of 3 months' duration. To qualify for the provisional diagnosis of BED, *DSM-IV* suggested that an individual must binge eat on at least 2 *days* per week, irrespective of the number of binge episodes that may occur per day. Also, *DSM-IV* suggested a 6-month duration of binge eating to qualify for the diagnosis of BED rather than the 3-month duration stipulated for BN.

It is understandable that *DSM-IV* provided different parameters for the frequency of binge eating in BN and BED. In the former, discrete binge-eating episodes are punctuated by self-induced vomiting, laxative abuse, or other compensatory behaviors, which makes it easy for the patient to recall binge episodes on a self-administered questionnaire. On the other hand, in BED, binge eating is not punctuated by any specific behavior and often occurs in the background of overeating. For that reason, it was felt that recalling binge-eating days rather than discrete episodes of binge eating helps the patient with BED to provide more accurate measurements on a self-administered questionnaire. It is also important to distinguish between BN, nonpurging type, and BED. The latter is characterized by the absence of the regular use of inappropriate nonpurging compensatory behaviors (such as fasting and excessive exercise) that are characteristic of BN, nonpurging type.

The Loss of Control

Loss of control can be defined as a situation where the patient violates his or her initial intent to eat a small or regular amount of food, which is followed by the inability of that patient to conform his or her action to the original intent. This definition of loss of control begs the following question: Do planned binges (i.e., binges that are anticipated and prepared for in advance) meet the criterion of loss of control? A planned binge violates the patient's dietary standards, and the patient is unable to alter the course of the binge once the decision and the planning for a binge were made. Also, a planned binge is followed by the same feelings of anguish and guilt experienced by the patient who spontaneously binges. To qualify for the parameter of loss of control, both spontaneous bingeing and planned binges are subjectively experienced by the patient as behavior out of control. In addition to the subjective feeling of loss of control, *DSM-IV* stipulates that at least three of the following five behavioral indicators of impaired control should be met: (1) eating very rapidly, (2) eating until feeling uncomfortably full, (3) eating large amounts of food when not hungry, (4) eating alone because of embarrassment over how much one is eating, and (5) feeling disgust, guilt, or depression after overeating.

It is worth noting that there is an impressive consensus about the loss of control as a necessary parameter to define binge eating compared to the other parameters (Garner, Shafer, & Rosen, 1992; Rossiter & Agras, 1990). If loss of control is present, then the quantity of food will differentiate between objective and subjective binge episodes. (1) If the quantity of food consumed is objectively large and there is a loss of control, then the episode is qualified as an *objective binge*. (2) If the quantity of food is not large and there is loss of control, then the episode qualifies as a *subjective binge*. Conversely, in the absence of loss of control, then the quantity of food consumed will differentiate between objective and subjective overeating (Fairburn & Wilson, 1993; van der

Ster Wallin, Norring, & Holmgren, 1994). (3) If the quantity of food is objectively large and there is no loss of control, the episode qualifies as *objective overeating*. (4) If the quantity of food is not objectively large but viewed as large by the subject, and there is loss of control, then the episode qualifies as a *subjective overeating*.

Diagnostic Significance of Purging

DSM-IV defines compensatory mechanisms as inappropriate efforts to achieve weight loss and/or to counteract the effect of binge eating (both objective and subjective binges). These compensatory mechanisms are divided into two categories: purging and nonpurging types. The latter includes dieting, overexercising, and the use of appetite suppressant medications, including psychostimulants. The purging type includes self-induced vomiting, misuse of laxatives and diuretics, and self-administered enemas.

The purging type of compensatory mechanisms is diagnostically significant in the subtyping of AN (binge/purge type) and BN (purging type). In addition, the absence of regular compensatory mechanisms, including regular purging, is a prerequisite for retaining the provisional diagnosis of a BED. It should be noted, however, that an occasional use of a laxative or a diuretic does not preclude the diagnosis of BED as long as the purging behavior is not repeated on a regular basis.

Parameters of Purging

DSM-IV diagnostic criteria call for assessment of the frequency of the purging behavior in the 3 months preceding the time the patient presented for the consultation. Purging behaviors, as enumerated above, are relatively easy for patients to report accurately in terms of frequency of the behavior—whether or not they have engaged in that behavior at least twice per week for the past 3 months—as stipulated by *DSM-IV* diagnostic criteria. Patients may also report if the purging

behavior was preceded by an objective binge or the patient engaged in purging for the purpose of body purification in the absence of any binge eating.

Self-Report Questionnaires

We now turn to assessment methods for binge eating and purging with a focus on self-report questionnaires and structured interviews. In the following section, self-report questionnaires that are most commonly used to assess binge eating or purging, and for which adequate psychometric properties exist, are detailed. We present a description of the measure, followed by evidence for reliability and validity, and conclude with a comment about availability of the tool.

Binge Eating Scale

Description

The Binge Eating Scale (BES; Gormally, Black, Daston, & Rardin, 1982) was developed as a self-report measure to assess the extent to which obese individuals experience binge-eating problems. The BES consists of 16 multiple-choice items, 8 items assessing the behavioral manifestations of a binge (e.g., eating in secret) and 8 items asking about thoughts and feelings that accompany binge eating (e.g., loss of control, guilt following a binge). Each item consists of four statements reflecting a range of severity (0 indicating no binge-eating problems and 3 indicating severe binge-eating problems). The statements were independently assigned weights of 0 to 3 by the authors. The BES yields a total score, by adding the individual values for all 16 items. Possible scores range from 0 to 46 (2 items were weighted from 0 to 2; Gormally et al., 1982). Marcus, Wing, and Lamparski (1985) established cutoff scores to assign respondents to one of three groups of binge-eating severity (mild or none, moderate, and severe). The cutoff for the severe category is ≥ 27, which they calculated by taking the mean of the BES score used by Gormally et al. (1982) for serious binge eaters and subtracting half the reported standard deviation. The cutoff for the mild or no binge-eating (BE) group was 17, calculated the same way based on the mean score in the Gormally et al. study for those with none or mild BE. Those with scores from 18 to 26 were considered to have moderate BE. This remains the acceptable scoring standard for the scale, although the reason for this method of determining the cutoffs remains unclear.

The BES has been widely used in research, both as a screening instrument and as a clinical tool to identify obese binge eaters (Freitas, Lopes, Appolinario, & Coutinho, 2006; Greeno, Marcus, & Wing, 1995; Malone & Alger-Mayer, 2004; Ricca et al., 2000). It has been translated into Dutch (Larsen et al., 2004) and Portuguese (Freitas et al., 2006), maintaining similar psychometric properties within these linguistic populations.

The BES has a broader focus than measuring specific bingeing and purging behaviors, as the global scale also measures attitudes associated with binge eating. These items may or may not contribute adequately to the classification of individuals as having BED (Celio, Wilfley, Crow, Mitchell, & Walsh, 2004). In addition, the measure does not specify a time frame or assess the *amount* of food consumed. Thus, it may be measuring other aspects related to BE, such as loss of control or negative cognitions and distress (Gladis, Wadden, Foster, Vogt, & Wingate, 1998; Timmerman, 1999). As Timmerman (1999) pointed out, users need to be cautious in using the BES in identifying objective binge-eating episodes (OBEs) as BES scores could be inflated due to subjective binge episode (SBE) severity. Thus, additional measures should be used with the BES when accurate assessment of OBEs is of interest. This scale can be easily administered, and it is quick and simple to score. Users also should keep in mind that the statements are weighted differently for scoring purposes.

Reliability

Stability. Two studies have measured the stability of the BES after a 2-week period. Timmerman (1999) found test-retest reliability for total BES

scores was $r = .87$ ($p \le .001$), using a subset of patients ($n = 34$) from her original sample ($N = 56$) of treatment-seeking female nonpurging binge eaters recruited for a research study. Freitas et al. (2006) assessed test-retest reliability with a Portuguese version of the BES in 121 participants (68% of original sample) of obese, treatment-seeking Brazilian women. A kappa statistic was calculated, $\kappa = 0.66$ (95% confidence interval [CI]: .48–.83), demonstrating good stability. Means and standard deviations for this replication sample were not reported.

Internal Consistency. For the validation sample, Gormally et al. (1982) determined internal consistency by comparing the participants' total scores with scores on each item. Using 65 participants from the original sample, a Kruskal-Wallis test of ranked data was performed. All chi-square tests of significance were above 9.1 ($p < .01$), indicating the individual ratings for each item were consistent with participants' overall ranked total score. Using Cronbach's alpha, Freitas et al. (2006) demonstrated high internal consistency for the Portuguese version of the scale (.89).

Validity

Concurrent Validity. Concurrent validity was assessed by Gormally et al. (1982) by comparing total BES scores with independent assessments of binge-eating severity level made by trained interviewers. Two independent samples of overweight individuals seeking treatment were utilized. Sample 1 ($N = 65$) was all female, ranging in age from 24 to 55 ($M_{age} = 39.3$ years, $SD = 8.1$), and Sample 2 ($N = 47$) consisted of 32 women and 15 men, ranging in age from 24 to 67 ($M_{age} = 41.2$ years, $SD = 11.6$), with average pretreatment weights of 178.1 pounds ($SD = 21.6$) and 209.9 pounds ($SD = 40.3$), respectively. Both samples were predominantly White and middle class. The means and standard deviations of the BES for both samples were similar (Sample 1: $M = 20.8$, $SD = 8.4$; Sample 2: $M = 21.4$, $SD = 9.2$). A one-way analysis of variance (ANOVA) showed that

BES scores were significantly different across interviewer-rated severity levels (no binge eating, moderate binge eating, and severe binge eating) for both samples of obese individuals ($p < .001$). Neumann-Keuls post hoc tests indicated means were different across all levels of severity at $p < .01$ for both samples, except for the first two levels of severity in Sample 1, which were nonsignificant (see Table 10.1). In this case, although the interviewer differentiated between no binge eating and moderate severity levels, the BES scores did not similarly reflect this as a significant difference. However, the BES scores did significantly differentiate between no binge eating and severe, as well as severe and moderate, severity levels.

Timmerman (1999) also tested concurrent validity of the BES by correlating total scores with a measure of binge-eating severity from 28-day food records in a sample of 68 healthy, treatment-seeking, binge-eating obese and normal-weight women (mean body mass index [BMI] = 32.7 kg/m², $SD = 9.3$, $M_{age} = 42.9$ years, $SD = 10.5$, and the sample was 91% White). BES scores showed a significant moderate association with food record measures of SBE (fewer than 1,000 calories consumed) and OBE (more than 1,000 calories consumed) severity, with correlations ranging from .29 to .40 ($p \le .05$). She also divided participants into three groups based on BES cutoff scores (mild, moderate, and severe binge eating) and conducted one-way ANOVAs to examine differences among the groups in average total binge calories (over the 28 days), binge days, and binge episodes. Significant differences were found between the severe BE group and the mild BE group on several outcomes, including (1) the average number of SBE calories consumed (severe BE: $M = 8,486$, $SD = 5,011$; mild BE: $M = 4,471$, $SD = 3,072$; $p < .05$), (2) the average number of subjective binge days (severe BE: $M = 12.5$, $SD = 6.1$; mild BE: $M = 6.9$, $SD = 4.8$; $p < .05$), and (3) SBEs (severe BE: $M = 17.1$, $SD = 10.1$; mild BE: $M = 8.5$, $SD = 6.9$; $p < .05$). These results showed the BES was able successfully to categorize severe and mild binge eaters who differed on uncontrolled eating episodes and overall caloric intake.

Celio et al. (2004) examined correlations between the BES (as a measure of severity) and frequency of BE as measured by the EDE (i.e., OBEs). Their multisite sample consisted of 157 self-referred, treatment-seeking adults. The sample was 86.6% female and predominantly White ($M_{age} = 41.9$ years, $SD = 11.3$, $M_{BMI} = 33.6$ kg/m², $SD = 5.3$). The BES correlated modestly with frequency of OBEs as measured by the EDE ($r = .24$, $p = .003$) and number of days with OBEs ($r = .24$, $p = .004$), but it was not significantly correlated with SBEs ($r = .11$, $p = .18$), SBE days ($r = .09$, $p = .29$), or objective overeating episodes ($r = .01$, $p = .89$).

Gladis et al. (1998) compared the BES to the Questionnaire of Eating and Weight Patterns (QEWP; Spitzer, Devlin, et al., 1992) with regards to classifying patients into bingers and non-bingers. The sample consisted of 128 obese women enrolled in a weight loss program ($M_{age} = 40.8$ years, $SD = 8.6$, $M_{BMI} = 97.9$ kg/m², $SD = 13.5$). To measure concordance between the scales, the authors calculated Cohen's kappa, yielding a kappa of .45, indicating a somewhat low agreement between the two measures. The authors argued that this difference may be a function of the degree to which the scales assess the critical aspects of binge eating. They suggest that the BES may also measure associated psychopathology (i.e., dysphoria and distress).

Predictive Validity. Sensitivity of an assessment measure is briefly defined as the probability of a positive test to identify those with a disease or condition, and specificity is briefly defined as the probability of a negative test among those without a disease or condition (Celio et al., 2004). Using a score of ≥ 27 to indicate severe binge eating, the BES yielded a sensitivity value of .85 and a specificity value of .20 in identifying individuals with severe binge eating (Celio et al., 2004) compared with the EDE as the diagnostic standard. Similarly, in a clinical sample of 344 (58 men and 286 women) obese treatment-seeking individuals ($M_{age} = 43.5$ years, $SD = 13.6$; $M_{BMI} = 35.8$ kg/m², $SD = 6.1$), Ricca et al. (2000) found (with the Structured Clinical Interview for *DSM-III-R*

Table 10.1   Binge Eating Scale (BES) Mean Scores and Standard Deviations for Three Severity
Levels (as Rated by a Structured Interview)

	Level of Severity		
	None	*Moderate*	*Severe*
Sample	*M* (SD)	*M* (SD)	*M* (SD)
1	14.9[a] (8.2)	19.6[a] (6.7)	28.9[b] (7.5)
(*N* = 65)	(*n* = 11)	(*n* = 40)	(*n* = 14)
2 Total	13.4[a] (5.2)	21.1[b] (7.0)	31.3[c] (6.6)
(*N* = 47)	(*n* = 14)	(*n* = 21)	(*n* = 12)
Men	14.4 (4.9)	17.5 (4.1)	26.0 (8.0)
(*n* = 15)	(*n* = 7)	(*n* = 4)	(*n* = 4)
Women	12.4 (5.6)	22.0 (7.4)	34.0 (3.9)
(*n* = 32)	(*n* = 7)	(*n* = 17)	(*n* = 8)

SOURCE: Data are from Gormally, Black, Daston, and Rardin (1982).

NOTE: Means across levels of severity with different superscripts are significantly different at $p < .01$.

[SCID] as the diagnostic criterion) that with a threshold of 17, the sensitivity of the BES was 84.8%, with a specificity 74.6% of identifying those with BED. Using a threshold of 27, sensitivity was 60.6% and specificity was 95.2%. These authors concluded that the threshold of 27 was too low for clinical purposes due to its low sensitivity. Freitas et al. (2006) compared scores on a Portuguese version of the BES to diagnosis on the SCID patient version (SCID-I/P; First, Gibbon, Spitzer, & Williams, 1995) using a clinical sample of 178 Brazilian women (M_{age} = 36.41 years, SD = 9.95, and M_{BMI} = 36.25 kg/m², SD = 3.76). In that sample, 51.69% was diagnosed with BED using the SCID-I/P compared to 75.84% using the BES. Sensitivity was 97.8% and specificity was 47.7 % at the cutoff of 17, indicating that the lower cutoff may lead to improved sensitivity. These authors concluded that the BES may be useful for identifying severe binge eating, as well as identifying nonbinge eaters (Freitas et al., 2006), but that supplementary assessments should be used when confirming a diagnosis of BED.

Sensitivity to Change

Malone and Alger-Mayer (2004) used the BES in a clinical sample of 109 obese gastric bypass surgery patients (18 men, 91 women, M_{age} = 46 years, SD = 10) to group patients according to BE status (none, moderate, severe). Data from 56 patients were collected at a 1-year follow-up, and the BES scores declined significantly postsurgery for each group ($p < .05$), indicating the BES is sensitive to change due to treatment. Effect sizes were not provided and could not be calculated with the information available.

Norms

The validation sample of the BES consisted of two samples of overweight individuals seeking treatment for obesity (Gormally et al., 1982, see Table 1). These data may be used as comparison data as there are presently no published norms for the BES. Marcus et al. (1985) gave the BES to a clinical sample of 432 obese women seeking a weight loss treatment. The women ranged in age from 17 to 65 (M_{age} = 39.3 years, SD = 10.1), and their average weight was 192.2 pounds (SD = 39.4). Scores on the 430 valid BESs ranged from 3 to 44 (M = 25.6, SD = 8.5), with 46% reporting serious BE, 36% moderate BE, and 17.9% mild or no BE problems.

Availability

A copy of the entire scale is reprinted in the paper by Gormally et al. (1982).

Binge Scale Questionnaire

Description

The Binge Scale Questionnaire (BSQ; Hawkins & Clement, 1980) consists of 19 items developed to measure the behavioral and attitudinal parameters of binge eating and vomiting. Nine of the 19 multiple-choice items can be added to yield a total BSQ score, reflecting the severity and intensity of the binge eating. Thus, although the measure does not assess specific diagnostic criteria, it provides a quick assessment of overall bingeing and vomiting behavior. The 9 items that combine to yield the total score do not ask for specific bingeing or vomiting frequency; rather, they require the user to choose between one of four responses corresponding to various frequencies of behaviors and attitudes that best describes their eating pattern. Each response is allotted a specific scoring weight (0 to 3) that was determined subjectively. The remaining 10 items aim to provide a clearer picture of the prevalence and characteristics of the binge eating. The scale does not include any items measuring other methods of purging other than vomiting, and it does not define the term *binge* for the user. The scale was

originally intended to measure binge-eating tendencies in a general college population. The measure is not frequently used, but it has been used profitably as a screening tool and as a treatment outcome measure in clinical research in the past (Bossert, Schmölz, Wiegand, Junker, & Krieg, 1992; Ordman & Kirschenbaum, 1985; Ortega, Waranch, Maldonado, & Hubbard, 1987).

There have been no revisions to the scale since its development; however, Hawkins and colleagues (personal communication, 2007) are in the process of updating the measure. The scale has been investigated cross-culturally, demonstrating good psychometric properties with Arabic women, but demonstrated poor internal validity with Arabic men (Dolan & Ford, 1991). An advantage of the scale is the administration and scoring, which is simple and quick.

Reliability

Stability. One month test-retest reliability for the total score was r = .88 (Hawkins & Clement, 1980), calculated on 48% of the original sample (described below). Mean differences for the retest administrations and effect size of the differences could not be calculated from the information provided in the paper. The validation sample was drawn from two undergraduate psychology classes at a large American university. The initial sample comprised 182 women and 65 men, and the replication sample consisted of 73 women and 45 men. An additional clinical sample of 26 overweight (mean excess weight of 40%) college women from a behavioral weight control program were included. There are no comparison data for a nonoverweight eating disorder sample. Means and standard deviations for the original and replication samples are provided in Tables 10.2 and 10.3.

Internal Consistency. A Cronbach's alpha of .68 was reported for the nine items comprising the total score using the initial validation sample (Hawkins & Clement, 1980), which is approaching the

Table 10.2   Binge Scale Questionnaire Mean Total Scores and Standard Deviations for Two
Validation Samples

Sample 1		Sample 2	
	Mean (SD)		Mean (SD)
Men (n = 65)	2.20 (2.72)	Men (n = 45)	2.84 (3.56)
Women (n = 182)	6.03 (4.52)	Women (n = 73)	5.89 (4.75)

SOURCE: Data are from Hawkins and Clement (1980).

Table 10.3   Binge Scale Mean Total Scores (Standard Deviations) for Male and Female Normal-
Weight and Overweight Participants

	Normal Weight	Overweight
Men	1.90 (2.55)	3.05 (3.09)
	n = 52	n = 18
Women	5.63 (4.37)	8.42 (4.76)
	n = 160	n = 26
Clinic-treated women		10.7 (4.4)
		n = 26
Control classroom women		8.9 (5.0)
		n = 26

SOURCE: Data are from Hawkins and Clement (1980).

acceptable range. In an independent sample of 160 Arabic undergraduate women and 58 Arabic undergraduate men, Dolan and Ford (1991) found an acceptable Cronbach's alpha at .70 for the women but a lower and unacceptable coefficient of .46 for the men.

Validity

Construct Validity. A principal components analysis (PCA) with a varimax rotation resulted in a two-component solution (Hawkins & Clement, 1980). One component representing guilt and concern about binge eating accounted for 71% of the variance. A second component, including items measuring duration and satiety feelings associated with the binge episodes, accounted for 16% of the variance. The first component was replicated in a study by Dolan and Ford (1991) in an exploratory factor analysis using 218 Arabic students (160 women and 58 men) in Egypt, accounting for 31% and 26% of the variance in the male and female groups, respectively. For the female group, the second factor that was identified accounted for 12% of the variance, but for men, this second factor did not emerge.

Criterion Validity

Concurrent Validity. Thelen, Farmer, Wonderlich, and Smith (1991) found the BSQ to be highly correlated with Smith and Thelen's (1984) Bulimia Test–Revised (BULIT-R; $r = .85$, $p < .001$), suggesting the two scales measure similar constructs, but there may be some redundancy between the measures.

Predictive Validity. There are no specific or recent studies of the predictive validity of the items on the BSQ. However, the BSQ has been used as a screening and assessment measure to identify binge eating and classify patients as either BED or not BED prior to bariatric surgery (Powers, Perez, Boyd, & Rosemurgy, 1999). One hundred sixteen patients (2 men, 114 women, M_{age} at surgery = 38.9 years, $SD = 9.3$, 73% White) were assessed, and follow-ups were completed on average 5.5 years postsurgery. Of these patients, 19 (16%) were classified with BED, which is a much lower percentage than is typically found among patients enrolled in weight control programs (i.e., 29%; Spitzer, Yanovski, Wadden, et al., 1993). The scale was developed prior to the elaboration of *DSM-IV* (APA, 1994) criteria for BED, which may have contributed to the lower than typical classification rate of BED in the Powers et al. (1999) study.

Sensitivity to Change

The BSQ has shown change from pre- to post-treatment when used in treatment outcome research (Bossert et al., 1992; Ordman & Kirschenbaum, 1985; Ortega et al., 1987). The results are somewhat mixed, however, as to where the change is most notable. In a clinical sample of 8 women with BN ($M_{age} = 22.1$ years; range, 17–32), Ortega et al. (1987) found that the total scores on the BSQ declined significantly post-treatment (using paired t test comparisons, $p < .05$, $d > .65$). They noted that the changes were in scale items that primarily addressed attitudes and feelings, rather than specific bingeing and purging

behaviors. In contrast, in a clinical sample of 31 treatment-seeking women with BN ($M_{age} = 22.9$ years, $SD = 4.1$), Bossert et al. (1992) examined only two items on the scale that assess frequency of bingeing and vomiting. They found a significant difference in scores pre- versus posttreatment in bingeing and vomiting ($p < .01$). Lang, Hauser, Buddeberg, and Klaghofer (2002) gave obese patients the BSQ before and after laparoscopic-adjustable gastric banding surgery. The sample consisted of 66 morbidly obese patients (87.9% female, $M_{age} = 38.1$ years, $SD = 11.2$, $M_{weight} = 132.9$ kg, $SD = 24.0$). Postsurgery, a repeated-measures ANOVA revealed a significant decrease in BSQ scores from baseline to 3-month follow-up ($p < .001$; effect size [ES] = .43), and a small but significant increase in BSQ scores from 3-month to 6-month follow-up ($p < .05$, ES = .06). The specific statistic for the effect size was not reported. The results were suggestive of the BSQ's sensitivity to change following medical treatment.

Norms

There are no published norms on the BSQ, but several studies provided means and standard deviations of clinical and nonclinical samples. In the initial validation sample, 79% of the women and 49% of the men reported binge-eating occurrences. Dolan and Ford (1991) reported similar means for their sample of Arabic undergraduate students. On the basis of these studies and further research, Hawkins (personal communication, 2007) suggested a total score of 10 to 15 as a cutoff score to identify a clinical sample of binge eaters and a score of 7 or below to reflect a "normal group."

Availability

A copy of the 9 scored items of the BSQ is available in the paper by Hawkins and Clement (1980). A copy of the entire 19-item scale is reprinted with kind permission from Elsevier Limited in the appendix at the end of this book. It is also available from Hawkins, who is at the

University of Texas at Austin (e-mail: Hawkins @psy.utexas.edu).

Bulimia Scale–Eating Disorders Inventory

Description

The Bulimia scale of the Eating Disorders Inventory (EDI) assesses one's thoughts and proclivity to engage in binge eating. Originally, there were 7 items in the scale for the EDI (Garner & Olmsted, 1984) and the EDI-2 (Garner, 1991). Six of the 7 items referred to binge eating thoughts or behaviors, and 1 item referred to thoughts of vomiting. In the EDI-3, Garner (2004) included an eighth item that was originally in the Interoceptive Awareness scale of the EDI-2. The entire EDI-3 contains 92 items. The EDI and subsequent generations of the inventory are arguably one of the most used measures to assess eating disorder behaviors and related psychopathology (Joiner & Heatherton, 1998). The Bulimia scale, like other EDI scales, is self-report and scored on a 6-point Likert-type scale. These responses are recoded into a 4-point scale with 0 assigned to the three least symptomatic responses. Raw scores are transformed into percentile scores, which can be compared to an adult female control sample. Raw scores are also transformed into T scores, which can be compared to an adult normal control sample and a "typical" clinical comparison sample. The computerized scoring program for the EDI-3 allows one to select which comparison groups one wishes to use (e.g., U.S. adult or adolescent, AN, BN, etc.).

Reliability

Stability. Rizvi, Stice, and Agras (1999) reported a test-retest Pearson correlation over a 6-year period among a community sample of 166 women to be .75. The Bulimia scale scores were not significantly different from Time 1 to Time 2, but the authors did not report the means and

standard deviations. In a longer term 10-year test-retest study among 509 female college students, Joiner, Heatherton, and Keel (1997) reported a lower Pearson correlation of .56. Joiner and colleagues also reported a decline in Bulimia scale scores from 14.36 ($SD = 5.14$) at Time 1 to 11.10 ($SD = 4.31$) at Time 2. However, the authors do not report significance testing for these repeated measurements.

Internal Consistency. Garner (2004) reported internal consistency by coefficient alpha to be high for the Bulimia scale for the EDI-2 and EDI-3 for 429 participants with BN (range, .82–.92). In an independent report including 144 women with BED and 152 women with BN, Tasca, Illing, Lybanon-Daigle, Bissada, and Balfour (2003) reported a lower coefficient alpha of .68 for the BED sample and .74 for the BN sample. However, Tasca and colleagues reported adequate mean interitem correlations of .20 and .30 for the two samples, respectively. Similarly, Rathner and Rumpold (1994) reported coefficient alpha of a German-language translation of the EDI. The sample included Austrian medical students, and the coefficient alpha for the Bulimia scale was .78 for the 133 women and .72 for the 195 men.

Validity

Construct Validity. Garner (2004) reported an exploratory factor analysis (EFA) for a U.S. adult clinical sample of 983 individuals using the items from the eating disorder risk scales of the EDI-3 (Drive for Thinness, Bulimia, Body Dissatisfaction). A principal axis extraction was used with promax rotation, but the exact method of arriving at a factor solution was not specified. The three-factor solution accounted for 63% of the variance. The 8 items of the Bulimia scale loaded on that scale, with Item 53, related to thoughts of vomiting, having the lowest factor loading of .36. Welch, Hall, and Norring (1990) conducted an EFA on the 64-item version of the original EDI on 271 eating disorder patients. The authors were not specific about what extraction method was used, but they did employ an orthogonal rotation and found an eight-factor solution. The amount of variance accounted for by the model was not reported. The original 7 items of the Bulimia scale each had factor loadings of greater than .48 with no cross-factor loadings. These EFA studies provide support for the construct validity of the Bulimia scale.

To assess the construct validity of the eating disorder symptom factor of the EDI, Tasca et al. (2003) conducted a confirmatory factor analysis (CFA) of a two-factor second-order model suggested by Garner and Olmsted (1984). The eating disorder symptom factor was hypothesized to include the Drive for Thinness, Bulimia, and Body Dissatisfaction scales. The personality traits factor was hypothesized to include the remaining five scales of the original EDI. Participants were 144 patients with BED and 152 patients with BN. The factor structure was supported for BED (comparative fit index [CFI] = .96, root mean square error of approximation [RMSEA] = .07) but not for BN (CFI = .82, RMSEA = .14). This CFA study provided some support for the construct validity of the Bulimia scale in its role in determining an eating disorder symptom factor for BED, but no such support was found for the BN sample.

Criterion Validity

Concurrent Validity. Garner (2004) reported a study in which a clinical group of 210 female adults completed the EDI-3 and the Eating Attitudes Test (EAT-26; Garner, Olmsted, Bohr, & Garfinkel, 1982), a measure of dieting, bulimia, food preoccupation, and oral control. Pearson correlation with the Bulimia scale was low at .25. Garner (2004) also reported on a nonclinical group of 543 women who completed the EDI-3 and the BULIT-R (Thelen et al., 1991), a measure of clinical aspects specific to BN. The Bulimia scale correlated highly, $r = .81$, with the BULIT-R. Tasca and colleagues (2003) correlated the Bulimia scale and the Eating Concerns scale of the Eating Disorder Examination–Questionnaire (EDE-Q; Fairburn & Beglin, 1994) among 296 patients with BED or BN. The Pearson correlation

between these scales was .57. Finally, Rathner and Rumpold (1994) reported correlations among EDI scales and the Anorexia Nervosa Inventory for Self Rating Scales (ANIS; Fichter & Keeser, 1980) among a sample of 133 German-speaking male and female medical students. The Pearson correlation between the EDI Bulimia scale and the ANIS Bulimia scale was .59. These studies provide mixed but overall positive evidence for the concurrent validity of the Bulimia scale.

Predictive Validity. Schoemaker, Verbraak, Breteler, and van der Staak (1997) assessed 78 patients with BN and 67 general psychiatric outpatients on the EDI-2. They conducted a stepwise discriminant function analysis with all 11 EDI-2 scales to predict group membership. The Bulimia scale was found to correctly classify 97% of all cases. Although this study provided excellent support for predictive validity of the Bulimia scale, the stepwise method used tends to capitalize on chance, and so the correct classification may be an overestimate.

Rosenvinge, Borgen, and Börresen (1999) compared 19 eating-disordered and 126 non-eating-disordered 15-year-old adolescents on the Bulimia scale of the EDI-2. The eating-disordered group had higher scores ($M = 5.3$, $SD = 4.32$) than the non-eating-disordered group ($M = 2.0$, $SD = 2.95$), $p < .001$, and the effect size was large ($d > .8$). Garner (2004) reported mean raw scores for 101 patients with AN restricting subtype (AN-R; $M = 2.86$, $SD = 3.38$) and 98 patients with BN ($M = 16.59$, $SD = 8.93$) on the Bulimia scale. An independent samples t test indicates that the difference in scores is statistically significant, $p < .001$, and the effect size is large ($d > .8$). These studies provide support for the Bulimia scale's predictive validity.

Sensitivity to Change

Esplen, Garfinkel, Olmsted, Gallop, and Kennedy (1998) reported that a 6-week randomized controlled trial of guided imagery treatment resulted in a mean reduction of bingeing and vomiting among a group of 24 individuals with

BN compared to 26 individuals with BN who received comparable contact with a therapist but no guided imagery. There was a significant group-by-time interaction for the Bulimia scale as well as for Drive for Thinness and Ineffectiveness scales. In another study, Laessle et al. (1991) used the EDI in their comparison of nutritional management versus stress management in the treatment of 55 patients with BN. There were significant improvements noted in the stress management compared to the nutritional management group on the Drive for Thinness, Bulimia, Body Dissatisfaction, Perfectionism, and Interoceptive Awareness scales. These studies indicate that the Bulimia scale may be sensitive to change due to psychotherapeutic treatment.

Norms

Garner (2004) provided extensive information about population and clinical norms in the EDI-3 manual. The following is based on norms for the U.S. adult combined clinical sample. For the Bulimia scale, a raw score of 19 to 32 (67th to 99th percentile, T score > 56) indicates frequent thoughts and behaviors consistent with binge eating (Garner, 2004). A raw score between 5 and 18 (25th to 66th percentile, T score = 42–55) indicates reporting of thoughts and behaviors consistent with binge eating (Garner, 2004). Finally, a raw score of less than or equal to 4 (1st to 24th percentile, T score < 41) occurs in only 3% of those with a diagnosis of BN (Garner, 2004).

Availability

The EDI-3 is a copyright test by Psychological Assessment Resources. The test, as well as the computer scoring and interpretive program, can be purchased from Psychological Assessment Resources (www.parinc.com). The EDI-3 can be hand scored or computer scored. Computer scoring allows one to generate interpretive statements with comparisons to several clinical and normative groups. The program will also generate raw scores based on the EDI-2.

The Bulimia Test–Revised

Description

The Bulimia Test–Revised (BULIT-R; Thelen et al., 1991) is a 36-item self-report, multiple-choice measure of bulimia that was originally based on *DSM-III* criteria. The BULIT-R is a brief, easily administered, cost-effective measure to screen and identify individuals who may meet criteria for bulimia in clinical and nonclinical populations of both adults and adolescents. The scale has also been validated using *DSM-IV* criteria to identify women with BN (Thelen, Mintz, & Vander Wal, 1996). The BULIT-R has also demonstrated good psychometric properties with adolescent populations (McCabe & Vincent, 2003; McCarthy, Simmons, Smith, Tomlinson, & Hill, 2002). Twenty-eight of the 36 items are summed to provide an overall score. The remaining 8 items are unscored and refer to specific weight control behaviors. The 28 scored items are rated using a 5-point Likert-type scale (5 = *extreme disturbance*, 1 = *absence of a disturbance*). The range of possible scores is 28 to 140, with a cutoff of 104 or higher indicating the presence of BN and a score below 104 being considered normal.

Reliability

Stability. A portion of the validation student sample ($n = 98$) scores on the BULIT-R was compared with their scores on a second administration of the BULIT-R 2 months later. Overall test-retest reliability was found to be .95 ($p < .001$) using the Pearson product-moment correlation (Thelen et al., 1991). Stability was also assessed by Brelsford, Hummel, and Barrios (1992) with a sample of 39 college women (age range 18–25 years, 92% of the sample was White), who completed the BULIT-R a second time after a 4- to 6-week interval. The measure demonstrated good stability after this interval, .83 ($p < .05$).

Internal Consistency. Using a sample of 23 women with BN ($M_{age} = 21.48$ years, $SD = 3.92$) and 124 controls who were female undergraduate students (M_{age} = 19.12 years, SD = 2.8), Thelen et al. (1996) reported a Cronbach's alpha coefficient of .98, indicating very high internal consistency of the scale. This is similar to a previous report of Cronbach's alpha of .97 (Thelen et al., 1991).

Validity

Construct Validity. Factor analyses were conducted in two validation samples described by Thelen et al. (1991). The first sample consisted of 23 treatment-seeking women with BN and 157 college female controls. The authors reported using a "principal factor analysis" on all 36 BULIT-R items, with iterative estimates of item communalities. A promax matrix (oblique) rotation was used because the factors were theoretically expected to correlate with each other. Using a criterion of an eigenvalue > 1.0, five factors emerged that accounted for 46.8% of the total variance (Thelen et al., 1991). The five factors contained items relating to the following: Factor 1 (bingeing and control), Factor 2 (general use of radical weight loss measures and body image), Factor 3 (four nonscored items about laxative and diuretic use), Factor 4 (vomiting), and Factor 5 (nonscored items related to exercise). The second sample consisted of 37 treatment-seeking women with BN and 124 female college students. Again, five factors emerged, explaining 41.6% of the total variance, producing a pattern similar to the first sample (Thelen et al., 1991).

Criterion Validity

Concurrent Validity. The BULIT-R demonstrated a positive relationship with the Binge Scale Questionnaire (Hawkins & Clement, 1980), indicating they are based on similar constructs, with some redundancy between the measures. The Pearson product-moment correlation was .85 ($p <$ .001). Brelsford et al. (1992) assessed concurrent validity by comparing BULIT-R scores to recorded symptom frequency on 21-day self-monitoring sheets in a sample of 39 undergraduate women

who scored 60 or higher on the BULIT-R. The average BULIT-R scores correlated significantly with the self-monitored reports of binge eating (r = .65, $p <$ .05) and purging (r = .60, $p <$ .05). Welch, Thompson, and Hall (1993) examined a sample of 243 female undergraduate students in New Zealand (M_{age} = 21.3 years, SD = 4.4; M_{BMI} = 22.1 kg/m^2, SD = 2.6; and the majority of the sample was of high socioeconomic status). The BULIT-R demonstrated high concurrent validity with the Bulimic Investigatory Test Edinburgh (BITE; Henderson & Freeman, 1987), r = .90, $p <$ .001, and good concurrent validity with a 21-item subscale from the EDI, composed of items from the original Drive for Thinness, Body Dissatisfaction, and Bulimia subscales (r = .75, $p <$ .001).

Predictive Validity. In a sample of 21 women with BN and 100 female controls (college psychology students), Thelen et al. (1991) found that BULIT-R scores were significantly different between BN (M = 117.95) and control (M = 57.50) groups (no standard deviations were reported), $t(46)$ = 16.41, $p <$ .001. In a sample of 161 female college students, the BULIT-R demonstrated ratings of specificity, positive predictive value, and negative predictive value of .82 or higher, and sensitivity was .62 (Thelen et al., 1991). These authors suggested that for research or screening purposes, it may be advantageous to use a cutoff lower than 104 to reduce the number of false negatives. Similarly, Thelen et al. (1996) in their sample (described above) found the BULIT-R to successfully differentiate those with BN, as the means of the two samples were significantly different ($p <$ .001). Mean BULIT-R scores for the BN participants were 119.26, and for controls, the mean was 53.31 (no standard deviations were reported). For this sample, sensitivity, specificity, and negative predictive values were all above .90.

Norms

There are no published norms for the BULIT-R, but the authors provide comparison data from clinical and nonclinical samples. Thelen et al.

(1991) administered the BULIT-R to 1,739 college women participating in psychology classes in large Midwestern universities. Fifty-three participants (3% of the sample) met the scale criterion for BN. Thelen et al. (1991) and Thelen et al. (1996) also reported data for three validation samples, for both BN and nonclinical participants. Means for these samples are in Table 10.4. Standard deviations were not reported.

Availability

The scale and scoring information is available through Mark H. Thelen (thelenm@missouri.edu). It was previously published with permission in the previous edition of this handbook (Williamson, Anderson, Jackman, & Jackson, 1995). The scale is reproduced in the appendix to Chapter 11 of this handbook.

Eating Disorder Diagnostic Scale

Description

The Eating Disorder Diagnostic Scale (EDDS; Stice, Telch, & Rizvi, 2000) is a brief self-report scale that is designed to provide diagnoses of AN, BN, and BED. The authors wished to create a scale that could be used in etiologic research, for research where relatively frequent measurements were required, or for clinical settings that require a brief screening for eating pathology (Stice et al., 2000). The EDDS was designed to correspond to *DSM-IV* (APA, 1994) diagnostic criteria for the eating disorders, including BED. Hence, there are three separate questions related to binge-eating days and frequencies over the past 3 months (for BN) and 6 months (for BED). Binges are explicitly defined in the EDDS as eating an unusually large amount of food and losing control, but no examples are provided. There are a further six questions about binge eating and its aftermath that are geared toward specifying a diagnosis. The EDDS also asks several questions regarding frequency of purging behaviors. The EDDS results in classifications of participants into one of the *DSM-IV* eating disorder categories or to a no-eating disorder category. It also provides an overall symptom composite designed for use in outcome studies. The main drawback to this scale is that it is new, though promising, and most psychometric research on the EDDS so far was conducted by the original author.

Table 10.4   Bulimia Test–Revised Means and Standard Deviations for Validation Samples

	n	*Mean*	*SD*
Bulimia nervosa			
Sample 1	21	117.95	NA
Sample 2	23	118.08	NA
Sample 3	21	119.26	NA
Nonclinical			
Sample 1	100	57.50	NA
Sample 2	157	59.62	NA
Sample 3	124	53.31	NA

SOURCE: Data are from Thelen, Farmer, Wonderlich, and Smith (1991) and Thelen, Mintz, and Vander Wal (1996).

NOTE: NA = not available.

Reliability

Stability. There are no test-retest reliability studies of the specific items regarding binge eating and purging. However, 1-week test-retest chance-corrected kappa coefficients were calculated for 367 participants (BN = 3, BED = 17, AN = 12, subthreshold eating disorder = 185, and mixed psychiatric patients = 150). Kappa coefficient was .71 for BN and .75 for BED (Stice et al., 2000). This provides some indirect evidence for moderate test-retest reliability for diagnostic classification that is based on items of binge eating and purging.

Criterion Validity

Concurrent Validity. Again, there are no specific studies of concurrent validity of specific EDDS items related to binge eating or purging. However, Stice and colleagues (2000) did test whether EDDS-identified diagnostic groups would differ from a non-eating-disordered control group. As predicted, those classified as BN (*n* = 39) or BED (*n* = 57) by the EDDS reported higher scale scores on all EDE-Q (Fairburn & Beglin, 1994) scales, except Restraint, compared to the non-eating-disordered controls (*n* = 103; *p* values not reported). Similarly, Stice, Fisher, and Martinez (2004) reported significant differences between those identified with BN by the EDDS (*n* = 80) compared to a non-eating-disordered group (*n* = 538) on a number of eating disorder measures, including the EDE (Fairburn & Cooper, 1993) symptom composite. Stice and colleagues (2004) also reported a Pearson correlation of .82 between the EDE symptom composite and the EDDS symptom composite.

Predictive Validity. There are also no specific studies of predictive validity of binge eating and purging behaviors as measured by the EDDS. Stice and colleagues (2000) did present data regarding specificity, sensitivity, and predictive value of EDDS-based classification. The 367 participants described earlier were diagnosed with the EDE interview (Fairburn & Cooper, 1993) or the SCID (Spitzer, Williams, Gibbon, & First, 1992). Kappa coefficient between structured interview and EDDS was .81 for BN and .74 for BED. Values for sensitivity, specificity, and predictive values for BN were all above .81, and for BED, they were all above .77.

Sensitivity to Change

There are no studies that specifically address sensitivity to change of the binge eating and purging questions of the EDDS. However, Stice and colleagues (2004) report two treatment studies that suggest that the EDDS composite score is sensitive to change as a result of psychoeducation and dissonance treatment. In the first study, Stice and colleagues (2004) enrolled 98 undergraduate women to examine a psychoeducational intervention for the prevention of disordered eating. Thirty-five women were in the intervention condition, and 63 women were matched based on EDDS symptom composite scores at pretreatment. A repeated-measures ANOVA indicated a time-by-treatment interaction in which intervention participants showed greater pre (*M* = 3.76, *SD* = 11.96) to post (*M* = 0.75, *SD* = 13.76) treatment change on the EDDS composite measure compared to the control condition (pre: *M* = –0.23, *SD* = 10.10; post: *M* = 0.89, *SD* = 11.69), *p* = .01.

In the second study, Stice and colleagues (2004) reported on an intervention for 181 adolescent girls, in which a dissonance treatment condition (*n* = 70) was compared to an "alternate" intervention condition (*n* = 59) and a no-treatment control condition (*n* = 47). The hypothesis was that the dissonance intervention condition would result in greater change in EDDS and EDE composite scores pre- to post-treatment. In a series of repeated-measures ANOVAs, Stice and colleagues found that both the EDDS and EDE symptom composites indicated positive change pre- to posttreatment for the dissonance condition compared to the other two study conditions.

Norms

There are no published norms for the EDDS composite score or for specific items of binge eating or purging.

Availability

A copy of the EDDS items is available in the appendix of the paper by Stice et al. (2000). There is a correction to those published items that appears in the subsequent issue of the same journal on page 252. A useful SPSS scoring syntax and algorithm appears in the appendix to the Stice et al. (2004) paper. The EDDS items are reproduced in Appendix 10.B at the end of this book.

Eating Disorder Examination–Questionnaire

Description

The Eating Disorder Examination–Questionnaire (EDE-Q; Fairburn & Beglin, 1994) is a 36-item self-report measure modeled on the EDE (Fairburn & Cooper, 1993) interview. Each item is taken from a corresponding EDE item with some modifications to the wording. Items addressing eating disorder attitudes are scored on a 7-point (0 to 6) Likert-type scale. Subscales (Restraint, Eating Concerns, Weight Concerns, Shape Concerns) and the total score are derived in the same way as for the EDE. Scores of 4 or higher on key items are considered to lie in the clinical range. Frequencies of eating-disordered behaviors are assessed in terms of number of episodes of each behavior occurring in the past 28 days. As with the EDE, OBEs (i.e., overeating and loss of control), SBEs (loss of control without overeating), and objective overeating (OEs; with no loss of control) can be differentiated by examining responses to several of the items on amount of food and loss of control. However, the EDE-Q does not provide examples of amounts of food or loss of control. Frequencies of other eating-disordered behaviors

such as laxative misuse, diuretic misuse, vomiting, and excessive exercise are also self-reported. The main advantage of the EDE-Q compared to the EDE is that the EDE-Q is easier and quicker to use and requires no reliability training. On the other hand, as indicated below, there are questions about the EDE-Q's validity with regard to recording of complex behaviors such as OBEs and SBEs.

This review will focus on binge eating (i.e., OBEs and SBEs) and on purging behaviors (i.e., vomiting, laxatives, diuretics) as measured by the EDE-Q. The vast majority of studies using the EDE-Q are with adults with eating disorders, and these will be discussed below. However, there are a few studies in which the EDE-Q was used among healthy female adolescents (Engelsen & Laberg, 2001), adolescents with AN (Passi, Bryson, & Lock, 2002), bariatric surgery candidates (Elder et al., 2006), and individuals who abuse substances (Black & Wilson, 1996).

Reliability

Stability. In a study of 139 female undergraduates, Luce and Crowther (1999) readministered the EDE-Q after 2 weeks. Pearson correlations (r) for frequencies and phi coefficients (φ) for OBEs were $r = .68$, $\varphi = .62$; for vomiting, $r = .92$, $\varphi = .66$; for laxative misuse, $r = .65$, $\varphi = .70$; and for diuretic misuse, $r = .54$, $\varphi = .57$. Given the frequency count and nonnormal distribution of these data in a normative sample, it is likely that the φ coefficient is a better indicator of test-retest reliability in this case. Longer term (median = 315 days) test-retest reliability of a community sample of 196 women was reported by Mond, Hay, Rodgers, Owen, and Beumont (2004). These authors reported Kendall's tau b for nonnormally distributed data and φ coefficient for occurrence between the two time points. Tau b for frequencies and phi coefficients (φ) for OBEs were tau b = .44, $\varphi = .44$; for SBEs, tau b = .28, $\varphi = .24$. These data suggest that the stability of measurement of OBEs and other eating disorder–specific behaviors is low among normative samples. It is possible that the very low frequency of these behaviors, especially of purging, may have affected the results in these samples. We found no stability studies of the EDE-Q measurement of these specific eating-disordered behaviors in clinical samples. This remains an understudied domain for the EDE-Q.

Criterion Validity

Concurrent Validity. The most extensive area of research on the EDE-Q has been in regard to its concurrent validity. A number of studies have assessed the concurrent validity of the EDE-Q scales and items related to specific eating-disorder behaviors compared to the EDE. In most of these studies, the EDE was considered the standard by which the EDE-Q was compared.

Several studies have examined the concurrent validity of the EDE-Q in assessing OBEs among patients with BED. OBEs have a particular importance for the assessment of BED, and assessing OBEs is complex because its definition includes evaluating what constitutes a large amount of food and judging oneself to be out of control. Grilo, Masheb, and Wilson (2001) administered the EDE-Q and the EDE to 82 participants with BED who were enrolled in a randomized controlled treatment trial. Using Wilcoxon's matched-pairs signed rank sum test, the authors found no significant differences ($p > .05$) between EDE and EDE-Q on OBEs (EDE: $M = 20.4$, $SD = 17.8$; EDE-Q: $M = 17.8$, $SD = 11.6$) and SBEs (EDE: $M = 4.8$, $SD = 9.4$; EDE-Q: $M = 4.3$, $SD = 8.1$). There was a significant difference ($p < .05$) for OEs (EDE: $M = 6.1$, $SD = 14.7$; EDE-Q: $M = 2.5$, $SD = 8.5$). The correlation for OBEs between EDE and EDE-Q assessments was significant but small in size, tau b = .29, $p < .001$. Correlations for SBEs (tau b = −.06) and OEs (tau b = −.11) were nonsignificant.

Goldfein, Devlin, and Kamenetz (2005) assessed 37 men and women with BED on the EDE-Q and EDE. They found no significant difference on measurement of OBEs using a *t* test (EDE: $M = 15.5$, $SD = 6.21$; EDE-Q: $M = 17.4$, $SD = 9.06$; $p > .05$). Pearson correlation indicated

a small and nonsignificant correlation between the EDE and EDE-Q measurement of OBEs ($r = .197$). Wilfley, Schwartz, Spurrell, and Fairburn (1997) also examined binge eating among 52 individuals with BED as measured by the EDE and EDE-Q. They defined binge eating as objective binge days (OBDs) as opposed to OBEs. OBDs are more consistent with *DSM-IV* (APA, 1994) criteria for BED. Using Wilcoxon's matched-pairs signed rank sum test, the authors found no significant differences ($p > .05$) between the EDE and EDE-Q on OBDs (EDE: $M = 17.4$, $SD = 7.0$; EDE-Q: $M = 13.4$, $SD = 8.5$), and the correlation was small and nonsignificant, tau b = .20.

The original EDE-Q study by Fairburn and Beglin (1994) reported on concurrent validity with the EDE in a community sample of 286 women and a patient sample of 36 women (BN = 23, AN = 13). That paper did not report means and standard deviations. Nonparametric tests were used to calculate correlations between the EDE and EDE-Q (tau b) and differences (Wilcoxon matched pairs test). For the community sample: OBE tau b = .45, p value for difference < .001; vomiting tau b = .88, p value for difference > .05; laxatives tau b = .60, p value for difference < .01. For the patient sample: OBE tau b = .60, p value for difference < .01; vomiting tau b = .91, p value for difference > .05; laxatives tau b = .89, p value for difference > .05.

Carter, Aimé, and Mills (2001) provide evidence for concurrent validity of the EDE-Q with the EDE among 60 women with BN. However, the EDE-Q was administered after the EDE, and thus participants effectively were given specific definitions for large amounts of food and loss of control. Analyses were with nonparametric tests. For OBEs: EDE mean episodes = 27.8, $SD = 24.4$, EDE-Q mean episodes = 23.7, $SD = 28.3$, tau b = .56, p for the difference < .01. For SBEs: EDE mean episodes = 16.7, $SD = 21.5$, EDE-Q mean episodes = 12.0, $SD = 15.0$, tau b = .45, p for the difference > .05. For vomiting: EDE mean frequency = 39.6, $SD = 46.2$, EDE-Q mean frequency = 26.0, $SD = 29.9$, tau b = .72, p for the difference < .01. For laxative misuse: EDE mean frequency = 5.5,

SD = 10.2, EDE-Q mean frequency = 4.6, SD = 8.6, tau b = .88, p for the difference > .05. For diuretic misuse: EDE mean frequency = 1.3, SD = 5.5, EDE-Q mean frequency = 1.4, SD = 5.6, tau b = .86, p for the difference > .05.

In a study of concurrent validity in 98 obese (BMI > 30) bariatric surgery patients, Kalarachian, Wilson, Brolin, and Bradley (2000) used nonparametric statistics to compare the EDE-Q to the EDE on OBEs. EDE M = 9.32, SD = 19.8; EDE-Q M = 5.71, SD = 12.7, tau b = .46, p for the difference > .05, suggesting that the two measures did not differ in their assessment of OBEs.

Finally, Grilo et al. (2001) provided evidence of concurrent validity of the EDE-Q with 28-day prospective daily self-monitoring assessment in which OBEs, SBEs, and OEs were explicitly defined. Outpatients (N = 82) with BED who were consecutively evaluated for a randomized controlled trial participated in the study. Correlations of the EDE-Q and self-monitoring, as well as differences, were assessed using nonparametric tests. Results were as follows: for OBEs, tau b = .60, p > .05 for the difference between the EDE-Q and self-monitoring; for SBEs, tau b = .49, p < .001 for the difference; OE tau b = .16, p < .001 for the difference. Hence, OBEs were not significantly different between the EDE-Q and self-monitoring, but there were significant differences between the two assessment methods for SBEs and OEs. As indicated, correlations were adequate for OBEs and SBEs but small though significant for OEs.

As seen in the above review, evidence for the concurrent validity of the EDE-Q for assessing bingeing and purging is mixed. Correlations between the EDE and EDE-Q for OBEs, SBEs, and OEs tend to be small to moderate. Correlations tend to be large for vomiting and laxative misuse. It is likely that the complex definition of binge eating (large amount of food and loss of control) contributes to the lower estimates of concurrent validity for the EDE-Q.

One recent solution to problems associated with the complex definition of binge eating in the EDE-Q has been to explicitly define and give examples of binges. Goldfein et al. (2005) provided a detailed definition of "a large amount of food" and "loss of control" to their participants. As well, several written examples were provided to participants (pp. 110–111). This version of the EDE-Q is commonly referred to as the EDE-Q with instruction (EDE-QI). Goldfein et al. (2005) reported Pearson correlations and t tests for their data for 89 men and women with BED. Of those, 57 received the EDE-Q, 37 received the EDE-QI, and all were given the EDE interview. The correlation for OBEs between the EDE-QI and the EDE was .54 (p < .001), and for the EDE-Q and EDE, the correlation was .20 and nonsignificant. OBE means were as follows: EDE-QI M = 16.2, SD = 7.76; EDE-Q M = 17.4, SD = 9.06; EDE for the sample receiving the EDE-QI M = 16.2, SD = 7.76; EDE for the sample receiving the EDE-Q M = 15.5, SD = 9.92. None of the mean differences were significant, and effects were small in size.

Similar positive findings for OBDs were reported by Celio et al. (2004) for 154 women with BED. The Goldfein et al. (2005) definitions of OBDs were "modified" by Celio et al. in an unspecified way. In the Celio et al. study, the EDE-QI and the EDE assessment of OBDs was correlated at r = .65, and t tests revealed no significant differences between the EDE-QI (M = 17.1, SD = 7.0) and the EDE (M = 16.8, SD = 8.0). The results from Goldfein et al. and Celio et al. suggest that the concurrent validity of OBEs measured by the EDE-Q may be meaningfully enhanced with instruction. A caveat to these results is that both studies used parametric tests on frequency data that in previous research appeared to be nonnormally distributed.

Predictive Validity. One study by Mond et al. (2004) provided evidence of predictive validity of the EDE-Q. A community-based sample of 208 women was assessed, and 13 met study criteria for a clinically significant eating disorder (referred to as "cases"). There was a significantly higher percentage of cases compared to noncases who reported OBEs (58% vs. 5.5%) and SBEs

(41% vs 13.2%), $p < .001$ by Mann-Whitney U test. The authors did not report means and standard deviations of these data.

Sensitivity to Change

Walsh, Fairburn, Mickley, Sysko, and Parides (2004) used the EDE and EDE-Q to assess change related to fluoxetine ($n = 20$) versus placebo ($n = 22$) in a randomized double-blind treatment study for BN. Using an analysis of covariance (ANCOVA) to compare the groups on the EDE-Q, no significant differences were noted for OBEs ($p = .16$) and laxative misuse ($p = .68$), but significant differences were noted for vomiting episodes ($p = .01$). However, the EDE did indicate significant differences for OBEs ($p = .03$), for laxative misuse ($p = .002$), and for vomiting episodes ($p = .004$). In a follow-up study with the same sample, Sysko, Walsh, and Fairburn (2005) reported that the Pearson correlation was .45 for change scores on OBEs for the EDE and EDE-Q, .97 for change in laxative misuse, and .93 for change in vomiting episodes. The results suggest that the EDE-Q was not as sensitive to change as the EDE for OBEs and was likely not as sensitive to change for laxative misuse, but there was evidence for EDE-Q sensitivity to change for vomiting episodes.

Norms

There are no published norms on the EDE-Q behavioral assessment of binge eating or purging behavior. However, several studies provide means and standard deviations of clinical samples, and these are reproduced in Table 10.5.

Availability

An updated version of the EDEQ is now available in a book by Fairburn (2008). The scale can be accessed at www.psychiatry.ox.ac.uk/research/researchunits/credo/assessment-measures-pdf-files/EDE-Q6.pdf. The instructions for the

EDE-QI are available in the appendix of the article by Goldfein et al. (2005).

The Eating Symptoms Inventory

Description

The Eating Symptom Inventory (ESI; Whitaker et al., 1989) is a self-report measure that was designed to measure symptoms related to AN and BN. It contains 24 sets of questions that inquire about the key features of AN and BN. Whereas some questions use a 5-point Likert-type scale, others are multiple choice, and others are short answer or fill in the blank (e.g., height, weight, etc.). The ESI defines a binge by specifying the 2-hour time frame required for a binge and providing examples of binges that vary in quantity. Individuals are asked to approximate the amount eaten in a typical binge and the frequency of binge-ing. However, loss of control, which is required for individuals to meet diagnostic criteria for an objective binge, is not assessed. Specific to purging, individuals are asked about the frequency of purging behaviors such as self-induced vomiting and laxative and diuretic use. A notable limitation of this instrument is that it only inquires about lifetime totals for binge eating, self-induced vomiting, and laxative and diuretic use, making it impossible to determine an accurate picture of current symptomatology or to determine a diagnosis of BN. As a result, this would not be an appropriate instrument to use to measure change in symptomatology over time or to include in a clinical trial.

In completing searches on PsycINFO and MEDLINE, no updated psychometric information was found on the ESI. One recent study (Basile, 2004) was found to use the ESI, but minimal information was available regarding the ESI's properties. The ESI does not appear to be a currently used measure for bingeing and purging. Interested readers should refer to the previous version of this chapter (Pike, Loeb, & Walsh, 1995) for more information.

Table 10.5 Means (Standard Deviations) of Features Assessed by the Eating Disorder Examination–Questionnaire Studies and Diagnostic Groups

Feature	BN[a]	Obese Bariatric[b]	BED[c]	BED[d]	BED EDE-QI[e]	BED EDE-QI[f]
OBE	23.7 (28.3)	9.32 (19.8)	NA	17.8 (11.6)	25.6 (19.7)	16.2 (7.76)
OBD	NA	NA	13.4 (8.5)	NA	17.1 (7.0)	NA
SBE	12.0 (15.0)	NA	NA	4.3 (8.1)	NA	NA
OE	NA	NA	NA	2.5 (8.5)	NA	NA
Vomiting	26.0 (29.9)	NA	NA	NA	NA	NA
Laxative	4.6 (8.6)	NA	NA	NA	NA	NA
Diuretic	1.4 (5.6)	NA	NA	NA	NA	NA

NOTE: OBE = objective binge episodes; OBD = objective binge days; SBE = subjective binge episodes; OE = overeating episodes. All episodes and numbers are for a 28-day period. NA = not assessed or not reported. EDE-QI = Eating Disorder Examination with instruction.

a. N = 57; BN = bulimia nervosa; data from Carter, Aimé, and Mills (2001).

b. N = 98; data from Kalarchian, Wilson, Brolin, and Bradley (2000).

c. N = 52; data from Wilfley, Schwartz, Spurrell, and Fairburn (1997).

d. N = 82; data from Grilo, Masheb, and Wilson (2001).

e. N = 157; data from Celio, Wilfley, Crow, Mitchell, and Walsh (2004).

f. N = 52; data from Goldfein, Devlin, and Kamenetz (2005).

Multifactorial Assessment of Eating Disorder Symptoms

Description

The Multifactorial Assessment of Eating Disorder Symptoms (MAEDS; Anderson, Williamson, Duchmann, Gleaves, & Barbin, 1999) is a self-report measure consisting of 56 items intended to measure six clusters of symptoms such as depression, fear of fatness, restrictive eating, avoidance of forbidden foods, and, of particular interest to this chapter, binge eating and purgative behavior. This measure was primarily designed as a treatment outcome measure for BN and AN. Individuals are asked to complete the questionnaire using a 7-point rating scale for each symptom cluster, ranging from *always* to *never*.

Two psychometric studies were found on the MAEDS, as well as one additional study that used this instrument. The available psychometric information is summarized below.

Reliability

Stability. Test-retest reliabilities over an average of 8 days (range, 5–21 days) for 15 female inpatients with eating disorders ranged from .89 for binge eating to .99 for purgative behaviors (Anderson et al., 1999).

Internal Consistency. Internal consistency was calculated based on completed questionnaires from

118 women (with and without eating disorders) as part of a multistudy research project. Cronbach alpha coefficients for subscales ranged from .80 for purgative behaviors to .92 for binge eating, indicating good internal consistency (Anderson et al., 1999).

Construct Validity

The initial development of the MAEDS included a total of 389 women, 295 college undergraduates, and 94 clinical inpatients or outpatients diagnosed with eating disorders (Anderson et al., 1999). The majority of women were between ages 18 and 25 years. The clinical group consisted of individuals with AN, BN, and EDNOS. The 90 questions (15 questions per symptom cluster) were evaluated for content validity by a panel of judges with expertise in the area of eating disorders. Initially, judges grouped the questions into one of six categories based on where they believed items should be assigned and rated items for fit within a specific category. When consensus between judges could not be reached as to the categorization of an item, the item was eliminated.

A PCA with an orthogonal varimax rotation was conducted on the items. The decision to retain items was based on a component loading of .40 or higher and if items loaded .40 or greater on only one component (Anderson et al., 1999). According to examination of the scree plot, the six component solutions accounted for 57.3% of the total variance. After the rotation and elimination of items not meeting above criteria, 53.2% of the total variance was accounted for, and 41 items were retained. Binge eating (8 items) and purgative behavior (8 items) accounted for 11.1% and 9.1% of the variance, respectively. The final version of the MAEDS contains 56 items.

Criterion Validity

Concurrent Validity. The relationship between the MAEDS and other commonly used eating disorder measures such as the EAT (Garner et al.,

1982), the EDI-2 (Garner, 1991), the BULIT-R (Thelen et al., 1991), and the Goldfarb Fear of Fatness Scale (GFFS; Goldfarb, Dykens, & Gerrard, 1985) was examined by Anderson and colleagues (1999). Both the binge eating and purgative behaviors subscales were significantly correlated with the EAT total score (.49 and .45, respectively), the EAT dieting factor (.45 and .42, respectively), the EAT bulimia factor (.67 and .35, respectively), the BULIT-R total score (.86 and .38, respectively), the EDI-2 Bulimia scale (.69 and .28, respectively), and the GFFS score (.62 and .42, respectively). Anderson et al. (1999) found that the binge-eating scale of the MAEDS significantly and negatively correlated ($r = -.30$) with the oral control factor of the EAT.

Predictive Validity. Martin, Williamson, and Thaw (2000) compared the subscale scores of the MAEDS across four eating disorder diagnoses (BN-purging type, AN-binge/purge type, AN-restricting type, and BED) among 177 treatment-seeking patients. The multivariate analysis of variance (MANOVA) indicated that the four diagnostic groups differed on subscales of the MAEDS based on whether patients had a full versus a partial syndrome ($p < .005$). Researchers collapsed syndrome type and directly compared four eating disorder subtypes (i.e., BN-purging type, AN-binge/purge type, AN-restricting type, and BED) by Tukey's HSD post hoc comparisons. Those with BN-purging type and BED scored higher ($M = 68.86, SD = 12.98, M = 73.41, SD = 6.53$, respectively) than the two AN groups (binge/purge type: $M = 51.22, SD = 14.01$; restricting type: $M = 42.50, SD = 6.63$) on the Binge Eating subscale ($p < .05$). Those with BN-purging type ($M = 80.17, SD = 13.04$) and AN-binge/purge type ($M = 74.19, SD = 19.47$) scored higher on the Purging subscale compared to the AN-restricting ($M = 53.36, SD = 12.40$) and BED ($M = 51.69, SD = 13.70$) groups ($p < .05$; Martin et al., 2000).

Discriminant Validity. Discriminant validity (Anderson et al., 1999) was shown by small correlations between measures of psychopathology (maturity fears, interpersonal distrust, and perfectionism on the EDI-2) and eating-related scales of the MAEDS. For example, there was no correlation ($r = .00$) between the binge-eating scale on the MAEDS and a measure of exercising on the BULIT-R (Thelen et al., 1991) and a small correlation ($r = .03$) between the Maturity Fears scale of the EDI-2 (Garner, 1991) and the purging scale of the MAEDS.

Norms

The standardization sample consisted of 178 college women with no eating disorders. The mean for all subscales is a T score of 50 with a standard deviation of 10; this translates into raw scores of 26 and 11 on the binge-eating and purgative behaviors subscales, respectively. For detailed norms, the reader is referred to the chapter on the assessment of eating-disordered thoughts, feelings, and behaviors that appears in this compendium.

Availability

Copies of the MAEDS and instructions for their use may be obtained from Dr. Drew A. Anderson, University at Albany, Department of Psychology, 369 Social Science, Albany NY 12222; telephone: (518) 442-4835; e-mail: drewa@csc.albany.edu. A copy is also available in Appendix 11.E at the end of this book.

Questionnaire of Eating and Weight Patterns–Revised

Description

The Questionnaire on Eating and Weight Patterns–Revised (QEWP-R: Spitzer, Devlin, et al., 1992; Spitzer, Yanovski, & Marcus, 1993) was initially developed to identify individuals with BED. Of particular relevance to this chapter, the QEWP-R asks individuals to self-report the presence and frequency of binge eating and purging within the past 6 months. Individuals are also asked about other symptoms such as dieting, distress related to eating, and weight. A 5-point Likert-type scale is used, asking individuals to rate their responses from *not at all* to *to an extreme degree*. This scale consists of 28 items, following *DSM-IV* criteria, and individuals may be diagnosed with BED or with BN, purging or nonpurging subtypes, after completion of the measure. Decision rules for scoring are available in Spitzer, Yanovski, Wadden, et al. (1993). This measure also captures individuals' age, gender, ethnic background, education, height, and weight.

Reliability

Stability. Nangle, Johnson, Carr-Nangle, and Engler (1994) found modest 3-week test-retest reliability ($\kappa = .58$) for a diagnosis of BED made using the original QEWP in a sample of 104 self-referred binge eaters and a comparison sample. Diagnosis of nonclinical bingeing (including subcategories of episodic overeating, binge eating, binge-eating syndrome, and binge eating syndrome and distress) and no diagnosis were modestly stable over a 3-week period with a kappa coefficient of .43. Nangle et al. (1994) also examined the stability of bingeing probability over a 3-week period. The mean probabilities of bingeing for BED and nonclinical binging groups did not change significantly over 3 weeks, but those with no diagnosis ($n = 4$) showed a trend toward a decrease in bingeing ($p = .057$). For individuals with BED, the probability of bingeing at Weeks 1 and 3 were significantly related ($r = .70, p < .001$), but this was not the case for the nonclinical bingeing group ($r = -.10, p = .78$).

Test-retest reliability was examined more recently (Johnson, Kirk, & Reed, 2001) in an adolescent school sample. Over a 3-week period, the QEWP-A (adolescent version) showed significant but modest levels of stability for a sample of 106 boys and girls ($\varphi = .42, p < .001$).

Validity

Construct Validity. This instrument does not include empirically derived factors apart from the diagnostic criteria that comprise BED.

Content Validity. Nangle et al. (1994) found the sensitivity and specificity of the original QEWP to detect binge eating to be 71.4% and 69.2%, respectively, for first week of the initial assessment. After a 3-week interval, sensitivity and specificity were 81.8% and 62.5%, respectively. For both time periods, the associations were significant ($p < .05$).

In a study assessing the concordance between the QEWP-R and the BES in 157 adults with and without BED, Celio et al. (2004) found a sensitivity value of .74 and a specificity value of .35, suggesting that while the QEWP-R is an adequate screening measure for BED, it may not be sufficient for diagnostic purposes due to the high percentage of misclassifications. The QEWP-R correctly identified the frequency of days binged over a period of 6 months for 63.2% of participants, using the EDE and EDE-QI as comparison measures (Celio et al., 2004).

Criterion Validity

Concurrent Validity. In terms of diagnosing BED, the patient-rated QEWP has been found to have modest convergence with the clinician-rated SCID for *DSM-III-R* in a sample of 100 obese women seeking weight loss treatment, with a kappa coefficient of .57 (de Zwann et al., 1993). Discrepancies between patient and clinician ratings were not solely due to the QEWP overestimating the prevalence of BED (de Zwaan et al., 1993). Authors suggested discrepancies may have been due to patients interpreting the questions differently, resistance to give correct information, or changes in reporting across contexts (de Zwaan et al., 1993). Celio et al. (2004) reported the correlation between the QEWP-R and the EDE to be good (Kendall's tau b = .53, $p < .001$).

Gladis et al. (1998) found moderate agreement between the Binge Eating Scale (BES) and the QEWP-R in 128 obese women enrolled in a weight loss program. When those with BED were compared to those without BED, a kappa coefficient of .45 was found. An improved kappa of .64

was found when subthreshold BED cases were removed from the analyses, and nonbingers were compared to those with BED. Celio and colleagues (2004) suggested discordance between the QEWP-R and BES could have been, in part, as a result of the former measure focusing on BED criteria and the latter measure assessing psychopathology related to binge eating.

Elder and colleagues (2006) assessed 249 gastric bypass candidates, the majority of whom were women, on the QEWP-R and the EDE-Q to compare the concordance of these two instruments. Although the instruments identified a comparable number of patients with recurrent binge eating, the overlap was low, with a kappa coefficient of .26. In terms of twice-weekly binge eating, the kappa coefficient was poor at .05. Authors concluded that while both measures identified individuals who binge eat, the QEWP-R was less good at differentiating between non- or infrequent bingers and recurrent binge eaters compared to the EDE-Q.

Predictive Validity. In a sample of binge eaters, Nangle and colleagues (1994) found the predictive efficiency values at Week 1 and 3 assessments to be 70.7% and 73.7%, respectively, for the original version of the QEWP. No studies were found using the QEWP-R to discriminate among BED, BN-purging type, and BN-nonpurging types.

Norms

This is not applicable.

Availability

The manual and the QEWP-R measure are available from the author, Dr. Robert Spitzer at the New York State Psychiatric Institute, Unit 60, 1051 Riverside Drive, New York City, NY 10533; telephone: 212–543–5524; e-mail: RLS8@ Columbia .edu. A copy of the scale is reprinted in Appendix 10.A at the end of this book.

Stirling Eating Disorder Scales

Description

The Stirling Eating Disorder Scales (SEDS; G.-J. Williams & Power, 1995) was designed as a measure of symptomatology for AN and BN. In particular, the SEDS was meant to address the limitations of existing eating disorder measures by assessing a range of anorexia- and bulimia-related cognitions and behaviors, as well as relevant psychological variables (Openshaw & Waller, 2005). It is an 80-item, paper-and-pencil, self-report questionnaire that instructs individuals to endorse either "true" or "false" on items about anorexic and bulimic dietary cognitions and dietary behavior (comprising four scales) and perceived external control, low assertiveness, low self-esteem, and self-directed hostility (comprising four scales). Each scale consists of 10 items. Individuals take approximately 15 to 20 minutes to complete the measure. This scale is intended to be used by clinicians and clinical researchers to screen for eating disorder behaviors and cognitions; it is not intended to be a diagnostic tool.

The SEDS has been widely used for clinical purposes in the United Kingdom but has not yet received similar recognition in North America. This may be because there are few studies detailing the reliability and validity of this measure, apart from the original validation study (G.-J. Williams et al., 1994). The available psychometrics are summarized below, and the reader will see that there are mixed results regarding the psychometric strengths of the SEDS. As noted by Openshaw and Waller (2005), more studies are required to confirm the SEDS strengths and to examine its limitations.

Reliability

Stability. Test-retest correlations for the eight SED scales were stable over a 3-week period for normal controls and eating disorder patients alike (Williams et al., 1994). Correlations ranged from .85 ($p < .001$) for Perceived External Control to .97 ($p < .001$) and .98 ($p < .001$) for Anorexic Dietary Cognitions and overall scores, respectively. Specific to this chapter, retest correlations for Anorexic Dietary Behavior and Bulimic Dietary Behavior subscales were .90 ($p < .001$) and .93 ($p < .001$), respectively.

Internal Consistency. Williams et al. (1994) found Cronbach's alphas for the eight SEDS to be high, ranging from .83 to .92 ($p < .001$). Split-half reliability coefficients were significant, ranging from .72 to .99 ($p < .001$). Campbell, Lawrence, Serpell, Lask, and Neiderman (2002) confirmed adequate internal consistency in their sample of adolescents with eating disorders and a nonpatient control group. All Cronbach alpha coefficients exceeded .70, indicating good to excellent internal consistency, and all coefficients were below .90, indicating that items were not redundant.

However, Openshaw and Waller (2005) noted some limitations to the SEDS. In assessing an adult sample of 40 women with BN ($M_{age} = 28.4$ years, $SD = 6.6$) using the SEDS, these researchers found mixed results for internal consistency. Whereas Cronbach's alpha for the total score was good (.84), alphas for individual subscales were much lower, with the majority falling below .70. Openshaw and Waller suggested that this pattern of results may be due to the SEDS only measuring one construct of eating and related pathology, rather than several distinct factors of eating and related pathology. When up to three items with the poorest alphas were removed to examine whether internal consistency for individual subscales could be improved, two of the eight Cronbach alphas improved to above .70 (including the Bulimic Dietary Behaviors subscale), but others remained low (Openshaw & Waller, 2005). These authors concluded that perhaps sample differences or issues related to comorbidity within the sample may have contributed to divergent findings in the above studies. They suggested that the SEDS required more psychometric evaluation with regard to its validity and reliability.

In a large sample of 241 patients (M_{age} = 26.8 years, SD = 7.8) diagnosed with AN, BN, or EDNOS, Gamble and colleagues (2006) found somewhat more promising results than Openshaw and Waller (2005) regarding internal consistency of the SEDS. However, they also noted that some internal consistencies for individual subscales appeared to vary depending on diagnosis (Gamble et al., 2006). Of specific relevance to this chapter, Cronbach alphas for bulimic behaviors ranged from .58 for the BN group to .85 for the AN group and .80 for the total sample, including EDNOS. Similar to Openshaw and Waller, some alphas could be raised to acceptable levels (i.e., ≥ .70) by deleting an item from the subscale (see Gamble et al., 2006, for details). Cronbach alphas for the overall SEDS for each diagnosis and the combined sample were consistently high, ranging from .86 to .91.

In general, research (Gamble et al., 2006; Openshaw & Waller, 2005) has suggested that perhaps the SEDS may be more reliable with certain eating disorder groups (e.g., AN and EDNOS) as compared to others (e.g., BN).

Validity

Construct Validity. G.-J. Williams and colleagues (1994) used a modified version of the Thurstone method of scale development to create the SEDS. Two hundred forty items were generated from four sources, such as a review of other standardized measures, interview data from 30 patients with AN and BN, research experience, and the eating disorders literature in general (G.-J. Williams et al., 1994). Items were grouped according to the eight intended scales to be measured. Items were checked for face validity and modified accordingly. Two hundred thirty-five items were submitted to a test by a panel of 40 psychologists and psychiatrists who were experts in the field of eating disorders. These experts rated each item on a scale of 1 (low) to 7 (high), to reflect the degree to which each item reflected

a given construct of interest. Final items were selected so as to include a range of different weights along the scale and low ambiguity as determined by the quartile deviation. The final 80 items were randomly presented to a second panel of experts, and they were asked to assign items to the scales that best represented the items (G.-J. Williams et al., 1994). Two items were revisited and replaced due to low agreement among the experts as to which scale they should be assigned.

Gamble and colleagues (2006) performed a CFA on the SEDS subscales, producing a goodness-of-fit index (GFI) of .80, indicating that the SEDS subscales accounted for 80% of the variance in the sample covariance. This analysis showed a poor CFI of .64, an RMSEA greater than .10 (RMSEA = .24), and a normative fit index (NFI) of less than .90 (NFI = .63), indicating a poor-fitting model (Gamble et al., 2006). Gamble and colleagues attempted to replicate the SEDS subscales by performing a PCA and a second CFA with the new subscales. Readers are directed to this article for details of these analyses. Overall, these researchers found that the new subscales derived from the PCA adequately modeled the data compared to the original SEDS subscales, as evidenced by a CFA conducted with the new scales (GFI = .96; CFI = .91; RMSEA = .13; NFI = .90).

Criterion Validity

Concurrent Validity. G.-J. Williams and colleagues (1994) correlated the SEDS with six subscales from the Eating Attitudes Test–40 (EAT-40) and the Bulimic Investigatory Test, Edinburgh (BITE; Henderson & Freeman, 1987). The authors found acceptable concurrent validity, with correlations between the SEDS and the EAT-40 and BITE ranging from .83 to .90.

Using a sample of 53 adolescent patients with eating disorders and 61 age-matched nonclinical controls, Campbell and colleagues (2002) correlated the four dietary SED subscales with the restraint, eating concern, weight concern, and shape concern subscales of the EDE (Fairburn & Cooper, 1993) to examine concurrent or criterion validity. All SED scales showed significant positive correlations with EDE scales, ranging from .27 ($p = .025$) to .56 ($p < .001$), with the exception of the relationship between bulimic dietary behaviors measured by the SEDS and restraint measured by the EDE, which was nonsignificant. In a separate study, Gamble et al. (2006) also found acceptable correlations between SEDS bulimic cognitions and behaviors scales with the EDE assessment of bulimic behaviors ($r = .47$, $p < .01$ and $r = .56$, $p < .01$, respectively) but small correlations between SEDS anorexic cognitions and behavior scales and the EDE restraint scale ($r = .11$, $p > .05$ and $r = .13$, $p < .05$, respectively). These suggest good evidence for concurrent validity of the bulimia scales but not for the anorexia scales of the SEDS.

Predictive Validity. Evidence for predictive validity was found by Campbell et al. (2002). The majority of their eating-disordered patients scored above the adult threshold on the anorexic dietary subscales of the SEDS (96.2% and 77.4% on cognitions and behaviors, respectively), whereas the majority of the nonclinical control group scored below the thresholds (72.1% and 96.7% on cognitions and behaviors, respectively). In terms of bulimic dietary behaviors, most of the participants (62.3% of patients and 82.0% of nonpatients) scored below the threshold. Patients scored significantly higher ($p < .001$) than the nonpatient group on all SEDS scales (Campbell et al., 2002).

Norms

Norms are available in the G.-J. Williams et al. (1994) paper, in which the authors present data on 38 patients with AN ($M_{age} = 24.7$, $SD = 5.3$), 36 patients with BN ($M_{age} = 25.0$, $SD = 6.1$), and 68 individuals no disorders ($M_{age} = 23.8$, $SD = 4.9$). Individuals in the AN group weighed significantly less than those in the other groups, but there were no age differences between groups. Both AN and BN groups were attending treatment for their eating disorders at the time of recruitment into the study (G.-J. Williams et al., 1994). The comparison group was recruited from a university student population and the community. Group means and between-group comparisons on the eight Stirling Eating Disorder Scales are presented in Table 10.6. Readers are directed to the manual for the SEDS (G.-J. Williams & Power, 1995) for detailed information on the standardization sample.

Table 10.6   Group Means (Standard Deviations) for Three Diagnostic Groups on the Anorexia- and Bulimia-Related Subscales of the Stirling Eating Disorder Scales (SEDS)

	Groups		
Scale	*Anorexia (n = 38)*	*Bulimia (n = 36)*	*Control (n = 68)*
Anorexic dietary cognitions	32.95[a] (12.5)	25.25[b] (10.9)	2.85[c] (5.5)
Anorexic dietary behaviors	22.16[a] (12.2)	11.51[b] (9.8)	1.94[c] (3.2)
Bulimic dietary cognitions	24.70[a] (14.8)	35.75[b] (7.7)	5.53[c] (8.8)
Bulimic dietary behaviors	21.57[a] (13.4)	34.54[b] (9.8)	3.79[c] (6.1)

SOURCE: Data are from G.-J. Williams et al. (1994, p. 40).

NOTE: Means across groups with different superscripts within each scale indicate significant differences (Scheffé's post hoc comparisons $p < .001$).

Availability

The SEDS manual, scales, and profile forms may be purchased through the publisher, Harcourt Assessment (England), 1 Procter Street, London WC1V 6EU, England; telephone: +44 (0)20 7911 1975; fax: +44 (0)20 7911 1961; Web site: www.harcourt-uk.com.

Survey for Eating Disorders

Description

The Survey of Eating Disorders (SEDs) is a new self-report measure developed by Götestam and Agras (1995). The scale provides eating disorder diagnoses based on *DSM-IV* criteria. It was developed out of a need for short and cost-effective instruments to diagnose eating disorders. The measure's psychometric properties have not yet been rigorously evaluated, but some preliminary data on reliability and validity were reported by Ghaderi and Scott (2002). The scale has been used in clinical research as a screening/assessment tool (de Man Lapidoth, Ghaderi, & Norring, 2006; Kjelsås, Bjornstrom, & Götestam, 2004). The measure consists of 39 questions, 18 of which are necessary for diagnosis, 4 of which are demographic, and the remaining questions provide information on age of onset of dieting, bingeing, and antecedents and triggers of dieting and bingeing. A definition of binge eating (per *DSM-IV*) is presented to the responders before the questions about binge eating. Purging questions are combined to cover occurrence, method, frequency, and duration. A main limitation to the scale is that it requires further psychometric validation, particularly from independent labs rather than the original author.

The SEDs shows good preliminary reliability and validity as a screening and diagnostic measure using *DSM-IV* criteria. The scale, overall, has demonstrated good psychometric properties, and this provides indirect evidence for its ability to assess parameters of bingeing and purging. It

is relatively brief and easy to administer, and the measure uses clear and simple words.

Reliability

There are no test-retest reliability studies of the specific items regarding bingeing and purging. However, full-scale test-retest reliability was examined by Ghaderi and Scott (2002) by comparing the derived diagnostic categories from a student sample ($n = 124$) for a 2-week period, using Wilcoxon matched pairs test. The entire sample was reclassified into their original categories when the second administration of the SEDs was coded, indicating a very high level of reliability (Ghaderi & Scott, 2002).

Criterion Validity

Concurrent Validity. There are no studies specifically investigating the validity of items related to bingeing and purging. However, the SEDs as a whole has demonstrated evidence of concurrent validity with the EDI-2 (Garner, 1991) on a student sample (Ghaderi & Scott, 2002). The sample consisted of 124 students (81% female, $M_{age} = 28.7$ years, $SD = 6.3$, 53% were single, $M_{BMI} = 22.2$ kg/m^2, $SD = 4.1$) recruited from clinical psychology master's programs. Students who met the diagnostic criteria for an eating disorder using the SEDs had significantly higher scores on all the EDI-2 subscales, except for Interpersonal Distrust. The mean total of the EDI-2 for students with a current eating disorder diagnosis on the SEDs was significantly higher than the mean score for students with a past history of an eating disorder and students with no eating disorder ($p < .001$). All three groups were significantly different from one another using Tukey's post hoc test, indicating concurrent and predictive validity of the measure.

Predictive Validity. There are no studies specifically assessing the predictive validity of the bingeing and purging items, but Ghaderi and Scott (2002) assessed predictive validity of the entire scale using a clinical sample of 45 treatment-seeking women recruited from the newspaper for binge eating (M_{age} = 27.6 years, SD = 10.0; M_{BMI} = 24.7 kg/m^2, SD = 6.0). Seventy percent of the sample was single. Wilcoxon matched pairs test showed no significant difference between the derived diagnosis from the SEDs when compared with the EDE (Fairburn & Cooper, 1993) based diagnosis (t = 186, z = .96, p = .34). The SEDs resulted in only two cases of false positives (Peterson & Miller, 2005), demonstrating a positive predictive value as high as .96. Thus, the sensitivity of the SEDs appears to be very good, although the specificity of the measure was not calculated due to the nature of the sample (non-eating-disordered participants were excluded).

Norms

This is not applicable.

Availability

A copy of the scale along with scoring information is available in the paper by Ghaderi and Scott (2002).

Other Self-Report Measures

Several self-report measures were touched upon in this chapter but not comprehensively reviewed. The EAT-40, also available as the EAT-26 and the EAT-12, is a standardized measure of symptoms and concerns characteristic of eating disorders (Garfinkel & Newman, 2001; Garner & Garfinkel, 1979). The EAT has been used as a screening tool in large-scale community studies of adolescents and adults. The TFEQ (Stunkard & Messick, 1985) has three subscales: Cognitive Restraint of Eating, Susceptibility to Hunger, and Disinhibition of Eating. The Disinhibition of Eating scale does address some aspects of disregulation of eating or emotional eating but not binge eating per se. Mazzeo, Aggen, Anderson, Tozzi, and Bulik (2003) failed to replicate the

factor structure of the TFEQ by CFA, and Tasca et al. (2006) found the internal consistency of the Disinhibition scale to be inadequate in a clinical sample of individuals with BED.

The BITE (Henderson & Freeman, 1987) was developed as the authors saw a need for a more sensitive measure to correctly identify clinical and subclinical cases of individuals with bulimic symptoms. The authors recommended the BITE for use as an epidemiological tool and as a screening measure. The BITE consists of two scales, a Symptom scale and a Severity scale. The Symptom scale is made of up 30 items relating to symptoms, behaviors, and dieting. The Severity scale is composed of 6 items, which provide an index of severity of bingeing and purging as defined by their frequency. Range of possible scores on the Symptom scale is 0 to 30, with a cutoff score of 20, and for the Severity scale, the range of possible scores is 0 to 39, with a cutoff score of 5. The two scales may be added to provide a total score, with a possible range of 0 to 69 and a cutoff of 25. A score at or above the cutoff suggests a bulimic disorder (Waller, 1992). The scale's original validation demonstrated a moderate to high test-retest reliability (r = .68–.86) and high internal consistency using Cronbach's alpha for the Symptom scale (.96). Cronbach's alpha was inadequate for the Severity scale (.62). Henderson and Freeman (1987) and also G.-J. Williams et al. (1994) demonstrated acceptable concurrent validity of the BITE with other similar measures, including the EAT-40, the EDI (Garner & Olmsted, 1984), and the SEDs (G.-J. Williams & Power, 1995). Henderson and Freeman found the BITE to correctly identify binge eaters versus control participants perfectly, but these results were not replicated by independent labs. Specifically, Waller (1992) found that the BITE was not as useful when classifying low-weight binge eaters or those with anorexia binge-purge subtype. Overall advantages to the BITE are that the scale requires less than 10 minutes to complete, and it is very good at identifying individuals with bulimia nervosa and bulimic symptoms. The main drawback to the scale is that it was standardized using women who met *DSM-III* (American Psychiatric Association, 1980) criteria for bulimia nervosa. The items on the scale may not reflect the diversity of binge eating, particularly with regard to anorexic individuals who binge and purge and those with binge-eating disorder. The scale may require updating in keeping with diagnostic changes since its development. A copy of the scale can be found in the original article by Henderson and Freeman (1987).

Structured Interviews

Several interviews have been developed for the assessment of eating disorders, particularly with subscales related to bingeing and/or purging behaviors. However, many of these interviews are not widely used, and preliminary or limited information is available regarding their reliability and validity. The previous version of this chapter by Pike et al. (1995) identified the Clinical Eating Disorder Rating Instrument (CEDRI) as lacking rigorous psychometric evaluation (Palmer, Christie, Cordle, Davies, & Kenrick, 1987). The current review found only one validation study that was conducted (Palmer, Roberston, Cain, and Black, 1996) using only a subset of the interview questions that measure eating pathology. No further validation has been conducted. The Rating of Anorexia and Bulimia Interview–Revised (RAB-R; Nevonen, Broberg, Clinton, & Norring, 2003) showed some promising preliminary reliability and validity, but it is not widely used at present. Thus, both of these instruments will not be reviewed in detail here. Rather, we will review in depth the interviews that have noteworthy updates and that are widely used in the field.

Eating Disorder Examination (EDE)

Description

The Eating Disorder Examination (EDE; Fairburn & Cooper, 1993) is a 62-item semistructured interview that was designed to assess the specific psychopathology of eating disorders. The measure includes specific measurement of the presence and frequency of specific eating-disordered behaviors: overeating, self-induced vomiting, laxative misuse, diuretic misuse, and intense exercise. Overeating is further defined as objective binge episodes (OBEs), subjective binge episodes (SBEs), and objective overeating episodes (OEs). OBEs are defined as eating a large amount of food within a 2-hour time period and having a sense of loss of control during that episode. SBEs include a sense of loss of control but not eating an objectively large amount of food. OEs are defined as eating a large amount of food but no loss of control. There are four scales measuring eating disorder attitudes and cognitions, including Eating Concerns, Weight Concerns, Shape Concerns, and Restraint. A global score of overall severity of eating disorder psychopathology can also be calculated. This review will focus on the measures of eating disorder behaviors related to binge eating (OBEs and SBEs) and purging (self-induced vomiting, laxative misuse, and diuretic misuse) only.

The advantage of the EDE for measuring eating disorder behaviors is that the interviewer can provide a specific definition of the complex behaviors in questions. This is particularly important for the assessment of OBEs and SBEs where the interviewee has to make decisions about the quantity of food and the aspect of loss of control. The total interview takes about 30 minutes to 1 hour to administer, and all questions refer to the 4 weeks preceding the interview. For each item, there is at least one probe question. Scale items are rated on a 7-point Likert-type scale, and items are rated according to the severity and frequency of behaviors. Items regarding OBEs, SBEs, and purging behaviors are coded for presence or absence and frequency of the behaviors for the past 28 days. Some researchers have relied on direct training from the scale developer, presumably to achieve adequate reliability (e.g., Beumont, Kopec-Schrader, Talbot, & Touyz, 1993).

The EDE is perhaps the most widely used semistructured interview for the assessment of the specific psychopathology of eating disorders. The measure was initially developed for adults with eating disorders, but the measure has been used with children (Watkins, Frampton, Lask, & Byrant-Waugh, 2005), and a Spanish-language version has been developed (Grilo, Lozano, & Elder, 2005).

Reliability

Stability. Several studies assessed the test-retest reliability of bingeing and purging behaviors as measured by the EDE in clinical samples. Rizvi, Peterson, Crow, and Agras (2000) reported retest correlations 2 to 7 days after the initial assessment where the reassessment was conducted by a different interviewer. Participants were 20 women with full syndrome or subthreshold eating disorders (AN = 4; BN = 10; BED = 6). Test-retest Spearman correlations were as follows: OBEs = .848, objective bulimic days (OBDs) = .825, SBEs = .335, subjective bulimic days (SBDs) = .401, vomit episodes = .970, and vomit days = .967. Grilo, Masheb, Lozano-Blanco, and Barry (2003) reported Spearman correlations across 6 to 14 days for women with BED: OBEs = .70, OBDs = .71, SBEs = .17, SBDs = .17. Nunally and Bernstein (1994) suggest a minimum acceptable retest correlation of .80. Hence, the short-term stability of the assessment of OBEs and OBDs was reported to be good for a mixed group of full and partial syndrome patients (Rizvi et al., 2000) but somewhat less than adequate for patients with BED (Grilo et al., 2003). The evidence is generally poor for stability of SBEs and SBDs and is good for vomit episodes and days of stability. There were no studies that we could find that reported retest reliability for laxative or diuretic misuse as measured by the EDE.

Interrater Reliability. Given that the EDE items are interviewer administered, interrater reliability is an important psychometric aspect to measure. Rizvi et al. (2000) reported interrater reliability for 19 of their 20 patients using Spearman correlation (see above). All correlations were above .91

(OBE = .995, OBD = .998, SBE = .916, SBD = .991, vomit episodes = 1.00, vomit days = 1.00). A preferred assessment of interrater reliability is the intraclass coefficient (ICC), which accounts not only for covariation of the two raters' judgments but also for concordance of judgments (Shrout & Fliess, 1979). Grilo et al. (2003) used the ICC to measure interrater reliability for their sample of 18 women with BED. ICCs for OBEs and SBEs were .99.

Criterion Validity

Concurrent Validity. There are very few studies on concurrent validity of binge eating and purging measured by the EDE, and results have been mixed. The EDE is a retrospective interview measure in which participants are asked to recall frequencies of and number of days in which a series of complexly defined behaviors (e.g., OBEs) occurred in the past 28 days. Friedman and deWinstanley (1998) argue that detailed characteristics of specific episodes may not be retained in memory for more than a few days. Stein and Corte (2003) provide a more detailed account of the episodic and semantic memory processes involved in reliably retrieving and counting specific instances of behavior. In their study of concurrent validity of the EDE, Stein and Corte included 16 patients with subthreshold AN and BN who recorded their eating disorder behaviors for 4 weeks using a handheld computer (e.g., ecologic momentary assessment [EMA] of eating-disordered behaviors). Participants were trained on the EMA procedures and device and given a 24-hour practice period. The number of errors in using the EMA appeared to be small; there was little evidence of reactivity to the EMA, as evidenced by no difference between recordings on the first versus second 2 weeks; and most participants self-reported that they missed few recordings of eating disorder behaviors. The EDE was administered immediately after the 28-day EMA. Using a Wilcoxon signed ranks test, OBEs were significantly higher for the EDE (*M* = 14.23, *SD* = 18.77) than for the EMA (*M* = 7.62,

$SD = 11.51$), $p = .023$. There were no differences in specific purging behaviors between the two methods, although the sum of all bingeing and purging behaviors was significantly different between the two methods, $p = .012$. Stein and Corte (2003) argued that even though the EDE interviewer provided detailed information defining an OBE, the lack of information available in participants' memories may result in an overestimation of episode frequency.

Predictive Validity. Beumont et al. (1993) assessed 116 patients seeking treatment for an eating disorder (AN = 50, BN = 28, and EDNOS = 38). Those with AN and EDNOS reported significantly fewer OBEs, OBDs, SBEs, and SBDs than the BN group ($p < .05$), but the statistic used for this test was not indicated. A review of the means provided in their table suggested that all differences between the BN group and the other two groups were at least medium in effect size ($d > .5$). However, the means reported by Beumont et al. appear to be too small for a 28-day period of assessment (e.g., mean OBEs for the BN group was 4.2 [$SD = 1.9$]).

Wilfley et al. (1997) reported on differences between 105 women with BED, 53 women with BN, 47 women with AN (subtypes were not indicated), 42 normal-weight non-eating-disordered women, and 15 obese (BMI > 30) nonbinge eaters. Table 10.7 reproduces the results regarding OBEs and vomiting episodes per month. The authors reported that the BN group had significantly more vomiting episodes per month than the AN group and that the BN and AN groups had more vomiting episodes than the BED group. The normal-weight and the obese comparison groups reported no vomiting episodes. The BN group reported the greatest number of OBEs, which were significantly higher than for the BED group, which had significantly more OBEs than the AN group. The normal-weight and obese comparisons reported no OBEs. Although these data represent the largest and most comprehensive samples to test OBEs and vomiting episodes measured by the EDE, aspects of the statistical analyses were problematic or incomplete. First, ANOVA was used when some of the data were likely nonnormally distributed (e.g., OBEs for BN) or had no distribution (e.g., OBEs and vomiting for the comparison samples). Second, overall F tests were reported, but no follow-up multiple comparison tests, such as Tukey's HSD, were reported so it is unclear how the between-group differences were analyzed. Third, effect sizes were not reported, and some differences appear to be small (e.g., for BED vs. BN on OBEs, $d = .35$).

Table 10.7   Comparison of Objective Binge Episodes (OBEs) and Vomiting Episodes in the Past 28 Days Measured by the Eating Disorder Examination

Subscale	BED (n = 105)	AN (n = 47)	BN (n = 53)	Controls (n = 42)	Obese (n = 15)
	M (SD)	M (SD)	M (SD)	M (SD)	M (SD)
Age	45.5 (10.1)[c]	25.5 (4.9)[a]	22.1 (4.9)[ab]	21.3 (6.9)[ab]	27.2 (4.1)[b]
OBEs	20.1 (11.1)[c]	10.4 (23.6)[b]	26.5 (27.8)[d]	0[a]	0[a]
Vomiting	0.04 (0.3)[a]	18 (40.8)[b]	30.8 (35.5)[c]	0[a]	0[a]

SOURCE: Data are from Wilfley et al. (1997).

NOTE: Different superscripts within each scale denote significant differences between groups at $p < .01$. BED = binge eating disordered; AN = anorexia nervosa; BN = bulimia nervosa; Controls = normal-weight controls; Obese = obese controls.

Sensitivity to Change

The EDE has been used in a number of randomized controlled trials to assess for OBEs and purging behaviors (e.g., Wilfley et al., 1993; Wilfley et al., 2002; Wilson, Fairburn, Agras, Walsh, & Kraemer, 2002). In two trials, Wilfley and her colleagues showed the EDE measurement of OBEs to be sensitive to measuring change in objective days binged following group treatment for BED. In the Wilfley et al. (1993) trial, the two treatment conditions showed significant reductions in days binged compared to the no-treatment control group, which showed no differences pre- to posttreatment. Similarly, Wilson et al. (2002) showed significant positive change in both vomiting episodes and OBEs during and following 20 weeks of individual treatment for 154 individuals with BN.

Norms

No formal norms are available for clinical or community samples for behavioral assessment of binge eating or purging using the EDE. The data available in Table 10.7 are taken from Wilfley et al. (1997) and represent the most comprehensive and largest samples of eating-disordered women on measures of OBEs and of vomiting. Wilfley et al. provide demographic data only for the 105 women with BED in their sample. The BED sample mean BMI was 37.0 ($SD = 5.5$); they had an average of 15.6 years of education ($SD = 2.3$) and reported an average household income of U.S.$55,000 ($SD = $23,000). The ethnic distribution of the sample was White = 93%, African American = 4%, Hispanic = 2%, and Native American = 1%. All patient participants met *DSM* criteria for BED, BN, or AN (subtypes were not indicated). Normal-weight controls were randomly drawn from a general practice register in Cambridge, England, and the obese control group was taken from a sample reported by Fairburn and Cooper (1993).

Availability

A new interview protocol for the 16th edition of the EDE is available in the book by Fairburn (2008). Training for interrater reliability may be available by contacting Christopher Fairburn at Oxford University, credo@medsci.ox.ac.uk. As indicated, some researchers have relied on the author of the EDE for training and for assessment of interrater reliability.

Interview for the Diagnosis of Eating Disorders–IV (IDED-IV)

Description

The Interview for the Diagnosis of Eating Disorders–IV (IDED-IV; Kutlesic, Williamson, Gleaves, Barbin, & Murphy-Eberenz, 1998; Williamson, 1990; Williamson, Anderson, & Gleaves, 1996) is a semistructured interview that was developed for the purpose of differential diagnosis using *DSM-IV* (APA, 1994) criteria, including BED and subthreshold diagnoses that fall in the EDNOS category. The measure has undergone two revisions, IDED-R and IDED-III, and it was revised a fourth time to reflect changes in *DSM-IV* for diagnosing eating disorders. Symptom ratings are directly related to *DSM-IV* diagnostic criteria, and questions are designed to allow the interviewer to assess the presence or absence of specific symptoms. The interview begins by requesting basic demographic information and then assessing eating disorder and psychiatric history, current eating pattern, and family information. This is followed by three subscales (Anorexia Nervosa, Bulimia Nervosa, and Binge Eating Disorder) that systematically assess for specific eating disorder symptoms. The interviewer rates 20 symptoms (per *DSM-IV*) on a 5-point Likert-type scale reflecting the presence of a criterion and its severity. A rating of 3 or higher indicates the presence of a diagnostic symptom, and the level of the rating indicates severity. Severity is determined by adding symptom ratings within a particular subscale. The results are used to complete a diagnostic checklist and construct a decision tree, which leads directly to differential diagnosis. Participants are diagnosed with AN, BN, or BED when all ratings within a subscale are rated with a score of 3 or higher (Kutlesic et al., 1998).

The interview could be useful for research that requires rigorous diagnostic assessment and for clinical practice (Kutlesic et al., 1998). The interview is limited in that it does not include specific definitions of binge eating or specific assessment of weight concerns. A one-page instruction sheet accompanies the interview, but the scoring instructions could be improved to be more user-friendly. In addition, given that the primary goal of the interview is differential diagnosis, it does not focus on obtaining frequency and severity information, which could be better captured by using the EDE (Grilo et al., 2005).

The interview is straightforward. Based on these preliminary findings, the interview appears to be reliable and valid when used for differential diagnosis of eating disorders, including BN and BED. However, further research is needed to compare the IDED with other widely used interviews for assessing eating disorders.

Reliability

Internal Consistency. Kutlesic et al. (1998) assessed internal consistency in a sample of treatment-seeking participants ($n = 96$; $M_{age} = 33.7$ years, $SD = 14.3$; 88.5% White, 11.5% African American; 92.3% middle to upper class) and community controls ($n = 80$; $M_{age} = 30.7$ years, $SD = 15.2$; 71.2% White, 20% African American; 70% were middle to upper class), comprising 162 women and 14 men. Cronbach's alpha was moderate to high for each of the subscales of the interview: .75 for the Anorexia Nervosa subscale, .96 for the Binge Eating Disorder subscale, and .75 for the Bulimia Nervosa subscale (Kutlesic et al., 1998). Item-total correlations were calculated to evaluate the

strength of the relationship between each rating and each subscale's total score. Item-total correlations were found to be high to very high (.83–.94) for the Binge Eating Disorder subscale and moderate to high (.50–.76) for the Bulimia subscale.

Interrater Reliability. In Kutlesic et al. (1998), a subsample (47%, $n = 82$) of participants from the larger validation sample ($N = 176$) agreed to have their interviews audiotaped for the purpose of assessing interrater reliability. Interviewers were eight predoctoral graduate students in clinical psychology and three postdoctoral clinical researchers, each with 2 to 4 years of experience working with eating disorders. The second rater was blind to the results of the first diagnostic interview. A kappa coefficient was calculated on the basis of diagnostic agreement between evaluators for 17 possible diagnoses. The kappa coefficient demonstrated excellent interrater reliability (diagnostic agreement for all diagnoses was .86). Kappa coefficients for the individual diagnostic categories were very high, 1.00 for AN, .87 for BED, .88 for obese controls, and .91 for normal-weight controls, with the exception of BN, which was adequate (.64). ICCs, kappas (for the presence of a symptom), and exact percent agreement for severity of symptoms were calculated for individual symptom ratings for each of the subscales. On the BED subscale, kappas were high (.73–.95), percent agreement was good (70.3–85.3), and ICCs were high (.82–.93). On the Bulimia subscale, kappas were moderate to high (.64–.95), percent agreement was moderate to high (59.2–93.8), and ICCs were moderate to high (.70–.93). Thus, it appears that these scales may be more reliable as diagnostic measures than as measures of symptom severity (Kutlesic et al., 1998).

Construct Validity

Content Validity. Content validity was assessed by a panel of 10 experts (with experience in eating disorders) who reviewed the content of the IDED-IV and responded to 12 questions using rating scales (range from 1 = *do not agree* to 7 = *strongly* agree). These 12 questions asked about the expert's agreement with statements about the stated purpose of the measure, clarity of instructions, and specificity of questions pertaining to *DSM-IV* (APA, 1994) criteria. The ratings were high for each feature of the IDED-IV that was evaluated (Kutlesic et al., 1998), indicating good content validity of the measure. The mean average expert rating for the 12 questions for characteristics of the Bulimia scale and the Binge Eating Disorder scale ranged from 6.2 to 6.7 (*SD* range .53–.84).

Criterion Validity

Concurrent Validity. Concurrent validity was evaluated by examining Pearson product moment correlations between the IDED-IV subscale scores and self-report measures of related and unrelated constructs in the validation sample described above (*N* = 176; Kutlesic et al., 1998). For the Bulimia subscale, significant positive Pearson correlations (*p* < .001) were found for the EAT (Garner & Garfinkel, 1979) Dieting scale (.60); the BULIT-R Binge Eating (.68), Radical Weight Loss (.76), Vomiting (.68), Laxative Abuse (.44), and Exercise (.30) subscales; the EDI-II Drive for Thinness (.45) and Body Dissatisfaction (.29) subscales; and the Body Image Assessment (BIA; Williamson, Davis, Bennett, Goreczny, & Gleaves, 1989) Current Body Size subscale (.39). The Binge Eating Disorder subscale was significantly negatively correlated with the EAT Oral Control scale (−.31) and positively correlated with the BULIT-R Binge Eating (.88), Radical Weight Loss (.53), and Vomiting (.47) subscales; the EAT-II Drive for Thinness (.31) and Body Dissatisfaction (.42) scales; and the BIA Current Body Size (.51) subscale.

Norms

This is not applicable.

Availability

For a copy of the interview and instructions, please contact Vesna Kutlesic, University of New Mexico Health Sciences Center, Children's Psychiatric Hospital, 1001 Yale Boulevard, NE, Albuquerque, NM 87131; e-mail: Kutlesicv@od.nih.gov. The interview protocol is reproduced in the appendix to Chapter 11 in this handbook.

The Mini International Neuropsychiatric Interview

Description

Both versions of the Mini International Neuropsychiatric Interview (MINI and the MINI Plus; Sheehan et al., 2003) are semistructured diagnostic interviews for individuals older than 16 years of age. These interviews yield current and lifetime diagnoses of the major Axis I psychiatric disorders in the *DSM-IV* and *ICD-10* (World Health Organization [WHO], 2007), as well as antisocial personality disorder. Like the SCID, the MINI/MINI Plus is not an eating disorder–specific measure and therefore cannot be considered a measure of binge eating or purging. However, it allows the interviewer to assess BN and AN, as well as its subtypes using the MINI Plus. Much like the SCID (First et al., 1995), the MINI is divided into modules for each disorder, and the interviewer is prompted to advance to the next module if patients fail to meet the basic level of symptomatology required to meet diagnostic criteria.

The focus of the MINI is primarily on assessing current psychopathology. The MINI Plus is a lengthier (45–60 minutes), more comprehensive version of the MINI that assesses both current and lifetime presence of most Axis I disorders. A major advantage of the MINI is the ease and speed of administration compared to that of other, longer clinical interviews, such as the SCID (Summerfeldt & Antony, 2002). The MINI takes approximately 15 minutes to administer, and limited training is required to administer the interview.

The MINI is a relatively new diagnostic interview and has not been widely used in North America. It is an internationally recognized interview and has been translated into 43 different languages. Versions of the MINI include the MINI-Kid for use with children and youth under the age of 17 and the MINI Screen, a 5-minute brief diagnostic screen. A patient-rated version of the MINI is also available, but it is not reviewed here.

Like the SCID (First et al., 1995), the MINI interviews measure binge-eating and purging behaviors indirectly through their assessment of AN and BN. Although the MINI and MINI Plus are relatively new diagnostic interviews, the psychometric data are promising. Research by an independent set of researchers would be important to further assess the reliability and validity of this interview with other samples.

Reliability

Stability. Sheehan and colleagues (1997) found kappa values for AN and BN to be .78 and 1.0, respectively, over a 1- to 2-day period (Sheehan et al., 1997). The majority of the reported kappa coefficients for other diagnoses were 0.75 or greater, indicating good test-retest reliability.

Interrater Reliability. In Lecrubier et al. (1997), 346 patients (with a variety of Axis I disorders) and nonpatients (no previous psychiatric disorders) from France and the United States were recruited for a reliability study comparing the MINI to the Composite International Diagnostic Interview (CIDI; World Health Organization [WHO], 1990). Interrater reliability for a subset of 42 patients was very high, with kappa coefficients ranging from .88 to 1.0. In the second validation study with 370 patients and nonpatients (40 of whom also participated in Lecrubier et al., 1997), Sheehan et al. (1997) also found excellent interrater reliability, with the majority of the reported kappa coefficients for Axis I disorders falling at 0.90 or higher. Kappas for AN and BN were both 1.0.

Construct Validity

Content Validity. Sensitivity was 0.70 or greater, and specificities, negative predictive values, and

efficiency scores were 0.85 or greater across all of the diagnoses (Sheehan et al., 1998). More recent research has also demonstrated good and very good sensitivity and specificity, respectively, in a Hungarian version of the MINI (Balazs & Bitter, 2000; article only available in Hungarian).

Criterion Validity

Concurrent Validity. Lecrubier et al. (1997) examined concordance between the MINI and the CIDI. They found kappa coefficients were good to very good for all diagnoses with the exception of BN (kappa = .53), social phobia (kappa = .54), simple phobia (kappa = .43), agoraphobia (kappa = .58), and generalized anxiety disorder (GAD; kappa = .36). These authors could not examine AN due to low prevalence within the sample.

Sheehan and colleagues (1997) examined concordance between the MINI and the SCID-P. They found kappa coefficients for AN and BN (lifetime) to be very high, .90, and high, .78, respectively. However, they suggested cautious interpretation of these values given that fewer than 5% of patients met SCID patient version (SCID-P) criteria for one of these eating disorders.

Norms

This is not applicable.

Availability

A complimentary copy of the MINI, the MINI-Plus, or the MINI-Kid may be obtained by contacting Dr. David V. Sheehan at the Institute for Research in Psychiatry, University of South Florida College of Medicine, 3515 East Fletcher Avenue, Tampa, FL 33613, or by accessing the Web site: www.medical-outcomes.com. Individuals may register for a free account online and have access to updated versions of the MINI. Electronic versions of the MINI are now also available at a cost.

Structured Clinical Interview for *DSM-IV* Axis I Disorders

Description

The patient version of the Structured Clinical Interview for *DSM-IV* Axis I Disorders (SCID for *DSM-IV*; First et al., 1995) is a clinician-administered, semistructured diagnostic interview that assesses frequently diagnosed Axis I *DSM-IV* disorders in adults; these include eating disorders BN and AN. Although the SCID prompts the interviewer to inquire about binge eating and purging, it cannot be considered a measure of these constructs. The SCID, however, does allow for the differentiation between subtypes of eating disorders, such as AN-restricting and binge/purge types, whereas the previous SCID for *DSM-III-R* did not include these specifiers. In the previous version, patients who met criteria for AN but who also binged and/or purged at least twice per month were given an additional diagnosis of BN.

The SCID is considered the gold standard of diagnostic interviews and is likely the most widely used diagnostic interview in North American research (Summerfeldt & Antony, 2002). It is composed of self-contained modules for each disorder, with each module listing all criteria required to meet a diagnosis. Interviewers are prompted to review essential criteria with patients, and then interviewers are instructed to proceed to the next item only if the patient endorses some level of symptomatology (a rating of subthreshold or threshold) on the essential criteria.

The SCID for *DSM-IV* is available in two versions: the SCID-CV (clinician version) (First, Spitzer, Gibbon, & Williams, 2002), which is the briefer of the two versions, and the SCID-I (research version; First et al., 1995). Whereas the research version is much longer and allows the interviewer to obtain information on a greater number of disorders and their subtypes, the clinician version is most practical for use in clinical settings and includes assessment of disorders most typically seen in these settings (Summerfeldt &

Antony, 2002). In addition, the research version contains assessment criteria for BED as an appendix category. The SCID-I is available in three standard versions—namely, the SCID-I/P (for identified patients), the SCID-I/P with Psychotic Screen (for those patients where there is unlikely to be a diagnosis of psychotic disorder and screening is sufficient), and the SCID-I/NP (nonpatient version).

The majority of psychometric information available on the SCID exists for the previous version, the SCID for *DSM-III-R*. PsychINFO and MEDLINE searches retrieved few psychometric studies for the SCID for *DSM-IV*.

Although the SCID is not an eating disorder–specific interview, solid psychometric data for the measure as a whole would suggest that one may reliably and validly assess for the presence of eating disorders, which indirectly assesses for the presence of binge-eating and purging behaviors.

Reliability

Stability. J. B. W. Williams et al. (1992) demonstrated test-retest reliability for the SCID-III-R with a sample of 592 individuals in four patient and nonpatient sites in the United States and Germany. One to 3-week test-retest reliabilities (kappas) for the majority of the diagnoses, current and lifetime, were above .60 for the patient subgroup. The overall weighed kappas were .61 and .68 for current and lifetime diagnoses, respectively. For eating disorders, however, there was very good agreement, with current and lifetime kappas for the total sample of .72 and .84, respectively, for AN, and .86 and .87, respectively, for BN.

In examining the SCID for *DSM-III-R*, Zanarini and Frankenburg (2001) reported 7- to 10-day, 2-year follow-up, and 4-year follow-up interval test-retest kappas. A test-retest kappa of .84 was found for EDNOS, but test-retest data were not available for diagnoses of BN and AN. Zanarini et al. (2000) found a good 7- to 10-day test-retest kappa coefficient of .64 ($n = 15$) for "any eating disorder," with kappa coefficients for other Axis I disorders ranging from .35 to .78.

Interrater Reliability. In general, few studies have examined interrater reliability for the eating disorder module of the SCID; even fewer have used the SCID for *DSM-IV* to do so. Among the few who examined interrater reliability for eating disorder categories, Zanarini et al. (2000) found an excellent kappa coefficient of .77 for any eating disorder (*n* = 5) and kappas ranging from .57 to 1.0 for other Axis I disorders. Zanarini and Frankenburg (2001) found a good baseline interrater reliability for BN using SCID for *DSM-III-R* (kappa = .73). Kurth, Krahn, Nairn, and Drewnowski (1995) found an excellent kappa score of .91 (using the nonpatient version of the SCID) for agreement on eating disorder diagnoses, including AN, BN, and EDNOS, when they reviewed 10% of their female college sample of 306 students.

Criterion Validity

Concurrent Validity. In comparing the SCID for *DSM-III-R* and *DSM-IV,* Sunday et al. (2001) found 79% agreement for diagnoses of AN, with kappa being poor (.485). In fact, less than 50% of the individuals who were diagnosed with AN-binge/purge type using *DSM-IV* were diagnosed with AN and BN using *DSM-III-R.* There was 100% agreement between versions of the SCID for diagnoses of BN, and all other Axis I disorders except alcohol abuse/dependence and substance abuse/dependence. In a study of obese women with BED, Freitas and colleagues (2006) found evidence for concurrent validity between the Portuguese version of the SCID for *DSM-IV* and the BES (Freitas et al., 2006). The SCID-Patient version identified 51.69% of the obese sample as having BED. Sensitivity, specificity, positive predictive values, and negative predictive values were 97.8%, 47.7%, 66.7%, and 95.3%, respectively.

Norms

This is not applicable.

Availability

The SCID for *DSM-IV* is readily available and must be purchased through the authors: SCID Orders, Biometrics Research Department/ Columbia University, 1051 Riverside Drive, Unit 60, New York, NY 10032; fax: (212) 543-5525. Training tapes may be ordered online, and additional information on the SCID is also available on the Web site: http://www.scid4.org/.

Structured Interview for Anorexic and Bulimic Syndromes

Description

The Structured Interview for Anorexic and Bulimic Syndromes (SIAB-EX) was first developed in 1991 by Fichter and colleagues, and since then, it has undergone several revisions. The current version of the SIAB-EX (Fichter, Herpertz, Quadflieg, & Herpertz-Dahlmann, 1998) produces data and diagnoses consistent with both *DSM-IV* and *ICD-10* classification systems. It was developed as a semistandardized interview for reliable and valid assessment of specific and general psychopathology of eating disorders (e.g., depression, phobias, anxieties, compulsions, sexual problems, social functioning) and for the assessment of familial interaction and pathology in eating disorders. Three of six of the SIAB-EX subscales specifically relate to assessing bingeing and purging behavior: Bulimic Symptoms; Inappropriate Compensatory Behaviors to Counteract Weight Gain, Fasting and Substance Abuse (Compensatory behavior); and Atypical Binges. The Atypical Binges subscale is new, and the authors consider this scale experimental until further validity is established (Fichter & Quadflieg, 2001). The SIAB-EX assesses present (in the past 3 months) and lifetime/past symptom expression and supplies present and past lifetime *DSM-IV* and *ICD-10* diagnoses.

The current version consists of 87 items, 67 of which assess severity or duration of eating disorder symptoms on a 5-point scale from 0 (no symptoms) to 4 (very severe symptom expression). The interview provides general probes for each item to determine if the item applies to the respondent. Operational criteria and examples are given in the manual for each rating code of any item. A rating code of 2, 3, or 4 of the item is counted toward meeting the criterion or part of the criterion for a diagnosis. The SIAB-EX assesses specific criteria for BN diagnoses and binges (adhering closely to *DSM-IV*), and it can be used (following a computer algorithm) to produce a BED diagnosis (Peterson & Miller, 2005). Length of the interview is between 30 and 60 minutes, depending on the need for exploration of responses. The interview is increasingly used in clinical trials (Keel et al., 2004; Shroff et al., 2006). The SIAB-EX is available in English, German, and Spanish.

The SIAB-EX covers a wide scope of symptoms that commonly occur alongside eating disorder diagnoses that are not assessed with most other interview measures. It is useful for diagnostic categorization of eating disorders. Intensive training is required by the user (with video and supervision) until an acceptable standard of interrater reliability is achieved. To assist the user, a 90-page manual is available with case examples. A computer algorithm for the diagnoses and sum scores is available from the authors.

Reliability

Internal Consistency. Fichter et al. (1998) assessed internal consistency of the entire scale in a clinical sample of 330 eating disorder patients (9 men, 321 women; M_{age} = 28.0 years, SD = 8.3; M_{BMI} = 24.0 kg/m^2, SD = 11.2) diagnosed with AN, BN, BED, or EDNOS. In addition, a sample of 148 treated AN patients (M_{age} = 26.2 years, SD = 6.8; M_{BMI} = 19.1 kg/m^2, SD = 3.0), a sample of 185 treated BN patients (M_{age} = 32 years, no SD reported; M_{BMI} = 22.3 kg/m^2, no SD reported), and a sample of 111 female community controls (M_{age} = 20.9 years, SD = 3.2; M_{BMI} = 20.3 kg/m^2, SD = 2.4) were also assessed. Cronbach's alpha for past/lifetime SIAB-EX version ranged between .64 and .89, and for the SIAB-EX current version, coefficient alphas ranged from .43 to .91. Specifically, Cronbach's alpha for past/lifetime symptoms was very good (.89) for the Bulimic Symptoms subscale, was low (.64) for Compensatory Behaviors, and was good (.82) for Atypical Binges. For the present symptoms, coefficient alpha was high for Bulimic Symptoms (.91), was poor for Compensatory Behaviors (.43), and was good for Atypical Binges (.80).

Interrater Reliability. Fichter and Quadflieg (2001) assessed interrater reliability with a sample of eating disorder inpatients (n = 31; demographic data not provided) whose interviews were recorded on videotape. Seven trained raters rated the tapes (up to two times), for a total of 116 complete interview ratings. Raters were blind to the previous findings. All interviewers were clinical psychologists who were trained in the use of the SIAB-EX. Kappa coefficients were calculated for each pair of interviews. Mean unweighted kappa values were .64 (current) and .63 (past) for the 5-point scales. Dichotomizing the ratings into 0 (score 0 = no symptoms or subthreshold symptoms) or 1 (ratings 2, 3, and 4 = clinically significant) resulted in mean kappa values of .81 (current) and .85 (past), demonstrating good interrater reliability. Fichter et al. (1998) also assessed interrater reliability on a subsample of 15 eating disorder patients, using an unadjusted intraclass correlation coefficient. For past/lifetime symptoms, rater agreement was high for the Bulimic Symptoms scale (M = .90, SD = .13) and Compensatory Behaviors scale (M = .88, SD = .09). For current symptoms, agreement was also high for the Bulimic Symptoms scale (M = .89, SD = .14) and Compensatory Behaviors scale (M = .96, SD = .05). Rater agreement was not assessed for the Atypical Binges scale.

Validity

Construct Validity. Fichter et al. (1998) conducted a PCA with varimax rotation on 61 of the 87 items using data from 346 eating-disordered patients and 111 community controls (described above). Most items excluded from the PCA were items with dichotomous ratings, yielding yes or no responses for the subclassification of eating disorders. The number of components was derived using an Eigenwert criterion > 1. A criterion of .4 was adopted as the cutoff for items loading on each component. For the items related to lifetime data, 16 components met the Eigenwert criterion and accounted for 64.2% of the total variance. The rotation of a forced solution with six components accounted for 42.8% of the variance. This approach was taken because it "produced the most meaningful pattern of item allocation to components" (Fichter et al., 1998, p.231). The components or subscales were as follows: (I) Body Image and Slimness Ideal; (II) General Psychopathology; (III) Sexuality and Social Integration; (IV) Bulimic Symptoms; (V) Measures to Counteract Weight Gain, Fasting, and Substance Abuse; and (VI) Atypical Binges. The first three components together accounted for 31.0% of the total variance. In the PCA for the current version (symptom expression at the time of assessment), 17 components fulfilled the Eigenwert criterion (> 1.0) and accounted for 64.4% of the total variance. A forced six-component solution was rotated (to keep factor structure similar to the lifetime data), which accounted for 40.5% of the total variance, with the first three components contributing to 29.2%. Factors I, IV, V, and VI remained the same, but the remaining two components were termed (II) General Psychopathology and Social Integration and (III) Sexuality.

Criterion Validity

Concurrent Validity. Fichter and Quadflieg (2001) compared the SIAB-EX to the EDE with a sample of 80 eating disorder inpatients diagnosed with AN, BN, BED, and EDNOS (77 women, 3 men;

$M_{age} = 28.8$ years, $SD = 9.5$; $M_{BMI} = 22.8$ kg/m^2, $SD = 11.0$). The authors found a high degree of agreement between the total scores of the two measures using Pearson's product moment correlation coefficient, $r = .77$; $p < .01$. The SIAB-EX Bulimic Symptoms scale was significantly moderately to highly correlated ($r = .28–.61$, $p < .05$) with all subscales of the EDE. The Compensatory Behaviors Scale was also significantly moderately to highly correlated with all scales of the EDE ($r = .35–.69$, $p < .05$). The Atypical Binges scale was moderately correlated to the EDE Eating Concerns scale ($r = .31$, $p < .01$).

Using a clinical sample of 377 treatment-seeking eating disorder inpatients (366 women, 11 men; $M_{age} = 29.1$ years, $SD = 9.3$; $M_{BMI} = 25.7$ kg/m^2, $SD = 11.7$) diagnosed with AN or BN, Fichter and Quadflieg (2001) assessed concurrent validity of the SIAB-EX with self-report measures EDI-2 (Garner, 1991) and the Three Factor Eating Questionnaire (TFEQ; Stunkard & Messick, 1985). The Bulimic Symptoms subscale correlated highly with the EDI-2 Bulimia and TFEQ Disinhibition scales ($r = .65$ and $r = .51$, respectively, $p < .01$). The Compensatory Behaviors subscale was moderately correlated with the EDI Drive for Thinness scale and the TFEQ Cognitive Control subscale ($r = .36$ and $r = .41$, respectively, $p < .01$). For a complete list of correlations, see Fichter and Quadflieg (2001). Overall, this evidence for concurrent validity is good.

Discriminant Validity. Fichter and Quadflieg (2001) also reported on evidence for the discriminant validity of the SIAB-EX. The Atypical Binges scale showed low and nonsignificant correlations with most EDE scales ($r = -.05$ to $.20$, $p > .05$; an exception is the Eating Concerns scale, see above), indicating very little overlap among these measures. As reported above, Fichter and Quadflieg administered the TFEQ to a clinical sample of 377 treatment-seeking eating disorder inpatients. With the same sample, Fichter and Quadflieg administered the Symptom Checklist 90 (SCL-90; Derogatis, Rickels, & Rock, 1976), the Beck Depression Inventory (BDI; Beck, Ward, Mendelson, Mock, &

Erbaugh, 1961), and the PERI Demoralization scale (PDS; Dohrenwend, Shrout, Egri, & Mendelsohn, 1980). The SIAB-EX Bulimic Symptoms had a low and nonsignificant correlation with the TFEQ Cognitive Control scale ($r = .07; p > .05$). The SIAB-EX Bulimic Symptoms, Compensatory Behaviors, and Atypical Binges scales had small correlations with the SCL-90 subscales ($r = .01–.14$). Some correlations between Bulimic Symptoms and Compensatory Behaviors with the BDI and the PDS were significant, but all were small in size ($r < .25$) except for the correlation between the BDI and Compensatory Behaviors ($r = .37, p < .01$). Overall, this evidence for the discriminant validity of these three SIAB-EX scales is good.

Norms

There are no published norms for the SIAB-EX, but the validation studies provide good comparison data. Fichter et al. (1998) provided means and standard deviations for individual items and subscales of their validation sample. Means and standard deviations are presented in Table 10.8 for *current* symptom expression for the total patient group, AN, BN, and controls for the Bulimic Symptoms, Compensatory Behaviors, and Atypical Binges subscales and individual items. For a complete table with norms for the follow-up AN and BN samples, please see the paper by Fichter et al. (1998).

Availability

Please contact the original author for information on obtaining a copy of the interview, Manfred M. Fichter, MD, Klinic Roseneck, affiliated with the University of Munich, Am Roseneck 6, D-83209 Prien, Germany; e-mail: MFichter@t-online.de. A German version has appeared in print; see Fichter and Quadflieg (1999).

Summary and Conclusions

In this chapter, we reviewed the assessment of binge eating and purging by self-report and by structured interview. Binge eating is a complex behavior to assess because of judgments required about what constitutes a large amount of food and how to define loss of control. There is a consensus that both are required to define a binge (Fairburn & Wilson, 1993). Assessment of binge eating by self-report is potentially problematic if OBEs are not defined explicitly and if examples are not provided to those being assessed. Some efforts by researchers, notably with the addition of instructions to the EDE-QI (Goldfein et al., 2005), address this potential shortcoming. Certainly, assessment of binge eating by trained interviewers who explicitly define a binge may yield more valid evaluations.

Both self-report and interview formats are limited by the participants' ability to accurately define and recall incidences of binge eating. This is potentially problematic since the *DSM-IV* (APA, 1994) requires a 6-month history of binge eating at least 2 days a week for a diagnosis of BED or a 3-month history of binge eating two times per week for a diagnosis of BN. The EDE (Fairburn & Cooper, 1993) asks about binge eating in the past 28 days, but even then, obtaining an accurate number may be limited by difficulties encountered by human memory systems when remembering complex affect-laden details (Friedman & deWinstanley, 1998). This may be especially problematic for research protocols where the exact number of OBEs or days binged is required. The use of EMAs (Stein & Corte, 2003) may represent an alternative to evaluating the validity of self-report or interview assessments of binge eating.

The assessment of purging behaviors tends to be more straightforward as the behaviors are not as complexly defined as in the case of binge eating. Purging by vomiting, for example, typically punctuates a binge-purge episode for someone with BN, and so the behavior is likely more easily or accurately recalled.

There were a number of statistical and methodological problems and inconsistencies encountered in the review of this literature. First, many studies did not report psychometric properties of scales

Table 10.8   SIAB-EX Average Mean Scores and Standard Deviations for the Current Symptom Expression

	Total Patient (n = 330)	AN[a] (n = 53)	BN[a] (n = 97)	Controls (n = 111)
	M (SD)	M (SD)	M (SD)	M (SD)
Bulimic symptoms				
Total scale	2.1 (1.1)	1.9 (1.3)	3.1 (0.5)	NA
Frequency of binge	2.0 (1.6)	1.6 (1.7)	3.4 (0.8)	NA
Bingeing (objective)	2.1 (1.6)	1.8 (1.8)	3.3 (0.7)	0.7 (0.8)
Bingeing (subjective)	2.3 (1.6)	1.8 (1.8)	3.5 (0.7)	NA
Loss of control	1.8 (1.3)	1.5 (1.3)	2.8 (0.7)	NA
Bingeing and distress	1.8 (1.5)	1.3 (1.5)	2.7 (1.1)	NA
Induced vomiting	1.7 (1.8)	1.5 (1.8)	3.0 (1.4)	0.1 (0.3)
Craving for food	2.0 (1.4)	1.9 (1.5)	2.6 (1.3)	NA
Global evaluation symptoms	3.4 (0.7)	3.7 (0.5)	3.6 (0.5)	0.1 (0.2)
Course of binge eating	NA	NA	NA	NA
Compensatory behaviors				
Total scale	0.4 (0.4)	0.5 (0.4)	0.6 (0.5)	NA
Appetite suppressants	0.1 (0.6)	0.0 (0.0)	0.3 (1.0)	NA
Excessive fasting	0.3 (0.8)	0.04 (0.3)	0.5 (1.1)	NA
Laxative abuse	0.5 (1.2)	0.6 (1.4)	0.9 (1.4)	0.2 (0.5)
Abuse of illegal drugs	0.04 (0.3)	0.0 (0.0)	0.1 (0.5)	NA
Autoaggressive behavior	0.2 (0.7)	0.3 (0.8)	0.3 (0.8)	NA
Abuse of diuretics	0.1 (0.4)	0.0 (0.0)	0.2 (0.6)	NA
Quantitative reduction food	1.7 (1.6)	2.9 (1.3)	1.8 (1.6)	0.5 (0.7)
Alcohol abuse	0.7 (0.7)	0.6 (0.7)	0.7 (0.7)	0.2 (0.5)
Abuse of thyroid medication	0.02 (0.1)	0.0 (0.0)	0.03 (0.2)	NA
Enemas	NA	NA	NA	NA
Ipecac abuse	NA	NA	NA	NA
Atypical binges				
Total scale	0.5 (0.9)	0.3 (0.7)	0.4 (0.7)	NA
Atypical binges	0.6 (1.2)	0.3 (0.8)	0.5 (1.1)	NA

	Total Patient (n = 330)	AN[a] (n = 53)	BN[a] (n = 97)	Controls (n = 111)
	M (SD)	M (SD)	M (SD)	M (SD)
Frequency of atypical binges	0.6 (1.2)	0.3 (0.8)	0.4 (1.0)	NA
Stress-induced eating	0.7 (1.4)	0.4 (1.1)	0.7 (1.3)	NA
Feeling uncomfortably full	0.2 (0.7)	0.2 (0.9)	0.1 (0.3)	NA

NOTE: AN = anorexia nervosa; BN = bulimia nervosa; NA = item not assessed.

a. Subsample of total patient group. Data are from Fichter, Herpertz, Quadflieg, and Herpertz-Dahlmann (1998).

used within their study sample. Typically, for example, simple measures of internal consistency (i.e., coefficient alpha and mean interitem correlation) were not reported. Researchers should not assume that a scale, especially when used with a population for which it was not originally validated, will retain its psychometric properties. Second, a number of research papers did not report means, standard deviations, and correlations among dependent variables. This was especially evident among early studies of the EDE-Q. Often, we resorted to cobbling together a table of "normative" data from a variety of sources as a result of this practice. This may be frustrating for a clinician who may be looking for an adequate comparison group for some indication of the meaning of a scale score. Third, a number of studies inappropriately used parametric tests for count/rank data or low-frequency data. Researchers are encouraged to assess for assumptions such as normality of distributions and to use nonparametric tests when appropriate. This was particularly problematic for studies in which the number of vomiting episodes, a low-frequency event in some samples, was the dependent variable. Fourth, with the exception of some research on the EDI, there was a paucity of research using CFA for scales that were originally constructed by exploratory methods. A CFA approach can be an important step to continue to evaluate the construct validity of scales. Fifth, effect sizes

(e.g., Cohen's d, r, partial eta-squared) were seldom reported in studies that compared samples or in studies that assessed change. The reporting of effect sizes is essential to evaluate the potential clinical meaningfulness of a statistically significant finding (Wilkinson & The Task Force on Statistical Inference, 1999).

Whether to use self-report or interview approaches is a decision often faced by researcher and clinician alike. In some respects, interview formats, such as the EDE or the SCID, may be more accurate, but they are time-consuming and labor intensive, require some training, and require an assessment of interrater reliability. In some contexts, interview formats can be impractical. Self-report methods are certainly easier to administer and provide the interviewee with the possibility of anonymity, and many questionnaires have adequate psychometric merits. Researchers and clinicians are encouraged to consider their requirements, as well as the needs of participants or patients, and to evaluate carefully the evidence for an assessment tool's psychometric strengths when choosing which approach to adopt in the research lab or the clinic.

References

American Psychiatric Association. (1980). *Diagnostic and statistical manual of mental disorders* (3rd ed.). Washington, DC: Author.

American Psychiatric Association. (1994). *Diagnostic and statistical manual of mental disorders* (4th ed.). Washington, DC: Author.

Anderson, D. A., Williamson, D. A., Duchmann, E. G., Gleaves, D. H., & Barbin, J. M. (1999). Development and validation of a multifactorial treatment outcome measure for eating disorders. *Assessment, 6,* 7–20.

Balazs, J., & Bitter, I. (2000). Study on construct validity of the M.I.N.I. Plus interview [abstract]. *Psychiatria Hungarica, 15,* 134–144.

Basile, B. (2004). Self-disclosure in eating disorders. *Eating and Weight Disorders, 9,* 217–223.

Beck, A. T., Ward, C. H., Mendelson, M., Mock, J., & Erbaugh, J. (1961). An inventory for measuring depression. *Archives of General Psychiatry, 4,* 561–571.

Beglin, S. J., & Fairburn, C. G. (1992). What is meant by the term binge? *American Journal of Psychiatry, 149,* 123–124.

Beumont, P. J. V., Kopec-Schrader, E. M., Talbot, P., & Touyz, S. W. (1993). Measuring the specific psychopathology of eating disorder patients. *Australian and New Zealand Journal of Psychiatry, 27,* 506–511.

Black, C. M. D., & Wilson, G. T. (1996). Assessment of eating disorders: Interview versus questionnaire. *International Journal of Eating Disorders, 20,* 43–50.

Boskind-White, M., & White, W. C. (1983). *Bulimarexia: The binge/purge cycle.* New York: Norton.

Bossert, S., Schmölz, U., Wiegand, M., Junker, M., & Krieg, J. C. (1992). Predictors of short-term treatment outcome in bulimia nervosa inpatients. *Behaviour Research and Therapy, 30,* 193–199.

Brelsford, T. N., Hummel, R. M., & Barrios, B. A. (1992). The Bulimia Test–Revised: A psychometric investigation. *Psychological Assessment, 4,* 399–401.

Campbell, M., Lawrence, B., Serpell, L., Lask, B., & Neiderman, M. (2002). Validating the Stirling Eating Disorders Scales (SEDS) in an adolescent population. *Eating Behaviors, 3,* 285–293.

Carter, J. C., Aimé, A. A., & Mills, J. S. (2001). Assessment of bulimia nervosa: A comparison of interview and self-report questionnaire methods. *International Journal of Eating Disorders, 30,* 187–192.

Celio, A. A., Wilfley, D. E., Crow, S. J., Mitchell, J., & Walsh, B. T. (2004). A comparison of the Binge Eating Scale, Questionnaire for Eating and Weight Patterns–Revised, and Eating Disorder Examination Questionnaire with instructions with the Eating Disorder Examination in the assessment of binge eating disorder and its symptoms. *International Journal of Eating Disorders, 36,* 434–444.

de Man Lapidoth, J., Ghaderi, A., & Norring, C. (2006). Eating disorders and disordered eating among patients seeking non-surgical weight-loss treatment in Sweden. *Eating Behaviors, 7,* 15–26.

de Zwann, M., Mitchell, J. E., Specker, S. M., Pyle, R. L., Mussell, M. P., & Seim, H. C. (1993). Diagnosing binge eating disorder: Level of agreement between self-report and expert-rating. *International Journal of Eating Disorders, 14,* 289–295.

Derogatis, L. R., Rickels, K., & Rock, A. F. (1976). The SCL-90 and the MMPI: A step in the validation of a new self-report scale. *British Journal of Psychiatry, 128,* 280–289.

Dohrenwend, B. P., Shrout, P. E., Egri, G., & Mendelsohn, F. S. (1980). Nonspecific psychological distress and other dimensions of psychopathology. *Archives of General Psychiatry, 37,* 1229–1236.

Dolan, B., & Ford, K. (1991). Binge eating and dietary restraint: A cross-cultural analysis. *International Journal of Eating Disorders, 10,* 345–353.

Elder, K. A., Grilo, C. M., Masheb, R. M., Rothschild, B. S., Burke-Martindale, C. H., & Brody, M. L. (2006). Comparison of two self-report instruments for assessing binge eating in bariatric surgery candidates. *Behaviour Research and Therapy, 44,* 545–560.

Engelsen, B. K., & Laberg, J. C. (2001). A comparison of three questionnaires (EAT-12, EDI, and EDE-Q) for assessment of eating problems in healthy female adolescents. *Nordic Journal of Psychiatry, 55,* 129–135.

Esplen, M. J., Garfinkel, P. E., Olmsted, M., Gallop, R. M., & Kennedy, S. (1998). A randomized controlled trial of guided imagery in bulimia nervosa. *Psychological Medicine, 28,* 1347–1357.

Fairburn, C. G. (1987). The definition of bulimia nervosa: Guidelines for clinicians and research workers. *Annals of Behavioral Medicine, 9,* 307.

Fairburn, C. G. (2008). *Cognitive behaviour therapy and eating disorders.* New York: Guilford.

Fairburn, C. G., & Beglin, S. J. (1994). Assessment of eating disorders: Interview or self-report questionnaire? *International Journal of Eating Disorders, 16,* 363–370.

Fairburn, C. G., & Cooper, Z. (1993). The Eating Disorder Examination (12th ed.). In C. G. Fairburn & G. T. Wilson (Eds.), *Binge eating: Nature, assessment and treatment* (pp. 317–360). New York: Guilford.

Fairburn, C. G., & Wilson, G. T. (1993). Binge eating: Definition and classification. In C. G. Fairburn & G. T. Wilson (Eds.), *Binge eating: Nature, assessment and treatment* (pp. 3–14). New York: Guilford.

Fichter, M. M., Elton, M., Engel, K., Meyer, A.-E., Mall, H., & Poustka, F. (1991). Structured Interview for Anorexia and Bulimia Nervosa (SIAB): Development of a new instrument for the assessment of eating disorders. *International Journal of Eating Disorders, 10,* 571–592.

Fichter, M. M., Herpertz, S., Quadflieg, N., & Herpertz-Dahlmann, B. (1998). Structured Interview for Anorexic and Bulimic Disorders for *DSM-IV* and ICD-10: Updated (third) revision. *International Journal of Eating Disorders, 24,* 227–249.

Fichter, M. M., & Keeser, W. (1980). Das Anorexia-nervosa-Inventar zur Selbstbeurteilung (ANIS) [The Anorexia Nervosa Inventory for Self-rating (ANIS)]. *Archiv für Psychiatrie und Nervenkrankheiten, 228,* 67–89.

Fichter, M. M., & Quadflieg, N. (1999). Six-year course and outcome of anorexia nervosa. *International Journal of Eating Disorders, 26,* 359–385.

Fichter, M. M., & Quadflieg, N. (2001). The Structured Interview for Anorexic and Bulimic Disorders for *DSM-IV* and ICD-10 (SIAB-EX): Reliability and validity. *European Psychiatry, 16,* 38–48.

First, M. B., Gibbon, M., Spitzer, R. L., & Williams, J. B. W. (1995). *Structured Clinical Interview for DSM-IV Axis I Disorders, Clinician Version (SCID-CV).* Washington, DC: American Psychiatric Press.

First, M. B., Spitzer, R. L., Gibbon M., & Williams, J. B. W. (2002). *Structured Clinical Interview for DSM-IV-TR Axis I Disorders, Research Version, Nonpatient Edition (SCID-I/NP).* New York: Biometrics Research, New York State Psychiatric Institute.

Freitas, S. R., Lopes, C. S., Appolinario, J. C., & Coutinho, W. (2006). The assessment of binge eating disorder in obese women: A comparison of the Binge Eating Scale with the Structured Clinical Interview for the *DSM-IV. Eating Behaviors, 7,* 282–289.

Friedman, W. J., & deWinstanley, P. A. (1998). Changes in the subjective properties in autobiographical memories with the passage of time. *Memory, 6,* 367–381.

Gamble, C., Bryant-Waugh, R., Turner, H., Jones, C., Mehta, R., & Graves, A. (2006). An investigation into the psychometric properties of the Stirling Eating Disorder Scales. *Eating Behaviors, 7,* 395–403.

Garfinkel, P. E., & Newman, A. (2001). The Eating Attitude Test: Twenty-five years later. *Eating and Weight Disorders, 6,* 1–24.

Garner, D. M. (1991). *Eating Disorder Inventory–2 professional manual.* Odessa, FL: Psychological Assessment Resources.

Garner, D. M. (2004). *Eating Disorder Inventory–3 professional manual.* Lutz, FL: Psychological Assessment Resources.

Garner, D. M., & Garfinkel, P. E. (1979). The eating attitude test: An index of the symptoms of anorexia nervosa. *Psychological Medicine, 9,* 273–279.

Garner, D. M., & Olmsted, M. P. (1984). *The Eating Disorder Inventory manual.* Odessa, FL: Psychological Assessment Resources.

Garner, D. M., Olmsted, M. P., Bohr, Y., & Garfinkel, P. E. (1982). The Eating Attitudes Test: Psychometric features and clinical correlates. *Psychological Medicine, 12,* 871–878.

Garner, D. M., Shafer, C. L., & Rosen, L. W. (1992). Critical appraisal of the *DSM-III-R* diagnostic criteria for eating disorders. In S. R. Hooper, G. W. Hynd, & R. E. Mattison (Eds.), *Child psychopathology: Diagnostic criteria and clinical assessment* (pp. 261–303). Hillsdale, NJ: Lawrence Erlbaum.

Ghaderi, A., & Scott, B. (2002). The preliminary reliability and validity of the Survey for Eating Disorders (SEDs): A self-report questionnaire for diagnosing eating disorders. *European Eating Disorders Review, 10,* 61–76.

Gladis, M. M., Wadden, T. A., Foster, G. D., Vogt, R. A., & Wingate, B. J. (1998). A comparison of two approaches to the assessment of binge eating in obesity. *International Journal of Eating Disorders, 23,* 17–26.

Goldfarb, L. A., Dykens, E. M., & Gerrard, M. (1985). The Goldfarb Fear of Fatness scale. *Journal of Personality Assessment, 49,* 329–332.

Goldfein, J. A., Devlin, M. J., & Kamenetz, C. (2005). Eating Disorder Examination–Questionnaire with and without instruction to assess binge eating in patients with binge eating disorder. *International Journal of Eating Disorders, 37,* 107–111.

Gormally, J., Black, S., Daston, S., & Rardin, D. (1982). The assessment of binge eating severity among obese persons. *Addictive Behaviors, 7,* 47–55.

Götestam, K. G., & Agras, W. S. (1995). General population-based epidemiological study of eating disorders in Norway. *International Journal of Eating Disorders, 18,* 119–126.

Greeno, C. G., Marcus, M. D., & Wing, R. R. (1995). Diagnosis of binge eating disorder: Discrepancies between a questionnaire and clinical interview. *International Journal of Eating Disorders, 17,* 153–160.

Grilo, C. M., Lozano, C., & Elder, K. A. (2005). Inter-rater and test-retest reliability of the Spanish language version of the Eating Disorder Examination Interview: Clinical and research implications. *Journal of Psychiatric Practice, 11,* 231–240.

Grilo, C. M., Masheb, R. M., Lozano-Blanco, C., & Barry, D. T. (2003). Reliability of the Eating Disorder Examination in patients with binge eating disorder. *International Journal of Eating Disorders, 35,* 80–85.

Grilo, C. M., Masheb, R. M., & Wilson, G. T. (2001). A comparison of different methods for assessing the features of eating disorders in patients with binge eating disorder. *Journal of Consulting and Clinical Psychology, 69,* 317–322.

Hawkins, R. C., & Clement, P. F. (1980). Development and construct validation of a self-report measure of binge eating tendencies. *Addictive Behaviors, 5,* 219–226.

Henderson, M., & Freeman, C. P. (1987). A self-rating scale for bulimia: The "BITE." *British Journal of Psychiatry, 150,* 18–24.

Johnson, W. G., Kirk, A. A., & Reed, A. E. (2001). Adolescent version of the Questionnaire of Eating and Weight Patterns: Reliability and gender differences. *International Journal of Eating Disorders, 29,* 94–96.

Joiner, T. E., Jr., & Heatherton, T. F. (1998). First- and second-order factor structure of five subscales of the Eating Disorder Inventory. *International Journal of Eating Disorders, 23,* 189–198.

Joiner, T. E., Jr., Heatherton, T. F., & Keel, P. K. (1997). Ten-year stability and predictive validity of five bulimia-related indicators. *American Journal of Psychiatry, 154,* 1133–1138.

Kalarachian, M. A., Wilson, G. T., Brolin, R. E., & Bradley, L. (2000). Assessment of eating disorders in bariatric surgery candidates: Self-report questionnaire versus interview. *International Journal of Eating Disorders, 28,* 465–469.

Keel, P. K., Fichter, M., Quadflieg, N., Bulik, C. M., Baxter, M.G., Thornton, L., et al. (2004). Application of a latent class analysis to empirically define eating disorder phenotypes. *Archives of General Psychiatry, 61,* 192–200.

Kjelsås, E., Bjornstrom, C., & Götestam, K. G. (2004). Prevalence of eating disorders in female and male adolescents (14–15 years), *Eating Behaviors, 5,* 13–25.

Kurth, C. L., Krahn, D. D., Nairn, K., & Drewnowski, A. (1995). The severity of dieting and binging behaviors in college women: Interview validation of survey data. *Journal of Psychiatric Research, 29,* 211–225.

Kutlesic, V., Williamson, D. A., Gleaves, D. H., Barbin, J. M., & Murphy-Eberenz, K. P. (1998). The Interview for the Diagnosis of Eating Disorders–IV: Application to *DSM-IV* diagnostic criteria. *Psychological Assessment, 10,* 41–48.

Laessle, R. G., Beumont, P. J. V., Butow, P., Lennerts, W., O'Connor, M., Pirke, K. M., et al. (1991). A comparison of nutritional management with stress management in the treatment of bulimia nervosa. *British Journal of Psychiatry, 159,* 250–261.

Lang, T., Hauser, R., Buddeberg, C., & Klaghofer, R. (2002). Impact of gastric binging on eating behavior and weight. *Obesity Surgery, 12,* 100–107.

Larsen, J. K., van Ramshorst, B., Geenen, R., Brand, N., Stroebe, W., & van Doornen, L. J. P. (2004). Binge eating and its relationship to outcome after laparoscopic adjustable gastric banding. *Obesity Surgery, 14,* 1111–1117.

Lecrubier, Y., Sheehan, D., Weiller, E., Amorim, P., Bonora, I., Sheehan, K., et al. (1997). The MINI International Neuropsychiatric Interview (M.I.N.I.). A short diagnostic structured interview: Reliability and validity according to the CIDI. *European Psychiatry, 12,* 224–231.

Liddell, H. G., & Scott, R. (1972). *Greek and English lexicon.* Oxford, UK: Clarendon.

Luce, K. H., & Crowther, J. H. (1999). The reliability of the Eating Disorder Examination–Self-Report Questionnaire Version (EDE-Q). *International Journal of Eating Disorders, 25,* 349–351.

Malone, M., & Alger-Mayer, S. (2004). Binge status and quality of life after gastric bypass surgery: A one-year study. *Obesity Research, 12,* 473–481.

Marcus, M. D., Wing, R. R., & Lamparski, D. M. (1985). Binge eating and dietary restraint in obese patients. *Addictive Behaviors, 10,* 163–168.

Martin, C. K., Williamson, D. A., & Thaw, J. M. (2000). Criterion validity of the Multiaxial Assessment of Eating Disorders Symptoms. *International Journal of Eating Disorders, 28,* 303–310.

Mazzeo, S. E., Aggen, S. H., Anderson, C., Tozzi, F., & Bulik, C. M. (2003). Investigating the structure of the eating inventory (Three-Factor Eating Questionnaire): A confirmatory approach. *International Journal of Eating Disorders, 34,* 255–264.

McCabe, M. P., & Vincent, M. A. (2003). The role of biodevelopmental and psychological factors in disordered eating among adolescent males and females. *European Eating Disorders Review, 11,* 315–328.

McCarthy, D. M., Simmons, J. R., Smith, G. T., Tomlinson, K. L., & Hill, K. K. (2002). Reliability, stability, and factor structure of the Bulimia Test–Revised and Eating Disorder Inventory–2 scales in adolescence. *Assessment, 9,* 382–389.

Mond, J. M., Hay, P. J., Rodgers, B., Owen, C., & Beumont, P. J. V. (2004). Temporal stability of the Eating Disorder Examination Questionnaire. *International Journal of Eating Disorders, 36,* 195–203.

Nangle, D. W., Johnson, W. G., Carr-Nangle, R. E., & Engler, L. B. (1994). Binge eating disorder and the proposed *DSM-IV* criteria: Psychometric analysis of the Questionnaire of Eating and Weight Patterns. *International Journal of Eating Disorders, 16,* 147–157.

Nevonen, L., Broberg, A. G., Clinton, D., & Norring, C. (2003). A measure for the assessment of eating disorders: Reliability and validity studies of the Rating of Anorexia and Bulimia interview–Revised version (RAB-R). *Scandinavian Journal of Psychology, 44,* 303–310.

Nunally, J. C., & Bernstein, I. H. (1994). *Psychometric theory* (3rd ed.). New York: McGraw-Hill.

Openshaw, C., & Waller, G. (2005). Psychometric properties of the Stirling Eating Disorder Scales with bulimia nervosa patients. *Eating Behaviors, 6,* 165–168.

Ordman, A. M., & Kirschenbaum, D. S. (1985). Cognitive-behavioral therapy for bulimia: An initial outcome study. *Journal of Consulting and Clinical Psychology, 53,* 305–313.

Ortega, D. F., Waranch, H. R., Maldonado, A. J., & Hubbard, F. A. (1987). A comparative analysis of self-report measures of bulimia. *International Journal of Eating Disorders, 6,* 301–311.

Palmer, R. (1979). The dietary chaos syndrome: A useful new term? *British Journal of Medical Psychology, 52,* 187–190.

Palmer, R., Christie, M., Cordle, C., Davies, D., & Kenrick, J. (1987). The Clinical Eating Disorder Rating Instrument (CEDRI): A preliminary description. *International Journal of Eating Disorders, 6,* 9–16.

Palmer, R., Robertson, D., Cain, M., & Black, S. (1996). The Clinical Eating Disorders Rating Instrument (CEDRI): A validation study. *European Eating Disorders Review, 4,* 149–156.

Passi, V. A., Bryson, S. W., & Lock, J. (2002). Assessment of eating disorders in adolescents with anorexia nervosa: Self-report questionnaire versus interview. *International Journal of Eating Disorders, 33,* 45–54.

Peterson, C. B., & Miller, K. B. (2005). Assessment of eating disorders. In S. Wonderlich, J. Mitchell, M. de Zwann, & H. Steiger (Eds.), *Eating disorders review part I* (pp. 105–126). Oxford, UK: Radcliffe Publishing Ltd.

Pike, K. M., Loeb, K., & Walsh, T. B. (1995). Binge eating and purging. In D. B. Allison (Ed.), *Handbook of assessment methods for eating behaviors and weight-related problems: Measures, theory, and research* (pp. 303–346). Thousand Oaks, CA: Sage.

Powers, P. S., Perez, A., Boyd, F., & Rosemurgy, A. (1999). Eating pathology before and after bariatric surgery: A prospective study. *International Journal of Eating Disorders, 25,* 293–300.

Rathner, G., & Rumpold, G. (1994). Convergent validity of the Eating Disorder Inventory and the Anorexia Nervosa Inventory for Self-rating in an Austrian nonclinical population. *International Journal of Eating Disorders, 16,* 381–393.

Ricca, V., Mannucci, E., Moretti, S., Di Bernardo, M., Zucchi, T., Cabras, P. L., et al. (2000). Screening for binge eating disorder in obese outpatients. *Comprehensive Psychiatry, 41,* 111–115.

Rizvi, S. L., Peterson, C. B., Crow, S. J., & Agras, W. S. (2000). Test-retest reliability of the Eating Disorder Examination. *International Journal of Eating Disorders, 28,* 311–316.

Rizvi, S. L., Stice, E., & Agras, W. S. (1999). Natural history of disordered eating attitudes and behaviors over a 6-year period. *International Journal of Eating Disorders, 26,* 406–413.

Rosenvinge, J. H., Borgen, J. S., & Börresen, R. (1999). The prevalence and psychological correlates of anorexia nervosa, bulimia nervosa and binge eating among 15-year-old students: A controlled epidemiological study. *European Eating Disorders Review, 7,* 382–391.

Rossiter, E. M., & Agras, W. S. (1990). An empirical test of the *DSM-III-R* definition of binge. *International Journal of Eating Disorders, 9,* 513–518.

Russell, G. F. M. (1979). Bulimia nervosa: An ominous variant of anorexia nervosa. *Psychological Medicine, 9,* 429–448.

Schoemaker, C., Verbraak, M., Breteler, R., & van der Staak, C. (1997). The discriminant validity of the Eating Disorder Inventory–2. *British Journal of Clinical Psychology, 36,* 627–629.

Sheehan, D. V., Janavs, J., Baker, R., Harnett-Sheehan, K., Knapp, E., Sheehan, M., et al. (2003). *Mini International Neuropsychiatric Interview (MINI Plus).* Jacksonville, FL: Sheehan & Lecrubier.

Sheehan, D. V., Lecrubier, Y., Harnett-Sheehan, K., Amorim, P., Janavs, J., Weiller, E., et al. (1998). The Mini International Neuropsychiatric Interview (M.I.N.I.): The development and validation of a structured diagnostic psychiatric interview. *Journal of Clinical Psychiatry, 59,* 22–33.

Sheehan, D. V., Lecrubier, Y., Harnett-Sheehan, K., Janavs, J., Weiller, E., Bonara, I., et al. (1997). Reliability and validity of the MINI International Neuropsychiatric Interview (M.I.N.I.): According to the SCID-P. *European Psychiatry, 12,* 232–241.

Shroff, H., Reba, L., Thornton, L. M., Tozzi, F., Klump, K. L., Berrettini, W. H., et al. (2006). Features associated with excessive exercise in women with eating disorders. *International Journal of Eating Disorders, 39,* 454–461.

Shrout, P. E., & Fliess, J. L. (1979). Intraclass correlations: Uses in assessing rater reliability. *Psychological Bulletin, 86,* 420–428.

Smith, M. C., & Thelen, M. H. (1984). Development and validation of a test for bulimia. *Journal of Consulting and Clinical Psychology, 52,* 863–872.

Spitzer, R. L., Devlin, M., Walsh, B. T., Hasin, D., Wing, R., Marcus, M., et al. (1992). Binge eating disorder: A multisite field trial of the diagnostic criteria. *International Journal of Eating Disorders, 11,* 191–203.

Spitzer, R. L., Williams, J. B., Gibbon, M., & First, M. B. (1992). The Structured Clinical Interview for *DSM-III-R* (SCID) I: History, rationale, and description. *Archive of General Psychiatry, 49,* 624–629.

Spitzer, R. L., Yanovski, S. Z., & Marcus, M. D. (1993). *The Questionnaire on Eating and Weight Patterns–Revised (QEWP-R, 1993).* (Available from the New York State Psychiatric Institute, 722 West 168th Street, New York, NY 10032)

Spitzer, R. L., Yanovski, S., Wadden, T., Wing, R., Marcus, M. D., Stunkard, A., et al. (1993). Binge eating disorder: Its further validation in a multisite study. *International Journal of Eating Disorders, 13,* 137–153.

Stein, K. F., & Corte, C. M. (2003). Ecologic momentary assessment of eating-disordered behaviors. *International Journal of Eating Disorders, 34,* 349–360.

Stice, E., Fisher, M., & Martinez, E. (2004). Eating Disorder Diagnostic Scale: Additional evidence of reliability and validity. *Psychological Assessment, 16,* 60–71.

Stice, E., Telch, C. F., & Rizvi, S. L. (2000). Development and validation of the Eating Disorder Diagnostic Scale: A brief self-report measure of anorexia, bulimia, and binge-eating disorder. *Psychological Assessment, 12,* 123–131.

Stunkard, A. J. (1959). Eating patterns and obesity. *Psychiatric Quarterly, 33,* 284–292.

Stunkard, A. J., & Messick, S. (1985). The three-factor eating questionnaire to measure dietary restraint, disinhibition and hunger. *Journal of Psychosomatic Research, 29,* 71–83.

Summerfeldt, L. J., & Antony, M. M. (2002). Structured and semistructured diagnostic interviews. In M. M. Antony & D. H. Barlow (Eds.), *Handbook of assessment and treatment planning for psychological disorders* (pp. 3–37). New York: Guilford.

Sunday, S. R., Peterson, C. B., Andreyka, K., Crow, S. J., Mitchell, J. E., & Halmi, K. A. (2001). Differences in *DSM-III-R* and *DSM-IV* diagnoses in eating disorder patients. *Comprehensive Psychiatry, 42,* 448–455.

Sysko, R., Walsh, B. T., & Fairburn, C. G. (2005). Eating Disorder Examination–Questionnaire as a measure of change in patients with bulimia nervosa. *International Journal of Eating Disorders, 37,* 100–106.

Tasca, G. A., Illing, V., Lybanon-Daigle, V., Bissada, H., & Balfour, L. (2003). Psychometric properties of the Eating Disorders Inventory–2 among women seeking treatment for binge eating disorder. *Assessment, 10,* 228–236.

Tasca, G. A., Ritchie, K., Conrad, G., Balfour, L., Gayton, J., Daigle, V., et al. (2006). Attachment scales predict outcome in a randomized controlled trial of two group therapies for Binge Eating Disorder: An aptitude by treatment interaction. *Psychotherapy Research, 16,* 106–121.

Thelen, M. H., Farmer, J., Wonderlich, S., & Smith, M. (1991). A revision of the Bulimia Test: The BULIT-R. *Psychological Assessment, 3,* 119–124.

Thelen, M. H., Mintz, L. B., & Vander Wal, J. S. (1996). The Bulimia Test–Revised: Validation with *DSM-IV* criteria for bulimia nervosa. *Psychological Assessment, 8,* 219–221.

Timmerman, G. M. (1999). Binge Eating Scale: Further assessment of validity and reliability. *Journal of Applied Biobehavioral Research, 4,* 1–12.

van der Ster Wallin, G., Norring, C., & Holmgren, S. (1994). Binge eating versus nonpurged eating in bulimics: Is there a carbohydrate craving after all? *Acta Psychiatrica Scandinavica, 89,* 376–381.

Waller, G. (1992). Bulimic attitudes in different eating disorders: Clinical utility of the BITE. *International Journal of Eating Disorders, 11,* 73–78.

Walsh, B. T., Fairburn, C. G., Mickley, D., Sysko, R., & Parides, M. K. (2004). Treatment of bulimia nervosa in a primary care setting. *American Journal of Psychiatry, 161,* 556–561.

Watkins, B., Frampton, I., Lask, B., & Byrant-Waugh, R. (2005). Reliability and validity of the child version of the Eating Disorder Examination: A preliminary investigation. *International Journal of Eating Disorders, 38,* 183–187.

Welch, G., Hall, A., & Norring, C. (1990). The factor structure of the Eating Disorder Inventory in a patient setting. *International Journal of Eating Disorders, 9,* 79–85.

Welch, G., Thompson, L., & Hall, A. (1993). The BULIT-R: Its reliability and clinical validity as a screening tool for *DSM-III-R* bulimia nervosa in a female tertiary education population. *International Journal of Eating Disorders, 14,* 95–105.

Whitaker, A., Davies, M., Shaffer, D., Johnson, J., Abrams, S., Walsh, T. B., et al. (1989). The struggle to be thin: A survey of anorexic and bulimic symptoms in a non-referred adolescent population. *Psychological Medicine, 19,* 143–163.

Wilfley, D. E., Agras, W. S., Telch, C. F., Rossiter, E. M., Schneider, J. A., Cole, A. G., et al. (1993). Group cognitive-behavioral therapy and group interpersonal psychotherapy for the nonpurging bulimic individual: A controlled comparison. *Journal of Consulting and Clinical Psychology, 61,* 296–305.

Wilfley, D. E., Schwartz, M. B., Spurrell, E. B., & Fairburn C. G. (1997). Assessing the specific psychopathology of binge eating disorder patients: Interview or self-report? *Behaviour Research and Therapy, 35,* 1151–1159.

Wilfley, D. E., Welch, R. R., Stein, R. I., Spurrell, E. B., Cohen, L. R., Saelens, B. E., et al. (2002). A randomized comparison of group cognitive-behavioral therapy and group interpersonal psychotherapy for the treatment of overweight individuals with binge-eating disorder. *Archives of General Psychiatry, 59,* 713–721.

Wilkinson, L., & The Task Force on Statistical Inference. (1999). Statistical methods in psychology journals: Guidelines and explanations. *American Psychologist, 54,* 594–604.

Williams, G.-J., & Power, K. (1995). *Stirling Eating Disorder Scales.* London: The Psychological Corporation.

Williams, G.-J., Power, K. G., Miller, H. R., Freeman, C. P., Yellowlees, A., Dowds, T., et al. (1994). Development and validation of the Stirling Eating Disorder Scales. *International Journal of Eating Disorders, 16,* 35–43.

Williams, J. B. W., Gibbon, M., First, M. B., Spitzer, R. L., Davies, M., Borus, J., et al. (1992). The Structured Clinical Interview for *DSM-III-R* (SCID) II. Multi-site test-retest reliability. *Archives of General Psychiatry, 49,* 630–636.

Williamson, D. A. (1990). *Assessment of eating disorders: Obesity, anorexia, and bulimia nervosa.* New York: Pergamon.

Williamson, D. A., Anderson, D. A., & Gleaves, D. H. (1996). Anorexia and bulimia nervosa: Structured interview methodologies and psychological assessment. In K. Thompson (Ed.), *Body image, eating disorders, and obesity: A practical guide for assessment and treatment* (pp. 205–223). Washington, DC: American Psychological Association.

Williamson, D. A., Anderson, D. A., Jackman, L. P., & Jackson, S. J. (1995). Assessment of eating disordered thoughts, feelings, and behaviours. In D. B. Allison (Ed.), *Handbook of assessment methods for eating behaviors and weight-related problems: Measures, theory, and research* (pp. 347–386). London: Sage.

Williamson, D. A., Davis, C. J., Bennett, S. M., Goreczny, A. J., & Gleaves, D. H. (1989). Development of a simple procedure for assessing body image disturbances. *Behavioral Assessment, 11*, 433–446.

Wilson, G. T., Fairburn, C. G., Agras, W. S., Walsh, B. T., & Kraemer, H. (2002). Cognitive-behavioral therapy for bulimia nervosa: Time course and mechanisms of change. *Journal of Consulting and Clinical Psychology, 70*, 267–274.

World Health Organization. (1990). *Composite International Diagnostic Interview.* Geneva, Switzerland: Author.

World Health Organization. (2007). *International statistical classification of diseases and related health problems, 10th revision (ICD-10).* Geneva, Switzerland: Author.

Zanarini, M. C., & Frankenburg, F. R. (2001). Attainment and maintenance of reliability of Axis I and II disorders over the course of a longitudinal study. *Comprehensive Psychiatry, 42*, 369–374.

Zanarini, M. C., Skodol, A. E., Bender, D., Dolan, R., Sanislow, C., Schaefer, E., et al. (2000). The Collaborative Longitudinal Personality Disorders Study: Reliability and the Axis I and II diagnoses. *Journal of Personality Disorders, 14*, 291–299.

CHAPTER 11

Assessment of Eating-Disordered Thoughts, Feelings, and Behaviors

Drew A. Anderson, Kyle P. De Young, and D. Catherine Walker

This chapter reviews a number of assessment measures that were generally designed to assess overall eating-related pathology. The particular measures were chosen for this chapter based on a number of criteria. First, measures were chosen on the basis of their popularity. A recent review of the research literature (Anderson & Paulosky, 2004a) and a recent survey of eating disorder professionals in clinical practice (Anderson & Paulosky, 2004b) found that a relative few of the many measures available are actually being used with any regularity; most of these measures are included in this chapter. We also conducted an informal literature review to identify measures used in multiple research studies that were not identified in these reviews, Second, we chose measures that, while not widely used in the research literature or clinical practice, had good psychometric properties and other advantages to their use. Third, we chose instruments designed specifically for eating disorders, not components of measures that are used for multiple disorders

(e.g., the Structured Clinical Interview for *DSM-IV* Axis I Disorders; First, Spitzer, Gibbon, & Williams, 1997). Finally, we emphasized measures that were designed for use in older adolescents and adults. Comprehensive reviews of measures designed for children and adolescents appear elsewhere (Anderson, Lavender, Milnes, & Simmons, 2008). The chapter is divided into two sections: interviews and self-report inventories. Wherever possible, copies of the measures are included as appendixes at the end of the book.

Interviews

The Eating Disorder Examination

The Eating Disorder Examination (EDE; Z. Cooper & Fairburn, 1987; Fairburn & Cooper, 1993) is a semistructured interview designed to assess the full range of specific psychopathology of eating disorders. The EDE was intended for use in research studies of eating disorder psychopathology and for treatment outcome research (Z. Cooper & Fairburn, 1987).

The EDE has been revised a number of times, and the 16th edition was recently released. It differs only slightly from the popular 12th edition (Fairburn & Cooper, 1993). Most published data on the psychometric properties of the EDE pertain to the earlier 12th edition.

The EDE has 62 items divided into four subscales: Dietary Restraint, Eating Concern, Weight Concern, and Shape Concern. The average scores of the subscales comprise the global EDE score. Each item consists of a required probe question and a number of additional probes to facilitate similar conceptualization of key concepts and comprehension of terminology between the interviewer and interviewee. Individual items are scored using a 7-point forced-choice format (0–6) with higher scores reflecting greater severity or frequency of eating disorder pathology and behavior.

The EDE assesses eating disorder psychopathology and behavior over the previous 4 weeks, with diagnostic items measuring these behaviors over the past 3 and/or 6 months.

Reliability

Internal Consistency. Both Z. Cooper, Cooper, and Fairburn (1989) and Stice and Fairburn (2003) found Cronbach's alpha coefficients for the EDE subscales to be good, ranging from .67 to .96, and Cooper and colleagues found the scales to have generally good item-subscale correlations. These data are summarized in Table 11.1.

Test-Retest Reliability. Overall, test-retest reliability of the EDE is good, although the reliability of subjective bulimic episodes is somewhat problematic. Rizvi, Peterson, Crow, and Agras (2000) found that the EDE subscales' test-retest reliability over a 2- to 7-day interval (median = 4 days) ranged from .71 to .76 among a sample of 20 adult women with a range of eating disorder psychopathology, and with the exception of subjective bulimic days and episodes, test-retest reliabilities of all eating disorder behavior

frequencies were over .83. Test-retest reliability ($M = 10.5$ days; $SD = 3.2$ days) in a sample of 18 adults with binge-eating disorder ranged from a Spearman's rho of .50 (Shape Concern) to .88 (Restraint; Grilo, Masheb, Lozano-Blanco, & Barry, 2004). Grilo and colleagues (2004) also found that Spearman's rho was good for objective bulimic episodes and objective bulimic days but was poor for subjective bulimic episodes and subjective bulimic days. Data pertaining to test-retest reliability are presented in Table 11.1.

Interrater Reliability. Psychometric studies of the EDE have demonstrated high interrater reliability, with correlations characteristically above .90 (Rizvi et al., 2000; Rosen, Vara, Wendt, & Leitenberg, 1990; Wilson & Smith, 1989). Grilo et al. (2004) reported that interrater reliability ranged from .65 to .99 (Spearman's rho) for EDE subscales, binge-eating behaviors, and the global EDE scale. Data pertaining to interrater reliability are summarized in Table 11.1.

Validity

Concurrent Validity. Rosen and colleagues (1990) found adequate correlations between EDE dietary restraint measures and food records ($r = -.39$ for daily caloric intake, $r = -.37$ for frequency of regular meals, and $r = -.22$ for frequency of snack foods). Correlations between the EDE overeating scale and food records were also adequate (ranging from .38 for total calories consumed per day to .56 for frequency of binge eating). Correlations between EDE measures of vomiting and behavior monitoring records were high, ranging from .81 for subjects with bulimia nervosa to .90 for all subjects. Rosen and colleagues (1990) also found good concurrent validity on the EDE Weight and Shape Concern subscales compared to the Body Shape Questionnaire (P. J. Cooper, Taylor, Cooper, & Fairburn, 1987). Fichter and Quadflieg (2001) found that correlations between individual EDE scales and the Structured Interview for Anorexic and Bulimic Disorders for *DSM-IV* and *ICD-10* (SIAB-EX) ranged from .48 (Weight

Table 11.1   EDE: Summary of Psychometric Data

A. Reliability

	Internal Consistency	Test-Retest Reliability		Interrater Reliability
		Spearman's Rho		
	Cronbach's Alpha	Median 4 Days[a]	Mean 10.5 Days[b]	Spearman's Rho
Subscale				
Dietary restraint	.92[c]/.75[d]	.762	.88	.953[a]/.96[b]
Bulimia	.90[d]	NA	NA	NA
Eating concern	.71[c]/.78[d]	.743	.51	.904[a]/.90[b]
Weight concern	.95[c]/.68[d]	.708	.52	.939[a]/.65[b]
Shape concern	.96[c]/.82[d]	.761	.50	.990[a]/.84[b]
Behaviors				
Objective bulimic days		.825	.71	.998[a]/.99[b]
Objective bulimic episodes		.848	.70	.995[a]/.98[b]
Subjective bulimic days		.401	.17	.991[a]/.91[b]
Subjective bulimic episodes		.335	.17	.916[a]/.91[b]
Vomit days		.967		1.000[a]
Vomit episodes		.970		1.000[a]
EDE global score		.71		.72[b]

B. Validity[e]

Concurrent Validity: Pearson's r						
	Dietary Restraint	Eating Concern	Weight Concern	Shape Concern	Overeating[f]	Vomiting
BSQ			.78	.78		
Eating record	−.39					.90
Total calories/day					.38	
Binge-eating frequency		.50			.56	
Calorie content of binges		.52			.54	

(Continued)

Table 11.1 (Continued)

Discriminant validity
Bulimia nervosa > controls, restrained eaters[d]
Anorexia nervosa > controls

C. Norms

	Dietary Restraint	Eating Concerns	Weight Concerns	Shape Concerns
	M (SD)	M (SD)	M (SD)	M (SD)
AN (N = 45)[g]	3.0 (2.0)	2.7 (1.7)	3.2 (1.8)	3.4 (1.9)
BN (N = 87)[g]	3.3 (1.6)	2.7 (1.4)	3.6 (1.5)	3.8 (1.4)
BED (N = 104)[g]	2.2 (1.3)	2.1 (1.3)	3.6 (1.1)	3.9 (1.1)
Partial AN (N = 47)[g]	2.8 (1.9)	1.9 (1.6)	2.8 (1.9)	3.0 (1.9)
Partial BN (N = 57)[g]	2.5 (1.6)	1.5 (1.4)	2.9 (1.6)	3.2 (1.5)
Partial BED (N = 45)[g]	1.9 (1.4)	1.9 (1.2)	3.1 (1.1)	3.3 (1.2)
BED (N = 52)[h]	2.0 (1.2)	1.7 (1.1)	3.4 (1.0)	3.8 (0.9)
Gastric bypass (N = 98)[i]	1.60 (1.5)	1.34 (1.4)	3.30 (1.1)	3.28 (1.4)

NOTE: BN = bulimia nervosa; AN = anorexia nervosa; BED = binge-eating disorder; BSQ = Body Shape Questionnaire; EDE = Eating Disorder Examination; NA = not available.

a. Rizvi, Peterson, Crow, and Agras (2000).

b. Grilo, Masheb, Lozano-Blanco, and Barry (2004).

c. Stice and Fairburn (2003).

d. Z. Cooper, Cooper, and Fairburn (1989).

e. Rosen, Vara, Wendt, and Leitenberg (1990).

f. This subscale is found in the 11th edition of the EDE.

g. Crow, Agras, Halmi, Mitchell, and Kraemer (2002).

h. Wilfley, Schwartz, Spurrell, and Fairburn (1997).

i. Kalarchian, Wilson, Brolin, and Bradley (2000).

Concern) to .72 (Eating Concern); the EDE total was highly correlated with the SIAB-EX (.77). Data are summarized in Table 11.1.

Wilson and Smith (1989) found that the EDE discriminated between bulimic and nonbulimic highly restrained eaters on all subscales except Restraint.

It should be noted that some treatment outcome studies have shown discrepancies between the EDE and other instruments in assessing the rate of binge eating, purgative episodes, and shape and weight concerns (Anderson & Maloney, 2001), which does raise some questions about the instrument's concurrent validity in the context of these variables.

Predictive Validity. No data on the predictive validity of the EDE are available.

Discriminant Validity. Cooper, Cooper, and Fairburn (1989) reported that the EDE discriminated well between women with and without eating disorders. Wilson and Smith (1989) found that four of the five subscales (all but the Restraint subscale) of the first version of the EDE* successfully discriminated between women with bulimia nervosa and control women who were restrained eaters.

Norms

Adult norms for several groups are summarized in Table 11.1.

Availability of Measure and Related Costs

The 16th edition of the EDE and instructions for its use are available (Fairburn, Cooper, & O'Connor, 2008); they may also be downloaded from http://www.psychiatry.ox.ac.uk/research/researchunits/credo. A Spanish version has also been developed (Grilo, Lozano, & Elder, 2005).

Special Issues/Considerations/ Pros and Cons

The authors of the EDE have suggested that the key features of the eating disorders are difficult to define and interpret (particularly binge eating), and allowing the interviewer, not the interviewee, to rate every eating episode as a binge or not allows for more objectivity and improved reliability and validity (Fairburn & Beglin, 1994; Fairburn & Cooper, 1993).

Susceptibility to Dissimulation. Because it is a semistructured interview with a number of probe questions, it has been suggested that the EDE may be less susceptible to dissimulation than other self-report formats, such as questionnaires (Z. Cooper & Fairburn, 1987). On the other hand, it has also been suggested that shame and other factors may lead individuals to minimize eating-related pathology in face-to-face interviews compared to other formats (Anderson, Simmons, Milnes, & Earleywine, 2007; French et al., 1998; Keel, Crow, Davis, & Mitchell, 2002). Also, it is not clear whether the amounts of food reported by interviewees are accurate, as large errors in the assessment of food intake are routine, and this can influence the assessment of binge eating (Anderson & Paulosky, 2004a). These issues have not yet been resolved.

Training. Z. Cooper and Fairburn (1987) asserted that "brief training in its use is required," and the authors note in the current version that training is "essential" if it is to be used for research purposes (Fairburn et al., 2008), although details concerning where to receive training for the EDE were not provided. Instructions for interviewers are provided with the current version of the measure, however (Fairburn et al, 2008).

Practicality. Because the EDE takes 30 to 60 minutes to complete and must be administered by a trained interviewer, it is less practical than many other self-report measures, which may be why it does not appear to be widely used in clinical contexts (Anderson & Paulosky, 2004b). On the other hand, it is routinely used in controlled clinical trials and other research studies (Anderson & Paulosky, 2004a).

To conclude, given its psychometric properties and interview-based format, the EDE is widely considered to be the "gold-standard" assessment instrument for the assessment of eating disorder symptomatology. While it does have some limitations, the EDE is a valuable assessment instrument, and its use is encouraged where it is practical.

Interview for the Diagnosis of Eating Disorders–IV

The fourth version of the Interview for Diagnosis of Eating Disorders (IDED-IV; Kutlesic, Williamson, Gleaves, Barbin, & Murphy-Eberenz, 1998) is a semistructured diagnostic interview based on the fourth edition of the *Diagnostic and Statistical Manual of Mental Disorders* (*DSM-IV*; American Psychiatric Association [APA], 1994) diagnostic criteria for anorexia nervosa (AN), bulimia nervosa (BN), and binge-eating disorder (BED). In addition to allowing for the diagnoses of AN, BN, BED, and eating disorders not otherwise specified (EDNOS), the IDED-IV assesses demographic variables, weight, family and treatment history, and associated medical problems.

The IDED contains three subscales that correspond to diagnoses of AN, BN, and BED, with summed subscale scores indicating the severity of symptoms. Twenty symptoms relating to *DSM-IV* diagnostic criteria each contain a separate set of questions rated on a 5-point scale with a rating of 3 or higher indicating the presence of that symptom. A checklist completed at the conclusion of the interview assists in making differential diagnoses.

Reliability

Internal Consistency. The subscales of the IDED-IV show good internal consistency with coefficient alpha values between .75 and .95 (Kutlesic et al., 1998). Table 11.2 summarizes these data.

Interrater Reliability. Interrater reliability was investigated using a subset of participants (*n* = 82) from the original sample, 38 of whom had an eating disorder diagnosis (14.6% AN; 19.8% BN; 39.6% BED; 26% EDNOS). Adequate to high agreement was found for each eating disorder diagnosis, as displayed in Table 11.2.

Validity

Concurrent Validity. Kutlesic and colleagues (1998) found the anorexia nervosa subscale to be associated with dieting as assessed by the Eating Attitudes Test, drive for thinness as assessed by the Eating Disorders Inventory–2, and exercise, vomiting, and radical weight loss measures as assessed by the Bulimia Test–Revised. The bulimia nervosa subscale was found to be associated with binge eating and inappropriate compensatory behaviors as assessed by the

Bulimia Test–Revised and body dissatisfaction and drive for thinness as assessed by the Eating Disorders Inventory–2, and the binge-eating disorder subscale was found to be most strongly associated with binge eating as assessed by the Bulimia Test–Revised. These correlations are shown in Table 11.2.

Discriminant Validity. Intercorrelations of the IDED-IV subscales with subscales of other symptom measures are presented in Table 11.2; these correlations generally show the expected pattern. Also, as can be seen in this table, correlations between the IDED-IV subscales show the expected patterns, with a moderate positive correlation between the AN and BN subscales, a moderately high positive correlation between the BN and BED subscale, and a low positive correlation between the AN and BED subscales (Kutlesic et al., 1998).

Norms

Norms are not available for the IDED-IV; however, because it was designed primarily for use as an aid to diagnosis, this does not represent a significant shortcoming.

Availability of Measure and Related Costs

A copy of the IDED-IV is included as Appendix 11.D at the end of the book.

Special Issues/Consideration/ Pros and Cons

Susceptibility to Dissimulation. Because symptom questions are based on *DSM-IV* criteria for anorexia nervosa, bulimia nervosa, and binge-eating disorder, they are face valid and therefore susceptible to symptom exaggeration or minimization. As noted in the discussion of the EDE, it is not clear to what degree interviews improve the validity of assessment of eating disorder symptoms.

Training. Interviewers in the validation studies of the IDED-IV had specific training in its use

Table 11.2   IDED-IV: Summary of Psychometric Data

A. Reliability

Internal Consistency	Subscale	Coefficient Alpha
	Anorexia nervosa	.75
	Binge-eating disorder	.96
	Bulimia nervosa	.75
Interrater Reliability	*Diagnosis*	*Kappa*
	All diagnoses	.86
	Anorexia nervosa	1.00
	Binge-eating disorder	.87
	Bulimia nervosa	.64

B. Validity

Content Validity

Ten doctoral-level psychologists in the eating disorders field rated the adequacy, representativeness, and clarity of each of subscales and the overall scale on a 7-point Likert-type scale where 1 was *do not agree* and 7 was *strongly agree*. Mean ratings ranged from 5.90 to 6.70.

Concurrent/Discriminant Validity

Correlation of IDED-IV Subscales With Self-Report Measures[a]			
	AN	*BN*	*BED*
EAT factors			
Dieting	.71*	.60*	.18
Oral control	.44*	.14	−.31*
BULIT-R factors			
Binge eating	.24	.68*	.88*
Radical weight loss	.66*	.76*	.53*
Vomiting	.33*	.68*	.47*
Laxative-diuretic abuse	.26	.44*	.23
Exercise	.33*	.30*	−.03

(Continued)

Table 11.2 (Continued)

Correlation of IDED-IV Subscales With Self-Report Measures[a]			
EDI-II subscales			
	AN	BN	BED
Drive for thinness	.48*	.45*	.31*
Body dissatisfaction	.19	.29*	.2*
BIA subscales			
Current body size	.12	.39*	.51*
Ideal body size	−.23	−.13	.10
IDED-IV Subscales			
AN	—	.63*	.22*
BN		—	.70*
Correlation of IDED-IV Subscales[b]			
AN	—	0.63	0.22
BN		—	0.70

a. Table adapted from Kutlesic, Williamson, Gleaves, Barbin, and Murphy-Eberenz (1998).

b. Kutlesic et al. (1998).

*$p < .001$.

(Kutlesic et al., 1998), although it does not appear that such training is needed for everyday use of the measure. General training in interviewing skills is presumably necessary to administer the IDED-IV, however.

Practicality. The checklist included with the IDED-IV aids in differential diagnosis, which increases the measure's practicality. Like other interviews, however, the IDED-IV takes longer to administer than most self-report questionnaires and requires that a trained individual administer the measure, which makes it somewhat less practical to use in some clinical contexts.

In sum, the IDED-IV was developed for the purpose of assisting trained interviewers in making eating disorder diagnoses, and it appears to be most useful in this context.

Structured Interview for Anorexic and Bulimic Disorders for *DSM-IV* and *ICD-10*

The Structured Interview for Anorexic and Bulimic Disorders for *DSM-IV* and *ICD-10* (SIAB-EX; Fichter, Herpertz, Quadflieg, & Herpertz-Dahlmann, 1998) is an 87-item semistructured interview developed to assess psychopathology specific to eating disorders, including diagnostic criteria, as well as a broader range of psychopathology common in eating disorder patients. The SIAB-EX assesses symptoms in both the present (previous 2 weeks) and past (worst lifetime episode). General probes are given for each item as well as additional probes to be used when responses to general probes do not offer sufficient information. Questions are rated on a 5-point forced-choice scale from 0 (symptom not present) to 4 (symptom very much/very severely present).

The SIAB has six subscales/factors: (1) Body Image and Slimness Ideal; (2) General Psychopathology; (3) Sexuality and Social Integration; (4) Bulimic Symptoms; (5) Measures to Counteract Weight Gain, Fasting, and Substance Abuse; and (6) Atypical Binges (Fichter et al., 1991; Fichter et al., 1998).

Reliability

Internal Consistency. High internal consistency was established for five of the six subscales of the SIAB-EX (lifetime), ranging from .78 to .91 (Fichter et al., 1998). Data are summarized in Table 11.3.

Test-Retest Reliability. There is no published test-retest reliability for the SIAB-EX to date.

Interrater Reliability. Psychometric studies of the SIAB-EX have demonstrated high interrater reliability (Fichter et al., 1991; Fichter et al., 1998); the unadjusted intraclass correlation coefficient ranged from .80 to .90 on ratings of past symptom expression and from .86 to .96 on ratings of current symptom expression (Fichter et al., 1998). Fichter and Quadflieg (2001) found mean kappa values of .81 and .85 for interrater reliability of current and past sections of the SIAB-EX. Data are summarized in Table 11.3.

Validity

Concurrent Validity. Fichter and colleagues (1991) found that the SIAB bulimic behavior component and the EDE Bulimia subscale (found on an earlier version of the EDE) to be highly correlated ($r = .53$), and the SIAB body image and slimness ideal component was highly correlated with all EDE subscales except Bulimia. More recently, Fichter and Quadflieg (2001) compared the SIAB-EX to the EDE and found high correlations between EDE items on Food Avoidance and Dietary Rules and SIAB-EX qualitative and quantitative reduction of food items. SIAB-EX and EDE items covering vomiting, laxative abuse, and loss of control over eating were also highly correlated; however, this relationship was not as robust for items assessing objective and subjective binges. The SIAB Atypical Binges subscale was not highly correlated with any EDE items, suggesting that it may tap into aspects of eating disorder psychopathology and behavior that are not assessed in the EDE (Fichter & Quadflieg, 2001).

Fichter et al. (1991) found that the Body Image and Slimness and Sexuality and Social Integration components of the SIAB for present symptom expression were highly correlated with most Anorexia Nervosa Inventory for Self-Rating (ANIS; Fichter & Keeser, 1980) subscales, and the SIAB marital dissatisfaction component (found on an earlier version of the SIAB) correlated strongly with ANIS's Feelings of Insufficiency and Bulimic Symptoms subscales. The SIAB bulimic behavior component did not correlate highly with the ANIS bulimic symptoms factor. Data pertaining to concurrent validity of the SIAB-EX are presented in Table 11.3.

The SIAB distinguishes between five levels of food restriction and five levels of excessive physical activity: In a sample of 11 inpatients with acute anorexia nervosa, serum leptin levels at admission showed a significant inverse correlation with both the level of quantitative food restriction ($r = -.73$) and level of physical activity ($r = -.66$), as measured by the SIAB-EX (Holtkamp, Hebebrand, & Herpertz-Dahlmann, 2004).

Predictive Validity. There is no published predictive validity information for the SIAB-EX to date; however, Fichter et al. (1998) recommend that the instrument be used for the assessment

Table 11.3   SIAB-EX: Summary of Psychometric Data

A. Reliability[a]

| Subscale | Internal Consistency | | Unadjusted Intraclass Correlation Coefficients | |
| | Past | Current | Past | Current |
	Cronbach's Alpha	Cronbach's Alpha	M (SD)	M (SD)
Body Image	.81	.85	.86 (.12)	.88 (.08)
General Psychopathology	.84	.86	.80 (.16)	.86 (.10)
Sexuality and Social Integration	.78	.78	.83 (.13)	.91 (.04)
Bulimic Symptoms	.89	.91	.90 (.13)	.89 (.14)
Counteracting	.64	.43	.88 (.09)	.96 (.05)
Atypical Binges	.82	.80	NA	NA

Factor Structure: five-factor structure for current, six factors for past.

B. Validity

Concurrent Validity[b]

	Slimness/ Body Image	Sexuality and Social Integration	Depression	Compulsion and Anxiety	Bulimic Behavior	Laxative Abuse	Marital Dissatisfaction	Achievement Orientation/ Performance Expectancy	Rigidity and Family Interaction	Family Closeness and Enmeshment
Correlation With Current SIAB-EX										
ANIS mean	.47**	.37**	.32**	.09	NA	.24*	.34**	.20	.20	.24*
EDE mean	.46*	-.13	.30*	-.03	.43*	.31*	.06	.42*	-.10	-.06
Restraint	.50**	.07	.38**	.30*	.08	.09	-.11	.32	-.35	.31
Bulimia	.21	-.26*	.19	-.14	.53**	.33**	.02	.27	.04	-.29
Eating concern	.61**	.11	.20	-.08	.26	.35**	.02	.29	-.16	.24
Weight concern	.47**	.06	.04	.16	-.11	.20	-.36	.29	-.31	.29
Shape concern	.55**	.08	.24*	.08	.10	.20	-.30	.22	-.10	.30
Correlation With Past SIAB-EX										
ANIS mean	.06	-.02	-.12	.17	.14	-.29*	.27*	.18	.14	.12

(Continued)

Table 11.3 (Continued)

Predictive Validity for the SIAB-S[c]

	Diagnostic Sensitivity	Diagnostic Specificity	Positive Predictive Value
Past symptom expression			
Cutoff score of 1.3	.79	.66	.86
Criterion C for AN and BN omitted	.73	.63	.58
Current symptom expression			
Cutoff score of 1.3	.72	.76	.89
Criterion C for AN and BN omitted	.60	.70	.59

C. Norms[a]

	Total Patient Group (n = 330)	AN Patients (n = 53)	BN Patients (n = 97)	Follow-Up Group AN (n = 148)	Follow-Up Group BN (n = 185)	Community Controls (n = 111)
	M (SD)	M (SD)	M (SD)	M (SD)	M (SD)	M (SD)
Past symptom expression						
Body Image	1.9 (.7)	2.5 (.4)	2.1 (.6)	1.5 (.7)	1.2 (.6)	NA
General Psychopathology	1.5 (.7)	1.7 (.6)	1.7 (.8)	1.1 (.7)	1.1 (.8)	NA
Sexuality and Social Integration	2.3 (.8)	2.7 (1.7)	1.9 (1.7)	1.8 (2.1)	1.6 (.8)	NA
Bulimic Symptoms	2.5 (1.1)	2.0 (1.4)	3.2 (.5)	1.3 (1.4)	0.7 (.7)	NA
Counteract	1.0 (.6)	1.0 (.5)	1.2 (.6)	0.5 (.4)	NA	NA
Atypical Binges	0.8 (1.1)	0.5 (.9)	0.6 (.9)	NA	NA	NA
Current symptom expression						
Body Image	1.5 (.6)	2.1 (.5)	1.5 (.6)	1.0 (.6)	0.8 (.5)	0.5 (.3)
General Psychopathology	1.2 (.6)	1.3 (.6)	1.3 (.7)	0.7 (.7)	0.6 (.7)	0.5 (.3)

Sexuality and Social Integration	2.2 (1.3)	3.2 (.9)	2.1 (1.2)	1.4 (1.3)	1.2 (1.2)	0.5 (.7)
Bulimic Symptoms	2.1 (1.1)	1.9 (1.3)	3.1 (.5)	0.9 (1.2)	1.2 (1.2)	NA
Counteract	0.4 (.4)	0.5 (.4)	0.6 (.5)	0.3 (.3)	0.4 (.5)	NA
Atypical Binges	0.5 (.9)	0.3 (.7)	0.4 (.7)	NA	NA	NA

NOTE: BN = bulimia nervosa; AN = anorexia nervosa; ANIS = Anorexia Nervosa Inventory for Self-Rating; EDE = Eating Disorder Examination; SIAB-EX = Structured Interview for Anorexic and Bulimic Disorders for DSM-IV and ICD-10; NA = not available.

a. Fichter, Herpertz, Quadflieg, and Herpertz-Dahlmann (1998).

b. Fichter et al. (1991).

c. Fichter and Quadflieg (2001).

*p < .01. **p < .001.

of eating-disordered patients over time in longitudinal studies and suggest that the subscales of the SIAB might also be used as possible predictors of the course of illness.

Discriminant Validity. Fichter and Quadflieg (2001) compared the SIAB-EX to the Beck Depression Inventory (BDI; Beck, Ward, Mendelson, & Erbaugh, 1961), Symptom Checklist (SCL-90; Derogatis, Rickels, & Rock, 1976), PERI Demoralization Scale (Dohrenwend, Shrout, Egri, & Mendelson, 1980), the Eating Disorder Inventory (EDI; Garner, Olmstead, & Polivy, 1983), and the Three Factor Eating Questionnaire (TFEQ; Stunkard & Messick, 1985). All SIAB-EX subscales except General Psychopathology and Social Integration were not significantly correlated with the SCL-90. Fichter and Quadflieg found low correlations between all SIAB-EX scales other than Atypical Binges when compared to the BDI and the PERI Demoralization Scale. Although the EDI Bulimia subscale was highly correlated with the SIAB-EX Bulimic Symptoms subscales, this relationship was not present when compared to the SIAB-EX Body Image and Slimness Ideal scale, suggesting that these two SIAB scales measure different constructs. The TFEQ Disinhibition and Hunger scales were only significantly correlated with SIAB-EX scales that assessed binge-eating behavior (Fichter & Quadflieg, 2001).

The SIAB-EX measures a broader array of psychopathology than the ANIS and the EDE and examines both past and present eating disorder symptoms. Because neither the EDE nor the ANIS assess general psychopathology and past symptom expression, as expected, SIAB-EX scales that assess those facets were not highly correlated with the EDE or ANIS (Fichter & Quadflieg, 2001; Fichter et al., 1991). Data are presented in Table 11.3.

Norms

Norms are available for each item of the second and third revisions of the SIAB-EX for clinical and nonclinical samples of adolescents and adults and are given for both past and present symptom

expression (Fichter et al., 1991; Fichter et al., 1998). Norms are summarized in Table 11.3.

Availability of Measure and Related Costs

The SIAB-EX is available in English, Spanish, Italian, and German versions. A detailed manual with extensive psychometric data and instructions for use is also available, as are scoring algorithms. All materials related to the SIAB-EX can be downloaded from http://www.epi.med.uni-muenchen.de/.

Special Issues/Consideration/ Pros and Cons

Susceptibility to Dissimulation. As an interview, the SIAB-EX has similar issues to the EDE and IDED-IV in terms of validity and maximization and minimization of symptoms.

Training. The SIAB-EX must be administered by an expert interviewer. A 90-page manual is available to facilitate interviewer training (Fichter & Quadflieg, 1999; see section on availability).

Practicality. The SIAB-EX can be used in practice and research for the quantitative assessment and diagnostic classification of eating disorders based on *DSM-IV* and *ICD-10* diagnoses such as anorexia nervosa, bulimia nervosa, binge-eating disorder, and eating disorder not otherwise specified, as well as in nonclinical cases with high shape and weight concern (Fichter & Quadflieg, 1999). It can also be used in longitudinal studies as an outcome measure (Fichter et al., 1998). The SIAB-EX has the additional advantages of assessing a wide range of psychopathology common among those with eating disorders as well as assessing both present and past symptom presentation to get a more complete picture of the underlying eating disorder psychopathology and course of the illness. The SIAB-EX does suffer from the same limits on practicality as other interviews—namely, that it requires a trained interviewer and takes time to administer.

Self-Report Questionnaires

The SCOFF

The SCOFF (Morgan, Reid, & Lacey, 1999), a five-item measure, was developed to serve as a simple, easy-to-remember screening instrument for eating disorders for use by nonspecialists such as general medical practitioners. Items were developed through focus groups with eating-disordered patients and specialists in the field (Morgan et al., 1999). Questions can be administered orally or in written format (Perry et al., 2002). "SCOFF" is an acronym developed from the items.

Each "yes" response to the five yes/no questions on the SCOFF is summed for the total score. Scores of 2 or greater were originally suggested as a cutoff point for maximum sensitivity to detect anorexia and bulimia nervosa (Morgan et al., 1999); however, Siervo, Boschi, Papa, Bellini, and Falconi (2005) found that a cutoff of 3 was the best compromise between sensitivity and specificity. Using a cutoff of 3 yielded a low area under the receiver operating characteristic (ROC) curve (.68), which Siervo et al. suggest may limit the application of the SCOFF in populations with low rates of eating disorders, such as was sampled in their study of women seeking diet therapy. The SCOFF questions use vernacular specific to the United Kingdom, but items have been adapted for use in the United States (Morgan at al., 1999; Parker, Lyons, & Bonner, 2005). Spanish and Japanese translations of the SCOFF have been developed as well (Garcia-Campayo, Sanz-Carillo, Ibañez, Solano, & Alda, 2005; Noma et al., 2006). Psychometric data pertaining to the SCOFF are summarized in Table 11.4.

Reliability

Internal Consistency. Perry et al. (2002) reported high correlations between item responses on oral and written administration of the SCOFF. Kappa coefficients ranged from 0.85 to 0.94 for the two forms of test administration.

Test-Retest Reliability. Garcia-Campayo et al. (2005) reported excellent test-retest reliability in a sample of 110 previously undiagnosed eating disorder patients over a 2-week interval (intraclass correlation coefficient = 0.97; 95% confidence interval: 0.96–0.98).

Validity

Concurrent Validity. Written administration of the SCOFF produces somewhat higher scores than verbal administration, as has been noted with other self-report eating disorder questionnaires (Black & Wilson, 1996; Fairburn & Beglin, 1994; Perry et al., 2002). Scores on a Japanese sample of 80 patients with eating disorders were highly correlated with the EAT-26 for all subjects and all eating disorders and subtypes (Noma et al., 2006). Data are summarized in Table 11.4.

Predictive Validity. Garcia-Campayo and colleagues (2005) found that using two positive responses as a threshold resulted in the highest predictive validity, yielding sensitivity and specificity of 97.7% and 94.4% overall. For bulimia nervosa, anorexia nervosa, and EDNOS, sensitivity scores were 97.8%, 93.1%, and 100%, respectively; specificity scores were 94.4% across eating disorder diagnoses; and the positive predictive value (PPV) was 82.2% (Garcia-Campayo et al., 2005). Luck et al. (2002) found sensitivity of 84.6%, specificity of 89.6%, PPV of 24.4%, and negative predictive value (NPV) of 99.3%. Parker et al. (2005) found lower estimates for predictive validity when compared to EDE-Q scores in a sample of graduate students who attended their university health center. In their sample, sensitivity was 53.3%, specificity was 93.2%, PPV was 66.7%, and the NPV was 88.7% using two positive responses as a cutoff. Comparing the Questionnaire for Eating Disorder Diagnosis (Mintz, O'Halloran, Mulholland, & Schneider, 1997), Cotton, Ball, and Robinson (2003) also also found lower predictive validity than was reported in the derivation study (Morgan et al.,

Table 11.4 SCOFF: Summary of Psychometric Data

A. Reliability

Cross-Method Reliability (* = Oral; + = Written)[a]							
		Consistent Responses		Discrepant Responses		Comparisons	
Question	n	*no, +no	*yes, +yes	*yes, +no	*no, +yes	Kappa	% Agreement
1	181	169 (93.4%)	10 (5.5%)	0 (0.0%)	2 (1.1%)	.903	98.9
2	182	133 (73.1%)	36 (19.8%)	6 (3.3%)	7 (3.8%)	.800	92.9
3	182	155 (85.2%)	24 (13.2%)	1 (0.5%)	2 (1.1%)	.932	98.3
4	179	138 (77.1%)	32 (17.9%)	3 (1.7%)	6 (3.4%)	.845	95.0
5	182	151 (83.0%)	28 (15.4%)	2 (1.1%)	1 (0.5%)	.939	98.3
Test-Retest Reliability[b]							
Interval Between Testing		Intraclass Correlation Coefficient (95% CI)					n
2 weeks (median = 13 days)		.97 (.96–.98)					110

B. Validity

Concurrent Validity			
	EAT-26	TFEQ	
	Pearson r	Pearson r	
SCOFF	.575[c]/.34[d]	.36[d]	

Predictive Validity				
	Sensitivity, %	Specificity, %	Positive Predictive Value, %	Negative Predictive Value, %
Bulimia nervosa (n = 47)[b]	97.8	94.4	NA	NA
Anorexia nervosa (n = 29)[b]	93.1	94.4	NA	NA
EDNOS (n = 55)[b]	100.0	94.4	NA	NA
Total (n = 203)[b]	NA	NA	82.2	NA
Total (n = 341)[e]	84.6	89.6	24.4	99.3
AN and BN (n = 53,[e] 116[f])	100.0[f]	87.5[f]	96.2[e]	NA
ANr (n = 13)[e]	NA	NA	84.6	NA
ANbp (n = 10)[e]	NA	NA	100.0	NA
BNp (n = 26)[e]	NA	NA	100.0	NA
BNnp (n = 4)[c]	NA	NA	100.0	NA
Total (n = 233)[g]	78	88	NA	NA
Nonclinical (n = 305, 162)[h]	53.3, 94	93.2, 21	66.7, NA	88.7, NA

C. Norms[c]

	M (SD)	Question 1, %	Question 2, %	Question 3, %	Question 4, %	Question 5, %
ANr (n = 13)	2.08 (.86)	7.7	61.5	15.4	46.2	76.9
ANbp (n = 10)	3.00 (.67)	100.0	90.0	0.0	30.0	80.0
BNp (n = 26)	3.12 (.65)	88.5	92.3	3.8	42.3	84.6
BNnp (n = 4)	2.25 (.50)	25.0	75.0	25.0	25.0	75.0
EDNOS (n = 27)	NA	22.2	63.0	7.4	18.5	55.6
Total (N = 80)	NA	51.3	76.3	7.5	32.5	72.5

Education (highest degree completed)	Nonclinical (n = 87), %	Bulimic EDNOS (n = 63), %	BED (n = 12), %
Secondary school	20.6	41.2	50
High school	71.2	52.3	50
Higher education	8.2	6.5	0

	M (SD)	M (SD)	M (SD)
Body mass index (kg/m²)	27.7 (5.2)	31.1 (6.5)	35.0 (8.5)
Age (years)	24.2 (5.2)	23.6 (4.4)	26.1 (4.7)
SCOFF	2.3 (1.2)	3.0 (.9)	3.3 (1.1)

NOTE: NA = not available; BN = bulimia nervosa; BNp = bulimia nervosa purging type; BNnp = bulimia nervosa nonpurging type; AN = anorexia nervosa; ANr = anorexia nervosa restricting type; ANbp = anorexia nervosa binge-purge type; BED = binge-eating disorder; EAT-26 = Eating Attitudes Test–26; EDNOS = eating disorders not otherwise specified; TFEQ = Three Factor Eating Questionnaire; CI = confidence interval.

a. Perry et al. (2002).

b. Garcia-Campayo et al. (2005).

c. Noma et al. (2006).

d. Siervo, Boschi, Papa, Bellini, and Falconi (2005).

e. Luck et al. (2002).

f. Morgan, Reid, and Lacey (1999).

g. Cotton, Ball, and Robinson (2003).

h. Parker, Lyons, and Bonner (2005).

1999), with sensitivity of 78% and specificity of 88%, using two abnormal responses as a cutoff. Data are summarized in Table 11.4.

Discriminant Validity. No data on the discriminant validity of the SCOFF have been published.

Norms

Normative data are available for adult patients with eating disorders as well as for nonclinical community samples. Norms are summarized in Table 11.4.

Availability of Measure and Related Costs. Copies of both the British and American versions of the SCOFF are included as an appendix.

Special Issues/Consideration/ Pros and Cons

Susceptibility to Dissimulation. As a self-report measure, the SCOFF is subject to dissimulation. For example, Luck and colleagues (2002) found the sensitivity of the SCOFF to be lower than reported elsewhere (Morgan et al., 1999; Perry et al., 2002) as a result of artificially low scores of two participants who did not disclose information to the assessor at the time.

Readability. The five items on the SCOFF were written in simple vernacular common among persons in the United Kingdom (Morgan at al., 1999) but have been adapted for comparable simplicity and readability for American use (Parker et al., 2005).

Practicality. The SCOFF was designed to be a brief, practical screening instrument to identify potential cases of eating disorders in an adult primary care context so that they might be examined in more detail. The SCOFF serves a particular need; it has been suggested that other eating disorder assessment tools have not been validated in primary care populations, are too lengthy to administer in this setting, and involve careful analysis to interpret (Cotton et al., 2003). While the SCOFF appears to overidentify individuals who might have an eating disorder, over-inclusion is acceptable for screening instruments designed for disorders with high rates of medical complications, especially since the instrument is exceedingly short and easy to administer (Luck et al., 2002). Thus, the SCOFF would be useful in any context in which a brief, easy to score screening measure is desired.

Eating Disorder Diagnostic Scale

The Eating Disorder Diagnostic Scale (EDDS; Stice, Telch, & Rizvi, 2000) is a 22-item questionnaire developed to assess anorexia nervosa, bulimia nervosa, and binge-eating disorder according to *DSM-IV* (APA, 1994) criteria. A continuous symptom score is also derivable from a subset of the items. The EDDS was developed on a sample of 367 women ranging in age from 13 to 61 years from both clinical and nonclinical populations with full threshold, subthreshold, and no eating disorders.

Reliability

Internal Consistency. The EDDS has been found to have good internal consistency, as shown in Table 11.5.

Test-Retest Reliability. With the EDDS, 367 participants in the original sample were classified into the following diagnostic categories: anorexia nervosa ($n = 18$), bulimia nervosa ($n = 39$), binge-eating disorder ($n = 57$), and non–eating disordered ($n = 253$). The 1-week test-retest reliability was very good for these diagnostic categories, as displayed in Table 11.5.

Concurrent Validity. Stice and colleagues (2000) found that the EDDS correlated moderately to highly with other measures of eating pathology, including the EDE, the Yale-Brown-Cornell Eating Disorders Scale (Mazure, Halmi, Sunday, Romano,

Table 11.5   EDDS: Summary of Psychometric Data

A. Reliability

Internal Consistency	
either Cronbach's Alpha for Symptom Composite Score or	
Mixed clinical/nonclinical sample of 367 females	.91[a]
Nonclinical sample of 728 adolescent females	.89[b]
Test-Retest Reliability[a]	
One-week correlation coefficient of symptom composite score (*n* = 55) equals .87.	
One-Week Kappa Coefficient for Diagnosis in a Sample of 55	
Anorexia nervosa	.95
Bulimia nervosa	.91
Binge-eating disorder	.75

B. Validity

Concurrent Validity	
Measure	*Pearson's r With EDDS Symptom Composite Score*
Eating Disorder Examination	
Restraint	.36
Eating concern	.54
Weight concern	.57
Shape concern	.66
Yale-Brown-Cornell	
Eating and weight preoccupations	.47
Eating and weight rituals	.36
Three Factor Eating Questionnaire	
Cognitive restraint	.10
Hunger	.53
Disinhibition	.63

(Continued)

Table 11.5 (Continued)

Predictive Validity[a]				
Eating Disorder	Sensitivity	Specificity	Positive Predictive Value	Negative Predictive Value
Anorexia nervosa	.93	1.00	.93	1.00
Bulimia nervosa	.81	.98	.86	.97
Binge-eating disorder	.77	.96	.80	.95

a. Stice, Telch, and Rizvi (2000).

b. Stice, Fisher, and Martinez (2004).

& Einhorn, 1994), and the TFEQ (Stunkard & Messick, 1985), as shown in Table 11.5. In addition, individuals identified by the EDDS as having a diagnosis of bulimia nervosa had significantly higher EDE composite scores, thin-ideal internalization, body dissatisfaction, dieting, negative affectivity, depressive symptoms, and social impairment than individuals without an eating disorder (Stice, Fisher, & Martinez, 2004).

Validity

Predictive Validity. The EDDS was found to have high sensitivity and specificity for identifying *DSM-IV* anorexia nervosa, bulimia nervosa, and binge-eating disorder (see Table 11.5; Stice et al., 2000).

Norms

No norms are available for the EDDS.

Availability of Measure and Related Costs

A copy of the EDDS is presented in Appendix 11.F at the end of the book. Syntax code for scoring the EDDS in a popular statistical package (i.e., SPSS) has been published by the developers (Stice et al., 2004).

Special Issues/Considerations/ Pros and Cons

The EDDS is a brief, self-report diagnostic instrument that allows for diagnoses of anorexia nervosa, bulimia nervosa, and binge-eating disorder. Diagnoses made with the EDDS are highly correlated with interview-based assessment methods and can be administered and scored by untrained individuals; thus, the EDDS can be useful in situations where diagnostic accuracy is desired but a full structured interview is not practical or possible.

Eating Attitudes Test and Eating Attitudes Test-26

The Eating Attitudes Test (EAT; Garner & Garfinkel, 1979) was arguably the first self-report questionnaire developed to assess eating disorder symptoms. It contained 40 questions answered on a 6-point Likert-type scale (1 = *never*, 6 = *always*) and was originally validated on a clinical sample of women with anorexia nervosa as defined by the criteria put forth by Feighner and colleagues in 1972. Since then, a shortened 26-item version (EAT-26) was developed by factor analyzing the 40-item version and selecting the items accounting for the most variance

(Garner, Olmsted, Bohr, & Garfinkel, 1982). Both versions are widely used as measures of symptom severity, and they have often been used as screening measures because they each have established cutoff values for probable anorexia nervosa. The EAT and EAT-26 are scored by summing scores for each individual item calculated by assigning 3 points for the most extreme response, 2 points for the next most extreme answer, 1 point for the next, and no points for the three least extreme responses. Typically, a cutoff score of 30 on the EAT or 20 on the EAT-26 is used to indicate the presence of clinically significant eating pathology (Garfinkel & Newman, 2001).

Reliability

Internal Consistency. The original factor analysis of the EAT suggested a three-factor solution (Garner et al., 1982), but since that time, other studies have suggested that a four-factor model with 20 items (Koslowsky et al., 1992) or a four-factor model with 16 items (Ocker, Lam, Jensen, & Zhang, 2007) is more appropriate. However, the EAT and the EAT-26 are most often used as unidimensional measures of symptom severity or for screening purposes. When used in this fashion, the potential variance of factor structure is not particularly problematic. Data on internal consistency are presented in Table 11.6.

Test-Retest Reliability. As shown in Table 11.6, the EAT-26 has good test-retest reliability.

Validity

Concurrent Validity. Table 11.6 provides details on concurrent validity of the EAT. Total scores on the EAT-26 correlate strongly with eating disorder status (Mintz & O'Halloran, 2000) and the Drive for Thinness and Bulimia subscales of the EDI (Brookings & Wilson, 1994; Miller, Schmidt, Vaillancourt, McDougall, & Laliberte, 2006). When used as a measure of symptom severity, the EAT-26 has been shown to correspond to full-threshold,

subthreshold, symptomatic, and asymptomatic diagnoses (Mintz & O'Halloran, 2000).

The EAT can successfully discriminate individuals with full or subthreshold eating disorders from those who have recovered (Steinhausen & Seidel, 1993). In females, the EAT has been shown to discriminate those with bulimia nervosa from women with no eating disorder (Gross, Rosen, Leitenberg, & Willmuth, 1986) but cannot discriminate between the restricting and binge-purge subtypes of anorexia nervosa using total scores (Thompson, 1988). The EAT can also differentiate males with anorexia or bulimia nervosa from those without an eating disorder (Garfinkel & Newman, 2001).

Discriminant Validity. Scores on the EAT-26 correlate weakly or only moderately with several subscales on the EDI (Brookings & Wilson, 1994), Eysenck Personality Questionnaire (Miller et al., 2006), and the Rutgers Alcohol Problems Index (Anderson, Simmons, Martens, Ferrier, & Sheehy, 2006), distinguishing it solely as a measure of disturbed eating behaviors and not as a measure of associated psychopathology (Garfinkel & Newman, 2001).

Predictive Validity. The cutoff score of 20 on the EAT-26 indicating probable anorexia nervosa is more likely to result in false positives than false negatives. Table 11.6 displays specific values of the EAT-26's screening properties.

Norms

Garner and colleagues (1982) published norms for the EAT-26 based on Feighner et al.'s (1972) definition of anorexia nervosa, as modified by Garfinkel and Garner (1982). This definition differs from that in current usage in the *DSM-IV* (APA, 2000) by not requiring a fear of fatness, undue influence of weight and shape on self-evaluation, and amenorrhea, although subjects may have had these symptoms. As a result, the norms they collected may differ from what researchers may obtain using current definitional

Table 11.6   EAT: Summary of Psychometric Data

A. Reliability

Internal Consistency	Cronbach's Alpha
Nonclinical	.90[a]
Males	.89[b]
Adolescent females	.87[c]

Test-Retest Reliability[c]		
Testing Interval	Pearson's r	Sample Size
4 to 5 weeks	.89	393

B. Validity

Concurrent Validity

Measure	r With EAT-26
Eating disorder status	.79[d]
EDI Drive for Thinness	.78[a]/.84[e]
EDI Bulimia	.66[a]

Discriminant Validity

Measure	r With EAT-26
EDI Ineffectiveness	.37[e]
EDI Perfectionism	.24[e]
EDI Interpersonal Distrust	.14[e]
EDI Interoceptive Awareness	.56[e]
EPQ Extraversion	−.24[a]
EPQ Neuroticism	.29[a]
RAPI	.28[f]

Predictive Validity[d]	
Sensitivity/specificity	.77/.94
Positive predictive value	.79
False-negative/false-positive rate	.23/.06
Negative predictive value	.94

C. Norms

	EAT-40	EAT-26	
	M (SD)	M (SD)	Sample Size
AN–restricting subtype[g]	50.1 (24.9)	33.7 (18.7)	77
AN–binge/purge subtype[g]	55.5 (21.0)	38.4 (15.0)	83
Female comparison subjects[g]	15.4 (11.0)	9.9 (9.2)	140

NOTE: EPQ = Eysenck Personality Questionnaire; EDI = Eating Disorder Inventory; RAPI = Rutgers Alcohol Problems Index; AN = anorexia nervosa; BN = bulimia nervosa; EDNOS = eating disorder not otherwise specified.

a. Miller, Schmidt, Vaillancourt, McDougall, and Laliberte (2006).

b. Russell and Keel (2002).

c. Banasiak, Wertheim, Koerner, and Voudouris (2001).

d. Mintz and O'Halloran (2000).

e. Brookings and Wilson (1994).

f. Anderson, Simmons, Martens, Ferrier, and Sheehy (2006).

g. Garner and Garfinkel (1982).

criteria. Table 11.6 lists those norms. In addition, norms for females in the community have been found to be between 11 and 15; typically, 10% to 15% of women screened with the EAT score above the cutoff (Garfinkel & Newman, 2001).

Availability of Measure and Related Costs

A copy of the EAT-26 can be found in Appendix 11.C at the end of this book. The EDE has also been translated into Spanish (Castro, Toro, Salamero, & Guimera, 1991), Urdu (Choudry & Mumford, 1992), Hebrew (Koslowsky et al., 1992), French (Leichner, Steiger, Puentes-Neuman, Perreault, & Gottheil, 1994), Arabic (Nasser, 1986), German (Neumärker, Dudeck, Vollrath, Neumärker, & Steinhausen 1992), Japanese (Ujiie & Kono, 1994), Turkish (Elal, Altug, Slade, & Tekcan, 2000), Korean (Ko & Cohen, 1998), Italian (Cuzzolaro & Petrilli, 1988), and Portuguese (Nunes, Camey, Olinto, & Mari,

2005), and a version for children has also been developed (Maloney, McGuire, & Daniels, 1988).

Special Issues/Considerations/ Pros and Cons

Because they appear to measure general eating-related pathology, the EAT and EAT-26 are recommended for use primarily as screening measures or as a way to track treatment progress over time (Garfinkel & Newman, 2001). These measures are some of the most widely used in both research and clinical contexts (Anderson & Paulosky, 2004a, 2004b) and can be used whenever a brief measure of eating-disordered symptoms is desired.

Eating Disorder Examination Questionnaire

The Eating Disorder Examination Questionnaire (EDE-Q; Fairburn & Beglin, 1994; 2008) is a 28-item measure of eating-disordered behaviors derived from the EDE interview (Fairburn & Cooper, 1993). The 6th edition was recently released (Fairburn & Beglin, 2008). Psychometric data reported here were collected using an earlier edition of the measure (Fairburn & Cooper, 1993), but there are only very minor changes between that edition and the 6th edition. The EDE-Q retains the same wording and initial probe question as the EDE; however, the questionnaire does not have the additional probes and definitions of key terms given when administering the semistructured interview. Like the EDE, the EDE-Q is scored using a 7-point, forced-choice rating scale (0–6) with scores of 4 or higher considered to be in the clinical range. The EDE-Q has four subscales: Restraint, Eating Concern, Weight Concern, and Shape Concern. Frequencies are based on number of days when specific behaviors occurred rather than number of episodes and are measured for the previous 28 days. Psychometric data pertaining to the EDE-Q are summarized in Table 11.7.

Reliability

Internal Consistency. Internal consistency in the EDE-Q has been shown to be good, with Cronbach's alpha coefficients ranging from .70 to .83 and from .78 to .93 in a clinical sample and general population sample, respectively (Luce & Crowther, 1999; Peterson et al., 2007). Mond, Hay, Rodgers, Owen, and Beumont (2004a) reported an alpha coefficient of .93 for the global scale. Using factor-analytic methods, Peterson et al. found that a three-factor solution may provide a more parsimonious fit for the EDE-Q in a sample of women with bulimia nervosa: Most EDE-Q Shape Concern and Weight Concern items appeared to load onto one factor, with most Eating Concern items loading on a second factor and most Restraint items loading on a third. Internal consistency data are summarized in Table 11.7.

Test-Retest Reliability. Luce and Crowther (1999) reported 2-week test-retest reliability of subscales that ranged from .81 to .94 in undergraduate women. Mond et al. (2004a) found Pearson correlations ranging from .57 (Restraint) to .77 (Eating Concern) over a test-retest period with a median of 315 days in a large general population sample of Australian women. These data are summarized in Table 11.7.

Validity

Concurrent Validity. Studies of the validity of the EDE-Q have demonstrated a high level of agreement between the EDE-Q and EDE in assessing core attitudinal features of eating disorder psychopathology in the general population (Elder & Grilo, 2007; Fairburn & Beglin, 1994; Mond, Hay, Rodgers, Owen, & Beumont, 2004b), among female substance abusers (Black & Wilson, 1996), in male and female bariatric surgery candidates (Kalarchian, Wilson, Brolin, & Bradley, 2000), in clinical samples of both bulimia nervosa and binge-eating disorder (Carter, Aime, & Mills, 2001; Wilfley, Schwartz, Spurrell, & Fairburn, 1997), and in adolescents with full and partial bulimia and anorexia nervosa (Binford, Le Grange, & Jellar, 2005). The EDE-Q tended to yield higher scores than the EDE across subscales. In addition, the EDE-Q Shape Concern subscale has been found to be highly correlated with the Body Shape Questionnaire ($r = .72$; Ghaderi & Scott, 2004).

Although studies of the EDE-Q have shown high levels of agreement between the EDE-Q and EDE in assessing core attitudinal features of eating disorder psychopathology in variegated samples (Mond, Hay, Rodgers, & Owen, 2006), the validity of the EDE-Q in assessing eating disorder behaviors is less clear. This difference stems from a difficulty in determining frequency of objective bulimic episodes (OBEs), subjective bulimic episodes (SBEs), and objective overeating episodes (OOEs). In the EDE, a trained investigator makes this determination, while on the EDE-Q, the respondent makes this determination. As there are differences in the definition of binge eating between researchers and laypersons (for a review, see Anderson, Lundgren, Shapiro, & Paulosky,

Table 11.7 EDE-Q: Summary of Psychometric Data

A. Reliability

Subscale	Internal Consistency			Test-Retest Reliability	
		Cronbach's Alpha[b]		Pearson's r	
	Cronbach's Alpha[a]	Time 1	Time 2	Median 315 days[c]	2 Weeks[b]
Dietary Restraint	.70	.84	.85	.57	.81
Eating Concern	.73	.89	.89	.77	.87
Weight Concern	.72	.78	.81	.73	.92
Shape Concern	.83	.93	.92	.75	.94
Global Score	.90				

Factor Structure: Three factors.[a]

B. Validity

Concurrent Validity

Correlation Between EDE and EDE-Q Subscales				
Subscale	Pearson r[d]	Pearson r[e]	Pearson r[f]	Pearson r[g]
Dietary Restraint	.81	.71	.60	.66
Eating Concern	NA	.68	.62	.69
Weight Concern	.79	.77	.71	.63
Shape Concern	.80	.78	.77	.69
Global Score	NA	.84	NA	NA

Predictive Validity[e]

Sensitivity	Specificity	Positive Predictive Value
.83	.96	.56

Discriminant Validity[h]

Correlation between EDE-Q and EDI-2 Subscales								
	Restraint		Eating Concern		Weight Concern		Shape Concern	
EDI-2 Subscales	BED	BN	BED	BN	BED	BN	BED	BN
Drive for Thinness	.41	.40	.42	.55	.53	.61	.49	.62
Bulimia	.24	.13	.49	.57	.37	.15	.32	.14
Body Dissatisfaction	.12	.23	.19	.35	.36	.55	.45	.73

(Continued)

Table 11.7 (Continued)

Correlation between EDE-Q and EDI-2 Subscales								
	Restraint		Eating Concern		Weight Concern		Shape Concern	
EDI-2 Subscales	BED	BN	BED	BN	BED	BN	BED	BN
Ineffectiveness	.02	.20	.22	.38	.28	.26	.28	.37
Perfectionism	.11	−.06	.15	.07	.20	.19	.18	.18
Interpersonal Distrust	.06	−.01	.09	.30	.14	.26	.15	.29
Interoceptive Awareness	.18	−.03	.27	.38	.30	.11	.18	.31
Maturity Fears	.01	.11	.16	.20	.18	.18	.15	.19
Asceticism	.06	.08	.19	.41	.29	.24	.30	.31
Impulse Regulation	.11	.16	.16	.33	.18	.21	.08	.25
Social Introversion	.07	.06	.15	.30	.19	.26	.17	.35

C. Norms

	Restraint	Eating Concern	Weight Concern	Shape Concern	Global Score
	M (SD)	M (SD)	M (SD)	M (SD)	M (SD)
18–45 years (N = 195)[e]	1.29 (1.27)	0.59 (0.84)	1.64 (1.31)	2.16 (1.44)	1.42 (1.04)
16–35 years (N = 243)[d]	1.25 (1.32)	0.62 (0.86)	1.59 (1.37)	2.15 (1.60)	1.55 (1.21)
18–22 years (N = 1,186)[i]	1.29 (1.31)	0.87 (1.13)	1.89 (1.60)	2.29 (1.68)	1.59 (1.32)
23–27 years (N = 908)[i]	1.34 (1.39)	0.81 (1.10)	1.84 (1.50)	2.24 (1.61)	1.56 (1.26)
28–32 years (N = 1,206)[i]	1.28 (1.37)	0.78 (1.07)	1.90 (1.51)	2.37 (1.65)	1.58 (1.23)
33–27 years (N = 928)[i]	1.20 (1.43)	0.69 (1.04)	1.64 (1.48)	2.10 (1.67)	1.42 (1.24)
38–42 years (N = 1,003)[i]	1.31 (1.38)	0.61 (0.94)	1.64 (1.48)	2.10 (1.67)	1.42 (1.24)

NOTE: NA = not available; BN = bulimia nervosa; BED = binge-eating disorder; EDI-2 = Eating Disorder Inventory–2.

a. Peterson et al. (2007).

b. Luce and Crowther (1999).

c. Mond, Hay, Rodgers, Owen, and Beumont (2004a).

d. Fairburn and Beglin (1994).

e. Mond, Hay, Rodgers, Owen, and Beumont (2004b).

f. Kalarchian, Wilson, Brolin, and Bradley (2000).

g. Wilfley, Schwartz, Spurrell, and Fairburn (1997).

h. Tasca, Illing, Lybanon-Daigle, Bissada, and Balfour (2003).

i. Mond, Hay, Rodgers, and Owen (2006).

2004), the relatively low correlation between the EDE and EDE-Q in the assessment of binge eating is not surprising. To help improve the EDE-Q's validity for assessing binge-eating behaviors, researchers devised a modified version of the EDE-Q with instructions (EDE-Q-I), which provides definitions and examples of "unusually large amount of food" and "sense of loss of control" (Goldfein et al., 2002, cited in Celio, Wilfley, Crow, Mitchell, & Walsh, 2004; Goldfein, Devlin, & Kamenetz, 2005). When the EDE was used as the criterion measure from which to compare the EDE-Q-I, Binge Eating Scale (BES; Gormally, Black, Daston, & Rardin, 1982), and the Questionnaire for Eating and Weight Patterns–Revised (QEWP-R; Yanovski, 1993), the EDE-Q-I had the highest criterion validity (Celio et al., 2004). Data concerning concurrent validity of the EDE-Q are summarized in Table 11.7.

Predictive Validity. Beglin and Fairburn (1992) demonstrated the predictive validity of a short form of the EDE-Q comprising nine EDE items that best discriminated cases of clinically significant eating disorders from nonclinical cases in a community sample of women ages 18 to 35. This short-form EDE-Q had better predictive validity than the EAT (Beglin & Fairburn, 1992). Mond et al. (2004b) performed a stepwise discriminant function analysis and pinpointed eight EDE-Q items that best distinguished clinical from nonclinical cases: frequency of OBEs, use of exercise as a means of weight control, use of self-induced vomiting, use of laxatives, guilt about eating, social eating, discomfort seeing body, and avoidance of exposure ($\chi^2 = 105.9$, $p < .01$). They found optimal validity coefficients (sensitivity = .83, specificity = .96, and positive predictive value = .56) when a score of 2.3 on the global scale, in addition to either the occurrence of any OBEs and/or use of exercise as a means of weight control, was used to predict eating disorder diagnosis (Mond et al., 2004b). Sysko, Walsh, and Fairburn (2005) found that the EDE-Q was sensitive to change in bulimic women receiving fluoxetine. Predictive validity data are presented in Table 11.7.

Discriminant Validity. Tasca, Illing, Lybanon-Daigle, Bissada, and Balfour (2003) provided correlations between EDI-2 and EDE-Q subscales, which are summarized in Table 11.7.

Norms

Normative data are available for a community sample of adult women (Mond et al., 2006), clinical samples of women with bulimia nervosa (Carter, Aime, & Mills, 2001; Sysko et al., 2005) and binge-eating disorder (Grilo, Masheb, & Wilson, 2001; Wilfley et al., 1997), and in morbidly obese bariatric surgery candidates (Kalarchian et al., 2000). Carter, Steward, and Fairburn (2001) recently published a modified form of the EDE-Q suitable for adolescents along with normative data for that age group. Adult norms are summarized in Table 11.7.

Availability of Measure

The 6th edition of the EDE-Q has been published (Fairburn & Beglin, 2008) and can also be found online at http://www.psychiatry.ox.ac.uk/research/researchunits/credo. Supplemental EDE-Q-I instructions can be obtained by request from Juli A. Goldfein, PhD, Eating Disorders Research Unit, New York State Psychiatric Institute—Unit 116, 1051 Riverside Drive, New York, NY 10032; e-mail: jag73@columbia.edu. A Spanish-language version of the EDE-Q has also been developed (Elder & Grilo, 2007).

Eating Disorder Inventory–2 and Eating Disorder Inventory–3

The Eating Disorder Inventory (EDI; Garner et al., 1983) was designed to assess psychological characteristics and symptoms common to anorexia and bulimia nervosa. The original EDI had 64 items that formed eight subscales (Drive for Thinness, Bulimia, Body Dissatisfaction, Ineffectiveness, Perfection, Interpersonal Distrust, Interoceptive Awareness, and Maturity Fears). A revised edition of the EDI, the Eating Disorder Inventory–2 (EDI-2; Garner, 1991), retained the original 64 items and eight subscales and added 27 items that formed three additional scales (Ascetism, Impulse Regulation, and Social Insecurity).

Recently, Garner (2004) published a second revision, the Eating Disorder Inventory–3 (EDI-3), which has retained the EDI-2's 91 items but has expanded its 11 scales to 12 scales and added six composite scores and three response style indicators, which gauge response style and profile validity. The EDI-3's scales and composite scores were developed from extensive research with the EDI-2 (Bennett & Stevens, 1997). Exploratory factor analysis yielded 3 eating disorder–specific scales (Drive for Thinness, Bulimia, Body Dissatisfaction) and 8 general psychological scales. The primary consideration in constructing the EDI-3 scales was clinical relevance (Garner, 2004), so concerns such as continuity with the EDI-2, content-based decisions, and comparative model fits found with confirmatory factor analysis led to the adoption of 9 psychological scales, rather than 8 (Low Self-Esteem, Personal Alienation, Interpersonal Insecurity, Interpersonal Alienation, Interoceptive Deficits, Emotional Dysregulation, Perfectionism, Ascetism, and Maturity Fears), that assess psychopathology common in eating disorder patients. It also yielded six composite scores: one that is eating disorder specific (Eating Disorder Risk) and five that are general integrative psychological constructs (Ineffectiveness, Interpersonal Problems, Affective Problems, Overcontrol, General Psychological Maladjustment). The three response-style indicators are Inconsistency, Infrequency, and Negative Impression.

The Professional Manual of the EDI-3 presents factor-analytic data on the measure. Data from the EDI-2 are summarized in Table 11.8 (section B). Tasca et al. (2003) performed confirmatory factor analysis on the EDI-2 and the original EDI for a sample of 152 women with bulimia nervosa–purging type and 144 women with BED. The factor structure of the EDI was tested with data from the BED sample and demonstrated a good fit (comparative fit index = 0.96); however, the factor structures hypothesized by the EDI and EDI-2 were not supported in the sample of bulimic patients using

the original EDI or the EDI-2 (Tasca et al., 2003). There is some inconsistency in the factor structure across adult American, adult international, and adolescent nonclinical comparison groups; however, factor analyses do offer suitable support for the EDI-3, suggesting that composite scale scores represent theoretically distinct higher order constructs (Cumella, 2006).

Items are scored using the 6-point, forced-choice format of the previous EDI versions but have been recalibrated to expand the range of scores possible and improve psychometric properties in nonclinical populations (Cumella, 2006). Respondents rate whether each item applies "always," "usually," "often," "sometimes," "rarely," or "never." Most of the published research pertaining to the psychometric properties of the EDI has been conducted using the EDI-2, but the EDI-3 manual provides ample psychometric data from large, diverse populations (Garner, 2004). Psychometric data pertaining to the EDI-2 and EDI-3 are summarized in Table 11.8.

Reliability

Internal Consistency. Internal consistency estimates for the 18 clinical and composite scales of the EDI-3 are available for the American adult, international adult, and American adolescent samples and, with rare exception, are approximately .80 (Garner, 2004). Unlike the EDI-2, internal consistency estimates for nonclinical comparison groups and item-total correlations are not available for the EDI-3.

Eating Disorder Risk composite reliability ranged from .90 to .97 (median = .94) across the clinical and nonclinical samples. Internal consistency coefficients were high for both the three eating disorder risk scales and the general psychopathology scales; eating disorder risk scales were in the high .80s to low .90s, and General Psychological Maladjustment reliability ranged from .93 to .97 (Garner, 2004). With one exception, all of the other EDI-3 composite reliabilities were in the .80s to .90s for the normative samples. Internal consistency data are presented in Table 11.8.

(Text continues on page 430)

Table 11.8 EDI-2 and EDI-3: Summary of Psychometric Data

A. Reliability[a]

Subscale/Composite	ANr			ANbp			BN			EDNOS			Test-Retest
	U.S. Adult	International Adult	U.S. Adolescent	U.S. Adult	International Adult	U.S. Adolescent	U.S. Adult	International Adult	U.S. Adolescent	U.S. Adult	International Adult	U.S. Adolescent	Pearson's r Mean 2.6 = Days
Drive for Thinness	.91	.91	.93	.86	.87	.93	.81	.82	.87	.89	.90	.88	.95
Bulimia	.63	.84	.63	.90	.85	.93	.88	.83	.92	.87	.87	.86	.94
Body Dissatisfaction	.91	.90	.93	.91	.89	.96	.91	.88	.91	.92	.92	.92	.95
ED Risk Composite	.90	.94	.91	.94	.92	.97	.93	.91	.95	.94	.95	.94	.98

Total	Pearson's r : Mean 2.6 Days		
	U.S. Adult	International Adult	U.S. Adolescent
Low Self-Esteem	.89	.81	.89
Personal Alienation	.84	.78	.87
Interpersonal Insecurity	.84	.73	.85
Interpersonal Alienation	.78	.69	.80
Interoceptive Deficits	.87	.79	.89
Emotional Dysregulation	.75	.67	.77
Perfectionism	.82	.74	.82
Asceticism	.75	.64	.80
Maturity Fears	.87	.82	.86
Ineffectiveness Composite	.92	.88	.93
Interpersonal Problems Composite	.88	.81	.90
Affective Problems Composite	.88	.82	.89
Overcontrol Composite	.85	.78	.88
General Psychological Maladjustment Composite	.96	.93	.97

(Continued)

Table 11.8 (Continued)

B. Validity
Concurrent/Discriminant Validity[a]

Correlation Between EDI and Select Measures

Subscale/Composite	EAT-26 Clinical	BULIT-R Nonclinical	DEBQ Clinical			DEBQ Nonclinical			SCL-90 Clinical	SCL-90 Nonclinical	RSES Nonclinical	CESD Nonclinical
			EmE	ExE	RE	EmE	ExE	RE				
Drive for Thinness	.72	.77	.46	.05	.06	.47	.54	.30	.42	.55	−.40	.42
Bulimia	.25	.81	.33	.54	.43	.48	.70	.42	.36	.55	−.48	.50
Body Dissatisfaction	.52	.64	.42	−.04	−.03	.41	.54	.41	.33	.44	−.44	.44
ED Risk Composite	.63	.83	.52	.23	.20	.50	.65	.42	.48	.56	−.50	.51
Low Self-Esteem	.30	.57	.58	.12	.09	.64	.38	.27	.53	.56	−.75	.77
Personal Alienation	.37	.55	.67	.19	.14	.71	.41	.27	.61	.66	−.45	.47
Interpersonal Insecurity	.17	.27	.40	−.07	−.13	.46	.23	.14	.26	.36	−.54	.64
Interpersonal Alienation	.18	.44	.45	.13	.09	.51	.32	.20	.35	.43	−.60	.67
Interoceptive Deficits	.36	.52	.57	.16	.12	.63	.37	.25	.56	.55	−.52	.62

Subscale/Composite	EAT-26 Clinical	BULIT-R Nonclinical	DEBQ Clinical			DEBQ Nonclinical			SCL-90 Clinical	SCL-90 Nonclinical	RSES Nonclinical	CESD Nonclinical
			EmE	ExE	RE	EmE	ExE	RE				
Emotional Dysregulation	.27	.45	.54	.14	.20	.58	.31	.33	.51	.51	-.13	.26
Perfectionism	.15	.15	.32	.17	.07	.41	.23	.17	.30	.38	-.48	.56
Asceticism	.50	.60	.57	.05	-.02	.54	.50	.31	.52	.59	-.40	.43
Maturity Fears	.27	.35	.26	-.17	-.17	.23	.12	.04	.18	.24	-.82	.78
Ineffectiveness Composite	.39	.59	.66	.17	.12	.72	.42	.29	.60	.64	-.57	.64
Interpersonal Problems Composite	.19	.41	.49	.04	-.01	.53	.30	.19	.35	.43	-.62	.71
Affective Problems Composite	.36	.53	.64	.17	.18	.71	.40	.34	.62	.62	-.35	.48
Overcontrol Composite	.38	.44	.52	.13	.03	.56	.43	.29	.49	.57	—	—
General Psychological Maladjustment	.42	.59	.73	.11	.06	.77	.47	.32	.64	.69	—	—

(Continued)

Table 11.8 (Continued)

Predictive Validity[b]

EDI-2 Subscale/Composite	Most Sensitive Cutoff	Sensitivity/Specificity	PPV/NPV	Most Specific Cutoff	Sensitivity/Specificity	PPV/NPV
Drive for Thinness	12	91.0/80.0	80.0/91.0	14	86.4/84.0	82.6/87.5
Bulimia	2	77.3/76.0	73.9/79.2	3	68.2/84.0	78.9/75.0
Body Dissatisfaction	11	86.4/72.0	73.1/85.7	14	77.3/80.0	77.3/80.0
Inadequacy	5	81.8/80.0	78.3/83.3	7	77.3/84.0	81.0/81.0
Perfectionism	9	72.2/68.0	66.7/73.4	11	68.2/76.0	71.4/73.1
Interpersonal Alienation	5	91.0/72.0	74.1/90.0	7	86.4/84.0	82.6/87.5
Maturity Fears	8	68.2/84.0	78.9/75.0	8	68.2/84.0	78.9/75.0
Asceticism	6	81.8/76.0	75.0/82.6	7	72.7/88.0	84.2/78.6
Emotional Dysregulation	8	86.4/68.0	70.4/85.0	11	77.3/80.0	77.3/80.0
Interpersonal Insecurity	5	91.0/72.0	74.1/90.0	6	77.3/84.0	81.0/80.8
Symptom Composite	10	91.0/80.0	80.0/91.0	11	81.8/92.0	90.0/85.2
Total	80	86.4/84.0	82.6/87.5	105	81.8/88.0	85.7/84.6

C. Norms for EDI Subscales

	Drive for Thinness	Bulimia	Body Dissatisfaction	Ineffectiveness	Perfectionism	Interpersonal Distrust	Interoceptive Awareness	Maturity Fears	Ascetism	Impulse Regulation	Social Insecurity
	M (SD)	M (SD)	M (SD)	M (SD)	M (SD)	M (SD)	M (SD)	M (SD)	M (SD)	M (SD)	M (SD)
Pretreatment (n = 34)[c]	14.9 (4.19)	9.2 (5.47)	17.0 (7.14)	10.6 (6.00)	6.3 (4.60)	5.0 (4.55)	13.4 (6.74)	7.8 (5.83)	8.2 (4.01)	6.2 (4.32)	6.0 (3.39)
Posttreatment (n = 34)[c]	12.1 (5.62)	5.8 (5.17)	14.4 (7.41)	8.8 (6.52)	4.7 (4.02)	4.0 (3.75)	9.6 (6.41)	5.9 (4.62)	5.6 (3.86)	5.4 (4.66)	5.2 (3.42)
Two-month follow-up (n = 31)[c]	11.7 (6.49)	6.1 (5.50)	14.7 (7.13)	9.1 (6.76)	4.6 (3.86)	3.9 (3.89)	9.5 (6.93)	6.2 (5.25)	6.3 (4.49)	5.8 (5.07)	5.5 (3.49)
ED patients (n = 978)[d]	13.4 (5.6)	8.0 (5.9)	17.3 (7.5)	11.6 (6.7)	6.1 (4.1)	4.6 (4.0)	12.2 (6.5)	5.5 (4.8)	6.9 (3.9)	6.0 (4.9)	7.6 (4.3)
Psychiatric OP (n = 106)[d]	6.5 (6.5)	2.4 (4.0)	13.7 (9.0)	10.8 (7.4)	5.1 (4.0)	4.7 (4.5)	7.6 (6.3)	4.8 (4.1)	4.9 (3.9)	5.7 (5.0)	7.6 (4.8)
Normal controls (n = 602)[d]	3.3 (4.6)	0.8 (2.0)	9.3 (7.6)	2.6 (3.7)	2.6 (3.4)	2.0 (2.8)	2.3 (3.4)	3.2 (3.1)	2.5 (2.1)	2.6 (3.5)	2.7 (3.0)
AN (n = 179)[d]	11.8 (6.0)	4.1 (5.4)	14.5 (6.4)	12.9 (7.3)	5.6 (3.7)	4.9 (4.1)	12.0 (6.6)	6.7 (5.1)	6.8 (4.2)	5.4 (4.1)	8.2 (4.4)
BN (n = 432)[d]	14.8 (4.9)	11.0 (5.1)	18.4 (7.3)	12.0 (6.2)	6.4 (4.0)	4.9 (4.1)	13.1 (6.3)	5.6 (4.9)	7.3 (3.7)	6.6 (4.9)	7.7 (4.2)
EDNOS (n = 367)[d]	12.6 (5.8)	6.3 (5.2)	17.4 (8.0)	10.7 (6.7)	6.0 (4.3)	4.3 (3.9)	11.3 (6.5)	4.7 (4.3)	6.5 (3.8)	5.7 (5.2)	7.2 (4.2)

NOTE: AN = anorexia nervosa; ANr = anorexia nervosa restricting type; ANbp = anorexia nervosa binge/purge type; BN = bulimia nervosa; BED = binge-eating disorder; EDNOS = eating disorder not otherwise specified; OP = outpatients; EmE = emotional eating; ExE = external eating; RE = restrained eating; PPV = positive predictive value; NPV = negative predictive value; EDI-2 = Eating Disorder Inventory–2; DEBQ = Dutch Eating Behaviors Questionnaire; SCL-90 = Symptom Checklist–90; BULIT-R = Bulimia Test–Revised; EAT-26 = Eating Attitudes Test–26; RSES = Rosenberg Self-Esteem Scale; CESD = Center for Epidemiologic Studies Depression Scale.

a. Garner (2004).

b. García-García, Vázquez-Velásquez, López-Albarenga, and Arcila-Martínez (2003).

c. Nevonen, Mark, Levin, Lindström, and Paulson-Karlsson (2006).

d. Nevonen, Clinton, and Norring (2006).

Test-Retest Reliability. Test-retest correlations ranged from $r = .67$ to $r = .82$ for all EDI-2 scales over a 16-week interval (Tasca et al., 2003). Test-retest reliability coefficients for the EDI-3 were excellent across scales, ranging from .93 to .98, but are only available in a small clinical sample (Cumella, 2006). Test-retest reliability for the EDI-3 Eating Disorder Risk and General Psychological Maladjustment Composites were .98 and .97, respectively (Garner, 2004).

Validity

Concurrent Validity. Correlations with six alternate reliable and valid measures of eating disorder behaviors and issues suggest acceptable convergent validity. The EDI-3's Eating Disorder Risk, Drive for Thinness, and Body Dissatisfaction scales are highly correlated (.96 and .97, respectively) with their EDI-2 counterparts for both the U.S. adult and adolescent clinical samples. The Professional Manual shows the EDI-3's relationships with a broad range of external instruments (Garner, 2004). These data are summarized in Table 11.8.

Predictive Validity. Data on the predictive validity of the EDI-3 were not provided in the EDI-3 manual; however, Weber, Davis, and McPhie (2006) found that the EDI-3 was sensitive to change in a group of women receiving treatment in a rural region of New South Wales. Similarly, all EDI-2 scales except for Ineffectiveness, Impulse Regulation, and Social Insecurity were significantly different following treatment in a sample of Swedish women (Nevonen, Mark, Levin, Lindström, & Paulson-Karlsson, 2006). The EDI-2 successfully discriminated between Mexican women with and without eating disorders (García-García, Vázquez-Velásquez, López-Albarenga, & Arcila-Martínez, 2003). Sensitivity, specificity, and predictive value are summarized in Table 11.8.

Discriminant Validity. Correlations with the Symptom Checklist–90 (Derogatis, 1977) and Millon Clinical Multiaxial Inventory–II (Millon,

1987) indicate reasonable discriminant validity for most subscales and composite scales. The Professional Manual for the EDI-3 shows its relationship to a broad range of external instruments (Garner, 2004). As hypothesized, Tasca et al. (2003) found a significantly larger correlation between the EDI eating disorder symptoms factor and the EDE-Q ($r = .59$) than with the Personality Assessment Inventory (PAI; Morey, 1991; $r = .37$). Similarly, the EDI personality traits factor had a significantly great correlation with the PAI ($r = .74$) than with the EDE-Q ($r = .33$), suggesting that the EDI factors appear to measure the intended constructs for those with BED (Tasca et al., 2003).

Availability of Measure and Related Costs

The EDI-3 can be obtained from Psychological Assessment Resources, Inc., 16204 North Florida Avenue, Lutz, FL 33549. At the time of publication, the EDI-3 SP (an unlimited-use computer-based scoring program that is also compatible with EDI-2 scores) was available for Windows for $270.00, the EDI-3 Introductory Kit (which includes the Professional Manual, Referral Form Manual, 25 Item Booklets, 25 Answer Sheets, 25 Percentile/ *T*-Score Profile Forms, 25 Symptom Checklists, and 25 Referral Forms) was available for $272.00, the EDI-3 Professional Manual was available for $68.00, a package of 25 EDI-3 Item Booklets was available for $42.00, a package of 25 EDI-3 Answer Sheets was available for $52.00, a package of 25 EDI-3 Percentile/ *T*-Score Profile Forms was available for $31.00, and a package of 25 EDI-3 Symptom Checklists was available for $44.00. These products can be purchased from the PAR, Inc. Web site: http://www3.parinc.com/products/product .aspx?Productid=EDI-3.

Special Issues/Considerations/ Pros and Cons

It should be noted that the Bulimia subscale of the EDI is not a diagnostic measure of the disorder.

Susceptibility to Dissimulation. As noted previously, one problem with self-report inventories is the risk that subjects can magnify or minimize symptom reports. The EDI is susceptible to this type of biased report.

Practicality. The EDI and its revisions are easy to administer and score; the EDI-3 can be completed in about 20 minutes. These instruments assess a wide range of problematic eating-related attitudes and behaviors and have good psychometric properties. For these reasons, the EDI family of instruments is used widely in both research and treatment contexts (Anderson & Paulosky, 2004a, 2004b).

While the EDI and its revisions can be used as a screening instrument to detect at-risk populations, there are briefer measures available for this purpose. Garner (2004) asserts that the EDI-3 is not intended as a diagnostic tool, but the EDI and its revisions appear to be useful in the context of assessing treatment outcome (Garner, 2004; Nevonen, Mark, et al., 2006), for generating treatment plans (Garner, 2004), and as a general measure of eating-related pathology.

Bulimia Test–Revised

The Bulimia Test was first published in 1984 by Smith and Thelen as a self-report questionnaire designed to assess bulimic symptoms and to screen for *DSM-III* (APA, 1980) bulimia nervosa. In 1991, the Bulimia Test–Revised (BULIT-R; Thelen, Farmer, Wonderlich, & Smith, 1991) was published in response to the alterations made to the criteria for bulimia nervosa in the *DSM-III-R* (APA, 1987). After the publication of the *DSM-IV* (APA, 1994), the BULIT-R was reevaluated to assess its utility as a screening tool and symptom measure based on the newest definitional criteria (Thelen, Mintz, & Vander Wal, 1996). Because the measure performed well, it remained in its revised 36-item, 5-point multiple-choice form. Total scores range from 28 to 140 and are calculated by summing 28 of the items,

18 of which are reverse scored. In addition to its English form, there are Korean (Ryu, Lyle, Galer-Unti, & Black, 1999) and Icelandic (Jonsdottir, Thornorsteinsdottir, & Smari, 2005) versions of the BULIT-R. Psychometric data for the BULIT-R are summarized in Table 11.9.

Reliability

Internal Consistency. Internal consistency for the BULIT-R is very high (α = .97–.98; Thelen et al., 1991; Thelen et al., 1996). Several researchers have investigated the internal consistency of the BULIT-R across ethnic groups; their findings are summarized in Table 11.9. In addition, Fernandez, Malcarne, Wilfley, and McQuaid (2006) performed factor analyses of the BULIT-R on samples of African American, White, Asian American, and Latino American women, finding differing six-factor solutions for each group. None of the solutions matched the five-factor solution originally posited by Thelen et al. (1991). In another study, men and women were found to share the same four-factor solution, which also differed from the original five factors (Boerner, Spillane, Anderson, & Smith, 2004). In addition, McCarthy, Simmons, Smith, Tomlinson, and Hill (2002) found a one-factor model fit both female and male adolescents very well.

Test-Retest Reliability. Researchers (Brelsford, Hummel, & Barrios, 1992; Thelen, et al., 1991) have found the BULIT-R to have very good test-retest reliability, as displayed in Table 11.9.

Validity

Concurrent Validity. Studies have found the BULIT-R to correlate highly with other measures of general eating pathology, bulimic symptoms, restraint, and disinhibition (see Table 11.9; Boerner et al., 2004; Brelsford, Hummel, & Barrios, 1992; Rogers & Petrie, 2001; Welch, Thompson, & Hall, 1993).

Predictive Validity. The clinical cutoff score of 104 for a probable diagnosis of bulimia nervosa is

Table 11.9   BULIT-R: Summary of Psychometric Data

A. Reliability

Internal Consistency

Ethnicity	Cronbach's Alpha	Gender	Cronbach's Alpha
Caucasian	.95[a]	Women	.94–.98[b–d]
African American	.90[e]/.92[a]	Men	.90[d]
Asian American	.93[a]		
Latino American	.92–.94[a,e]		

Test-Retest Reliability

Testing Interval	Pearson's r	Sample Size
2 months[c]	.95	98
4–6 weeks[g]	.83	39

B. Validity

Concurrent Validity

Measure	r With BULIT-R	Behavior	r With BULIT-R
EAT-40	.70[d]/.76[h]	Binge-eating frequency	.65[g]
TFEQ Disinhibition	.71[d]	Purging frequency	.60[g]
RS	.69[d]		
BITE	.90[i]		

Predictive Validity[b]

Sensitivity/specificity	.91/.98	Positive predictive value	.81
False-negative/false-positive rate	.08/.04	Negative predictive value	.98

Discriminant Validity

r with Beck Depression Inventory = .48[i]	r with body mass index = .16[h]

C. Norms

Group	M	SD	Sample Size
Bulimia nervosa	117.95[c]/118.08[c]/119.26[b]	NA	21/23/23
EDNOS	91.00[b]	NA	21
Control	45.63[b]	NA	103

Group	M	SD	Sample Size
Nonclinical	57.50[c]/59.62[c]/63.86[d]	NA/NA/21.09	100/157/215
Caucasian	54.64[a]	20.68	1,463
African Americans	50.08[a]	17.72	192
Latino Americans	52.54[a]	18.59	632
Asian Americans	51.80[a]	18.31	384
Men	55.11[d]	15.71	214

NOTE: Statistics are from all female samples unless otherwise stated. NA = none available; BITE = Bulimia Investigatory Test, Edinburgh; EAT = Eating Attitudes Test; EDNOS = eating disorders not otherwise specified; TFEQ = Three-Factor Eating Questionnaire; RS = Restraint Scale; BULIT-R = Bulimia Test–Revised.

a. Fernandez, Malcarne, Wilfley, and McQuaid (2006).

b. Thelen, Mintz, and Vander Wal (1996).

c. Thelen, Farmer, Wonderlich, and Smith (1991).

d. Boerner, Spillane, Anderson, and Smith (2004).

e. Lester and Petrie (1998).

f. Joiner and Kashubeck (1996).

g. Brelsford, Hummel, and Barrios (1992).

h. Rogers and Petrie (2001).

i. Welch, Thompson, and Hall (1993).

j. Friedman and Whisman (1998).

highly sensitive at a value of .91 and specific at a value of .96 for detecting *DSM-IV* bulimia nervosa (see Table 11.9; Thelen et al., 1996). It is also sensitive to therapeutic change, as demonstrated by a reduction in total scores after an 8-week trial of sertraline in 18 women with bulimia nervosa (Sloan, Mizes, Helbok, & Muck, 2004).

Discriminant Validity. Rogers and Petrie (2001) found the BULIT-R to be weakly correlated with body mass index, and Friedman and Whisman (1998) found it to be moderately correlated with a widely used measure of depression (see Table 11.9).

Norms

Normative data for women from nonclinical populations, controls, women with bulimia nervosa, and women with various eating disorders not otherwise specified, as well as data from men and Caucasian, African American, Asian American, and Latino American women, can be found in Table 11.9.

Availability of Measure and Related Costs

A copy of the BULIT-R has been included as Appendix 11.B at the end of this book.

Special Issues/Considerations/ Pros and Cons

The BULIT-R is a brief self-report measure that can be administered by untrained research assistants. It takes little time to complete, and its directions are easily understood. It is a highly effective screening instrument when using the cutoff score of 104. Due to questions regarding its factor structure, however, only total scores should be interpreted.

Multifactorial Assessment of Eating Disorder Symptoms

The Multifactorial Assessment of Eating Disorder Symptoms (MAEDS; Anderson, Williamson, Duchmann, Gleaves, & Barbin, 1999) was developed as a self-report inventory to assess the domains of eating disorder symptoms necessary for successful treatment. The MAEDS has 56 items and six subscales: Depression, Binge Eating, Purgative Behavior, Fear of Fatness, Restrictive Eating, and Avoidance of Forbidden Foods, each containing between 7 and 11 items.

Reliability

Internal Consistency. Each of the six subscales of the MAEDS has been shown to be highly internally consistent with coefficient alphas ranging from .85 to .92 (Anderson, et al., 1999), as displayed in Table 11.10.

Test-Retest Reliability. Fifteen inpatients with diagnoses of AN, BN, or EDNOS completed the MAEDS an average of 8 days apart. The correlations of the subscales between the two administrations ranged from .89 to .99 (Anderson, et al., 1999), as displayed in Table 11.10.

Validity

Concurrent/Discriminant Validity. Specific MAEDS scales are highly correlated with other measures of similar constructs such as the BDI, EAT, BULIT-R, EDI-2, and the Goldfarb Fear of Fatness Scale and are not highly correlated with scales that are not theoretically associated with one another. These data are presented in Table 11.10.

Predictive Validity. Martin, Williamson, and Thaw (2000) found the Binge Eating scale of the

MAEDS to differentiate women with full bulimia nervosa–purging subtype from those with subthreshold bulimia nervosa–purging subtype; also, the Avoidance of Forbidden Foods scale differentiated women with full anorexia nervosa–restricting subtype from those with subthreshold anorexia nervosa–restricting subtype. In addition, Reas, Williamson, Martin, and Zucker (2000) defined recovery using the MAEDS as no subscale *T* score elevations over 70 and found women defined as recovered from bulimia nervosa using the MAEDS to have significantly lower EAT and BDI scores at 9-year follow-up compared to initial assessment.

Norms

Norms collected by Martin et al. (2000) for women with bulimia nervosa–purging subtype, anorexia nervosa–binge/purge subtype and restricting subtype, and binge-eating disorder are presented in Table 11.10. Unpublished norms developed by the first author are also presented in Table 11.10.

Availability of Measure and Related Costs

A copy of the MAEDS is included in Appendix 11.E at the end of this book.

Special Issues/Considerations/ Pros and Cons

Although the MAEDS is somewhat longer than other self-report questionnaires measuring eating pathology, it provides more information than a unidimensional total summed score of general eating pathology. Six major domains of eating and associated pathology are assessed and can be individually interpreted using the MAEDS. It has also been shown to be sensitive to changes in symptoms and may be ideally suited for the purposes of tracking progress and evaluating recovery.

Table 11.10   MAEDS: Summary of Psychometric Data

A. Reliability[a]

Subscale	Internal Consistency: Cronbach's Alpha	Test-Retest Reliability: Pearson's r
Depression	.90	.90
Binge eating	.92	.89
Purgative behavior	.80	.99
Fear of fatness	.90	.93
Restrictive eating	.85	.96
Avoidance of forbidden foods	.87	.94

B. Validity

	Concurrent/Discriminant Validity: Pearson's r[a]					
	Binge Eating	Purgative Behavior	Avoidance of Forbidden Foods	Restrictive Eating	Fear of Fatness	Depression
BDI	.58	.42	.06	.35	.56	.84
EAT	.49	.45	.42	.51	.78	.44
BULIT-R	.86	.38	.19	.37	.77	.61
GFFS	.62	.42	.45	.48	.86	.58
EDI-2						
DT	.51	.37	.42	.48	.84	.49
BUL	.69	.28	.03	.18	.57	.51
BD	.70	.20	.32	.31	.66	.55

C. Norms[b]

	Binge Eating	Purgative Behavior	Avoidance of Forbidden Foods	Restrictive Eating	Fear of Fatness	Depression
	M (SD)	M (SD)	M (SD)	M (SD)	M (SD)	M (SD)
BNp (n = 35)	68.86 (12.98)	80.17 (13.04)	55.59 (11.64)	67.64 (13.72)	61.94 (9.22)	67.15 (12.78)
ANbp (n = 16)	51.22 (14.01)	74.19 (19.47)	64.69 (13.24)	70.08 (17.36)	61.31 (9.11)	67.69 (13.69)

(Continued)

Table 11.10 (Continued)

	Binge Eating	Purgative Behavior	Avoidance of Forbidden Foods	Restrictive Eating	Fear of Fatness	Depression
	M (SD)	M (SD)	M (SD)	M (SD)	M (SD)	M (SD)
ANr (n = 18)	42.50 (6.63)	53.36 (12.40)	63.41 (10.12)	67.23 (16.15)	59.41 (7.42)	63.13 (13.92)
BED (n = 17)	73.41 (6.53)	51.69 (13.70)	45.83 (9.25)	52.66 (8.94)	55.59 (10.18)	66.00 (10.66)

NOTE: BNp = bulimia nervosa–purging subtype; ANbp = anorexia nervosa–binge/purge subtype; ANr = anorexia nervosa–restricting subtype; BED = binge-eating disorder; BDI = Beck Depression Inventory; EAT = Eating Attitudes Test; BULIT-R = Bulimia Test–Revised; GFFS = Goldfarb Fear of Fatness Scale; EDI-2 = Eating Disorders Inventory, 2nd Edition; DT = Drive for Thinness subscale; BUL = Bulimia subscale; BD = Body Dissatisfaction subscale.

a. Anderson, Williamson, Duchmann, Gleaves, and Barbin (1999).

b. Martin, Williamson, and Thaw (2000).

Bulimia Investigatory Test, Edinburgh

The Bulimia Investigatory Test, Edinburgh (BITE; Henderson & Freeman, 1987) is a 33-item self-report questionnaire developed to assess attitudes and behaviors associated with bulimia nervosa as well as the severity of these behaviors, as measured by the frequency of binge eating and purging. Individuals are directed to answer the questions on the BITE in regards to their feelings and behaviors over the past 3 months. Thirty items assess symptoms, behavior, and dieting, and these items compose the Symptom subscale with a maximum score of 30. Six items measure the severity of disordered eating behavior by assessing its frequency. These items make up the Severity subscale and have a maximum score of 39. A clinical cutoff score of 20 or more on the Symptom scale is considered to be indicative of a probable DSM-III (APA, 1980) bulimia diagnosis. A cutoff score of 5 on the Severity scale and a total score of 25 indicate clinically significant symptoms. In addition to the 33 items comprising the BITE, a supplementary page of 16 optional items may be administered that assess demographic information, weight history, ideal weight, weight perception, eating patterns, and eating disorder history.

Reliability

Internal Consistency. The Symptom scale of the BITE has been found to have very good internal consistency, while the Severity scale has only moderately good internal consistency, as shown in Table 11.11 (Henderson & Freeman, 1987).

Test-Retest Reliability. The test-retest reliability for the BITE is adequate; Henderson and Freeman (1987) tested a group of controls 1 week apart and a group of women with DSM-III (APA, 1980) bulimia 15 weeks apart and found scores on the measure to be relatively stable for the time intervals elapsed (see Table 11.11).

Validity

Concurrent Validity. Henderson and Freeman (1987) found the BITE to correlate highly with other measures of eating pathology, including the Eating Attitudes Test and the Eating Disorders Inventory Drive for Thinness and

Table 11.11 BITE: Summary of Psychometric Data

A. Reliability[a]

Internal Consistency
Coefficient alpha = .96 for Symptom subscale
Coefficient alpha = .62 for Severity subscale

Test-Retest Reliability

Groups	Interval Between Testing	r	Sample Size
Controls	At least 1 week	.86	30
Bulimics	15 weeks	.68	10

B. Validity

Concurrent/Discriminant Validity	
Measure	r *With BITE*
EAT	.70[a]
EDI Drive for Thinness	.59[a]
EDI Bulimia	.68[a]
EDI Perfectionism	.14[a]
EDI Interpersonal Distrust	.23[a]
BDI	.39[b]
STAI State/Trait	.35[e]/.43[b]

Predictive Validity[c]			
Sensitivity/specificity	1.00/.96	Positive predictive value	.93
False-negative/false-positive rate	0.00/.04	Negative predictive value	1.00

C. Norms

	Symptom		Severity		Total	
	M (SD)	n	M (SD)	n	M (SD)	n
Nonclinical	7.55 (7.40)	63[d]	2.20 (3.05)	63[d]	9.75 (10.1)	63[d]
Nonclinical					9.33 (7.81)	61[e]
Nonclinical					8.54 (7.97)	125[f]
Controls	2.94 (2.94)	32[a]	.44 (.29)	32[a]	5.7 (3.3)	25[g]

(Continued)

Table 11.11 (Continued)

	Symptom		Severity		Total	
	M (SD)	n	M (SD)	n	M (SD)	n
Men					3.99 (3.33)	125[f]
Anorexia nervosa	14.1 (8.0)	134[h]			23.5 (9.7)	21[i]
Anorexia nervosa					19.9 (9.0)	21[g]
Bulimia nervosa	26.03 (2.25)	32[a]	10.16 (3.63)	32[a]	36.19 (4.47)	32[a]
Bulimia nervosa	23.6 (4.9)	198[h]			38.2 (7.6)	21[i]
Bulimia nervosa					36.6 (7.6)	32[g]
Binge-eating disorder					34.0 (8.5)	14[g]

NOTE: EAT = Eating Attitudes Test; EDI = Eating Disorders Inventory; STAI = State-Trait Anxiety Inventory; BDI = Beck Depression Inventory.

a. Henderson and Freeman (1987).

b. Ricca et al. (2000).

c. Freeman and Henderson (1988).

d. Calam and Waller (1998).

e. Meyer, Leung, Feary, and Mann (2001).

f. Meyer et al. (2005).

g. Monteleone, Di Lieto, Tortorella, Longobardi, and Maj (2000).

h. Bussolotti et al. (2002).

i. Maes et al. (2001).

Bulimia subscales (see Table 11.11). Freeman and Henderson (1988) evaluated the sensitivity and specificity of the BITE in a sample of 1,333 students (53% female) and found the measure to perform very well at the task of identifying eating disorders, as displayed in Table 11.11.

Predictive Validity. No data on predictive validity are available.

Discriminant Validity. Researchers (Henderson & Freeman, 1987; Ricca et al., 2000) found that the BITE has moderate to low correlations with unrelated measures such as the BDI, State-Trait Anxiety Inventory (Spielberger, 1968), and EDI

Perfectionism and Interpersonal Distrust subscales (see Table 11.11).

Norms

The BITE has been in use for nearly two decades and has been administered to a variety of populations. Norms for the total scale score and symptom and severity scales are presented in Table 11.11.

Availability of Measure and Related Costs

A copy of the BITE can be found in Appendix 11.A at the end of this book. Spanish (Moya, Bersabe, &

Jimenez, 2004), Hungarian (Resch, 2003), and Italian (Orlandi, Mannucci, Cuzzolaro, & SISDCA–Study Group on Psychometrics, 2005) versions of the BITE have also been developed.

Special Issues/Considerations/ Pros and Cons

The BITE is a brief self-report measure that can be administered by untrained individuals. It is best used as a screening tool for probable bulimia nervosa. Because it was developed to reflect *DSM-III* (APA, 1980) criteria, the content and wording of some questions may be somewhat dated. However, it appears to still be useful as an assessment instrument.

Suggestions for Future Research/Comments

As noted earlier in this chapter, a recent review of the assessment literature (Anderson & Paulosky, 2004a) and a survey of clinicians (Anderson & Paulosky, 2004b) found that relatively few assessment measures appear to be used in the eating disorders field. As Anderson and Paulosky (2004a) note, this can be considered both a strength and a weakness. The use of a small number of instruments allows for direct comparisons of treatment effectiveness across research studies, which is an improvement over the situation described in the first edition of this text (Williamson, Anderson, Jackman, & Jackson, 1995). However, the reliance on only a few measures has also led to a situation where not all the domains thought to be central to the maintenance of eating disorders are routinely assessed (e.g., Anderson & Maloney, 2001). Thus, improvements in current assessment instruments and/or the development of more comprehensive assessment batteries may broaden our understanding of the critical factors associated with the development and treatment of eating disorders.

Also, technological advances such as pagers, palmtop computers, personal data assistants, mobile phones, and other text-messaging devices have allowed for the assessment of behavior and psychological states in the natural environment, a procedure known as ecological momentary assessment (EMA; Stone & Shiffman, 1994). At the present time, EMA is still primarily a method of administration rather than a specific assessment protocol, program, or measure, although such protocols and measures undoubtedly will be developed and disseminated in the future. Finally, as noted earlier in this chapter, there have been important questions raised about the presumed superiority of interviews over self-report inventories in the assessment of eating disorders and related constructs, and research is needed to investigate the systematic differences in response rates found between these assessment modalities (Anderson & Maloney, 2001; Anderson et al., 2007; French et al., 1998; Keel et al., 2002).

References

American Psychiatric Association. (1980). *Diagnostic and statistical manual of mental disorders* (3rd ed.). Washington, DC: Author.

American Psychiatric Association. (1987). *Diagnostic and statistical manual of mental disorders* (3rd ed., rev.). Washington, DC: Author.

American Psychiatric Association. (1994). *Diagnostic and statistical manual of mental disorders* (4th ed.). Washington, DC: Author.

American Psychiatric Association. (2000). *Diagnostic and statistical manual of mental disorders* (4th ed., text revision). Washington, DC: Author.

Anderson, D. A., Lavender, J. M., Milnes, S. M. & Simmons, A. M. (2009). Assessment of eating disturbances in children and adolescents. In J. K. Thompson & L. Smolak (Eds.), *Body image, eating disorders, and obesity in youth* (2nd ed., pp. 193–213). Washington, DC: American Psychological Association.

Anderson, D. A., Lundgren, J. D., Shapiro, J. R., & Paulosky, C. A. (2004). Clinical assessment of eating disorders: Review and recommendations. *Behavior Modification, 28,* 763–782.

Anderson, D. A., & Maloney, K. C. (2001). The efficacy of cognitive-behavioral therapy on the core symptoms of bulimia nervosa. *Clinical Psychology Review, 21,* 971–988.

Anderson, D. A., & Paulosky, C. A. (2004a). Psychological assessment of eating disorders and related features. In J. K. Thompson (Ed.), *Handbook of eating disorders and obesity* (pp. 112–129). New York: John Wiley.

Anderson, D. A., & Paulosky, C. A. (2004b). A survey of the use of assessment instruments by eating disorder professionals in clinical practice. *Eating and Weight Disorders, 9,* 238–241.

Anderson, D. A., Simmons, A. M., Martens, M. P., Ferrier, A. G., & Sheehy, M. J. (2006). The relationship between disordered eating behavior and drinking motives in college-age women. *Eating Behaviors, 7,* 419–422.

Anderson, D. A., Simmons, A. M., Milnes, S., M., & Earleywine, M. (2007). The effect of response format on endorsement of eating disordered attitudes and behaviors. *International Journal of Eating Disorders, 40,* 90–93.

Anderson, D. A., Williamson, D. A., Duchmann, E. G., Gleaves, D. H., & Barbin, J. M. (1999). Development and validation of a multifactorial treatment outcome measure for eating disorders. *Assessment, 6,* 7–20.

Banasiak, S. J., Wertheim, E. H., Koerner, J., & Voudouris, N. J. (2001). Test-retest reliability and internal consistency of a variety of measures of dietary restraint and body concerns in a sample of adolescent girls. *International Journal of Eating Disorders, 29,* 85–89.

Beck, A. T., Ward, C., Mendelson, J. M., & Erbaugh, J. (1961). An inventory for measuring depression. *Archives of General Psychiatry, 4,* 561–571.

Beglin, S. J., & Fairburn, C. G. (1992). Evaluation of a new instrument for the detection of eating disorders in community samples. *Psychiatry Research, 44,* 191–201.

Bennett, K., & Stevens, R. (1997). The internal structure of the Eating Disorder Inventory. *Health Care for Women International, 18,* 495–504.

Binford, R. B., Le Grange, D., & Jellar, C. C. (2005). Eating Disorders Examination versus Eating Disorders Examination–Questionnaire in adolescents with full and partial-syndrome bulimia nervosa and anorexia nervosa. *International Journal of Eating Disorders, 37*(1), 44–49.

Black, C. M. D., & Wilson, G. T. (1996). Assessment of eating disorders: Interview versus questionnaire. *International Journal of Eating Disorders, 20,* 43–50.

Boerner, L. M., Spillane, N. S., Anderson, K. G., & Smith, G. T. (2004). Similarities and differences between women and men on eating disorder risk factors and symptom measures. *Eating Behaviors, 5,* 209–222.

Brelsford, T. N., Hummel, R. M., & Barrios, B. A. (1992). The Bulimia Test–Revised: A psychometric investigation. *Psychological Assessment, 4,* 399–401.

Brookings, J. B., & Wilson, J. F. (1994). Personality and family-environment predictors of self-reported eating attitudes and behaviors. *Journal of Personality Assessment, 63,* 313–326.

Bussolotti, D., Fernandez-Aranda, F., Solano, R., Jimenez-Murcia, S., Turon, V., & Vallejo, J. (2002). Marital status and eating disorders: An analysis of its relevance. *Journal of Psychosomatic Research, 53,* 1139–1145.

Calam, R., & Waller, G. (1998). Are eating and psychological characteristics in early teenage years useful predictors of eating characteristics in early adulthood? A 7-year longitudinal study. *International Journal of Eating Disorders, 24,* 351–362.

Carter, J. C., Aime, A. A., & Mills, J. S. (2001). Assessment of bulimia nervosa: A comparison of interview and self-report questionnaire methods. *International Journal of Eating Disorders, 30,* 187–192.

Carter, J. C., Steward, D. A., & Fairburn, C. G. (2001). Eating Disorder Examination Questionnaire: Norms for young adolescent girls. *Behavior Research and Therapy, 39,* 625–632.

Castro, J., Toro, J., Salamero, M., & Guimera, E. (1991). The Eating Attitudes Test: Validation of the Spanish version. *Evaluacion Psicologica, 7,* 175–189.

Celio, A. A., Wilfley, D. E., Crow, S. J., Mitchell, J., & Walsh, B. T. (2004). A comparison of the Binge Eating Scale, Questionnaire for Eating and Weight Patterns–Revised, and Eating Disorder Examination Questionnaire with Instructions with the Eating Disorder Examination in the assessment of binge eating disorder and its symptoms. *International Journal of Eating Disorders, 36,* 434–444.

Choudry, I. Y., & Mumford, D. B. (1992). A pilot study of eating disorders in Mirpur (Pakistan) using an Urdu version of the Eating Attitudes Test. *International Journal of Eating Disorders, 11,* 243–251.

Cooper, P. J., Taylor, M. J., Cooper, Z., & Fairburn, C. G. (1987). The development and validation of the Body Shape Questionnaire. *International Journal of Eating Disorders, 6,* 485–494.

Cooper, Z., Cooper, P. J., & Fairburn, C. G. (1989). The validity of the Eating Disorder Examination and its subscales. *British Journal of Psychiatry, 154,* 807–812.

Cooper, Z., & Fairburn, C. G. (1987). The Eating Disorder Examination: A semi-structured interview for the assessment of the specific psychopathology of eating disorders. *International Journal of Eating Disorders, 6,* 1–8.

Cotton, M., Ball, C., & Robinson, P. (2003). Four simple questions can help screen for eating disorders. *Journal of General Internal Medicine, 18,* 53–56.

Crow, S. J., Agras, W. S., Halmi, K., Mitchell, J. E., & Kraemer, H. C. (2002). Full syndrome versus subthreshold anorexia nervosa, bulimia nervosa, and binge eating disorder: A multicenter study. *International Journal of Eating Disorders, 32,* 309–318.

Cumella, E. J. (2006). Review of the Eating Disorder Inventory–3. *Journal of Personality Assessment, 87,* 116–117.

Cuzzolaro, M., & Petrilli, A. (1988). Validazione della versione italiana dell'EAT 40 [Validation of the Italian version of EAT 40]. *Psichiatria dell'infanzia e dell'Adolescenza, 55,* 209–217.

Derogatis, L. R. (1977). *The SCL-90 manual: Scoring, administration, and procedures for the SCL-90.* Towson, MD: Clinical Psychometric Research.

Derogatis, L. R., Rickels, K., & Rock, A. F. (1976). The SCL-90 and the MMPI: A step in the validation of new self-report scale. *British Journal of Psychiatry, 128,* 280–289.

Dohrenwend, B. P., Shrout, P. E., Egri, G., & Mendelson, F. S. (1980). Nonspecific psychological distress and other dimensions of psychopathology. *Archives of General Psychiatry, 37,* 1129–1236.

Elal, G., Altug, A., Slade, P., & Tekcan, A. (2000). Factor structure of the Eating Attitudes Test (EAT) in a Turkish university sample. *Eating and Weight Disorders, 5,* 46–50.

Elder, K. A., & Grilo, C. M. (2007). The Spanish language version of the Eating Disorder Examination Questionnaire: Comparison with the Spanish language version of the eating disorder examination and test-retest reliability. *Behaviour Research and Therapy, 145,* 1369–1377.

Fairburn, C. G., & Beglin, S. J. (1994). Assessment of eating disorders: Interview or self-report questionnaire? *International Journal of Eating Disorders, 16,* 363–370.

Fairburn, C. G., & Beglin, S. (2008). Eating Disorder Examination Questionnaire (EDE-Q 6.0). In C. G. Fairburn (Ed.), *Cognitive behavior therapy and eating disorders* (pp. 309–313). New York: Guilford.

Fairburn, C. G., & Cooper, Z. (1993). The Eating Disorder Examination (12th ed.). In C. G. Fairburn & G. T. Wilson (Eds.), *Binge eating: Nature, assessment, and treatment* (pp. 317–360). New York: Guilford.

Fairburn, C. G., Cooper, Z., & O'Connor, M. E. (2008). Eating Disorder Examination (Edition 16.0D). In C. G. Fairburn (Ed.), *Cognitive behavior therapy and eating disorders* (pp. 265–308). New York: Guilford.

Feighner, J. P., Robins, E., Guze, S. B., Woodruff, R. A., Winokru, G., & Munoz, R. (1972). Diagnostic criteria for use in psychiatric research. *Archives of General Psychiatry, 26,* 57–63.

Fernandez, S., Malcarne, V. L., Wilfley, D. E., & McQuaid, J. (2006). Factor structure of the Bulimia Test–Revised in college women from four ethnic groups. *Cultural Diversity and Ethnic Minority Psychology, 12,* 403–419.

Fichter, M. M., Elton, M., Engel, K., Meyer, A., Mall, H., & Poustka, F. (1991). Structured Interview for Anorexia and Bulimia Nervosa (SIAB): Development of a new instrument for the assessment of eating disorders. *International Journal of Eating Disorders, 10,* 571–592.

Fichter, M. M., Herpertz, S., Quadflieg, N., & Herpertz-Dahlmann, B. (1998). Structured Interview for Anorexic and Bulimic Disorders for *DSM-IV* and *ICD-10:* Updated (third) revision. *International Journal of Eating Disorders, 24,* 227–249.

Fichter, M. M., & Keeser, W. (1980). Das Anorexia-nervosa-Inventar zur Selbstbeurteilung (ANIS) [The Anorexia Nervosa Inventory for Self-Rating (ANIS)]. *Archiv für Psychiatrie und Nervenkrankheiten, 228,* 67–89.

Fichter, M. & Quadflieg, N. (1999). SIAB Professional Manual: Structured Inventory for Anorexic and Bulimic Eating Disorders (SIAB). Questionnaire (SIAB-S) and Expert-rating (SIAB-EX) according to DSM-IV and ICD-10. Retrieved August 28, 2007, from http://www.epi.med.uni-muenchen.de/

Fichter, M. M., & Quadflieg, N. (2001). The structured interview for anorexic and bulimic disorders for DSM-IV and ICD-10 (SIAB-EX): Reliability and validity. *European Psychiatry, 16,* 38-48.

First, M. B., Spitzer, R. L., Gibbon, M., & Williams, J. B. W. (1997). *Structured clinical interview for*

DSM-IV-TR Axis I disorders, Research Version, Patient Edition (SCID-I/P). New York: Biometrics Research, New York State Psychiatric Institute.

Freeman, C. P., & Henderson, M. (1988). The BITE: Indices of agreement. *British Journal of Psychiatry, 152,* 575–577.

French, S. A., Peterson, C. B., Story, M., Anderson, N, Mussell, M. P., & Mitchell, J. E. (1998). Agreement between survey and interview measures of weight control practices in adolescents. *International Journal of Eating Disorders, 23,* 45–56.

Friedman, M. A., & Whisman, M. A. (1998). Sociotropy, autonomy, and bulimic symptomatology. *International Journal of Eating Disorders, 23,* 439–442.

Garcia-Campayo, J., Sanz-Carillo, C., Ibañez, L. S., Solano, V., & Alda, M. (2005). Validation of the Spanish version of the SCOFF questionnaire for the screening of eating disorders in primary care. *Journal of Psychometric Research, 59,* 51–55.

García-García, E., Vázquez-Velásquez, V., López-Albarenga, J. C., & Arcila-Martínez, D. (2003). Validez interna y utilidad diagnóstica del Eating Disorders Inventory en mujeres mexicanas [Internal validity and diagnostic utility of the Eating Disorders Inventory in Mexican women.]. *Salud Pública de México, 45,* 206–210.

Garfinkel, P. E., & Garner, D. M. (1982). *Anorexia nervosa: A multidimensional perspective.* New York: Brunner/Mazel.

Garfinkel, P. E., & Newman, A. (2001). The eating attitudes test: Twenty-five years later. *Eating and Weight Disorders, 6,* 1–24.

Garner, D. M. (1991). *Eating Disorder Inventory–2 professional manual.* Odessa, FL: Psychological Assessment Resources.

Garner, D. M. (2004). *EDI-3 Eating Disorder Inventory–3 professional manual.* Odessa, FL: Psychological Assessment Resources.

Garner, D. M., & Garfinkel, P. E. (1979). The Eating Attitudes Test: An index of the symptoms of anorexia nervosa. *Psychological Medicine, 9,* 273–279.

Garner, D. M., & Garfinkel, P. E. (1982). *Anorexia nervosa: A multidimensional perspective.* New York: Brunner/Mazel.

Garner, D. M., Olmsted, M. P., Bohr, Y., & Garfinkel, P. E. (1982). The Eating Attitudes Test: Psychometric features and clinical correlates. *Psychological Medicine, 12,* 871–878.

Garner, D. M., Olmstead, M. P., & Polivy, J. (1983). Development and validation of a multidimensional eating disorder inventory of anorexia nervosa and bulimia. *International Journal of Eating Disorders, 2,* 14–34.

Ghaderi, A., & Scott, B. (2004). The reliability and validity of the Swedish version of the Body Shape Questionnaire. *Scandinavian Journal of Psychology, 45,* 319–324.

Goldfein, J. A., Devlin, M. J., & Kamenetz, C. (2005). Eating Disorder Examination–Questionnaire with and without instruction to assess binge eating in patients with binge eating disorder. *International Journal of Eating Disorders, 37,* 107–111.

Gormally, J., Black, S., Daston, S., & Rardin, D. (1982). The assessment of binge eating severity among obese persons. *Addictive Behaviors, 7,* 47–55.

Grilo, C. M., Lozano, C., & Elder, K. A. (2005). Inter-rater and test-retest reliability of the Spanish language version of the eating disorder examination interview: Clinical and research implications. *Journal of Psychiatric Practice, 11,* 231–240.

Grilo, C. M., Masheb, R. M., Lozano-Blanco, C., & Barry, D. T. (2004). Reliability of the Eating Disorder Examination in patients with binge eating disorder. *International Journal of Eating Disorders, 35,* 80–85.

Grilo, C. M., Masheb, R. M., & Wilson, G. T. (2001). A comparison of different methods for assessing the features of eating disorders in patients with binge eating disorder. *Journal of Consulting and Clinical Psychology, 69,* 317–322.

Gross, J., Rosen, J. C., Leitenberg, H., & Willmuth, M. E. (1986). Validity of the eating attitudes test and the eating disorders inventory in bulimia nervosa. *Journal of Consulting and Clinical Psychology, 54,* 875–876.

Henderson, M., & Freeman, C. P. (1987). A self-rating scale for bulimia: The 'BITE.' *British Journal of Psychiatry, 150,* 18–24.

Holtkamp, K., Hebebrand, J., & Herpertz-Dahlmann, B. (2004). The contribution of anxiety and food restriction on physical activity levels in acute anorexia nervosa. *International Journal of Eating Disorders, 36,* 163–171.

Joiner, G. W., & Kashubeck, S. (1996). Acculteration, body image, self-esteem, and eating-disorder symptomatology in adolescent Mexican American women. *Psychology of Women Quarterly, 20,* 419–435.

Jonsdottir, S. M., Thornorsteinsdottir, G., & Smari, J. (2005). Reliability and validity of the Icelandic version of the Bulimia Test–Revised (BULIT-R) [in Icelandic]. *Laeknabladid, 91,* 923–928.

Kalarchian, M. A., Wilson, G. T., Brolin, R. E., & Bradley, L. (2000). Assessment of eating disorders in bariaric surgery candidates: Self report questionnaire versus interview. *International Journal of Eating Disorder, 28,* 465–459.

Keel, P. K., Crow, S., Davis, T. L., & Mitchell, J. E. (2002). Assessment of eating disorders: Comparison of interview and questionnaire data from a long-term follow-up study of bulimia nervosa. *Journal of Psychosomatic Research, 53,* 1043–1047.

Ko, C., & Cohen, H. (1998). Intraethnic comparison of eating attitudes in native Korean and Korean American using a Korean translation of the eating attitudes test. *Journal of Nervous and Mental Disease, 186,* 631–636.

Koslowsky, M., Scheinberg, Z., Bleich, A., Mark, M., Apter, A., Danon, Y., et al. (1992). The factor structure and criterion validity of the short form of the Eating Attitudes Test. *Journal of Personality Assessment, 58,* 27–35.

Kutlesic, V., Williamson, D. A., Gleaves, D. H., Barbin, J. M., & Murphy-Eberenz, K. P. (1998). The Interview for the Diagnosis of Eating Disorders–IV: Application to *DSM-IV* diagnostic criteria. *Psychological Assessment, 10,* 41–48.

Leichner, P., Steiger, H., Puentes-Neuman, G., Perreault, M., & Gottheil, N. (1994). Validation of the Eating Attitudes Test (EAT-26) in a French-speaking population of Quebec. *Canadian Journal of Psychiatry, 39,* 49–54.

Lester, R., & Petrie, T. A. (1998). Physical, psychological, and societal correlates of bulimic symptomatology among African American college women. *Journal of Counseling Psychology, 45,* 315–321.

Luce, K. H., & Crowther, J. H. (1999). The reliability of the Eating Disorder Examination—self-report questionnaire version (EDE-Q). *International Journal of Eating Disorders, 25,* 349–351.

Luck, A. J., Morgan, J. F., Reid, F., O'Brien, A., Brunton, J., Price, C., et al. (2002). The SCOFF questionnaire and clinical interview for eating disorders in general practice: Comparative study. *British Medical Journal, 325,* 755–756.

Maes, M., Monteleone, P., Bencivenga, R., Goossens, F., Maj, M., van West, D., et al. (2001). Lower serum activity of prolyl endopeptidase in anorexia and bulimia nervosa. *Psychoneuroendocrinology, 26,* 17–26.

Maloney, M. J., McGuire, J. B., & Daniels, S. R. (1988). Reliability testing of a children's version of the Eating Attitudes Test. *Journal of the American Academy of Child and Adolescent Psychiatry, 27,* 541–543.

Martin, C. K., Williamson, D. A., & Thaw, J. M. (2000). Criterion validity of the Multiaxial Assessment of Eating Disorders Symptoms. *International Journal of Eating Disorders, 28,* 303–310.

Mazure, C. M., Halmi, K. A., Sunday, S. R., Romano, S. J., & Einhorn, A. M. (1994). The Yale-Brown-Cornell Eating Disorder Scale: Development, use, reliability and validity. *Journal of Psychiatric Research, 28,* 425–445.

McCarthy, D. M., Simmons, J. R., Smith, G. T., Tomlinson, K. L., & Hill, K. K. (2002). Reliability, stability, and factor structure of the Bulimia Test–Revised and Eating Disorder Inventory–2 scales in adolescence. *Assessment, 9,* 382–389.

Meyer, C., Leung, N., Feary, R., & Mann, B. (2001). Core beliefs and bulimic symptomatology in non-eating-disordered women: The mediating role of borderline characteristics. *International Journal of Eating Disorders, 30,* 434–440.

Meyer, C., Leung, N., Waller, G., Perkins, S., Paice, N., & Mitchell, J. (2005). Anger and bulimic psychopathology: Gender differences in a nonclinical group. *International Journal of Eating Disorders, 37,* 69–71.

Miller, J. L., Schmidt, L. A., Vaillancourt, T., McDougall, P., & Laliberte, M. (2006). Neuroticism and introversion: A risky combination for disordered eating among a non-clinical sample of undergraduate women. *Eating Behaviors, 7,* 69–78.

Millon, T. (1987). *Millon Clinical Multiaxial Inventory–II manual.* Bloomington, MN: Pearson Education.

Mintz, L. B., & O'Halloran, M. S. (2000). The Eating Attitudes Test: Validation with *DSM-IV* eating disorder criteria. *Journal of Personality Assessment, 74,* 489–503.

Mintz, L. B., O'Halloran, M. S., Mulholland, A. M., & Schneider, P. A. (1997). Questionnaire for Eating Disorder Diagnosis: Reliability and validity of operationalizing *DSM-IV* criteria into a self-report format. *Journal of Counseling Psychology, 44,* 63–79.

Mond, J. M., Hay, P. J., Rodgers, B., & Owen, C. (2006). Eating Disorder Examination Questionnaire (EDE-Q): Norms for young adult women. *Behaviour Research and Therapy, 44,* 53–62.

Mond, J. M., Hay, P. J., Rodgers, B., Owen, C., & Beumont, P. J. V. (2004a). Temporal stability of the Eating Disorder Examination Questionnaire. *International Journal of Eating Disorders, 36,* 195–203.

Mond, J. M., Hay, P. J., Rodgers, B., Owen, C., & Beumont, P. J. V. (2004b). Validity of the Eating Disorder Examination Questionnaire (EDE-Q) in screening for eating disorders in community samples. *Behaviour Research and Therapy, 42,* 551–567.

Monteleone, P., Di Lieto, A., Tortorella, A., Longobardi, N., & Maj, M. (2000). Circulating leptin in patients with anorexia nervosa, bulimia nervosa or binge-eating disorder: Relationship to body weight, eating patterns, psychopathology and endocrine changes. *Psychiatry Research, 94,* 121–129.

Morey, L. (1991). *Personality Assessment Inventory: Professional manual.* Odessa, FL: Psychological Assessment Resources.

Morgan, J. F., Reid, F., & Lacey, H. (1999). The SCOFF questionnaire: Assessment of a new screening tool for eating disorders. *British Medical Journal, 319,* 1467–1468.

Moya, T. R., Bersabe, R., & Jimenez, M. (2004). Fiabilidad y validez del test de investigacion bulimica de edimburgo (BITE) en una muestra de adolescents espanoles [Reliability and validity of the Bulimic Investigatory Test, Edinburgh (BITE) in a sample of Spanish adolescents.]. *Psicologia Conductual, 12,* 447–461.

Nasser, M. (1986). The validity of the Eating Attitudes Test in a non-Western population. *Acta Psychiatrica Scandinavica, 73,* 109–110.

Neumärker, U., Dudeck, U., Vollrath, M., Neumärker, K. J., & Steinhausen, H. C. (1992). Eating attitudes among adolescent anorexia nervosa patients and normal subjects in former West and East Berlin: A transcultural comparison. *International Journal of Eating Disorders, 12,* 281–289.

Nevonen, L., Clinton, D., & Norring, C. (2006). Validating the EDI-2 in three Swedish female samples: Eating disorders patients, psychiatric outpatients and normal controls. *Nordic Journal of Psychiatry, 60,* 44–50.

Nevonen, L., Mark, M., Levin, B., Lindström, M., & Paulson-Karlsson, G. (2006). Evaluation of a new Internet-based self-help guide for patients with bulimic symptoms in Sweden. *Nordic Journal of Psychiatry, 60,* 463–468.

Noma, S., Nakai, Y., Hamagaki, S., Uehara, M., Hayashi, A., & Hayashi, T. (2006). Comparison between the SCOFF questionnaire and the Eating Attitudes Test in patients with eating disorders. *International Journal of Psychiatry in Clinical Practice, 10,* 27–32.

Nunes, M. A., Camey, S., Olinto, M. T. A., & Mari, J. J. (2005). The validity and 4-year test-retest reliability of the Brazilian version of the Eating Attitudes Test–26. *Brazilian Journal of Medical and Biological Research, 38,* 1655–1662.

Ocker, L. B., Lam, E. T. C., Jensen, B. E., & Zhang, J. J. (2007). Psychometric properties of the Eating Attitudes Test. *Measurement in Physical Education and Exercise Science, 11,* 25–48.

Orlandi, E., Mannucci, E., Cuzzolaro, M., & SISDCA–Study Group on Psychometrics (2005). Bulimic Investigatory Test, Edinburgh (BITE): A validation study of the Italian version. *Eating and Weight Disorders, 10,* e14–e20.

Parker, S. C., Lyons, J., & Bonner, J. (2005). Eating disorders in graduate students: Exploring the SCOFF questionnaire as a simple screening tool. *Journal of American College Health, 54,* 103–107.

Perry, L., Morgan, J., Reid., F., Brunton, J., O'Brien, A., Luck, A., et al. (2002). Screening for symptoms of eating disorders: Reliability of the SCOFF screening tool with written compared to oral delivery. *International Journal of Eating Disorders, 32,* 466–472.

Peterson, C. B., Crosby, R. D., Wonderlich, S. A., Joiner, T., Crow, S. J. Mitchell, J. E., et al. (2007). Psychometric properties of the Eating Disorder Examination–Questionnaire: Factor structure and internal consistency. *International Journal of Eating Disorders, 40,* 386–389.

Reas, D. L., Williamson, D. A., Martin, C. K., & Zucker, N. L. (2000). Duration of illness predicts outcome for bulimia nervosa: A long-term follow-up study. *International Journal of Eating Disorders, 27,* 428–434.

Resch, M. (2003). Employment and effectiveness of the BITE questionnaire in screening for eating disorders [in Hungarian]. *Orvosi hetilap, 144,* 2277–2281.

Ricca, V., Mannucci, E., Moretti, S., Di Bernardo, M., Zucchi, T., Cabras, P. L., et al. (2000). Screening for binge eating disorder in obese outpatients. *Comprehensive Psychiatry, 41,* 111–115.

Rizvi, S. L., Peterson, C. B., Crow, S. G., & Agras, W. S. (2000). Test-retest reliability of the Eating Disorder Examination. *International Journal of Eating Disorders, 28,* 311–316.

Rogers, R. L., & Petrie, T. A. (2001). Psychological correlates of anorexia and bulimic symptomatology. *Journal of Counseling and Development, 79,* 178–187.

Rosen, J. C., Vara, L., Wendt, S., & Leitenberg, H. (1990). Validity studies of the Eating Disorder Examination. *International Journal of Eating Disorders, 9,* 519–528.

Russell, C. J., & Keel, P. K. (2002). Homosexuality as a specific risk factor for eating disorders in men. *International Journal of Eating Disorders, 31,* 300–306.

Ryu, H. R., Lyle, R. M., Galer-Unti, R. A., & Black, D. R. (1999). Cross-cultural assessment of eating disorders: Psychometric characteristics of a Korean version of the Eating Disorder Inventory–2 and the Bulimia Test–Revised. *Eating Disorders: The Journal of Treatment and Prevention, 72,* 109–122.

Siervo, M., Boschi, V., Papa, A., Bellini, O., & Falconi, C. (2005). Application of the SCOFF, Eating Attitudes Test 26 (EAT 26) and Eating Inventory (TFEQ) Questionnaires in young women seeking diet-therapy. *Eating and Weight Disorders, 10,* 76–82.

Sloan, D. M., Mizes, J. S., Helbok, C., & Muck, R. (2004). Efficacy of sertraline for bulimia nervosa. *International Journal of Eating Disorders, 36,* 48–54.

Smith, M. C., & Thelen, M. H. (1984). Development and validation of a test for bulimia. *Journal of Consulting and Clinical Psychology, 52,* 863–872.

Spielberger, C. D. (1968). *State Trait Anxiety Inventory.* Mountain View, CA: Consulting Psychologists Press.

Steinhausen, H. C., & Seidel, R. (1993). Correspondence between the clinical assessment of eating-disordered patients and findings derived from questionnaires at follow-up. *International Journal of Eating Disorders, 14,* 367–374.

Stice, E., & Fairburn, C. G. (2003). Dietary and dietary-depressive subtypes of bulimia nervosa show differential symptom presentation, social impairment, comorbidity, and course of illness. *Journal of Consulting and Clinical Psychology, 71,* 1090–1094.

Stice, E., Fisher, M., & Martinez, E. (2004). Eating disorder diagnostic scale: Additional evidence of reliability and validity. *Psychological Assessment, 16,* 60–71.

Stice, E., Telch, C. F., & Rizvi, S. L. (2000). Development and validation of the Eating Disorder Diagnostic Scale: A brief self-report measure of anorexia, bulimia, and binge-eating disorder. *Psychological Assessment, 12,* 123–131.

Stone, A., & Shiffman, S. (1994). Ecological momentary assessment (EMA) in behavioral medicine. *Annals of Behavioral Medicine, 16,* 199–202.

Stunkard, A. J., & Messick, S. (1985). The Three Factor Eating Questionnaire to measure dietary restraining, disinhibition, and hunger. *Journal of Psychosomatic Research, 29,* 71–81.

Sysko, R., Walsh, B. T., & Fairburn, C. G. (2005). Eating Disorder Examination–Questionnaire as a measure of change in patients with bulimia nervosa. *International Journal of Eating Disorders, 37,* 100–106.

Tasca, G. A., Illing, V., Lybanon-Daigle, V., Bissada, H., & Balfour, L. (2003). Psychometric properties of the Eating Disorders Inventory–2 among women seeking treatment for binge eating disorder. *Assessment, 10,* 228–236.

Thelen, M. H., Farmer, J., Wonderlich, S., & Smith, M. (1991). A revision of the Bulimia Test: The BULIT-R. *Psychological Assessment, 3,* 119–124.

Thelen, M. H., Mintz, L. B., & Vander Wal, J. S. (1996). The Bulimia Test–Revised: Validation with *DSM-IV* criteria for bulimia nervosa. *Psychological Assessment, 8,* 219–221.

Thompson, J. K. (1988). Similarities among bulimia nervosa patients categorized by current and historical weight: Implications for the classification of eating disorders. *International Journal of Eating Disorders, 7,* 185–189.

Ujiie, T., & Kono, M. (1994). Eating attitudes test in Japan. *Japanese Journal of Psychiatry and Neurology, 48,* 557–565.

Weber, M., Davis, K., & McPhie, L. (2006). Narrative therapy, eating disorders and groups: Enhancing outcomes in rural NSW. *Australian Social Work, 59,* 391–405.

Welch, G., Thompson, L., & Hall, A. (1993). The BULIT-R: Its reliability and clinical validity as a screening tool for *DSM-III-R* bulimia nervosa in a female tertiary education population. *International Journal of Eating Disorders, 14,* 95–105.

Wilfley, D. E., Schwartz, M. B., Spurrell, E. B., & Fairburn, C. G. (1997). Assessing the specific psychopathology of binge eating disorder patients: Interview or self-report? *Behaviour Research and Therapy, 35,* 1151–1159.

Williamson, D. A., Anderson, D. A., Jackman, L. P., & Jackson, S. R. (1995). Assessment of eating disordered thoughts, feelings, and behaviors. In D. B. Allison (Ed.), *Handbook of assessment methods for eating behaviors and weight-related problems: Measures, theory, and research* (pp. 347–386). Thousand Oaks, CA: Sage.

Wilson, G. T., & Smith, D. (1989). Assessment of bulimia nervosa: An evaluation of the Eating Disorder Examination. *International Journal of Eating Disorder, 8,* 173–179.

Yanovski, S. (1993). Binge eating disorder: Current knowledge and future directions. *Obesity Research, 1,* 306–324.

CHAPTER 12

Assessment of Eating and Weight-Related Problems in Children

Tanja V. E. Kral, Myles S. Faith, and Angelo Pietrobelli

The continuing increase worldwide in the prevalence of overweight among children and adolescents is alarming. To better understand the mechanisms underlying this excessive weight gain, one must effectively study children's attitudes and behaviors surrounding eating and weight. The assessment of these behaviors and attitudes, however, has often been challenging due to methodological difficulties and limitations of current measures. These difficulties include issues related to the accuracy of parental dietary recalls, portion size estimation, variability in children's intake, and children's cognitive abilities and memory (Livingstone & Robson, 2000; Livingstone, Robson, & Wallace, 2004). Another problematic issue that can affect the accuracy of self-reported dietary intake is parent and/or child bias. For example, children's and/or parents' weight status may affect the degree to which underreporting of dietary intake occurs (Champagne, Baker, DeLany, Harsha, & Bray, 1998; Fiorito, Ventura, Mitchell, Smiciklas-Wright, & Birch, 2006; Garaulet et al., 2000;

Heitmann & Lissner, 1995; R. C. Klesges, Hanson, Eck, & Durff, 1988). Hence, it is important for researchers to refine existing dietary assessment methods and develop new tools for use in children and adolescents.

Different assessment methods can be used to measure children's eating habits and food intake. As is the case with adults, each method has its advantages and limitations. When deciding on a particular assessment method, investigators should consider the specific study objectives as well as children's developmental stage and cognitive abilities. Some methods of dietary assessment (e.g., self-report measures) may require the assistance of parents and caretakers to ensure a high quality of the data that are being collected (Livingstone & Robson, 2000; Livingstone et al., 2004; McPherson, Hoelscher, Alexander, Scanlon, & Seruda, 2002). These and other issues merit special consideration when deciding upon specific assessment tools for use with children.

The aim of the present chapter is to provide an overview of current assessment methods that are available to study eating behavior and eating/weight attitudes in children and adolescents. The first section describes methods that are being used to assess children's eating behavior in the laboratory. The second section briefly discusses other behavioral methods for assessing children's eating behavior and related physical and social environmental variables. The third section discusses ordinal and continuous tools that are being used in the laboratory to assess children's hunger and satiety. The fourth section describes measures that were developed to assess children's food preferences and palatability. The fifth section outlines self-report methods (i.e., food records, 24-hour dietary recalls, food frequency questionnaires) used to assess children's dietary intake and eating patterns in the free-living environment. The sixth section describes assessment tools that are being used to examine eating-related problems in children. This section discusses both relevant questionnaires, as well as structured and semistructured interviews. The seventh section provides an overview of assessment tools available to assess weight-related problems (e.g., body image dissatisfaction) in children. The chapter concludes with a general discussion of ways to help improve existing methods to assess eating behavior and weight-related problems in children.

Assessment of Children's Eating Behavior in the Laboratory

The study of human ingestive behavior in the laboratory has a longstanding history with adult populations (Kissileff, Klingsberg, & Van Itallie, 1980; Rodin, 1975; Rolls et al., 1981; Rozin, Ebert, & Schall, 1982; Schachter, 1968; Stunkard, 1968). The systematic assessment of eating behavior in children and adolescents in the laboratory has been the scientific focus of fewer researchers in the past (Birch, 1989; Birch, Billman, & Richards, 1984; Birch, McPhee, Bryant, & Johnson, 1993; Birch, McPhee, Shoba, Pirok, & Steinberg, 1987; Fisher & Birch, 1995, 1999; S. L. Johnson & Birch, 1994; S. L. Johnson,

McPhee, & Birch, 1991) but has gained considerable attention in more recent years. Table 12.1 provides an overview of common laboratory assessment protocols that have been conducted to study children's eating behavior.

Laboratory studies of human eating behavior can be challenging and require sophisticated skills and knowledge on the part of the researcher. The laboratory conditions under which children's eating behavior is being assessed must be child-friendly. Likewise, the methods and designs used to study eating behavior ought to take into consideration children's level of comprehension and their more limited attention span.

The following strategies can be used to make children feel comfortable in the laboratory and facilitate their cooperation with study procedures when participating in eating experiments:

- Decorate the laboratory in child-friendly ways (e.g., posters, pictures, bright colors).

- Provide age-appropriate reading materials (e.g., books, cartoon books) and games to occupy the child/adolescent during waiting times.

- Employ experienced staff who interact well with children.

- Consider having parents/primary caretakers present during the eating protocol.

- Have children eat in groups with other children rather than eating alone.

- Allow ample time to complete a particular task.

- Thoroughly explain all procedures to the child and verify comprehension.

Despite these strategies being helpful and necessary at times, some of them also may carry the risk of affecting children's eating behavior (e.g., presence of parent/caretaker in the room). It will depend on the type of assessment and on the child's age for the investigator to decide which of these strategies he or she may want to use to ensure child compliance with the procedures and thus improve the quality of the measurement.

Table 12.1   Examples of Experimental Procedures Used to Assess Eating Behavior and Taste Preferences in Children and Adolescents

Environmental factors	Effects of the portion size of foods on intake (Fisher, 2007; Fisher, Arreola, Birch, & Rolls, 2007; Fisher, Liu, Birch, & Rolls, 2007; Orlet Fisher, Rolls, & Birch, 2003; Rolls, Engell, & Birch, 2000)
	Effects of social influences on eating (Addessi, Galloway, Visalberghi, & Birch, 2005; Birch, 1980a, 1980b; Lumeng & Hillman, 2007; Salvy, Romero, Paluch, & Epstein, 2007)
	Effects of olfactory and visual food stimuli on intake (Epstein et al., 2003; Epstein, Saad, Giacomelli, & Roemmich, 2005)
	Effects of television watching on eating behavior (Francis, Lee, & Birch, 2003; Temple, Giacomelli, Kent, Roemmich, & Epstein, 2007)
Properties of foods	Effects of energy density on intake (Birch, McPhee, Bryant, & Johnson, 1993; Leahy, Roe, Birch, & Rolls, 2006; Leahy, Birch, & Rolls, 2008a, 2008b; Leahy, Birch, Fisher, & Rolls, 2008)
	Effects of changes in the glycemic index of foods on intake (Ball et al., 2003; Gilbertson, Thorburn, Brand-Miller, Chondros, & Werther, 2003; Warren, Henry, & Simonite, 2003)
Eating behaviors related to eating regulation	Assessment of eating in the absence of hunger (Birch, Fisher, & Davison, 2003; Cutting, Fisher, Grimm-Thomas, & Birch, 1999; Faith et al., 2006; Fisher & Birch, 2002)
	Assessment of caloric compensation (Birch & Deysher, 1985, 1986; Birch & Fisher, 1997; Birch, Johnson, Jones, & Peters, 1993; Birch, McPhee, & Sullivan, 1989; Faith et al., 2004)
	Assessment of food preferences and acceptance in children (Birch, 1989, 1992, 2002; Birch, Billman, & Richards, 1984; Birch, Birch, Marlin, & Kramer, 1982; Birch, McPhee, Shoba, Pirok, & Steinberg, 1987; Borzekowski & Robinson, 2001; Hendy & Raudenbush, 2000; Pelchat & Pliner, 1995)
"Abnormal" eating behaviors	Assessment of eating behavior among adolescents who report binge eating (Mirch et al., 2006)
Taste	Assessment of children's taste preferences (Liem & de Graaf, 2004; Liem, Mars, & de Graaf, 2004; Liem & Mennella, 2003; Liem, Westerbeek, Wolterink, Kok, & de Graaf, 2004; Mennella, Kennedy, & Beauchamp, 2006)
	Strategies to reduce food neophobia (Addessi et al., 2005; Birch et al., 1987; Cooke, Carnell, & Wardle, 2006; Loewen & Pliner, 1999; Pliner & Stallberg-White, 2000)
Genetic taste markers	Assessment of sensitivity to bitter compound 6-n-propylthiouracil (PROP) (Goldstein, Daun, & Tepper, 2007; Keller, Steinmann, Nurse, & Tepper, 2002; Keller & Tepper, 2004; Mennella, Pepino, & Reed, 2005; Turnbull & Matisoo-Smith, 2002)
Food reinforcement	Assessment of reinforcing value of food (i.e., measure of motivation to eat) using a computer-generated choice task (Epstein, Smith, Vara, & Rodefer, 1991; Lappalainen & Epstein, 1990; Smith & Epstein, 1991)

Many of the existing methodologies have been successfully applied to study children's eating behavior. In order to further advance our understanding of the mechanisms that underlie children's eating behavior and integrate knowledge from different fields of research, we must refine existing assessment tools and apply new, innovative designs. The advancement of such assessment strategies presents a unique opportunity for an interdisciplinary team of researchers to integrate behavioral, genetic, and physiologic measures in the study of child eating behavior and the development and treatment of childhood obesity.

Other Methods for Behavioral Assessment of Children's Eating Behavior

This section reviews other standardized test procedures that are currently available to assess children's eating behavior in the laboratory.

Behavioral Eating Test (BET). The Behavioral Eating Test (BET) was designed to assess actual food and beverage consumption in children using a standardized test meal in the laboratory (Jeffrey et al., 1980). During this test meal, which lasts 8 minutes, children are given access to a tray of 12 equal-sized foods and beverages, 6 of which are considered nutritious (e.g., cheese, carrots, apples, orange juice) and 6 of which are considered less nutritious (e.g., candy, chocolate, soda; Jeffrey, McLellarn, & Fox, 1982). Children are instructed to sample the different foods and beverages and eat as much or as little as they want. Once the test is completed, children's food intake is measured, and energy intake is computed. The test-retest reliability coefficients for the 12 foods and beverages ranged from .04 to .88 (Bridgwater, Jeffrey, Walsh, Dawson, & Peterson, 1984; Jeffrey et al., 1982). Other studies using the BET replicated the inconsistent reliability coefficients for consumption of the individual foods (Fox, Jeffrey, Dahlkoetter, McLellarn, & Hickey,

1980; Lemnitzer et al., 1979). The use of total score variables (e.g., total calories pro-nutrition foods and beverages, total calories low-nutrition foods and beverages) only moderately improved test-retest coefficients (range, .51–.85). A subsequent refinement of the BET (i.e., reducing the number of foods from 12 to 6, increasing eating time from 8 to 10 minutes, selecting foods with more similar nutrient properties) resulted in only moderate improvements in the psychometric properties of the test. With the modified BAT, test-retest reliability coefficients improved for both individual foods (.44–.74) and total food scores (.65–.76; Bridgwater et al., 1984).

Bob and Tom's Method of Assessing Nutrition (BATMAN). Bob and Tom's Method of Assessing Nutrition (BATMAN) is an observational assessment designed to record children's eating behavior and related physical and social environmental variables (R. C. Klesges et al., 1983). The assessment also records parent behavior (e.g., physical or verbal discouragement or encouragement) as parental variables, and parent-child interactions which may influence children's eating behavior. The BATMAN uses a partial interval time-sampling system (Cone & Foster, 1982) to record behavior. With this procedure, children and parents are observed for 10 seconds, followed by a 10-second recording period during which observers code all of children's behavior. Parental behaviors, such as prompts to eat or food offers, were significantly related to children's relative weight status (Klesges et al., 1983). The BATMAN method has also been used to examine the microstructure of eating (e.g., number of bites, number of chews, number of sips) in obese and nonobese children (Drabman, Hammer, & Jarvie, 1977). Test-retest reliability coefficients ranged from .61 to .94 (mean $r = .84$) for child and adult mealtime behaviors when assessed in children ranging in age from 12 to 36 months (R. C. Klesges et al., 1983). The test has not been validated for use in eating-disordered children (Netemeyer & Williamson, 2001).

Assessment of Child-Reported Hunger and Fullness in the Laboratory

The systematic study of hunger and fullness in children in the laboratory has become an important and evolving field of research. As has been said about laboratory measures in general, the tools and measures to assess these sensations need to be age appropriate. Currently, few measures exist to measure sensations of hunger and fullness in children, and the tools that do exist often have not been formally validated. The following section outlines both ordinal scale and continuous measures to assess perceptions of hunger and fullness in children.

Ordinal Scale Measures

Cartoon Figures

Birch and colleagues developed three cartoon figures (Figure 12.1) to assist children with their assessment of hunger and fullness (Birch & Fisher, 2000; Fisher & Birch, 2000).

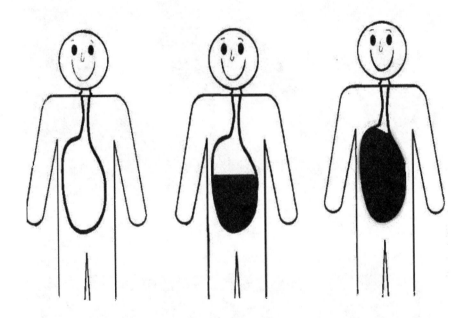

Figure 12.1   Cartoon Figures to Assess Hunger and Fullness in Children

SOURCE: Fisher and Birch (2000). Copyright Elsevier (2000).

During this assessment, children are asked to indicate the extent to which they are hungry using the cartoon figures, which depict an empty stomach ("hungry"), a half-empty stomach ("half-full"), and a full stomach ("full"). The figures have been used in preschool children. Self-report scales with cartoon drawings have been used to rate pain in children as young as 3 years of age (Belter, McIntosh, Finch, & Saylor, 1988; Fanciullo, Cravero, Mudge, McHugo, & Baird, 2007; Stanford, Chambers, & Craig, 2006). Only a few of these scales have been validated for use in children (Beyer, Denyes, & Villarruel, 1992; Beyer & Knott, 1998; Villarruel & Denyes, 1991).

Dolls With Attached Stomachs

The aim of an intervention study by S. L. Johnson (2000) was to investigate whether preschool-age children could be taught to focus on internal cues of hunger and fullness and to consequently improve their ability to regulate energy intake. The investigator used an age-appropriate doll prototype with a mouth, esophagus, and place for stomach on the exterior of the doll abdomen to help children identify feelings of hunger and satiety (see Figure 12.2).

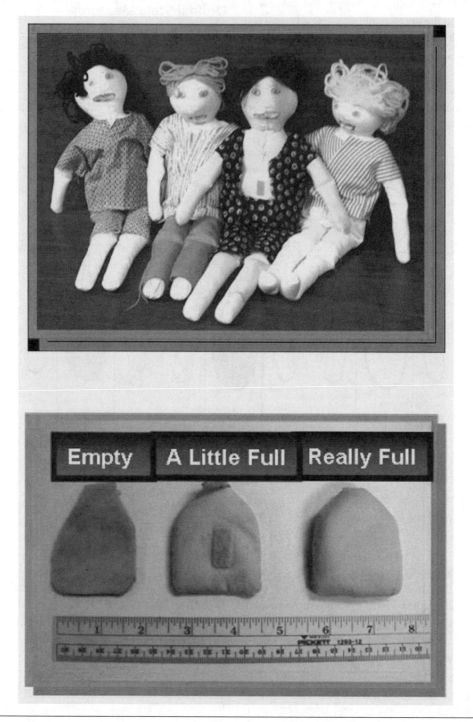

Figure 12.2   Dolls With Attachable Stomachs to Assess Hunger and Fullness in Children

The dolls were modified from a previously developed doll prototype by Birch and investigators and constructed to be androgynous and to represent different hair, eye, and skin colors. Three sets of stomachs were developed from nylon material that could be attached to the dolls by Velcro strips. The stomachs were filled to varying degrees with salt to represent an empty stomach that was hungry, a stomach that was a little full, and another stomach that was very full. Children were asked to place their hand over their own stomach and report to the investigators whether they were hungry, a little full, or very full and to identify the appropriate doll stomach. This task was repeated after the consumption of food to train children on how to determine their own hunger state. Using this approach, children were successfully trained in assessing feelings of hunger and satiety. The

results of the study showed that children's ability to self-regulate energy intake significantly improved as a result of the intervention.

Thus, using age-appropriate dolls as a training tool to teach young children how to identify and adhere to internal hunger and satiety cues has been shown to improve children's compensation ability.

Silhouettes

Faith, Kermanshah, and Kissileff (2002) developed a set of gender-specific pictorial silhouettes that can be used with preschool-age children to communicate feelings of fullness. The five silhouettes (see Figure 12.3) depict full-child profiles with incremental amounts of jelly beans in their stomachs.

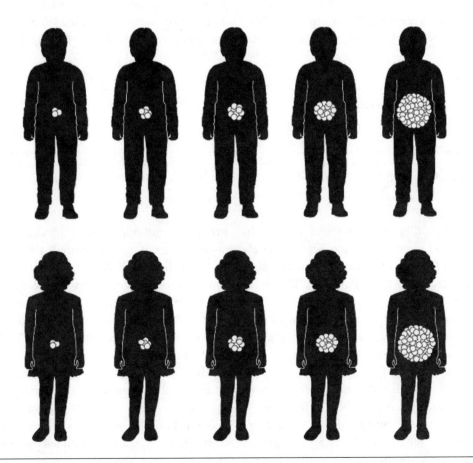

Figure 12.3   Silhouettes for the Assessment of Hunger and Fullness in Children

SOURCE: Faith, Kermanshah, and Kissileff (2002). Copyright Elsevier (2000).

The increasing numbers of circles over the abdominal region serve to indicate increasing levels of fullness. Investigators assigned scores to the silhouettes in increasing numbers of circles, thus yielding a 1 to 5 ordinal scale with higher scores denoting greater satiety. Investigators used an "imagined eating procedure" as a preliminary validation of the scale in which children used the silhouettes to indicate how full they would feel during three hypothetical situations associated with hunger, partial satiety, or satiety. Prior to indicating their sensations of fullness using the silhouettes, children received training with specially constructed puppet dolls whose bellies were salt shakers where the increasing amount of rice in their translucent bellies was designed to denote increasing satiety. The scale has undergone only preliminary testing and no formal validation at this point. This preliminary testing provided evidence for the silhouettes' validity by virtue of the fact that children reported greater

fullness when they imagined having completed dinner compared to how full they would feel before dinner or when interrupted in the middle of a meal. The outcome of this study showed that young children appeared to have the capacity to report, quantitatively, internal feelings of satiety by means of a five-level categorical scale.

Continuous Measures

Visual Analog Scales

Visual analog scales (VAS) are widely used to assess hunger and fullness and perceived palatability of foods in adults (M. Hetherington & Rolls, 1987). Subjects are instructed to answer a question (e.g., "How hungry are you right now?") by marking a line (typically 100 mm in length) that is anchored on the left by *not at all* and on the right by *extremely* (see Figure 12.4).

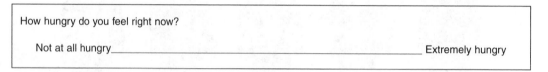

How hungry do you feel right now?

Not at all hungry_____ Extremely hungry

Figure 12.4   Example of a Hunger Rating Completed Using a Visual Analog Scale

Several studies have used VAS in children (ages 10 and 11 years) and adolescents to assess hunger and fullness (Anderson, Saravis, Schacher, Zlotkin, & Leiter, 1989; Barkeling, Ekman, & Rössner, 1992; Ludwig et al., 1999; Rolls & McDermott, 1991). VAS have also been successfully used in children as young as 6 years of age in the assessment of pain (Clark, Plint, Correll, Gaboury, & Passi, 2007).

The accurate use of rating scales, such as VAS, has been reported to be a difficult developmental task for young children (Chambers & Johnston, 2002). The ability for children to seriate their perceptions from small to large is

believed to not appear until the child reaches about 7 years of age (Ginsburg & Opper, 1969; E. M. Hetherington & Parke, 1979). Whereas some authors suggested that VAS can be reliably used in children age 5 years and older (McGrath, 1989; McGrath, de Veber, & Hearn, 1985), others (Beyer & Aradine, 1988; Erickson, 1990) proposed that young children (i.e., children younger than 7 years of age) may have difficulty translating subjective sensory experiences into a linear VAS format and thus may not have the cognitive ability to use this instrument. A study conducted by Shields and colleagues (Shields, Palermo, Powers,

Grewe, & Smith, 2003) found that only 42% of kindergarten children, ages 5 to 6.8 years, could accurately complete VAS and that children's age (≥ 5.6 years), combined with their estimated intelligence quotient (≥ 100), was the best predictor of a child's ability to use a VAS with 88% accuracy.

Analog Scaling Device

Keller and colleagues (2006) designed an analog scaling device for measuring fullness in children. The device, a pictorial analog scale, was developed in the shape of a doll, named "Freddy," which has a 150-mm long rectangular stomach, with protruding head, arms, and feet (see Figure 12.5).

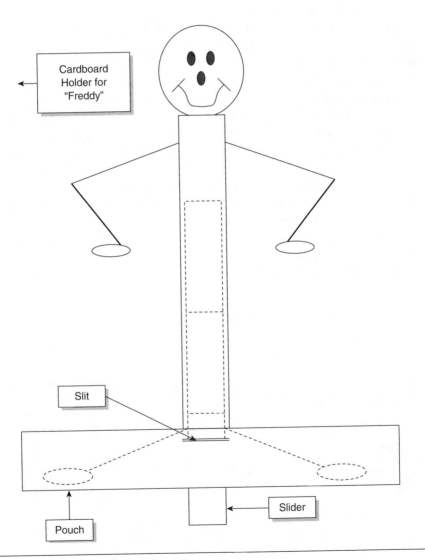

Figure 12.5   Analog Scaling Device "Freddy"

SOURCE: Keller et al. (2006). Copyright Elsevier (2000).

Data sheets were placed in a cardboard folder with a pouch attached to the bottom of a folder. A slit was cut in the middle of the pouch large enough to allow children to slide a rectangle. This scale was tested in 4- to 5-year-old normal-weight children. Children were trained to push a sliding rectangle in a vertical direction, the entire length of Freddie's stomach, to communicate fullness in response to viewing different-sized portions of foods on photographs. Preliminary findings suggest that young children can be trained to use an analog scaling device to rate fullness levels on a doll in simulated eating situations. The authors suggest, however, that the scale should be used by children 5 years and older, as younger children showed some degree of difficulty with the scaling method.

In summary, the tools described above can be used to quantify hunger and fullness in children. They can also be used as training tools to teach children to adhere to their internal cues of hunger and fullness and thereby improve their ability to regulate energy intake. Future studies ought to continue developing similarly innovative measures, refine existing tools, and further assess their reliability and validity in a diverse group of children of different ages, weights, and ethnicities.

Assessment of Child-Reported Food Preferences and Palatability in the Laboratory

When assessing children's eating behavior and food intake in the laboratory, it is important to ensure that children like the food items that they are being offered. The following tools are currently available to conduct taste preference assessments.

Ordinal Measures

Cartoon Faces

A rank-order taste preference procedure was developed by Birch (1979). During this assessment, children are shown three cartoon faces: A smiling face is described to the child as "yummy," a neutral face is described as "just okay," and a frowning face is described as "yucky" (see Figure 12.6; Fisher & Birch, 1995).

The child is presented with small samples of foods and is asked to taste each food and place the sample in front of the face that represents his or her liking or disliking of that food. Once children have tasted all foods and assigned a

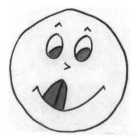 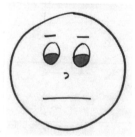 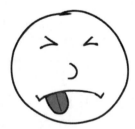

Figure 12.6   Cartoon Faces for Rank-Order Taste Preference Assessment

SOURCE: Fisher and Birch (2000). Copyright Elsevier (2000).

preference rating, rank-order preference scores are assigned as foods for each face are sequentially ranked and removed. This rank-order preference procedure has been used in preschool-age children and shown to yield reliable and valid data on young children's food preferences (Birch 1980a, 1980b; Birch & Sullivan, 1991).

More recently, Jaramillo and colleagues (2006) developed a computerized, interactive food preference assessment tool (see Figure 12.7) using the cartoon figures developed by Birch (1979).

The computerized test, available in English and Spanish, can be accessed at http://www .bcm.edu/cnrc/faculty/nicklas.htm. The tool was shown to have adequate internal consistency when tested in African American and Hispanic preschool children. The internal

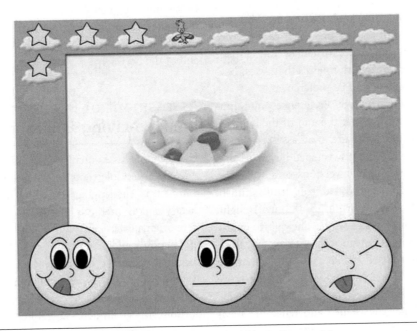

Figure 12.7   Interactive Computerized Fruit and Vegetable Preference Measure

SOURCE: Jaramillo et al. (2006).

reliability coefficient for overall fruit, juice, and vegetable (FJV) preference was .87. Cronbach's alphas for fruit, fruit juice, and vegetable subscales were .77, .58, and .82, respectively (Jaramillo et al., 2006). Test-retest reliability coefficients for the fruit, fruit juice, and vegetable subscales were .49, .37, and .73, respectively. The overall test-retest correlation coefficient for the tool was .73 (Jaramillo et al., 2006).

Visual Analog Scales

When conducting studies with older children, VAS can be used to assess the pleasantness of taste of foods or beverages. Similar to hunger and fullness ratings, subjects are instructed to answer a question (e.g., "How pleasant is the taste of this food right now?") by marking a 100-mm line that is anchored with *not at all pleasant* and *extremely pleasant* (see Figure 12.8).

How pleasant is the taste of this food *right now?*

Not at all pleasant_____ Extremely pleasant

Figure 12.8   Example of a Taste Rating Completed Using a Visual Analog Scale

Questionnaires

The Girls Health Enrichment Multisite Studies (GEMS), a series of weight gain prevention intervention studies for female youth, made use of self-report questionnaires that assess beverage preferences and FJV preferences.

The GEMS Beverage Preferences questionnaire (Appendix 12.A at the end of the book) is an 11-item questionnaire that assesses preferences for the following sweetened beverages and water: regular and diet versions of soft drinks, Kool-Aid, Snapple, iced tea, fruit drinks, punch, Powerade/Gatorade, Fruitopia, Sunny Delight, Capri Sun, and bottled water. The questionnaire includes response categories ("I do not like this," "I like this a little," "I like this a lot") that are coded as 1, 2, or 3, respectively. A higher score indicates a higher preference (L. M. Klesges et al., 2004). Internal consistency and reliability measures showed that the beverage preferences questionnaire had substantial internal consistency (Cronbach's alpha of 0.71) and adequate test-retest reliability (intraclass correlations of .79) when administered to 8- to 10-year old African American girls (Cullen et al., 2004).

The GEMS FJV Preferences questionnaire was designed to measure fruit and vegetable preferences among fourth- and fifth-grade students (Domel et al., 1993). The questionnaire assesses children's preferences for frequently consumed fruits, 100% fruit juices, and frequently consumed vegetables using three response categories ("I do not like this," "I like this a little," "I like this a lot"). The original version of the questionnaire showed acceptable internal consistency (.65–.95) and adequate test-retest reliability (.65–.84) when administered to a sample of fourth- and fifth-grade students from an elementary school (Domel et al., 1993). The questionnaire has recently been revised to include a greater number of FJV (see Appendix 12.B at the end of the book).

Assessment of Eating in the Free-Living Environment

The accurate assessment of habitual intake of children and adolescents in the free-living environment is challenging. For one, most of the dietary survey methods that are available today were originally constructed for adult populations. In addition, children's cognitive development can affect their concept of time, memory skills, and attention span. Also, young children's knowledge of the names of foods and capability of estimating portion size is limited. Therefore, parents and caretakers play an important role by assisting their children with these assessment methods, which enhances the quality and accuracy of the assessment. Livingstone and Robson (2000; Livingstone et al., 2004) provide a detailed discussion about issues related to the measurement of dietary intake in children and adolescents. In this section, we briefly summarize select quantitative diet assessment methods that can be used to ascertain habitual dietary intake in children and adolescents. At the end of this section, we outline advantages and disadvantages of each method (see Table 12.2). As with adults, there may exist substantial error in children's self-report of food intake with each of the described measures. Specifically, children and adolescents are prone to underreport their daily food intake. The magnitude of underreporting tends to increase with children's age and weight status (Bandini, Schoeller, Cyr, & Dietz, 1990; Livingstone et al., 2004). In the following sections, we present information on the validity of self-reported food intakes from food records, dietary recalls, and food frequency questionnaires when compared to data on children's total energy expenditure (TEE) using the doubly labeled water method. For a detailed review of validation studies that compared children's self-reported intakes to other measures, we refer the interested reader to recent reviews (McPherson et al., 2002; Serdula, Alexander, Scanlon, & Bownan, 2001).

Food Records

Food records, also known as food diaries, can be used to assess intake of foods and beverages that are consumed in a defined period of time (i.e., usually 1 to 7 days). Due to considerable intraindividual variation in intake among children and adolescents, multiple days of records are needed to determine intake that is representative of usual or habitual intake (Smiciklas-Wright, Mitchell, & Harris, 2002). Portion sizes of foods and beverages may be either weighed or estimated. Weighing foods and beverages may increase accuracy, but it also increases subject burden. For children who are younger than 9 years of age (McPherson et al., 2002), it is recommended that the parents or caretakers assist the child with these tasks. When portion sizes are estimated, tools such as household measures (e.g., measuring cups and spoons), food models (e.g., food replicas), pictures (e.g., two-dimensional portion shape drawings, portion photos of popular foods), or food labels (e.g., nutrition facts label) can be used to help with the estimations. Once the records are returned, they should be reviewed for completion. With so-called interviewer-assisted food records, the person reviewing the records can ask probing questions that may be used to clarify ambiguities (Smiciklas-Wright et al., 2002). Several studies (Bandini et al., 1990; Bandini et al., 2003; Bandini, Cyr, Must, & Dietz, 1997;

Rockett & Colditz, 1997) tested the accuracy of self-reported dietary intake in children and adolescents using food records.

Davies and colleagues (Davies, Coward, Gregory, White, & Mills, 1994) assessed the accuracy of self-reported daily energy intake in a cohort of children ages 1.5 to 4.5 years. Four-day weighed food records were completed by children's mothers or guardians, and children's TEE was measured using the doubly labeled water method. The percent difference between reported daily energy intake and energy expenditure was 3%. Correlation coefficients between children's energy intake and expenditure (expressed as kJ/d and kJ/kg) were .41 and .36 ($p < .05$).

In a cross-sectional investigation by Bandini et al. (1997), girls between the ages of 8 and 12 years kept food records for 7 days. Investigators used the doubly labeled water technique to assess the girls' energy expenditure for a 2-week period. Results showed that the percent difference between girls' self-reported energy intake and measured energy expenditure was 22%. The magnitude of error reporting increased with children's age, and their total daily energy expenditure indicating that subjects who consumed more total energy (as reflected by doubly labeled water estimates of energy expenditure) tended to report their energy intake less accurately, and older children showed more reporting error than did younger children.

Results from a longitudinal study in girls 10 to 15 years of age (Bandini et al., 2003) also confirmed that as girls got older, they tended to report their energy intake less accurately. Compared to data from the doubly labeled water method, the average accuracy was 88% ± 13% at age 10 years, 77% ± 21% at age 12 years, and 68% ± 17% at age 15 years.

An earlier investigation by Bandini and colleagues (1990) assessed the accuracy of self-reported energy intake in nonobese and obese 12- to 18-year-old adolescents. Adolescents were instructed to complete food records over a period of 2 weeks and have their TEE measured. The results showed that self-reported daily energy

Table 12.2   Summary of Advantages and Disadvantages of 24-Hour Dietary Recalls, Food Records, and Food Frequency Questionnaires

Method	Study Design Applications	Advantages	Disadvantages
24-hour dietary recall	Cross-sectional Intervention Monitoring Clinical Epidemiologic	Short administration time Defined recall time Intake can be quantified Procedure does not alter habitual dietary patterns Low respondent burden Can be telephone administered Procedure can be automated	Recall depends on memory Portion size difficult to estimate Trained interviewer required Expensive to collect and code
Food record	Cross-sectional Intervention Monitoring Clinical Epidemiologic	Record does not rely on memory Defined record time Intake can be quantified Training can be group administered Procedure can be automated	Recorder must be literate High respondent burden Food eaten away from home less accurately recalled Procedure may alter habitual dietary patterns Validity may decrease as recording days increase Expensive to collect and code
Food frequency questionnaire	Cross-sectional Intervention Monitoring Epidemiologic	Trained interviewers not needed Interviewer or self-administered Relatively inexpensive to collect Procedure may not alter habitual dietary habits Low respondent burden Total diet or selected foods or nutrients can be assessed Can be used to rank according to nutrient intake Procedure can be automated	Recall depends on memory Period of recall imprecise Quantification of intake imprecise because of poor recall or use of standard portion sizes Specific food descriptions not obtained

SOURCE: Adapted from McPherson, Hoelscher, Alexander, Scanlon, and Seruda (2002).

intake did not differ between obese and nonobese adolescents. However, in both groups, self-reported energy intake was found to be significantly lower than their TEE measured by the doubly labeled water method. Specifically, reported energy intake as a percentage of adolescents' TEE was significantly lower in the obese than the nonobese group (58.7% ± 23.6% vs. 80.6% ± 18.7%, respectively). Also, children's body weight was found to be independently correlated with reported energy intake as a percentage of their TEE ($r = -.48$; $p < .001$), suggesting that recording errors may increase with increasing body size.

In summary, the accuracy of self-reported intake from food records seems highest for young children for whom their parents report (and measure) their intake. The accuracy of food records has been shown to decline with increasing age and weight status in children. Several factors may explain the decline in accuracy of self-reported intakes as children get older. One, younger children may be more likely to receive help from their parents when completing food records. As children get older, they become more independent from their parents. They spend more time away from home and consume a greater proportion of meals and snacks in schools and restaurants, which likely complicates their reporting of intake. In addition, adolescents, especially females, often become more preoccupied with their weight, which may affect the way they think about food and the accuracy with which they report their intake (Bandini et al., 1997).

Dietary Recalls

Dietary recalls are a retrospective record of intake over a defined period of time (i.e., typically 24 hours; Smiciklas-Wright et al., 2002). Multiple recalls are needed to establish habitual intake. It is preferable for these recalls to be completed on random, nonconsecutive days. Nelson and colleagues provide an overview of the number of recording days that are needed to estimate intakes of specific nutrients for children and adolescents (Nelson, Black, Morris, & Cole, 1989). The

number of days needed for dietary recalls depends on the nutrient(s) that are being assessed (Nelson et al., 1989). The recommended minimum number of days for dietary recalls is 3 days, which typically include 2 weekdays and 1 weekend day (Fiorito, Mitchell, Smiciklas-Wright, & Birch, 2006a, 2006b; Fiorito et al., 2006; Nelson et al., 1989). Depending on the nutrient(s) to be assessed, more days may be necessary, but conducting recalls over more than 3 days has shown not to necessarily improve data accuracy (Nelson et al. 1989). The recalls can be completed either in person or be telephone administered. In either case, it is important that trained interviewers conduct these recalls. Interviewers typically administer the recall using the multiple-pass method, which was originally developed by the U.S. Department of Agriculture (USDA)—Human Nutrition Information Services (Guenther, DeMaio, Ingwersen, & Berlin, 1995). This multiple-pass method uses three distinct passes to garner information about the subjects' intake during the preceding 24 hours (R. K. Johnson, Driscoll, & Goran, 1996). The first pass is termed *quick list*. Here the respondent (i.e., parent and/or child) recalls everything the subject ate the previous day. During the second pass, termed *detailed description,* the respondent clarifies any foods or beverages that were mentioned in the previous pass. Here the respondent details the type and amount of the food/beverages that were consumed. The third pass is termed *review.* Here the interviewer reviews the list of foods and beverages that were reported during passes one and two, probes the respondent for additional eating occasions, and clarifies portion sizes. For the estimation of portion sizes, tools similar to the ones described for food records can be used (e.g., household measures, food models, pictures, or food labels). Dietary recalls were shown to be valid for group estimates in 4- to 7-year-old children when tested against energy expenditure data obtained by the doubly labeled water method but were less precise for individual measurements of energy intake (R. K. Johnson et al., 1996).

A study by Lindquist, Cummings, and Goran (2000) tested the use of self-report of dietary intake in children by tape recorders to document children's intake immediately upon consumption and to compare this method with the traditional 24-hour multipass dietary recall technique. Children, ages 6.5 to 11.6 years, completed three 24-hour dietary recalls and three tape-recorded food records. For the tape-recorded records, children were instructed to record all foods and beverages that they consumed, using a handheld tape recorder. Two-dimensional food models were provided to the children to help estimate portion sizes, and children were given detailed verbal and written instructions specifying the degree of detail required in the record. Children's total energy expenditure was measured over a 14-day period using the doubly labeled water method to assess the accuracy of the dietary assessments. Overall, the results of this study revealed poor within-subject agreement and thus poor validity of the tape recorder method to assess children's energy intake. The data also showed that older children and children with higher adiposity were more likely to misreport their intake using the tape recorder method. The authors suggested that based on the finding that younger and leaner children reported their intakes more accurately, the tape recorder method possibly may be used for these sub-groups of children of the general population.

Ventura and colleagues (Ventura, Loken, Mitchell, Smiciklas-Wright, & Birch, 2006) con-ducted a study to describe patterns of bias in self-reported dietary recall data of 11-year-old girls classified as underreporters, plausible reporters, and overreporters. Children completed three 24-hour dietary recalls; reporting accuracy was assessed using age- and gender-specific cutoffs for the reported energy intake (rEI)/predicted energy requirements (pER) ratio (Huang, Howarth, Lin, Roberts, & McCrory, 2004; Huang, Roberts, Howarth, & McCrory, 2005; McCrory, Hajduk, & Roberts, 2002). Results showed that girls identified as underreporters had a higher weight status, higher levels of weight concern,

and higher levels of dietary restraint. In addition, findings revealed that their underreporting tended to be selective in that underreporters reported fewer servings from food groups and subgroups with higher energy density and lower nutrient densities and fewer snacks per day. Hence, these results indicate that underreporting was prevalent in children as young as 11 years of age and that the dietary patterns of children who underreport were similar to those previously seen in adult underreporters (Horner et al., 2002; R. K. Johnson, Goran, & Poehlman, 1994; Lichtman, Goran, & Poehlman, 1992; Livingstone & Black, 2003; Tooze et al., 2004).

A study by R. K. Johnson et al. (1996) deter-mined the accuracy of the multiple-pass 24-hour dietary recall method for estimating energy intake in preschool children, ages 4 to 7 years, by com-paring it with children's TEE measured using the doubly labeled water technique. The data showed that 24-hour dietary recalls underestimated mean energy intake in this cohort of preschool child-ren by 3%. The correlation ($r = .25$) between children's daily energy intake and TEE was not statistically significant, which indicates that on an individual basis, the ability to predict energy intake from energy intake was poor.

For more detailed information on the validity of dietary recalls in comparison to other meth-ods (e.g., observed intake, food records, etc.), we refer the interested reader to reviews by Serdula et al. (2001) and McPherson et al. (2002).

Food Frequency Questionnaire

Food frequency questionnaires (FFQs) are designed to obtain information about usual food consumption patterns of individuals. They pro-vide an estimate on intake over a specified period of time, which can last from 1 week to 1 year (McPherson et al., 2002; Smiciklas-Wright et al., 2002). The questionnaire can be self-administered or conducted with individual or group assistance. In contrast to dietary recalls and food records, FFQs assess the frequency of consumption of a certain food or beverage. Sometimes, portion sizes response categories are given for a defined list of foods (Smiciklas-Wright et al., 2002).

An aim of a study by Kaskoun, Johnson, and Goran (1994) was to assess the validity of a semi-quantitative FFQ to estimate daily energy intake in young children by comparison with TEE, which was determined by the doubly labeled water method. Mothers of children between 4.2 and 6.9 years of age were asked to complete a FFQ to document children's usual intake over the last year. The findings of this study showed a significant difference between reported total energy intake and children's TEE. The FFQ overestimated children's daily energy intake by 3.39 ± 2.45 MJ/d (or 59%), with misreporting ranging from an overestimation of 9.57 MJ/d to an underestimation of 1.58 MJ/d.

Rockett and colleagues modified the Nurses' Health Study semiquantitative FFQ, which has been validated for adult populations, to develop a FFQ for older children and adolescents. This Youth/Adolescent Questionnaire (YAQ) has been modified to include more youth-specific food choices (e.g., snack foods) and to make the format easier to complete by youth (Rockett, Wolf, & Colditz, 1995; Rockett et al., 1997). Perks and colleagues (2000) validated energy intake estimated by the YAQ in a sample of boys and girls, ages 8.6 to 16.2 years, against the youths' TEE measured by doubly labeled water. The results of the study showed that the individual accuracy of estimated energy intake ranged from a 6.39-MJ/d underestimation to a 6.65-MJ/d overestimation compared to the youths' TEE. The correlation between TEE and estimated energy intake by YAQ was not significant ($r = .22$, $p = .13$). The authors concluded that while the YAQ provided an adequate estimation of the mean energy intake of prepubertal and pubertal boys and girls as a group, it did not for an individual, as they found significant individual variability in reporting accuracy.

In conclusion, there exist several tools to assess intake in children in the free-living environment. These tools, for the most part, are adapted versions of those available for intake assessment in adult populations. The accuracy with which children self-report their intakes with each of these assessment methods depends on factors such as the child's cognitive development and weight status. Accuracy can be greatly improved when assistance of parents and other caretakers becomes available. As it is the case for the assessment of other behaviors, there is a need for existing intake measures to be improved and new tools to be developed to further increase the accuracy of self-reported intake and facilitate the ease with which this assessment can be completed by children of various ages and ethnic backgrounds.

Assessment of Eating-Related Problems

The assessment of eating-related problems is facilitated through self-report measures or structured or semistructured interviews. As with the dietary intake measures (e.g., 24-hour recalls, food records), the assistance of parents or guardians may be essential to ensure a high quality of the data that are being collected. A reliable diagnosis of eating disorders in children and adolescents is best accomplished through structured interviews (Netemeyer & Williamson, 2001). The following section provides an overview of questionnaire measures and structured and semistructured interviews that are currently in use for the assessment of eating-related problems in children and adolescents.

Questionnaire Measures

Kid's Eating Disorders Survey. The Kid's Eating Disorders Survey (KEDS; see Appendix 12.C at the end of the book) was originally developed by Childress and colleagues (Childress, Brewerton, Hodges, & Jarrell, 1993) to assess current disordered eating tendencies in children. Specifically, the survey is composed of 12 items that assess weight dissatisfaction and restricting/purging behaviors in children (Childress, Jarrell, &

Brewerton, 1992). The survey also includes Body Image Silhouettes (BIS), which consist of eight child drawings for each gender depicting children who range in size from very thin to severely overweight (see "Assessment of Weight-Related Problems").

When tested in children who attended Grades 5 to 8, the internal consistency of the questionnaire was good. Cronbach's alpha for the group as a whole was .73. Cronbach's alphas were similar for boys and girls (.70 and .73, respectively). A 4-month test-retest measure showed good to adequate reliability. Test-retest coefficients were .83 for the entire group, .85 for boys, and .77 for girls, respectively (Childress, Jarrell, & Brewerton, 1993). For younger children, an interview format can be used to help interpret questions (Childress et al., 1992; Childress, Brewerton, et al., 1993).

McKnight Risk Factor Survey III. The McKnight Risk Factor Survey III (MRFS-III) was designed to assess risk and protective factor domains for disordered-eating tendencies for preadolescent and adolescent girls (Shisslak et al., 1999). The survey was recently revised (MRFS-IV) to assess demographics, age at onset of menstrual period and dating, appearance appraisal, effect of body changes, confidence, depressed mood, emotional eating, media modeling, concern with weight/shape, parental and peer concern with thinness, teasing, negative life events, perfectionism, changing eating around peers, substance use, support from others, dieting behaviors, "activities that make you feel good about yourself," participation in high-risk activities, perceived mother's and father's maximum scores on the Figure Rating Scale of Stunkard (Stunkard, Sørensen, & Schulsinger, 1983), and other miscellaneous items (The McKnight Investigators, 2003). The survey is available in an elementary school version (Grades 4–5) and middle and high school version (Grades 6–12).

Test-retest reliability coefficients for the scales (items combined) for the MRFS-III were higher in high school students (range $r = .59$–1.00) than in elementary students (range $r = .31$–$.90$). Several individual items indicated very low test-retest

reliability in elementary school children (Shisslak et al., 1999). The internal consistency of the MRFS-III was shown to be appropriate, with most Cronbach's alpha coefficients being above $r > .60$ for high school students (Shisslak et al., 1999).

Dutch Eating Behavior Questionnaire. The Dutch Eating Behavior Questionnaire (DEBQ) was developed by van Strien and colleagues (van Strien, Frijters, Bergers, & Defares, 1986) to measure restrained eating, emotional eating, and external eating in individuals.

When tested in obese and nonobese adults, the DEBQ showed high internal consistency (van Strien, Frijters, van Staveren, Defares, & Deurenberg, 1986). Cronbach's alphas for the individual subscales were .95 for restrained eating, .86 to .94 for the three subscales of emotional eating, and .80 for external eating, respectively. The DEBQ subscales also showed high validity for food consumption and high convergent and discriminative validity (van Strien, 2002). Regarding reliability measures, Allison, Kalinsky, and Gorman (1992) found the test-retest reliability of the DEBQ restraint subscale (DEBQ-R) to be .92 when tested over a 2-week period (Allison et al., 1992).

The questionnaire, whose reading level is between the fifth and eighth grades (Allison & Franklin, 1993), has been used in studies with children and adolescents (Hill, Draper, & Stack, 1994; Snoek, van Strien, Janssens, & Engels, 2007; Wardle & Beales, 1986; Wardle & Marsland, 1990; Wardle et al., 1992). When tested in ninth-grade female adolescents, the DEBQ-R showed a Cronbach's alpha of .94 (range, .65–.84; Banasiak, Wertheim, Koerner, & Voudouris, 2001). The test-retest reliability of the DEBQ-R in female adolescents was .85 when tested over a 4- to 5-week period (Banasiak et al., 2001). It is important to note that the DEBQ-R is not considered a valid indicator of actual dietary restriction as the scale, as well as other self-report measures of dietary restraint, failed to show significant inverse correlations with objective measures of short-term or longer term caloric intake (e.g., Bathalon et al., 2000; Rolls et al., 1997; Stice, Fisher, & Lowe, 2004).

A parent version of the Dutch Eating Behavior Questionnaire (DEBQ-P) was developed (Braet & van Strien, 1997) to overcome the difficulties (i.e., low validity of self-reports) that are associated with assessing psychological factors of overeating in children and adolescents (Bandini et al., 1990; Miotto, De Coppi, Frezza, Rossi, & Preti, 2002). The three subscales on this revised version of the questionnaire showed adequate dimensional stability, with Cronbach's alpha coefficients for a group of normal-weight and overweight children (ages 9–12 years) and their parents ranging from .79 to .86 (Braet & van Strien, 1997).

Dietary Intent Scale. The Dietary Intent Scale (DIS; see Appendix 12.D at the end of the book) was developed by Stice (1998a, 1998b). It is a nine-item measure of dietary behaviors that includes three subscales assessing reduced intake of food, abstaining from eating, and consumption of low-calorie foods. Participants are instructed to respond to the items on 5-point scales ranging from *never* to *always*. When tested in a pilot study with adolescents, the DIS showed good internal consistency with Cronbach's alphas ranging from .94 for the overall scale, .94 for the reduced intake subscale, .93 for the abstinence subscale, to .91 for the low-calorie subscale, respectively. The test-retest reliability coefficients for these scales were .92, .87, .91, and .90, respectively, when tested over a period of 1 month (Stice, 1998a, 1998b).

The scale was also found to be strongly correlated with the Dutch Restraint Scale ($r = .92$; van Strien, Frijters, Bergers, et al., 1986; van Strien, Frijters, van Staveren, et al., 1986) and the Restraint Scale ($r = .82$; Herman & Polivy, 1980; van Strien, Frijters, Bergers, et al., 1986; van Strien, Frijters, van Staveren, et al., 1986) and to predict a behaviorally based measure of eating (Stice, 1998a, 1998b).

Emotional Eating Scale. The Emotional Eating Scale (EES) was originally developed for use in obese adults with binge-eating disorder (BED). Respondents rate their desire to eat in response to different emotions on a 5-point scale. Three distinct subscales are being generated reflecting the urge to eat in response to anger/frustration, anxiety, and depression (Arnow, Kenardy, & Agras, 1995). Tanofsky-Kraff and colleagues (2007) recently adapted the scale for use in children and adolescents ages 8 to 17 years (EES-C; see Appendix 12.E at the end of the book). The authors slightly adapted the language of the questionnaire to increase comprehension and added a question to the right of the five-scale options inquiring about the frequency with which children engage in eating in response to specific emotions. A factor analysis generated three subscales that were (a) eating in response to anxiety, anger, and frustration (EES-C-AAF); (b) depressive symptoms (EES-C-DEP); and (c) feeling unsettled (EES-C-UNS).

When tested in children and adolescents, all three subscales demonstrated good internal consistency. Cronbach's alphas for the three subscales EES-C-AAF, EES-C-DEP, and EES-C-UNS were .95, .92, and .83, respectively (Tanofsky-Kraff et al., 2007). Furthermore, children reporting recent loss of control (LOC) eating episodes scored higher on all three subscales compared to children without LOC, indicating that the EES-C demonstrated good convergent validity with LOC eating. There was also evidence for good discriminant validity for the EES-C-AAF and EES-C-UNS subscales and adequate discriminant validity for EES-C-DEP. Test-retest reliability coefficients for EES-C-AAF, EES-C-DEP, and EES-C-UNS were .59, .74, and .66, respectively, suggesting good temporal stability of the three subscales (Tanofsky-Kraff et al., 2007).

Eating Attitudes Test. The Eating Attitudes Test (EAT) was developed by Garner and Garfinkel (1979) and is a 40-item (EAT-40) self-report inventory to measure attitudes, thoughts, and behaviors associated with anorexia nervosa. The questionnaire's internal consistency was found to be satisfactory (.79; Garner, Olmsted, Bohh, & Garfinkel, 1982) as was the test-retest reliability (.84; Carter & Moss, 1984). Content, criterion, and construct validity were established for the questionnaire. The original 40-item version was shortened to a 26-item version (EAT-26; Garner et al., 1982). The subscales of the EAT-26 were designed to assess restrictive attitudes and behaviors (dieting), bulimic attitudes and behaviors (bulimia), and personal and social control over intake (oral control). EAT-40 and EAT-26 scores were found to be highly correlated (Garner & Garfinkel, 1979; Williamson, Anderson, & Gleaves, 1996). The questionnaire has been used with adolescents (Gila, Castro, Cesena, & Toro, 2005; Jonat & Birmingham, 2004; Lynch, Eppers, & Sherrodd, 2004; Toro et al., 2006); norms for use of the scale in adolescents were published (A. Wood, Waller, Miller, & Slade, 1992). The reading level of the original scale (EAT) is fifth grade. An adapted language version of the EAT (A-EAT) was created with a third-grade reading level (Vacc & Rhyne, 1987).

Children's Eating Attitudes Test. The Children's Eating Attitudes Test (ChEAT; see Appendix 12.F at the end of the book) was developed by Maloney, McGuire, and Daniels (1988) from the 26-item Eating Attitudes Test (Garner et al., 1982) and was modified for use in preadolescents. The questionnaire was designed to assess eating and weight control habits in children. Factor-analytic studies (Williamson et al., 1997) of the ChEAT identified the following four factors: (1) dieting, (2) overconcern with eating, (3) social pressure to increase body weight, and (4) extreme weight control practices. Two subscales of the ChEAT, the Dieting subscale and the Social Pressure to Increase Body Weight subscale, were significantly correlated with measures of adiposity. When tested in children ages 8 to 13 years, the instrument showed good internal reliability with an overall Cronbach's alpha coefficient of .76. Across school Grades 3, 4, 5, and 6, Cronbach's alpha coefficients were .80, .77, .68, and .76, respectively. The scale also showed good test-retest reliability with an overall coefficient of .81. Test-retest coefficients appeared consistent across Grades 3 (.84), 4 (.88), 5 (.75), and 6 (.85), respectively (Maloney et al., 1988). These test-retest and internal reliability coefficients are comparable to those obtained for the EAT (Garner, Rockert, Olmsted, Johnson, & Coscina, 1985; Maloney et al. 1988). The factor structure of a revised version of the ChEAT with a different scoring system and factor model has been empirically tested more recently (Anton et al., 2006; Lynch & Eppers-Reynolds, 2005).

Children's Eating Behavior Inventory. The Children's Eating Behavior Inventory (CEBI; see Appendix 12.G at the end of the book) is a 40-item parent-report instrument that assesses eating and mealtime problems across a broad age span in a wide variety of medical and developmental disorders (Archer, Rosenbaum, & Streiner, 1991). The items are grouped into questions pertaining to the child and to the parent and family system, respectively. The child domain is intended to assess children's food preferences, motor skills, and behavioral compliance, whereas the parent domain is intended to assess parent-child behavior controls, cognitions, and feelings about feeding one's child and interactions between family members. The CEBI yields a total eating problems score, as well as the frequency of the problem listed. The instrument was tested in a sample of children, ages 2 to 12 years, who were referred for assessment and treatment of an identified or anticipated eating problem due to developmental or medical disorders.

When tested in a clinic and nonclinic sample of children who were 2 to 12 years of age, the instrument showed adequate test-retest reliability. The intraclass correlation coefficients for the total eating problem score and the percentage of items perceived to be a problem were .87 and .84, respectively (Archer et al., 1991). Internal reliability coefficients for the most part were within acceptable limits for different parent/child subgroups. Specifically, Cronbach's alphas for two parents with two or more children, two parents with one child, single parent with two or more children, and single parent with one child were .76, .71, .58, and .76, respectively. Preliminary analyses also confirmed the construct validity of the CEBI (Archer et al., 1991).

Archer and Szatmari (1990) confirmed the instrument's ability to reflect improvement in eating and mealtime problems after an intervention and suggested that the CEBI may also serve as a companion questionnaire to be administered in conjunction with the Children's Eating Attitudes Test (Maloney et al., 1988).

Eating Disorder Inventory–2. The Eating Disorder Inventory–2 (EDI-2) is a 91-item self-report measure of cognitive and behavioral characteristics of anorexia and bulimia nervosa (Garner, 1991a). It was expanded from the original 64-item EDI (Garner, Olmsted, & Polivy, 1983). The EDI-2 contains 11 scales that include (a) drive for thinness, (b) body dissatisfaction, (c) ineffectiveness, (d) perfectionism, (e) bulimia, (f) interoceptive awareness, (g) interpersonal distrust, (h) asceticism, (i) impulse regulation, (j) social insecurity, and (k) maturity fears. The reading level of the EDI-2 is fifth grade (Williamson, Anderson, Jackman, & Jackson, 1995). The questionnaire is intended for use in adolescents ages 12 and older (Garner, 1991a). When a subset of the scales (i.e., drive for thinness, body dissatisfaction, ineffectiveness, perfectionism, and interpersonal trust) was tested in a sample of young adolescents (ages 12–15 years), the scales showed acceptable internal consistency (coefficient alphas ranged from .69–.92) and stability over time (McCarthy, Simmons, Smith, Tomlinson, & Hill, 2002).

Eating Disorder Inventory–C. The Eating Disorder Inventory–C (EDI-C) is a child version of the Eating Disorder Inventory–2 (Garner, 1991b). The wording of the questionnaire was edited to better suit younger respondents. The EDI-C also contains 91 items and uses the same 11 subscales as the EDI-2.

The psychometric properties of the EDI-C were found to be comparable to the properties of the EDI-2 (Thurfjell, Edlund, Arinell, Hägglöf, & Engström, 2003). The internal consistency of the EDI-C was reported to be adequate. When tested in two populations of adolescents, an eating-disordered group and a normal group, Cronbach's alphas for the two groups ranged from .70 to .91 (alpha coefficient for total EDI-C was .94) and .52 to .92 (alpha coefficient for total EDI-C was .93), respectively (Thurfjell et al., 2003). Eleven factors with an eigenvalue > 2.2 explained 56% of the total variance. They showed satisfying correspondence to the proposed constructs of the inventory. A discriminant analysis between subject groups classified 85.6% of the cases correctly (86.9% of the normal group and 72.6% of the eating-disordered group; Thurfjell et al., 2003). The use of a modified subscale structure was proposed more recently (Eklund, Paavonen, & Almqvist, 2005), which would improve the reliability of the scales.

Assessment of Weight-Related Problems

As is the case with assessing children's eating behavior and intake, assessing children's body satisfaction and dissatisfaction adequately is equally difficult. For one, young children's ability to understand and respond to measures of dissatisfaction may depend on the type of measure that is being used. Also, children and teenagers may be unable or unwilling to answer questions concerning their preferred body weight and shape.

The development of measures of weight-related problems in children often included adapting well-established paper-and-pencil tests that were used in adults and adolescents into instruments that effectively measure body image satisfaction and dissatisfaction in younger children. The two kinds of measures of body image (dis)satisfaction that currently exist include questionnaires and figure drawings, some of which are described in the following section.

Body Rating Scale. The Body Rating Scale (BRS; see Appendix 12.H at the end of the book) was developed by Sherman, Iacono, and Donnelly (1995) to assess body image satisfaction in preadolescent and adolescent females. The scale comes in two sets of line drawings, each consisting of nine figures ranging from thin to obese. One series of drawings, developed for use in 11-year-old children, depicts "preadolescent" females; the second series of drawings, developed for use in 17-year-old adolescents, depicts older "adolescent" females. Except for differences in body size, the figures kept all other features (e.g., face, hair). The BRS and Figure Rating Scale (Stunkard et al., 1983) were administered to three age groups: 11-year-olds, 17-year-olds, and their mothers (Sherman et al., 1995). Pearson product correlations among the body scales were high both for intraobserver ratings and self-ratings ranging from .81 to .95. Interrater correlations were high for mothers (.78) but lower for 17-year-olds (.54) and 11-year-olds (.64). Correlations between body mass index (BMI) and body scale ratings were .84 for mothers, .59 for 17-year-olds, and .78 for 11-year-olds, respectively. The BRS was found to be a reliable and valid measure of body image satisfaction in adolescent females.

Children's Body Image Scale. The Children's Body Image Scale (CBIS; see Appendix 12.I at the end of the book) was developed by Truby and Paxton (2002), and examines perception and satisfaction with body size in young children. The CBIS is a gender-specific pictorial scale of prepubescent children. The male and female versions of the scale contain seven body pictures that represent standard percentile curves for BMI for children ranging from the 3rd to the 97th National Center for Health Statistics percentile. When administered to children, each child is asked to identify the body figure that is most like his or her own (perceived figure). The child is then asked to nominate the body figure he or she would most like to have (ideal figure). The difference between the category scores of children's perceived and ideal figures is used as a measure of body size dissatisfaction (i.e., perceived-ideal discrepancy). Besides a directional score, the scale also generates an absolute discrepancy score (i.e., perceived minus ideal), which provides a nondirectional indicator of body dissatisfaction. Correlations between children's actual BMI and perceived BMI category for ages 8 to 12 were between .50 and .60 for girls and .34

and .35 for boys, respectively. The CBIS is a reliable measure of body size perception in girls and an adequate measure in boys age 8 years and older. Preliminary testing, however, showed that the scale provides only a moderate indication of actual body size in boys age 8 years and older and was judged not to be a reliable measure of body size in 7-year-old boys. To date, no test-retest reliability data are available (Truby & Paxton, 2002).

Figure Drawings. The figure drawings (see Appendix 12.J at the end of the book) developed by Collins (1991) are a pictorial instrument to examine the perceptions of body figure in preadolescent children. The adult figure drawings developed by Stunkard et al. (1983) were used as a template to develop the child figures. The drawings were developed to depict seven male and female child and adult figures that illustrate body weight ranging from very thin to obese. Subjects are instructed to make five figure selections to rate the following: (a) self, (b) ideal-self, (c) ideal other child, (d) ideal adult, and (e) ideal other adult. When tested in preadolescent children, test-retest coefficients for figure selections were .71 for Self, .59 for Ideal Self, and .38 for Ideal Other Child. Correlations showed more stability in figure selections related to subjects' own gender; those for other-gender selections were often low. Criterion-related validity was assessed through comparison of pictorial figure selections with actual weight and BMI. Coefficients were .36 ($p < .05$) for pictorial self and weight and .37 ($p < .05$) for pictorial self and BMI (Collins, 1991).

KEDS Body Image Silhouettes. The KEDS Body Image Silhouettes (BIS; see Appendix 12.K at the end of the book) were developed by Childress, Jarrell, and Brewerton (1993) to assess body image in children. The figure drawings were based on adult silhouettes that were initially created by Stunkard et al. (1983). When administering the scale to children, they are asked to examine the eight silhouettes and circle the one they think looks most like themselves (Perceived Body Size) and to underline the one that represents how they would most like to look (Desired Body Size). BIS Dissatisfaction scores are then computed by subtracting the number corresponding to the silhouette, which represents children's desired body size, from the number that corresponds with the silhouette that represents children's perceived body size. When tested in 9- to 12-year-old children, test-retest reliability coefficients were, across age groups, .77 for perceived body size, .74 for desired body size, and .82 for body size dissatisfaction, respectively (Candy & Fee, 1998). Pearson product moment correlations indicated a moderately strong correlation between children's BMI and BIS Perceived Body Size scores (.54, $p < .001$), a moderate correlation between BMI and BIS Body Image Dissatisfaction (.65, $p < .001$), and a low correlation between BMI and BIS Desired Body Size (.18, $p < .05$; Candy & Fee, 1998).

Body-Esteem Scale. The Body-Esteem Scale (BE; see Appendix 12.L at the end of the book) was originally developed by Mendelson and White (1982). It is a self-report instrument for children to investigate the relation between body-esteem and self-esteem in normal-weight and overweight children. The instrument contains 24 items that assess how children value their appearance and body and how they believe they are being evaluated by others. These simple statements, only four of which directly relate to weight, fatness, or thinness, require a yes/no response. The BE scale is suitable for second-grade readers. In a study with children between the ages of 7 and 12 years, the scale demonstrated adequate split-half reliability (.85) and construct validity (.67; Mendelson & White, 1982, 1985).

Body-Esteem Scale for Adolescents and Adults. The Body-Esteem Scale for Adolescents and Adults (BESAA) is an extension of the above-described Body-Esteem Scale (Mendelson, Mendelson, & White, 2001). This revised scale contains 23 items. Respondents rate the degree of agreement with each statement using a 5-point Likert scale ranging from 0 (*never*) to 4 (*always*). A factor analysis

of this scale identified the following three subscales: (1) general feelings of appearance, (2) weight satisfaction, and (3) attributions of positive evaluations about one's body and appearance to others. When tested in males and females between the ages of 12 and 25 years, the original 30-item scale showed good internal consistency, with Cronbach's alpha coefficients for the three subscales ranging between .81 and .95. Three-month test-retest reliability ranged between .83 and .92. The scale thus is suggested to be a valid and reliable instrument to assess self-evaluations of body or appearance in adolescents of a wide age range. The scale can be administered to youth as young as 12 years of age and to individuals well into adulthood (Mendelson et al., 2001).

Body Dissatisfaction Scale of the Eating Disorder Inventory. The Body Dissatisfaction Scale of the Eating Disorder Inventory (EDI-BD) is one of the eight subscales of the EDI. This nine-item scale was designed to measure adults' and adolescents' beliefs that various parts of the body are too large or are associated with fatness (Garner et al., 1983). The EDI-BD has been widely used in eating disorders and body image research. In a sample of 11- to 18-year-old teens, Shore and Porter (1990) determined the coefficients of internal consistency (standardized alpha) for the EDI-BD to be .91 for girls and .86 for boys, respectively.

Wood and colleagues (K. C. Wood, Becker, & Thompson, 1996) made small revisions to the scale to develop a version for use in preadolescent children (Revised EDI-BD). When tested in children between the ages of 8 and 10 years, the Revised EDI-BD demonstrated test-retest reliability coefficients between .71 and .88 across gender and age groups except for 9-year-old boys (.66). The revised scale showed good internal consistency with coefficient alphas ranging from .73 and .95 (K. C. Wood et al., 1996).

Summary and Conclusion

For a considerable amount of time, the focus of dietary assessment methods has been on adults.

Sophisticated methods were developed to help improve reporting accuracy while reducing systematic reporting bias (e.g., underreporting). Now this focus has widened to include the development of new assessment methods and the refinement of existing tools for use in children and adolescents. While some instruments that were initially developed for use in adults may be effectively revised for use in children and adolescents, there also are respondent and observer considerations that are specific to pediatric populations (e.g., cognitive abilities) that make it necessary to tailor the assessment tool to the needs of children and their caretakers.

As demonstrated in this chapter, there currently exists a multitude of innovative tools that were designed to assess children's eating behaviors and weight-related problems. The majority of these tools have undergone satisfactory validity and reliability testing, which confirmed good psychometric properties of these methods for use in children and adolescents. At the same time, different assessment methods require different approaches to establish the validity and reliability of a respective measure. It is important to remember that the question of a method's "validity" requires understanding valid *for what purpose?* For example, most conventional psychometric tests (e.g., internal consistency, convergent and discriminant validities, reliability, readability) will often be appropriate and informative for most questionnaire measures under most circumstances. The doubly labeled water technique may be the "gold standard" for validating tools purporting to estimate total energy intake, but the method may not meaningfully measure broader eating patterns, styles, or tendencies. For experimental procedures conducted in the laboratory, the most useful information on validity may be test-retest reliability and associations with self-report instruments purporting to assess the same eating domain. Thus, validity depends on valid for what research purpose.

Across the range of approaches reviewed in this chapter, more standardized assessment tools are needed, especially for experimental research,

to enhance validity and reliability assessments. To achieve these improvements in both the assessment and validation of eating behaviors and weight-related problems in children, researchers will need to employ trained interviewers who follow standardized procedures and guidelines when administering the assessments to children and their guardians.

References

Addessi, E., Galloway, A. T., Visalberghi, E., & Birch, L. L. (2005). Specific social influences on the acceptance of novel foods in 2–5-year-old children. *Appetite, 45,* 264–271.

Allison, D. B., & Franklin, R. D. (1993). The readability of three measures of dietary restraint. *Psychotherapy in Private Practice, 12,* 53–57.

Allison, D. B., Kalinsky, L. B., & Gorman, B. S.. (1992). The comparative psychometric properties of three measures of dietary restraint. *Psychological Assessment, 4,* 391–398.

Anderson, G. H., Saravis, S., Schacher, R., Zlotkin, S., & Leiter, L. A. (1989). Aspartame: Effect on lunchtime food intake, appetite and hedonic response in children. *Appetite, 13,* 93–103.

Anton, S. D., Han, H., Newton, R. L., Jr., Martin, C. K., York-Crowe, E., Stewart, T. M., et al. (2006). Reformulation of the Children's Eating Attitudes Test (ChEAT): Factor structure and scoring method in a non-clinical population. *Eating and Weight Disorders, 11,* 201–210.

Archer, L. A., Rosenbaum, P. L., & Streiner, D. L. (1991). The children's eating behavior inventory: Reliability and validity results. *Journal of Pediatric Psychology, 16,* 629–642.

Archer, L. A., & Szatmari, P. (1990). Assessment and treatment of food aversion in a four year old boy: A multidimensional approach. *Canadian Journal of Psychiatry, 35,* 501–505.

Arnow, B., Kenardy, J., & Agras, W. S. (1995). The Emotional Eating Scale: The development of a measure to assess coping with negative affect by eating. *International Journal of Eating Disorders, 18,* 79–90.

Ball, S. D., Keller, K. R., Moyer-Mileur, L. J., Ding, Y. W., Donaldson, D., & Jackson, W. D. (2003). Prolongation of satiety after low versus moderately high glycemic index meals in obese adolescents. *Pediatrics, 111,* 488–494.

Banasiak, S. J., Wertheim, E. H., Koerner, J., & Voudouris, N. J. (2001). Test-retest reliability and internal consistency of a variety of measures of dietary restraint and body concerns in a sample of adolescent girls. *International Journal of Eating Disorders, 29,* 85–89.

Bandini, L. G., Cyr, H., Must, A., & Dietz, W. H. (1997). Validity of reported energy intake in preadolescent girls. *American Journal of Clinical Nutrition, 65*(Suppl.), 1138S–1141S.

Bandini, L. G., Must, A., Cyr, H., Anderson, S. E., Spadano, J. L., & Dietz, W. H. (2003). Longitudinal changes in the accuracy of reported energy intake in girls 10–15 y of age. *American Journal of Clinical Nutrition, 78,* 480–484.

Bandini, L. G., Schoeller, D. A., Cyr, H. N., & Dietz, W. H. (1990). Validity of reported energy intake in obese and nonobese adolescents. *American Journal of Clinical Nutrition, 52,* 421–425.

Barkeling, B., Ekman, S., & Rössner, S. (1992). Eating behaviour in obese and normal weight 11-year-old children. *International Journal of Obesity and Related Metabolic Disorders, 16,* 355–360.

Bathalon, G. P., Tucker, K. L., Hays, N. P., Vinken, A. G., Greenberg, A. S., & McCrory, M. A. (2000). Psychological measures of eating behavior and the accuracy of 3 common dietary assessment methods in healthy postmenopausal women. *American Journal of Clinical Nutrition, 71,* 739–745.

Belter, R. W., McIntosh, J. A., Finch, A., & Saylor, C. F. (1988). Preschoolers' ability to differentiate levels of pain: Relative efficacy of three self-report measures. *Journal of Clinical Child Psychology, 17,* 329–335.

Beyer, J. E., & Aradine, C. R. (1988). Convergent and discriminant validity of a self-report measure of pain intensity for children. *Journal of the Association for the Care of Children's Health, 16,* 274–282.

Beyer, J. E., Denyes, M. J., & Villarruel, A. M. (1992). The creation, validation, and continuing development of the Oucher: A measure of pain intensity in children. *Journal of Pediatric Nursing, 7,* 335–346.

Beyer, J. E., & Knott, C. B. (1998). Construct validity estimation for the African-American and Hispanic versions of the Oucher Scale. *Journal of Pediatric Nursing, 13,* 20–31.

Birch, L. L. (1979). Preschool children's food preferences and consumption patterns. *Journal of Nutrition Education, 11,* 189–192.

Birch, L. L. (1980a). Effects of peer models' food choices and eating behaviors on preschoolers' food preferences. *Child Development, 51,* 489–496.

Birch, L. L. (1980b). The relationship between children's food preferences and those of their parents. *Journal of Nutrition Education, 12,* 14–18.

Birch, L. L. (1989). Effects of experience on the modification of food acceptance patterns. *Annals of the New York Academy of Science, 561,* 209–216.

Birch, L. L. (1992). Children's preferences for high-fat foods. *Nutrition Review, 50,* 249–255.

Birch, L. L. (2002). Acquisition of food preferences and eating patterns in children. In C. G. Fairburn & K. D. Brownell (Eds.), *Eating disorders and obesity* (pp. 75–79). New York: Guilford.

Birch, L. L., Billman, J., & Richards, S. S..(1984). Time of day influences food acceptability. *Appetite, 5,* 109–116.

Birch, L. L., Birch, D., Marlin, D. W., & Kramer, L. (1982). Effects of instrumental consumption on children's food preference. *Appetite, 3,* 125–134.

Birch, L. L., & Deysher, M. (1985). Conditioned and unconditioned caloric compensation: Evidence for self-regulation of food intake by young children. *Learning and Motivation, 16,* 341–355.

Birch, L. L., & Deysher, M. (1986). Caloric compensation and sensory specific satiety: Evidence for self regulation of food intake by young children. *Appetite, 7,* 323–331.

Birch, L. L., & Fisher, J. O. (1997). Food intake regulation in children: Fat and sugar substitutes and intake. *Annals of New York Academy of Science, 819,* 194–220.

Birch, L. L., & Fisher, J. O. (2000). Mothers' child-feeding practices influence daughters' eating and weight. *American Journal of Clinical Nutrition, 71,* 1054–1061.

Birch, L. L., Fisher, J. O., & Davison, K. K. (2003). Learning to overeat: Maternal use of restrictive feeding practices promotes girls' eating in the absence of hunger. *American Journal of Clinical Nutrition, 78,* 215–220.

Birch, L. L., Johnson, S. L., Jones, M. B., & Peters, J. C. (1993). Effects of a nonenergy fat substitute on children's energy and macronutrient intake. *American Journal of Clinical Nutrition, 58,* 326–333.

Birch, L. L., McPhee, L. S., Bryant, J. L., & Johnson, S. L. (1993). Children's lunch intake: Effects of mid-morning snacks varying in energy density and fat content. *Appetite, 20,* 83–94.

Birch, L. L., McPhee, L., Shoba, B. C., Pirok, E., & Steinberg, L. (1987). What kind of exposure reduces children's food neophobia? Looking vs. tasting. *Appetite, 9,* 171–178.

Birch, L. L., McPhee, L., & Sullivan, S. (1989). Children's food intake following drinks sweetened with sucrose or aspartame: Time course effects. *Physiology & Behavior, 45,* 387–395.

Birch, L. L., & Sullivan, S. A. (1991). Measuring children's food preferences. *Journal of School Health, 61,* 212–214.

Borzekowski, D. L., & Robinson, T. N. (2001). The 30-second effect: An experiment revealing the impact of television commercials on food preferences of preschoolers. *Journal of the American Dietetic Association, 101,* 42–46.

Braet, C., & van Strien, T. (1997). Assessment of emotional, externally induced and restrained eating behaviour in nine to twelve-year-old obese and non-obese children. *Behavior Research and Therapy, 35,* 863–873.

Bridgwater, C. A., Jeffrey, D. B., Walsh, J. A., Dawson, B., & Peterson, P. (1984). Measuring children's food consumption in the laboratory: A methodological refinement of the behavioral eating test. *Behavioral Assessment, 6,* 357–364.

Candy, C. M., & Fee, V. E. (1998). Reliability and concurrent validity of the Kids' Eating Disorders Survey (KEDS) body image silhouettes with preadolescent girls. *Eating Disorders, 6,* 297–308.

Carter, P. I., & Moss, R. A. (1984). Screening for anorexia and bulimia nervosa in a college population: Problems and limitations. *Addictive Behaviors, 9,* 417–419.

Chambers, C. T., & Johnston, C. (2002). Developmental differences in children's use of rating scales. *Journal of Pediatric Psychology, 27,* 27–36.

Champagne, C. M., Baker, N. B., DeLany, J. P., Harsha, D. W., & Bray, G. A. (1998). Assessment of energy intake underreporting by doubly labeled water and observations on reported nutrient intakes in children. *Journal of the American Dietetic Association, 98,* 426–433.

Childress, A. C., Brewerton, T. D., Hodges, E. L., & Jarrell, M. P. (1993). The Kids' Eating Disorders Survey (KEDS): A study of middle school students. *Journal of the American Academy of Child and Adolescent Psychiatry, 32,* 843–850.

Childress, A. C., Jarrell, M. P., & Brewerton, T. (1992, April). *The Kid's Eating Disorder Survey (KEDS): Internal consistency, component analysis, and test-retest reliability.* Paper presented at the Fifth International Conference on Eating Disorders, New York.

Childress, A. C., Jarrell, M. P., & Brewerton, T. (1993). The Kids' Eating Disorders Survey (KEDS): Internal consistency, component analysis, and reliability. *Eating Disorders, 1,* 123–133.

Clark, E., Plint, A. C., Correll, R., Gaboury, I., & Passi, B. (2007). A randomized, controlled trial of acetaminophen, ibuprofen, and codeine for acute pain relief in children with musculoskeletal trauma. *Pediatrics, 119,* 460–467.

Collins, M. S. (1991). Body figure perceptions and preferences among preadolescent children. *International Journal of Eating Disorders, 10,* 199–208.

Cone, J., & Foster, S. L. (1982). Direct observation in clinical psychology. In P. Kendall (Ed.), *Research design in clinical psychology.* New York: John Wiley.

Cooke, L., Carnell, S., & Wardle, J. (2006). Food neophobia and mealtime food consumption in 4–5 year old children. *International Journal of Behavioral Nutrition and Physical Activity, 3,* 14.

Cullen, K. W., Klesges, L. M., Sherwood, N. E., Baranowski, T., Beech, B., Pratt, C., et al. (2004). Measurement characteristics of diet-related psychosocial questionnaires among African-American parents and their 8- to 10-year-old daughters: results from the Girls' Health Enrichment Multi-site Studies. *Preventive Medicine, 38*(Suppl.), S34–S42.

Cutting, T. M., Fisher, J. O., Grimm-Thomas, K., & Birch, L. L. (1999). Like mother, like daughter: Familial patterns of overweight are mediated by mothers' dietary disinhibition. *American Journal of Clinical Nutrition, 69,* 608–613.

Davies, P. S., Coward, W. A., Gregory, I., White, A., & Mills, A. (1994). Total energy expenditure and energy intake in the pre-school child: A comparison. *British Journal of Nutrition, 72,* 13–20.

Domel, S. B., Baranowski, T., Davis, H., Leonard, S. B., Riley, P., & Baranowski, J. (1993). Measuring fruit and vegetable preferences among 4th- and 5th-grade students. *Preventive Medicine, 22,* 866–879.

Drabman, R. S., Hammer, D., & Jarvie, G. J. (1977). Eating styles of obese and nonobese Black and White children in a naturalistic setting. *Addictive Behaviors, 2,* 83–86.

Eklund, K., Paavonen, E. J., & Almqvist, F. (2005). Factor structure of the Eating Disorder Inventory–C. *International Journal of Eating Disorders, 37,* 330–341.

Epstein, L. H., Saad, F. G., Giacomelli, A. M., & Roemmich, J. N. (2005). Effects of allocation of attention on habituation to olfactory and visual food stimuli in children. *Physiology & Behavior, 84,* 313–319.

Epstein, L. H., Saad, F. G., Handley, E. A., Roemmich, J. N., Hawk, L. W., & McSweeney, F. K. (2003). Habituation of salivation and motivated responding for food in children. *Appetite, 41,* 283–289.

Epstein, L. H., Smith, J. A., Vara, L. S., & Rodefer, J. S. (1991). Behavioral economic analysis of activity choice in obese children. *Health Psychology, 10,* 311–316.

Erickson, C. J. (1990). Pain measurement in children: Problems and directions. *Journal of Developmental and Behavioral Pediatrics, 11,* 135–137; discussion 138–139.

Faith, M. S., Berkowitz, R. I., Stallings, V. A., Kerns, J., Storey, M., & Stunkard, A. J. (2006). Eating in the absence of hunger: A genetic marker for childhood obesity in prepubertal boys? *Obesity Research, 14,* 131–138.

Faith, M. S., Keller, K. L., Johnson, S. L., Pietrobelli, A., Matz, P. E., Must, S., et al. (2004). Familial aggregation of energy intake in children. *American Journal of Clinical Nutrition, 79,* 844–850.

Faith, M. S., Kermanshah, M., & Kissileff, H. R. (2002). Development and preliminary validation of a silhouette satiety scale for children. *Physiology & Behavior, 76,* 173–178.

Fanciullo, G. J., Cravero, J. P., Mudge, B. O., McHugo, G. J., & Baird, J. C. (2007). Development of a new computer method to assess children's pain. *Pain Medicine, 8*(Suppl. 3), S121–S128.

Fiorito, L. M., Mitchell, D. C., Smiciklas-Wright, H., & Birch, L. L. (2006a). Dairy and dairy-related nutrient intake during middle childhood. *Journal of the American Dietetic Association, 106,* 534–542.

Fiorito, L. M., Mitchell, D. C., Smiciklas-Wright, H., & Birch, L. L. (2006b). Girls' calcium intake is associated with bone mineral content during middle childhood. *Journal of Nutrition, 136,* 1281–1286.

Fiorito, L. M., Ventura, A. K., Mitchell, D. C., Smiciklas-Wright, H., & Birch, L. L. (2006). Girls' dairy intake, energy intake, and weight status. *Journal of the American Dietetic Association, 106,* 1851–1855.

Fisher, J. O. (2007). Effects of age on children's intake of large and self-selected food portions. *Obesity (Silver Spring), 15,* 403–412.

Fisher, J. O., Arreola, A., Birch, L. L., & Rolls, B. J. (2007). Portion size effects on daily energy intake in low-income Hispanic and African American children and their mothers. *American Journal of Clinical Nutrition, 86,* 1709–1716.

Fisher, J. O., & Birch, L. L. (1995). Fat preferences and fat consumption of 3- to 5-year-old children are related to parental adiposity. *Journal of the American Dietetic Association, 95,* 759–764.

Fisher, J. O., & Birch, L. L. (1999). Restricting access to foods and children's eating. *Appetite, 32,* 405–419.

Fisher, J. O., & Birch, L. L. (2000). Parents' restrictive feeding practices are associated with young girls' negative self-evaluation of eating. *Journal of the American Dietetic Association, 100,* 1341–1346.

Fisher, J. O., & Birch, L. L. (2002). Eating in the absence of hunger and overweight in girls from 5 to 7 y of age. *American Journal of Clinical Nutrition, 76,* 226–231.

Fisher, J. O., Liu, Y., Birch, L. L., & Rolls, B. J. (2007). Effects of portion size and energy density on young children's intake at a meal. *American Journal of Clinical Nutrition, 86,* 174–179.

Fox, D. T., Jeffrey, D. B., Dahlkoetter, J., McLellarn, R. W., & Hickey, J. S. (1980, September). *How television commercials affect children's attitudes and eating behavior.* Paper presented at the meeting of the American Psychological Association, Montreal, Canada.

Francis, L. A., Lee, Y., & Birch, L. L. (2003). Parental weight status and girls' television viewing, snacking, and body mass indexes. *Obesity Research, 11,* 143–151.

Garaulet, M., Martínez, A., Victoria, F., Pérez-Llamas, F., Ortega, R. M., & Zamora, S. (2000). Difference in dietary intake and activity level between normal-weight and overweight or obese adolescents. *Journal of Pediatric Gastroenterology and Nutrition, 30,* 253–258.

Garner, D. M. (1991a). *Eating Disorder Inventory–2 professional manual.* Odessa, FL: Psychological Assessment Inventory.

Garner, D. M. (1991b). *Eating Disorders Inventory–C.* Lutz, FL: Psychological Assessment Resources.

Garner, D. M., & Garfinkel, P. E. (1979). The Eating Attitudes Test: An index of the symptoms of anorexia nervosa. *Psychological Medicine, 9,* 273–279.

Garner, D. M., Olmsted, M. P., Bohh, Y., & Garfinkel, P. E. (1982). The eating attitudes test: Psychometric features and clinical correlates. *Psychological Medicine, 12,* 871–878.

Garner, D. M., Olmsted, M. P., & Polivy, J. (1983). Development and validation of a multidimensional eating disorder inventory for anorexia nervosa and bulimia. *International Journal of Eating Disorders, 2,* 15–34.

Garner, D. M., Rockert, W., Olmsted, M. P., Johnson, C. L., & Coscina, D. V. (1985). Psychoeducational principles in the treatment of bulimia and anorexia nervosa. In D. E. Garner & P. E. Garfinkel (Eds.), *Handbook of psychotherapy for anorexia nervosa and bulimia* (pp. 513–572). New York: Guilford.

Gila, A., Castro, J., Cesena, J., & Toro, J. (2005). Anorexia nervosa in male adolescents: Body image, eating attitudes and psychological traits. *Journal of Adolescent Health, 36,* 221–226.

Gilbertson, H. R., Thorburn, A. W., Brand-Miller, J. C., Chondros, P., & Werther, G. A. (2003). Effect of low-glycemic-index dietary advice on dietary quality and food choice in children with type 1 diabetes. *American Journal of Clinical Nutrition, 77,* 83–90.

Ginsburg, H., & Opper, S. (1969). *Piaget's theory of intellectual development.* Englewood Cliffs, NJ: Prentice Hall.

Goldstein, G. L., Daun, H., & Tepper, B. J. (2007). Influence of PROP taster status and maternal variables on energy intake and body weight of preadolescents. *Physiology & Behavior, 90,* 809–817.

Guenther, P. M., DeMaio, T. J., Ingwersen, L. A., & Berlin, M. (1995, January). The multiple-pass approach for the 24-hour recall in the Continuing Survey of Food Intakes by Individuals (CSFII) 1994–1996. Paper presented at the International Conference on Dietary Assessment Methods, Boston.

Heitmann, B. L., & Lissner, L. (1995). Dietary underreporting by obese individuals—is it specific or nonspecific? *British Medical Journal, 311,* 986–989.

Hendy, H. M., & Raudenbush, B. (2000). Effectiveness of teacher modeling to encourage food acceptance in preschool children. *Appetite, 34,* 61–76.

Herman, C. P., & Polivy, J. (1980). Restrained eating. In A. Stunkard (Ed.), *Obesity* (pp. 208–225). Philadelphia: W. B. Saunders.

Hetherington, E. M., & Parke, R. D. (1979). *Child psychology: A contemporary viewpoint* (2nd ed.). New York: McGraw-Hill.

Hetherington, M., & Rolls, B. J. (1987). Methods of investigating human eating behavior. In F. M. Toates & N. E. Rowland (Eds.), *Feeding and drinking* (pp. 77–109). Amsterdam: Elsevier.

Hill, A. J., Draper, E., & Stack, J. (1994). A weight on children's minds: Body shape dissatisfactions at 9-years old. *International Journal of Obesity and Related Metabolic Disorders, 18,* 383–289.

Horner, N. K., Patterson, R. E., Neuhouser, M. L., Lampe, J. W., Beresford, S. A., & Prentice, R. L. (2002). Participant characteristics associated with errors in self-reported energy intake from the Women's Health Initiative food-frequency questionnaire. *American Journal of Clinical Nutrition, 76,* 766–773.

Huang, T. T., Howarth, N. C., Lin, B.-H., Roberts, S., & McCrory, M. (2004). Energy intake and meal portions: Associations with BMI percentile in U.S. children. *Obesity Research, 12,* 1875–1885.

Huang, T. T., Roberts, S. B., Howarth, N. C., & McCrory, M. A. (2005). Effect of screening out implausible energy intake reports on relationships between diet and BMI. *Obesity Research, 13,* 1205–1217.

Jaramillo, S. J., Yang, S. J., Hughes, S. O., Fisher, J. O., Morales, M., & Nicklas, T. A. (2006). Interactive computerized fruit and vegetable preference measure for African-American and Hispanic preschoolers. *Journal of Nutrition Education and Behavior, 38,* 352–359.

Jeffrey, D. B., Lemnitzer, N. B., Hickey, J. S., Hess, M. J., McLellarn, R. W., & Stroud, J. M. (1980). The development of a behavioral eating test and its relationship to a self-report food attitude scale in young children. *Behavioral Assessment, 2,* 87–98.

Jeffrey, D. B., McLellarn, R. W., & Fox, D. T. (1982). The development of children's eating habits: The role of television commercials. *Health Education Quarterly, 9,* 174–189.

Johnson, R. K., Driscoll, P., & Goran, M. I. (1996). Comparison of multiple-pass 24-hour recall estimates of energy intake with total energy expenditure determined by the doubly labeled water method in young children. *Journal of the American Dietetic Association, 96,* 1140–1144.

Johnson, R. K., Goran, M. I., & Poehlman, E. T. (1994). Correlates of over- and underreporting of energy intake in healthy older men and women. *American Journal of Clinical Nutrition, 59,* 1286–1290.

Johnson, S. L. (2000). Improving preschoolers' self-regulation of energy intake. *Pediatrics, 106,* 1429–1435.

Johnson, S. L., & Birch, L. L. (1994). Parents' and children's adiposity and eating style. *Pediatrics, 94,* 653–661.

Johnson, S. L., McPhee, L., & Birch, L. L. (1991). Conditioned preferences: Young children prefer flavors associated with high dietary fat. *Physiology & Behavior, 50,* 1245–1251.

Jonat, L. M., & Birmingham, C. L. (2004). Disordered eating attitudes and behaviours in the high-school students of a rural Canadian community. *Eating and Weight Disorders, 9,* 285–289.

Kaskoun, M. C., Johnson, R. K., & Goran, M. I. (1994). Comparison of energy intake by semiquantitative food-frequency questionnaire with total energy expenditure by the doubly labeled water method in young children. *American Journal of Clinical Nutrition, 60,* 43–47.

Keller, K. L., Assur, S. A., Torres, M., Lofink, H. E., Thornton, J. C., Faith, M. S., et al. (2006). Potential of an analog scaling device for measuring fullness in children: Development and preliminary testing. *Appetite, 47,* 233–243.

Keller, K. L., Steinmann, L., Nurse, R. J., & Tepper, B. J. (2002). Genetic taste sensitivity to 6-n-propylthiouracil influences food preference and reported intake in preschool children. *Appetite, 38,* 3–12.

Keller, K. L., & Tepper, B. J. (2004). Inherited taste sensitivity to 6-n-propylthiouracil in diet and body weight in children. *Obesity Research, 12,* 904–912.

Kissileff, H. R., Klingsberg, G., & Van Itallie, T. B. (1980). Universal eating monitor for continuous recording of solid or liquid consumption in man. *American Journal of Physiology, 238,* R14–R22.

Klesges, L. M., Baranowski, T., Beech, B., Cullen, K., Murray, D. M., Rochon, J., & Pratt, C. (2004). Social desirability bias in self-reported dietary, physical activity and weight concerns measures in 8- to 10-year-old African-American girls: Results from the Girls Health Enrichment Multisite Studies (GEMS). *Preventive Medicine, 38*(Suppl.), S78–S87.

Klesges, R. C., Coates, T. J., Brown, G., Sturgen-Tillisch, J., Moldenhauer-Kleges, L. M., Holzer, B., et al. (1983). Parental influences on children's eating behavior and relative weight. *Journal of Applied Behavior Analysis, 16,* 371–378.

Klesges, R. C., Hanson, C. L., Eck, L. H., & Durff, A. C. (1988). Accuracy of self-reports of food intake in obese and normal-weight individuals: Effects of parental obesity on reports of children's dietary intake. *American Journal of Clinical Nutrition, 48,* 1252–1256.

Lappalainen, R., & Epstein, L. H. (1990). A behavioral economics analysis of food choice in humans. *Appetite, 14,* 81–93.

Leahy, K. E., Birch, L. L., & Rolls, B. J. (2008a). Reducing the energy density of an entrée decreases children's energy intake at lunch. *Journal of the American Dietetic Association, 108,* 41–48.

Leahy, K. E., Birch, L. L., & Rolls, B. J. (2008b). Reducing the energy density of multiple meals decreases the energy intake of preschool-age children. *American Journal of Clinical Nutrition, 88,* 1459–1468.

Leahy, K. E., Birch, L. L., Fisher, J. O., & Rolls, B. J. (2008). Reductions in entrée energy density increase children's vegetable intake and reduce energy intake. *Obesity, 16,* 1559–1565.

Leahy, K. E., Roe, L. S., Birch, L., & Rolls, L. (2006). Does the energy density of an entree influence children's energy intake? *Obesity, 14,* A19.

Lemnitzer, N. B., Jeffrey, D. B., Hess, M. J., Hickey, J. S., & Stroud, J. M. (1979). *Television food advertising: Does it affect children's food consumption?* Paper presented at the meeting of the Society for Research on Child Development, San Francisco.

Lichtman, S. W., Pisarska, K., Berman, E. R., Perstone, M., Dowling, H., Offenbacher, E., et al. (1992). Discrepancy between self-reported and actual caloric intake and exercise in obese subjects. *New England Journal of Medicine, 327,* 1893–1898.

Liem, D. G., & de Graaf, C. (2004). Sweet and sour preferences in young children and adults: Role of repeated exposure. *Physiology & Behavior, 83,* 421–429.

Liem, D. G., Mars, M., & de Graaf, C. (2004). Sweet preferences and sugar consumption of 4- and 5-year-old children: Role of parents. *Appetite, 43,* 235–245.

Liem, D. G., & Mennella, J. A. (2003). Heightened sour preferences during childhood. *Chemical Senses, 28,* 173–180.

Liem, D. G., Westerbeek, A., Wolterink, S., Kok, F. J., & de Graaf, C. (2004). Sour taste preferences of children relate to preference for novel and intense stimuli. *Chemical Senses, 29,* 713–720.

Lindquist, C. H., Cummings, T., & Goran, M. I. (2000). Use of tape-recorded food records in assessing children's dietary intake. *Obesity Research, 8,* 2–11.

Livingstone, M. B., & Black, A. E. (2003). Markers of the validity of reported energy intake. *Journal of Nutrition, 133*(Suppl. 3), 895S–920S.

Livingstone, M. B., & Robson, P. J. (2000). Measurement of dietary intake in children. *Proceedings of the Nutrition Society, 59,* 279–293.

Livingstone, M. B., Robson, P. J., & Wallace, J. M. (2004). Issues in dietary intake assessment of children and adolescents. *British Journal of Nutrition, 92*(Suppl. 2), S213–S222.

Loewen, R., & Pliner, P. (1999). Effects of prior exposure to palatable and unpalatable novel foods on children's willingness to taste other novel foods. *Appetite, 32,* 351–366.

Ludwig, D. S., Majzoub, J. A., Al-Zahrani, A., Dallal, G. E., Blanco, I., & Roberts, S. B. (1999). High glycemic index foods, overeating, and obesity. *Pediatrics, 103,* E26.

Lumeng, J. C., & Hillman, K. H. (2007). Eating in larger group increases food consumption. *Archives of Disease in Childhood, 92,* 384–387.

Lynch, W., Eppers, K., & Sherrodd, J. (2004). Eating attitudes of Native American and white female adolescents: A comparison of BMI- and age-matched groups. *Ethnicity & Health, 9,* 253–266.

Lynch, W. C., & Eppers-Reynolds, K. (2005). Children's Eating Attitudes Test: Revised factor structure for adolescent girls. *Eating and Weight Disorders, 10,* 222–235.

Maloney, M. J., McGuire, J. B., & Daniels, S. R. (1988). Reliability testing of a children's version of the Eating Attitude Test. *Journal of the American Academy of Child and Adolescent Psychiatry, 27,* 541–543.

McCarthy, D. M., Simmons, J. R., Smith, G. T., Tomlinson, K. L., & Hill, K. K. (2002). Reliability, stability, and factor structure of the Bulimia Test–Revised and Eating Disorder Inventory–2 scales in adolescence. *Assessment, 9,* 382–389.

McCrory, M. A., Hajduk, C. L., & Roberts, S. B. (2002). Procedures for screening out inaccurate reports of dietary energy intake. *Public Health Nutrition, 5,* 873–882.

McGrath, P. A. (1989). Evaluating a child's pain. *Journal of Pain and Symptom Management, 4,* 198–214.

McGrath, P. A., de Veber, L. L., & Hearn, M. (1985). Multidimensional pain assessment in children. *Advances in Pain Research and Therapy, 9.* 387–393.

The McKnight Investigators. (2003). Risk factors for the onset of eating disorders in adolescent girls: Results of the McKnight longitudinal risk factor study. *American Journal of Psychiatry, 160,* 248–254.

McPherson, R. S., Hoelscher, D. M., Alexander, M., Scanlon, K., & Seruda, M. l. (2002). Validity and reliability of dietary assessment in school-age children. In C. D. Berdanier (Ed.), *Handbook of nutrition and food* (pp. 495–522). Boca Raton, FL: CRC Press.

Mendelson, B. K., Mendelson, M. J., & White, D. R. (2001). Body-esteem scale for adolescents and adults. *Journal of Personality Assessment, 76,* 90–106.

Mendelson, B. K., & White, D. R. (1982). Relation between body-esteem and self-esteem of obese and normal children. *Perceptual and Motor Skills, 54,* 899–905.

Mendelson, B. K., & White, D. R. (1985). Development of self-body esteem in overweight youngsters. *Developmental Psychology, 21,* 90–96.

Mennella, J. A., Kennedy, J. M., & Beauchamp, G. K. (2006). Vegetable acceptance by infants: Effects of formula flavors. *Early Human Development, 82,* 463–468.

Mennella, J. A., Pepino, M. Y., & Reed, D. R. (2005). Genetic and environmental determinants of bitter perception and sweet preferences. *Pediatrics, 115,* e216–e222.

Miotto, P., De Coppi, M., Frezza, M., Rossi, M., & Preti, A. (2002). Social desirability and eating disorders: A community study of an Italian school-aged sample. *Acta Psychiatrica Scandinavica, 105,* 372–377.

Mirch, M. C., McDuffie, J. R., Yanorski, S. Z., Schollnberger, M., Tanofsky-Kraff, M., & Theim, K. R., et al. (2006). Effects of binge eating on satiation, satiety, and energy intake of overweight children. *American Journal of Clinical Nutrition, 84,* 732–738.

Nelson, M., Black, J. R., Morris, J. A., & Cole, T. J. (1989). Between- and within-subject variation in nutrient intake from infancy to old age: Estimating the number of days required to rank dietary intakes with desired precision. *American Journal of Clinical Nutrition, 50,* 155–167.

Netemeyer, S., & Williamson, D. (2001). Assessment of eating disturbance in children and adolescents with eating disorders and obesity. In J. Thompson & L. Smolak (Eds.), *Body image, eating disorders, and obesity in youth.*(pp. 215–233). Washington, DC: American Psychological Association.

Orlet Fisher, J., Rolls, B. J., & Birch, L. L. (2003). Children's bite size and intake of an entree are greater with large portions than with age-appropriate or self-selected portions. *American Journal of Clinical Nutrition, 77,* 1164–1170.

Pelchat, M. L., & Pliner, P. (1995). Try it. You'll like it. Effects of information on willingness to try novel foods. *Appetite, 24,* 153–165.

Perks, S. M., Roemmich, J. N., Sandow-Pajewski, M., Clark, P. A., Thomas, E., Weltman, A., et al.

(2000). Alterations in growth and body composition during puberty. IV. Energy intake estimated by the youth-adolescent food-frequency questionnaire: Validation by the doubly labeled water method. *American Journal of Clinical Nutrition, 72*, 1455–1460.

Pliner, P., & Stallberg-White, C. (2000). Pass the ketchup, please: Familiar flavors increase children's willingness to taste novel foods. *Appetite, 34*, 95–103.

Rockett, H. R., Breitenbach, M., Frazier, A. L., Witschi, J., Wolf, A. M., Field, A. E., Colditz, G. A. (1997). Validation of a youth/adolescent food frequency questionnaire. *Preventive Medicine, 26*, 808–816.

Rockett, H. R., & Colditz, G. A. (1997). Assessing diets of children and adolescents. *American Journal of Clinical Nutrition, 65*(Suppl.), 1116S–1122S.

Rockett, H. R., Wolf, A. M.., & Colditz, A. M. (1995). Development and reproducibility of a food frequency questionnaire to assess diets of older children and adolescents. *Journal of the American Dietetic Association, 95*, 336–340.

Rodin, J. (1975). Effects of obesity and set point on taste responsiveness and ingestion in humans. *Journal of Comparative Physiological Psychology, 89*, 1003–1009.

Rolls, B. J., Castellanos, V. H., Shide, D. J., Miller, D. L., Pelkman, C. L., Thorwart, M. L., et al. (1997). Sensory properties of a nonabsorbable fat substitute did not affect regulation of energy intake. *American Journal of Clinical Nutrition, 65*, 1375–1383.

Rolls, B. J., Engell, D., & Birch, L. L. (2000). Serving portion size influences 5-year-old but not 3-year-old children's food intakes. *Journal of the American Dietetic Association, 100*, 232–234.

Rolls, B. J., & McDermott, T. M. (1991). Effects of age on sensory-specific satiety. *American Journal of Clinical Nutrition, 54*, 988–996.

Rolls, B. J., Rowe, E. A., Rolls, E. J., Kingston, B., Megson, A., & Gunary, R. (1981). Variety in a meal enhances food intake in man. *Physiology & Behavior, 26*, 215–221.

Rozin, P., Ebert, L., & Schall, J. (1982). Some like it hot: A temporal analysis of hedonic responses to chili pepper. *Appetite, 3*, 13–22.

Salvy, S. J., Romero, N., Paluch, R., & Epstein, L. H. (2007). Peer influence on pre-adolescent girls' snack intake: Effects of weight status. *Appetite, 49*, 177–182.

Schachter, S. (1968). Obesity and eating: Internal and external cues differentially affect the eating behavior of obese and normal subjects. *Science, 161*, 751–756.

Serdula, M. K., Alexander, M. P., Scanlon, K. S., & Bowman, B. A. (2001). What are preschool children eating? A review of dietary assessment. *Annual Review of Nutrition, 21*, 475–498.

Sherman, D. K., Iacono, W. G., & Donnelly, J. M. (1995). Development and validation of body rating scales for adolescent females. *International Journal of Eating Disorders, 18*, 327–333.

Shields, B. J., Palermo, T. M., Powers, J. D., Grewe, S. D., & Smith, G. A. (2003). Predictors of a child's ability to use a visual analogue scale. *Child: Care, Health and Development, 29*, 281–290.

Shisslak, C. M., Renger, R., Sharpe, T., Crago, M., McKnight, K. M., Gray, N., et al. (1999). Development and evaluation of the McKnight Risk Factor Survey for assessing potential risk and protective factors for disordered eating in preadolescent and adolescent girls. *International Journal of Eating Disorders, 25*, 195–214.

Shore, R., & Porter, J. (1990). Normative and reliability data for 11 to 18 year olds for the Eating Disorder Inventory. *International Journal of Eating Disorders, 9*, 201–208.

Smiciklas-Wright, H., Mitchell, D. C., & Harris, J. (2002). Dietary intake assessment: Methods for adults. In C. D. Berdanier (Ed.), *Handbook of nutrition and food* (pp. 477–493). Boca Raton, FL: CRC Press.

Smith, J. A., & Epstein, L. H. (1991). Behavioral economic analysis of food choice in obese children. *Appetite, 17*, 91–95.

Snoek, H. M., van Strien, T., Janssens, J. M., & Engels, R. C. (2007). Emotional, external, restrained eating and overweight in Dutch adolescents. *Scandinavian Journal of Psychology, 48*, 23–32.

Stanford, E. A., Chambers, C. T., & Craig, K. D. (2006). The role of developmental factors in predicting young children's use of a self-report scale for pain. *Pain, 120*, 16–23.

Stice, E. (1998a). Prospective relation of dieting behaviors to weight change in a community sample of adolescents. *Behavior Therapy, 29*, 277–297.

Stice, E. (1998b). Relations of restraint and negative affect to bulimic pathology: A longitudinal test of three competing models. *International Journal of Eating Disorders, 23*, 243–260.

Stice, E., Fisher, M., & Lowe, M. R. (2004). Are dietary restraint scales valid measures of acute dietary restriction? Unobtrusive observational data suggest not. *Psychological Assessment, 16*, 51–59.

Stunkard, A. J. (1968). Environment and obesity: Recent advances in our understanding of regulation of food intake in man. *Federal Proceedings, 27*, 1367–1373.

Stunkard, A. J., Sørensen, T., & Schulsinger, F. (1983). Use of the Danish Adoption Register for the study of obesity and thinness. *Research Publications—Association for Research in Nervous and Mental Diseases, 60*, 115–120.

Tanofsky-Kraff, M., Theim, K. R., Yanovski, S. Z., Bassett, A. M., Burns, N. P., & Ranzenhofer, L. M. (2007). Validation of the emotional eating scale adapted for use in children and adolescents (EES-C). *International Journal of Eating Disorders, 40*, 232–240.

Temple, J. L., Giacomelli, A. M., Kent, K. M., Roemmich, J. N., & Epstein, L. H. (2007). Television watching increases motivated responding for food and energy intake in children. *American Journal of Clinical Nutrition, 85*, 355–361.

Thurfjell, B., Edlund, B., Arinell, H., Hägglöf, B., & Engström, I. (2003). Psychometric properties of Eating Disorder Inventory for Children (EDI-C) in Swedish girls with and without a known eating disorder. *Eating and Weight Disorders, 8*, 296–303.

Tooze, J. A., Subar, A. F., Thompson, F. E., Troiano, R., Schatzkin, A., & Kipnis, V. (2004). Psychosocial predictors of energy underreporting in a large doubly labeled water study. *American Journal of Clinical Nutrition, 79*, 795–804.

Toro, J., Gomez-Peresmitré, G., Sentis, J., Vallés, A., Casulà, V., Castro, J. et al. (2006). Eating disorders and body image in Spanish and Mexican female adolescents. *Social Psychiatry and Psychiatric Epidemiology, 41*, 556–565.

Truby, H., & Paxton, S. J. (2002). Development of the Children's Body Image Scale. *British Journal of Clinical Psychology, 41*(Pt. 2), 185–203.

Turnbull, B., & Matisoo-Smith, E. (2002). Taste sensitivity to 6-n-propylthiouracil predicts acceptance of bitter-tasting spinach in 3–6-y-old children. *American Journal of Clinical Nutrition, 76*, 1101–1105.

Vacc, N. A., & Rhyne, M. (1987). The Eating Attitudes Test: Development of an adapted language form for children. *Perceptual and Motor Skills, 65*, 335–336.

van Strien, T. (2002). *Dutch Eating Behavior Questionnaire manual.* Bury St. Edmunds, UK: Thames Valley Test Company.

van Strien, T., Frijters, J. E., Bergers, G. P. A., & Defares, P. B. (1986). The Dutch Eating Behavior Questionnaire (DEBQ) for assessment of restrained, emotional, and external eating behavior. *International Journal of Eating Disorders, 5*, 295–315.

van Strien, T., Frijters, J. E., van Staveren, W. A., Defares, P. B., & Deurenberg, P. (1986). The predictive validity of the Dutch Restrained Eating Scale. *International Journal of Eating Disorders, 5*, 747–755.

Ventura, A. K., Loken, E., Mitchell, D. C., Smiciklas-Wright, H., & Birch, L. L. (2006). Understanding reporting bias in the dietary recall data of 11-year-old girls. *Obesity (Silver Spring), 14*, 1073–1084.

Villarruel, A. M., & Denyes, M. J. (1991). Pain assessment in children: Theoretical and empirical validity. *Advances in Nursing Science, 14*, 32–41.

Wardle, J., & Beales, S. (1986). Restraint, body image and food attitudes in children from 12 to 18 years. *Appetite, 7*, 209–217.

Wardle, J., & Marsland, L. (1990). Adolescent concerns about weight and eating: A social-development perspective. *Journal of Psychosomatic Research, 34*, 377–391.

Wardle, J., Marsland, L., Sheikh, Y., Quinn, M., Fedoroff, I., & Ogden, J. (1992). Eating style and eating behaviour in adolescents. *Appetite, 18*, 167–183.

Warren, J. M., Henry, C. J., & Simonite, V. (2003). Low glycemic index breakfasts and reduced food intake in preadolescent children. *Pediatrics, 112*, e414.

Williamson, D. A., Anderson, D. A., & Gleaves, D. H. (1996). Anorexia and bulimia nervosa: Structured interview methodologies and psychological assessment. In K. Thompson (Ed.), *Body image, eating disorders, and obesity: A practical guide for assessment and treatment* (pp. 205–223). Washington, DC: American Psychological Association.

Williamson, D. A., Anderson, D. A., Jackman, L. P., & Jackson, S. R. (1995). Assessment of eating disordered thoughts, feelings, and behaviors. In D. B. Allison (Ed.), *Methods for the assessment of eating behaviors and weight related problems* (pp. 347–386). Newbury Park, CA: Sage.

Williamson, D. A., DeLany, J. P., Bentz, B. G., Bray, G. A., Champagne, C. M., & Harsha, D. W. (1997).

Gender and racial differences in dieting and social pressures to gain weight among children. *Journal of Gender, Culture, and Health, 2,* 231–243.

Wood, A., Waller, G., Miller, J., & Slade, P. (1992). The development of eating attitudes test scores in adolescence. *International Journal of Eating Disorders, 11,* 279–282.

Wood, K. C., Becker, J. A., & Thompson, J. K. (1996). Body image dissatisfaction in preadolescent children. *Journal of Applied Developmental Psychology, 17,* 85–100.

CHAPTER 13

Assessment of Human Body Composition

Dympna Gallagher and Fahad Javed

Overview of Phenotyping in Human Body Composition

The measurement of human body composition in living persons involves using available techniques to provide information acquired in vivo on tissues and/or organs that make up the body. Some of the information acquired is an estimate and not a direct measurement of any given tissue. A direct measurement would require invasively extracting tissue, which is typically not feasible and certainly not desirable in living persons but is possible in cadavers, or using neutron activation analysis, which involves high radiation exposure. Measuring body composition in humans is often inspired by the need to describe either deficiencies or excesses of a component that is thought or known to be related to health risk. Understanding how the quantity and distribution of body fat and the composition of fat-free mass (FFM) varies as a function of sex, race, and age or changes with growth, weight gain, or weight loss (Forbes, 1987; Sopher, Shen, & Pietrobelli, 2005) are examples of

areas of interest that require human body composition phenotyping.

The available measurement methods range from simple to complex, with all methods having limitations and some degree of measurement error. The clinical significance of the body compartment to be measured should first be determined before a measurement method is selected since the more advanced techniques are less accessible and more costly. The interest in or need to understand the composition of the human body has grown over the past several decades in part due to the steady increase in overweight and obesity and the metabolic consequences (e.g., insulin resistance) associated with high and low levels of body fat and where the fat is distributed, in addition to many other clinical conditions where chemical content in body tissues is known to be altered. While much progress has been made in developing and applying techniques for the noninvasive assessment of tissues and organs in vivo, a complete characterization of the human body is far from having been accomplished.

AUTHORS' NOTE: This work was supported by Grants HD42187 and DK72507 from the National Institutes of Health.

The assessment of body composition in an individual can occur at a simple level where anthropometric measures, such as weight, height, waist, and hip circumference as well as skinfold thicknesses are measured, or at an advanced level where multiple organs and tissues are measured. Whether the interest in assessing body composition arises from the need to quantify the amount of excess fat or the degree to which too little fat is present, the tools are available to make these assessments. It is not well understood what "normal" or "healthy" body fat percentages are. The healthy fat ranges proposed by the American College of Sports Medicine (2001) are 8% to 22% in men and 20% to 35% in women, and average values based on risk are presented in Table 13.1. The body composition parameters and characteristics put forth for the "Reference Man" and "Reference Woman" (Snyder et al., 1975) are as follows:

Reference man: ages 20–24; height 68.5 in; weight 154 lb; total fat 23.1 lb (15%) of which storage fat is 18.5 lb (12%) and essential fat is 4.6 lb (3%); muscle 69 lb (44.8%); bone 23 lb (14.9%); remainder 38.9 lb (25.3%)

Reference woman: ages 20–24; height 64.5 in; weight 125 lb; total fat 33.8 lb (27%) of which storage fat is 18.5 lb (15%) and essential fat is 15 lb (12%); muscle 45 lb (36%); bone 15 lb (12%); remainder 31.2 lb (25%)

There is a lack of equivalent data in children of all ages, including newborns. Published data for fat and fat-free mass based on bioelectrical impedance values are available for 3- to 11-year-old healthy Japanese children (Nakao & Komiya, 2003). An evaluation of the usefulness of body mass index (BMI) and age-, gender-adjusted BMI and gender-specific percentiles of BMI as surrogate measures of body fatness in 5- to 18.7-year-old (Field et al., 2003) U.S. children found that all of the aforementioned BMI indices had similar associations with body fatness, but age- and gender-specific percentiles of BMI were the least accurate. A BMI *z* score of 1, a BMI percentile of 85, and a BMI of 20 kg/m² were all applicable for identifying children who may be overfat.

Importance of Body Composition Measurements in Clinical Practice

The higher prevalence of obesity in minority populations and individuals with lower income and education levels contributes to excess disease and mortality rates among these groups. Research has shown that obesity in childhood tracks into adulthood (Dietz, 1998) and is associated with increased susceptibility to hypertension, dyslipidemia, and glucose intolerance. Race/ethnic differences in the prevalence of type 2 diabetes in adults in the United States are well established. The significant increase in the prevalence of childhood obesity over the past 30 years has coincided with a notable increase in the incidence of type 2 diabetes among adolescents. Substantial progress has been made toward identifying population-based risk factors for the development of type 2 diabetes that might lead to these race-ethnic disparities, including total body fatness or adiposity, central adiposity, duration of obesity, high caloric intake, physical inactivity, and genetic predisposition. While all race/ethnic groups are at risk for type 2 diabetes, the way in which some groups respond to specific risk factors may predispose them to a greater risk of diabetes. Therefore, the inclusion of body fat and/or body fat distribution measurements in clinical practice could assist in the identification and treatment of persons at risk for comorbid conditions.

Historical Background

The study of body composition as it is known today actively evolved during the latter half of the 19th and throughout the 20th centuries and has been comprehensively chronicled by Shen, St-Onge, Wang, and Heymsfield (2005).

Assessment Issues Related to Assumptions and Population Being Assessed

An example of a classical assumption in body composition assessment that has a significant

Table 13.1   Average Percent Body Fat Values in Adult Men and Women

	Males (%)	Females (%)
Average	15–17	23
Above average	17–23	24–31
At risk	24 and above	32 and above

SOURCE: Heyward and Stolarczyk (1996).

impact on body fat estimation is that the densities of fat (0.9007 g/cm³) and FFM (1.100 g/cm³) are stable across all adults irrespective of age, race/ethnicity, and disease. A second area of debate is whether the water fraction of FFM changes with age as many assessment approaches assume a constant hydration of FFM (73%). Since approximately 25% of adipose tissue is water, adipose tissue water contributes to FFM and may contribute to a higher hydration of the FFM in obese persons (Deurenberg, Leenen, Van der Kooy, & Hautvast, 1989; Waki et al., 1991). The latter would imply a lower density of FFM in obese people.

Sex

As documented in Table 13.1, the average percent body fat is greater in females than in males. This sexual dimorphism in body fat is evident as early as birth and extends throughout the life span (Fomon, Haschke, Ziegler, & Nelson, 1982). As reported by Greil (2006), girls are shorter at birth but increase in length at higher rates than boys and overgrow boys up to age 12 years, after which males demonstrate 6% to 9% more length by adult years. There are only small differences between the sexes for body circumferences up to the age of 13 years, after which female circumferences tend to be smaller across the remainder of the life span. The developmental pattern of sexual dimorphism in weight and BMI is similar to that for length measurements, while subcutaneous fat

and total body fat content are always higher in females. These findings highlight that sexual dimorphism develops at different paces for the various components of the body. The implication therefore is that assessment methods that assume constant proportions with increasing age in children are flawed and will provide inaccurate body composition results.

Race/Ethnicity

For the same total fat mass, race differences in fat distribution are evident as early as prepuberty (He et al., 2002) and remain throughout adulthood. Smaller hip circumferences have been documented in Asian females at all pubertal stages compared with Whites and Hispanics (Hammer et al., 1991), and trunk subcutaneous fat is greater in Asian females compared with Whites (Malina, Huang, & Brown, 1995). Differences in subcutaneous fat mass and fat distribution in Asian compared with White adults (J. Wang et al., 1994) and race differences in the course of sex-specific fat distribution with the progression of puberty (He et al., 2004) have been described. Differences between Blacks and Whites in the distribution of subcutaneous adipose tissue and in the density of FFM (1.113 g/cm³ vs. 1.100 g/cm³ in Blacks and Whites, respectively) reduce the validity of some body fat measurement techniques (Dioum, Gartner, Maire, Delpeuch, & Wade, 2005), including anthropometry, hydrodensitometry, and air displacement plethysmography.

Aging

An important component of understanding obesity is determining what a normal body fat content is and how this may change with age. Many studies investigating the relationship between body fat and aging have reported either an increase in body fat until early old age, followed by a decrease thereafter, or a pattern of steadily increasing body fat with aging (Coin et al., 2008; Going, Williams, & Lohman, 1995; Mott et al., 1999; Silver, Guillen, Kahl, & Morley, 1993). Some previous studies of the relation between age and fatness used two-compartment models of body composition based on hydrodensitometry (Durnin & Womersley, 1974) or measurement of total body potassium (Flynn, Nolph, Baker, Martin, & Krause, 1989) where these models are dependent on assumptions such as a constant density of FFM across the adult age span or a constant potassium concentration in the FFM. However, these assumptions have been shown to have poor validity (Heymsfield et al., 1993; Mazariegos et al., 1994) as both the density and the potassium content of the FFM have been shown to change with age (Bergsma-Kadijk, Baumeister, & Deurenberg, 1996; Heymsfield et al., 1993).

Special Populations

Distinct changes in body composition occur following spinal cord injury (SCI). Specifically, there is a reduction in FFM and an increase in fat mass, a paradigm that has been compared to premature aging (Evans, 1995; Spungen, Bauman, Wang, & Pierson, 1995). Persons with SCI were found to be fatter for any body mass index, with less lean and more adipose tissues for any given age compared with controls (Spungen et al., 2003). In a study of monozygotic twins where one twin has SCI, Spungen et al. (2003) reported a steady loss of leg lean tissue that was directly correlated with duration of injury (Spungen et al., 2003), while the level of SCI, with successively higher, more complete spinal cord lesions

was associated with decreased FFM and body cell mass (Nulicek et al., 1988). The latter demonstrate that some basic assumptions inherent in body composition assessment methods are not true in special populations such as those with SCI; persons with certain genetic disorders such as Down syndrome, Turner syndrome, Prader-Willi syndrome, and cystic fibrosis; and patients with certain diseases such as end-stage renal disease and Duchenne muscular dystrophy.

Obesity

Many currently available body composition measurement techniques are unable to accommodate very large-sized persons (e.g., dual-energy X-ray absorptiometry [DXA], total body potassium, magnetic resonance imaging [MRI], computed tomography [CT]). Moreover, some techniques have low or questionable (e.g., bioimpedance analysis) validity in very obese persons (Alvarez et al., 2007; Chouinard et al., 2007). Reference will be made throughout this chapter to assessment issues in obese individuals.

The feasibility of some methods is also affected by specific conditions; for example, it is difficult to perform underwater weighing with small children, nonambulatory elderly, or patients with lung diseases.

In the subsequent sections, additional consideration by the way of examples is given to how sex, race, age, and special conditions affect the underlying assumptions of *specific* body composition assessment methods.

Measurement Approaches in Body Composition

The use of models in body composition assessment (see Table 13.2) allows for an indirect estimation of a specific body component such as fat. Typically, a compartment is homogeneous in composition (e.g., fat), but the simpler the model, the greater the assumptions made and the greater the likelihood of error. However, the converse can also be true in that the more complex the model and the greater the number of independent measurements, the greater the potential for cumulative, propagated errors. The sum of components in each model should be equivalent to body weight. These models generally make assessments at the whole-body level and do not provide for regional or specific organ/tissue assessments.

Two-Compartment Model

The two-compartment (2C) models partition the body into FFM and FM and are the most widely used approaches to estimate body composition in adults (see Table 13.2). For example, Behnke's two-compartment model assumes known and constant proportions of FFM as water, protein, and mineral (Behnke, Feen, & Welham, 1942). It was from these assumed proportions, as well as the assumed density of each chemical component, that the density of FFM was derived as 1.100 g/cm³ (Brozek, Grande, Anderson, & Keys, 1963). When the assumptions that form the basis for the 2C model are not met, body composition estimates will be inaccurate. This may occur systematically with characteristics such as in aging, pregnancy, maturation, weight reduction in obese people, and various disease states. The 2C model approach is not ideal for

Table 13.2   Two- and Multicompartment Body Composition Models for Measuring Percentage Fat (%Fat)

Model	Equations for %Fat	Reference
2C	100 × (4.971/Db − 4.519)	Behnke, Feen, and Welham (1942)
2C	100 × (4.95/Db − 4.50)	Siri (1956)
2C	100 × (4.570/Db − 4.142)	Brozek, Grande, Anderson, and Keys (1963)
3C	100 × [2.118/Db − 0.78 × (TBW/W) 1.354]	Siri (1961)
3C	100 × [6.386/Db − 3.961 × M − 6.090]	Lohman (1986)
4C	100 × [2.747/Db − 0.714 × (TBW/W) + 1.129 × (TBBM/W) − 2.037]	Sellinger (1977)
4C	100 × [2.748/Db − 0.6744 × (TBW/W) + 1.4746 × (TBBM/W) − 2.051]	Heymsfield et al. (1990)
4C	100 × [2.513/Db − 0.739 × (TBW/W) + 0.947 × (TBBM/W) − 1.790]	Withers, Smith, Chatterton, Schultz, and Gaffney (1992)

NOTE: Db = body density (in kg/L); TBW = total body water (in kg); W = body weight (in kg); TBBM = total body bone mineral (osseous + nonosseous, in kg).

measuring fat mass or FFM in infants and young children as the proportions of FFM as water, protein, and mineral are changing with growth. The two-compartment model does not give information regarding the nutritionally important total body protein and mineral components.

Three- and Four-Compartment Models

A three-compartment (3C) model consists of fat, fat-free solids, and water (see Table 13.2) and includes measurements of body weight, volume, and water. The 3C model attempts to control for variability in the components of FFM (water, protein, bone mineral, and nonbone mineral; Withers, Laforgia, & Heymsfield, 1999). The water content of FFM is assumed to range between 70% and 76%, with a steady-state average of ~73% for most species. Results from several cross-sectional studies suggest that this assumption is generally robust over a broad age range in healthy adult humans (Chumlea et al., 2001; Visser et al., 1997; Z. Wang, Deurenberg, & Heymsfield, 2000). The fat-free solids component of FFM refers to minerals (including bone) and proteins. The Siri 3C model (Siri, 1961) is based on the assumption that the relationship between protein and mineral is constant, which it is not (Baumgartner, Heymsfield, Lichtman, Wang, & Pierson, 1991). The 3C approach involves the measurement of body density (usually by hydrodensitometry) and total body water by a tracer dilution technique. Assumptions are made that both the hydration of FFM and the solids portion of FFM are constant. Since bone mineral content is known to decrease with age, the 3C approach is limited in its accuracy in persons or populations where these assumptions are incorrect, such as the elderly and persons with osteopenia and osteoporosis.

A four-compartment (4C) model (see Table 13.2) involves the additional measure of bone mineral content by DXA to the 3C components of body density (for fat), total body water, and residual (residual = body weight − [fat + water + bone]; Heymsfield et al., 1990; Sellinger, 1977; Withers, Smith, Chatterton, Schultz, & Gaffney, 1992). This model allows for the assessment of several assumptions that are central to the 2C model. An advantage of the 4C model is that it takes into account deviations in the composition of FFM; for example, in children, with maturation, hydration of FFM decreases, whereas bone mineral increases with age (Slaughter, Christ, Stillman, & Boileau, 1993). The 4C approach is frequently used as the criterion method against which new body composition methods are compared in both children and adults.

An alternative 4C model (Cohn, Vaswani, Yasumura, Yuen, & Ellis, 1984) involves neutron activation methods for the measurement of total body nitrogen and total body calcium, where total body fat = body weight − total body protein (from total body nitrogen) + total body water (dilution volume) + total body ash (from total body calcium). However, the availability of neutron activation facilities is limited, and therefore the latter model is not readily obtainable by most researchers.

A six-compartment model (Heymsfield et al., 1991; Z. Wang, Ma, Pierson, & Heymsfield, 1993) can be calculated as follows: fat mass (measured from total body carbon) = body weight − (total body protein + total body water + bone mineral + soft tissue mineral [from a combination of total body potassium, total body nitrogen, total body chloride, total body calcium] + glycogen [total body nitrogen] + unmeasured residuals). Again, the availability of neutron activation facilities is limited, and therefore the latter model is not readily obtainable by most researchers.

Five-Level Model

At the organizational level, a five-level model (Wang, Pierson, & Heymsfield, 1992) was developed where the body can be characterized at five levels, thus providing a structural framework for studying human body composition that goes beyond an individual compartment or level. Each level and its components are distinct. The following are the levels and their constituents: atomic = oxygen, carbon, hydrogen, and other (Level 1); molecular = water, lipid, protein, and other (Level 2); cellular = cell mass, extracellular fluid, and extracellular solids (Level 3); tissue system level = skeletal muscle, adipose tissue, bone, blood, and other (Level 4); and whole body (Level 5).

Assessment Methods

Body composition measurement methods vary in complexity and precision and range from simple field-based methods (anthropometry, bioimpedance analysis) to more technically challenging laboratory-based methods (DXA; hydrostatic weighing; air plethysmography; whole-body counting for [40]K, deuterium, and bromide dilutions; and imaging). The choice of a body composition measurement method greatly depends on which body component is being investigated. (It also depends on issues such as study design, cost, and feasibility.) Each assessment method will be described, and the reliability (i.e., test-retest) of each method as reported in the published literature is reported in Table 13.3. The second column contains correlation reliability estimates, either Pearson product moment or interclass coefficients. The third column in Table 13.3 presents within-person coefficients of variation (CVs), where the CV is defined as the ratio of the within-person standard deviation to the mean. Smaller CVs indicate greater reliability. "Validity" coefficients that represent correlations among different methods of measuring fat can be found in Table 13.4. The numbers in parentheses next to the coefficients indicate the reference number of the corresponding source, which can be found in Table 13.5. For a method to be considered accurate (valid), the standard error of the estimate for percent fat should be less than 3%. Errors between 3% and 4% demonstrate limited validity, and errors greater than 4% suggest that variability is too high (Lohman, 1992a, 1992b, 1992c).

Anthropometry

Anthropometry is the study of human body measurements that yields information on fat, muscle, and bone dimensions. Anthropometry is composed of physical measurements that include stature, weight, and regional dimensions, including circumference measurements, skinfold thicknesses, bone breaths, and bone lengths. Anthropometry is inexpensive and noninvasive.

Stature, Body Weight, and Body Mass Index

Stature or standing height is measured using a calibrated stadiometer. The subject stands erect with feet positioned on the floor board of the stadiometer, arms by sides (palms facing legs), and back vertical to the back board of the stadiometer such that the heels, buttocks, and back of head make contact with the back board. The measurement bar is lowered to contact the skull (hair should be flat) as the subject is asked to take a deep breath in and at the end of expiration; stature is recorded to within 0.01 cm.

Body weight is measured using a calibrated scale. The subject stands on the center of scale with weight equally balanced on both feet, wearing minimal clothing and no footwear. Weight is recorded when the subject is standing motionless to within 0.01 kg.

Body mass index or Quetelet's index was an attempt by the 19th-century mathematician to describe the relationship between body weight and stature in humans (Quetelet, 1842/1973) and is calculated by dividing body weight (in kilograms) by height (in meters) squared (wt/ht^2). Today, BMI is a widely used index of adiposity or fatness due largely to the well-established relationship between BMI and fatness (Keys, Fidanza, Karvonen, Kimura, & Taylor, 1972; Khosla & Lowe, 1967). Similar adult body weight standards for diagnosing overweight and obesity based on BMI have been adopted by the National Institutes of Health and the World Health

Table 13.3   Reliability Coefficients for Selected Body Fat Measurement Methods

Method	r_{xx}	CV
Body mass index	>.99 (unpublished) > .99 (73)	< 1% (42)
Skinfolds	.91 (64) .96 (42) .93 (78) .98 (19) .81 to .95 (67) for individual skinfolds .98 (4)	6% (42) 4% (56) 3% (4)
Bioimpedance analysis	.96 (64) .96 (42) .93 (78) .96 (19)	6% (42) 1% (14) (within 1day) 2% (14) (within 1 week) 2% to 5% (11) 2% (57)
Dual-energy X-ray absorptiometry	.97 (59) .99 (42)	1% (70) 1% (41) 3% (41) 1% (42) 4% (66) 3% (66) 6% (3) 2% (55) 2% (9) < 1% (39)
Hydrodensitometry	.95 (29) .97 (42) .97 (19)	1% (42) 5% (56) 4% (4)
Isotope dilution	.97 (42) .996 (9) .95 (78)	2% (42) 2% (55) 2% (65) 1% (61) 2% (13) 1% (21) 2% (12)
Total body potassium	.33 (42) .96 (65)	7% (42) 4% (55) 3% (61) 3% (21) 3% (22)

Method	r_{xx}	CV
In vivo neutron activation	.99 (2)	1% to 3% (2) 3% (44) 3% (33) 3% (72) 2% (12)
Air displacement plethysmography (ADP)	(10) .98 (34)	1.7% to 4.5% (5)[a] 3.7% (25)[a] 1.7% (43)[a] 1.7% to 4.5% (48)[a] 1.7% to 4.5% (60)[a] 2.0% to 2.3% (35)[b] 2.0% to 2.3% (48)[b] 0.83% (80) 0.99% (80)
PEA POD	.96 (38)	−0.50% ± 1.21% (38)[b] 0.16% ± 1.44% (38)[a]
Three-dimensional photonic scanning	>.97 (76)	< 4.5% (76) 4.1% (81)
Magnetic resonance imaging	.99 (16)	1.7% (16) 2.3% (16) 5.9% (16) 3% (17)
Computed tomography scan	.99 (40)	−0.34% to 0.59% (40)

a. Within 1 day.

b. Between days.

Organization and are presented in Table 13.6. Since body fatness varies as a function of age, sex, and ethnicity/race, the application of fixed BMI ranges as proxies for adiposity/fatness is associated with some degree of systematic error or bias. A major assumption is that BMI represents adiposity, independent of age, sex, and ethnicity. That is, the use of BMI assumes that after adjusting a person's body weight for stature, all individuals have the same relative fatness regardless of their age, sex, or ethnicity. There have been few investigations of the validity of the assumption. Moreover, those studies that examined the relationships between BMI, fatness, aging, sex, and ethnicity usually relied on potentially biased methods for estimating fatness. Bias can be introduced into adipose tissue/fat measurements if a method makes assumptions related to body composition proportions and characteristics that are inaccurate across different populations. Among these methodological concerns are the following observations: hydration of fat-free body mass

(*Text continues on page 496*)

Table 13.4 Validity Coefficients for Selected Methods of Measuring Body Fat in Vivo

	BMI	Skinfolds	BIA	DXA/DPA	UWW	CT Scan	3-DPS	TBW	TBK	MRI
BMI Skinfold	.76 (62) .70 (68) .80 (23) .80 (32) .49 (36) .80 (20) .49 (71) .64 (71)									.88 (6)
BIA	.63 (36) > .62 (51)	.60 (28) .74 (42) .61 (42) .51 (7) .89 (59) .81 (36) > .62 (51)		.84 (58) .70 (58)				.66 (51) .87 (51) .88 (51) .93 (51)		.92 (17)
DXA	.57 (36)	.89 (64) .55 (69) .80 (36) .87 (48) .85 (49)	.77 (28) .98 (55) .83 (42) .74 (42) .49 (7) .88 (36) .84 (15) .81 (52)			.95 (75)				
UWW	.60 (73) .82 (73) .71 (73) .70 (73) .75 (19) .94 (9) .54 (31) .71 (45) .89 (23)	.81 (28) .65 (42) .77 (42) .92 (56) .90 (79) .90 (19) .77 (31)	.58 (28) .98 (53) .72 (42) .77 (42) .72 (19) .81 (31) .83 (11) .96 (24)	.86 (28) .76 (26) .66 (26) .82 (42) .78 (42) .87 (56) .92 (79) .86 (79) .97 (3) .84 (31)(25)						

	BMI	Skinfolds	BIA	DXA/DPA	UWW	CT Scan	3-DPS	TBW	TBK	MRI
ADP	.83 (50)		> .90 (35) .74 (15)	.95 (7) .84–.95 (54) .90–.93 (54) > .90 (35)	.78–.94 (36) .94 (18) > .90 (35)					
3-DPS					.65 (76)					
TBW	.43 (36) .80 (49) .93 (46) .99 (46)	.74 (42) .65 (42) .73 (7) .55 (36)	.70 (42) .68 (42) .59 (7) .56 (36)	.70 (42) .81 (42) .81 (7)| .83 (35) .65 (36)	.72 (42) .73 (42) .71 (26) .63 (36)					.92 (17) .91 (17)
TBK		.65 (42) .68 (42) .53 (7)	.67 (42) .68 (42) .33 (7)	.74 (42) .76 (42) .63 (7) .91 (3) .87 (39)	.73 (42) .76 (42) .78 (26)			.71 (42) .79 (42) .69 (7) .83 (32)		
IVNA		.80 (77) .78 (7)	.79 (77) .63 (7) > .62 (81) .77 (30) .90 (76) .87 (76)	.92 (77) .82 (7) .94 (39) .98 (22)	.86 (77) .90 (22)	.83 (75)		.97 (77) .97 (7)	.92 (77) .68 (7)	
WC					.76 (40) .83 (40)					.68 (6) .70 (31) .87 (31) .77 (31)
PEA POD								.76 (38)		

NOTE: BMI = body mass index; BIA = bioelectrical impedance analysis; DXA/DPA = dual-energy X-ray absorptiometry; UWW = underwater weighing; ADP = air displacement plethysmography; 3-DPS = three-dimensional photonic scan; TBW = total body weight; TBK = total body potassium; IVNA = in vivo neutron activation analysis; WC = waist circumference.

Table 13.5   Sources of Reliability and Validity Coefficients

Study	Mean Age	n	% Male/% Female	Mean BMI
Abdel-Malek, Mukherjee, and Roche (1985)	6–51	458	52%/48%	NA
Albu et al. (1992)	48 ± 3	10	100% F	43 ± 1
Bellisari, Roche, and Siervogel (1993)	18–62	35	49%/51%	26.0 ± 4.2 M 25.0 ± 5.3 F
Biaggi et al. (1999)	33 ± 8.7 M 30.7 ± 7.2 F	47	49%/51%	%BF 20.2 ± 6.3 M %BF 27.5 ± 7.4 W
Brambilla et al. (2006)	11.8 ± 1.8	407	53% M 47% F	26 ± 6.5
Cochran et al. (1988)	23–58	20	50%/50%	NA
Cohn, Vaswani, Yasumura, Yuen, and Ellis (1984)	27–70	137	50%/50%	NA
Demerath et al. (2002)	18–69 adults 8–17 children	126	NA	NA
Eckerson, Housh, and Johnson (1992a, 1992b)	22 ± 3	68	100% M	%BF 9.1 ± 2.2
Eckerson, Housh, and Johnson (1992a, 1992b)	23 ± 5	35	100% M	%BF 9.6 ± 2.3
Flakoll et al. (2004)	52 ± 2.3	85	51%/49%	26.7 ± 0.95
Gallagher et al. (2005)	21–70 F 20–71 M	338	70% F 30% M	NA
Gerard et al. (1991)	25.4 ± 1.1	5	100% F	NA
Ginde et al. (2005)	46.5 ± 16.9	123	70%/30%	31.5 ± 7.3
Haarbo, Gotfredsen, Hassager, and Christiansen (1991)	23–41	25	40%/60%	NA
Hergenroeder (1991)	11–25	1656	56%/44%	NA
Heymsfield and Wang (1994)	60.1 ± 21.1	13	38%/62%	22.6 ± 1.6
Heymsfield et al. (1989)	NA	13	38%/62%	NA
Heymsfield et al. (1990)	NA	4	NA	NA
Heymsfield et al. (1990)	58 ± 20	31	58%/42%	23.4 ± 2.6
Iwaoka et al. (1998)	31–44	7	NA	NA

Study	Mean Age	n	% Male/% Female	Mean BMI
Jackson, Pollock, Graves, and Mahar (1988)	28–45	68	35%/65%	20–28
Jackson et al. (1988)	31 ± 11	331	100% F	%BF 24 ± 7
Johansson et al. (1993)	37 ± 10.2	23	100% M	NA
Abu Khaled et al. (1988)	24.9 ± 3.1	56	69%/31%	21.7 ± 3.7
Kotler, Burastero, Wang, and Pierson (1996)	NA	NA	NA	NA
Kullberg et al. (2007)	14–70	336	NA	NA
Kushner and Schoeller (1986)	28.6–53.7	58	NA	20.8–35.6
Kyere et al. (1982)	NA	6	83%/16%	%BF 3.84 ± 14.5
Le Carvennec et al. (2007)	54 ± 13	10	50%/50%	39.3 ± 2.8
Levenhagen et al. (1999)	31.1 ± 1.8	20	50%/50%	25.2 ± 0.9
Lohman (1992c)	(review article)			
Lukaski and Johnson (1985)	28.8 ± 7.1	37	100% M	%BF 20.2 ± 7.6
Ma et al. (2004)	7.6 ± 7.2 weeks	36	54% M 46% F	%BF −0.50 ± 1.21 %BF 0.16 ± 1.44
Marks, Habicht, and Mueller (1989)	38–54	229	41%/59%	NA
Maurovich-Horvat et al. (2007)	37–83	100	49% F 51% M	NA
Mazess, Barden, Bisek, and Hanson (1990)	NA	12	50%/50%	NA
Mazess, Peppler, and Gibbons (1984)	23–61	18	22%/88%	8.3–45.7
McCrory, Gomez, Bernauer, and Mole (1995)	20–56	68	62%/38%	NA
Mernagh, Harrison, and McNeill (1977)	(review article)			
Michielutte, Diseker, Corbett, Schey, and Ureda (1984)	5–12	1668	50%/50%	NA

(Continued)

Table 13.5 (Continued)

Study	Mean Age	n	% Male/% Female	Mean BMI
Minten, Lowik, Deurenberg, and Kok. (1991)	65–79	515	51%/49%	25.5 ± 2.9 M 27.1 ± 4.3 F
Miyatake, Nonaka, and Fujii (1999)	NA	NA	NA	NA
Nicholson et al. (2001)	9.8 ± 1.7	119	47%/53%	%BF 39.2 ± 11.7
Ode, Pivarnik, Reeves, and Knous (2007)	NA	439	NA	NA
Papathakis, Rollins, Brown, Bennish, and Van Loan (2005)	25.7 ± 3.9	68	100% F	26.2 ± 3.7
Pateyjohns, Brinkworth, Buckley, Noakes, and Clifton (2006)	25–60	43	100% M	28–43
Pierson et al. (1991)	19–94	389[a]	40%/60%	21.2–25.7
Radley et al. (2003)	14 ± 1.65	69	71%/29%	31.3 ± 5.6 %BF 42.5 ± 8.4
Rammohan and Aplasca (1992)	52–70	56	50%/50%	22–32
Revicki and Israel (1986)	20–70	474	100% M	38.3
Rising, Swinburn, Larson, and Ravussin (1991)	30 ± 8	156	58%/42%	%BF 34 ± 9
Rush, Chandu, and Plank (2006)	19–74	211	52% M 48% F	NA
Russell-Aulet, Wang, Thornton, and Pierson (1991)	45 ± 17	81	51%/49%	23±3
Sardinha, Lohman, Teixeira, Guedes, and Going (1998)	37.6 ± 2.9	62	100% M	%BF 23.4 ± 7.0
Schoeller et al. (1980)	NA	10	70%/30%	NA
Smalley, Kneer, Kendrick, Colliver, and Owen (1990)	34.6 ± 12	36	41%/59%	%BF 24 ± 9.1

Study	Mean Age	n	% Male/% Female	Mean BMI
Steijaert, Deurenberg, Van Gaal, and De Leeuw (1997)	NA	45	NA	NA
Svendsen, Haarbo, Heitmann, Gotfredsen, and Christiansen (1991)	75	46	50%/50%	25.0 ± 3.4 M 25.9 ± 4.3 F
Tzen and Wu (1989)	33–45	7	71%/29%	NA
Van Itallie (1986)	(review article)			
Van Loan and Mayclin (1987)	18–35	40	50%/50%	%BF 14.46 M %BF 24.42 F
Vartsky, Ellis, and Cohn (1979)	(review article)			
Venkataraman and Ahluwalia (1992)	1.46 ± 12 days	28	NA	NA
Volz and Ostrove (1984)	18–26	66	100% F	%BF 22.8 ± 4.54
J. Wang et al. (2006)	6–83	92	52%/48%	NA
J. Wang, Kotler, et al. (1992)	41 ± 10	18	100% M	20 ± 2
J. Wang, Pierson, and Kelly (1973)	27–69	10	70%/30%	NA
Z. M. Wang et al. (1996)	35 ± 13	25	100% M	24.3 ± 3.0 %BF 16.6 ± 6.7
Ward et al. (1975)	NA	259	86%/14%	NA
Wells and Fuller (2001)	22–48 M 24–42 F 5–14 Boys 5–16 Girls	58	50%/50%	NA
Wells, Douros, Fuller, Elia, and Dekker (2000)	31.1 ± 7.8 adults 10.0 ± 2.4 children	32	50%/50%	21.8 ± 2.5 adults 16.9 ± 1.8 children

NOTE: BF = body fat; BMI = body mass index; M = male; F = female; NA = not available.

a. The reliability data from this article are based on only 5 of 389 subjects.

b. These include data from the introduction.

changes with age and differs across ethnic groups (Cohn, Vaswani, Yasumura, Yuen, & Ellis, 1985; Gerace et al., 1994, Mazariegos et al., 1994), the density of fat-free body mass changes with age and differs between men and women (He et al., 2003; Heymsfield et al., 1993), and total body potassium decreases with age (He et al., 2003) and fatness (Pierson, Lin, & Phillips, 1974) and differs between Blacks and Whites (He et al., 2003; Ortiz et al., 1992). These between-group differences influence the absolute accuracy of methods for estimating fatness such as the two-compartment total body water, underwater weighing, and total body potassium methods (Heymsfield et al., 1991). Gallagher, Kovera et al. (2000) have shown that percentage body fat prediction models differed by age and ethnicity terms when grouped by BMI category (see Table 13.7), thereby highlighting a critical concern regarding population specificity.

Another concern is that relative extremity length, independent of total stature, may influence the association between fatness and BMI (Garn, Leonard, & Hawthorne, 1986; Quaade, 1956). Due to kyphosis and osteoporotic degeneration of vertebral bodies, older subjects reportedly have a higher proportion of stature contributed by the lower extremities and pelvis than do young subjects (Chumlea & Guo, 1992; Miller, Schmatz, & Schultz, 1988; Prothro & Rosenbloom, 1993; Trotter & Gleser, 1958). Similarly, the lower extremity to stature ratio is reportedly greater in Blacks than in Whites (Gerace et al., 1994; Ortiz et al., 1992) and in Whites than in Mexican Americans (Malina, Brown, & Zavaleta, 1987).

In childhood, BMI changes significantly with increasing age (Rolland-Cachera et al., 1991) and is influenced by developmental patterns of change in body weight, height, and body composition (Horlick, 2001; see CDC charts in Figure 13.1). As noted earlier, these patterns are sex and race specific and must be taken into consideration, or they may introduce bias in the use of BMI as an index of body fatness. In the United States, the 85th and 95th centiles of BMI for age and sex based on nationally representative survey data (see Figure 13.1) are used as cutoff points to identify overweight and obesity (Barlow & Dietz, 1998). Alternative age- and sex-based cutoff points based on data pooled from several nationally representative children data sets have been proposed as more internationally based, where centile curves were drawn so that age 18 years passed through the widely used cutoff points of 25 and 30 kg/m^2 for adult overweight and obesity. The resulting curves

Table 13.6   Adult BMI Categories

Category	Mean
Underweight	Below 18.5
Normal weight	18.5 to 24.9
Overweight	25 to 29.9
Obese: Class I	30 to 34.9
Obese: Class II	35 to 39.9
Extreme obesity: Class III	40 or more

SOURCE: Adapted from Expert Panel on the Identification, Evaluation, and Treatment of Overweight in Adults (1998).

Table 13.7   Predicted Percentage Body Fat by Sex and Ethnicity Based on Four-Compartment Estimates of Percentage Body Fat

Age (Years) and BMI	Females			Males		
	African American	Asian	White	African American	Asian	White
20–39						
BMI < 18.5	20	25	21	8	13	8
BMI ≥ 25	32	35	33	20	23	21
BMI ≥ 30	38	40	39	26	28	26
40–59						
BMI < 18.5	21	25	23	9	13	11
BMI ≥ 25	34	36	35	22	24	23
BMI ≥ 30	39	41	41	27	29	29
60–79						
BMI < 18.5	23	26	25	11	14	13
BMI ≥ 25	35	36	38	23	24	25
BMI ≥ 30	41	41	43	29	29	31

SOURCE: Gallagher, Heymsfield, et al. (2000). Reprinted with permission.

were averaged to provide age- and sex-specific cutoff points from 2 to 18 years (Cole, Bellizzi, Flegal, & Dietz, 2000) that would allow for internationally comparable prevalence rates of overweight and obesity in children (see Table 13.8). BMI cutoffs to define thinness in children and adolescents have been published recently (Cole, Flegal, Nicholls, & Jackson, 2007).

The advantages of BMI as an index of fatness in children and adults include simple to acquire, inexpensive, good for health risk stratification that is suitable for large-scale studies. However, BMI does not provide qualitative information on body composition (i.e., amount of fat, fat-free mass, or distribution of fat and FFM).

Reliability. The reliability for both measured height and weight measures approaches 1.0 when proper measurement procedures are followed (especially important for height) and the stadiometer and scale are calibrated properly.

Accuracy and Validity. The correlation between BMI and common measures of fat mass ranges from 0.5 to 0.8 (see Table 13.4). Since fat and FFM are highly correlated, BMI has poor discriminant validity. BMI is more highly correlated with FFM in thin children and fat mass in fatter children (Freedman et al., 2005), and the same is true in adults, as reported in a number of studies involving athletes (Ode, Pivarnik, Reeves, & Knous, 2007; Sempolska & Stupnicki, 2007).

Considerations. Since most adults can self-report their height and weight, many epidemiological studies rely on these self-reported values as it is a

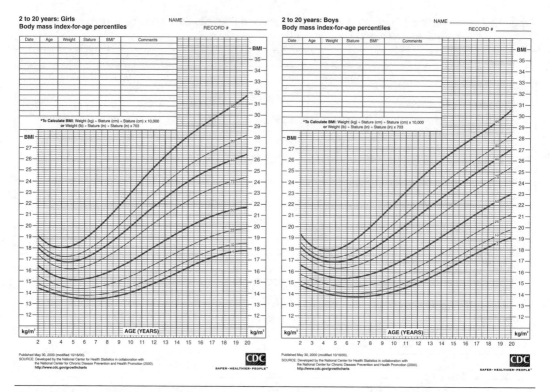

Figure 13.1   Body Mass Index for Age Percentiles

SOURCE: Developed by the National Center for Health Statistics in collaboration with the National Center for Chronic Disease and Health Promotion (http://www.cdc.gov/nchs/about/major/nhanes/growthcharts/charts.htm).

low-cost, quick, and easy approach for sampling large numbers of persons. In general, body weight tends to be underestimated in women (−0.1 to −6.5 kg) and men (−0.1 to −3.2 kg; Ziebland, Thorogood, Fuller, & Muir, 1996). With regards to height, mean error between self-report and directly measured values ranges from 0.6 to 7.5 cm (Gorber, Tremblay, Moher, & Gorber, 2007), with a greater tendency to overestimate height within each sex.

Circumference Measurements

Circumferences are measured using a tape, preferably a tension-calibrated measuring tape with minimal pressure applied to the skin so that the soft tissue is not compressed. Each measurement is performed twice, and the average of the two readings is used. Commonly measured sites include waist, hip, upper arm, thigh, and calf. Careful attention must be given to identifying the point or level to be measured, which ideally should involve bony landmarks relative to the measurement site (Lohman, Roche, & Martorell, 1988). The latter allows for greater precision and reproducibility when longitudinal measures are being acquired. The measurement location for limb sites should be identified using a measuring tape and the skin marked with a marking pen. Circumferences at the waist, hip, and thigh are used to estimate upper and lower body fat distribution. Waist circumference is highly correlated with visceral fat (Janssen, Heymsfield, Allison, Kotler, & Ross, 2002; Pouliot et al., 1994) and is included as a clinical risk factor in the definition of the metabolic syndrome in adults and children (Cruz & Goran, 2004; Hirschler, Aranda,

Table 13.8   International Cutoff Points for Body Mass Index for Overweight and Obesity by Sex Between 2 and 18 years, Defined to Pass Through Body Mass Index of 25 and 30 kg/m^2 at Age 18, Obtained by Averaging Data From Brazil, Great Britain, Hong Kong, Netherlands, Singapore, and the United States

| Age (Years) | Body Mass Index 25 kg/m^2 | | Body Mass Index 30 kg/m^2 | |
	Males	Females	Males	Females
2	18.41	18.02	20.09	19.81
2.5	18.13	17.76	19.8	19.55
3	17.89	17.56	19.57	19.36
3.5	17.69	17.4	19.39	19.23
4	17.55	17.28	19.29	19.15
4.5	17.47	17.19	19.26	19.12
5	17.42	17.15	19.3	19.17
5.5	17.45	17.2	19.47	19.34
6	17.55	17.34	19.78	19.65
6.5	17.71	17.53	20.23	20.08
7	17.92	17.75	20.63	20.51
7.5	18.16	18.03	21.09	21.01
8	18.44	18.35	21.6	21.57
8.5	18.76	18.69	22.17	22.18
9	19.1	19.07	22.77	22.81
9.5	19.46	19.45	23.39	23.46
10	19.84	19.86	24	24.11
10.5	20.2	20.29	24.57	24.77
11	20.55	20.74	25.1	25.42
11.5	20.89	21.2	25.58	26.05
12	21.22	21.68	26.02	26.67
12.5	21.56	22.14	26.43	27.24
13	21.91	22.58	26.84	27.76
13.5	22.27	22.98	27.25	28.2
14	22.62	23.34	27.63	28.57
14.5	22.96	23.66	27.98	28.87

(Continued)

Table 13.8 (Continued)

Age (Years)	Body Mass Index 25 kg/m²		Body Mass Index 30 kg/m²	
	Males	Females	Males	Females
15	23.29	23.94	28.3	29.11
15.5	23.6	24.17	28.6	29.29
16	23.9	24.37	28.88	29.43
16.5	24.19	24.54	29.14	29.56
17	24.46	24.7	29.41	29.69
17.5	24.73	24.85	29.7	29.84
18	25	25	30	30

SOURCE: Cole, Bellizzi, Flegal, and Dietz (2000). Reproduced with permission.

Calcagno, Maccalini, & Jadzinsky, 2005). Waist circumference values based on currently acceptable guidelines have limited clinical application when BMI and obesity-related cardiometabolic risk factors are already available (Klein et al., 2007). Waist circumference has also been criticized as an index of visceral fat due to limitations associated with the underlying assumption that the anatomic site being measured (there are four commonly used sites) best represents overall visceral adiposity.

Commonly measured waist sites (see Figure 13.2) include (a) immediately below the lower most rib, (b) at the narrowest waist, (c) the midpoint between the lowest rib and iliac crest, and (d) immediately above the iliac crest (J. Wang et al., 2003). Note that three of the aforementioned sites include a reference to at least one bony landmark. Waist circumference measured at "the narrowest waist" based on visual inspection is problematic when measuring obese persons where a discernible "narrowest waist" is not visible. Moreover, when acquiring longitudinal assessments where weight loss or weight gain

occurs, the "narrowest waist" may change in anatomic location, and therefore follow-up measures will not be acquired at the same location as baseline measures.

The ratio of waist circumference to hip circumference is a commonly used index of fat distribution as it relates to health risk. A ratio of < 0.90 for men and < 0.80 for women is considered desirable (Dobbelsteyn, Joffres, MacLean, & Flowerdew, 2001). A high waist/hip ratio indicates that excessive fat is stored in the central part of the body, which increases risk for certain metabolic diseases (e.g., diabetes, heart disease, and high blood pressure), whereas a low waist/hip ratio indicates a lower propensity for developing these health problems as it suggests that fat is stored in the femoral-gluteal area (hips; Dalton et al., 2003).

Reliability. The reproducibility of waist circumference measurements performed in triplicate at four sites for males and females ($N = 93$) was high (J. Wang et al., 2003). The intraclass correlations ranged from $r = .996$ to .998 in males and $r = .998$ to $r = .999$ in females.

a

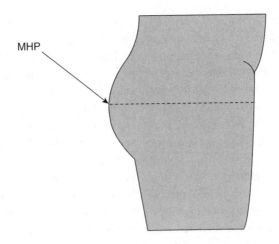

MHP

b

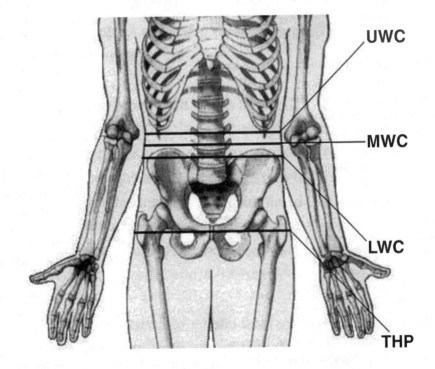

UWC

MWC

LWC

THP

Figure 13.2   Commonly Used Sites for the Measurement of Waist and Hip Circumferences

NOTE: Upper waist circumference (UWC) is taken immediately below the end of the lowest rib on the mid-axillary line; mid-waist circumference (MWC) is taken at the midpoint between the lowest rib and the iliac crest on the mid-axillary line; lower waist circumference (LWC) is taken immediately above the iliac crest and on the mid-axillary line; trochanteric hip protuberance (THP) is taken at the level of the greater trochanter of the femoral bone that is palpated laterally and approximately coincides with level of the symphysis pubis; maximum hip protuberance (MHP) is taken at the maximum posterior protuberance of the buttocks at the end of normal expiration and as the technician faces the right side of the participant.

Accuracy and Validity. The accuracy of waist circumference (WC) compared to subcutaneous adipose tissue (SAT) volume and visceral adipose tissue (VAT) volume by computerized topography (CT) in White adults showed *r*s of .83 and .76, respectively (Maurovich-Horvat et al., 2007). The correlations reported for WC versus VAT at the L4-L5 level were $r = .794$ (young females), $r = .70$ (elderly females), and $r = .87$ (young females) and .77 (males) (Kullberg et al., 2007). In children, Brambilla and colleagues (2006) pooled data from several laboratories to investigate the relationship between waist circumference and MRI-derived VAT and SAT from a single abdominal slice from which they developed VAT and SAT prediction equations with error of 13 cm² and 57 cm², respectively.

Norms. Waist circumferences ≥ 102 cm (40 in.) in men and ≥ 88 cm (35 in.) in women are suggestive of elevated risk (National Institutes of Health, 1998). Much discussion surrounds whether "norms" or cutoff values should be developed specific to other ethnic/race groups and for different age groups. Proposed cutoffs for waist circumference in specific populations include a waist circumference cutoff of 80 cm (and a BMI cutoff of ≥ 24 kg/m²) for both men and women for the identification of Chinese patients at high risk of cardiovascular disease (Wildman, Gu, Reynolds, Duan, & He, 2004), a waist circumference ≥ 90 cm in men and ≥ 85 cm in women for South Koreans (Park, Yun, Park, Kim, & Choi, 2003), a waist circumference ≥ 78 cm in men and ≥ 72 cm in women for Asian Indians (Misra et al., 2006), and a waist circumference ≥ 85 cm in men and ≥ 90 cm in women for Japanese (Miyatake et al., 2007).

Availability and Costs. Cost of tape measure is minimal (less than $27). Tester training is required, but the level of skill is significantly less than that required for skinfold measures.

Skinfolds

Skinfold thicknesses are measured using plastic or metal skinfold calipers. A calibration block is available to check the accuracy of the more reputable calipers (e.g., Lange, Harpenden, Holtain). The latter is a check to ensure that the gap width and jaw pressure being exerted by the calipers are accurate.

Skinfold thicknesses measure the thickness of the subcutaneous fat that underlies the skin at a specific site. Skinfolds measurements are most often used to estimate percentage body fat. The primary assumptions on which the technique are based include that (a) more than 50% of total body fat is located subcutaneously, (b) fat content of the site measured does not vary, and (c) the sites being measured are representative of overall body fat distribution. All of these assumptions have questionable validity. There are numerous equations that use skinfold thicknesses to predict body density (see Table 13.9). Each equation is specific to the population in which it was developed. The value for body density (Db in kg/L) is transformed to a percent body fat using an equation (Brozek et al., 1963; Siri, 1961).

As the subject stands relaxed, the tester pinches the skin at the appropriate site to raise a double layer of skin along with subcutaneous tissue that underlies the skinfold, which is picked up firmly between thumb and forefinger of the left hand and pulled away from the underlying muscle. With a few exceptions, the skinfold is pinched in a vertical line. The calipers are then applied 1.0 cm below the thumb and forefinger and at a right angle to the pinch, and a reading is taken (after 2–3 seconds of caliper pressure) to the nearest 0.1 mm. The mean of three measurements that falls within 2.0 mm of each other is acceptable. Depending on the specific regression equation used, a weighted combination of skinfolds and often other characteristics such as age and sex are summed, and body density and percent body fat are calculated.

The skinfold method is safe, requires little time to administer, requires little subject participation, and is relatively inexpensive and suitable for large-scale studies. The primary disadvantage is that the technician must be trained and regression equations must be used to calculate percent body fat. With measurements usually acquired on the right side of the body,

Table 13.9   Equations to Estimate Percent Body Fat From Skinfold Thicknesses

Measurement	Sex	Equation
Triceps + calf $(\Sigma)^a$	Black and White Boys Girls	% BF = 0.735 (Σ) + 1.0 % BF = 0.610 (Σ) + 5.1
Triceps + subscapular (> 35 mm) $(\Sigma)^a$	Black and White Boys Girls	% BF = 0.783 (Σ) + 1.6 % BF = 0.546 (Σ) + 9.7
Triceps + subscapular (> 35 mm) $(\Sigma)^a$	Prepubescent males—White Prepubescent males—Black Pubescent males—White Pubescent males—Black Postpubescent males—White Postpubescent males—Black All females	%BF = 1.21 (Σ) − 0.008 $(\Sigma)^2$ − 1.7 %BF = 1.21 (Σ) − 0.008 $(\Sigma)^2$ − 3.2 %BF = 1.21 (Σ) − 0.008 $(\Sigma)^2$ − 3.4 %BF = 1.21 (Σ) − 0.008 $(\Sigma)^2$ − 5.2 %BF = 1.21 (Σ) − 0.008 $(\Sigma)^2$ − 5.5 %BF = 1.21 (Σ) − 0.008 $(\Sigma)^2$ − 6.8 %BF = 1.33 (Σ) − 0.013 $(\Sigma)^2$ − 2.5
Sum of triceps + biceps + subscapular + suprailliac	Prepubescent males[b] Prepubescent females[b] Adolescent males[c] Adolescent females[c]	BD = 1.1690 − 0.0788 log sum of 4 skinfolds BD = 1.2063 − 0.0999 log sum of 4 skinfolds %BF = ([4.95/BD] − 4.5) 100 BD = 1.1533 − 0.0643 log sum of 4 skinfolds BD = 1.1369 − 0.0598 log sum of 4 skinfolds %BF = ([4.95/BD] − 4.5) 100
Sum of triceps + biceps + subscapular + iliac crest	Adult males[d] Adult females[d]	BD = 1.1765 − 0.0744 log sum of 4 skinfolds BD = 1.1567 − 0.0717 log sum of 4 skinfolds %BF = ({4.95/BD} − 4.5) 100
Sum of triceps + subscapular + suprailiac + mid-thigh	Adult males[e] Adult females[e]	%BF = 20.94878 + (age × 0.1166) − (Ht × 0.11666) + (sum of 4 skinfolds × 0.42696) − ([sum of 4 skinfolds]^2 × 0.00159) %BF = 22.18945 + (age × 0.06368) + (BMI × 0.60404) − (Ht × 0.14520) + (sum of 4 skinfolds × 0.30919) − ([sum of 4 skinfolds]^2 × 0.00099562)

NOTE: Σ = sum of skinfolds (mm); %BF = percent body fat; BD = body density; Ht = height; BMI = body mass index.

a. Slaughter et al. (1988).

b. Brook (1971).

c. Durnin et al. (1967).

d. Durnin and Womersley (1974).

e. Peterson, Czerwinski, and Siervogel (2003).

Table 13.10   Selected Single-Frequency BIA Equations for Predicting Fat-Free Mass (Fat Mass = Body Weight – Fat-Free Mass)

Study	Reference Method	n	Age	Equation	R^2	SEE	Comments
Children							
Deurenberg, Vanderkooy, Leenen, Weststrate, and Seidell (1991)	Db	166	7–15	$0.406 (S^2/R) + 0.36 (W) + 5.58 (S) + 0.56 (Sex) – 6.48$	0.97	1.68	Split-sample cross validation FFM by age-adjusted Db equations
Houtkooper, Lohman, Going, and Hall (1989)	3C	53 M, 41 F	10–14	$0.83 (S^2/R) + 4.43$	0.88	2.60	Model based on deuterium dilution and Db
Adults							
Baumgartner, Heymsfield, Lichtman, Wang, and Pierson (1991)	4C	35 M, 63 F	65–94	$0.28 (S^2/R) + 0.27 (W) + 4.5 (S) +0.31(Thigh C) – 1.732$	0.91	2.47	Model based on tritium dilution, Db, and dual photon absorptiometry; elderly-specific equation
Deurenberg et al. (1991)	Db	661	16–83	$0.34 (S^2/R) – 0.127 (Age) + 0.273 (W) + 4.56 (Sex) + 15.34 (S) – 12.44$	0.93	2.63	Split-sample cross-validation
	Db	498 F		$0.0011 (S^2) – 0.021 (R) + 0.232 (W) – 0.068 (Age) + 14.595$	0.89	2.43	Cross-validated
Sun et al. (2004)	3C	669 M	12–94	$FFM = –10.68 + 0.65 (S)^2/(R) + 0.26 (W) + 0.02 (R)$	0.90	3.9	FFM was estimated with a multicomponent model based on densitometry, isotope dilution, and dual-energy -ray absorptiometry.

(Continued)

Table 13.10 (Continued)

		944 F		FFM = −9.53 + 0.69 $(S)^2/(R)$ + 0.17 (W) + 0.02 (R)	0.83	2.9	

SOURCE: Adapted from Baumgartner (1996, p. 92). Reprinted with permission.

NOTE: FFM = fat-free mass; Db = body density; 3C, 4C = three- and four-component models, respectively; M = male; F = female; R = resistance; S = statue; Thigh C = thigh circumference; W = body weight.

skinfolds are obtained at 3 to 9 standard anatomical sites (subscapular, tricep, biceps, suprailiac, abdomen, etc.) around the body. Skinfold thicknessess acquired at different sites have been shown to correlate differently with percent body fat and total fat where triceps skinfolds were found to have a better correlation with percent body fat while subscapular skinfolds correlated better with total body fat mass (Slaughter et al., 1988). A study of mortality rate as a function of weight loss and fat loss (measured by skinfolds) showed that among nonseverely obese individuals, weight loss is associated with increased mortality and fat loss with decreased mortality rate (Allison et al., 1999).

Reliability. There can be a large degree of between-tester variability with skinfold measurements. Proper technician training and hands-on tester experience greatly increase the likelihood of reliable data. As evident in Table 13.3, the rs are > .90. The interobserver reliability of anthropometric measurements is lower among the elderly and varies by sex (Chumlea, Roche, & Rogers, 1984). Both the reliability and feasibility of skinfold measurements are diminished in the obese. Some skinfolds are too large to be measured using conventional calipers.

Accuracy and Validity. The accuracy of skinfold measurements for estimating percent body fat shows rs that range from .49 to .80 (see Table 13.4). Validity is influenced by experience and skill of tester(s).

Norms. Since percentage body fat is the outcome measure, the norms would be consistent with the values presented in Table 13.1.

Availability and Costs. Cost of skinfold calipers ($8 to $400) is low compared to many of the other body fat measurement instruments. Technician training is required.

Bioimpedance Analysis

Bioelectrical impedance analysis (BIA) is a commonly used method for estimating body composition based on a 2C body composition model. In very simple terms, BIA measures the impedance or resistance to a small electrical current as it travels through the body's water pool. Total body BIA is the sum of resistance and reactance in the four limbs (arms and legs) and trunk. The impedance of the whole body is dependent on the length and cross-sectional area of each limb/trunk component and the signal frequency (Nyboer, 1972). Since the body's configuration is constant and a fixed signal frequency is used (most single-frequency analyzers operate at a current frequency of 50 kHz), the body's impedance to current flow can be related to its volume since conductor volume equals the cross-sectional area × length or height.

Since fat is relatively anhydrous, the electrical current is conducted by the water and electrolyte-rich FFM compartment and is resisted or impeded by the anhydrous fat compartment. An estimate of total body water (TBW) is acquired from which total body FFM is calculated using the assumption that 73% of the body's FFM is water (Sheng & Huggins, 1979). The difference between body weight and FFM is equivalent to total body fat. Table 13.10 presents some examples of equations.

Conventional single-frequency BIA systems transmit and receive electrical signals through electrodes placed on the body where the body is considered to be a single cylinder-shaped form. Single-frequency BIA is most commonly used for assessing TBW and FFM but is limited in its ability to distinguish the distribution of TBW into its intra- and extracellular compartments. The arm-to-leg electrical pathway approach requires two gel electrodes placed on the right side of the body at distal upper and two at corresponding lower extremity sites. Single frequency is passed between surface electrodes placed on the right hand and right foot. The leg-to-leg pressure contact BIA approach has the potential of simplifying impedance measurements by eliminating the need for gel electrodes, and the electrical current passes between surface electrodes that both feet stand onto (foot to foot). Body weight is provided simultaneously with impedance measurements in the leg-to-leg pressure contact BIA and is less time-consuming for health care practitioners in medical offices or in settings where time and/or technician experience is at a premium (Nuñez et al., 1997).

Multifrequency BIA allows for the differentiation of TBW into intracellular water (ICW) and extracellular water (ECW) compartments, which is useful to describe fluid shifts and fluid balance and to explore variations in levels of hydration (Chumlea & Guo, 1994; Thomas, Ward, & Cornish, 1998). In addition to providing information on fat mass, multifrequency BIA (frequencies up to 300 kHz) may have an added advantage over single-frequency BIA (50 kHz) for evaluating leg skeletal muscle (Pietrobelli et al., 1998). Now, multisegmental BIA is available in both single- and multifrequency systems. The multisegmental approach assumes that the body is made up of a group of cylinders as opposed to one cylinder only. The impedance of the left and right arms, the left and right legs, and the total body is measured. The summed value for the four limbs is subtracted from the total body to derive the impedance of the trunk.

The advantages of BIA include its portability and ease of use, relatively low cost, minimal participant participation required, and safety (not recommended for participants with a pacemaker), thus making it attractive for large-scale studies.

Reliability. The measurement of TBW and FFM using a tetrapolar system showed a .99 test-retest correlation coefficient (Lukaski, Bolonchuk, Hall, & Siders, 1986; Lukaski, Johnson, Bolonchuk, & Lykken, 1985). For resistance measurements acquired on 5 successive days, the coefficients of variation for resistance values ranged from 0.9% to 3.4%, and the average precision was 2%. Test-retest correlation coefficient was .99 for a single-resistance measurement, and the reliability coefficient for a single-resistance measurement over 5 days was .99 (Lukaski et al., 1985). Overall, the reliability of BIA has test-retest *r*s of .93 to .96 and within-person CVs between 1% and 6%.

Accuracy and Validity. The accuracy of body fat measures is considered to be within 3.5% to 5.0% (Baumgartner, 1996) when conditions such as ambient temperature, participant hydration status, position of participant, correct electrode placement, use of appropriate equations, and eating and drinking that can affect total body water are regulated. Validity of BIA is also influenced by sex, age, disease state (Kotler, Burastero, Wang, & Pierson, 1996); race/ethnicity (Rush, Chandu, & Plank, 2006); level of fatness (Steijaert, Deurenberg, Van Gaal, & De Leeuw, 1997), where TBW and relative extracellular water are greater in obese subjects compared with normal-weight individuals (Waki et al., 1991); and type of BIA system, where single-frequency BIA was found to have better absolute agreement than multifrequency BIA when compared to DXA as a criterion measure for fat and FFM estimates in overweight and obese men (Pateyjohns, Brinkworth, Buckley, Noakes, & Clifton, 2006). Most BIA applications incorporate a prediction equation approach, like skinfolds, that includes other measurements such as weight and length and characteristics such as age, sex, and race. These equations tend to be population specific, and their validity is also limited by that of the criterion measure used in their calibration. A study involving HIV-negative and HIV-positive breastfeeding South African mothers reported that multifrequency BIA (or bioimpedance spectroscopy, as referred to in the study) provided values that compared favorably to values obtained by the dilution technique for TBW, FFM, and fat mass, whereas BMI did not (Papathakis, Rollins, Brown, Bennish, & Van Loan, 2005).

Norms. Since percentage body fat is the outcome measure, the norms would be consistent with the values presented in Table 13.1.

Availability and Costs. There are many BIA devices available with a wide range in cost: home devices (below $130) and research devices (up to $22,000).

Hydrodensitometry

Hydrodensitometry or underwater weighing (UWW) involves measuring a person's body weight while submersed underwater when all air has been expelled from the lungs. It is based on the Archimedes principle that states that the weight of an object in water is proportional to the amount of water displaced by that object. The density of the human body is equivalent to the ratio of its mass and volume. The density (expressed as g/cc) of fat (0.9007 g/cm^3) differs from the density of fat-free or lean tissue (1.100 g/cm^3) and is assumed stable across all adults irrespective of age, race/ethnicity, and disease. A formula is used to compute the relative density of the submersed body:

Body density (g/cc) = body weight/
(body weight – weight in water).

The derived body density value is then incorporated into a formula (see Table 13.2) used to estimate percent body fat. Many textbooks in the past have referred to the hydrostatic weighing technique as the "gold standard" or reference method for estimating body fat. However, limitations associated with this technique, combined with the development of newer techniques, have resulted in reduced use. Limitations include subject discomfort with having to submerge one's body, including head, underwater while exhaling maximally; the assumption that residual lung volume estimate is accurate and if residual lung volume is measured prior to submersion, the value obtained is similar to the value when the subject is submerged and has exhaled maximally; and accessing the water tank for persons with physical function limitations.

The hydrostatic weighing device consists of a large tank of water with the water temperature maintained at approximately 37°C. The system has a seat or platform that is attached to a scale. The subject is positioned on the seat or platform and is submerged underwater while expelling maximally all air from the lungs. Residual lung volume makes a sizable contribution to total body volume (1 to 2 liters), and it is therefore important to measure residual lung volume prior to or during the underwater weighing procedure. Disadvantages of this technique include total submersion underwater, which can be especially difficult for nonswimmers. Climbing steps and descending into a tank of water can be difficult for many obese and elderly persons.

Accuracy and Validity. The accuracy of UWW compared to DXA averages .83 and .88 compared to in vivo neutron activation analysis (IVNA; see Table 13.4). Issues related to the validity of the assumptions underlying UWW have been described above.

Reliability. The technical error for between-day test-retest is approximately 1.1% fat in males and 1.2% fat in females (Jackson, Pollock, Graves, & Mahar, 1988). Within-day test-retest is 1% fat

(Going et al., 1995). The greatest source of error in the measurement of body density relates to residual lung volume (RV) where a 100-mL error in RV translates to a 100-g error in underwater weight of subject and a 1% error in fat.

Norms. Since percentage body fat is the outcome measure, the norms would be consistent with the values presented in Table 13.1.

Availability and Costs. Hydrostatic weighing systems are typically custom built, and an estimated cost is $25,000.

Air Plethysmography

Air displacement plethysmography (ADP) is an alternative to hydrostatic weighing for the determination of body volume/body density and uses air displacement instead of water displacement to measure body volume. A commercially available system is the BOD POD (Life Measurement Instruments, Inc., Concord, CA), which can be used in persons weighing between 35 and 200 kg. This system consists of a front test chamber and a rear reference chamber. The subject sits in the front chamber. Body volume is derived from the ratio of the pressure in the reference and test chambers based on Boyle's law, where volume varies inversely with pressure when temperature is constant (Dempster & Aitkens, 1995). A diaphragm mounted on the common wall oscillates during testing under computer control. When the volume is increased in one of the chambers, it is decreased by the same amount in the other chamber and vice versa. The pressure in each of the two chambers responds immediately to this volume change or perturbation, and the magnitude of the pressure changes indicates the relative size of each chamber. A lung volume measurement is performed during the test that requires the subject to breathe through a disposable tube, which, when cued by the technician, performs gentle puffs. Pressure in the breathing tube changes as the subject's diaphragm contracts and expands, which, combined with

chamber pressure changes, allows for an estimation of lung volume.

Subjects are required to wear a tight-fitting bathing suit, and an acrylic cap covers the head so that trapped air within the hair is minimal. Loose-fitting clothes, scalp hair, and facial hair can introduce error such that percent fat is underestimated (Higgins, Fields, Gower, & Hunter, 2001). The BOD POD weight scale on which the subject is weighed must be calibrated daily using a 20-kg weight. Before subject evaluation, a 2-point chamber calibration is performed using the empty chamber and a 50.218-liter calibration cylinder. Two trials are performed on a subject, and the volumes are averaged when within 150 mL (Fields, Goran, & McCrory, 2002). The ADP measurement is quicker to perform and more subject friendly than hydrostatic weighing. The disadvantages of ADP include the following: a breathing maneuver may be difficult for some, claustrophobic persons may be unable to tolerate the chamber, and extremely large persons may not fit within the chamber.

Reliability. Between-day test-retest correlation coefficients for body density and percent fat are $r = .95$ in adults and $r = .90$ in children (Demerath et al., 2002).

Accuracy and Validity. The accuracy of percent body fat measures is within –4.0% to 1.9% when ADP is compared to UWW (Demerath et al., 2002; Fields et al., 2002; Ginde et al., 2005; Nuñez et al., 1999) for adults. Comparing ADP to DXA, the accuracy of percent body fat measures is between –3.0% and 1.7% (Fields et al., 2002; Levenhagen et al., 1999; Nuñez et al., 1999; Sardinha, Lohman, Teixeira, Guedes, & Going, 1998)

Specifically in relation to overweight and obese, ADP was compared to UWW in persons with a maximum BMI of 58.4 kg/m^2 (Ginde et al., 2005), 37.2 kg/m^2 (Vescovi et al., 2001), and 58.8 kg/m^2 (Petroni et al., 2003). In the study by Ginde et al. (2005), a Bland-Altman analysis showed no significant bias between D(b) measured by UWW and ADP, and percent fat estimates from UWW and ADP using the two-compartment Siri equation were highly correlated ($r = .94$, standard error of the estimate = 3.58%, $p < .001$). Limitations are similar to those outlined for UWW and include the assumption that the density of FFM or lean is stable across all adults irrespective of age, race/ethnicity, and disease and that lung volume measures are correctly estimated.

Norms. Since percentage body fat is the outcome measure, the norms would be consistent with the values presented in Table 13.1.

Availability and Costs. The BOD POD system is available at a cost of $39,577, and a full yearly service contract costs $3,500.

An infant ADP system (PEA POD; Life Measurement Instruments Inc., Concord, CA) is available for the assessment of body composition in infants up to a maximum weight of 8 kg, as recommended by the manufacturer. A movable cart houses the reference chamber and calibration volume, and the test chamber is mounted on the cart's top surface. A volume-perturbing diaphragm is located between the test and reference chambers, and a pneumatic valve (calibration valve) allows the test chamber to be connected to the calibration volume (Urlando, Dempster, & Aitkens, 2003). Infant length is first measured with a length board, and all subsequent measures are acquired with the infant naked, except for a nylon head stocking that is used to remove the effect of trapped air among the hairs. Alternatively, the hair can be smoothed flat using oil. Infant weight is measured on the ADP electronic scale while a system volume calibration is in progress. The infant is then positioned on a tray that slides into a clear acrylic test chamber. When the chamber door closes, pressure changes are measured over a 2-minute period. The test ends with the door opening automatically, and results are displayed on the computer monitor. Prior to each measurement, a volume calibration is run using a certified aluminum cylinder (5 L), and the weight scale is calibrated using a certified NIST weight (5 kg).

Reliability. In this study by Ma et al. (2004), there were no significant differences between days

($-0.50\% \pm 1.21\%$) or within days ($0.16\% \pm 1.44\%$) for percent fat. The mean between- and within-day test-retest standard deviations were 0.69% and 0.72% fat, respectively. In this study, it was reported that percent fat measurements were not significantly influenced by infant behavioral state such as activity and/or crying (Ma et al., 2004).

Accuracy and Validity. There are relatively few published studies thus far using the PEA POD. In 36 full-term infants (Ma et al., 2004), percent fat by ADP did not differ significantly from ^2H_2O dilution (20.32% vs. 20.39%; $R^2 = 0.76$; standard error estimate [SEE] = 3.26%), and the 95% limits of agreement were -6.84% to 6.71% fat. Individual differences between the two methods were not influenced by either body mass or fatness.

Norms. Unpublished data collected in our laboratory on healthy infants born at term (> 37 weeks' gestation) to mothers with no medical condition who were tested between 1 and 4 days of age had a range in body fat from 8% to 24%.

Availability and Costs. The only available infant ADP system (PEA POD) costs $87,000, and the annual service contract cost is ~$9,000.

Three-Dimensional Photonic Scanning

The use of a digitized optical method and computer to generate a three-dimensional photonic scan (3-DPS) image of an object in humans was developed more than four decades ago (Hertzberg, Dupertuis, & Emanual, 1957) and has more recently been applied for the measurement of whole-body surface anthropometry, whole-body and regional volumes, and body fat (Robinette, Daanen, & Paquet, 1999). The 3-DPS is a noninvasive optical method that uses high-speed digital cameras and triangular mathematics to detect the position of eye-safe Class 1 laser light points (664 nm) projected onto the surface of an object and reflected to the cameras. Software connects the points to generate a 3-D image from which values for total and regional body volumes and dimensions, such as body circumferences, lengths, widths, and thicknesses, can be obtained (J. Wang et al., 2006). The measurement accuracy and precision of the 3-DPS is directly related to the number of data points obtained on an object's surface. The greater the number of data points, the higher the resolution or precision. The software can also calculate the volume of any specified region of the body. The 3-DPS has potential application in the prevention, classification, and monitoring of disease treatments that relate to body shape, size, or degree of fatness, as well as in growth and development, aging, weight management, and fitness management. The 3-DPS has important application in the measurement of extreme obesity and in studies of before and following bariatric surgery. The 3-DPS can accommodate the maximum adult body size and is therefore without body size constraints. Presented in Figure 13.3 are 3-DPS images of an adult woman (175.9 kg; 66.4 kg/m²; 55.3% fat) from front (A), side (B), and back (C) views with corresponding total and regional body volume

information. The lines visible on the body images delineate examples of circumference and distance measurements that can be performed by the system software. Presented in Figure 13.4 are body outlines generated from a 3-DPS of an adult woman from a side view before and after bariatric surgery–induced weight loss. Information is provided on circumference changes of the chest, waist, hip, and mid-thigh as determined by the 3-DPS for this specific subject. The baseline scan report is also provided showing the anthropometric, body volume, and percent fat information.

Validation studies for total body volume from the 3-DPS have been conducted in children and adults using underwater weighing and air displacement plethysmography techniques as standards (Dekker, Douros, Buxton, & Treleaven, 1999; J. Wang et al., 2006; Wells, Douros, Fuller, Elia, & Dekker, 2000). This technique is easy to perform, fast, and accurate for determining total and regional body volumes and dimensions in persons tested to date with a maximum weight of 182 kg and a maximum BMI of 63 kg/m² (J. Wang et al., 2006).

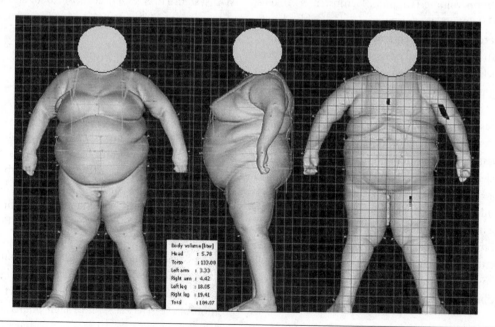

Figure 13.3   Three-Dimensional Photonic Scan Images of an Adult Woman (175.9 kg; 66.4 kg/m2; 55.3% fat) from (A) Front, (B) Side, and (C) Back Views With Corresponding Total and Regional Body Volume Information

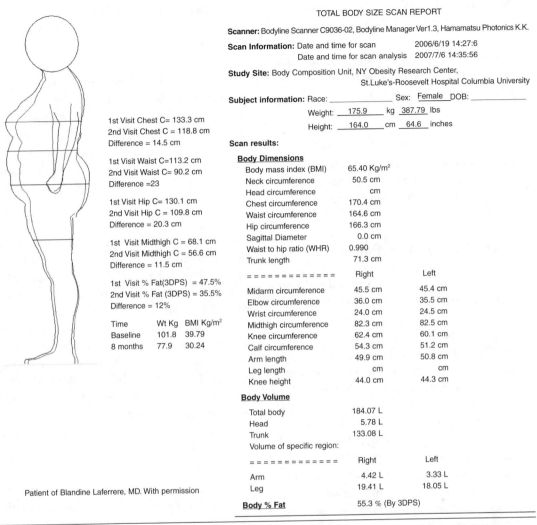

TOTAL BODY SIZE SCAN REPORT

Scanner: Bodyline Scanner C9036-02, Bodyline Manager Ver1.3, Hamamatsu Photonics K.K.

Scan Information: Date and time for scan   2006/6/19 14:27:6
                     Date and time for scan analysis   2007/7/6 14:35:56

Study Site: Body Composition Unit, NY Obesity Research Center,
                St.Luke's-Roosevelt Hospital Columbia University

Subject information: Race: _____   Sex: Female DOB: _____
                        Weight: __175.9__ kg _387.79_ lbs
                        Height: __164.0__ cm _64.6_ inches

Scan results:

1st Visit Chest C= 133.3 cm
2nd Visit Chest C = 118.8 cm
Difference = 14.5 cm

1st Visit Waist C=113.2 cm
2nd Visit Waist C= 90.2 cm
Difference =23

1st Visit Hip C= 130.1 cm
2nd Visit Hip C = 109.8 cm
Difference = 20.3 cm

1st Visit Midthigh C = 68.1 cm
2nd Visit Midthigh C = 56.6 cm
Difference = 11.5 cm

1st Visit % Fat(3DPS) = 47.5%
2nd Visit % Fat (3DPS) = 35.5%
Difference = 12%

Time	Wt Kg	BMI Kg/m²
Baseline	101.8	39.79
8 months	77.9	30.24

Body Dimensions

Body mass index (BMI)	65.40 Kg/m²
Neck circumference	50.5 cm
Head circumference	cm
Chest circumference	170.4 cm
Waist circumference	164.6 cm
Hip circumference	166.3 cm
Sagittal Diameter	0.0 cm
Waist to hip ratio (WHR)	0.990
Trunk length	71.3 cm

= = = = = = = = = = = = =	Right	Left
Midarm circumference	45.5 cm	45.4 cm
Elbow circumference	36.0 cm	35.5 cm
Wrist circumference	24.0 cm	24.5 cm
Midthigh circumference	82.3 cm	82.5 cm
Knee circumference	62.4 cm	60.1 cm
Calf circumference	54.3 cm	51.2 cm
Arm length	49.9 cm	50.8 cm
Leg length	cm	cm
Knee height	44.0 cm	44.3 cm

Body Volume

Total body	184.07 L
Head	5.78 L
Trunk	133.08 L
Volume of specific region:	

= = = = = = = = = = = = =	Right	Left
Arm	4.42 L	3.33 L
Leg	19.41 L	18.05 L

Body % Fat   55.3 % (By 3DPS)

Patient of Blandine Laferrere, MD. With permission

Figure 13.4   Body Outlines Generated From a Three-Dimensional Photonic Scan of an Adult Woman From a Side View Before and After Bariatric Surgery–Induced Weight Loss

NOTE: Information is provided on circumference changes of the chest, waist, hip, and mid-thigh as determined by the 3-DPS. The baseline (presurgery) report generated from a 3-DPS scan is also presented documenting the anthropometric and volume information that is generated.

Reliability. The reliability of the measurements for volumes, circumferences, and length obtained by the 3-DPS in 61 human subjects on whom triplicate measures were acquired shows intraclass correlations coefficients > .97 for all measures. The CV was < 0.9 for circumferences and < 1.1 for partial thigh length. The CVs for volumes were < 1.9 (head), < 3.0 (left arm), < 1.94 (right arm), < 4.4 (left leg), < 4.5 (right leg), and < 1.9 (torso). For total body volume, the CV was < 0.4, and the standard deviation was .33.

Accuracy and Validity. In 92 children and adults (6–82 years), J. Wang et al. (2006) found that body volume values obtained with the 3-DPS were slightly but significantly greater than those obtained with UWW for body volume (81.9 ± 4.0 L vs. 81.5 ± 4.0 L, $p < .0001$) and those obtained with a tape measure for circumferences ($p < .001$), but the values for percentage body fat were not significantly different between 3-DPS and UWW ($p = .65$). (Again, it would appear that the limitations to underlying assumptions would be the same as any technique based on total body volume; i.e., UWW or ADP.)

Norms. Since percentage body fat is the outcome measure, the norms would be consistent with the values presented in Table 13.1.

Availability and Costs. To our knowledge, there are a number of systems being developed and validated for the measurement of body composition. However, we are unclear of the costs of any commercially available systems at this time.

Tracer Dilution Techniques

Water is an important constituent in the body. Changes in the body's total body water (TBW) will affect body composition, especially when body composition estimates are acquired based on TBW assumptions. The volume of water in the body can be measured by the stable isotope dilution tracer technique of deuterium oxide (D_2O) and oxygen-18 labeled water ($H_2^{18}O$). The tracer sodium bromide (NaBr) can be used for the measurement of extracellular water space (ECW). The D_2O-derived TBW measurement method was proposed by Hevesy and Hofer (1934); improved by J. Wang, Pierson, and Kelly (1973); and later revised by Lukaski and Johnson (1985). The estimated ratios of TBW.D_2O and TBW/$H_2^{18}O$ are .97 and .99, respectively (Schoeller, Kushner, Taylor, Dietz, & Bandini, 1985), and concentrations are assayed by high-performance liquid chromatography (HPLC; Wong et al., 1989). Plasma or saliva samples are obtained at baseline and 3 hours after administering the tracers in adults and 2 hours after in children. D_2O has been widely used for the measurement of TBW in humans for more than four decades with doses from 40 to 100 g (i.e., using 0.1g/kg body weight). With this dose, the D_2O concentration at equilibrium is less than 0.03% of TBW. Administration of these tracers and collection of samples are easy, but these methods are unpractical for large-scale studies and studies in

very small children, particularly newborns. Fat mass is calculated in the TBW method as body weight minus FFM.

Reliability. The reliability of the TBW measurement is influenced by the analytical method used and the amount of tracer administered to a subject. Precision for TBW is considered to be 1% to 3% as estimated from repeat measurements (Schoeller et al., 1985; Speakman, Nair, & Goran, 1993) and the comparison of two isotopes (Racette et al., 1994).

Accuracy and Validity. Fat mass by isotope dilution techniques versus DXA/DPA values shows average correlations of .70 to .80 (see Table 13.4). The main limiting assumptions of TBW and ECW dilution techniques have been well summarized by Schoeller (2005) and include the following: (a) The tracer is distributed only in body water or ECW, (b) the tracer is equally distributed in all anatomical water compartments or ECW, (c) the rate of equilibration of the tracer is rapid, and (d) neither the tracer nor body water/ECW are metabolized during the time of tracer equilibration.

Norms. Since percentage body fat is the outcome measure, the norms would be consistent with the values presented in Table 13.1.

Availability and Costs. The isotope deuterium oxide is available from vendors (ICON and Fischer Scientific) and is relatively inexpensive ($10 per subject for deuterium oxide). The sodium bromide is widely available, and the dose solution can be easily prepared. However, the equipment and labor required for sample analyses are significant.

Practical Considerations. Due to ionizing radiation associated with the tracer tritium, this previously commonly used tracer for TBW is used less today and was never an option in children and pregnant women.

Dual Energy X-Ray Absorptiometry

DXA systems provide whole-body and regional estimates of three main components: bone mineral, bone-free FFM, and fat (Pietrobelli, Formica, Wang, & Heymsfield, 1996). The DXA technique is generally accepted as a noninvasive measurement method that can be applied in humans of all ages. An invisible beam of low-dose X-rays with two distinct low- and high-energy peaks is transmitted through the body. The measured attenuation of DXA's two main energy peaks is used to estimate each pixel's fraction of fat and lean. Fat and lean components are quantified over regions devoid of bone. The radiation exposure from a whole-body DXA scan ranges from 0.04 to 0.86 mrem (instrument and subject size dependent), which is equivalent to between 1% and 10% of a chest X ray. The subject, wearing a hospital gown and with all metal removed from the body, lies flat on the DXA stretcher, with feet in a prone position secured with a Velcro strap and arms by the side. Persons whose body size extends to the field-of-view limit are wrapped securely in a bed sheet so as to retain all of the soft tissue within the field of view. Shown in Figure 13.5 is a whole-body DXA scan acquired in an obese woman whose soft tissue extends to the instrument's field-of-view limits.

The advantages of DXA include good accuracy and reproducibility, providing for the assessment of regional body composition and nutritional status in disease states and growth disorders. Disadvantages of DXA include the following: There is a small amount of radiation, the scanning bed or stretcher has an upper weight limit (all Hologic systems < 136–159 kg [300–350 lbs]; GE Lunar Prodigy: < 136–159 kg [300–350 lbs]; GE Lunar iDXA: < 182kg [400 lbs]), and the whole-body field of view cannot accommodate very large persons. DXA estimates of fat mass are influenced by "trunk thickness," with the error increasing as the subject's trunk thickness increases (Roubenoff, Kehayias, Dawson-Hughes, & Heymsfield, 1993).

DXA is considered the gold-standard technique for the diagnosis of osteopenia and osteoporosis. The diagnosis is made when the bone mineral density *T* score is less than or equal to 2.5 standard deviations below that of a young adult reference population. The World Health Organization has established diagnostic guidelines where a *T* score –1.0 or greater is "normal," a *T* score between –1.0 and –2.5 is "low bone mass" (or "osteopenia"), and –2.5 or below is osteoporosis.

Reliability. Reliability of whole-body DXA is high (see Table 13.3). The currently available systems from GE Lunar and Hologic are fan beam technology. An important consideration is that differences in soft tissue and bone estimates are apparent within the same subject scanned on different systems and within the same subject scanned on the same system but with various software used for analyses.

Accuracy and Validity. DXA estimates of fat mass compare highly with other established methods such as IVNA (average *r* = .95) and UWW (*r* = .85; see Table 13.4). Assumptions associated with DXA include (a) the assumed constant attenuation (R) of fat (R = 1.21) and of bone mineral content, (b) minimal effects of hydration on lean tissue estimates, and (c) lack of an effect of variations in regional (e.g., chest, leg, arm) thickness on soft tissue estimates (Jebb, Goldberg, Jennings, & Elia, 1995; Kohrt, 1998; Salamone et al., 2000) and that the fat content of the area being analyzed (non-bone-containing area/pixels) is comparable to the fat content of the unanalyzed area (bone-containing area or pixels; Lohman & Chen, 2005). The limitations associated with these assumptions when these assumptions are not met include errors in the estimation of fat, lean, and bone in both regional and whole-body values.

Norms. Since percentage body fat is the outcome measure, the norms would be consistent with the values presented in Table 13.1.

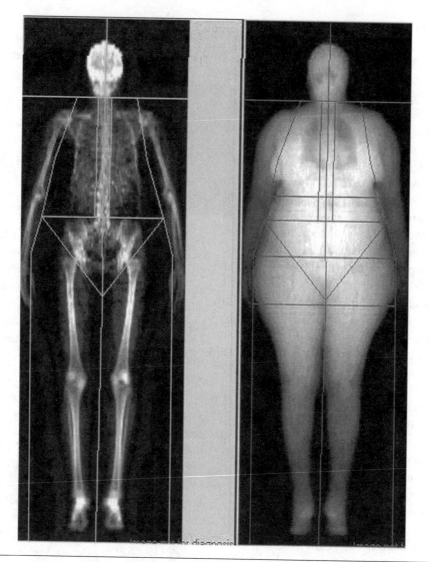

Figure 13.5   Whole-Body DXA Scan (iDXA GE Lunar) in a Woman (98.3 kg) Showing the Regional Cut Points for Fat Distribution

Availability and Costs. DXA scanners cost between $80,000 and $320,000. The annual service contract costs range from $8,000 to $13,000. A radiology technician or physician is required to operate the scanner, as ionizing radiation is being administered. DXA scans for osteoporosis screening and diagnosis are widely available and are reimbursable through health insurance. A whole-body DXA scan for the determination of body composition is primarily available at research laboratories at an average cost of only $200.

In Vivo Neutron Activation Analysis and Whole-Body Counting

Nitrogen, carbon, hydrogen, phosphorus, sodium, chlorine, calcium, and oxygen are all measurable in vivo by methods known as neutron activation analysis. A source emits a neutron stream that interacts with body tissues. The resulting decay products of activated elements can be counted by detectors and elemental mass established. C, N, and Ca can be used to estimate total body fat, protein, and bone mineral mass using established equations. Neutron activation analysis is uniquely valuable in body composition research as there are no known age or sex effects of currently applied equations. However, facilities that provide these techniques are limited, and radiation exposure is variable depending on the system being used (Dilmanian et al., 1990).

Whole-Body ^{40}K Counting Technique. A small constant percentage (0.0118%) of total body potassium (TBK) is radioactive (^{40}K) and emits a γ-ray. With appropriate shielding from background, this γ-ray can be counted using different types of detectors. As the ratio of ^{40}K to ^{39}K is known and constant, ^{39}K or "total body potassium" can be estimated accordingly. All of the body's potassium is within the FFM compartment, and the proportion of the body FFM compartment TBK/FFM ratio is reasonably stable in the same subject over time and between different subjects. However, with increasing age or when comparing young versus elderly, the TBK to FFM ratio decreases. Body cell mass (BCM) can also be estimated from TBK with the assumptions that the intracellular K is 150 mmol/L and that 25% of cell mass is intracellular solid. BCM derived from TBK was proposed by Moore et al. (1963) to be a superior index of the body's metabolically active tissue mass:

$$FFM \text{ (kg)} = TBK \text{ (mmols)} \times 0.011.$$

$$BCM \text{ (kg)} = TBK \text{ (mmols)} \times 0.0083.$$

Reliability. Precision for TBK counting in adults ranges from 2% to 5% (Cohn & Parr, 1985). In our laboratory, the CV for measured TBK in healthy human volunteers ranged from 3.8% at low body weights to 0.8% at high body weights (mean CV of 2.3%: Schneider et al., 2004). Precision for IVNA measures reported from Brookhaven National Laboratories (Heymsfield et al., 1993) are ±3.0% for carbon, ±3.0% for nitrogen, ±1.5% for calcium, ±0.7% for potassium, and ±1.6% for sodium.

Accuracy and Validity. The accuracy of TBK estimates of fat mass compared to other methods is variable such that $r = .92$ for IVNA and is lower (average $r = .75$) for UWW, DXA, and TBW (see Table 13.4). The accuracy of IVNA in healthy weight-stable men and women is reported to be excellent ($r = .97$) for IVNA-measured body weight (from the sum of six total body components: water, protein bone, soft tissue, lipid, and glycogen) compared to actual body weight (Heymsfield et al., 1993). The main assumptions for IVNA analysis are that the proportions of carbon, nitrogen, and calcium are known and constant within lipid, protein, and bone mineral. When skeletal muscle mass by IVNA was compared to that by CT scans, the standard error of the estimate was larger by IVNA (4.4 kg) compared to DXA (1.6 kg; Z. M. Wang et al., 1996).

Norms. Since percentage body fat is the outcome measure, the norms would be consistent with the values presented in Table 13.1.

Availability and Costs. IVNA and ^{40}K techniques are largely used for research purposes. The systems are very costly, which prohibits their widespread use.

Imaging Techniques

Imaging methods are considered to be among the most accurate approaches for the in vivo quantification of body composition. Imaging methods, specifically MRI and CT, allow for the estimation of adipose tissue, skeletal muscle, and other internal tissues and organs. Their primary application has been in quantifying the distribution of adipose tissue into visceral, subcutaneous, and intermuscular depots (Gallagher et al., 2005). A secondary application of MRI in body composition assessment has been to dissect the FFM compartment for the quantification of specific high metabolic rate organs in vivo (e.g., liver, kidneys, heart, spleen, and brain) with application to improving our understanding of resting energy expenditure (Gallagher et al.,

1998; Gallagher et al., 2006; Illner, Brinkmann, Heller, Bosy-Westphal, & Müller, 2000).

Magnetic Resonance Imaging (MRI)

MRI allows for the quantification of body composition at the organ-tissue level. The subject lies within the scanner's magnetic field, and a series of axial images is acquired based on the relaxation properties of excited hydrogen nuclei in water and lipids. Differentiating between different tissues within the body is based on the different relaxation times between organs and tissues. Imaging analysis software is used to quantify the area and thus volume of a specific tissue. A certain amount of analyst subjectivity is required to identify or trace the tissue boundary of interest.

A number of research laboratories today use a whole-body MRI protocol (Ross, 1996; Song et al., 2004) to quantify whole-body adipose tissue and skeletal muscle mass. A series of axial images (e.g., slice thickness 10 mm and interslice gap 40 mm) is acquired across the body. Thereafter, the tissue area between the slices is integrated to produce a tissue volume and converted to mass using assumed tissue/organ-specific density factors (Snyder et al., 1975). This protocol allows for the quantification of adipose tissue distribution—namely, visceral, subcutaneous, and intermuscular adipose tissue depots—and can be applied in children and adults. A significant advantage of MRI over CT is that MRI is free of ionizing radiation. The limitations of MRI include high costs due to scan acquisition and post-processing of data, large subjects cannot fit within field of view, and claustrophobic persons cannot be scanned. As an example, Figure 13.6 shows a three-dimensional volume rendering of total visceral adipose tissue (VAT) acquired from a whole-body magnetic resonance image scan in a woman age 67 years before (A) and after (B) a 16-week weight loss program (Gallagher, Kovera, et al., 2000). The total amount of VAT lost was 34.5%.

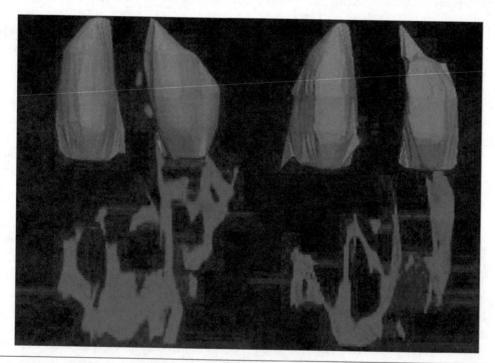

Figure 13.6 A Three-Dimensional Volume Rendering of Visceral Adipose Tissue (VAT) Acquired From a Whole-Body Magnetic Resonance Image Scan in a Woman Age 67 Years (left) Before and (right) After a 16-Week Weight Loss Program

NOTE: Total VAT loss was 34.5%. Total weight loss was 10.2 kg (11.1% of baseline) of which 9.4 kg was total adipose tissue. The solid structures in the upper half of the figure are the lungs.

Computerized Tomography (CT)

CT allows for the quantification of body composition at the organ-tissue level. The CT emits X-rays, the receiver detects the attenuated X-ray, and an image is reconstructed. The X-ray attenuation is expressed in CT number, which is a measure of the tissue attenuation relative to air and water. The CT numbers for air and water are −1,000 and 0 Hounsfield units (HU), respectively. The CT ranges for adipose tissue and skeletal muscle are −190 to −30 HU and 30 to 100 HU, respectively. The tissue area (cm^2) for a specific tissue (e.g., visceral or subcutaneous adipose tissue, skeletal muscle) on each cross-sectional CT image is determined. CT use has been predominantly confined to single-slice studies of abdomen and thigh. The disadvantages of CT for clinical research include high radiation exposure (~1,000 mrem for a single abdominal slice compared to a chest X-ray of 2 to 4 mrem (http://hps.org/documents/meddiagimaging.pdf), high cost, and larger subjects not being able to fit within field of view.

Validity. For the quantification of adipose tissue distribution, the validity of MRI and CT is considered high based on the comparison of MRI and CT with tissue biopsy samples. For example, skeletal muscle lipid content by CT versus muscle biopsy had an *r* of .58 (Goodpaster, Kelley, Thaete, He, & Ross, 2000). See an extensive review by Ross and Jannsen (2005).

Reliability. The intraobserver error or reproducibility for MRI abdominal scans ranges from 5.5% to 9.0% for VAT and 1.1% to 3.0% for SAT (Abate, Burns, Peshock, Garg, & Grundy, 1994; Gerard et al., 1991; Ross, Leger, Morris, de Guise, & Guardo, 1992; Staten, Totty, & Kohrt, 1989). The technical errors for four repeated readings of the same four whole-body scans by the same observer of MRI-derived SAT, VAT, and IMAT volumes in our laboratory are 1.7%, 2.3%, and 5.9%, respectively (Gallagher et al., 2005).

Availability and Costs. Scan acquisition can cost from $250 to over $1,000. Scan analysis costs are variable with some analysis software available for free (ImageJ) and others (SliceOMatic, Tomovision, CA) costing $4,000. An analyst is also required, and a whole-body MRI scan can require 3 hours to 4.5 hours of analyst time.

For both CT and MRI measurements of soft tissue, it is assumed that the information obtained from the slice(s) being analyzed is representative of the volume of the tissue of interest in its entirety. For example, a single abdominal slice at L4-L5 for VAT or a single mid-thigh slice for skeletal muscle or IMAT estimations is assumed to be a valid surrogate measure for total tissue volume irrespective of age, sex, and race/ethnicity, which may not be the case (Shen et al., 2007). Neither of these techniques is capable of accommodating very large persons (BMI > 40 kg/m²) where the field of view for most MRI scanners is limited to 48 × 48 cm. The latter is a significant limitation when the need arises to image persons before treatments such as bariatric surgery, which typically involves persons who have BMIs greater than 40 kg/m².

Future Directions

Our knowledge of what constitutes "normal" or altered body composition at birth and the early years of life, as well as extreme old age, is limited in part by the lack of adequate methodologies appropriate for use in these age groups. There is a need to better understand how body composition changes with growth and senescence. These gaps need to be filled. As more and more children are becoming obese and these obese children are likely to be obese as adults, accurate serial phenotyping is desirable. The proportion of elders > 75 years of age is expected to double over the next two decades, and the consequences of obesity and muscle loss in old age are still not well established. The available assessment methods applicable for the measurement of body composition in the severely obese individual are also limited, and more validated assessment methods are needed. There has been an increased interest in and need to understand the role played by ectopic fat depots (fat accumulation in the liver, skeletal muscle, pancreatic beta cells, epicardial). Improvement in the in vivo measurement methods of ectopic depots is needed. Body composition assessment is growing in importance as the efficacy of new drugs (e.g., for weight loss) is tested in clinical trials.

References

Abate, N., Burns, D., Peshock, R. M., Garg, A., & Grundy, S. M. (1994). Estimation of adipose tissue mass by magnetic resonance imaging: Validation against dissection in human cadavers. *Journal of Lipid Research, 35,* 1490–1496.

Abdel-Malek, A. K., Mukherjee, D., & Roche, A. F. (1985). A method of constructing an index of obesity. *Human Biology, 57,* 415–430.

Abu Khaled, M., McCutcheon, M. J., Reddy, S., Pearman, P. L., Hunter, G. R., & Weinsier, R. L. (1988). Electrical impedance in assessing human body composition: The BIA method. *American Journal of Clinical Nutrition, 47,* 789–792.

Albu, J., Smolowitz, J., Lichtman, S., Heymsfield, S. B., Wang, J., Pierson, R. N., Jr., et al. (1992). Composition of weight loss in severely obese women: A new look at old methods. *Metabolism, 41,* 1068–1074.

Allison, D. B., Zannolli, R., Faith, M. S., Heo, M., Pietrobelli, A., Van Itallie, T. B., et al. (1999). Weight loss increases and fat loss decreases all-cause mortality rate: Results from two independent cohort studies. *International Journal of Obesity and Related Metabolic Disorders, 23,* 603–611.

Alvarez, V. P., Dixon, J. B., Strauss, B. J., Laurie, C. P., Chaston, T. B., & O'Brien, P. E. (2007). Single frequency bioelectrical impedance is a poor method for determining fat mass in moderately obese women. *Obesity Surgery, 17,* 211–221.

American College of Sports Medicine. (2001). *ACSM resource manual for guidelines for exercise testing and prescription* (4th ed.). Baltimore: Lippincott Williams & Wilkins.

Barlow, S. E., & Dietz, W. H. (1998). Obesity evaluation and treatment: Expert Committee recommendations. The Maternal and Child Health Bureau, Health Resources and Services Administration and the Department of Health and Human Services. *Pediatrics, 2,* E29.

Baumgartner, R. N. (1996). Electrical impedance and total body electrical conductivity. In A. F. Roche, S. B. Heymsfield, & T. G. Lohman (Eds.), *Human body composition* (pp. 79–102). Champaign, IL: Human Kinetics.

Baumgartner, R. N., Heymsfield, S. B., Lichtman, S., Wang, J., & Pierson, R.N., Jr. (1991). Body composition in elderly people: Effect of criterion estimates on predictive equations. *American Journal of Clinical Nutrition, 53,* 1345–1353.

Behnke, A. R., Jr., Feen, B. G., & Welham, W. C. (1942). The specific gravity of healthy men. *Journal of the American Medical Association, 118,* 495–498.

Bellisari, A., Roche, A. F., & Siervogel, R. M. (1993). Reliability of B-mode ultrasonic measurements of subcutaneous adipose tissue and intra-abdominal depth: Comparisons with skinfold thicknesses. *International Journal of Obesity and Related Metabolic Disorders, 17,* 475–480.

Bergsma-Kadijk, J. A., Baumeister, B., & Deurenberg, P. (1996). Measurement of body fat in young and elderly women: Comparison between a four-compartment model and widely used reference methods. *British Journal of Nutrition, 75,* 649–657.

Biaggi, R. R., Vollman, M. W., Nies, M. A., Brener, C. E., Flakoll, P. J., Levenhagen, D. K., et al. (1999). Comparison of air-displacement plethysmography with hydrostatic weighing and bioelectrical impedance analysis for the assessment of body composition in healthy adults. *American Journal of Clinical Nutrition, 69,* 898–903.

Brambilla, P., Bedogni, G., Moreno, L. A., Goran, M. I., Gutin, B., Fox, K. R., et al. (2006). Cross validation of anthropometry against magnetic resonance imaging for the assessment of visceral and subcutaneous adipose tissue in children [Review]. *International Journal of Obesity (London), 30,* 23–30.

Brook, C. G. D. (1971). Determination of body composition of children from skinfold measurements. *Archives of Disease in Childhood, 46,* 182–184.

Brozek, J., Grande, F., Anderson, J. T., & Keys, A. (1963). Densitometric analysis of body composition: Revision of some quantitative assumptions. *Annals of the New York Academy of Sciences, 110,* 113–140.

Chouinard, L. E., Schoeller, D. A., Watras, A. C., Clark, R. R., Close, R. N., & Buchholz, A. C. (2007). Bioelectrical impedance vs. four-compartment model to assess body fat change in overweight adults. *Obesity (Silver Spring), 15*, 85–92.

Chumlea, W. C., & Guo, S. (1992). Equations for predicting stature in white and black elderly individuals. *Journal of Gerontology, 47*, M197–M203.

Chumlea, W. C., & Guo, S. S. (1994). Bioelectrical impedance and body composition: Present status and future directions. *Nutrition Reviews, 52*, 123–131.

Chumlea, W. C., Guo, S. S., Zeller, C. M., Reo, N. V., Baumgartner, R. N., Garry, P. J., et al. (2001). Total body water reference values and prediction equations for adults. *Kidney International, 59*, 2250–2258.

Chumlea, W. C., Roche, A. F., & Rogers, E. (1984). Replicability for anthropometry in the elderly. *Human Biology, 56*, 329–337.

Cochran, W. J., Wong, W. W., Fiorotto, M. L., Sheng, H. P., Klein, P. D., & Klish, W. J. (1988). Total body water estimated by measuring total-body electrical conductivity. *American Journal of Clinical Nutrition, 48*, 946–950.

Cohn, S. H., & Parr, R. M. (Eds.). (1985). Nuclear based techniques for the in vivo study of human body composition. *Clinical Physics and Physiological Measurements, 6*, 275–301.

Cohn, S. H., Vaswani, A. N., Yasumura, S., Yuen, K., & Ellis, K. J. (1984). Improved models for determination of body fat by in vivo neutron activation. *American Journal of Clinical Nutrition, 40*, 255–259.

Cohn, S. H., Vaswani, A. N., Yasumura, S., Yuen, K., & Ellis, K. J. (1985). Assessment of cellular mass and lean body mass by noninvasive nuclear techniques. *Journal of Laboratory and Clinical Medicine, 105*, 305–311.

Coin, A., Sergi, G., Minicuci, N., Giannini, S., Barbiero, E., Manzato, E., et al. (2008). Fat-free mass and fat mass reference values by dual-energy X-ray absorptiometry (DEXA) in a 20–80 year-old Italian population. *Clinical Nutrition, 27*, 87–94.

Cole, T. J., Bellizzi, M. C., Flegal, K. M., & Dietz, W. H. (2000). Establishing a standard definition for child overweight and obesity worldwide: International survey. *British Medical Journal, 320*, 1240–1243.

Cole, T. J., Flegal, K. M., Nicholls, D., & Jackson, A. A. (2007). Body mass index cut offs to define thinness in children and adolescents: International survey. *British Medical Journal, 335*, 194.

Cruz, M. L., & Goran, M. I. (2004). The metabolic syndrome in children and adolescents [Review]. *Current Diabetes Reports, 4*, 53–62.

Dalton, M., Cameron, A. J., Zimmet, P. Z., Shaw, J. E., Jolley, D., Dunstan, D. W., et al. (2003). Waist circumference, waist-hip ratio and body mass index and their correlation with cardiovascular disease risk factors in Australian adults. *Journal of Internal Medicine, 254*, 555–563.

Dekker, L., Douros, I., Buxton, B. F., & Treleaven, P. (1999). Building symbolic information for 3D human body modeling from range data: Second International Conference on 3-D imaging and modeling. *Institute of Electrical and Electronic Engineers*, pp. 388–397.

Demerath, E. W., Guo, S. S., Chumlea, W. C., Towne, B., Roche, A. F., & Siervogel, R. M. (2002). Comparison of percent body fat estimates using air displacement plethysmography and hydrodensitometry in adults and children. *International Journal of Obesity and Related Metabolic Disorders, 26*, 389–397.

Dempster, P., & Aitkens, S. (1995). A new air displacement method for the determination of human body composition. *Medicine & Science in Sports & Exercise, 27*, 1692–1697.

Deurenberg, P., Leenen, R., Van der Kooy, K., & Hautvast, J. G. (1989). In obese subjects the body fat percentage calculated with Siri's formula is an overestimation. *European Journal of Clinical Nutrition, 43*, 569–575.

Deurenberg, P., Vanderkooy, K., Leenen, R., Weststrate, J., & Seidell, J. (1991). Sex and age specific prediction formulas for estimating body composition from bioelectrical impedance: A cross-validation study. *International Journal of Obesity and Related Metabolic Disorders, 15*, 17–25.

Dietz, W. H. (1998). Health consequences of obesity in youth: Childhood predictors of adult disease. *Pediatrics, 101*, 518–525.

Dilmanian, F. A., Weber, D. A., Yasumura, S., Kamen, Y., Lidofsky, L., Heymsfield, S. B., et al. (1990). Performance of the delayed- and prompt-gamma neutron activation systems at Brookhaven National Laboratory. *Basic Life Science, 55*, 309–315.

Dioum, A., Gartner, A., Maire, B., Delpeuch, F., & Wade, S. (2005). Body composition predicted from skinfolds in African women: A cross-validation study using air-displacement plethysmography and a Black-specific equation. *British Journal of Nutrition, 93*, 973–979.

Dobbelsteyn, C. J., Joffres, M. R., MacLean, D. R., & Flowerdew, G. (2001). A comparative evaluation of waist circumference, waist-to-hip ratio and body mass index as indicators of cardiovascular risk factors. The Canadian Heart Health Surveys. *International Journal of Obesity and Related Metabolic Disorders, 25,* 652–661.

Durnin, J. V., & Womersley, J. (1974). Body fat assessed from total body density and its estimation from skinfold thickness: Measurements on 481 men and women aged from 16 to 72 yr. *British Journal of Nutrition, 32,* 77–97.

Eckerson, J. M., Housh, T. J., & Johnson, G. O. (1992a). Validity of bioelectrical impedance equations for estimating fat-free weight in lean males. *Medicine & Science in Sports & Exercise, 24,* 1298–1302.

Eckerson, J. M., Housh, T. J., & Johnson, G. O. (1992b). The validity of visual estimations of percent body fat in lean males. *Medicine & Science in Sports & Exercise, 24,* 615–618.

Evans, W. J. (1995). What is sarcopenia? *Journal of Gerontology, 50A,* 5–8.

Expert Panel on the Identification, Evaluation, and Treatment of Overweight in Adults. (1998). Clinical guidelines on the identification, evaluation, and treatment of overweight and obesity in adults: Executive summary. *American Journal of Clinical Nutrition, 68,* 901.

Field, A. E., Laird, N., Steinberg, E., Fallon, E., Semega-Janneh, M., & Yanovski, J. A. (2003). Which metric of relative weight best captures body fatness in children? *Obesity Research, 11,* 1345–1352.

Fields, D. A., Goran, M. I., & McCrory, M. A. (2002). Body-composition assessment via air-displacement plethysmography in adults and children: A review. *American Journal of Clinical Nutrition, 75,* 453–467.

Flakoll, P. J., Kent, P., Neyra, R., Levenhagen, D., Chen, K. Y., & Ikizler, T. A. (2004). Bioelectrical impedance vs air displacement plethysmography and dual-energy X-ray absorptiometry to determine body composition in patients with end-stage renal disease. *Journal of Parenteral and Enteral Nutrition, 28,* 13–21.

Flynn, M. A., Nolph, G. B., Baker, A. S., Martin, W. M., & Krause, G. (1989). Total body potassium in aging humans: A longitudinal study. *American Journal of Clinical Nutrition, 50,* 713–717.

Fomon, S. J., Haschke, F., Ziegler, E. E., & Nelson, S. E. (1982). Body composition of reference children from birth to age 10 years. *American Journal of Clinical Nutrition, 35,* 1169–1175.

Forbes, G. (1987). *Human body composition.* New York: Springer-Verlag.

Freedman, D. S., Wang, J., Maynard, L. M., Thornton, J. C., Mei, Z., Pierson, R. N, et al. (2005). Relation of BMI to fat and fat-free mass among children and adolescents. *International Journal of Obesity, 29,* 1–8.

Gallagher, D., Albu, J., He, Q., Heshka, S., Boxt, L., Krasnow, N., et al. (2006). Small organs with a high metabolic rate explain lower resting energy expenditure in African American than in white adults. *American Journal of Clinical Nutrition, 83,* 1062–1067.

Gallagher, D., Belmonte, D., Deurenberg, P., Wang, Z., Krasnow, N., Pi-Sunyer, F. X., et al. (1998). Organ-tissue mass measurement allows modeling of REE and metabolically active tissue mass. *American Journal of Physiology, 275*(Pt. 1), E249–E258.

Gallagher, D., Heymsfield, S. B., Heo, M., Jebb, S. A., Murgatroyd, P. R., & Sakamoto, Y. (2000). Healthy percentage body fat ranges: An approach for developing guidelines based on body mass index. *American Journal of Clinical Nutrition, 72,* 699.

Gallagher, D., Kovera, A. J., Clay-Williams, G., Agin, D., Leone, P., Albu, J., et al. (2000). Weight loss in postmenopausal obesity: No adverse alterations in body composition and protein metabolism. *American Journal of Physiology—Endocrinology and Metabolism, 279,* E124–E131.

Gallagher, D., Kuznia, P., Heshka, S., Albu, J., Heymsfield, S. B., Goodpaster, B., et al. (2005). Adipose tissue in muscle: A novel depot similar in size to visceral adipose tissue. *American Journal of Clinical Nutrition, 81,* 903–910.

Garn, S. M., Leonard, W. R., & Hawthorne, V. M. (1986). Three limitations of the body mass index. *American Journal of Clinical Nutrition, 44,* 996–997.

Gerace, L., Aliprantis, A., Russell, M., Allison, D. B., Buhl, K. M., Wang, J., et al. (1994). Skeletal differences between black and white men and their relevance to body composition estimates. *American Journal of Human Biology, 6,* 255–262.

Gerard, E. L., Snow, R. C., Kennedy, D. N., Frisch, R. E., Guimaraes, A. R., Barbieri, R. L., et al. (1991). Overall body fat and regional fat distribution in young women: Quantification with MR imaging. *American Journal of Roentgenology, 157,* 99–104.

Ginde, S. R., Geliebter, A., Rubiano, F., Silva, A. M., Wang, J., Heshka, S., et al. (2005) Air displacement plethysmography: Validation in overweight and obese subjects. *Obesity Research, 13,* 1232–1237.

Going, S., Williams, D., & Lohman, T. (1995). Aging and body composition: Biological changes and methodological issues. *Exercise and Sport Sciences Reviews, 23,* 411–458.

Goodpaster, B. H., Kelley, D. E., Thaete, F. L., He, J., & Ross, R. (2000). Skeletal muscle attenuation determined by computed tomography is associated with skeletal muscle lipid content. *Applied Physiology, 89,* 104–110.

Gorber, S. C., Tremblay, M., Moher, D., & Gorber, B. (2007). A comparison of direct vs. self-report measures for assessing height, weight and body mass index: A systematic review. *Obesity Review, 8,* 307–326.

Greil, H. (2006). Patterns of sexual dimorphism from birth to senescence. *Collegium Antropologicum, 30,* 637–641.

Haarbo, J., Gotfredsen, A., Hassager, C., & Christiansen, C. (1991). Validation of body composition by dual energy X-ray absorptiometry (DEXA). *Clinical Physiology, 11,* 331–341.

Hammer, L. D., Wilson, D. M., Litt, I. F., Killen, J. D., Hayward, C., Miner, B., et al. (1991). Impact of pubertal development on body fat distribution among White, Hispanic, and Asian female adolescents. *Journal of Pediatrics, 118,* 975–980.

He, Q., Heo, M., Heshka, S., Wang, J., Pierson, R. N., Jr., Albu, J., et al. (2003). Total body potassium differs by sex and race across the adult age span. *American Journal of Clinical Nutrition, 78,* 72–77.

He, Q., Horlick, M., Thornton, J., Wang, J., Pierson, R. N., Jr., Heshka, S., et al. (2002). Sex and race differences in fat distribution among Asian, African-American, and Caucasian prepubertal children. *Journal of Clinical Endocrinology & Metabolism, 87,* 2164–2170.

He, Q., Horlick, M., Thornton, J., Wang, J., Pierson, R. N., Jr., Heshka, S., et al. (2004). Sex-specific fat distribution is not linear across pubertal groups in a multiethnic study. *Obesity Research, 12,* 725–733.

Hergenroeder, A. C. (1991). Obesity and body-mass index. *American Journal of Diseases of Children, 145,* 972.

Hertzberg, H. T., Dupertuis, C. W., & Emanual, I. (1957). Stereophotogrammetry as an anthropometric tool. *Photogrammetric Engineering, 23,* 942–947.

Hevesy, G., & Hofer, E. (1934). Elimination of water from the human body. *Nature, 134,* 879.

Heymsfield, S. B., Lichtman, S., Baumgartner, R. N., Wang, J., Kamen, Y., Aliprantis, A., et al. (1990). Body composition of humans: Comparison of two improved four-compartment models that differ in expense, technical complexity, and radiation exposure. *American Journal Clinical Nutrition, 52,* 52–58.

Heymsfield, S. B., Waki, M., Kehayias, J., Lichtman, S., Dilmanian, F. A., Kamen, Y., et al. (1991). Chemical and elemental analysis of humans in vivo using improved body composition models. *American Journal of Physiology, 261*(Pt. 1), E190–E198.

Heymsfield, S. B., Wang, J., Kehayias, J., Heshka, S., Lichtman, S., & Person, R. N., Jr. (1989). Chemical determination of human body density in vivo: Relevance to hydrodensitometry. *American Journal of Clinical Nutrition, 50,* 1280–1289.

Heymsfield, S. B., Wang, Z., Baumgartner, R. N., Dilmanian, F. A., Ma, R., & Yasumura, S. (1993). Body composition and aging: A study by in vivo neutron activation analysis. *Journal of Nutrition, 123*(Suppl.), 432–437.

Heymsfield, S. B., & Wang, Z. M. (1994). *The future of body composition research.* Cambridge, UK: Cambridge University Press.

Heyward, V. H., & Stolarczyk, L. M. (1996). *Applied body composition assessment.* Champaign, IL: Human Kinetics.

Higgins, P. B., Fields, D. A., Gower, B. A., & Hunter, G. R. (2001). The effect of scalp and facial hair on body fat estimates by the BOD POD. *Obesity Research, 9,* 326–330.

Hirschler, V., Aranda, C., Calcagno, Mde. L., Maccalini, G., & Jadzinsky, M. (2005). Can waist circumference identify children with the metabolic syndrome? *Archives of Pediatric and Adolescent Medicine, 159,* 740–744.

Horlick, M. (2001). Body mass index in childhood-measuring a moving target. *Journal of Clinical Endocrinology and Metabolism, 86,* 4059–4060.

Houtkooper, L. B., Lohman, T. G., Going, S. B., & Hall, M. C. (1989). Validity of bioelectric impedance for body composition assessment in children. *Journal of Applied Physiology, 66,* 814–821.

Illner, K., Brinkmann, G., Heller, M., Bosy-Westphal, A., & Müller, M. J. (2000). Metabolically active components of fat free mass and resting energy expenditure in nonobese adults. *American Journal of Physiology—Endocrinology & Metabolism, 278,* E308–E315.

Iwaoka, H., Yokoyama, T., Nakayama, T., Matsumura, Y., Yoshitake, Y., Fuchi, T., et al. (1998). Determination of percent body fat by the newly developed sulfur hexafluoride dilution method and air displacement plethysmography. *Journal of Nutritional Science and Vitaminology (Tokyo), 44,* 561–568.

Jackson, A. S., Pollock, M. L., Graves, J., & Mahar, M. T. (1988). Reliability and validity of bioimpedance in determining body composition. *Journal of Applied Physiology, 64,* 529–534.

Janssen, I., Heymsfield, S. B., Allison, D. B., Kotler, D. P., & Ross, R. (2002). Body mass index and waist circumference independently contribute to the prediction of nonabdominal, abdominal subcutaneous, and visceral fat. *American Journal of Clinical Nutrition, 75,* 683–688.

Jebb, S. A., Goldberg, G. R., Jennings, G., & Elia, M. (1995). Dual-energy X-ray absorptiometry measurements of body composition: Effects of depth and tissue thickness, including comparisons with direct analysis. *Clinical Science (London), 88,* 319–324.

Johansson, A. J., Forslund, A., Sjodin, A., Mallmin, H., Hambraeus, L., & Ljunghall, S. (1993). Determination of body composition: A comparison of dual-energy X-ray absorptiometry and hydrodensitometry. *American Journal Clinical Nutrition, 57,* 323–326.

Keys, A., Fidanza, F., Karvonen, M. J., Kimura, N., & Taylor, H. L. (1972). Indices of relative weight and obesity. *Journal of Chronic Diseases, 25,* 329–343.

Khosla, T., & Lowe, R. (1967). Indices of obesity derived from body weight and height. *British Journal of Preventive and Social Medicine, 21,* 122–128.

Klein, S., Allison, D. B., Heymsfield, S. B., Kelley, D. E., Leibel, R. L., Nonas, C., et al. (2007). Waist circumference and cardiometabolic risk: A consensus statement from Shaping America's Health: Association for Weight Management and Obesity Prevention; NAASO, the Obesity Society; the American Society for Nutrition; and the American Diabetes Association [Review]. *Obesity (Silver Spring), 5,* 1061–1067.

Kohrt, W.M. (1998). Preliminary evidence that DEXA provides an accurate assessment of body composition. *Journal of Applied Physiology, 84,* 372–377.

Kotler, D. P., Burastero, S., Wang, J., & Pierson, R. N, Jr. (1996). Prediction of body cell mass, fat-free mass, and total body water with bioelectrical impedance analysis: Effects of race, sex, and disease. *American Journal of Clinical Nutrition, 64,* 489S–497S.

Kullberg, J., von Below, C., Lönn, L., Lind, L., Ahlström, H., & Johansson, L. (2007). Practical approach for estimation of subcutaneous and visceral adipose tissue. *Clinical Physiology and Functional Imaging, 27,* 148–153.

Kushner, R. F., & Schoeller, D. A. (1986). Estimation of total body water by bioelectric impedance analysis. *American Journal of Clinical Nutrition, 144,* 417–424.

Kyere, K., Oldroyd, B., Oxby, C. B., Burkinshaw, L., Ellis, R. E., & Hill, G. L. (1982). The feasibility of measuring total body carbon by counting neutron inelastic scatter gamma rays. *Physics in Medicine and Biology, 27,* 805–817.

Le Carvennec, M., Fagour, C., Adenis-Lamarre, E., Perlemoine, C., Gin, H., & Rigalleau, V. (2007). Body composition of obese subjects by air displacement plethysmography: The influence of hydration. *Obesity (Silver Spring),15,* 78–84.

Levenhagen, D. K., Borel, M. J., Welch, D. C., Piasecki, J. H., Piasecki, D. P., Chen, K. Y., et al. (1999). A comparison of air displacement plethysmography with three other techniques to determine body fat in healthy adults. *Journal of Parenteral and Enteral Nutrition, 23,* 293–299.

Lohman, T. G. (1986). Applicability of body composition techniques and constants for children and youths. *Exercise and Sports Sciences Reviews, 14,* 325–257.

Lohman, T. G. (1992a). *Advances in body composition assessment.* Champaign, IL: Human Kinetics.

Lohman, T. G. (1992b). Advances in body composition techniques and constants for children and youth. *Exercise and Sports Sciences Reviews, 14,* 325–357.

Lohman, T. G. (1992c). Exercise training and body composition in childhood [Review]. *Canadian Journal of Sport Science, 17,* 284–287.

Lohman, T. G., & Chen, Z. (2005). Dual-energy X-ray absorptiometry. In S. B. Heymsfield & T. G. Lohman (Eds.), *Human body composition: Methods and findings* (pp. 63–77). Champaign, IL: Human Kinetics.

Lohman, T. G., Roche, A. F., & Martorell, R. (Eds.). (1988). *Anthropometric standardization reference manual.* Champaign, IL: Human Kinetics.

Lukaski, H. C., Bolonchuk, W. W., Hall, C. B., & Siders, W. (1986). Validation of tetrapolar bioelectrical impedance method to assess human body composition. *Journal of Applied Physiology, 60,* 1327–1332.

Lukaski, H. C., & Johnson, P. E. (1985). A simple, inexpensive method of determining total body water using a tracer dose of D_2O and infrared absorption of biological fluids. *American Journal Clinical Nutrition, 41,* 363–370.

Lukaski, H. C., Johnson, P. E., Bolonchuk, W. W., & Lykken, G. I. (1985). Assessment of fat free mass using bio-electrical impedance measurements of the human body. *American Journal of Clinical Nutrition, 41,* 810–817.

Ma, G. S., Yao, M., Liu, Y., Lin, A., Zou, H., Urlando, A., et al. (2004). Validation of a new pediatric air displacement plethysmograph for assessing body composition in infants. *American Journal of Clinical Nutrition, 79,* 653–660.

Malina, R. M., Brown, K. H., & Zavaleta, A. N. (1987). Relative lower extremity length in Mexican American and in American Black and White youth. *American Journal of Physical Anthropology, 72,* 89–94.

Malina, R. M., Huang, Y. C., & Brown, K. H. (1995). Subcutaneous adipose tissue distribution in adolescent girls of four ethnic groups. *International Journal of Obesity and Related Metabolic Disorders, 19,* 793–797.

Marks, G. C., Habicht, J. P., & Mueller, W. H. (1989). Reliability, dependability, and precision of anthropometric measurements. The Second National Health and Nutrition Examination Survey 1976–1980. *American Journal of Epidemiology, 130,* 578–587.

Maurovich-Horvat, P., Massaro, J., Fox, C. S., Moselewski, F., O'Donnell, C. J., & Hoffmann, U. (2007). Comparison of anthropometric, area- and volume-based assessment of abdominal subcutaneous and visceral adipose tissue volumes using multi-detector computed tomography. *International Journal of Obesity (London), 31,* 500–506.

Mazariegos, M., Wang, Z., Gallagher, D., Baumgartner, R. N., Allison, D. B., Wang, J., et al. (1994). Differences between young and old females in the five levels of body composition and their relevance to the two-compartment chemical model. *Journal of Gerontology, 49,* M201–M208.

Mazess, R. B., Barden, H. S., Bisek, J. P., & Hanson, J. (1990). Dual-energy X-ray absorptiometry for total-body and regional bone-mineral and soft-tissue composition. *American Journal of Clinical Nutrition, 51,* 1106–1112.

Mazess, R. B., Peppler, W. W., & Gibbons, M. (1984). Total body composition by dual-photon (153Gd) absorptiometry. *American Journal of Clinical Nutrition, 40,* 834–839.

McCrory, M. A., Gomez, T. D., Bernauer, E. M., & Mole, P. A. (1995). Evaluation of a new air displacement plethysmograph for measuring human body composition. *Medicine & Science in Sports & Exercise, 27,* 1686–1691.

Mernagh, J. R., Harrison, J. E., & McNeill, K. G. (1977). In vivo determination of nitrogen using Pu-Be sources. *Physics in Medicine and Biology, 22,* 831–835.

Michielutte, R., Diseker, R. A., Corbett, W. T., Schey, H. M., & Ureda, J. R. (1984). The relationship between weight-height indices and the triceps skinfold measure among children age 5 to 12. *American Journal of Public Health, 74,* 604–606.

Miller, J. A. A., Schmatz, C., & Schultz, A. B. (1988). Lumbar disc degeneration: Correlation with age, sex, and spine level in 600 autopsy specimens. *Spine, 13,* 173–178.

Minten, V. K., Lowik, M. R., Deurenberg, P., & Kok, F. J. (1991). Inconsistent associations among anthropometric measurements in elderly Dutch men and women. *Journal of the American Dietetic Association, 91,* 1408–1412.

Misra, A., Vikram, N. K., Gupta, R., Pandey, R. M., Wasir, J. S., & Gupta, V. P. (2006). Waist circumference cut-off points and action levels for Asian Indians for identification of abdominal obesity. *International Journal of Obesity (London), 30,* 106–111.

Miyatake, N., Nonaka, K., & Fujii, M. (1999). A new air displacement plethysmograph for the determination of Japanese body composition. *Diabetes, Obesity, and Metabolism, 1,* 347–351.

Miyatake, N., Wada, J., Matsumoto, S., Nishikawa, H., Makino, H., & Numata, T. (2007). Re-evaluation of waist circumference in metabolic syndrome: A comparison between Japanese men and women. *Acta Medica Okayama, 61,* 167–169.

Moore, F. D., Olsen, K. H., McMurray, J. D., Parker, H. V., Ball, M. R., & Boyden, C. M. (1963). *The body cell mass and its supporting environment: Body composition in health and disease.* Philadelphia: W. B. Saunders.

Mott, J. W., Wang, J., Thornton, J. C., Allison, D. B., Heymsfield, S. B., & Pierson, R. N., Jr. (1999).

Relation between body fat and age in 4 ethnic groups. *American Journal of Clinical Nutrition, 69,* 1007–1013.

Nakao, T., & Komiya, S. (2003). Reference norms for a fat-free mass index and fat mass index in the Japanese child population. *Journal of Physiological Anthropology and Applied Human Science, 22,* 293–298.

National Institutes of Health, National Heart, Lung and Blood Institute. (1998). Clinical guidelines on the identification, evaluations, and treatment of overweight and obesity in adults: The evidence report. *Obesity Research, 6*(Suppl. 2), 51S–209S.

Nicholson, J. C., McDuffie, J. R., Bonat, S. H., Russell, D. L., Boyce, K. A., McCann, S., et al. (2001). Estimation of body fatness by air displacement plethysmography in African American and White children. *Pediatric Research, 50,* 467–473.

Nulicek, D. N., Spurr, G. B., Barboriak, J. J., Rooney, C. B., el Ghatit, A. Z., & Bongard, R. D. (1988). Body composition of patients with spinal cord injury. *European Journal of Clinical Nutrition, 42,* 765–773.

Nuñez, C., Gallagher, D., Visser, M., Pi-Sunyer, F. X., Wang, Z., & Heymsfield, S. B. (1997). Bioimpedance analysis: Evaluation of leg-to-leg system based on pressure contact footpad electrodes. *Medicine & Science in Sports & Exercise, 29,* 524–531.

Nuñez, C., Kovera, A. J., Pietrobelli, A., Heshka, S., Horlick, M., Kehayias, J. J., et al. (1999). Body composition in children and adults by air displacement plethysmography. *European Journal of Clinical Nutrition, 53,* 382–387.

Nyboer, J. (1972). Workable volume and flow concepts of biosegments by electrical impedance plethysmography. *T.I.T. Journal of Life Sciences, 2,* 1–13.

Ode, J. J., Pivarnik, J. M., Reeves, M. J., & Knous, J. L. (2007). Body mass index as a predictor of percent fat in college athletes and nonathletes. *Medicine & Science in Sports & Exercise, 39,* 403–409.

Ortiz, O., Russell, M., Daley, T. L., Baumgartner, R. N., Waki, M., Lichtman, S., et al. (1992). Differences in skeletal muscle and bone mineral mass between Black and White females and their relevance to estimates of body composition. *American Journal of Clinical Nutrition, 55,* 1–6.

Papathakis, P. C., Rollins, N. C., Brown, K. H., Bennish, M. L., & Van Loan, M. D. (2005). Comparison of isotope dilution with bioimpedance spectroscopy and anthropometry for assessment of body composition in asymptomatic HIV-infected and HIV-uninfected breastfeeding mothers. *American Journal of Clinical Nutrition, 82,* 538–546.

Park, H. S., Yun, Y. S., Park, J. Y., Kim, Y. S., & Choi, J. M. (2003). Obesity, abdominal obesity, and clustering of cardiovascular risk factors in South Korea. *Asia Pacific Journal of Clinical Nutrition, 12,* 411–418.

Pateyjohns, I. R., Brinkworth, G. D., Buckley, J. D., Noakes, M., & Clifton, P. M. (2006). Comparison of three bioelectrical impedance methods with DXA in overweight and obese men. *Obesity (Silver Spring), 14,* 2064–2070.

Peterson, M. J., Czerwinski, S. A., & Siervogel, R. M. (2003). Development and validation of skinfold-thickness prediction equations with a 4-compartment model. *American Journal of Clinical Nutrition, 77,* 1186–1191.

Petroni, M. L., Bertoli, S., Maggioni, M., Morini, P., Battezzati, A., Tagliaferri, M. A., et al. (2003). Feasibility of air plethysmography (BOD POD) in morbid obesity: A pilot study. *Acta Diabetol, 40*(Suppl. 1), S59–S62.

Pierson, R. N., Jr., Lin, D. H. Y., & Phillips, R. A. (1974). Total-body potassium in health: Effects of age, sex, height, and fat. *American Journal of Physiology, 226,* 206–221.

Pierson, R. N., Jr., Wang, J., Heymsfield, S. B., Russell-Aulet, M., Mazariegos, M., Tierney, M., et al. (1991). Measuring body fat: Calibrating the rulers: Inter-method comparisons in 389 normal Caucasian subjects. *American Journal of Physiology, 261*(Pt. 1), E103–E108.

Pietrobelli, A., Formica, C., Wang, Z., & Heymsfield, S. B. (1996). Dual-energy X-ray absorptiometry body composition model: Review of physical concepts. *American Journal of Physiology, 271,* E941–E951.

Pietrobelli, A., Morini, P., Battistini, N., Chiumello, G., Nuñez, C., & Heymsfield, S. B. (1998). Appendicular skeletal muscle mass: Prediction from multiple frequency segmental bioimpedance analysis. *European Journal of Clinical Nutrition, 52,* 507–511.

Pouliot, M. C., Despres, J. P., Lemieux, S., Moorjani, S., Bouchard, C., Tremblay, A., et al. (1994). Waist circumference and abdominal sagittal diameter: Best simple anthropometric indexes of abdominal visceral adipose tissue accumulation and related cardiovascular risk in men and women. *American Journal of Cardiology, 73,* 460–468.

Prothro, J. W., & Rosenbloom, C. A. (1993). Physical measurements in an elderly Black population: Knee height as the dominant indicator of stature. *Journal of Gerontology, 48,* M15–M18.

Quaade, F. (1956). Influence of hereditary and environment upon stature in school children. *Acta Paediatrica, 45,* 523–533.

Quetelet, L. A. J. (1973). A treatise on man and the development of his faculties. In *Comparative statistics in the 19th century.* Farnborough, UK: Gregg International Publishers. (Original work published 1842)

Racette, S. B., Schoeller, D. A., Luke, A. H., Shay, K., Hnilicka, J., & Kushner, R. F. (1994). Relative dilution spaces of 2H- and 18O-labeled water in humans. *American Journal of Physiology, 267*(Pt. 1), E585–E590.

Radley, D., Gately, P. J., Cooke, C. B., Carroll, S., Oldroyd, B., & Truscott, J. G. (2003). Estimates of percentage body fat in young adolescents: A comparison of dual-energy X-ray absorptiometry and air displacement plethysmography. *European Journal of Clinical Nutrition, 57,* 1402–1410.

Rammohan, M., & Aplasca, E. C. (1992). Caliper method vs bioelectrical impedance analysis for determining body fat in patients undergoing chronic dialysis and in healthy individuals. *Journal of the American Dietetic Association, 92,* 1395–1397.

Revicki, D. A.,& Israel, R. G. (1986). Relationship between body mass indices and measures of body adiposity. *American Journal of Public Health, 76,* 992–994.

Rising, R., Swinburn, B., Larson, K., & Ravussin, E. (1991). Body composition in Pima Indians: Validation of bioelectrical resistance. *American Journal of Clinical Nutrition, 53,* 594—598.

Robinette, K. M., Daanen, H., & Paquet, E. (1999). The Caesar Project: A 3-D surface anthropometry survey. *Institute of Electrical and Electronic Engineers,* pp. 380–385.

Rolland-Cachera, M. F., Cole, T. J., Sempe, M., Tichet, J., Rossignol, C., & Charraud A. (1991). Body mass index variations: Centiles from birth to 87 years. *European Journal of Clinical Nutrition, 45,* 13–21.

Ross, R. (1996). Magnetic resonance imaging provides new insights into the characterization of adipose and lean tissue distribution. *Canadian Journal of Clinical Pharmacology, 74,* 778–785.

Ross, R., & Jannsen, I. (2005). Computed tomography and magnetic resonance imaging. In S. B. Heymsfield, T. G. Lohman, Z. Wang, & S. B. Going (Eds.), *Human body composition* (pp. 89–108). Champaign, IL: Human Kinetics.

Ross, R., Leger, L., Morris, D., de Guise, J., & Guardo, R. (1992). Quantification of adipose tissue by MRI: Relationship with anthropometric variables. *Journal of Applied Physiology, 72,* 787–795.

Roubenoff, R., Kehayias, J. J., Dawson-Hughes, B., & Heymsfield, S. B. (1993). Use of dual-energy X-ray absorptiometry in body-composition studies: Not yet a "gold standard" [Review]. *American Journal of Clinical Nutrition, 58,* 589–591.

Rush, E. C., Chandu, V., & Plank, L. D. (2006). Prediction of fat-free mass by bioimpedance analysis in migrant Asian Indian men and women: A cross validation study. *International Journal of Obesity (London), 30,* 1125–1131.

Russell-Aulet, M., Wang, J., Thornton, J., & Pierson, R. N., Jr. (1991). Comparison of dual-photon absorptiometry systems for total-body bone and soft tissue measurements: Dual-energy X-rays versus gadolinium 153. *Journal of Bone and Mineral Research, 6,* 411–415.

Salamone, L. M., Fuerst, T., Visser, M., Kern, M., Lang, T., Dockrell, M., et al. (2000). Measurement of fat mass using DEXA: A validation study in elderly adults. *Journal of Applied Physiology, 89,* 345–352.

Sardinha, L. B., Lohman, T. G., Teixeira, P. J., Guedes, D. P., & Going, S. B. (1998). Comparison of air displacement plethysmography with dual-energy X-ray absorptiometry and 3 field methods for estimating body composition in middle-aged men. *American Journal of Clinical Nutrition, 68,* 786–793.

Schneider, B., Wang, J., Thornton, J. C., Arbo, J., Horlick, M., Heymsfield, S., et al. (2004). Accuracy, reproducibility and normal total body potassium (TBK) measured using renovated whole body ^{40}K counter at St. Luke's-Roosevelt Hospital. *International Journal of Body Composition Research, 2,* 1–10.

Schoeller, D. A. (2005). Hydrometry. In S. B. Heymsfield, T. G. Lohman, & Z. Wang (Eds.), *Human body composition: Methods and findings* (pp. 35–49). Champaign, IL: Human Kinetics.

Schoeller, D. A., Kushner, R. F., Taylor, P., Dietz, W. H., & Bandini, L. (1985). Measurement of total body water: Isotope dilution techniques. In A. F. Roche (Ed.), *Body composition assessments in youth and adults: Sixth Ross conferences on medical research* (pp. 124–129). Columbus, OH: Ross Laboratories.

Schoeller, D. A., Van Santen, E., Peterson, D. W., Dietz, W. H., Jaspan, J., & Klen, P. D. (1980). Total body water measurement in humans with ^{18}O and ^2H labeled water. *American Journal of Clinical Nutrition, 33,* 2686–2693.

Sellinger, A. (1977). *The body as a three component system.* Unpublished doctoral dissertation, University of Illinois, Urbana.

Sempolska, K., & Stupnicki, R. (2007). Relative fat content in young women with normal BMI but differing in the degree of physical activity. *Rocz Panstw Zakl Hig, 58,* 333–338.

Shen, W., Punyanitya, M., Chen, J., Gallagher, D., Albu, J., Pi-Sunyer, X., et al. (2007). Visceral adipose tissue: Relationships between single slice areas at different locations and obesity-related health risks. *International Journal of Obesity (London), 31,* 763–769.

Shen, W., St-Onge, M. P., Wang, Z., & Heymsfield, S. (2005). Study of body composition: An overview. In S. B. Heymsfield, T. G. Lohman, Z. Wang, & S. B. Going (Eds.), *Human body composition* (pp. 3–14). Champaign, IL: Human Kinetics.

Sheng, H. P., & Huggins, R. A. (1979). A review of body composition studies with emphasis on total body water and fat. *American Journal of Clinical Nutrition, 32,* 630–647.

Silver, A. J., Guillen, C. P., Kahl, M. J., & Morley, J. E. (1993). Effect of aging on body fat. *Journal of the American Geriatrics Society, 41,* 211–213.

Siri, W. E. (1956). The gross composition of the body. *Advances in Biological and Medical Physics, 4,* 239–280.

Siri, W. E. (1961). Body composition from fluid spaces and density: Analysis of methods. In J. Brozek & A. Henschel (Eds.), *Techniques for measuring body composition* (pp. 223–244). Washington, DC: National Academy of Sciences.

Slaughter, M. H., Christ, C. B., Stillman, R. J., & Boileau, R. A. (1993). Mineral and water content of the fat-free body: Effects of gender, maturation, level of fatness, and age. *Obesity Research, 1,* 40–49.

Slaughter, M. H., Lohman, T. G., Boileau, R. A., Horswill, C. A., Stillman, R. J., & Van Loan, M. D. (1988). Skinfold equations for estimation of body fatness in children and youth. *Human Biology, 60,* 709–723.

Smalley, K. J., Knerr, A. N., Kendrick, Z. V., Colliver, J. A., & Owen, O. E. (1990). Reassessment of body mass indices. *American Journal of Clinical Nutrition, 52,* 405–408.

Snyder, W. S., Cook, M. J., Nasset, E. S., Karhausen, L. R., Howells, G. P., & Tipton, I. H. (1975). *Report of the Task Group on Reference Man.* Oxford, UK: Pergamon.

Song, M. Y., Ruts, E., Kim, J., Janumala, I., Heymsfield, S., & Gallagher D. (2004). Sarcopenia and increased adipose tissue infiltration of muscle in elderly African American women. *American Journal of Clinical Nutrition, 89,* 874–880.

Sopher, A., Shen, W., & Pietrobelli, A. (2005). Pediatric body composition methods. In S. B. Heymsfield, T. G. Lohman, & Z. Wang (Eds.), *Human body composition: Methods and findings* (pp. 129–139). Champaign, IL: Human Kinetics.

Speakman, J. R., Nair, K. S., & Goran, M. I. (1993). Revised equations for calculating CO_2 production from doubly labeled water in humans. *American Journal of Physiology, 264,* E912–E917.

Spungen, A. M., Adkins, R. H., Stewart, C. A., Wang, J., Pierson, R. N., Jr., Waters, R. L., et al. (2003). Factors influencing body composition in persons with spinal cord injury: A cross-sectional study. *Journal of Applied Physiology, 95,* 2398–2407.

Spungen, A. M., Bauman, W. A., Wang, J., & Pierson, R. N., Jr. (1995). Measurement of body fat in individuals with tetraplegia: A comparison of eight clinical methods. *Paraplegia, 33,* 402–408.

Staten, M. A., Totty, W. G., & Kohrt, W. M. (1989). Measurement of fat distribution by magnetic resonance imaging. *Investigative Radiology, 24,* 345–349.

Steijaert, M., Deurenberg, P., Van Gaal, L., & De Leeuw, I.(1997). The use of multi-frequency impedance to determine total body water and extracellular water in obese and lean female individuals. *International Journal of Obesity and Related Metabolic Disorders, 21,* 930–934.

Sun, S. S., Chumlea, W. C., Heymsfield, S. B., Lukaski, H. C., Schoeller, D., Friedl, K., et al. (2004). Development of bioelectrical impedance analysis prediction equations for body composition with the use of a multicomponent model for use in epidemiologic surveys. *American Journal of Clinical Nutrition, 79,* 335–336; author reply 336–337.

Svendsen, O. L., Haarbo, J., Heitmann, B. L., Gotfredsen, A., & Christiansen, C. (1991).

Measurement of body fat in elderly subjects by dual-energy X-ray absorptiometry, bioelectrical impedance, and anthropometry. *American Journal of Clinical Nutrition, 53,* 1117–1123.

Thomas, B. J., Ward, L. C., & Cornish, B. H. (1998). Bioimpedance spectrometry in the determination of body water compartments: Accuracy and clinical significance [Review]. *Applied Radiation and Isotopes, 49,* 447–455.

Trotter, M., & Gleser, G. C. (1958). A re-evaluation of estimation of stature based on measurements of stature taken during life and of long bones after death. *American Journal of Physical Anthropology, 16,* 79–123.

Tzen, K. Y., & Wu, C. (1989). Quality assurance and precision of dual photon absorptiometry in bone mineral measurement. *Zhonghua Yi Xue Za Zhi (Taipei), 43,* 1–8.

Urlando, A., Dempster, P., & Aitkens, S. (2003). A new air displacement plethysmograph for the measurement of body composition in infants. *Pediatric Research, 3,* 486–492.

Van Itallie, T. B. (1986). Bad news and good news about obesity. *New England Journal of Medicine, 314,* 239–240.

Van Loan, M., & Mayclin, P. (1987). A new TOBEC instrument and procedure for the assessment of body composition: Use of Fourier coefficients to predict lean body mass and total body water. *American Journal of Clinical Nutrition, 45,* 131–137.

Vartsky, D., Ellis, K. J., & Cohn, S. H. (1979). In vivo measurement of body nitrogen by analysis of prompt gammas from neutron capture. *Journal of Nuclear Medicine, 20,* 1158–1165.

Venkataraman, P. S., & Ahluwalia, B. W. (1992). Total bone mineral content and body composition by x-ray densitometry in newborns. *Pediatrics, 90,* 767–770.

Vescovi, J. D., Zimmerman, S. L., Miller, W. C., Hildebrandt, L., Hammer, R. L., & Fernhall, B. (2001). Evaluation of the BOD POD for estimating percentage body fat in a heterogeneous group of adult humans. *European Journal of Applied Physiology, 85,* 326–332.

Visser, M., Gallagher, D., Deurenberg, P., Wang, J., Pierson, R. N., Jr., & Heymsfield, S. B. (1997). Density of fat-free body mass: Relationship with race, age, and level of body fatness. *American Journal of Physiology, 272*(Pt. 1), E781–E787.

Volz, P. A., & Ostrove, S. M. (1984). Evaluation of a portable ultrasonoscope in assessing the body composition of college-age women. *Medicine & Science in Sports & Exercise, 16,* 97–102.

Waki, M., Kral, J. G., Mazariegos, M., Wang, J., Pierson, R. N., Jr., & Heymsfield, S. B. (1991). Relative expansion of extracellular fluid in obese vs. nonobese women. *American Journal of Physiology, 261*(Pt. 1), E199–E203.

Wang, J., Gallagher, D., Thornton, J. C., Yu, W., Horlick, M., & Pi-Sunyer, F. X. (2006). Validation of a 3-dimensional photonic scanner for the measurement of body volumes, dimensions, and percentage body fat. *American Journal of Clinical Nutrition, 83,* 809–816.

Wang, J., Kotler, D. P., Russell, M., Burastero, S., Mazariegos, M., Thornton, J., et al. (1992). Body-fat measurement in patients with acquired immunodeficiency syndrome: Which method should be used? *American Journal of Clinical Nutrition, 56,* 963–967.

Wang, J., Pierson, R. N., Jr., & Kelly, W. G. (1973). A rapid method for the determination of deuterium oxide in urine: Application to the measurement of total body water. *Journal of Laboratory and Clinical Medicine, 82,* 170–178.

Wang, J., Thornton, J. C., Bari, S., Williamson, B., Gallagher, D., Heymsfield, S. B., et al. (2003). Comparisons of waist circumferences measured at 4 sites. *American Journal of Clinical Nutrition, 77,* 379–384.

Wang, J., Thornton, J. C., Russell, M., Burastero, S., Heymsfield, S., & Pierson, R. N., Jr. (1994). Asians have lower body mass index (BMI) but higher percent body fat than do Whites: Comparisons of anthropometric measurements. *American Journal of Clinical Nutrition, 60,* 23–28.

Wang, Z., Deurenberg, P., & Heymsfield, S. B. (2000). Cellular-level body composition model: A new approach to studying fat-free mass hydration. *Annals of the New York Academy of Science, 904,* 306–311.

Wang, Z., Ma, R., Pierson, R. N., Jr., & Heymsfield, S. (1993). Five level model: Reconstruction of body weight at atomic, molecular, cellular, and tissue-system levels from neutron activation analysis. In K. J. Ellis & J. D. Eastman (Eds.), *Human body composition, in vivo methods, models, and assessment* (pp. 125–128). New York: Plenum.

Wang, Z. M., Pierson, R. N., Jr., & Heymsfield, S. B. (1992). The five-level model: A new approach to organizing body-composition research. *American Journal of Clinical Nutrition, 56,* 19–28.

Wang, Z. M., Visser, M., Ma, R., Baumgartner, R. N., Kotler, D., Gallagher, D., et al. (1996). Skeletal muscle mass: Evaluation of neutron activation and dual-energy X-ray absorptiometry methods. *Journal of Applied Physiology, 80,* 824–831.

Ward, G. M., Krzywicki, H. T., Rahman, D. P., Quaas, R. L., Nelson, R. A., & Consolazio, C. F. (1975). Relationship of anthropometric measurements to body fat as determined by densitometry, potassium-40, and body water. *American Journal of Clinical Nutrition, 28,* 162–169.

Wells, J. C., Douros, I., Fuller, N. J., Elia, M., & Dekker, L. (2000). Assessment of body volume using three-dimensional photonic scanning. *Annals of the New York Academy of Science, 904,* 247–254.

Wells, J. C., & Fuller, N. J. (2001). Precision of measurement and body size in whole-body air-displacement plethysmography. *International Journal of Obesity and Related Metabolic Disorders, 25,* 1161–1167.

Wildman, R. P., Gu, D., Reynolds, K., Duan, X., & He, J. (2004). Appropriate body mass index and waist circumference cutoffs for categorization of overweight and central adiposity among Chinese adults. *American Journal of Clinical Nutrition, 80,* 1129–1136.

Withers, R. T., Laforgia, J., & Heymsfield, S. B. (1999). Critical appraisal of the estimation of body composition via two-, three-, and four-compartment models. *American Journal of Human Biology, 11,* 175–185.

Withers, R. T., Smith, D. A., Chatterton, B. E., Schultz, C. G., & Gaffney, R. D. (1992). A comparison of four methods of estimating the body composition of male endurance athletes. *European Journal of Clinical Nutrition, 46,* 773–784.

Wong, W. W., Sheng, H. P., Morkeberg, J. C., Kosanovich, J. L., Carke, L. L., & Klein, P. D. (1989). Measurement of extracellular water volume by bromide ion chromatography. *American Journal of Clinical Nutrition, 50,* 1290–1294.

Ziebland, S., Thorogood, M., Fuller, A., & Muir, J. (1996). Desire for the body normal: Body image and discrepancies between self-reported and measured height and weight in a British population. *Journal of Epidemiology and Community Health, 50,* 105–106.

CHAPTER 14

Measurement of Energy Expenditure

James A. Levine and Ann M. Harris

Overview of Measurement of Energy Expenditure

Historical Background

The desire to understand and quantitate human energy expenditure has existed since the mid-18th century. A variety of devices of varying complexity have been developed initially for animal studies and then subsequentially for human energy expenditure assessment. A detailed review of the history of energy expenditure measurement can be found elsewhere (Ainslie, Reilly, & Westerterp, 2003; McLean & Tobin, 1987; Webb, 1991). Currently, with the obesity epidemic, the prevalence of malnutrition worldwide, and the management of increasingly complex medical illnesses, the requirement to understand and assess human energy expenditure is crucial.

We would like to acknowledge that some of the information presented in this chapter has been published previously (Levine, 2005).

Nature of the Condition and/or Phenotype

There are three components to energy expenditure in humans: basal metabolic rate, thermic effect of food, and the energy expenditure of activity (activity thermogenesis).

Basal metabolic rate is the energy expended when an individual is laying at complete rest, in the morning after sleep in the postabsorptive state. In individuals with sedentary occupations, basal metabolic rate accounts for approximately 60% of total daily energy expenditure (Ravussin & Bogardus, 1992) and is highly predicted by lean body mass within and across species (Deriaz, Fournier, Tremblay, Despres, & Bouchard, 1992; Ford, 1984). Resting energy expenditure, in general, is within 10% of basal metabolic rate (Danforth, 1985) and is measured in subjects at complete rest in the postabsorptive state.

Thermic effect of food is the increase in energy expenditure associated with the digestion,

AUTHORS' NOTE: Supported by grants DK56650, DK63226, DK66270, DK50456 (Minnesota Obesity Center), and RR-0585 from the U.S. Public Health Service and by the Mayo Foundation.

absorption, and storage of food and accounts for approximately 10% of total daily energy expenditure (Horton, 1983; Ravussin & Bogardus, 1992); many believe there to be facultative as well as fixed components.

Activity thermogenesis is the thermogenesis that accompanies physical activities and can be divided into exercise and nonexercise activity thermogenesis. Most individuals do not partake in purposeful sporting exercise, and so their exercise-related activity thermogenesis is zero; for those who do exercise regularly, exercise-related energy expenditure is generally ~10% of total daily energy expenditure (Jakicic, Wing, Butler, & Robertson, 1995). Nonexercise activity thermogenesis, or the energy expenditure of spontaneous physical activity, encompasses the combined energy costs of the physical activities of daily living, fidgeting, spontaneous muscle contraction, and maintaining posture when not recumbent and accounts for the remainder of total daily energy expenditure for most individuals (Levine et al., 2005).

Other thermogenic variables may also need to be considered such as the energetic costs of altered temperature, medications, and emotion.

Each of these components of energy expenditure is highly variable, and the sum effect of these variances determines the variability in daily energy expenditure between individuals. Also, measurements of energy expenditure can be used to assess the *relative* thermic effects of different foods, nutrient compositions, beverages, medications, and psychological components.

Fundamental Assessment Issues or Special Concerns in Assessing Energy Expenditure

Standardization of Protocols

Adhering to standardized protocols has several advantages; first, it allows comparisons to be made between different laboratories, and, second, it enables databases to be generated to explore the variance in the components of energy expenditure

and better characterize the energy expenditure of physical activities and free-living physical activity in different individuals and populations.

Basal Metabolic Rate. Basal metabolic rate should be measured between 6 and 9 in the morning in individuals who have slept at the site of measurement overnight. The individuals should not have consumed food or energy-containing beverage for 12 hours prior to the measurement but may have consumed water. The measurement should be performed with the patient supine. A single pillow may support the subject's head and/or the head of the bed should be at a 10-degree vertical tilt. The subject should be in thermal comfort (68–74°F), and the room should not be brightly lit. Subjects should be instructed to lie motionless and should not be allowed to talk or have other potentially stimulating distractions during the measurement. The measurement period should last for 20 to 40 minutes.

Resting Energy Expenditure. Resting energy expenditure should be performed in the postprandial state, at least 6 hours after consumption of any calories or performing any rigorous activity. Subjects should be fully rested while supine for 60 minutes prior to the measurement. The measurement is otherwise as described for basal metabolic rate.

Thermic Effect of Food. Optimally, a measurement of basal metabolic rate should be performed first. Then subjects should be provided with a meal. The energy content of the meal should be known precisely and should be of 400 kcal or greater. Energy expenditure should then be measured for at least 360 minutes postmeal (Reed & Hill, 1996) or optimally 480 minutes (Reed & Hill, 1996) or until energy expenditure falls to within 5% of the basal metabolic rate (Levine et al., 2005). For those using hood-based systems (with response time < 2 minutes), energy expenditure can be measured for every 15 minutes out of 30 minutes to avoid subject agitation (Piers, Soares, Makan, & Shetty, 1992). The thermic effect of food for the meal provided is calculated from the area under the energy expenditure above the basal metabolic rate versus time curve.

Energy Expenditure of Physical Activities. Points of reference are important. Resting energy expenditure should be measured first. Then the energy expenditure of the posture of reference should be measured while the subject is motionless. For example, for measuring the energy expenditure of secretarial work, sitting energy expenditure should be measured as the point of reference, whereas for measuring the energy expenditure of scything, standing energy expenditure should be measured as the point of reference. Measurement of energy expenditure during the performance of the activity of interest should be performed for 10 to 20 minutes if the calorimeter has a response time of < 2 minutes. Where calorimeter response times are longer, the measurement period needs to be prolonged so that steady-state energy expenditure is reached. The energy expenditure for the activity can be calculated as the steady-state energy expenditure for that activity minus (or divided by) either the energy expenditure of the posture of reference or resting energy expenditure.

Validation and Calibration of Techniques to Measure Energy Expenditure

Regardless of which measurement approach is selected, it is necessary to adhere to rigorous validation and calibration protocols.

Calorimetry

Validation involves burning a measured mass of a standard of known energy equivalent within the calorimeter and ascertaining what proportion of this standard is detected by the calorimeter. Examples of such standards include ultra- pure butane and ethanol. These chemical validations should be performed monthly and have been simplified by the availability of commercially

available equipment. When optimum precision for a calorimeter is within 3% of what has been predicted, this goal is readily achievable with careful attention to technique and detail.

Calibration should be performed before each measure and at intervals during the measurement period to protect against sensor drift. An indirect calorimeter calibration involves the use of standard gases. It is recommended that two span gases be used that cover the spectrum of oxygen and/or carbon dioxide concentrations that occur during human measurements. With improved sensor linearity, many systems employ a single span gas with 100% nitrogen as the second calibration gas. It is critical to ensure that the composition of the calibration gases is guaranteed; the accepted standard for calibration gases is to what is termed *primary gas standard*. Flow sensor calibration is more challenging, and some systems allow verification of flow sensor validity by displacing fixed volumes of gas through the system using a gas syringe of several liter capacity. Another approach is to use detachable flow sensors that can be shipped to the manufacturer for verification of precision. For direct calorimeters, calibration is performed before each measurement using a heat emitter of known energy dissipation. By adopting rigorous standards of validation and calibration, data will be more reliable and so readily disseminated and exchanged between laboratories.

Doubly Labeled Water

Validation involves analyzing a sample of the dose O^{18} and D_2 with mass spectrometry. This sample may be taken from a premixed batch of D_2O^{18} or following aliqouting the subject's dose by accurately measuring and then storing the sample for analysis at the time that the subject's urine/saliva or blood samples are analyzed.

Sample Analysis Interval

Sample interval (breath by breath vs. seconds to minutes) is important in indirect calorimetry techniques. The shorter the sample interval, the greater the variability in the energy expenditure data collected (Myers, Walsh, Sullivan, & Froelicher, 1990). In general, if the total sample period is appropriate (due to averaging of the results for the individual sample intervals), this effect may be minimized.

Assessment Issues Related to the Population(s) Being Assessed

Practical Recommendations for Measurement Techniques

The choice of measurement technique is determined by the objective of the assessment, the resources available, and the ability and willingness of the subjects to partake. Each investigator needs to define what components of energy expenditure are to be measured (Table 14.1), in what setting, and with how much resource.

Laboratory Setting

To provide precise and accurate short-term (several hours) measurements of energy expenditure in the laboratory, researchers should use well-validated and frequently calibrated indirect or direct calorimeters. The instruments can be used for measurements of basal metabolic rate and resting energy expenditure. Measurements of the energy expenditure of specific activities (e.g., hair brushing or walking) and even VO_2 max measurements can be made if the calorimeter's flow rate is adequate to prevent CO_2 accumulation and if the accuracy and precision of flow rate measurements are maintained at higher oxygen consumptions.

Recently, open circuit expiratory collection calorimeters have been produced with adequate precision for basal metabolic rate, resting energy expenditure measurements, and the determination of the energy costs of specific activities. These instruments may allow widespread measurements of these

variables (Dobrosielski, Brubaker, Berry, Ayabe, & Miller, 2002; Mendelsohn, Connelly, Overend, & Petrella, 2007; Phillips & Ziuraitis, 2004; Piccinini et al., 2007; Schmitz et al., 2005; Slawinski & Billat, 2004), and their true application will become apparent over the next several years.

Where investigators wish to make laboratory-based determinations of total daily energy expenditure, a room calorimeter can be built to provide accurate measurements of energy expenditure over the longer term (1–2 days). It should be recognized that this is a major undertaking. Unless the application of the investigator argues against it, constructing an indirect room calorimeter is simpler and less costly than a direct calorimeter. Room/chamber calorimeters require dedicated space, should be equipped with some means of detecting and quantifying physical activity within the room/chamber, and will necessitate at least one full-time, highly skilled technician to maintain, validate, calibrate, and use the instrument. Even with maximum precision, it should be noted that subjects within these chambers are confined and are unable to perform the activities of daily living.

Field Setting

Calorimeter Techniques. There is a paucity of high-quality data relating to activity-related energy expenditure (FAO/WHO Ad Hoc Committee of Experts, 1973). Modern tools may allow this concern to be readdressed. Several precise, portable expiratory collection open-circuit indirect calorimeters have been developed recently (as modifications of older devices such as the Kofranyi-Michaelis respirometer; Consolazio, 1971), and these may facilitate field-based measurements of energy expenditure at rest and with routine activities. Douglas bags can be used in the field for measuring basal metabolic rate, resting energy expenditure, and, in particular, the energy expenditure of physical activities. Conceptually, "metabolic carts" can be used in the field, but this rarely occurs because of constraints such as terrain and electricity supply.

Table 14.1   Applications for Commonly Used Energy Expenditure Measurement Systems

Approach	Specific Method	Basal Metabolic Rate	Resting Energy Expenditure	Thermic Effect of Food	Energy Expenditure of Specific Activities	Total Daily Energy Expenditure
Direct calorimeter		Yes	Yes	Yes	Yes	Yes (confined subject)
Indirect calorimeter	Room open circuit	Yes	Yes	Yes	Yes	Yes (confined subject)
	Hood/canopy open circuit	Yes	Yes	Yes	Yes	No
	Open-circuit expiratory collection	Yes	Yes	Yes	Yes	No
	Total collection Douglas bag	Yes	Yes	Yes	Yes	No
Noncalorimeter methods	Doubly labeled water	No	No	No	No	Yes

NOTE: "Yes" represents where a technique can be used to perform the respective measurement and "No" where it cannot.

Noncalorimeter Methods. Field-based measurements of total daily energy expenditure over 7 to 21 days can be obtained using doubly labeled water. Often, indirect calorimetry is used to measure basal metabolic rate in conjunction with the total daily energy expenditure measurements obtained using doubly labeled water. Activity thermogenesis can thereby be calculated (the thermic effect of food is generally assumed to equal 10% of total daily energy expenditure).

The major advantage of doubly labeled water measurements is that accurate measurements of total daily energy expenditure are obtained in truly free-living individuals. There are important limitations, however. First, no information is obtained regarding the components of activity thermogenesis. Second, the thermic effect of food is not measured and is known to be variable (most believe this to introduce only small error). Third, O^{18} is expensive (~$300/subject), thereby potentially limiting the number of subjects that can be studied. Fourth, isotope ratio mass spectrometers are expensive to purchase and maintain, and skilled staff are needed for their use; hence, collaboration is encouraged between field investigators and laboratories where these instruments are in routine use.

Logging physical activity and multiplying the nature and duration of these activities by the metabolic equivalents of these activities has been widely used to estimate activity thermogenesis. Overall, this approach is potentially of value, particularly as the components of activity thermogenesis are detailed. The precision and accuracy of the approach are highly variable, however, and depend on how precisely the subjects' activities are recorded and how accurately these are transformed to energy expenditures. It is important to note that the errors of this approach are additive. Where maximum precision is needed in small studies, trained enumerators might be used and measurements made of the energy expenditures of typical activities in representative individuals using calorimeters. Where less precision is acceptable and where study populations are larger, activity diaries combined with meaningful (e.g., gender-specific) tables of energy equivalents for representative activities are likely to provide useful group data, particularly for following population trends.

Review of Assessment Methods

Energy expenditure can be measured using one of three approaches:

1. In direct calorimetry, the rate of heat loss from the subject to the calorimeter is measured.

2. In indirect calorimetry, oxygen consumption and/or carbon dioxide production are measured and converted to energy expenditure using formulas (Cunningham, 1990; Weir, 1949).

3. A number of noncalorimeter techniques have been used to predict energy expenditure by extrapolation from physiological measurements and observations.

The accuracy, reproducibility, and reliability of the measurements obtained using these various techniques vary enormously as do the complexity and cost of the techniques themselves. Please note that unless stated otherwise, the information reported for each device's reliability and validity applies to that device's measurement of energy expenditure and not gas (CO_2 and O_2) measurements.

Direct Calorimetry

Description of Method/Instrument

Direct calorimeters measure the heat lost from the body. Radiative and convective heat losses account for approximately 80% of total heat loss, while evaporative heat loss accounts for the remainder. Conductive heat loss is negligible in humans. There are three principal types of direct calorimetry: isothermal, heat sink, and convection systems. These approaches have on occasion been used in combination.

An *isothermal calorimeter* consists of a chamber lined with a layer of insulating material. The inner aspect of the layer is in thermal equilibrium with the inside of the chamber, and the outside aspect of the layer is in thermal equilibrium with the chamber wall, which is maintained at a constant temperature using circulating fluid. The temperature gradient across the insulating layer is proportional to the nonevaporative heat loss from the subject in the calorimeter. The response time of these instruments can be < 5 minutes, and the period of measurement is 0.3 to 2 hours (Spinnler, Jequier, Favre, Dolivo, & Vannotti, 1973).

Heat sink or adiabatic systems consist of a chamber from which heat lost by the subject is extracted by a liquid-cooled heat exchanger. The rate of heat extraction is regulated so that the temperatures of the inner and outer chamber walls are equal, producing a zero temperature gradient wall. The response time of these instruments is 15 to 60 minutes, and the period of measurement is 2 to 72 hours (Dauncey, Murgatroyd, & Cole, 1978; Faber, Lammert, Johansen, & Garby, 1998; Jacobsen, Johansen, & Garby, 1985; Webb, Annis, & Troutman, 1980; Webster, Welsh, Pacy, & Garrow, 1986). Theses may be used in combination with indirect calorimeters (Faber et al., 1998).

A suit calorimeter was devised based on this principal. The suit weighed < 10 kg and could be worn by a subject for up to 33 hours (Webb et al., 1980; Webb, Annis, & Troutman, 1972).

Convection direct calorimeters consist of an insulated chamber ventilated with an airflow at a known rate. Heat lost by a subject inside the chamber is calculated from the flow rate, the specific heat capacity of the air, and the increase in temperature of ventilating air leaving the chamber. The response time of these instruments is 10 to 20 minutes, and the period of measurement is 2 to 48 hours (Snellen, 2000; Snellen, Chang, & Smith, 1983).

Reliability

All three types of direct calorimetry techniques are highly reliable (Jacobsen et al., 1985; Snellen et al., 1983; Spinnler et al., 1973).

Validity

Measurement error is 0.5% to 1% for the three types of direct calorimeters (Jacobsen et al., 1985; Snellen et al., 1983; Spinnler et al., 1973) and up to 23% for the portable adiabetic system during days of energy imbalance (Webb et al., 1980).

Normative Information

Not available; the data collected are specific to the individual.

Availability of Measure and Related Costs

The instruments are extremely expensive to build (> $1,000,000) and run requiring at least one full-time technician. Direct calorimeters require enormous expertise to establish and maintain. The systems need a dedicated site of installation, with the exception of the suit adiabetic system and a heat flux transducer combination direct calorimeter.

Special Issues/Considerations/Pros and Cons

Subjects are confined during the measurement period. In general, direct calorimeters offer little to the majority of investigators beyond less expensive and complex indirect calorimeters. Thus, application of direct calorimetry is in the domain of highly specialized laboratories where direct heat loss measurements are of specific value.

Indirect Calorimetry

There are four principal approaches to the measurement of energy expenditure using indirect calorimetry.

Total Collection Systems

Here, expired air is collected in either an airtight rigid structure or a portable flexible bag.

Rigid Total Collection System

Description of Method/Instrument. The Tissot Gasometer is an example of a rigid total collection system (Jette & Inglis, 1975; J. Tissot, 1904). It comprises a 100- to 1,000-liter capacity inverted glass bell fitted with an internal circulation fan suspended over water. The bell is emptied of air. The subject then expires through a mouthpiece and nonreturn valve into the bell, which gradually fills with expired air and so progressively rises above the water seal. The height reached by the bell is recorded every minute, and the composition of expired air is measured from the bell periodically to determine oxygen consumption and/or carbon dioxide production. The response time of this instrument is < 5 minutes, and the period of measurement is 30 minutes (McLean & Tobin, 1987).

Reliability and Validity. These are good, providing there is technique precision and accurate gas analysis.

Normative Information. Not available; the data collected are specific to the individual.

Availability of Measure and Related Costs. Until recently, Tissot Gasometers were rarely used, but with the desire to optimize control over the data collected and reduced cost (compared to highly automated indirect calorimeters), popularity is increasing among scientists (Novitsky, Segal, Chatr-Aryamontri, Guvakov, & Katch, 1995).

Special Issues/Considerations/Pros and Cons. The apparatus is not easily portable and is relatively complex to construct and operate. Total collection systems allow maximal operator control over the data collected and their interpretation.

Flexible Total Collection System

Description of Method/Instrument. The Douglas bag (de Groot, Schreurs, & van Ingen Schenau, 1983; Douglas, 1911; Lum, Saville, & Venkataraman, 1998; Macfarlane, 2001; Yoshida, Nagata, Muro, Takeuchi, & Suda, 1981) is an example of a flexible total collection system. It comprises a polyvinyl chloride (or other leak-proof material) bag of typically a 100- to 150-liter capacity. The top of the bag is connected by tubing to a three-way valve that may be rotated to seal the bag, admit atmospheric air, or admit expired air via tubing attached to a respiratory valve. To use this approach, the three-way valve is first rotated to open the circuit to atmospheric air, the bag is rolled up to expel its contents, and the three-way valve is then rotated to seal the bag. The subject breathes through a mouthpiece, and the three-way valve is rotated to allow entry of expired air for 10 to 20 minutes. After the timed collection period, the three-way valve is turned to seal the bag. An alternative valve system employs two valves, one at the mouthpiece and the other proximal to the bag. Several bags can be used to prolong the total measurement period (Daniels, 1971). After collection of the expired air, the volume of expired air in the bag is measured (e.g., using a mass flow meter) and a sample analyzed to determine oxygen and/or carbon dioxide concentrations. The response time of this instrument is 15 to 20 minutes, and the period of measurement is 2 to 30 minutes depending on the intensity of the subject's activity (limited by the capacity of the collection bag; McLean & Tobin, 1987).

Reliability and Validity. Under optimal conditions, the error of energy expenditure measurements undertaken with Douglas bags may be very small (< 1%; McLean & Tobin, 1987). The major sources of error with Douglas bags are leaks from the bag (which can readily be assessed), diffusion of gas from the bag (almost eliminated if the gas is analyzed within 10–15 minutes of collection; McLean & Tobin, 1987), gas analytical errors, and poor operator technique.

Normative Information. Not available; the data collected are specific to the individual.

Availability of Measure and Related Costs. Until recently, Douglas bags were rarely used, but with the desire to optimize control over the data collected and reduced cost (compared to highly automated indirect calorimeters), popularity is increasing among scientists (Bassett et al., 2001; Bredbacka, Kawachi, Norlander, & Kirk, 1984; Brehm, Harlaar, & Groepenhof, 2004; Foss & Hallen, 2005; King, McLaughlin, Howley, Bassett, & Ainsworth, 1999; McLaughlin, King, Howley, Bassett, & Ainsworth, 2001; Nieman et al., 2006; Nieman et al., 2007; Nieman, Trone, & Austin, 2003; Raurich, Ibanez, & Marse, 1989; Rietjens, Kuipers, Kester, & Keizer, 2001; S. Tissot et al., 1995). Douglas bags, however, may not necessarily be inexpensive. There are the combined costs of purchasing and maintaining high-quality bags, the costs of high-precision sensors for volume and gas concentration measurements, and, because the technique is highly operator dependent, skilled technicians are needed to obtain high-quality data using this approach.

Special Issues/Considerations/Pros and Cons. Flexible total collection systems are portable, allowing for field measurements of energy expenditure. Total collection systems thus allow maximal operator control over the data collected and their interpretation.

Open-Circuit Indirect Calorimeter Systems

These devices are the most common energy expenditure measuring devices used in research and clinical practice. They can produce accurate and reproducible results and are reliable, providing their limitations are acknowledged, they are maintained well, and they are used by trained staff familiar with the specific device.

These systems usually comprise the combination of the following:

1. Mechanism to collect the sample from the subject (e.g., canopy, mask, mouthpiece)

2. Collection receptacle

3. Accurate and precise flow measurement (this is in fact the most difficult of the analysis elements)

4. Drier technique, for removing the moisture from the gas sample ($Mg(ClO_4)_2$ appears to be optimal)

5. Sample pump to take a known volume and frequency of gas sample

6. Gas sensors, oxygen (cell or paramagnetic) and carbon dioxide (infrared absorptiometry)

7. Computer to record and analyze the obtained data

8. Power supply, less commonly a battery

Data collected from open-circuit systems usually include VO_2, VCO_2, respiratory quotient (RQ), O_2 in, CO_2 in, and flow rate. These data are then often within internal software computed to calculate heat using the Weir equation (Weir, 1949).

Ventilated Open-Circuit Systems

Description of Method/Instrument. The method of collecting expired air in ventilated open-circuit systems varies considerably. The least complex approach is for expired air to be collected using a mouthpiece, mask, transparent hood, or canopy (Levine, Schleusner, & Jensen, 2000; Sorkin, Rapoport, Falk, & Goldring, 1980; Weissman, Damask, Askanazi, Rosenbaum, & Kinney, 1985; Wilmore, Davis, & Norton, 1976). A more complex approach is for the subject to be placed inside of a room/chamber of known volume in which there are often sophisticated sensing devices to quantify physical activity (Sun & Hill, 1993).

Regardless of how the expired air is collected, the basic components of ventilated open-circuit indirect calorimeters are similar. Expired air is drawn out of the collection device using a pump; it is critical to accurately measure this flow rate. The expired air is then mixed using a fan and/or mixing chamber, and a sample of the expired air is dried and analyzed for oxygen and/or carbon dioxide concentrations. Oxygen is generally analyzed using paramagnetic analyzers and carbon dioxide using infrared analyzers; alternatively, a mass spectrometer can be used to measure the gas concentrations. Burning known masses of chemical standards, such as butane or ethanol, within the system and ascertaining what proportion of the burned mass is detected by the calorimeter can verify the precision of these calorimeters (MacKay, Loiseau, Poivre, & Huot, 1991; Moon, Jensen, & Butte, 1993).

Depending on software, air mixing, and room volume, response times for a room/chamber system can vary from 1 to 30 minutes (Jequier & Schutz, 1983; Sun, Reed, & Hill, 1994); for a ventilated hood or canopy, 2 to 10 minutes (Sorkin et al., 1980); and for a mask/mouthpiece, < 30 seconds (Levine, Melanson, Westerterp, & Hill, 2001). Period of measurement is up to 36 hours for the room/chamber system (Dallosso & James, 1984; Jequier & Schutz, 1983) and 0.2 to 8 hours for the hood/canopy/mask-based systems, in our experience. Hood/canopy/mask-based systems are often configured as a "metabolic cart" whereby the equipment can be moved on a wheeled cart (Davis et al., 2006; Dobratz et al., 2007; Levine et al., 2000; Levine et al., 2005).

Reliability and Validity. Well-calibrated devices can achieve reproducible results (within 2%) and precision of > 98% using alcohol burns (Levine et al., 2005).

Normative Information. Not available; the data collected are specific to the individual.

Availability of Measure and Related Costs. These systems are moderately complex and expensive (U.S.$15,000–40,000) to construct and operate—each greater with a chamber system.

Special Issues/Considerations/Pros and Cons. It is important that inspired carbon dioxide should not exceed 1% (Weissman et al., 1985) as concentrations in excess of this may increase respiratory effort. It is vital here also to ensure the technician is aware of the CO_2 sensor's range; standard sensors often only detect to 0.9% or 1.0% CO_2 and thus could be falsely reassuring. A chamber system needs a dedicated site and is limited by the need to confine the subject. A nonchamber system is portable. These instruments are fully automated and simple for a technician with moderate skill to use, validate, and calibrate.

Expiratory Collection Open-Circuit Systems

Description of Method/Instrument. There are several expiratory collection open-circuit systems. The advantage of this approach is that the calorimeter can be designed as a portable device so that energy expenditure can be measured in free-living individuals. In general, these devices comprise a mouthpiece or a mask connected to a one-way valve whereby expired air enters the instrument. The flow rate of expired air through the valve is measured, and a small proportion of the expired air is diverted to a gas storage reservoir that is analyzed at the end of each measurement period. Technological advance (Maiolo, Melchiorri, Iacopino, Masala, & De Lorenzo, 2003; McLaughlin et al., 2001; Pinnington, Wong, Tay, Green, & Dawson, 2001; Rietjens et al., 2001) has resulted in the design of more precise, robust, and dependable portable calorimeters that are likely to provide useful field data in the future. Rapidity of response is < 2 minutes (Eisenmann, Brisko, Shadrick, & Welsh, 2003), and period of measurement is up to 6 hours.

Reliability and Validity. Overall average test-retest reliability and validity data are published (Duffield, Dawson, Pinnington, & Wong, 2004; McNaughton, Sherman, Roberts, & Bentley, 2005; Pinnington et al., 2001). Despite the major advantage of this technique—portability—the reliability and validity for this system are, in general, not as good as that available for a ventilated open-circuit system.

Normative Information. Not available; the data collected are specific to the individual.

Availability of Measure and Related Costs. These devices are widely available at a reasonable expense (U.S.$10,000–20,000).

Special Issues/Considerations/Pros and Cons. Reduced complexity of construction and operation permit wide free-living use. These devices have been designed with the goal of portability.

Confinement Systems

Description of Method/Instrument. The subject is placed inside a gas-tight sealed container of known volume, and oxygen consumption and carbon dioxide production are estimated from changes in the concentrations of these gases in the chamber air over time (Aulick, Arnhold, Hander, & Mason, 1983). The period of observation may be prolonged by periodically flushing the chamber with fresh air. A number of confinement systems have been constructed with response times of 15 to 20 minutes (Henning, Lofgren, & Sjostrom, 1996; Nguyen, de Jonge, Smith, & Bray, 2003). These systems can have periods of measurement from 1 to 36 hours (Henning et al., 1996; Nguyen et al., 2003; Toubro, Christensen, & Astrup, 1995; Vasilaras, Raben, & Astrup, 2001; Westerterp, Wilson, & Rolland, 1999), but up to 72 hours is possible (Schrauwen, van Marken Lichtenbelt, & Westerterp, 1997).

Reliability and Validity. A number of confinement systems have been constructed with errors of ~2% (Charbonnier et al., 1990; Nguyen et al., 2003) and good reliability.

Normative Information. Not available; the data collected are specific to the individual.

Availability of Measure and Related Costs. Confinement systems are rarely used currently. These systems are expensive and complex to construct and operate and thus are only available at dedicated centers.

Special Issues/Considerations/Pros and Cons. Confinement systems require a dedicated site and are unable to collect data on free-living individuals.

Closed-Circuit Systems

Description of Method/Instrument. Closed-circuit systems consist of a sealed respiratory gas circuit in which gaseous concentrations are measured over time (Benedict, 1909; Dechert et al., 1985; Dechert et al., 1988; Stock, 1979). Carbon dioxide and water vapor are absorbed and then oxygen reintroduced into the air stream, which reenters the chamber. Energy expenditure is calculated from the quantities of carbon dioxide absorbed and oxygen reintroduced. A smaller scale application of this approach is to use a spirometer. A spirometer consists of an oxygen-containing bell from which the subject inspires; expired carbon dioxide and water vapor are absorbed before the expired air is reintroduced to the bell. The bell is suspended over water so that its height descends at a rate proportional to oxygen consumption. Period of measurement is hours for the respiratory chamber and 10 to 20 minutes for the spirometer (McLean & Tobin, 1987).

Reliability and Validity. The respiratory chamber is very accurate (> 99%; McLean & Tobin, 1987). The spirometer, however, only has modest accuracy (~5%; Dechert et al., 1988).

Normative Information. Not available; the data collected are specific to the individual.

Availability of Measure and Related Costs. Closed-circuit systems are rarely used at present. Respiratory chambers are both expensive and complex to construct and operate. Spirometers, however, in comparison are inexpensive and simple to construct and operate.

Special Issues/Considerations/Pros and Cons. Respiratory chambers require a dedicated site and confine the subject. Spirometers are portable.

Noncalorimeter Methods for Measuring Energy Expenditure

Noncalorimeter methods estimate energy expenditure by extrapolation from variables that relate to energy expenditure. These methods are often standardized against calorimetric methods.

Isotope Dilution, "Doubly Labeled Water"

Description of Method/Instrument. In the doubly labeled water method, both the hydrogen and oxygen of water are labeled or "tagged" using stable, nonradioactive isotopes (D_2O^{18}; Black, Coward, 1998; Coward, Cole, & Prentice, 1996; Coward, Roberts, & Cole, 1988; Goran, Poehlman, Nair, & Danforth, 1993; Kurpad, Borgonha, & Shetty, 1997; Schoeller, 1987). Elimination of administered D_2O^{18} may be used to estimate carbon dioxide production and subsequently energy expenditure.

The principal of this technique is as follows. In body water, the O_2 of expired CO_2 is in equilibrium with the O_2:

$$CO_2 + H_2O \leftrightarrow H_2CO_3$$

Thus, if the O_2 in body water is tagged with the tracer O^{18}, the label will distribute not only in body water but also in circulating H_2CO_3 and in expired CO_2. Over time, the concentration of the O_2 label in body water will decrease as CO_2 is expired and body water is lost in urine, perspiration, and respiration. If the H_2 in body water is tagged with the tracer D_2, the label will distribute solely in the circulating H_2O and H_2CO_3. Over time, the concentration of the H_2 label will decrease as body water is lost (some of the hydrogen can become portioned into body protein or fat, however). Thus, if both the O_2 and H_2 in body water are tagged, with known amounts of tracers at the same time, the differences in the elimination rates of the O_2 and H_2 tracers will represent the elimination rate of CO_2.

Subjects are usually given doubly labeled water orally after baseline samples of urine, saliva, or blood have been collected. Time is allowed for complete mixing of isotopes to occur within the body water space, and then samples of urine, saliva, or blood are collected over 7 to 21 days. Some investigators recommend daily sample collection, whereas others collect samples before and after the collection period. Specimens are readily transportable; they are not radioactive, and stable isotopes do not decay over time. Thus, as long as the samples are well sealed, measurement of enrichments can be performed even in another country at any time after collection.

These samples are used for measurements of D_2 and O^{18} enrichments using mass spectroscopy. Changes in D_2 and O^{18} concentrations in body water are then calculated over time and CO_2 production and energy expenditure calculated.

Reliability and Validity. Energy expenditure can be measured using this technique with an error of ~6% to 8%. This error can be decreased to a small degree by collecting samples repeatedly over the measurement period rather than by collecting samples only before and after the measurement period. The doubly labeled water technique is considered the gold standard for measuring free-living energy expenditure (Seale, 1995; Seale & Rumpler, 1997; Seale, Rumpler, Conway, & Miles, 1990; Webb, 1991).

Normative Information. The recommended dose of D_2 and O^{18} to be given to the subject varies depending on the specific research laboratory's protocol. Most important, it is essential that the dose be accurately measured and recorded. The data collected during a study are specific to the individual.

Availability of Measure and Related Costs. With the reducing cost of O^{18} (~$10/g to ~ $3/g over the past 5 years), availability of this technique is improving. If a mass spectrometer is available, the average cost per study may range $400 to $600 per subject. A mass spectrometer is expensive and requires dedicated staff. Thus, doubly labeled water assessment of total daily energy expenditure is limited to researchers who have direct or indirect (through collaborations) access to a mass spectrometer and the required support team.

Special Issues/Considerations/Pros and Cons. This technique is not complex but is expensive. The subject is not confined—this technique's major advantage is that it can be used easily in the free-living state.

Physiological Measurements

Heart Rate Monitoring

Description of Method/Instrument. Heart rate monitors are portable, nonrestraining, and unobtrusive, and measurements can be carried out over several days. A number of devices of varying complexity have been used to record heart rate in free-living subjects (Beghin et al., 2000; Ceesay et al., 1989; Dauncey & James, 1979; Kalkwarf, Haas, Belko, Roach, & Roe, 1989; Kashiwazaki, 1999; Macfarlane, Lee, Ho, Chan, & Chan, 2006; Maffeis et al., 1995; Rafamantanantsoa et al., 2002; Rennie, Hennings, Mitchell, & Wareham, 2001). The conceptual limitation of this approach is that energy expenditure and heart rate are not linearly related for an individual in part because cardiac stroke volume changes with changing heart rate and even posture. Usable data are collected on commencement of the device, and measurement periods are generally 1 to 27 hours (Dauncey & James, 1979; Kashiwazaki, 1999), but up to 7 days (Macfarlane et al., 2006) is possible.

Reliability and Validity. At best, the mean (± 95% confidence limits) error for estimating energy expenditure using heart rate monitoring is 3% ± 11% during light activity and –3% ± 7% for moderate activity (Dauncey & James, 1979) in comparison to room calorimetry-measured energy expenditure. Group accuracies of 1% (Ceesay et al., 1989) to –3% (Kashiwazaki, 1999) have been reported with errors in estimating individual energy expenditure ranging from –39% to 56% (Kalkwarf et al., 1989). Accuracies of up to 6% ± 5% have been reported in children (Maffeis et al., 1995). Thus, the use of heart rate monitoring to predict energy expenditure is limited to group assessments (not individual).

Normative Information. Not available; the data collected are specific to the individual.

Availability of Measure and Related Costs. Heart rate monitoring is an inexpensive and non-complex technique in design and operation. Not currently in clinical use.

Special Issues/Considerations/Pros and Cons. There is substantial interindividual variance for relationships between heart rate and energy expenditure in terms of slope, intercept, and curve characteristics. Furthermore, variance in covariables that affect heart rate such as emotion also affects the heart rate–energy expenditure relationship. Hence, precision of heart rate prediction of energy expenditure is improved where a separate regression equation is derived to relate heart rate to energy expenditure for each individual. Some investigators use multiple regression equations for each subject. Heart rate monitoring is portable.

Pulmonary Ventilation Volume

Description of Method/Instrument. Measurement of pulmonary ventilation volume (direct measurement of the volume of gas exchanged over time) may provide an estimate of energy expenditure, but this technique is impractical for use other than for very short periods of time (Malhotra, Ramaswamy, Joseph, & Sen Gupta, 1972; Young, Fenton, & McLean, 1984).

Reliability and Validity. A PubMed literature review did not identify any data.

Normative Information. Not available; the data collected are specific to the individual.

Availability of Measure and Related Costs. Not currently in clinical use. Relatively expensive and complex to set up and operate. Not easily portable.

Special Issues/Considerations/Pros and Cons. Until there is further development and validation of the pulmonary ventilation volume technique to assess energy expenditure, its use will be limited to specialized research laboratories.

Integrated EMG

Description of Method/Instrument. Muscular activity is a component of energy expenditure and can be measured using integrated electromyography (EMG; Pinnington, Lloyd, Besier, & Dawson, 2005). Here, cumulative electrical muscle activity from several muscle fibers is measured and the data accumulated over the measurement period. However, strength-force relationships differ for different muscle groups and fibers, and multiple muscle groups need to be measured to gain a representative assessment of whole-body activity. These limitations make this technique impractical (deVries, Burke, Hopper, & Sloan, 1976; Selliger, Dolejs, & Karas, 1980).

Reliability and Validity. A PubMed literature review did not identify any data.

Normative Information. Not available; the data collected are specific to the individual.

Availability of Measure and Related Costs. Not available for routine use. Complex and expensive to construct and operate.

Special Issues/Considerations/Pros and Cons. Until there is further development and validation of the integrated EMG technique to assess energy expenditure, its use will be limited to specialized research laboratories.

Thermal Imaging

Description of Method/Instrument. Limited precision and accuracy and the complexity of data processing complicated the early studies that employed thermal imaging to detect human heat loss to the environment. More recent studies have employed automated, high-resolution, rapid-response thermal imaging (Levine, Pavlidis, & Cooper, 2001) and offer promise for future studies, particularly in the area of thermoregulation (Shuran & Nelson, 1991).

Reliability and Validity. A PubMed literature review did not identify any data.

Normative Information. Not available; the data collected are specific to the individual.

Availability of Measure and Related Costs. Not available to routine use. Very expensive.

Special Issues/Considerations/Pros and Cons. Complex construction and operation. Until there is further development and validation of the thermal imaging technique to assess energy expenditure, its use will be limited to specialized research laboratories.

Physiological Observations

Activity Recall and Time and Motion Studies

Description of Method/Instrument. Nonspecific information about daily energy expenditure can be obtained using questionnaires, interviews, or time-and-motion studies. These approaches can be used for following trends in certain activities, particularly with relation to occupational practices (Pelto, Pelto, & Messer, 1989).

Reliability and Validity. Predictably, substantial errors are introduced through inaccurate recall, inadequate data recording, and the use of standardized energy expenditure of activity tables (Bonnefoy et al., 2001; Conway, Seale, Jacobs, Irwin, & Ainsworth, 2002; Lof & Forsum, 2004; Mahabir et al., 2006; Washburn, Jacobsen, Sonko, Hill, & Donnelly, 2003).

Normative Information. Not available; the data collected are specific to the individual.

Availability of Measure and Related Costs. Readily available at minimal cost.

Special Issues/Considerations/Pros and Cons. There are many questionnaires available; the user must carefully review the literature on the specific questionnaire for the population of interest to be able to select the questionnaire most reliable and valid. In general, activity and time-and-motion studies at best provide a general idea of daily energy expenditure in a population (not for an individual).

Activity Logs and the Factoral Method

Description of Method/Instrument. This is a frequently used approach for estimating activity thermogenesis in free-living individuals. First, a subject's physical activities are logged over the time period of interest (e.g., 1 week; Ainsworth, Bassett, et al., 2000). The energy equivalent of each of these activities is measured or estimated using a calorimeter or tables, respectively. The time spent in each activity is then multiplied by the energy equivalent for that activity. These values are then summed to derive an estimate of activity thermogenesis. This determination of activity thermogenesis is often combined with information on basal metabolic rate (measured or calculated) to estimate total daily energy expenditure (Blair & Buskirk, 1987; Borel, Riley, & Snook, 1984; Brun, Webb, de Benoist, & Blackwell, 1985; Geissler, Dzumbira, & Noor, 1986; Leonard, Katzmarzyk, Stephen, & Ross, 1995; Spurr, Dufour, & Reina, 1996; Warwick & Baines, 1996; Warwick, Edmundson, & Thomson, 1988).

Reliability and Validity. Group validation of 1% to 2% for group results and −17% to +25% for individuals has been reported (Geissler et al., 1986; Warwick et al., 1988).

There are two potential sources of error for the factoral approach for measuring activity thermogenesis. First, errors may result from inaccurate recording of activities and, second, from inaccurate determinations of the energy costs of the activities. To log activity, subjects are often asked to record in a diary the nature and amount of time spent performing each of their activities throughout the day (Ferro-Luzzi, Scaccini, Taffese, Aberra, & Demeke, 1990; Warwick & Baines, 1996). This has several limitations; subjects may be illiterate or enumerate, may report their activities inaccurately or incompletely, and/or may alter their normal activity patterns during periods of assessment. To limit these sources of error, one approach is to have trained enumerators follow subjects and objectively record their activities (Pelto et al., 1989). This approach is time-consuming and expensive but potentially a valuable source of accurate and objective data. Newer image-gathering technologies may be useful in the future for this purpose (Terrier, Ladetto, Merminod, & Schutz, 2001). To determine the energy costs of physical activities, researchers often use standard tables (Ainsworth, Haskell, et al., 2000). However, these may introduce substantial (albeit systematic) errors. First, the tables may not include the precise activity the subject performed. Second, the energy cost for a given activity is highly variable between subjects, even independent of gender. Third, calorimeter methods for measuring the energy costs of activities have not been standardized between investigators so that precision and accuracy of data in the activity tables cannot always be ensured. To limit these errors, researchers can measure the energy costs of each or most of the activities that the subjects of interest perform using calorimeters, as described above. At best, the energy costs for each subject's activities would be measured, but clearly, this is rarely practical except for small studies. In general, population-, gender-, and age-specific group means for the majority of the studied subjects' activities represent a standard that is worth achieving where optimum precision is warranted.

Normative Information. Not available; the data collected are specific to the individual.

Availability of Measure and Related Costs. This is limited to specialized research laboratories due mainly to the time and financial commitment required to carry out these studies.

Special Issues/Considerations/Pros and Cons. Has the potential to allow individual energy expenditure assessment with variable accuracy.

Kinematic Measurements

Description of Method/Instrument. In kinematic measurements, a subject's movements are quantified, and these measurements are usually performed in conjunction with other measures of energy expenditure. These tools are used primarily to estimate the energy cost of non-exercise activity thermogenesis (spontaneous physical activity).

Some techniques are specific for confined spaces such as radar tracking and cine photography (Schutz, Ravussin, Diethelm, & Jequier, 1982). Other techniques have been used in free-living individuals and generally focus on pedometers and accelerometers of varying sophistication. Pedometers typically detect the displacement of a subject with each stride. Accelerometers detect body displacement electronically with varying degrees of sensitivity—uniaxial accelerometers in one axis and triaxial accelerometers in three axes. Portable uniaxial accelerometer units have been widely used to detect physical activity (Bassett et al., 2000; Crouter, Schneider, Karabulut, & Bassett, 2003; Melanson & Freedson, 1995; Pambianco, Wing, & Robertson, 1990). The utility of motion tracking using approaches such as Global Positioning Systems has not been fully defined for human studies (Terrier et al., 2001).

Reliability and Validity. Pedometers tend to lack sensitivity because they do not quantify stride length or total body displacement and overall, therefore, become poor predictors of activity thermogenesis (Crouter et al., 2003; Foster et al., 2005). Careful evaluation demonstrates that these instruments in general are not sufficiently sensitive to quantify the physical activity of a given free-living subject, but rather they are more valuable for comparing activity levels between groups of subjects. Greater precision ($r = 0.86$–0.96 for accelerometer output vs. energy expenditure from indirect calorimetry [Bouten, Westerterp, Verduin, & Janssen, 1994]; 90% ± 5% of energy expenditure of activity [Chen et al., 2003]) and reliability (coefficient of variation [CV] < 2%; Levine, Baukol, & Westerterp, 2001) have been obtained using triaxial accelerometers. In free-living subjects, data from these devices correlate well with total daily energy expenditure, measured using doubly labeled water, divided by basal metabolic rate (Bouten, Verboeket–van de Venne, Westerterp, Verduin, & Janssen, 1996).

Normative Information. Not available; the data collected are specific to the individual.

Availability of Measure and Related Costs. Widely available at variable cost depending on the sophistication of the device used.

Special Issues/Considerations/Pros and Cons. In general, the greater the device complexity, the more likely the group data obtained are valid.

Suggestions for Future Research/Comments

There are a number of areas for future research with respect to energy expenditure measurements.

- *Integration of data on energy expenditure.* With standardization of technical standards and techniques, it would be advantageous to develop international databases on basal metabolic rate, resting energy expenditure, energy expenditure of specific activities, and total daily energy expenditure measured using doubly labeled water. This would facilitate validation of energy requirement recommendations and allow cross-cultural investigation into metabolic rate variance.

- *Doubly labeled water collaborative agreements.* It is recommended to establish a collaborative environment for analyses of doubly labeled water determinations. It is proposed to identify laboratories where isotope enrichments can be analyzed so that studies can be performed by other investigators lacking the necessary instruments.

- *Noncalorimeter methods.* The role of newer technologies such as thermal imaging or global positioning remains to be determined but should be explored.

- *Anaerobic energy expenditure assessment.* Most currently available, commonly used energy expenditure assessment techniques (particularly indirect calorimetry) do not directly assess anaerobic metabolism (Scott, 2005). The contribution of anaerobic metabolism to total daily energy expenditure warrants further investigation.

Summary

Measurement of energy expenditure in humans is required to assess metabolic needs and fuel utilization, as well as to assess the relative thermic effect of different food, drink, drug, and emotional components. Indirect and direct calorimeter and noncalorimeter methods for measuring energy expenditure have been reviewed, and their relative value for measurement in the laboratory and field settings has been assessed. Where high accuracy is required and sufficient resources are available, an open-circuit indirect calorimeter can be used. Open-circuit indirect calorimeters can employ a mask, hood, canopy, or room/chamber for collection of expired air. For short-term measurements, mask, hood, or canopy systems suffice. A detailed section on open-circuit indirect calorimetry systems has been included as this is the most common calorimeter method used in both the clinical and research setting. Chamber-based systems may be more accurate for the longer term measurement of specified activity patterns, but behavior constraints mean they do not reflect real life. Where resources are limited and/or optimum precision can be sacrificed, flexible total collection systems and noncalorimetric methods are potentially useful if the limitations of these methods are appreciated. The use of the stable isotope technique, doubly labeled water, enables total daily energy expenditure to be measured accurately in free-living subjects. The factoral method for combining activity logs and data on the energy costs of activities also can provide detailed information on free-living subjects.

References

Ainslie, P., Reilly, T., & Westerterp, K. (2003). Estimating human energy expenditure: A review of techniques with particular reference to doubly labelled water. *Sports Medicine, 33*, 683–698.

Ainsworth, B. E., Bassett, D. R., Jr., Strath, S. J., Swartz, A. M., O'Brien, W. L., Thompson, R. W., et al. (2000). Comparison of three methods for measuring the time spent in physical activity. *Medicine & Science in Sports & Exercise, 32*(Suppl.), S457–S464.

Ainsworth, B. E., Haskell, W. L., Whitt, M. C., Irwin, M. L., Swartz, A. M., Strath, S. J., et al. (2000).

Compendium of physical activities: an update of activity codes and MET intensities. *Medicine & Science in Sports & Exercise, 32*(Suppl.), S498–S504.

Aulick, L. H., Arnhold, H., Hander, E. H., & Mason, A. D., Jr. (1983). A new open and closed respiration chamber. *Quarterly Journal of Experimental Physiology, 68,* 351–357.

Bassett, D. R., Jr., Ainsworth, B. E., Swartz, A. M., Strath, S. J., O'Brien, W. L., & King, G. A. (2000). Validity of four motion sensors in measuring moderate intensity physical activity. *Medicine & Science in Sports & Exercise, 32*(Suppl.), S471–S480.

Bassett, D. R., Jr., Howley, E. T., Thompson, D. L., King, G. A., Strath, S. J., McLaughlin, J. E., et al. (2001). Validity of inspiratory and expiratory methods of measuring gas exchange with a computerized system. *Journal of Applied Physiology, 91,* 218–224.

Beghin, L., Budniok, T., Vaksman, G., Boussard-Delbecque, L., Michaud, L., Turck, D., et al. (2000). Simplification of the method of assessing daily and nightly energy expenditure in children, using heart rate monitoring calibrated against open circuit indirect calorimetry. *Clinical Nutrition, 19,* 425–435.

Benedict, F. G. (1909). An apparatus for studying the respiratory exchange. *American Journal of Physiology, 24,* 345–374.

Black, A. E., Coward, W. A., Cole, T. J., & Prentice, A. M. (1996). Human energy expenditure in affluent societies: An analysis of 574 doubly-labelled water measurements. *European Journal of Clinical Nutrition, 50,* 72–92.

Blair, D., & Buskirk, E. R. (1987). Habitual daily energy expenditure and activity levels of lean and adult-onset and child-onset obese women. *American Journal of Clinical Nutrition, 45,* 540–550.

Bonnefoy, M., Normand, S., Pachiaudi, C., Lacour, J. R., Laville, M., & Kostka, T. (2001). Simultaneous validation of ten physical activity questionnaires in older men: A doubly labeled water study. *Journal of the American Geriatric Society, 49,* 28–35.

Borel, M. J., Riley, R. E., & Snook, J. T. (1984). Estimation of energy expenditure and maintenance energy requirements of college-age men and women. *American Journal of Clinical Nutrition, 40,* 1264–1272.

Bouten, C. V., Verboeket–van de Venne, W. P., Westerterp, K. R., Verduin, M., & Janssen, J. D. (1996). Daily physical activity assessment: comparison between movement registration and doubly labeled water. *Journal of Applied Physiology, 81,* 1019–1026.

Bouten, C. V., Westerterp, K. R., Verduin, M., & Janssen, J. D. (1994). Assessment of energy expenditure for physical activity using a triaxial accelerometer. *Medicine & Science in Sports & Exercise, 26,* 1516–1523.

Bredbacka, S., Kawachi, S., Norlander, O., & Kirk, B. (1984). Gas exchange during ventilator treatment: A validation of a computerized technique and its comparison with the Douglas bag method. *Acta Anaesthesiologica Scandinavica, 28,* 462–468.

Brehm, M. A., Harlaar, J., & Groepenhof, H. (2004). Validation of the portable VmaxST system for oxygen-uptake measurement. *Gait and Posture, 20,* 67–73.

Brun, T., Webb, P., de Benoist, B., & Blackwell, F. (1985). Calorimetric evaluation of the diary-respirometer technique for the field measurement of the 24-hour energy expenditure. *Human Nutrition—Clinical Nutrition, 39,* 321–334.

Ceesay, S. M., Prentice, A. M., Day, K. C., Murgatroyd, P. R., Goldberg, G. R., Scott, W., et al. (1989). The use of heart rate monitoring in the estimation of energy expenditure: A validation study using indirect whole-body calorimetry. *British Journal of Nutrition, 61,* 175–186.

Charbonnier, A., Jones, C. D., Schutz, Y., Murgatroyd, P. R., Whitehead, R. G., Jequier, E., et al. (1990). A whole body transportable indirect calorimeter for human use in the tropics. *European Journal of Clinical Nutrition, 44,* 725–731.

Chen, K. Y., Acra, S. A., Majchrzak, K., Donahue, C. L., Baker, L., Clemens, L., et al. (2003). Predicting energy expenditure of physical activity using hip- and wrist-worn accelerometers. *Diabetes Technology & Therapeutics, 5,* 1023–1033.

Consolazio, C. F. (1971). Energy expenditure studies in military populations using Kofranyi-Michaelis respirometers. *American Journal of Clinical Nutrition, 24,* 1431–1437.

Conway, J. M., Seale, J. L., Jacobs, D. R., Jr., Irwin, M. L., & Ainsworth, B. E. (2002). Comparison of energy expenditure estimates from doubly labeled water, a physical activity questionnaire, and physical activity records. *American Journal of Clinical Nutrition, 75,* 519–525.

Coward, W. A. (1998). Contributions of the doubly labeled water method to studies of energy balance in the Third World. *American Journal of Clinical Nutrition, 68,* 962S–969S.

Coward, W. A., Roberts, S. B., & Cole, T. J. (1988). Theoretical and practical considerations in the doubly-labelled water (2H2(18)O) method for the measurement of carbon dioxide production rate in man. *European Journal of Clinical Nutrition, 42,* 207–212.

Crouter, S. E., Schneider, P. L., Karabulut, M., & Bassett, D. R., Jr. (2003). Validity of 10 electronic pedometers for measuring steps, distance, and energy cost. *Medicine & Science in Sports & Exercise, 35,* 1455–1460.

Cunningham, J. J. (1990). Calculation of energy expenditure from indirect calorimetry: Assessment of the Weir equation. *Nutrition, 6,* 222–223.

Dallosso, H. M., & James, W. P. (1984). Whole-body calorimetry studies in adult men: 2. The interaction of exercise and over-feeding on the thermic effect of a meal. *British Journal of Nutrition, 52,* 65–72.

Danforth, E., Jr. (1985). Diet and obesity. *American Journal of Clinical Nutrition, 41*(Suppl.), 1132–1145.

Daniels, J. (1971). Portable respiratory gas collection equipment. *Journal of Applied Physiology, 31,* 164–167.

Dauncey, M. J., & James, W. P. (1979). Assessment of the heart-rate method for determining energy expenditure in man, using a whole-body calorimeter. *British Journal of Nutrition, 42,* 1–13.

Dauncey, M. J., Murgatroyd, P. R., & Cole, T. J. (1978). A human calorimeter for the direct and indirect measurement of 24 h energy expenditure. *British Journal of Nutrition, 39,* 557–566.

Davis, K. A., Kinn, T., Esposito, T. J., Reed, R. L., II, Santaniello, J. M., & Luchette, F. A. (2006). Nutritional gain versus financial gain: The role of metabolic carts in the surgical ICU. *Journal of Trauma, 61,* 1436–1440.

de Groot, G., Schreurs, A. W., & van Ingen Schenau, G. J. (1983). A portable lightweight Douglas bag instrument for use during various types of exercise. *International Journal of Sports Medicine, 4,* 132–134.

Dechert, R., Wesley, J., Schafer, L., LaMond, S., Beck, T., Coran, A., et al. (1985). Comparison of oxygen consumption, carbon dioxide production, and resting energy expenditure in premature and full-term infants. *Journal of Pediatric Surgery, 20,* 792–798.

Dechert, R., Wesley, J., Schafer, L., LaMond, S., Nicks, J., Coran, A. G., et al. (1988). A water-sealed indirect calorimeter for measurement of oxygen consumption (VO_2), carbon dioxide production (VCO_2), and energy expenditure in infants. *Journal of Parenteral and Enteral Nutrition, 12,* 256–259.

Deriaz, O., Fournier, G., Tremblay, A., Despres, J. P., & Bouchard, C. (1992). Lean-body-mass composition and resting energy expenditure before and after long-term overfeeding. *American Journal of Clinical Nutrition, 56,* 840–847.

deVries, H. A., Burke, R. K., Hopper, R. T., & Sloan, J. H. (1976). Relationship of resting EMG level to total body metabolism with reference to the origin of "tissue noise." *American Journal of Physical Medicine, 55,* 139–147.

Dobratz, J. R., Sibley, S. D., Beckman, T. R., Valentine, B. J., Kellogg, T. A., Ikramuddin, S., et al. (2007). Predicting energy expenditure in extremely obese women. *Journal of Parenteral and Enteral Nutrition, 31,* 217–227.

Dobrosielski, D. A., Brubaker, P. H., Berry, M. J., Ayabe, M., & Miller, H. S. (2002). The metabolic demand of golf in patients with heart disease and in healthy adults. *Journal of Cardiopulmonary Rehabilitation, 22,* 96–104.

Douglas, C. G. (1911). A method for determining the total respiratory exchange in man. *Journal of Physiology, 42,* 17–18.

Duffield, R., Dawson, B., Pinnington, H. C., & Wong, P. (2004). Accuracy and reliability of a Cosmed K4b2 portable gas analysis system. *Journal of Science and Medicine in Sport, 7,* 11–22.

Eisenmann, J. C., Brisko, N., Shadrick, D., & Welsh, S. (2003). Comparative analysis of the Cosmed Quark b2 and K4b2 gas analysis systems during submaximal exercise. *Journal of Sports Medicine and Physical Fitness, 43,* 150–155.

Faber, P., Lammert, O., Johansen, O., & Garby, L. (1998). A fast responding combined direct and indirect calorimeter for human subjects. *Medical Engineering & Physics, 20,* 291–301.

FAO/WHO Ad Hoc Committee of Experts. (1973). *Energy and protein requirements: FAO and WHO.* Rome Author.

Ferro-Luzzi, A., Scaccini, C., Taffese, S., Aberra, B., & Demeke, T. (1990). Seasonal energy deficiency in Ethiopian rural women. *European Journal of Clinical Nutrition, 44*(Suppl. 1), 7–18.

Ford, L. E. (1984). Some consequences of body size. *American Journal of Physiology, 247*(Pt. 2), H495–H507.

Foss, O., & Hallen, J. (2005). Validity and stability of a computerized metabolic system with mixing chamber. *International Journal of Sports Medicine, 26,* 569–575.

Foster, R. C., Lanningham-Foster, L. M., Manohar, C., McCrady, S. K., Nysse, L. J., Kaufman, K. R., et al. (2005). Precision and accuracy of an ankle-worn accelerometer-based pedometer in step counting and energy expenditure. *Preventive Medicine, 41,* 778–783.

Geissler, C. A., Dzumbira, T. M., & Noor, M. I. (1986). Validation of a field technique for the measurement of energy expenditure: Factorial method versus continuous respirometry. *American Journal of Clinical Nutrition, 44,* 596–602.

Goran, M. I., Poehlman, E. T., Nair, K. S., & Danforth, E. (1993). Deuterium exchange in humans: effect of gender, body composition and age. *Basic Life Science, 60,* 79–81.

Henning, B., Lofgren, R., & Sjostrom, L. (1996). Chamber for indirect calorimetry with improved transient response. *Medical & Biological Engineering & Computing, 34,* 207–212.

Horton, E. S. (1983). Introduction: an overview of the assessment and regulation of energy balance in humans. *American Journal of Clinical Nutrition, 38,* 972–977.

Jacobsen, S., Johansen, O., & Garby, L. (1985). A 24-m3 direct heat-sink calorimeter with on-line data acquisition, processing, and control. *American Journal of Physiology, 249*(Pt. 1), E416–E432.

Jakicic, J. M., Wing, R. R., Butler, B. A., & Robertson, R. J. (1995). Prescribing exercise in multiple short bouts versus one continuous bout: Effects on adherence, cardiorespiratory fitness, and weight loss in overweight women. *International Journal of Obesity and Related Metabolic Disorders, 19,* 893–901.

Jequier, E., & Schutz, Y. (1983). Long-term measurements of energy expenditure in humans using a respiration chamber. *American Journal of Clinical Nutrition, 38,* 989–998.

Jette, M., & Inglis, H. (1975). Energy cost of square dancing. *Journal of Applied Physiology, 38,* 44–45.

Kalkwarf, H. J., Haas, J. D., Belko, A. Z., Roach, R. C., & Roe, D. A. (1989). Accuracy of heart-rate monitoring and activity diaries for estimating energy expenditure. *American Journal of Clinical Nutrition, 49,* 37–43.

Kashiwazaki, H. (1999). Heart rate monitoring as a field method for estimating energy expenditure as evaluated by the doubly labeled water method. *Journal of Nutritional Science and Vitaminology (Tokyo), 45,* 79–94.

King, G. A., McLaughlin, J. E., Howley, E. T., Bassett, D. R., Jr., & Ainsworth, B. E. (1999). Validation of Aerosport KB1-C portable metabolic system. *International Journal of Sports Medicine, 20,* 304–308.

Kurpad, A. V., Borgonha, S., & Shetty, P. S. (1997). Measurement of total energy expenditure by the doubly labelled water technique in free living Indians in Bangalore city. *Indian Journal of Medical Research, 105,* 212–219.

Leonard, W. R., Katzmarzyk, P. T., Stephen, M. A., & Ross, A. G. (1995). Comparison of the heart rate-monitoring and factorial methods: Assessment of energy expenditure in highland and coastal Ecuadoreans. *American Journal of Clinical Nutrition, 61,* 1146–1152.

Levine, J. A. (2005). Measurement of energy expenditure. *Public Health Nutrition, 8,* 1123–1132.

Levine, J. A., Baukol, P. A., & Westerterp, K. R. (2001). Validation of the Tracmor triaxial accelerometer system for walking. *Medicine & Science in Sports & Exercise, 33,* 1593–1597.

Levine, J. A., Lanningham-Foster, L. M., McCrady, S. K., Krizan, A. C., Olson, L. R., Kane, P. H., et al. (2005). Interindividual variation in posture allocation: possible role in human obesity. *Science, 307,* 584–586.

Levine, J. A., Melanson, E. L., Westerterp, K. R., & Hill, J. O. (2001). Measurement of the components of nonexercise activity thermogenesis. *American Journal of Physiology and Endocrinology Metabolism, 281,* E670–E675.

Levine, J. A., Pavlidis, I., & Cooper, M. (2001). The face of fear. *Lancet, 357,* 1757.

Levine, J. A., Schleusner, S. J., & Jensen, M. D. (2000). Energy expenditure of nonexercise activity. *American Journal of Clinical Nutrition, 72,* 1451–1454.

Lof, M., & Forsum, E. (2004). Validation of energy intake by dietary recall against different methods to assess energy expenditure. *Journal of Human Nutrition and Dietetics, 17,* 471–480.

Lum, L., Saville, A., & Venkataraman, S. T. (1998). Accuracy of physiologic deadspace measurement in intubated pediatric patients using a metabolic monitor: Comparison with the Douglas bag method. *Critical Care Medicine, 26,* 760–764.

Macfarlane, D. J. (2001). Automated metabolic gas analysis systems: a review. *Sports Medicine, 31,* 841–861.

Macfarlane, D. J., Lee, C. C., Ho, E. Y., Chan, K. L., & Chan, D. (2006). Convergent validity of six methods to assess physical activity in daily life. *Journal of Applied Physiology, 101,* 1328–1334.

MacKay, S. J., Loiseau, A., Poivre, R., & Huot, A. (1991). Calibration method for small animal indirect calorimeters. *American Journal of Physiology, 261*(Pt. 1), E661–E664.

Maffeis, C., Pinelli, L., Zaffanello, M., Schena, F., Iacumin, P., & Schutz, Y. (1995). Daily energy expenditure in free-living conditions in obese and non-obese children: Comparison of doubly labelled water (2H2(18)O) method and heart-rate monitoring. *International Journal of Obesity and Related Metabolic Disorders, 19,* 671–677.

Mahabir, S., Baer, D. J., Giffen, C., Clevidence, B. A., Campbell, W. S., Taylor, P. R., et al. (2006). Comparison of energy expenditure estimates from 4 physical activity questionnaires with doubly labeled water estimates in postmenopausal women. *American Journal of Clinical Nutrition, 84,* 230–236.

Maiolo, C., Melchiorri, G., Iacopino, L., Masala, S., & De Lorenzo, A. (2003). Physical activity energy expenditure measured using a portable telemetric device in comparison with a mass spectrometer. *British Journal of Sports Medicine, 37,* 445–447.

Malhotra, M. S., Ramaswamy, S. S., Joseph, N. T., & Sen Gupta, J. (1972). Functional capacity and body composition of different classes of Indian athletes. *Indian Journal of Physiology and Pharmacology, 16,* 301–308.

McLaughlin, J. E., King, G. A., Howley, E. T., Bassett, D. R., Jr., & Ainsworth, B. E. (2001). Validation of the COSMED K4 b2 portable metabolic system. *International Journal of Sports Medicine, 22,* 280–284.

McLean, J. A., & Tobin, G. (1987) *Animal and human calorimetry.* Cambridge, UK: Cambridge University Press.

McNaughton, L. R., Sherman, R., Roberts, S., & Bentley, D. J. (2005). Portable gas analyser Cosmed K4b2 compared to a laboratory based mass spectrometer system. *Journal of Sports Medicine and Physical Fitness, 45,* 315–323.

Melanson, E. L., Jr., & Freedson, P. S. (1995). Validity of the Computer Science and Applications, Inc. (CSA) activity monitor. *Medicine & Science in Sports & Exercise, 27,* 934–940.

Mendelsohn, M. E., Connelly, D. M., Overend, T. J., & Petrella, R. J. (2007). Reliability and validity of responses to submaximal all-extremity semirecumbent exercise in older adults. *Journal of Aging and Physical Activity, 15,* 184–194.

Moon, J. K., Jensen, C. L., & Butte, N. F. (1993). Fast-response whole body indirect calorimeters for infants. *Journal of Applied Physiology, 74,* 476–484.

Myers, J., Walsh, D., Sullivan, M., & Froelicher, V. (1990). Effect of sampling on variability and plateau in oxygen uptake. *Journal of Applied Physiology, 68,* 404–410.

Nguyen, T., de Jonge, L., Smith, S. R., & Bray, G. A. (2003). Chamber for indirect calorimetry with accurate measurement and time discrimination of metabolic plateaus of over 20 min. *Medical & Biological Engineering & Computing, 41,* 572–578.

Nieman, D. C., Austin, M. D., Benezra, L., Pearce, S., McInnis, T., Unick, J., et al. (2006). Validation of Cosmed's FitMate in measuring oxygen consumption and estimating resting metabolic rate. *Research in Sports Medicine, 14,* 89–96.

Nieman, D. C., Lasasso, H., Austin, M. D., Pearce, S., McInnis, T., & Unick, J. (2007). Validation of Cosmed's FitMate in measuring exercise metabolism. *Research in Sports Medicine, 15,* 67–75.

Nieman, D. C., Trone, G. A., & Austin, M. D. (2003). A new handheld device for measuring resting metabolic rate and oxygen consumption. *Journal of the American Dietetic Association, 103,* 588–592.

Novitsky, S., Segal, K. R., Chatr-Aryamontri, B., Guvakov, D., & Katch, V. L. (1995). Validity of a new portable indirect calorimeter: The AeroSport TEEM 100. *European Journal of Applied Physiology and Occupational Physiology, 70,* 462–467.

Pambianco, G., Wing, R. R., & Robertson, R. (1990). Accuracy and reliability of the Caltrac accelerometer for estimating energy expenditure. *Medicine & Science in Sports & Exercise, 22,* 858–862.

Pelto, G. H., Pelto, P. J., & Messer, E. (Eds.). (1989). *Research methods in nutritional anthropology.* New York: United Nations Publications.

Phillips, W. T., & Ziuraitis, J. R. (2004). Energy cost of single-set resistance training in older adults. *Journal of Strength and Conditioning Research, 18,* 606–609.

Piccinini, L., Cimolin, V., Galli, M., Berti, M., Crivellini, M., & Turconi, A. C. (2007). Quantification of energy expenditure during gait in children affected by cerebral palsy. *Eura Medicophys, 43,* 7–12.

Piers, L. S., Soares, M. J., Makan, T., & Shetty, P. S. (1992). Thermic effect of a meal: 1. Methodology and variation in normal young adults. *British Journal of Nutrition, 67,* 165–175.

Pinnington, H. C., Lloyd, D. G., Besier, T. F., & Dawson, B. (2005). Kinematic and electromyography analysis of submaximal differences running on a firm surface compared with soft, dry sand. *European Journal of Applied Physiology, 94,* 242–253.

Pinnington, H. C., Wong, P., Tay, J., Green, D., & Dawson, B. (2001). The level of accuracy and agreement in measures of FE02, FEC02 and VE between the Cosmed K4b2 portable, respiratory gas analysis system and a metabolic cart. *Journal of Science and Medicine in Sport, 4,* 324–335.

Rafamantanantsoa, H. H., Ebine, N., Yoshioka, M., Higuchi, H., Yoshitake, Y., Tanaka, H., et al. (2002). Validation of three alternative methods to measure total energy expenditure against the doubly labeled water method for older Japanese men. *Journal of Nutritional Science and Vitaminology (Tokyo), 48,* 517–523.

Raurich, J. M., Ibanez, J., & Marse, P. (1989). Validation of a new closed circuit indirect calorimetry method compared with the open Douglas bag method. *Intensive Care Medicine, 15,* 274–278.

Ravussin, E., & Bogardus, C. (1992). A brief overview of human energy metabolism and its relationship to essential obesity. *American Journal of Clinical Nutrition, 55*(Suppl.), 242S–245S.

Reed, G. W., & Hill, J. O. (1996). Measuring the thermic effect of food. *American Journal of Clinical Nutrition, 63,* 164–169.

Rennie, K. L., Hennings, S. J., Mitchell, J., & Wareham, N. J. (2001). Estimating energy expenditure by heart-rate monitoring without individual calibration. *Medicine & Science in Sports & Exercise, 33,* 939–945.

Rietjens, G. J., Kuipers, H., Kester, A. D., & Keizer, H. A. (2001). Validation of a computerized metabolic measurement system (Oxycon-Pro) during low and high intensity exercise. *International Journal of Sports Medicine, 22,* 291–294.

Schmitz, K. H., Treuth, M., Hannan, P., McMurray, R., Ring, K. B., Catellier, D., et al. (2005). Predicting energy expenditure from accelerometry counts in adolescent girls. *Medicine & Science in Sports & Exercise, 37,* 155–161.

Schoeller, D. A., & Taylor, P. B. (1987). Precision of the doubly labelled water method using the two-point calculation. *Human Nutrition—Clinical Nutrition, 41,* 215–223.

Schrauwen, P., van Marken Lichtenbelt, W. D., & Westerterp, K. R. (1997). Energy balance in a respiration chamber: Individual adjustment of energy intake to energy expenditure. *International Journal of Obesity and Related Metabolic Disorders, 21,* 769–774.

Schutz, Y., Ravussin, E., Diethelm, R., & Jequier, E. (1982). Spontaneous physical activity measured by radar in obese and control subject studied in a respiration chamber. *International Journal of Obesity, 6,* 23–28.

Scott, C. B. (2005). Contribution of anaerobic energy expenditure to whole body thermogenesis. *Nutrition & Metabolism (London), 2,* 14.

Seale, J. L. (1995). Energy expenditure measurements in relation to energy requirements. *American Journal of Clinical Nutrition, 62*(Suppl.), 1042S–1046S.

Seale, J. L., & Rumpler, W. V. (1997). Comparison of energy expenditure measurements by diet records, energy intake balance, doubly labeled water and room calorimetry. *European Journal of Clinical Nutrition, 51,* 856–863.

Seale, J. L., Rumpler, W. V., Conway, J. M., & Miles, C. W. (1990). Comparison of doubly labeled water, intake-balance, and direct- and indirect-calorimetry methods for measuring energy expenditure in adult men. *American Journal of Clinical Nutrition, 52,* 66–71.

Seliger, V., Dolejs, L., & Karas, V. (1980). A dynamometric comparison of maximum eccentric, concentric, and isometric contractions using EMG and energy expenditure measurements. *European Journal of Applied Physiology and Occupational Physiology, 45,* 235–244.

Shuran, M., & Nelson, R. A. (1991). Quantitation of energy expenditure by infrared thermography. *American Journal of Clinical Nutrition, 53,* 1361–1367.

Slawinski, J. S., & Billat, V. L. (2004). Difference in mechanical and energy cost between highly, well, and nontrained runners. *Medicine & Science in Sports & Exercise, 36,* 1440–1446.

Snellen, J. W. (2000). An improved estimation of mean body temperature using combined direct calorimetry and thermometry. *European Journal of Applied Physiology, 82,* 188–196.

Snellen, J. W., Chang, K. S., & Smith, W. (1983). Technical description and performance characteristics of a human whole-body calorimeter. *Medical and Biological Engineering and Computing, 21,* 9–20.

Sorkin, B., Rapoport, D. M., Falk, D. B., & Goldring, R. M. (1980). Canopy ventilation monitor for quantitative measurement of ventilation during sleep. *Journal of Applied Physiology, 48,* 724–730.

Spinnler, G., Jequier, E., Favre, R., Dolivo, M., & Vannotti, A. (1973). Human calorimeter with a new type of gradient layer. *Journal of Applied Physiology, 35,* 158–165.

Spurr, G. B., Dufour, D. L., & Reina, J. C. (1996). Energy expenditure of urban Colombian women: A comparison of patterns and total daily expenditure by the heart rate and factorial methods. *American Journal of Clinical Nutrition, 63,* 870–878.

Stock, M. J. (1979). Use of an automatic closed-circuit calorimeter for short-term measurements of resting oxygen consumption [Proceedings]. *Journal of Physiology, 291,* 11P–12P.

Sun, M., & Hill, J. O. (1993). A method for measuring mechanical work and work efficiency during human activities. *Journal of Biomechanics, 26,* 229–241.

Sun, M., Reed, G. W., & Hill, J. O. (1994). Modification of a whole room indirect calorimeter for measurement of rapid changes in energy expenditure. *Journal of Applied Physiology, 76,* 2686–2691.

Terrier, P., Ladetto, Q., Merminod, B., & Schutz, Y. (2001). Measurement of the mechanical power of walking by satellite positioning system (GPS). *Medicine & Science in Sports & Exercise, 33,* 1912–1918.

Tissot, J. (1904). Nouvelle methode de mesure et d'inscription du debit et des movements respiratories de l'homme et des animaux. *Journal of Physiology and Pathology General, 6,* 688–700.

Tissot, S., Delafosse, B., Bertrand, O., Bouffard, Y., Viale, J. P., & Annat, G. (1995). Clinical validation of the Deltatrac monitoring system in mechanically ventilated patients. *Intensive Care Medicine, 21,* 149–153.

Toubro, S., Christensen, N. J., & Astrup, A. (1995). Reproducibility of 24-h energy expenditure, substrate utilization and spontaneous physical activity in obesity measured in a respiration chamber. *International Journal of Obesity and Related Metabolic Disorders, 19,* 544–549.

Vasilaras, T. H., Raben, A., & Astrup, A. (2001). Twenty-four hour energy expenditure and substrate oxidation before and after 6 months' ad libitum intake of a diet rich in simple or complex carbohydrates or a habitual diet. *International Journal of Obesity and Related Metabolic Disorders, 25,* 954–965.

Warwick, P. M., & Baines, J. (1996). Energy expenditure in free-living smokers and nonsmokers: Comparison between factorial, intake-balance, and doubly labeled water measures. *American Journal of Clinical Nutrition, 63,* 15–21.

Warwick, P. M., Edmundson, H. M., & Thomson, E. S. (1988). Prediction of energy expenditure: Simplified FAO/WHO/UNU factorial method vs continuous respirometry and habitual energy intake. *American Journal of Clinical Nutrition, 48,* 1188–1196.

Washburn, R. A., Jacobsen, D. J., Sonko, B. J., Hill, J. O., & Donnelly, J. E. (2003). The validity of the Stanford Seven-Day Physical Activity Recall in young adults. *Medicine & Science in Sports & Exercise, 35,* 1374–1380.

Webb, P. (1991). The measurement of energy expenditure. *Journal of Nutrition, 121,* 1897–1901.

Webb, P., Annis, J. F., & Troutman, S. J., Jr. (1972). Human calorimetry with a water-cooled garment. *Journal of Applied Physiology, 32,* 412–418.

Webb, P., Annis, J. F., & Troutman, S. J., Jr. (1980). Energy balance in man measured by direct and indirect calorimetry. *American Journal of Clinical Nutrition, 33,* 1287–1298.

Webster, J. D., Welsh, G., Pacy, P., & Garrow, J. S. (1986). Description of a human direct calorimeter, with a note on the energy cost of clerical work. *British Journal of Nutrition, 55,* 1–6.

Weir, J. B. (1949). New methods for calculating metabolic rate with special reference to protein metabolism. *Nutrition, 6,* 213–221.

Weissman, C., Damask, M. C., Askanazi, J., Rosenbaum, S. H., & Kinney, J. M. (1985). Evaluation of a noninvasive method for the measurement of metabolic rate in humans. *Clinical Science (Colch), 69,* 135–141.

Westerterp, K. R., Wilson, S. A., & Rolland, V. (1999). Diet induced thermogenesis measured over 24h in a respiration chamber: effect of diet composition. *International Journal of Obesity and Related Metabolic Disorders, 23,* 287–292.

Wilmore, J. H., Davis, J. A., & Norton, A. C. (1976). An automated system for assessing metabolic and respiratory function during exercise. *Journal of Applied Physiology, 40,* 619–624.

Yoshida, T., Nagata, A., Muro, M., Takeuchi, N., & Suda, Y. (1981). The validity of anaerobic threshold determination by a Douglas bag method compared with arterial blood lactate concentration. *European Journal of Applied Physiology and Occupational Physiology, 46,* 423–430.

Young, B. A., Fenton, T. W., & McLean, J. A. (1984). Calibration methods in respiratory calorimetry. *Journal of Applied Physiology, 56,* 1120–1135.

Appendices

Chapter 2

Appendix 2.A Obesity and Weight-Loss Quality-of-Life (OWLQOL) 17-Item Questionnaire

1. Because of my weight, I try to wear clothes that hide my shape.

2. I feel frustrated that I have less energy because of my weight.

3. I feel guilty when I eat because of my weight.

4. I am bothered by what other people say about my weight.

5. Because of my weight, I try to avoid having my photograph taken.

6. Because of my weight, I have to pay close attention to personal hygiene.

7. My weight prevents me from doing what I want to do.

8. I worry about the physical stress that my weight puts on my body.

9. I feel frustrated that I am not able to eat what others do because of my weight.

10. I feel depressed because of my weight.

11. I feel ugly because of my weight.

12. I worry about the future because of my weight.

13. I envy people who are thin.

14. I feel that people stare at me because of my weight.

15. I have difficulty accepting my body because of my weight.

16. I am afraid that I will gain back any weight that I lose.

17. I get discouraged when I try to lose weight.

Response scale: 0 = not at all; 1 = hardly; 2 = somewhat; 3 = moderately; 4 = a good deal; 5 = a great deal; 6 = a very great deal.

SOURCE: Reprinted with permission from The Obesity Society. Patrick, D. L., Bushnell, D. M.,& Rothman, M. (2004), Performance of two self-report measures for evaluating obesity and weight loss. *Obesity Research, 12,* 48–57.

Appendix 2.B The 20-Item Weight-Related Symptom Measure (WRSM)

Shortness of breath, tiredness, sleep problems, sensitivity to cold, increased thirst, increased irritability, back pain, frequent urination, pain in the joints, water retention, foot problems, sensitivity to heat, snoring, increased appetite, leakage of urine, lightheadedness, increased sweating, loss of sexual desire, decreased physical stamina, skin irritation.

Response scale: yes/no for frequency; 0 = not at all; 1 = hardly; 2 = somewhat; 3 = moderately; 4 = a good deal; 5 = a great deal; 6 = a very great deal bothersomeness.

SOURCE: The OWLQOL and WRSM can be obtained at http://www.seaqolgroup.org. The instruments are copyrighted and cannot be used without permission.

© Reprinted with permission from The Obesity Society. Patrick, D. L., Bushnell, D. M., & Rothman, M. (2004). Performance of two self-report measures for evaluating obesity and weight loss. *Obesity Research, 12*, 48–57.

Appendix 2.C Obesity-Related Problems Scale (OP)

Does your body weight or body shape bother you in the following situations?

Read each statement and mark the alternative that best applies to you.

Examples of items
Private gatherings in a friend's or relative's home
Going to community activities, courses, etc.
Bathing in public places (beach, public pool, etc.)
Intimate relations
Response categories
Definitely bothered/Mostly bothered/Not so bothered/Definitely not bothered

SOURCE: Reprinted with permission from HRQL Group, Göteborg University on Campus Company, Göteborg, Sweden. Permission to use the OP Scale may be obtained by written request.

Appendix 2.D IWQOL-Lite

SAMPLE ITEMS
Impact of Weight on Quality of Life Questionnaire–Lite Version (IWQOL-Lite)

Please answer the following statements by circling the number that best applies to you *in the past week.* Be as open as possible. There are no right or wrong answers.

Physical Function	ALWAYS TRUE	USUALLY TRUE	SOMETIMES TRUE	RARELY TRUE	NEVER TRUE
Because of my weight I have trouble picking up objects.	5	4	3	2	1
Self-Esteem	ALWAYS TRUE	USUALLY TRUE	SOMETIMES TRUE	RARELY TRUE	NEVER TRUE
Because of my weight I am self-conscious.	5	4	3	2	1
Sexual Life	ALWAYS TRUE	USUALLY TRUE	SOMETIMES TRUE	RARELY TRUE	NEVER TRUE
Because of my weight I do not enjoy sexual activity.	5	4	3	2	1
Public Distress	ALWAYS TRUE	USUALLY TRUE	SOMETIMES TRUE	RARELY TRUE	NEVER TRUE
Because of my weight I experience ridicule, teasing, or unwanted attention.	5	4	3	2	1
Work (Note: For homemakers and retirees, answer with respect to your daily activities.)	ALWAYS TRUE	USUALLY TRUE	SOMETIMES TRUE	RARELY TRUE	NEVER TRUE
Because of my weight I have trouble getting things accomplished or meeting my responsibilities.	5	4	3	2	1

Appendix 2.E Moorehead-Ardelt Quality of Life Questionnaire II (MA II)

Moorehead-Ardelt Quality of Life Questionnaire II (MA II)
Self Esteem and Activity Levels
Please make a check in the box provided to show your answer.

1. Usually I Feel . . .

❑   ❑   ❑   ❑   ❑   ❑   ❑   ❑   ❑   ❑

Very Badly
About Myself

Very Good
About Myself

2. I Enjoy Physical Activities . . .

❑   ❑   ❑   ❑   ❑   ❑   ❑   ❑   ❑   ❑

Not At All

Very Many

3. I Have Satisfactory Social Contacts . . .

❑   ❑   ❑   ❑   ❑   ❑   ❑   ❑   ❑   ❑

None

Very Many

4. I Am Able to Work . . .

❑   ❑   ❑   ❑   ❑   ❑   ❑   ❑   ❑   ❑

Not At All

Very Much

5. The Pleasure I get Out Of Sex Is . . .

❑   ❑   ❑   ❑   ❑   ❑   ❑   ❑   ❑   ❑

Not At All

Very Much

6. The Way I Approach Food Is . . .

❑   ❑   ❑   ❑   ❑   ❑   ❑   ❑   ❑   ❑

I Live to Eat

I Eat to Live

Appendix 2.E The M.A QoL QII scoring key

Self Esteem and Activity Levels
SCORING KEY

1. Usually I Feel . . .

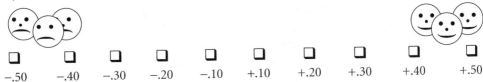

❏   ❏   ❏   ❏   ❏   ❏   ❏   ❏   ❏   ❏
−.50   −.40   −.30   −.20   −.10   +.10   +.20   +.30   +.40   +.50

2. I Enjoy Physical Activities . . .

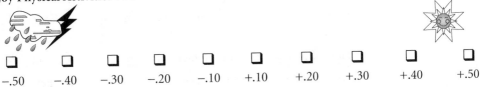

❏   ❏   ❏   ❏   ❏   ❏   ❏   ❏   ❏   ❏
−.50   −.40   −.30   −.20   −.10   +.10   +.20   +.30   +.40   +.50

3. I Have Satisfactory Social Contacts . . .

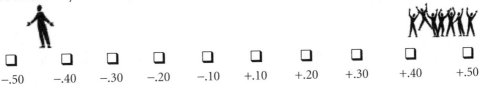

❏   ❏   ❏   ❏   ❏   ❏   ❏   ❏   ❏   ❏
−.50   −.40   −.30   −.20   −.10   +.10   +.20   +.30   +.40   +.50

4. I Am Able to Work . . .

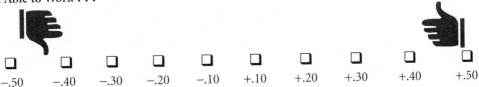

❏   ❏   ❏   ❏   ❏   ❏   ❏   ❏   ❏   ❏
−.50   −.40   −.30   −.20   −.10   +.10   +.20   +.30   +.40   +.50

5. The Pleasure I get Out Of Sex Is . . .

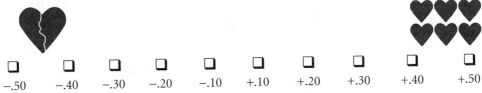

❏   ❏   ❏   ❏   ❏   ❏   ❏   ❏   ❏   ❏
−.50   −.40   −.30   −.20   −.10   +.10   +.20   +.30   +.40   +.50

6. The Way I Approach Food Is . . .

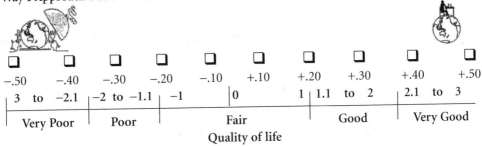

❏   ❏   ❏   ❏   ❏   ❏   ❏   ❏   ❏   ❏
−.50   −.40   −.30   −.20   −.10   +.10   +.20   +.30   +.40   +.50

3 to −2.1	−2 to −1.1	−1	0	1 1.1 to 2	2.1 to 3
Very Poor	Poor		Fair	Good	Very Good

Quality of life

SOURCE: Reprinted with permission from Springer Licensing Department. From Moorehead, M. K., Ardelt-Gattinger, E., Lechner, H., & Oria, H. E. (2003). The validation of the Moorehead-Ardelt Quality of Life Questionnaire II. *Obesity Surgery, 13*, 684–692.

Appendix 2.F Eating Disorder Quality of Life (EDQOL)

Psychological:

INSTRUCTIONS: Please answer the following statements according to how well they describe you in the last 30 days. Please be as open as possible. There are no right or wrong answers. Fill in the circle in the appropriate column. For those items that do not apply to you, please leave them blank.

In the last 30 days . . .

| Never | Rarely | Sometimes | Often | Always |

Psychological

1. How often has your eating/weight resulted in you feeling embarrassed or "different"?

2. How often has your eating/weight made you feel worse about yourself?

3. How often has your eating/weight made you not want to be with people?

4. How often has your eating/weight resulted in you believing that you will never get better?

5. How often has your eating/weight made you feel lonely?

6. How often has your eating/weight resulted in less interest or pleasure in activities?

7. How often has your eating/weight led you to not care about yourself?

8. How often has your eating/weight made you feel odd, weird, or unusual?

9. How often has your eating/weight resulted in avoiding eating in front of others?

Physical/Cognitive

10. How often has your eating/weight caused cold hands or feet?

11. How often has your eating/weight caused frequent headaches?

12. How often has your eating/weight caused weakness?

14. How often has your eating/weight affected your ability to comprehend some verbal and written information?

13. How often has your eating/weight affected your ability to pay attention when you wanted to?

15. How often has your eating/weight reduced your ability to concentrate?

Financial

16. How often has your eating/weight led to problems with treatment provider(s) regarding cost of treatment?

17. How often has your eating/weight led to you having difficulty paying monthly bills?

18. How often has your eating/weight resulted in significant financial debt?

19. How often has your eating/weight led to the need to spend money from savings or use your credit card frequently?

20. How often has your eating/weight resulted in the need to borrow money?

Work/School

21. How often has your eating/weight led to a leave of absence from work?

22. How often has your eating/weight led to low grades?

23. How often has your eating/weight resulted in reduced hours at work?

24. How often has your eating/weight resulted in you losing a job or dropping out of school?

25. How often has your eating/weight led to failure in a class or classes?

SOURCE: Copyright © 2005. Neuropsychiatric Research Institute and Scott Engel. Direct all correspondence to Scott G. Engel, PhD, Neuropsychiatric Research Institute, 120 Eighth Street South, Fargo, ND 58107. Not to be used without permission from Dr. Engel. Reprinted with permission from Scott G. Engel, PhD, and James E. Mitchell, MD, Neuropsychiatric Research Institute.

Appendix 2.G The Bariatric Quality of Life (BQL) Questionnaire

Part 1

Do you suffer from:

vomiting . . . . Yes ☐0   No ☐0.5

sour belching . . . . Yes ☐0   No ☐0.5

heartburn. . . . . Yes ☐0   No ☐0.5

nausea . . . . Yes ☐0   No ☐0.5

diarrhea . . . . Yes ☐0   No ☐0.5

flatulence (gassing) . . . . Yes ☐0   No ☐0.5

foul-odor feces . . . . Yes ☐0   No ☐0.5

bladder problems /

urinary incontinence . . . . Yes ☐0   No ☐0.5

hair loss . . . . Yes ☐0   No ☐0.5

gallstones

(or gallbladder removed) . . . . Yes ☐0   No ☐0.5

diabetes . . . . Yes ☐0   No ☐0.5

high blood pressure/hypertension

(also if treated) . . . . Yes ☐0   No ☐0.5

asthma / sleep apnea . . . . Yes ☐0   No ☐0.5

arthrosis / joint pain . . . . Yes ☐0   No ☐0.5

gout . . . . Yes ☐0   No ☐0.5

others: _____

**Do you take any medication
regularly?** . . . . Yes ☐0   No ☐0.5
If yes, what kind of medication do you take?
- antidiabetics . . . . Yes ☐   No ☐
- insulin . . . . Yes ☐   No ☐
- antihypertensives . . . . Yes ☐   No ☐
- antidepressants . . . . Yes ☐   No ☐
- appetite suppressants . . . . Yes ☐   No ☐
- diuretics . . . . Yes ☐   No ☐
- pain killers . . . . Yes ☐   No ☐
others:_____

Part 2

1. I like my weight.

☐1   ☐2   ☐3   ☐4   ☐5
absolutely wrong   wrong   half/half   true   absolutely right

2. I can accept my weight.

☐1   ☐2   ☐3   ☐4   ☐5
absolutely wrong   wrong   half/half   true   absolutely right

3. How is your actual quality of life?

☐1   ☐2   ☐3   ☐4   ☐5
very bad   bad   OK   good   very good

4. I exercise regularly.

☐1   ☐2   ☐3   ☐4   ☐5
absolutely wrong   wrong   half/half   true   absolutely right

5. I am participating in social activities (theatre, etc.).

☐1   ☐2   ☐3   ☐4   ☐5
absolutely wrong   wrong   half/half   true   absolutely right

6. I often meet friends or family.

☐1   ☐2   ☐3   ☐4   ☐5
absolutely wrong   wrong   half/half   true   absolutely right

7. I feel excluded from social life.

☐1   ☐2   ☐3   ☐4   ☐5
absolutely wrong   wrong   half/half   true   absolutely right

8. I feel under pressure because of my weight.

☐1   ☐2   ☐3   ☐4   ☐5
absolutely wrong   wrong   half/half   true   absolutely right

9. Sometimes, I feel depressed.

☐1   ☐2   ☐3   ☐4   ☐5
absolutely wrong   wrong   half/half   true   absolutely right

10. All in all, I feel satisfied in my life.

☐1   ☐2   ☐3   ☐4   ☐5
absolutely wrong   wrong   half/half   true   absolutely right

11. I feel restricted because of my weight.

a) at home

☐1
absolutely wrong ☐2
wrong ☐3
half/half ☐4
true ☐5
absolutely right

b) at work

☐1
absolutely wrong ☐2
wrong ☐3
half/half ☐4
true ☐5
absolutely right

c) privately

☐1
absolutely wrong ☐2
wrong ☐3
half/half ☐4
true ☐5
absolutely right

12. I feel self-confident.

☐1
absolutely wrong ☐2
wrong ☐3
half/half ☐4
true ☐5
absolutely right

SOURCE: Reprinted with permission from Springer Licensing Department. From Weiner, S., Sauerland, S., Fein, M., Blanco, R., Pomhoff, I., & Weiner, R. A. (2005). The Bariatric Quality of Life index: A measure of well-being in obesity surgery patients. *Obesity Surgery, 15,* 538–545.

Appendix 2.H IWQOL-Kids Sample Items

IWQOL-Kids

Please answer the following statements by circling the number that best applies to you *in the past seven days.* Be as open as possible. There are no right or wrong answers.

		ALWAYS TRUE	USUALLY TRUE	SOMETIMES TRUE	RARELY TRUE	NEVER TRUE
Physical Comfort						
1.	Because of my weight I avoid using stairs whenever possible.	1	2	3	4	5
Body Esteem		ALWAYS TRUE	USUALLY TRUE	SOMETIMES TRUE	RARELY TRUE	NEVER TRUE
7.	Because of my weight I am ashamed of my body.	1	2	3	4	5
Social Life		ALWAYS TRUE	USUALLY TRUE	SOMETIMES TRUE	RARELY TRUE	NEVER TRUE
16.	Because of my weight people tease me or make fun of me.	1	2	3	4	5
Family Relations		ALWAYS TRUE	USUALLY TRUE	SOMETIMES TRUE	RARELY TRUE	NEVER TRUE
25.	Because of my weight my parents aren't proud of me.	1	2	3	4	5

Appendix 2.1 Web Sites for Generic Measures of HRQOL

SF-36	http://www.qualitymetric.com
Nottingham Health Profile	https://www.cebp.nl/media/m83.pdf
Sickness Impact Profile	http://www.atsqol.org/sections/instruments/pt/pages/sick.html
General Health Questionnaire	http://www.proqolid.org/instruments/general_health_questionnaire_ghq

Chapter 3

Appendix 3.A Descriptors Used in Adjectival and Semantic Differential Anti-Fat Measurement (Staffieri, 1967)

Smart*	Ugly* **
Stupid*	Quiet*
Healthy*	Loud*
Sick*	Best friend**
Neat*	Kind**
Sloppy*	Helps others
Many friends*	Polite
Few friends*	Powerless
Strong*	Fights
Weak*	Unsound
Works hard*	Cheats
Lazy* **	Nervous
Nice*	Argues
Mean*	Dirty
Happy*	Spiritless
Sad*	Worrisome
Doesn't get teased*	Lonely**
Gets teased* **	Sneaky
Brave*	Tired
Afraid*	Undecided
Good looking (cute*)	

* These adjectives were employed by Brylinsky and Moore (1994).

** These adjectives were employed by Kraig and Keel (2001).

References

Brylinsky, J. A., & Moore, J. C. (1994). The identification of body build stereotypes in young children. *Journal of Research in Personality, 28,* 170–181.

Kraig, K. A., & Keel, P. K. (2001). Weight-based stigmatization in children. *International Journal of Obesity, 25,* 1661–1666.

Staffieri, J. R. (1967). A study of social stereotype of body image in children. *Journal of Personality & Social Psychology, 7,* 101–104.

Appendix 3.B F Scale (Bacon, Scheltema, & Robinson, 2001)

Directions: Listed below are 14 pairs of adjectives sometimes used to describe obese or fat people. For each adjective pair, please place an X on the line closest to the adjective that you feel best describes your feelings and beliefs.

1. lazy   ___ ___ ___ ___ ___   industrious

2. no will power   ___ ___ ___ ___ ___   has will power

3. attractive   ___ ___ ___ ___ ___   unattractive

4. good self-control   ___ ___ ___ ___ ___   poor self-control

5. fast   ___ ___ ___ ___ ___   slow

6. having endurance   ___ ___ ___ ___ ___   having no endurance

7. active   ___ ___ ___ ___ ___   inactive

8. weak   ___ ___ ___ ___ ___   strong

9. self-indulgent   ___ ___ ___ ___ ___   self-sacrificing

10. dislikes food   ___ ___ ___ ___ ___   likes food

11. shapeless   ___ ___ ___ ___ ___   shapely

12. undereats   ___ ___ ___ ___ ___   overeats

13. insecure   ___ ___ ___ ___ ___   secure

14. low self-esteem   ___ ___ ___ ___ ___   high self-esteem

F-Scale Scoring Instructions

Step 1:

For items 3, 4, 5, 6, 7, 10, and 12, score as follows: 1, 2, 3, 4, and 5.

Step 2:

For items 1, 2, 8, 9, 11, 13, and 14, score as follows: 5, 4, 3, 2, and 1.

Step 3:

Add up the score for each item to get the total score. Then divide by 14 (or the number of items answered, whichever is less). The range of scores is 1–5. Higher scores denote greater "fat phobia."

NOTE: This scale could be used in experimental studies designed to assess whether beliefs about "thin" versus "fat" targets differ. In this case, we recommend the directions be modified as follows: *Listed below are 14 pairs of adjectives. Based on your impression of the picture (drawing) that you have just seen, place an X on the line closest to the adjective that you feel best describes your feelings and beliefs.*

Reference

Bacon, J. G., Scheltema, K. E., & Robinson, B. E. (2001). Fat Phobia Scale revisited: The short form. *International Journal of Obesity, 25,* 252–257.

Appendix 3.C Anti-Fat Attitudes Scale (AFA; Crandall, 1994; Quinn & Crocker, 1999)

Directions: For the following questions, circle a number between 0 and 9 to indicate how much you agree or disagree with each of the following statements.

Dislike of Fat People Subscale

1. I really don't like fat people much.

2. I don't have many friends that are fat.

3. I tend to think that people who are overweight are a little untrustworthy.

4. Although some fat people are surely smart, in general, I think they tend not to be quite as bright as normal weight people.

5. I have a hard time taking fat people too seriously.

6. Fat people make me feel somewhat uncomfortable.

7. If I were an employer looking to hire, I might avoid hiring a fat person.

8. I feel repulsed when I see a fat person.

9. Fat people disgust me.

10. I have an immediate negative reaction when I meet a fat person.

Willpower Subscale

1. People who weigh too much could lose at least some part of their weight through a little exercise.

2. Some people are fat because they have no willpower.

3. Fat people tend to be fat pretty much through their own fault.

4. Fat people can lose weight if they really want to.

5. Through a combination of exercise and dieting, anyone can lose weight and keep it off indefinitely.

6. The medical problems that overweight people have are their own fault.

7. Overweight people are responsible for their own problems.

8. Weight is something which is under a person's control.

Fear of Fat Subscale

1. I feel disgusted with myself when I gain weight.

2. One of the worst things that could happen to me would be if I gained 25 pounds of fat.

3. I worry about becoming fat.

Each item is accompanied by the following response format:

0 1 2 3 4 5 6 7 8 9 (where 0 = very strongly disagree and 9 = very strongly agree). Total subscale scores are computed by summing responses and then dividing by the number of subscale items. The possible range for each subscale is 0 to 9.

NOTE: We do not recommend that researchers compute a total scale score as this combines dislike of fat people and beliefs about the controllability of weight, which are interrelated, yet distinct, constructs (Crandall, 1994). In addition, as it assesses the personal fear of becoming fat rather than negative attitudes toward obese persons, we do not recommend that individuals use the Fear of Fat subscale. It should be noted that Items 8 through 10 (Dislike) and 4 through 8 (Willpower) were generated by Quinn and Crocker (1999) for the purposes of improving reliability. Finally, to avoid possible sequencing effects, the Dislike and Willpower items should be interspersed.

References

Crandall, C. S. (1994). Prejudice against fat people: Ideology and self-interest. *Journal of Personality and Social Psychology, 66,* 882–894.

Quinn, D. M., & Crocker, J. (1999). When ideology hurts: Effects of belief in the Protestant ethic and feeling overweight on the psychological well-being of women. *Journal of Personality and Social Psychology, 77,* 402–414.

Appendix 3.D Anti-Fat Attitudes Scale (AFAS; Morrison & O'Connor, 1999)

Directions: For the following questions, select the response option that corresponds with your opinion. Please note that there are no right or wrong answers. Therefore, try to answer each question as honestly as possible.

1. Fat people are less sexually attractive than thin people.

2. I would never date a fat person.

3. On average, fat people are lazier than thin people.

4. Fat people only have themselves to blame for their weight.

5. It is disgusting when a fat person wears a bathing suit at the beach.

Each item is accompanied by the following response format: 1 = strongly disagree; 2 = disagree; 3 = neither agree nor disagree; 4 = agree; 5 = strongly agree. Total scale scores are computed by summing all items, and can range from 5 to 25.

Reference

Morrison, T. G., & O'Connor, W. E. (1999). Psychometric properties of a scale measuring negative attitudes toward overweight individuals. *Journal of Social Psychology, 139,* 436–445.

Appendix 3.E Anti-Fat Attitudes Test
(AFAT; Lewis, Cash, Jacobi, & Bubb-Lewis, 1997)

Directions: For each statement, select the response option that corresponds to your opinion.

Social/Character Disparagement Subscale

1. If fat people don't get hired, it's their own fault.

2. Fat people don't care about anything except eating.

3. I'd lose respect for a friend who started getting fat.

4. Most fat people are boring.

5. Society is too tolerant of fat people.

6. When fat people exercise, they look ridiculous.

7. Fat people are just as competent in their work as anyone.

8. Being fat is sinful.

9. I prefer not to associate with fat people.

10. Most fat people are moody and hard to get along with.

11. If bad things happen to fat people, they deserve it.

12. Most fat people don't keep their surroundings neat and clean.

13. Society should respect the rights of fat people.

14. Fat people are unclean.

15. It's hard to take fat people seriously.

Physical/Romantic Unattractiveness Subscale

1. If I were single, I would date a fat person.

2. Fat people are physically unattractive.

3. Fat people shouldn't wear revealing clothing in public.

4. I can't believe someone of average weight would marry a fat person.

5. It's disgusting to see fat people eating.

6. It's hard not to stare at fat people because they are so unattractive.

7. I would not want to continue in a romantic relationship if my partner became fat.

8. I don't understand how someone could be sexually attracted to a fat person.

9. People who are fat have as much physical coordination as anyone.

10. Fat people should be encouraged to accept themselves the way they are.

Weight Control/Blame Subscale

1. There's no excuse for being fat.

2. Most fat people buy too much junk food.

3. Most fat people are lazy.

4. If fat people really wanted to lose weight, they could.

5. Fat people have no will power.

6. The idea that genetics causes people to be fat is just an excuse.

7. If fat people knew how bad they looked, they would lose weight.

8. Most fat people will latch onto almost any excuse for being fat.

9. Fat people do not necessarily eat more than other people.

Filler Items

1. Jokes about fat people are funny.

2. If someone in my family were fat, I'd be ashamed of him or her.

3. I can't stand to look at fat people.

4. Fat people are disgusting.

5. If I have the choice, I'd rather not sit next to a fat person.

6. I hate it when fat people take up more room then they should in a theater or on a bus or a plane.

7. Most fat people don't care about anyone but themselves.

8. Fat people don't care about their appearance.

9. If I owned a business, I would not hire fat people because of the way they look.

10. I'd feel self-conscious being seen in public with a fat person.

11. The existence of organizations to lobby for the rights of fat people in our society is a good idea.

12. Fat people obviously have a character flaw otherwise they wouldn't become fat.

13. It makes me angry to hear anybody say insulting things about people because they are fat.

Each item is accompanied by the following response format: 1 = definitely disagree; 2 = mostly disagree; 3 = neither agree nor disagree; 4 = mostly agree; 5 = definitely agree. The following items are reverse scored: Items 7 and 13 (Social/Character Disparagement subscale); Items 1, 9, and 10 (Physical/Romantic

Unattractiveness subscale); Item 9 (Weight Control/Blame subscale); and Items 11 and 13 (Filler). Total scale scores are computed by summing all items and then dividing by the total number of items. This scoring method can be used for each subscale as well. Total scores can range from 1 to 5, with higher scores denoting stronger antifat attitudes.

Finally, when using the AFAT, items should be interspersed rather than grouped by subscale.

Reference

Lewis, R. J., Cash, T. F., Jacobi, L., & Bubb-Lewis, C. (1997). Prejudice toward fat people: The development and validation of the Anti-fat Attitudes Test. *Obesity Research, 5,* 297–307.

Appendix 3.F Attitudes Toward Obese Persons Scale (ATOP; Allison, Basile, & Yuker, 1991)

Directions: Please mark each statement below in the left margin, according to how much you agree or disagree with it. Please do not leave any blank.

1. _____ Obese people are as happy as non-obese people.

2. _____ Most obese people feel that they are not as good as other people.

3. _____ Most obese people are more self-conscious than other people.

4. _____ Obese workers cannot be as successful as other workers.

5. _____ Most non-obese people would not want to marry anyone who is obese.

6. _____ Severely obese people are usually untidy.

7. _____ Obese people are usually sociable.

8. _____ Most obese people are not dissatisfied with themselves.

9. _____ Obese people are just as self-confident as other people.

10. _____Most people feel uncomfortable when they associate with obese people.

11. _____ Obese people are often less aggressive than non-obese people.

12. _____ Most obese people have different personalities than non-obese people.

13. _____ Very few obese people are ashamed of their weight.

14. _____ Most obese people resent normal weight people.

15. _____ Obese people are more emotional than other people.

16. _____ Obese people should not expect to lead normal lives.

17. _____ Obese people are just as healthy as non-obese people.

18. _____ Obese people are just as sexually attractive as non-obese people.

19. _____ Obese people tend to have family problems.

20. _____ One of the worst things that could happen to a person would be for him or her to become obese.

The ATOP uses the following response format: −3 = I strongly disagree; −2 = I moderately disagree; −1 = I slightly disagree; +1 = I slightly agree; +2 = I moderately agree; + 3 = I strongly agree.

ATOP Scoring Instructions:

Step 1:

For Items 2 through 6, 10 through 12, 14 through 16, and 19 through 20, multiply the response by −1.

Step 2:

Sum the response to all items.

Step 3:

Add 60 to the value obtained in Step 2. The resultant score should fall between 0 and 120, with *higher* scores denoting *less* antifat prejudice.

NOTE: There are no published studies specifying which items are associated with the three dimensions identified by Allison et al. (1991). Individuals wishing to use subscale scores in their research should obtain these details from the authors.

Reference

Allison, D. B., Basile, V. C., & Yuker, H. E. (1991). The measurement of attitudes toward and beliefs about obese persons. *International Journal of Eating Disorders, 10,* 599–607.

Chapter 10

Appendix 10. A Questionnaire on Eating and Weight Patterns–Revised (QEWP-R)

Robert L. Spitzer, Susan Z. Yanovski, Marsha D. Marcus

Last name_____   First name_____

MI ____

Date_____   I.D. Number _____

Thank you for completing this questionnaire. Please circle the appropriate number or response, or write in information where asked. You may skip any question you do not understand or do not wish to answer.

1. Age ___ ___ years

2. Sex: 1   Male   2   Female

3. What is you ethnic/racial background?

    1. Black (not Hispanic)
    2. Hispanic
    3. White (not Hispanic)
    4. Asian
    5. Other (please specify)_____

4. How far did you get in school?

    1. Grammar school, junior high school or less
    2. Some high school
    3. High school graduate or equivalency (GED)
    4. Some college or associate degree
    5. Completed college

5. How tall are you?

    ____ feet ___ ___ in.

6. How much do you weigh now?

    _____ lbs

7. What has been your highest weight ever (when not pregnant)?

    _____ lbs

8. Have you ever been overweight by at least 10 lbs as a child or 15 lbs as an adult (when not pregnant)?

   1 Yes   2 No or not sure

   IF YES: How old were you when you were first overweight (at least 10 lbs as a child or 15 lbs as an adult)? If you are not sure, what is your best guess?

   _____ ___ years

9. How many times (approximately) have you lost 20 lbs or more—when you weren't sick—and then gained it back?

   1. Never
   2. Once or twice
   3. Three or four times
   4. Five times or more

10. During the past **six** months, did you often eat within any two hour period what most people would regard as an unusually large amount of food?

    1 Yes   2 No

    IF NO: SKIP TO QUESTION 15

11. During the times when you ate this way, did you often feel you couldn't stop eating or control what or how much you were eating?

    1 Yes   2 No

    IF NO: SKIP TO QUESTION 15

12. During the past **six** months, how often, on average, did you have times when you ate this way—that is, large amounts of food **plus** the feeling that your eating was out of control? (There may have been some weeks when it was not present—just average those in.)

    1. Less than one day a week
    2. One day a week
    3. Two or three days a week
    4. Four or five days a week
    5. Nearly every day

13. Did you **usually** have any of the following experiences during these occasions?

a. Eating much more rapidly than usual?	Yes No
b. Eating until you felt uncomfortably full?	Yes No
c. Eating large amounts of food when you didn't feel physically hungry?	Yes No
d. Eating alone because you were embarrassed by how much you were eating?	Yes No
e. Feeling disgusted with yourself, depressed, or feeling very guilty after overeating?	Yes No

14. Think about a typical time when you ate this way—that is, large amounts of food **plus** the feeling that your eating was out of control.

   a. What time of day did the episode start?
   1. Morning (8 AM to 12 Noon)
   2. Early afternoon (12 Noon to 4 PM)
   3. Late afternoon (4 PM to 7 PM)
   4. Evening (7 PM to 10 PM)
   5. Night (After 10 PM)

   b. Approximately how long did this episode of eating last, from the time you started to eat to when you stopped and didn't eat again for at least two hours?

   _____ hours _____ minutes

   c. As best you can remember, please list everything you might have eaten or drunk during that episode. If you ate for more than two hours, describe the foods eaten and liquids drunk during the two hours that you ate the most. Be specific—include brand names where possible, and amounts as best you can estimate. (For example: 7 ounces Ruffles potato chips; 1 cup Breyer's chocolate ice cream with 2 teaspoons hot fudge; 2 8-ounce glasses of Coca-Cola, 1 & 1/2 ham and cheese sandwiches with mustard)

   d. At the time this episode started, how long had it been since you had previously finished eating a meal or snack?

   _____ hours _____ minutes

15. In general, during the past **six** months, how upset were you by overeating (eating more than you think is best for you)?
   1. Not at all
   2. Slightly
   3. Moderately
   4. Greatly
   5. Extremely

16. In general, during the past **six** months, how upset were you by the feeling that you couldn't stop eating or control what or how much you were eating?
   1. Not at all
   2. Slightly
   3. Moderately
   4. Greatly
   5. Extremely

17. During the past **six** months, how important has your weight or shape been in how you feel about or evaluate yourself as a person—as compared to other aspects of your life, such as how you do at work, as a parent, or how you get along with other people?

    1. Weight and shape were **not very important**
    2. Weight and shape **played a part** in how you felt about yourself
    3. Weight and shape **were among the main things** that affected how you felt about yourself
    4. Weight and shape **were the most important things** that affected how you felt about yourself

18. During the past **three** months, did you ever make yourself vomit in order to avoid gaining weight after binge eating?

    1 Yes 2 No

    IF YES: How often, **on average**, was that?

    1. Less than once a week
    2. Once a week
    3. Two or three times a week
    4. Four or five times a week
    5. More than five times a week

19. During the past **three** months, did you ever take more than twice the recommended dose of laxatives in order to avoid gaining weight after binge eating?

    1 Yes 2 No

    IF YES: How often, **on average**, was that?

    1. Less than once a week
    2. Once a week
    3. Two or three times a week
    4. Four or five times a week
    5. More than five times a week

20. During the past **three** months, did you ever take more than twice the recommended dose of diuretics (water pills) in order to avoid gaining weight after binge eating?

    1 Yes 2 No

    IF YES: How often, **on average**, was that?

    1. Less than once a week
    2. Once a week
    3. Two or three times a week
    4. Four or five times a week
    5. More than five times a week

21. During the past **three** months, did you ever fast—not eat anything at all for at least 24 hours—in order to avoid gaining weight after binge eating?

    1 Yes   2 No

    IF YES: How often, **on average**, was that?

    1. Less than one day a week
    2. One day a week
    3. Two or three days a week
    4. Four or five days a week
    5. Nearly every day

22. During the past **three** months, did you ever exercise for more than an hour **specifically** in order to avoid gaining weight after binge eating?

    1 Yes   2 No

    IF YES: How often, **on average**, was that?

    1. Less than once a week
    2. Once a week
    3. Two or three times a week
    4. Four or five times a week
    5. More than five times a week

23. During the past **three** months, did you ever take more than twice the recommended dose of a diet pill in order to avoid gaining weight after binge eating?

    1 Yes   2 No

    IF YES: How often, **on average**, was that?

    1. Less than once a week
    2. Once a week
    3. Two or three times a week
    4. Four or five times a week
    5. More than five times a week

24. During the past **six** months, did you go to any meetings of an organized weight control program? (e.g., Weight Watchers, Optifast, Nutrisystem) or a self-help group (e.g., TOPS, Overeaters Anonymous)?

    1 Yes   2 No

    IF YES: Name of program_____

25. Since you have been an adult—18 years old— how much of the time have you been on a diet, been trying to follow a diet, or in some way been limiting how much you were eating in order to lost weight or keep from regaining weight you had lost? Would you say . . . ?

    1. None or hardly any of the time
    2. About a quarter of the time

   3. About half of the time
   4. About three-quarters of the time
   5. Nearly all of the time

26. SKIP THIS QUESTION IF YOU NEVER LOST AT LEAST 10 LBS BY DIETING:

   How old were you the first time you lost at least 10 lbs by dieting, or in some way limiting how much you ate? If you are not sure, what is your best guess?
   ___ ___ years

27. SKIP THIS QUESTION IF YOU'VE NEVER HAD EPISODES OF EATING UNUSUALLY LARGE AMOUNTS OF FOOD ALONG WITH THE SENSE OF LOSS OF CONTROL:

   How old were you when you first had times when you ate large amounts of food and felt that your eating was out of control? If you are not sure, what is your best guess?
   ___ ___ years

28. Please take a look at these silhouettes. Put a circle around the silhouettes which most resemble the body build of your natural father and mother at **their heaviest.** If you have no knowledge of your biological father and/or mother, don't circle anything for that parent.

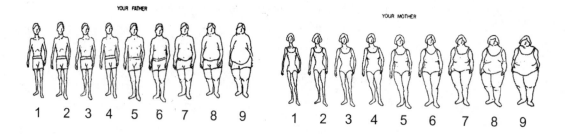

DECISION RULES FOR DIAGNOSING BINGE EATING DISORDER USING THE QUESTIONNAIRE ON EATING AND WEIGHT PATTERNS–Revised

(FOR EXAMINER'S USE ONLY)

DIAGNOSIS OF BED

QUESTION NUMBER	RESPONSE
10 AND 11	1 (BINGE EATING)
12	3, 4, OR 5 (AT LEAST 2 DAYS PER WEEK FOR SIX MONTHS)
13 a through e	3 OR MORE ITEMS MARKED "YES" (AT LEAST 3 ASSOCIATED SYMPTOMS DURING BINGE EATING EPISODES)
15 OR 16	4 OR 5 (MARKED DISTRESS REGARDING BINGE EATING)

DIAGNOSIS OF BED REQUIRES ALL OF THE ABOVE ALONG WITH THE ABSENCE OF PURGING OR NON-PURGING BULIMIA NERVOSA, AS DEFINED BELOW.

DIAGNOSIS OF PURGING BULIMIA NERVOSA

10 AND 11	1 (SAME AS BED)
12	3, 4, OR 5 (AT LEAST 2 DAYS PER WEEK FOR SIX MONTHS) Note: This is an approximation of the DSM-IV criterion of at least 2 episodes/week for three months).
17	3 OR 4 (OVERVALUATION OF WEIGHT/SHAPE)
18, 19, OR 20	ANY RESPONSE 3, 4, OR 5 (PURGING AT LEAST 2 TIMES PER WEEK FOR THREE MONTHS)

DIAGNOSIS OF NON-PURGING BULIMIA NERVOSA

10, 11, 12, 17	SAME AS PURGING BULIMIA NERVOSA
18, 19, AND 20	NO RESPONSE 3, 4, OR 5 (NO FREQUENT COMPENSATORY PURGING)
21, 22, OR 23	ANY RESPONSE 3, 4, OR 5 (COMPENSATORY NON-PURGING BEHAVIOR AT LEAST TWO TIMES PER WEEK FOR THREE MONTHS)

QUESTION FOR RESEARCH PURPOSES ONLY
(NOT TO BE USED FOR DIAGNOSIS OF BED OR
BULIMIA NERVOSA, PURGING OR NON-PURGING TYPE)

14 a through d	EXAMINER'S JUDGMENT THAT AMOUNT OF FOOD DESCRIBED IS UNUSUALLY LARGE GIVEN CIRCUMSTANCES (I.E., TIME OF DAY, HOURS SINCE PREVIOUS MEAL) YES____ NO____UNSURE____

Spitzer RL, Yanovski SZ, Marcus MD. (HaPI Record). 1994; Pittsburgh PA: Behavioral Measurement Database Services (Producer). McLean, VA: BRS Search Service (Vendor).

The following individuals contributed to the development of previous versions of the QEWP. Stewart Agras, Michael Devlin, Deborah Hasin, James Mitchell, Cathy Nonas, Albert Stunkard, Thomas Wadden, B. Timothy Walsh, Rena Wing.

Silhouettes from: Stunkard AJ, Sorensen T, Schulsinger F. *Use of the Danish Adoption Register for the Study of Obesity and Thinness.* In: Kety SS, Roland LP, Sidman RL, Matthysse S.W., eds. *The Genetics of Neurological and Psychiatric Disorders.* Raven Press: New York. 1983:119. Used by permission.

Appendix 10.B Eating Disorder Diagnostic Scale

Eating Screen
Please carefully complete **all** questions.

Over the <u>past 3 months</u> . . .	Not at all	Slightly	Moderately	Extremely
	0	1	2 3	4 5 6

1. Have you felt fat?

    0   1   2   3   4   5   6

2. Have you had a definite fear that you might gain weight or become fat?

    0   1   2   3   4   5   6

3. Has your weight influenced how you think about (judge) yourself as a person?

    0   1   2   3   4   5   6

4. Has your shape influenced how you think about (judge) yourself as a person?

    0   1   2   3   4   5   6

5. During the past **6 months** have there been times when you felt you have eaten what other people would regard as an unusually large amount of food (e.g., a quart of ice cream) given the circumstances? . . . .

    YES   NO

6. During the times when you ate an unusually large amount of food, did you experience a loss of control (feel you couldn't stop eating or control what or how much you were eating)? . . . . .

    YES   NO

7. How many **DAYS per week** on average over the **past 6 MONTHS** have you eaten an unusually large amount of food and experienced a loss of control?

    0   1   2   3   4   5   6   7

8. How many **TIMES per week** on average over the **past 3 MONTHS** have you eaten an unusually large amount of food and experienced a loss of control?

    0   1   2   3   4   5   6   7   8   9   10   11   12   13   14

During these episodes of overeating and loss of control did you. . .

9. Eat much more rapidly than normal? . . . .

    YES   NO

10. Eat until you felt uncomfortably full?. . . . .

    YES   NO

11. Eat large amounts of food when you didn't feel physically hungry?
....

YES   NO

12. Eat alone because you were embarrassed by how much you were eating?..

YES   NO

13. Feel disgusted with yourself, depressed, or very guilty after overeating?.
....

YES   NO

14. Feel very upset about your uncontrollable overeating or resulting weight gain?...

YES   NO

15. How many **times per week** on average over the past **3 months** have you made yourself vomit to prevent weight gain or counteract the effects of eating?

0   1   2   3   4   5   6   7   8   9   10   11   12   13   14

16. How many **times per week** on average over the past **3 months** have you used laxatives or diuretics to prevent weight gain or counteract the effects of eating?

0   1   2   3   4   5   6   7   8   9   10   11   12   13   14

17. How many **times per week** on average over the past **3 months** have you fasted (skipped at least 2 meals in a row) to prevent weight gain or counteract the effects of eating?

0   1   2   3   4   5   6   7   8   9   10   11   12   13   14

18. How many **times per week** on average over the past **3 months** have you engaged in excessive exercise specifically to counteract the effects of overeating episodes?

0   1   2   3   4   5   6   7   8   9   10   11   12   13   14

19. How much do you weigh? If uncertain, please give your best estimate.

____ lbs.

20. How tall are you? _Please specify in inches (5 ft.= 60 in.)___ in.

21. Over the past **3 months**, how many menstrual periods have you missed?
    0   1   2   3   n/a

22. Have you been taking birth control pills during the past **3 months**?
....

YES   NO

SOURCE: Stice, E., Telch, C.F., & Rizvi, S.L. (2000). Development and validation of the Eating Disorder Diagnostic Scale: A brief self-report measure of anorexia, bulimia, and binge eating disorder. *Psychological Assessment, 12,* 123–131.

Appendix 10.C Binge Scale Questionnaire

Binge Scale

Instructions: This questionnaire is designed to gather information about binge eating. Binge eating involves periods of uncontrolled, excessive eating. If you respond <u>no</u> to the first item, "Do you ever binge eat?", please answer only items 10, 13, and 14. If you respond <u>yes</u> to item 1, please answer all questions. For each item, circle only one answer unless otherwise specified. This questionnaire is confidential.

1. Do you ever binge eat?

    a. yes
    b. no

2. How often do you binge eat?

    a. seldom
    b. once or twice a month
    c. once a week
    d. almost every day

3. What is the average length of a binge eating episode?

    a. less than 15 minutes
    b. 15 minutes to one hour
    c. one hour to four hours
    d. more than four hours

4. Which of the following statements best applies to your binge eating?

    a. I eat until I have had enough to satisfy me.
    b. I eat until my stomach feels full.
    c. I eat until my stomach feels painfully full.
    d. I eat until I can't eat anymore.

5. Do you ever vomit after a binge?

    a. never
    b. sometimes
    c. usually
    d. always

6. Which one of the following best applies to your eating behavior when bingeing?

    a. I eat more slowly than usual.
    b. I eat about the same as I normally do.
    c. I eat very rapidly.

7. When you binge, which statement best describes your choice of food?

    a. I crave a particular food. or type of food. (If so, what food or type of food do you usually choose?) _____
    b. I don't crave any particular food or type of food but I eat high calorie foods that I wouldn't otherwise eat.
    c. I eat any type of food that's handy.

8. How much are you concerned about your binge eating?

   a. not bothered at all
   b. bothers me a little
   c. moderately concerned
   d. a major concern

9. Which best describes your feelings during a binge?

   a. I feel that I could control the eating if I chose.
   b. I feel that I have at least some control.
   c. I feel completely out of control.

10. How often are you bothered by unwanted thoughts of food or eating?

    a. never
    b. occasionally
    c. frequently
    d. almost constantly

11. Which of the following best describes your feelings after a binge?

    a. I feel fairly neutral, not too concerned.
    b. I am moderately upset.
    c. I just hate myself.

12. Which best describes your binge-eating behavior?

    a. I will binge if other people are around.
    b. I will binge eat only if I am alone.
    c. I make sure no one knows I have been binge eating.

13. When you look at yourself without clothes in the mirror, what is your reaction?

    a. I feel I look pretty good.
    b. I am slightly dissatisfied with the way I look.
    c. I am very dissatisfied with the way I look.
    d. I am really disgusted with the way I look.
    e. I never look at myself in the mirror because I'm too self-conscious.

14. How often are you on a diet?

    a. rarely
    b. sometimes
    c. usually
    d. always

15. How often is binge eating associated with each of the following (circle all that apply)?

    a. pressure from school or work
    b. going off a strict diet
    c. problems in personal relationships
    d. can't say – doesn't really seem to be connected with anything

16. Which most accurately describes your feelings after a binge?

    a. not depressed at all
    b. mildly depressed
    c. moderately depressed
    d. very depressed

17. At what age did you begin binge eating?

    a. younger than 10 years old
    b. 11 to 15 years old
    c. 16 to 20 years old
    d. 21 or older

18. To which of the following places would you go to binge eat?

    a. home
    b. in the car
    c. a restaurant
    d. all of these
    e. no particular places

19. Which best describes your frame of mind when binge eating?

    a. really enjoy the experience
    b. don't really enjoy the food – don't know why I do it
    c. no particular thoughts or attitude
    d. other (please describe_____)

Chapter 11

Appendix 11.A BITE

Optional front data sheet

1. What is your sex?

   MALE 1   FEMALE 2   (*please circle number*)

2. Are you:

   MARRIED 1 SINGLE 2 DIVORCED 3 SEPARATED 4 WIDOWED 5

3. What is your occupation? _____

4. If married, what is your spouse's occupation? _____

5. What is your age? _____years

6. What is your height? _____feet _____inches, or _____cm

7. What is your weight? _____stone _____pounds, or _____kg

8. What is the most that you have ever weighed?   _____stone _____pounds, or _____kg

9. What is the least that you have weighed at your present height? _____stone _____pounds, or _____kg

10. What would your ideal weight be if you could choose it? _____stone _____pounds, or _____kg

11. Do you consider yourself to be

VERY OVERWEIGHT	5
OVERWEIGHT	4 (*please*
AVERAGE	3 *circle*
UNDERWEIGHT	2 *number)*
VERY UNDERWEIGHT	1

12. Do you have regular periods? (if applicable)   YES 1   NO 2

13. How often, on average, do you eat the following meals? (*circle number*)

	EVERYDAY	5/7 DAYS	3/7 DAYS	1/7 DAYS	NEVER
BREAKFAST	1	2	3	4	5
LUNCH	1	2	3	4	5
DINNER	1	2	3	4	5
BETWEEN MEAL SNACKS	1	2	3	4	5

14. Have you ever consulted someone in a professional capacity for advice on dieting/eating?

    YES 1 NO 2

15. Have you ever been a member of a slimming club?

    YES 1 NO 2

16. Have you ever suffered from any type of eating disorder?

    YES 1 NO 2

    …………if yes, please give details over:

Bulimia Investigatory Test, Edinburgh

1. Do you have a regular daily eating pattern?

   YES   NO

2. Are you a strict dieter?

   YES   NO

3. Do you feel a failure if you break your diet once?

   YES   NO

4. Do you count calories of everything you eat, even when not on a diet?

   YES   NO

5. Do you ever fast for a whole day?

   YES   NO

6. If yes, how often is this?

   EVERY SECOND DAY 5   2-3 TIMES A WEEK 4

   ONCE A WEEK   3   NOW AND THEN   2   HAVE ONCE 1

7. Do you do any of the following to help you lose weight? *(circle number)*

	Never	Occasionally	Once a Week	2-3 Times Week	Daily	2-3 Times a Day	5+ Times a Day
TAKE DIET PILLS	0	2	3	4	5	6	7
TAKE DIURETICS	0	2	3	4	5	6	7
TAKE LAXATIVES	0	2	3	4	5	6	7
MAKE YOURSELF VOMIT	0	2	3	4	5	6	7

8. Does your pattern of eating severely disrupt your life?

   YES   NO

9. Would you say that food dominates your life?

   YES   NO

10. Do you ever eat and eat until you are stopped by physical discomfort?

    YES   NO

11. Are there times when all you can think about is food?

    YES   NO

12. Do you eat sensibly in front of others and make up in private?

    YES   NO

13. Can you always stop eating when you want to?

    YES   NO

14. Do you ever experience *overpowering* urges to eat and eat and eat?

    YES   NO

15. When you are feeling anxious do you tend to eat a lot?

    YES   NO

16. Does the thought of becoming fat *terrify* you?

    YES   NO

17. Do you ever eat large amounts of food rapidly (not a meal)?

    YES   NO

18. Are you ashamed of your eating habits?

    YES   NO

19. Do you worry that you have no control over how much you eat?

    YES   NO

20. Do you turn to food for comfort?

    YES   NO

21. Are you able to leave food on the plate at the end of a meal?

    YES   NO

22. Do you deceive other people about how much you eat?

    YES   NO

23. Does how hungry you feel determine how much you eat?

    YES   NO

24. Do you ever binge on large amounts of food?

    YES   NO

25. If yes, do such binges leave you feeling miserable?

    YES   NO

26. If you do binge, is this only when you are alone?

    YES   NO

27. If you do binge, how often is this?

    HARDLY EVER 1   ONCE A MONTH   2
    ONCE A WEEK 3   2-3 TIMES A WEEK 4
    DAILY   5   2-3 TIMES A DAY   6

28. Would you go to great lengths to satisfy an urge to binge?

    YES   NO

29. If you overeat, do you feel *very* guilty?

    YES   NO

30. Do you ever eat in secret?

    YES   NO

31. Are your eating habits what you would consider to be normal?

    YES   NO

32. Would you consider yourself to be a compulsive eater?

    YES   NO

33. Does your weight fluctuate by more than 5 pounds in a week?

    YES   NO

SOURCE: Used with permission of Dr. Chris Freeman.

Appendix 11.B BULIT-R

Answer each question by filling in the appropriate circle on the computer answer sheet. Please respond to each item as honestly as possible; remember all of the information you provide will be kept strictly confidential.

1. I am satisfied with my eating patterns.

    1. agree
    2. neutral
    3. disagree a little
    4. disagree
    5. disagree strongly

2. Would you presently call yourself a "binge eater"?

    1. yes, absolutely
    2. yes
    3. yes, probably
    4. yes, possibly
    5. no, probably not

3. Do you feel you have control over the amount of food you consume?

    1. most or all of the time
    2. a lot of the time
    3. occasionally
    4. rarely
    5. never

4. I am satisfied with the shape and size of my body.
   1. frequently or always
   2. sometimes
   3. occasionally
   4. rarely
   5. seldom or never

5. When I feel that my eating behavior is out of control, I try to take rather extreme measures to get back on course (strict dieting, fasting, laxatives, diuretics, self-induced vomiting, or vigorous exercise).
   1. always
   2. almost always
   3. frequently
   4. sometimes
   5. never or my eating behavior is never out of control

6. I use laxatives or suppositories to help control my weight.
   1. once a day or more
   2. 3-6 times a week
   3. once or twice a week
   4. 2-3 times a month
   5. once a month or less (never)

7. I am obsessed about the size and shape of my body.
   1. always
   2. almost always
   3. frequently
   4. sometimes
   5. seldom or never

8. There are times when I rapidly eat a very large amount of food.
   1. more than twice a week
   2. twice a week
   3. once a week
   4. 2–3 times a month
   5. once a month or less (or never)

9. How long have you been binge eating (eating uncontrollably to the point of stuffing yourself)?
   1. not applicable; I don't binge eat
   2. less than 3 months
   3. 3 months–1 year
   4. 1–3 years
   5. 3 or more years

10. Most people I know would be amazed if they knew how much food I can consume at one sitting.
   1. without a doubt
   2. very probably
   3. probably
   4. possibly
   5. no

11. I exercise in order to burn calories.

    1. more than 2 hours per day
    2. about 2 hours per day
    3. more than 1 but less than 2 hours per day
    4. one hour or less per day
    5. I exercise but not to burn calories or I don't exercise

12. Compared with women your age, how preoccupied are you about your weight and body shape?

    1. a great deal more than average
    2. much more than average
    3. more than average
    4. a little more than average
    5. average or less than average

13. I am afraid to eat anything for fear that I won't be able to stop.

    1. always
    2. almost always
    3. frequently
    4. sometimes
    5. seldom or never

14. I feel tormented by the idea that I am fat or might gain weight.

    1. always
    2. almost always
    3. frequently
    4. sometimes
    5. seldom or never

15. How often do you intentionally vomit after eating?

    1. 2 or more times a week
    2. once a week
    3. 2–3 times a month
    4. once a month
    5. less than once a month or never

16. I eat a lot of food when I'm not even hungry.

    1. very frequently
    2. frequently
    3. occasionally
    4. sometimes
    5. seldom or never

17. My eating patterns are different from the eating patterns of most people.

    1. always
    2. almost always
    3. frequently
    4. sometimes
    5. seldom or never

18. After I binge eat I turn to one of several strict methods to try to keep from gaining weight (vigorous exercise, strict dieting, fasting, self-induce vomiting, laxatives, or diuretics).
    1. never or I don't binge eat
    2. rarely
    3. occasionally
    4. a lot of the time
    5. most or all of the time

19. I have tried to lose weight by fasting or going on strict diets.
    1. not in the past year
    2. once in the past year
    3. 2–3 times in the past year
    4. 4–5 times in the past year
    5. more than 5 times in the past year

20. I exercise vigorously and for long periods of time in order to burn calories.
    1. average or less than average
    2. a little more than average
    3. more than average
    4. much more than average
    5. a great deal more than average

21. When engaged in an eating binge, I tend to eat foods that are high in carbohydrates (sweets and starches).
    1. always
    2. almost always
    3. frequently
    4. sometimes
    5. seldom, or I don't binge

22. Compared to most people, my ability to control my eating behavior seems to be:
    1. greater than others' ability
    2. about the same
    3. less
    4. much less
    5. I have absolutely no control

23. I would presently label myself a "compulsive eater" (one who engages in episodes of uncontrolled eating).
    1. absolutely
    2. yes
    3. yes, probably
    4. yes, possibly
    5. no, probably not

24. I hate the way my body looks after I eat too much.
    1. seldom or never
    2. sometimes
    3. frequently
    4. almost always
    5. always

25. When I am trying to keep from gaining weight, I feel that I have to resort to vigorous exercise, strict dieting, fasting, self-induced vomiting, laxatives, or diuretics.

    1. never
    2. rarely
    3. occasionally
    4. a lot of the time
    5. most or all of the time

26. Do you believe that it is easier for you to vomit than it is for most people?

    1. yes, it's no problem at all for me
    2. yes, it's easier
    3. yes, it's a little easier
    4. about the same
    5. no, it's less easy

27. I use diuretics (water pills) to help control my weight.

    1. never
    2. seldom
    3. sometimes
    4. frequently
    5. very frequently

28. I feel that food controls my life.

    1. always
    2. almost always
    3. frequently
    4. sometimes
    5. seldom or never

29. I try to control my weight by eating little or no food for a day or longer.

    1. never
    2. seldom
    3. sometimes
    4. frequently
    5. very frequently

30. When consuming a large quantity of food, at what speed do you usually eat?

    1. more rapidly than most people have ever eaten in their lives
    2. a lot more rapidly than most people
    3. a little more rapidly than most people
    4. about the same rate as most people
    5. more slowly than most people (or not applicable)

31. I use laxatives or suppositories to help control my weight.

    1. never
    2. seldom
    3. sometimes
    4. frequently
    5. very frequently

32. Right after I binge eat I feel:

    1. so fat and bloated I can't stand it
    2. extremely fat
    3. fat
    4. a little fat
    5. OK about how my body looks or I never binge eat

33. Compared to other people of my sex, my ability to always feel in control of how much I eat is:

    1. about the same or greater
    2. a little less
    3. less
    4. much less
    5. a great deal less

34. In the last 3 months, on the average how often did you binge eat (eat uncontrollably to the point of stuffing yourself)?

    1. once a month or less (or never)
    2. 2–3 times a month
    3. once a week
    4. twice a week
    5. more than twice a week

35. Most people I know would be surprised about how fat I look after I eat a lot of food.

    1. yes, definitely
    2. yes
    3. yes, probably
    4. yes, possibly
    5. no, probably not or I never eat a lot of food

36. I use diuretics (water pills) to help control my weight.

    1. 3 times a week or more
    2. once or twice a week
    3. 2–3 times a month
    4. once a month
    5. never

SOURCE: Used with permission of Dr. Mark H. Thelan, University of Missouri. Contact rights holder for purchase for use.

Appendix 11.C Eating Attitudes Test–26 (EAT-26)

Please check a response for each of the following questions						
	Always	Usually	Often	Sometimes	Rarely	Never
1. Am terrified about being overweight.	O	O	O	O	O	O
2. Avoid eating when I am hungry.	O	O	O	O	O	O

Please check a response for each of the following questions	Always	Usually	Often	Sometimes	Rarely	Never
3. Find myself preoccupied with food.	O	O	O	O	O	O
4. Have gone on eating binges where I feel I may not be able to stop.	O	O	O	O	O	O
5. Cut my food into small pieces.	O	O	O	O	O	O
6. Aware of calorie content of foods that I eat.	O	O	O	O	O	O
7. Particularly avoid food with a high carbohydrate content (i.e., bread, rice, potatoes, etc.)	O	O	O	O	O	O
8. Feel that others would prefer if I ate more.	O	O	O	O	O	O
9. Vomit after I have eaten.	O	O	O	O	O	O
10. Feel extremely guilty after eating.	O	O	O	O	O	O
11. Am preoccupied with a desire to be thinner.	O	O	O	O	O	O
12. Think about burning calories when I am exercising.	O	O	O	O	O	O
13. Other people think that I am too thin.	O	O	O	O	O	O
14. Am preoccupied with the thought of having fat on my body.	O	O	O	O	O	O
15. Take longer than others to eat my meals.	O	O	O	O	O	O
16. Avoid foods with sugar in them.	O	O	O	O	O	O
17. Eat diet foods.	O	O	O	O	O	O
18. Feel that food controls my life.	O	O	O	O	O	O
19. Display self-control around food.	O	O	O	O	O	O
20. Feel that others pressure me to eat.	O	O	O	O	O	O
21. Give too much time and thought to food.	O	O	O	O	O	O

Appendix 11.C (Continued)

Please check a response for each of the following questions						
	Always	Usually	Often	Sometimes	Rarely	Never
22. Feel uncomfortable after eating sweets.	O	O	O	O	O	O
23. Engage in dieting behaviors.	O	O	O	O	O	O
24. Like my stomach to be empty.	O	O	O	O	O	O
25. Enjoy trying new rich foods.	O	O	O	O	O	O
26. Have the impulse to vomit after eating.	O	O	O	O	O	O

SOURCE: Garner, D. M., Olsted, M. P., Bohr, Y., & Garfinkel, P. E. (1982), *Psychological Medicine*, 12. Used with permission.

Appendix 11.D Interview for Diagnosis of Eating Disorders-IV (IDED-IV)

Section 1: Demographic Information

DATE: _____

NAME: _____

AGE: _____ RACE: _____

DATE OF BIRTH _____

HEIGHT _____ WEIGHT _____

ADDRESS_____

HOME PHONE _____ WORK PHONE _____

(*If adolescent, ask for mother or father's occupations and education)

OCCUPATION _____ EDUCATION _____

SPOUSE'S OCCUPATION _____ SPOUSE EDUCATION _____

REFERRED BY _____

GENERAL PHYSICIAN _____

PSYCHIATRIST _____

THERAPIST(S) _____

MEDICATION (S) _____

    Prescription _____

    Nonprescription _____

INSURANCE _____

PREVIOUS TREATMENT

Professional / Affiliation	Treatment Period	Issues Addressed
1.	1.	1.
2.	2.	2.
3.	3.	3.
4.	4.	4.

Section 2: Detailed Instruction for Administering the IDED-IV

The IDED-IV begins with an overview section that follows the general structure of a clinical diagnostic interview. First, basic demographic information is obtained. This section is followed by an open-ended history of eating-disordered symptoms, a description of the chief complaint, and general questions about current functioning. Beginning with non-threatening demographic questions allows the interviewer and opportunity to establish rapport. The subject is then encouraged to describe the history of the present illness, which lays the groundwork for the more structured diagnostic sections that follow the overview. The overview concludes with general questions about current functioning which refocuses the subject on his or her current condition and provides a natural transition to the diagnostic sections. By the time the overview is completed, the interviewer should have obtained enough information to make a tentative differential diagnosis before systematically inquiring about specific symptoms in the diagnostic sections that follow.

The diagnostic sections each begin with a heading intended to cue the interviewer with regard to the DSM-IV diagnostic criterion being rated at the end of each set of questions. Ratings should be made based on subjects' responses to the questions that precede each diagnostic criterion. The majority of items are rated on a 5 point scale, on which either frequency or severity is rated. Ratings should be made as the interview proceeds (although the interviewer has the option to revise ratings if conflicting data are found later in the interview). A rating of 3 or more on each of the symptoms is the operational definition of that diagnostic symptom.

Due to the overlap in symptomatology across eating disorder diagnostic categories, some ratings have been replaced with instructions for transferring information to the diagnostic checklist found at the end of the interview schedule. In order to reduce redundancy in the interview's content and any related inconvenience to the subject, the interviewer is responsible for completing the diagnostic checklist according to the instructions provided throughout the interview and summarized within the diagnostic checklist. To promote the flow of the interview, it is recommended that transfer of information from the interview to the DSM-IV diagnostic checklist (located at the end of the interview protocol) be completed after the interview has been completed.

Please refer to the appendix for a decision-tree that can be used to translate symptom ratings into diagnoses using the DSM-IV criteria.

Section 3: Brief Instructions for Administering the IDED-IV

Interview the subject using each of the questions in the structured interview. Make note of the subject's answers. As you proceed with the interview, score each of the rating scales by circling the number of the description that best matches the subject's answers to your questions. If there is some doubt as to the best rating, you should ask additional questions to clarify your doubt. After completing the interview, use the eating disorder symptom checklists for the DSM-IV diagnostic criteria in order to establish a diagnosis. A rating of 3 or more on each of the symptoms is the operational definition for concluding that the person has endorsed the presence of the diagnostic symptom.

Section 4: History of Eating Disorder Symptoms

In order to understand the course of your weight and eating problems since early childhood, we will review the ages at which you experienced significant weight changes, and any life events that may have affected your eating pattern.

(To complete the table below, ask each of the following questions for each development period listed in the table. For example, begin with):

a. "During your childhood years, what weight changes did you experience?" (Note significant ages, and overall highest and lowest adult weight.)
b. "What life events may have affected these weight changes?"
c. "How did these life events affect your eating pattern?"

Period	Age/Weight	Life Events	Effects on Eating
Childhood (Birth–12 yrs)			
Adolescence (12–19 yrs)			
Young Adulthood (20–34 yrs)			

Period	Age/Weight	Life Events	Effects on Eating

Middle Adulthood
(35–49 yrs)

_____

Late Adulthood
(50 yrs & older)

_____

Section 5: Current Status of Eating Disorder Symptoms

A. Eating Pattern

1. What are your current concerns regarding your eating and your weight?

2. Would you describe an example of the types and amounts of foods you might eat in a typical day? While dieting?

	Typical Day	While Dieting

Breakfast:

Snack:

Lunch:

Snack:

Dinner:

Snack:

B. Medical Problems

1. Have you had any medical problems?

   Y   N   (Check for dizziness, LBP, HBP, thyroid problems, diabetes.)

2. Have you had any dental problems?

   Y   N   (e.g., tooth erosion)   (If yes, describe.)

C. Family Information

1. How many members are there in your household?

2. Do they know about your eating problems?

   Y   N   (If yes, how do they react/feel about your eating disorder?)

3. Who would be available to participate in your treatment?

4. Has anyone in your family had an eating disorder? Weight problems? Obesity?

     (If yes, describe.)

5. Has anyone in your family experienced psychiatric problems?

     (If yes, describe.)

Section 6: Questions for the Diagnosis of Anorexia Nervosa

Prior to the interview, the subject's height and weight should be measured and recorded on the front sheet of the IDED-IV. We have generally converted height and weight into body mass index (weight (Kg)/height (m)^2). We selected a BMI less than 18 as the criterion for maintaining a body weight that is 15% below normal.

A. Refusal to Maintain Normal Body Weight

1. Do you currently go periods of time without eating (starvation) to control your weight?

   Y   N   (If yes, describe.)

2. When did you first begin to lose weight by restricting your eating?

3. Are there any factors/situations which seem to <u>increase</u> your periods of restrictive eating?

4. Are there any factors/situations which seem to <u>decrease</u> your periods of restrictive eating?

5. What is your goal weight?

(Rating of 3 or higher meets criterion.)

A. Refusal to Maintain Appropriate Weight for Height (you may use height/weight charts to assist in making this rating)
   1. Weight is less than 9% below normal/or is normal or above normal
   2. Maintains weight that is 9 to 14% below normal
   3. Maintains weight that is 15 to 20% below normal
   4. Maintains weight that is 21 to 26% below normal
   5. Weight is greater than 26% below normal weight

B. Fear of Weight Gain
   1. Do you feel that your weight is normal?

      Y   N   (Describe.)

   2. How often do you weigh yourself?

   3. What emotional reaction would you have if you gained

   2 lbs?
   5 lbs?
   10 lbs?

(Rating of 3 or higher meets criterion.)

B. Intense Fear of Weight Gain
   1. Minimal fear
   2. Moderate fear

3. Intense fear
4. Extreme fear
5. Debilitating fear

C. Disturbance of Body Image
1. Do you wish to be thinner than you are now?

Y   N   (If yes, ask what body areas should be thinner.)

2. Do you think or worry a lot about your weight and body size?

Y   N   (Describe.)

3. Do you ever feel fat?

Y   N   (If yes, ask when do you feel fat?)

(Rating of 3 or higher meets criterion.)

C. Disturbance of Body Image
1. Body image disturbance: Feels "fat" even if not significantly overweight
1. Never or not applicable*
2. Sometimes
3. Often
4. Very often
5. All of the time

*For obese persons who feel fat, the rating of one is often most appropriate.

4. How often does your body size affect the way you feel about yourself?

(Rating of 3 or higher meets criterion.)

C. Disturbance of Body Image
2. Undue influence of body weight/shape on self-evaluation
1. Minimal influence
2. Influenced some of the time
3. Influenced most of the time

4. Influenced almost all of the time

5. Influenced all of the time

5. Do you feel that your current weight is creating any problems for you? (e.g., medical, emotional, family)

(Rating of 3 or higher meets criterion.)

C. Disturbance of Body Image

3. Denial of seriousness of current low body weight

1. No denial or not applicable

2. Some denial

3. Moderate denial

4. Strong denial

5. Extreme denial

D. Menstrual Irregularities

1. When was your last menstrual period?

2. Have you experienced any menstrual irregularities (skipped period, lighter flow, shorter number of days)?

Y   N   (If yes, describe type of irregularity and for how long.)

3. If yes, are there any medical reasons for these menstrual irregularities? (Describe.)

4. Are you taking any hormonal medication (e.g., birth control pills, estrogen)?

Y   N   (If yes, ask how long have you been taking this medication?)

5. Have you found that your menstrual periods cease when you stop taking birth control pills or hormone replacement medication?

Y   N   (Describe.)

6. For how many consecutive months have you not had your menstrual period?

(Rating of 3 or higher meets criterion.)

E. Amenorrhea

1. Very regular/N/A if male/medical reasons
2. Missed 1 or 2 cycles in past 3 months
3. Missed 3 consecutive cycles in past 3 months
4. Missed 4 or 5 consecutive cycles in past 5 months
5. Missed 6 or more consecutive cycles

Section 7: Questions for Binge Eating Disorder

A. Binge Eating (Recurrent Episodes)

1. Do you ever binge (rapidly consume a large amount of food in a discrete period of time)?

   Y   N

2. What kind of foods do you eat during a binge and how much?

3. Do you ever feel as though you have overeaten when you eat small portions of certain fattening foods?

   Y   N   (Describe.)

4. When do your binge eating episodes occur?

   (during meals, after meals, throughout day, etc.)

5. How long does each binge usually last?

(Rating of 3 or higher meets criterion.)

A. Recurrent Episodes of Binge Eating

1. Eating a large amount of food in a discrete period of time
   1. Doesn't binge
   2. Amount of binge food is average for meals and snacks
   3. Amount of binge food is typically larger than normal
   4. Amount of binge food is very large for almost every binge
   5. Amount of food is enormous for almost every binge

A. Binge Eating (Loss of Control)

  1. Do you feel you can stop eating once a binge has begun?

     Y   N   (Describe.)

  2. How often do you feel out of control of your eating during a binge?

(Rating of 3 or more meets criterion.)

A. Recurrent Binge Eating Episodes

  2. Feeling of loss of control of eating during a binge
    1. Always in control
    2. Occasional loss of control
    3. Frequent loss of control
    4. Almost always out of control
    5. Never in control

B. Behavioral Indicators

  1. When binge eating, do you feel your eating is more rapid than normal?

     Y   N   (Describe.)

(Rating of 3 or higher meets criterion.)

B. Behavioral Indicator

  1. Rapid eating during binges
    1. Doesn't binge
    2. Eating pace is reasonable
    3. Eating is much more rapid than average
    4. Eating pace is frantic
    5. Eating can be described as gorging

  2. When binge eating, how often do you eat enough to feel uncomfortably full?
                    (Describe.)

(Rating of 3 or higher meets criterion.)

B. Behavioral Indicator

   2. Eating until feeling uncomfortably full when bingeing
     1. Doesn't binge
     2. Usually eats until satisfied and then stops binge
     3. Feels uncomfortably full after 50% to 75% of binges
     4. Feels uncomfortably full after 75% to 95% of binges
     5. Always feels uncomfortably full after binges

   3. How often do you eat large amounts of food when you don't really feel hungry? (Describe.)

(Rating of 3 or higher meets criterion.)

B. Behavioral Indicator

   3. Eating large amounts of food when not hungry
     1. Seldom eats when not hungry
     2. 1–7 days/month
     3. 2 days–week
     4. 2–6 days/week
     5. At least once/day

---

   4. How often do you binge alone, or in a secret? Why? (Check for embarrassment.)

(Rating of 3 or higher meets criterion.)

B. Behavior Indicator

   4. Eating alone while bingeing due to embarrassment
     1. No binge eating
     2. Overeats or binges with friends or family
     3. Rarely binges with anyone else present
     4. Binges only when alone
     5. Binges and eats meals only when alone

---

   5. Are there any factors that appear to <u>increase</u> the frequency of your binge eating?

6. Are there any factors that appear to <u>decrease</u> the frequency of your binge eating?

7. What emotions do you typically experience before, during, and after a binge? (check for disgust, depression, guilt)

a. Before

b. During

c. After

(Rating of 3 or higher meets criterion.)

B   Behavioral Indicator
  5. Negative affect (disgusted, depression, very guilty) after binge eating
    1. Doesn't binge
    2. Minimal negative affect post-binge
    3. Moderate negative affect post-binge
    4. Severe negative affect post-binge
    5. Debilitating negative affect post-binge

C. Marked Distress
  1. How distressed are you about binge eating or the struggle to avoid binge eating?

(Rating of 3 or higher meets criterion.)

C. Distress Regarding Binge Eating
    1. Doesn't binge
    2. Mild distress

3. Marked distress
4. Severe distress
5. Debilitating distress

D. Frequency of Binge Eating

1. On average, how frequently do you binge, and how long have you been bingeing at that rate?

	Frequency	Time Frame
a. Per day?		
b. Per week?		
c. Per month?		

2. How long have you been bingeing at least two days per week?

D. Frequency of Binge Eating

1. If individual bingeing two days a week or more, for 6 or more months, endorse Criterion D for binge eating disorder on the attached diagnostic checklist.

2. If individual bingeing two days per week or more, for 3 or more months, endorse Criterion C for Bulimia Nervosa on the attached diagnostic checklist.

E. To Meet the Criteria for Binge Eating Disorder, Patient Must Have Absence of:

1. Inappropriate Compensatory (1 or 2) Behavior

(Rating 1 for rating B (1, 2, 3, & 4) meets this criterion. Transfer value to diagnostic checklist, Criterion E for Binge Eating Disorder)

2. Bulimia Nervosa (derived from results of diagnostic checklist)

3. Anorexia Nervosa (derived from results of diagnostic checklist)

Section 8: Bulimia Nervosa

(To make rating see rating A (1).)

A. Recurring Binge Eating Episodes

1. Eating large amounts of food in a discrete period of time (approximately 2 hours)
   1. Doesn't binge
   2. Amount of food is average for meals and snacks
   3. Amount of food is typically larger than normal
   4. Amount of food is very large for almost every binge
   5. Amount of food is enormous for almost every binge

(To make rating see rating A (2))

A. Recurrent Binge Eating Episodes

2. Feeling of loss of control of eating during a binge
   1. Always in control
   2. Occasional loss of control
   3. Frequent loss of control
   4. Almost always out of control
   5. Never in control

B. Compensatory Behavior

1. Do you purge after meals or after a binge (vomit, abuse laxatives or diuretics)?

   Y   N

2. When did you first begin to purge?

3. Are there any factors that appear to <u>increase</u> the frequency of purging?

4. Are there any factors that appear to <u>decrease</u> the frequency of purging?

5. Do you purge by vomiting?

   Y   N

   (If yes, ask how often do you purge by vomiting?)

(Rating of 3 or higher meets criterion.)

B. Compensatory Behavior

1. Self-induced vomiting
   1. None
   2. Vomits a few times/year
   3. Vomits several times/month
   4. Vomits several times/week
   5. Vomits 1 or more times/day

6. Do you purge by using laxatives?

   Y   N

(If yes, ask what types and how often)

7. Do you purge by using diuretics (i.e., water pills)?

   Y   N

(If yes, ask what type and how often.)

(Rating of 3 or higher meets criterion.)

B. Compensatory Behavior

2. Laxative/diuretic abuse (an episode is defined as taking 1 or more pills during a short time interval to rid body of food)
   1. None
   2. A few times/year
   3. Several times/month
   4. Several times/week
   5. Several times/day

---

8. Do you often go on strict diets (rigid eating, skipping meals, eating virtually nothing on a given day)? (Describe)

9. Do you use pills to lose weight?

   Y   N

(If yes, ask what type and how often.)

10. When was the last time you took a diet pill?

11. How often do you engage in strict dieting?

(Rating of 3 or higher meets criterion.)

_____

B. Compensatory Behavior

  3. Dieting/fasting
      1. Never diet
      2. Diet occasionally
      3. Diet/fast about two days/week
      4. Diet/fast several days/week
      5. Fasts almost every day

  12. Do you engage in vigorous exercise to control your weight? (Intense
       exercise which is compulsive or obligatory from person's description
       aimed at ridding body of food/calories.)

       Y   N   (If yes, ask what type and how often.)

(Rating of 3 or higher meets criterion.)

_____

B. Compensatory Behavior

  3. Vigorous exercise (exercise which is compulsive or obligatory from per-
      son's description aimed at ridding body of food/calories)
      1. Exercises to promote health
      2. Exercises to lose weight
      3. Exercises to rid body of food/calories 2-4 days per week
      4. Exercises to rid body of food/calories 5-7 days per week
      5. Exercises more than once on most days

_____

C. Frequency of Binge Eating Over Past 3 Months

See individual's response to Criterion D, question 2. If individual meets criterion
indicate on diagnostic checklist (Criterion C).

_____

(To make rating see Rating C(2).)

_____

D. Undue Influence of Body Weight/Shape on Self-Evaluation
   1. Minimal influence
   2. Moderate influence
   3. Influenced most of the time
   4. Influenced almost all of the time
   5. Influenced all of the time

Section 9: Eating Disorder Not Otherwise Specified

A–C. For Eating Disorder Not Otherwise Specified categories 1, 2, 3, see instructions for each category.

D. Purging Small Amounts of Food

   1. Do you ever purge (i.e., vomit, use laxatives/diuretics, exercise excessively) after eating small amounts of food (e.g., two cookies)?

      Y   N   (Describe.)

   2. If yes, how often do you purge small amounts of food, and for how long have you engaged in this behavior?

(If patient is normal weight, response to question A1 is "yes", and response to question A2 is "at least two days per week, for at least 3 months", endorse ED NOS eating pattern number 4.)

E. Tasting

   1. Have you ever attempted to control your weight by chewing, spitting out, and not swallowing large amounts of food?   Y   N (Describe.)

   2. If yes, how often do you purge small amounts of food, and for how long have you engaged in this type of behavior?

(If response to question B1 is "yes," and response to question B2 is "a least two days per week, for at least 3 months," endorse ED NOS eating pattern number 5.)

Section 10: Other Eating Problems

A. Night Bingeing

   1. Do you have a problem with binge eating primarily late in the evening?

      Y   N   (Describe.)

2. Do you awaken and binge during the night? Y   N (Describe.)

3. When bingeing during the evening, do you find yourself in a conscious or semi-conscious state? (Describe.)

4. How often do you binge at night, and for how long has this been a problem for you?

(If response to question A1 OR A2 is "yes," and response to question A4 is "at least two days per week, for at least 3 months" endorse Night Bingeing.)

Section 11: Diagnostic Checklists for the Eating Disorders

To derive the relevant eating disorder diagnoses, detach the following checklists, and review the ratings made within the IDED-IV interview. Check each criterion rated 3 or more on the rating scale pertaining to each symptom, and/or see special instructions where noted.

307.10 Anorexia Nervosa

_____ A. Refusal to maintain body weight at or above a minimally normal weight for age and height (e.g., weight loss leading to maintenance of body weight less than 85% of that expected; or failure to make expected weight gain during periods of growth, leading to body weight less than 85% of that expected).

_____ B. Intense fear of gaining weight or becoming fat, even though underweight.

_____ C. Disturbance in the way in which one's body weight or shape is experienced; undue influence of body weight or shape on self-evaluation, or denial of the seriousness of the current low body weight.

_____ D. In post-menarcheal females, amenorrhea, i.e., the absence of at least three consecutive menstrual periods. (A woman is considered to have amenorrhea if her periods occur only following hormone, e.g., estrogen, administration.)

(**Meets this criterion if rating 3 or higher for rating D, OR if "yes" response to question 5.)

Specify type:

(If person meets criteria for Anorexia Nervosa, check the type which is most descriptive.)

_____ Restricting type: During the episode of Anorexia Nervosa, the person does not regularly engage in binge eating or purging behavior (i.e., self-induced vomiting or the misuse of laxatives or diuretics).

(**Look for rating of 2 or lower on Ratings A1 and A2 AND on Ratings B1 and B2.)

_____ Binge Eating/Purging type: During the episode of Anorexia Nervosa, the person regularly engages in binge eating or purging behavior (i.e., self-induced vomiting or the misuse of laxatives or diuretics).

(**Look for rating of 3 or more on Ratings A1 and A2 OR on Ratings B1 and B2.)

Binge Eating Disorder

(Check symptoms that were rated 3 or more on the rating scales pertaining to each symptom. **See special instructions where noted.)

_____ A. Recurrent episodes of binge eating. An episode of binge eating is characterized by both of the following:

_____ (1) eating, in a discrete period of time (e.g., within any 2 hour period), an amount of food that is definitely larger than most people would eat during a similar period of time under similar circumstances, and,

_____ (2) a sense of lack of control over eating during the episode (e.g., a feeling that one cannot stop eating or control what or how much one is eating).

_____ B. The binge eating episodes are associated with at least three of the following:

_____(1) eating much more rapidly than normal;

_____(2) eating until feeling uncomfortably full;

_____(3) eating large amounts of food when not feeling physically hungry;

_____(4) eating alone because of being embarrassed by how much one is eating;

_____(5) feeling disgusted with oneself, depressed, or very guilty after overeating.

_____ C. Marked distress regarding binge eating.

_____ D. The binge eating occurs, on average, at least 2 days a week for 6 months.

(**To endorse criterion, see response to question D1.)

_____ E. The binge eating is not associated with the use of inappropriate compensatory behaviors (e.g., purging, fasting, excessive exercise), and does not occur exclusively during the course of Anorexia Nervosa or Bulimia Nervosa.

(**To meet criterion, look for rating of 1 for Ratings B (1, 2, 3, AND 4). In addition, see checklist to determine whether criteria for Anorexia Nervosa and Bulimia Nervosa have been met.)

307.51 Bulimia Nervosa

(Check symptoms that were rated 3 or more on the rating scales pertaining to each symptom. **See special instructions where noted.)

_____ A. Recurrent episodes of binge eating. An episode of binge eating is characterized by both of the following:

(Meets criteria, if (1) & (2) below were rated 3 or more.)

_____ (1) eating, in a discrete period of time (e.g., within any 2 hour period), an amount of food that is definitely larger than most people would eat during a similar period of time and under similar circumstances, and,

(**Rating of 3 or higher on Rating A (1) meets criterion.)

_____ (2) a sense of lack of control over eating during the episode (e.g., a feeling that one cannot stop eating or control what or how much one is eating.)

(**Rating of 3 or higher on Rating A (2) meets criterion.)

_____ B. Recurrent inappropriate compensatory behavior in order to prevent weight gain, such as: self-induced vomiting; misuse of laxatives, diuretics, or other medications; fasting; or excessive exercise.

(**Rating of 3 or higher on Ratings B (1, 2, 3, OR 4) meets criterion.)

_____ C. The binge eating and inappropriate compensatory behaviors both occur, on average, at least 2 days per week for 3 months.

(**See response to Criterion D2.)

_____ D. Self-evaluation is unduly influenced by body shape and weight.

(**Rating of 3 or higher on Rating C (2), meets criterion.)

_____ E. The disturbance does not occur exclusively during episodes of Anorexia Nervosa.

(**See results of diagnostic checklists.)

Specify type:

(If the person meets criteria for Bulimia Nervosa, check the type which is most descriptive.)

_____ Purging type: the person regularly engages in self-induced vomiting or the misuse of laxatives or diuretics.

(**Look for rating of 3 or higher on Rating B (1), OR Rating B(2).)

_____ Nonpurging type: the person uses other inappropriate compensatory behaviors such as fasting or excessive exercise, but does not regularly engage in self-induced vomiting or the misuse of laxatives or diuretics.

(**Look for rating of 3 or higher on Rating B (3) and Rating B (4) AND rating of 2 or less on on Rating B (1) and, Rating B (2).)

307.50 Eating Disorder Not Otherwise Specified (ED NOS)

If the subject does not meet the criteria for a diagnosis of anorexia nervosa, bulimia nervosa, or binge eating disorder, determine whether any of the following descriptions of Eating Disorders NOS apply.

This category is for disorders of eating that do not meet the criteria for any specific Eating Disorder. Examples include:

_____ (1) all of the criteria for Anorexia Nervosa are met except the individual has regular menses

_____ (2) all of the criteria for Anorexia Nervosa are met except that, despite significant weight loss, the individual's current weight is in the normal range

_____ (3) all the criteria for Bulimia Nervosa are met except binges occur at a frequency of less than twice a week or for the duration of less than three months

_____ (4) an individual of normal body weight who regularly engages in inappropriate compensatory behavior after eating a small amount of food (e.g., self-induced vomiting after the consumption of two cookies).

(**Meets criterion if response to question D1 is "yes" and response to D2 is "for at least 2 days per week, for at least 3 months", and individual is of normal weight.)

Other Eating Problems:

_____ Night Eating: an individual who binges late in the evening, or awakens repeatedly to binge, while in either a conscious or semi-conscious state.

(**Meets criterion if response to question A1 or A2 is "yes" and response to A4 is "for at least two days per week, for at least 3 months".)

Criteria

A) 15% below average body weight of greater	Yes	No (e.g., but significant weight loss)	Yes	Yes	Yes
B) fear weight gain	Yes	Yes	No (e.g., denial of fear of weight gain)	Yes	Yes
C) body image disturbance	Yes	Yes	Yes	No (e.g., recognizes underweight)	Yes
D) amenorrhea	Yes	Yes	Yes	Yes	No (has menses)

**ED NOS
Subclinical Anorexia
Nervosa**

ED NOS Type 1

ED NOS Type 2

Anorexia Nervosa

**ED NOS
Subclinical
Anorexia Nervosa**

Figure 1   Decision Tree for Making DSM-IV Anorexia Nervosa Diagnosis and Its Subclinical Variations Subsumed Under Eating Disorders Not Otherwise Specified (ED NOS)

SOURCE: Used with permission of Dr. Donald Williamson.

Appendix 11.E Multifactorial Assessment of Eating Disorder Symptoms (Revised 10/94)

Name: _____

Date: _____

Instructions: Using the scale below, please rate the following items on a scale from 1 to 7. Please answer as truthfully as possible.

1 = never
2 = very rarely

3 = rarely
4 = sometimes
5 = often
6 = very often
7 = always

1-----------2------------3------------4------------5------------6------------7
Never   Very Rarely   Rarely   Sometimes   Often   Very Often   Always

1. Fasting is a good way to lose weight.
      1   2   3   4   5   6   7

2. My sleep isn't as good as it used to be.
      1   2   3   4   5   6   7

3. I avoid eating for as long as I can.
      1   2   3   4   5   6   7

4. Certain foods are "forbidden" for me to eat.
      1   2   3   4   5   6   7

5. I can't keep certain foods in my house because I will binge on them.
      1   2   3   4   5   6   7

6. I can easily make myself vomit.
      1   2   3   4   5   6   7

7. I feel that being fat is terrible.
      1   2   3   4   5   6   7

8. I avoid greasy foods.
      1   2   3   4   5   6   7

9. It's okay to binge and purge once in a while.
      1   2   3   4   5   6   7

10. I don't eat certain foods.
      1   2   3   4   5   6   7

11. I think I am a good person.
      1   2   3   4   5   6   7

12. My eating is normal.
      1   2   3   4   5   6   7

13. I can't seem to concentrate lately.
      1   2   3   4   5   6   7

14. I try to diet by fasting.
      1   2   3   4   5   6   7

15. I vomit to control my weight.
      1   2   3   4   5   6   7

16. Lately nothing seems enjoyable anymore.
    1   2   3   4   5   6   7

17. Laxatives help keep you slim.
    1   2   3   4   5   6   7

18. I don't eat red meat.
    1   2   3   4   5   6   7

19. I eat so rapidly I can't even taste my food.
    1   2   3   4   5   6   7

20. I do everything I can to avoid being overweight.
    1   2   3   4   5   6   7

21. When I feel bloated, I must do something to rid myself of that feeling.
    1   2   3   4   5   6   7

22. I overeat too frequently.
    1   2   3   4   5   6   7

23. It's okay to be overweight.
    1   2   3   4   5   6   7

24. Recently I have felt that I am a worthless person.
    1   2   3   4   5   6   7

25. I would be very upset if I gained 2 pounds.
    1   2   3   4   5   6   7

26. I crave sweets and carbohydrates.
    1   2   3   4   5   6   7

27. I lose control when I eat.
    1   2   3   4   5   6   7

28. Being fat would be terrible.
    1   2   3   4   5   6   7

29. I have thought seriously about suicide lately.
    1   2   3   4   5   6   7

30. I don't have any energy anymore.
    1   2   3   4   5   6   7

31. I eat small portions to control my weight.
    1   2   3   4   5   6   7

32. I eat 3 meals a day.
    1   2   3   4   5   6   7

33. Lately I have been easily irritated.
    1   2   3   4   5   6   7

34. Some food should be totally avoided.
    1   2   3   4   5   6   7

35. I use laxatives to control my weight.

    1   2   3   4   5   6   7

36. I am terrified by the thought of being overweight.

    1   2   3   4   5   6   7

37. Purging is a good way to lose weight.

    1   2   3   4   5   6   7

38. I avoid fatty foods.

    1   2   3   4   5   6   7

39. Recently I have felt pretty blue.

    1   2   3   4   5   6   7

40. I am obsessed with becoming overweight.

    1   2   3   4   5   6   7

41. I don't eat fried foods.

    1   2   3   4   5   6   7

42. I skip meals.

    1   2   3   4   5   6   7

43. Fat people are unhappy.

    1   2   3   4   5   6   7

44. People are too concerned with the way I eat.

    1   2   3   4   5   6   7

45. I feel good when I skip meals.

    1   2   3   4   5   6   7

46. I avoid foods with sugar.

    1   2   3   4   5   6   7

47. I hate it when I feel fat.

    1   2   3   4   5   6   7

48. I am too fat.

    1   2   3   4   5   6   7

49. I eat until I am completely stuffed.

    1   2   3   4   5   6   7

50. I hate to eat.

    1   2   3   4   5   6   7

51. I feel guilty about a lot of things these days

    1   2   3   4   5   6   7

52. I'm very careful of what I eat.

    1   2   3   4   5   6   7

53. I can "hold off" and not eat even if I am hungry.

    1   2   3   4   5   6   7

54. I eat even when I am not hungry.

    1   2   3   4   5   6   7

55. Fat people are disgusting.

    1   2   3   4   5   6   7

56. I wouldn't mind gaining a few pounds.

    1   2   3   4   5   6   7

Appendix 11.F SCOFF

British Version

1. Do you ever make yourself **Sick** because you feel uncomfortably full?

2. Do you worry you have lost **Control** over how much you eat?

3. Have you recently lost more than **One** stone in a 3 month period?

4. Do you believe yourself to be **Fat** when others say you are too thin?

5. Would you say that **Food** dominates your life?

American Version

1. Do you make yourself **Sick** because you feel uncomfortably full?

2. Do you worry you have lost **Control** over how much you eat?

3. Do you believe yourself to be fat when **Others** say you are too thin?

4. Have you recently lost more than **Fourteen** pounds in a 3-month period?

5. Would you say that **Food** dominates your life?

SOURCE: Morgan, Reid, & Lacey (1999). Used with permission.

Chapter 12

Appendix 12.A GEMS Beverage Preferences Questionnaire

GEMS ID	Initials	Date of EvalUation	
☐☐☐☐☐	☐☐☐☐	☐☐ ☐☐ ☐☐☐☐	

Month   Day   Year

GEMS Food Preferences Questionnarie
December 18, 2000
Page 1 of 1

GEMS What Foods Do You Like?
(Food Preferences Questionnaire)

We would like to know how much you like the following drinks. Please put an "X" in the box below your response. The responses are: I do not like this; I like this a little; I like this a lot.

Drinks							
1. Soft drinks, regular, diet	I do not like this ☐	I like this a little ☐	I like this a lot ☐	**6. Snapple, diet, regular**	I do not like this ☐	I like this a little ☐	I like this a lot ☐
2. Koolaid, regular, diet	I do not like this ☐	I like this a little ☐	I like this a lot ☐	**7. Iced tea regular, diet**	I do not like this ☐	I like this a little ☐	I like this a lot ☐
3. Fruit drink	I do not like this ☐	I like this a little ☐	I like this a lot ☐	**8. Fruitopia**	I do not like this ☐	I like this a little ☐	I like this a lot ☐
4. Punch	I do not like this ☐	I like this a little ☐	I like this a lot ☐	**9. Sunny Delight**	I do not like this ☐	I like this a little ☐	I like this a lot ☐
5. Powerade/ Gatorade	I do not like this ☐	I like this a little ☐	I like this a lot ☐	**10. Capri Sun**	I do not like this ☐	I like this a little ☐	I like this a lot ☐
				11. Bottled Water	I do not like this ☐	I like this a little ☐	I like this a lot ☐

SOURCE: Accessed at http://www.bcm.edu/cnrc/faculty/Survey_documents/GEMSQnrs(01-02)/GIRLSFORMS/GEMS-BEV-P.pdf on 11/28/2007.

Appendix 12.B GEMS Fruit, Juice, and Vegetable Preference Questionnaire

GEMS ID	Initials	Date of Evaluation	BCM-GEMS FJV Prefer ?'naire

month   day   year

January 22 2001

Page 1 of 1

GEMS WHAT FOODS DO YOU LIKE?
(Food Preferences Questionnaire)

We would like to know how much you like the following foods. Please put an "X" in the box below your response. The responses are: I do not like this; I like this a little; I like this a lot.

Foods							
1. 100% Orange juice	I do not like this ☐	I like this a little ☐	I like this a lot ☐	**11. Plums**	I do not like this ☐	I like this a little ☐	I like this a lot ☐
2. 100% Apple juice	I do not like this ☐	I like this a little ☐	I like this a lot ☐	**12. Kiwi**	I do not like this ☐	I like this a little ☐	I like this a lot ☐
3. 100% Grape juice	I do not like this ☐	I like this a little ☐	I like this a lot ☐	**13. Strawberries**	I do not like this ☐	I like this a little ☐	I like this a lot ☐
4. Other 100% juice	I do not like this ☐	I like this a little ☐	I like this a lot ☐	**14. Pineapple**	I do not like this ☐	I like this a little ☐	I like this a lot ☐
5. Bananas	I do not like this ☐	I like this a little ☐	I like this a lot ☐	**15. Grapefruit**	I do not like this ☐	I like this a little ☐	I like this a lot ☐
6. Apples	I do not like this ☐	I like this a little ☐	I like this a lot ☐	**16. Fruit salad or Fruit cocktail**	I do not like this ☐	I like this a little ☐	I like this a lot ☐
7. Cantaloupe or Musk melon	I do not like this ☐	I like this a little ☐	I like this a lot ☐	**17. Applesauce**	I do not like this ☐	I like this a little ☐	I like this a lot ☐
8. Grapes	I do not like this ☐	I like this a little ☐	I like this a lot ☐	**18. Watermelon**	I do not like this ☐	I like this a little ☐	I like this a lot ☐
9. Oranges	I do not like this ☐	I like this a little ☐	I like this a lot ☐	**19. Raisins**	I do not like this ☐	I like this a little ☐	I like this a lot ☐
10. Pears	I do not like this ☐	I like this a little ☐	I like this a lot ☐	**20. Dried fruit**	I do not like this ☐	I like this a little ☐	I like this a lot ☐

SOURCE: Accessed at http://www.bcm.edu/cnrc/faculty/Survey_documents/GEMSQnrs(01-02)/GIRLSFORMS/GEMS-FJV-P.pdf on 11/28/2007.

Foods							
21. Peaches	I do not like this □	I like this a little □	I like this a lot □	**31. Tomatoes**	I do not like this □	I like this a little □	I like this a lot □
22. Carrots	I do not like this □	I like this a little □	I like this a lot □	**32. Broccoli**	I do not like this □	I like this a little □	I like this a lot □
23. Celery	I do not like this □	I like this a little □	I like this a lot □	**33. Lettuce**	I do not like this □	I like this a little □	I like this a lot □
24. Greens	I do not like this □	I like this a little □	I like this a lot □	**34. Green beans**	I do not like this □	I like this a little □	I like this a lot □
25. Spinach	I do not like this □	I like this a little □	I like this a lot □	**35. Cole slaw**	I do not like this □	I like this a little □	I like this a lot □
26. French fried potatotes	I do not like this □	I like this a little □	I like this a lot □	**36. Cooked beans (pinto, black eye peas, pork 'n beans)**	I do not like this □	I like this a little □	I like this a lot □
27. Potato salad	I do not like this □	I like this a little □	I like this a lot □	**37. Sweet potatoes**	I do not like this □	I like this a little □	I like this a lot □
28. Other white potatoes	I do not like this □	I like this a little □	I like this a lot □	**38. Cabbage**	I do not like this □	I like this a little □	I like this a lot □
29. Corn	I do not like this □	I like this a little □	I like this a lot □	**39. Okra**	I do not like this □	I like this a little □	I like this a lot □
30. Green peas	I do not like this □	I like this a little □	I like this a lot □				

For Coordinating Center use:

GEMS ID   Initials   Date of Evaluation

□□□□□   □□□□□   □□   □□   □□□□

                             month   day   year

Appendix 12.C Kids' Eating Disorders Survey

Teacher_____   Age_____   Student Number_____

School_____   Grade_____

(Circle)   Boy   Girl   Race: Black   White   Other

How much do you weigh now?_____

How much would you like to weigh?_____

How tall are you now?_____

CIRCLE THE BEST ANSWER BELOW. IF YOU ARE NOT SURE, CIRCLE THE
QUESTION MARK.

1. Do you want to lose weight now?	yes	no	?
2. Have you *ever* thought that you looked fat to other people?	yes	no	?
3. Have you *ever* been afraid to eat because you thought you would gain weight?	yes	no	?
4. Have you *ever* tried to lose weight by *dieting*? (Dieting means eating at least some food, but less than you usually eat.)	yes	no	?
5. Have you *ever* tried to lose weight by *fasting*? (Fasting means eating no solid food for at least 24 hours.)	yes	no	?
6. Have you *ever* made yourself throw up (*vomit*) to lose weight?	yes	no	?
7. Have you *ever exercised a lot* to lose weight? (A lot means more than one hour a day everyday.)	yes	no	?
8. Have you *ever* taken *diet pills* to lose weight?	yes	no	?
9. Have you *ever* taken *diuretics or water pills* to lose weight?	yes	no	?
10. Have you *ever* taken *laxatives* to lose weight?	yes	no	?

11. Circle the example below that is similar to the largest amount of food you have ever eaten in less than two hours (even if you did not eat exactly the same foods).

Example 1: Less food than in Example 2.
Example 2: Two doughnuts and a cup of ice cream and two cookies.
Example 3: Four doughnuts and a pint of ice cream or five cookies.
Example 4: Six doughnuts and a quart of ice cream and ten cookies.
Example 5: Eight doughnuts and a half gallon of ice cream and fifteen cookies.
Example 6: More food than in Example 5.

12. How many times have you *ever* eaten *the amount of food you circled above?*
   1 or 2 times only   3 to 12 times   13 to 24 times
   25 to 50 times   more than 50 times

SOURCE: Childress, A. C. et al., 1993.

Appendix 12.D Dietary Intent Scale

Please circle the response that best describes your eating behaviors in the past 6 months:

	Never	Seldom	Sometimes	Often	Always
1. I take small helpings in an effort to control my weight	1	2	3	4	5
2. I hold back at meals in an attempt to prevent weight gain	1	2	3	4	5
3. I limit the amount of food I eat in an effort to control my weight	1	2	3	4	5
4. I sometimes avoid eating in an attempt to control my weight	1	2	3	4	5
5. I skip meals in an effort to control my weight	1	2	3	4	5
6. I sometimes eat only one or two meals a day to try to limit my weight	1	2	3	4	5
7. I eat diet foods in an effort to control my weight	1	2	3	4	5
8. I count calories to try to prevent weight gain	1	2	3	4	5
9. I eat low-calorie foods in an effort to avoid weight gain	1	2	3	4	5

SOURCE: Stice (1998). Copyright 1998 by John Wiley & Sons, Inc. Reprinted with permission of John Wiley & Sons, Inc.

Appendix 12.E Emotional Eating Scale Adapted for Children and Adolescents (EES-C)

We all react to different feelings in different ways. Some types of feelings make us want to eat. Please let us know how much the following feelings make you want to eat by checking the appropriate box.

EXAMPLE

WHEN I FEEL THIS WAY	I have no desire to eat	I have a small desire to eat	I have a moderate desire to eat	I have a strong desire to eat	I have a very strong desire to eat	On average, how many days a week do you eat because you feel this way? (0–7)
Starving					x	3
Resentful						

WHEN I FEEL THIS WAY	I have no desire to eat	I have a small desire to eat	I have a moderate desire to eat	I have a strong desire to eat	I have a very strong desire to eat	On average, how many days a week do you eat because you feel this way? (0–7)
Discouraged						
Shaky						
Worn out						
Not doing enough						
Excited						
Disobedient						
Down						
Stressed out						
Sad						
Uneasy						
Irritated						
Jealous						
Worried						
Frustrated						
Lonely						
Furious						
On edge						
Confused						
Nervous						
Angry						
Guilty						
Bored						
Helpless						
Upset						
Happy						

SOURCE: From Tanofsky-Kraff, M. et al. (2007, April), "Validation of the Emotional Eating Scale Adapted for Use in Children and Adolescents (EES-C)." *International Journal Eating Disorders,* 40(3): 232-240. Reprinted with permission from John Wiley & Sons.

Appendix 12.F Children's Version of the Eating Attitudes Test (ChEAT)

Instructions: Please place an X under the word which best applies to the statements below.

Sample item: I like to eat vegetables

Always   Very Often   Often   Sometimes   Rarely   Never

1. I am scared about being overweight.
2. I stay away from eating when I am hungry.
3. I think about food a lot of the time.
4. I have gone on eating binges where I feel that I might not be able to stop.
5. I cut my food into small pieces.
6. I am aware of the energy (calorie) content in foods that I eat.
7. I try to stay away from foods such as breads, potatoes, and rice.
8. I feel that others would like me to eat more.
9. I vomit after I have eaten.
10. I feel very guilty after eating.
11. I think a lot about wanting to be thinner.
12. I think about burning up energy (calories) when I exercise.
13. Other people think I am too thin.
14. I think a lot about having fat on my body.
15. I take longer than others to eat my meals.
16. I stay away from foods with sugar in them.
17. I eat diet foods.
18. I think that food controls my life.
19. I can show self-control around food.
20. I feel that others pressure me to eat.
21. I give too much time and thought to food.
22. I feel uncomfortable after eating sweets.
23. I have been dieting.
24. I like my stomach to be empty.
25. I enjoy trying new rich foods.
26. I have the urge to vomit after eating.

SOURCE: Maloney et al., 1988.

Appendix 12.G Children's Eating Behavior Inventory (CEBI)

Child's Name_____ Age_____ / _____ Sex M F
Years   Months

HOW OFTEN DOES THIS HAPPEN?

	NEVER	SELDOM	SOMETIMES	OFTEN	ALWAYS	Is this a problem for you?
1. My child chews food as expected for his/her age	1	2	3	4	5	YES NO
2. My child helps to set the table	1	2	3	4	5	YES NO
3. My child watches TV at meals	1	2	3	4	5	YES NO
4. I feed my child if he/she doesn't eat	1	2	3	4	5	YES NO
5. My child takes more than half an hour to eat his/her meals	1	2	3	4	5	YES NO
6. Relatives complain about my child's eating	1	2	3	4	5	YES NO
7. My child enjoys eating	1	2	3	4	5	YES NO
8. My child asks for food which he/she shouldn't have	1	2	3	4	5	YES NO
9. My child feeds him/her self as expected for his/her age	1	2	3	4	5	YES NO
10. My child gags at mealtimes	1	2	3	4	5	YES NO
11. I feel confident my child eats enough	1	2	3	4	5	YES NO
12. I find our meals stressful	1	2	3	4	5	YES NO
13. My child vomits at mealtime	1	2	3	4	5	YES NO

14. My child takes food between meals without asking

| 1 | 2 | 3 | 4 | 5 | YES NO |

15. My child comes to the table 1 or 2 minutes after I call

| 1 | 2 | 3 | 4 | 5 | YES NO |

16. My child chokes at mealtimes

| 1 | 2 | 3 | 4 | 5 | YES NO |

17. My child eats quickly

| 1 | 2 | 3 | 4 | 5 | YES NO |

18. My child makes foods for him/her self when not allowed

| 1 | 2 | 3 | 4 | 5 | YES NO |

19. I get upset when my child doesn't eat

| 1 | 2 | 3 | 4 | 5 | YES NO |

20. At home my child eats food he/she shouldn't have

| 1 | 2 | 3 | 4 | 5 | YES NO |

21. My child eats foods that taste different

| 1 | 2 | 3 | 4 | 5 | YES NO |

22. I let my child have snacks between meals if he/she doesn't eat at meals

| 1 | 2 | 3 | 4 | 5 | YES NO |

23. My child uses cutlery as expected for his/her age

| 1 | 2 | 3 | 4 | 5 | YES NO |

24. At friends' homes my child eats food he/she shouldn't eat

| 1 | 2 | 3 | 4 | 5 | YES NO |

25. My child asks for food between meals

| 1 | 2 | 3 | 4 | 5 | YES NO |

26. I get upset when I think about our meals

| 1 | 2 | 3 | 4 | 5 | YES NO |

27. My child eats chunky foods

| 1 | 2 | 3 | 4 | 5 | YES NO |

28. My child lets food sit in his/her mouth

| 1 | 2 | 3 | 4 | 5 | YES NO |

29. At dinner I let my child choose the foods he/she wants from what is served

| 1 | 2 | 3 | 4 | 5 | YES NO |

If You are a Single Parent Skip to Number 34

30. My child's behavior at meals upsets my spouse

    1   2   3   4   5   YES NO

31. I agree with my spouse about how much our child should eat

    1   2   3   4   5   YES NO

32. My child interrupts conversations with my spouse at meals

    1   2   3   4   5   YES NO

33. I get upset with my spouse at meals

    1   2   3   4   5   YES NO

34. My child eats when upset

    1   2   3   4   5   YES NO

35. My child says he/she is hungry

    1   2   3   4   5   YES NO

36. My child says she/he'll get fat if she/he eats too much

    1   2   3   4   5   YES NO

37. My child helps to clear the table

    1   2   3   4   5   YES NO

38. My child hides food

    1   2   3   4   5   YES NO

39. My child brings toys or books to the table

    1   2   3   4   5   YES NO

If you have Only One Child Skip Number 40

40. My child's behavior at meals upsets our other children

    1   2   3   4   5   YES NO

PLEASE CHECK TO SEE THAT YOU HAVE ANSWERED *ALL* THE ITEMS.

HAVE YOU CIRCLED A YES OR NO FOR EACH ITEM? THANK YOU.

SOURCE: Archer, L. A. et al., 1991.

Appendix 12.H Body Rating Scale (BRS)

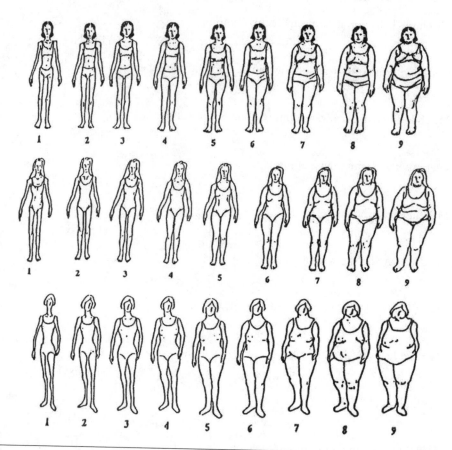

Figure 1   Nine silhouettes of the Body Rating Scale for 11-year-olds and the Body Rating Scale for 17-year-olds (top and center) representing adolescent females and the Figure Rating Scale silhouettes of adult females (bottom). (FRS from "Use of the Danish Adoption Register for the Study of Obesity and Thinness" by A. Stunkard, T. Sorenson, and F. Schlusinger, in *The genetics of neurological and psychiatric disorder,* edited by S. Kety, 1980, p. 119. Copyright 1983 by Raven Press. Reproduced by permission.)

SOURCE: Sherman, Iacono, and Donnelly (1995). Copyright (1995) John Wiley & Sons, Inc. Reprinted with permission of John Wiley & Sons, Inc.

Appendix 12.I Children's Body Image Scale (CBIS)

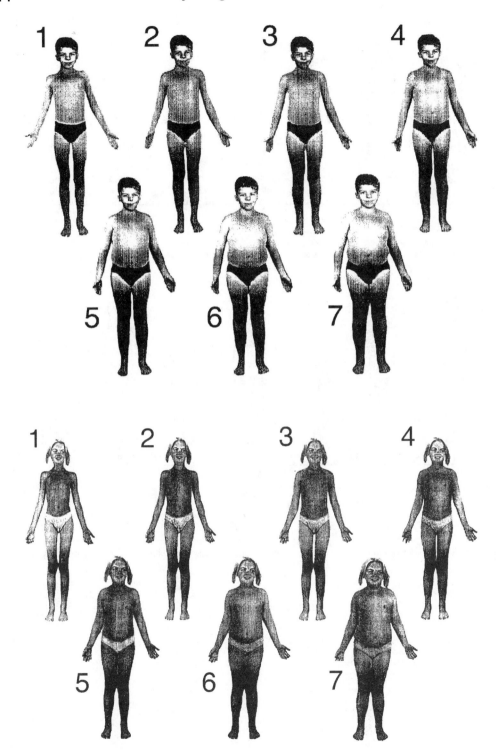

Appendix 12.J Figure Drawings

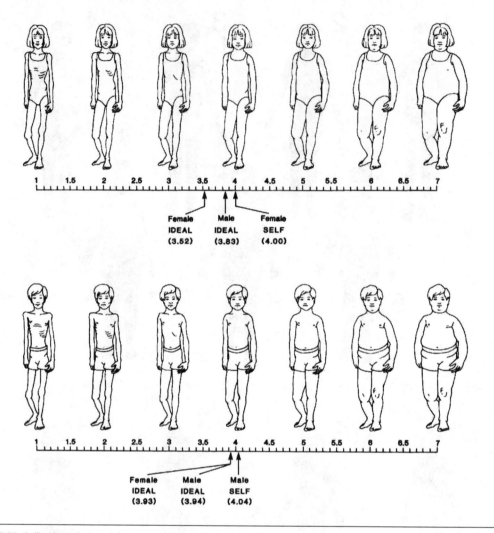

SOURCE: Collins (1991). Copyright © 1991 by John Wiley & Sons, Inc. Reprinted with permission of John Wiley & Sons, Inc.

Appendix 12.K KEDS Body Image Silhouettes (BIS)

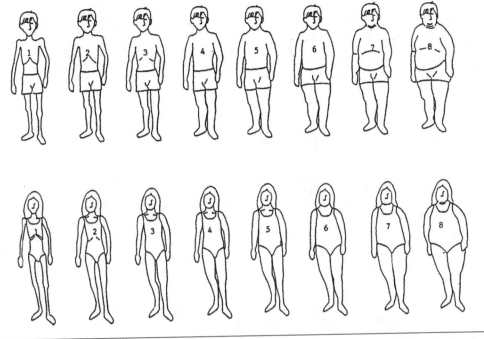

Figure 3   Instructions: "<u>Circle</u> the drawing that <u>most looks like you,</u> then <u>underline</u> the drawing you <u>would most like to look like.</u>"

SOURCE: Childress, A. C. et al., 1993.

Appendix 12.L Body-Esteem Scale (BE)

1. I like what I look like in pictures.	Yes*	No
2. Kids my own age like my looks.	Yes*	No
3. I'm pretty happy about the way I look.	Yes*	No
4. Most people have a nicer body than I do.	Yes	No*
5. My weight makes me unhappy.	Yes	No*
6. I like what I see when I look in the mirror.	Yes*	No
7. I wish I were thinner.	Yes	No*
8. There are lots of things I'd change about my looks if I could.	Yes	No*
9. I'm proud of my body.	Yes*	No
10. I really like what I weigh.	Yes*	No
11. I wish I looked better.	Yes	No*
12. I often feel ashamed of how I look.	Yes	No*
13. Other people make fun of the way I look.	Yes	No*
14. I think I have a good body.	Yes*	No
15. I'm looking as nice as I'd like to.	Yes*	No
16. It's pretty tough to look like me.	Yes	No*
17. I wish I were fatter.	Yes	No*
18. I often wish I looked like someone else.	Yes	No*
19. My classmates would like to look like me.	Yes*	No
20. I have a high opinion about the way I look.	Yes*	No
21. My looks upset me.	Yes	No*
22. I'm as nice looking as most people.	Yes*	No
23. My parents like my looks.	Yes*	No
24. I worry about the way I look.	Yes	No*

* High body-esteem response.

SOURCE: Mendelson & White, 1982.

Index

Aaby, P., 274
Aadahl, M., 221
Aaron, D. J., 193t–196t, 239
Aaronson, N. K., 35, 36
Abate, N., 517
Abbey, D. E., 221
Abdalla, M. I., 39
Abdel-Malek, A. K., 492t–495t
Abell, N., 96
Aberra, B., 545
Abetz, L., 59
Abraham, S., 66
Abramowitz, R. H., 116t–125t, 126
Abu Khaled, M., 492t–495t
Accelerometers
    best practices for using, 216–217
    biaxial, 210–211
    cutoff points and, 216
    data analysis for, 216–217
    described, 210
    epoch length and, 216
    identification of wearing period and, 217
    monitor placement and, 213, 215
    number of days for monitoring using, 215–216
    reproducibility and, 211–212
    triaxial, 211
    uniaxial, 210
    validity of, 212–213, 214t, 215t
Acebo, C., 224, 225
Acklin, M. W., 11
ACS (attributions of controllability scale), 85
Actigraphy method, 226–227
Activity logs, and physiological observations, 545–546
Activity recall, and physiological observations, 544–545
Adair, C. E., 65
Adami, G. F., 54
Adams, G. R., 85
Adams, H. E., 2

Adang, E. M., 40
Addessi, E., 449
Ader, M., 187
Ades, P. A., 221
Adeyanju, M., 80
Adolescents. *See also* Children; Explicit anti-fat
        attitudes of adolescents and adults
    AFA for measuring explicit anti-fat attitudes of,
        88–90, 106–107nn6–7, 567–568
    AFAS for measuring explicit anti-fat attitudes of,
        90–91, 568
    AFAT for measuring explicit anti-fat attitudes of,
        91–92, 569–571
    ATOP for measuring explicit anti-fat attitudes of,
        92–94, 107nn8–9, 571–572
    BESAA for, 469
    EES-C for, 465, 626–627
    food intake measurement in free-living
        populations and, 272–273
    FSQ for measuring explicit anti-fat attitudes
        of, 94
    measurement of explicit anti-fat attitudes of, 95t,
        106n4
    obesity disease-specific instruments for HRQOL
        assessment of, 59–62
    ranking tasks, and measurement of explicit anti-fat
        attitudes of, 87–88
    semantic differential measures of explicit anti-fat
        attitudes of, 106n5
Adolph, A. L., 213
ADP. *See* Air displacement plethysmography
Adults. *See also* Explicit anti-fat attitudes of
        adolescents and adults
    AFA for measuring explicit anti-fat attitudes of,
        88–90, 106–107nn6–7, 567–568
    AFAS for measuring explicit anti-fat attitudes of,
        90–91, 568
    AFAT for measuring explicit anti-fat attitudes of,
        91–92, 569–571

ATOP for measuring explicit anti-fat attitudes of, 92–94, 107nn8–9, 571–572

BESAA for, 469

Expert Panel on the Identification, Evaluation and Treatment of Overweight in Adults, 496

FSQ for measuring explicit anti-fat attitudes of, 94

measurement of explicit anti-fat attitudes of, 95t, 106n4

ranking tasks, and measurement of explicit anti-fat attitudes of, 87–88

semantic differential measures of explicit anti-fat attitudes of, 106n5

AFA (Anti-Fat Attitudes Questionnaire), 88–90, 106–107nn6–7, 567–568

AFAS (Anti-Fat Attitudes Scale), 90–91, 568

AFAT (Anti-Fat Attitudes Test), 91–92, 569–571

Affective measures, for body image assessment, 126–127

Age, and Herman and Polivy's Restraint Scale, 147

Aggen, S., 163, 175

Agras, W. S., 168, 348, 349, 357, 374, 377, 379, 398, 400, 465

Ahern, A. L., 99, 102t–105t

Ahlawat, K. S., 164

Ahluwalia, B. W., 492t–495t

Ahrén, A. M., 259

Aime, A. A., 364, 367, 420, 423

Aimé, A. A., 420, 423

Ainslie, P., 529

Ainsworth, B. E., 190, 208, 221, 537, 544, 545

Ainsworth, B. E. F., 222

Air displacement plethysmography
  accuracy and validity of, 508–509
  availability and costs of, 509
  described, 508
  norms for, 509
  reliability of, 508

Air plethysmography. See Air displacement plethysmography

Aitchison, T. A., 215

Aitkens, S., 308, 509

Akesson, A., 272

Albanes, D., 221

Albu, J., 492

Alexander, M., 447, 460t

Alexander, M. P., 459

Alger-Mayer, S., 351, 353

Algina, J., 148

Alindogan, J., 116t–125t, 130

Allen, D. G., 88

Allison, D. B., 81, 86t, 92, 95, 142, 145t–146t, 147, 149t–151t, 159, 169, 174, 328, 464, 498, 505

Allison, D. R., 256

Allor, K. M., 213

Almeras, N., 300

Almqvist, F., 467

Altabe, M. N., 116t–125t, 126

Altepeter, T. S., 9

Altug, A., 419

Alvarez, V. P., 484

Alverdy, J., 56

American College of Sports Medicine, 482

American Psychiatric Association, 347, 348, 356, 361, 364, 376, 379, 381, 387, 414, 417, 431, 436, 439

American Society for Bariatric Surgery, Allied Health Section Ad Hoc Behavioral Health Committee, 39, 58, 68

Ames-Frankel, J., 2

Ampudia, A., 5

Amrani, R., 304

AN. See Anorexia nervosa

Analytic issues relevant in obesity. See Obesity and relevant analytical issues

Anand, J., 267

Anastasi, A., 64

Ancoli-Israel, S., 225, 226

Andersen, L. B., 217

Andersen, R. E., 37

Anderson, A. S., 305, 306, 401

Anderson, C., 163, 175

Anderson, C. B., 230

Anderson, D. A., 116t–125t, 265, 361, 367, 368, 379, 397, 400, 401, 417, 419, 431, 434, 436, 439, 467

Anderson, G. H., 40, 454

Anderson, J. P., 42

Anderson, J. T., 485, 485t

Anderson, K. G., 145t–146t, 147, 162t, 431, 433

Anderson, L. H., 230

Andresen, E. M., 42

Andresen, M., 230

Andrianopoulos, G. D., 17

Andronikof, A., 11

Andrykowski, M. A., 193t–196t

Anesbury, T., 81, 83, 85, 86, 106n3

Aneshensel, C. S., 116t–125t

Angelopoulos, T. J., 20

ANIS (Anorexia Nervosa Inventory for Self Rating Scales), 358

Annis, J. F., 535

Anorexia nervosa. See also Binge Eating Scale; Binge eating scale; Eating disorders; Structured Interview for Anorexic and Bulimic Disorders
  ANIS and, 358
  purging and, 347, 350
  RAB-R and, 376

Anti-fat attitude measurement. See also Explicit anti-fat attitudes of adolescents and adults
  implicit measures and, 96–106, 99f, 100f, 102t–105t, 107nn11–16
  obesity defined, 79

passive obesity and, 79
summary of, 79–81, 106, 106nn1–2
Antipatis, V. J., 79
Anton, S. D., 466
Antony, M. M., 18, 381, 383
APA (American Psychiatric Association), 347, 348, 356, 361, 364, 376, 379, 381, 387, 414, 417, 431, 436, 439
Apajasalo, M., 65
Aplasca, E. C., 494
Apolone, G., 36
Aponte, J. F., 4
Appel, L. J., 222
Appetite studies, description of, 283–284, 284f. *See also* Food intake measurement in laboratory; Subjective measures of appetite
Applegate, K. L., 55
Appleton, K., 300
Appolinario, J. C., 15, 351
Aradine, C. R., 454
Araiza, P., 205, 208
Aranda, C., 498
Archer, L. A., 466, 467
Archer, R. P., 10, 16
Arcila-Martínez, D., 430
Ardelt-Gattinger, E., 43t–51t, 52, 559
Argyle, M., 40
Arinell, H., 129, 467
Arkes, H. R., 107n13
Armstrong, C. A., 202
Armstrong, J., 116t–125t
Arnau, R. C., 14
Arnhold, H., 540
Arnow, B., 465
Arostegui, I., 63
Arreola, A., 449
Arroll, B., 221
Aruguete, M. S., 90
Arvaniti, K., 308
Asbeck, I., 257
Åsberg, M., 5t–7t
ASDA Report, 225
Aserinsky, E., 223
Askanazi, J., 538
Assessment issues in energy expenditure measurement
  basal metabolic rate and, 530
  energy expenditure of physical activities and, 531
  resting energy expenditure and, 530
  standardization of protocols for, 530–531
  thermic effect of food and, 530–531
  validation and calibration of techniques for, 531
Assunçao, J., 328
Astrup, A., 291, 300, 540
Atger, F., 2

Atienza, A. A., 228, 229, 237
Atkinson, M., 270, 271
Atlas, J., 162t, 163, 164, 165, 168
Attitudes Toward Obese Persons Scale (ATOP), 92–94, 107nn8–9, 571–572
Augustinsson, L. E., 41
Aulick, L. H., 540
Austrheim-Smith, I. T., 53
Automated food measuring systems
  described, 311
  development of, 313–315, 314f, 316f
  microstructure of feeding behavior and, 312–313
  observation and, 313
  reliability of, 315
  UEM and, 306–307, 313–315, 314f, 316f
  validity of, 315
Ayabe, M., 532
Ayas, N. T., 223

Babbit, R. L., xiii
Bacharach, V. R., x
Backhaus, J., 193t–196t
Bacon, J. G., 86, 87
Badman, M. K., 286
Baecke, J., 227
Bailey, R., 204
Baines, J., 545
Baird, J. C., 451
Bak, J., 83
Baker, A. S., 484
Baker, N. B., 447
Balazs, J., 382
Balfour, L., 357, 422, 423
Ball, C., 411, 413
Ball, R., 14
Ball, S. D., 449
Ballantyne, G. H., 58
Ballard-Barbash, R., 257
Banaji, J. R., 99
Banaji, M. R., 96, 101
Banasiak, S., 171t, 172, 419, 464
Banasiak, S. J., 149t–151t
Bandini, L., 512
Bandini, L. G., 155, 273, 459, 461, 465
Banks, M., 80, 102t–105t
Banzet, M., 36, 43t–51t
Baranowski, T., 189, 205t–206t, 230
Barbe, P., 129
Barbin, J. M., 128, 379, 401, 404, 434, 436
Barden, H. S., 493
Bariatric Analysis and Reporting Outcome System, 42, 52–53
Bariatric Quality of Life Questionnaire, 561–563
Barkeling, B., 13, 300, 312, 313, 315, 454
Barker-Collo, S. L., 4

Barlow, S. E., 496
Barnette, J. J., 85
Barnhart Miller, A., 84
Barnowski, T., 193t–196t, 200, 201, 205t–206t
Baroffio, J. R., 10
Barofsky, I., 33, 35, 37
Baron, R. B., 270
Baron, R. M., 329
BAROS (Bariatric Analysis and Reporting Outcome
    System), 42, 52–53
Barrett-Connor, E., 42
Barrington, E., 221
Barrios, B. A., 359, 431, 433
Barron, F., 193t–196t, 202, 205t–206t
Barry, D. T., 377, 398, 400
Barthlow, D. L., 9
Bartlett, S. J., 34, 35, 37, 68
Basco, M. R., 16
Basdevant, A., 36, 43t–51t
Basile, B., 366
Basile, V. C., 86t, 92, 95
Bass, S. L., 229
Bassett, D. R., 204, 207
Bassett, D. R., Jr., 204, 207, 209, 221, 228, 537,
    545, 546
Bathalon, G., 162, 166
Bathalon, G. P., 464
Bathurst, K., 5
BATMAN (Bob and Tom's Method of Assessing
    Nutrition), 450
Batterham, M. J., 258t–259t
Batterham, R. L., 304
Baukol, P. A., 546
Bauman, A., 230
Bauman, W. A., 484
Baumeister, B., 484
Baumgartner, R. N., 486, 504t–505t, 505, 506
Bayon, C., 13
BCM (body cell mass), 515
BDD (body dysmorphic disorder), 128
BDI-II. *See* Beck Depression Inventory–II inventory
BE (Body-Esteem Scale), 469, 636
Beales, S., 145t–146t, 173, 464
Beasley, J., 265
Beatty, W. W., 328
Beauchamp, G. K., 449
Beck, A. T., 14, 15, 64, 67, 386, 410
Beck, J. G., 18
Beck, S., 327
Beck Depression Inventory–II inventory
    availability, 15
    limitations, 15
    norms, 15
    overview, 14
    reliability of, 14–15

research applications, 15
    validity, 15
Becker, E., 313
Becker, J. A., 469
BED. *See* Binge-eating disorder
Bedimo-Rung, A. L., 230
Beets, M. W., 208
Beghin, L., 209
Beglin, S., 63, 175, 358, 363, 364, 401, 411, 419, 420,
    422, 423
Beglin, S. J., 63, 175, 348, 358, 363, 364, 401, 411, 419,
    420, 422, 423
Behavior Eating Test, 450
Behnke, A. R., Jr., 485, 485t
Beiseigel, J., 166, 167
Belahsen, R., 130
Belko, A. Z., 542
Bell, E. A., 331
Bell, R., 327
Bell, R. C., 208
Bell, S. K., 83
Bellini, O., 413
Bellisari, A., 492t–495t
Bellisle, F., 161, 165, 166, 290, 304, 313
Bellizzi, M. C., 497, 500
Bellocco, R., 221
Bellwoar, V., 139
Belter, R. W., 451
Bender, S., 332
Bene, C. R., 145t–146t, 147, 148, 149t–151t, 155
Benedict, F. G., 540
Bengtsson, C., 256
Benjamin, A. B., 16
Bennett, H. W., 193t–196t, 221
Bennett, K., 424
Bennett, S. M., 381
Bennish, M. L., 492t–495t, 507
Ben-Porath, Y. S., 8, 9
Bentley, D. J., 539
Berenson, G. S., 261
Berg, C., 270
Berger, B., 20
Bergeron, D., 116t–125t
Bergers, G. P. A., 138, 149t–151t, 171t, 172,
    174, 465
Bergman, R. N., 187
Bergner, M., 41
Bergsma-Kadijk, J. A., 484
Bergstrom, A., 221
Berkman, L. F., 223
Berlin, M., 261, 461
Berman, S. R., 226
Bernauer, E. M., 492t–495t
Bernstein, I. H., 377
Bernstein, L., 187

Berridge, K. C., 303

Berry, C. C., 202

Berry, M. J., 532

Berry, S. L., 328

Berryman, D. E., 80

Bersabe, R., 439

Bertéus Forslund, H., 266

Berthoud, H. -R., 286

BES. *See* Binge eating scale

BESAA (Body-Esteem Scale for Adolescents and Adults), 469

Besier, T. F., 543

Bessenoff, G. R., 97

BET (Behavior Eating Test), 450

Beumont, P., 156

Beumont, P. J., 63

Beumont, P. J. V., 156, 376, 378, 420, 422

Beveridge, S. K., 202

Beyer, J. E., 451, 454

BIA. *See* Bioelectrical impedance analysis

Biaggi, R. R., 492t–495t

Biaxial accelerometers, 210–211

Bieberich, A., 83

Bieling, P. J., 18

Biertho, L., 52

Billat, V. L., 532

Billington, C., 80, 102t–105t

Billman, J., 448, 449

Binder, L. M., 19

Binford, R. B., 420

Binge-eating disorder. *See also* Binge eating scale; Binge Eating Scale Questionnaire

  clinical diagnosis criteria for, 348

  defined, 347–348

  described, 347, 387, 389

  DSM-IV and, 349

  EDE and, 348–349

  frequency and duration of, 349

  key symptoms in eating disorders and, 347

  loss of control and, 349–350

  parameters of, 348–350

  size of binge and, 348–349

Binge eating scale

  availability of, 354

  described, 350–351

  norms for, 353–354

  reliability of, 351

  sensitivity to change and, 353

  validity of, 351–353, 353t

Binge Eating Scale Questionnaire

  availability of, 356–357

  construct validity of, 355

  criterion validity of, 356

  norms for, 356

  reliability of, 354–355, 355t

  sensitivity to change and, 356

  validity of, 355

Bingham, S., 256, 260

Bingham, S. A., 269

Binkhorst, R. A., 227

Bioelectrical impedance analysis

  accuracy and validity of, 505–506

  availability and costs for, 506

  described, 504–505

  norms for, 506

  reliability of, 505

Bioimpedance analysis. *See* Bioelectrical impedance analysis

Birch, L., 449

Birch, L. L., 86t, 93, 94, 142, 307, 327, 329, 447, 448, 449, 451, 451f, 456, 456f, 457, 461, 462

Birmingham, C. L., 433

Biron, S., 35

BIS (KEDS Body Image Silhouettes), 468–469, 635

Bisek, J. P., 493

Bissada, H., 357, 422, 423

BITE. *See* Bulimia Investigatory Test

Bitter, I., 382

Bjornstrom, C., 374

Bjorntorp, P., 41

Black, A. E., 256, 462

Black, D. R., 431

Black, J. R., 461

Black, S., 350, 353, 376, 423

Blackwell, F., 545

Blair, D., 545

Blair, S. N., 80, 102t–105t, 212, 213, 221

Blais, M. A., 21

Blanchard, F. A., 148, 152, 153

Blanco, R., 563

Blanton, H., 107n13

Blix, A. G., 130

Blix, G. G., 130

Block, G., 156, 259, 270

Bloks, H., 3

Bloom, S. R., 304

Blouin, A. G., 4, 15

Bluemke, M., 107n10

Blundell, E., 294

Blundell, J. E., 175, 283, 285, 291, 296, 297, 298, 300, 302, 308, 309, 311, 312, 313, 315

Blundell, J. E., 284, 293

BMI. *See* Body mass index

BN. *See* Bulimia nervosa

Boan, J., 56

Boarnet, M. G., 230

Bob and Tom's Method of Assessing Nutrition, 450

Bobbitt, R. A., 41

Bobroff, E. M., 304

Bodenhausen, G. V., 81

Body cell mass, 515

Body composition assessment. *See* Human body composition assessment

Body Dissatisfaction Scale of the Eating Disorder Inventory, 469

Body dysmorphic disorder, 128

Body-Esteem Scale, 469, 636

Body-Esteem Scale for Adolescents and Adults, 469

Body fat values, 483, 483t

Body Image: An International Journal of Research, 115

Body image assessment
   BDD and, 128
   behavioral assessment and, 127
   cognitive measures for, 127
   interview scales for, 127–128
   measurement categories for, 126–127
   methodological issues and, 129–130
   recent advances in, 128–129
   subjective and affective measures for, 126–127
   summary of, 115–126, 116t–125t, 130–131

Body Image Silhouettes, 468–469, 635

Body mass index
   described, 487, 488t–489t, 489, 490t–495t, 496–497, 496t, 497t, 498f, 499t–500t
   measurement issues and techniques for, vii
   obesity defined and, 79

Body Rating Scale, 467–468, 632

Body's total body water, 512

Body weight, description of, 487, 488t–489t, 489, 490t–495t, 496–497, 496t, 497t, 498f

Boerner, L. M., 145, 145t–146t, 147, 148, 149t–151t, 152, 154, 156, 162t, 163, 164, 165, 168, 175, 176t, 431, 433

Bogardus, C., 529, 530

Bohh, Y., 358, 465

Bohr, Y., 417

Boileau, R. A., 221, 486

Boland, G. C., 5

Boll, V., 53

Bolonchuk, W. W., 506

Bond, M. J., 149t–151t, 163

Bonnefoy, M., 221, 544

Bonner, J., 411, 413

Bonsel, G. J., 35

Bonynge, E. R., 17

Booth, D. A., 304

Booth, M. L., 229

Boots, J. M., 169

Borel, M. J., 545

Borgen, J. S., 358

Borgonha, S., 541

Bornstein, R. F., 2, 11, 12

Bornstein, S. R., 15

Borowiecki, J., 116t–125t, 126

Börresen, R., 358

Borrud, L. G., 261

Borzekowski, D. L., 449

Bosaeus, I., 258, 260

Boschi, V., 413

Boskind-White, M., 348

Bossert, S., 354, 356

Bosy-Westphal, A., 516

Bothwell, S., 64

Bouchard, C., 529

Bourne, S. K., 156

Boutelle, K. N., 260

Bouten, C. V., 546

Bowling, A., 40, 41

Bowman, B. A., 459

Boyd, C., 66

Boyd, F., 356

Boyd, S., 20

BQL (Bariatric Quality of Life) Questionnaire, 561–563

Bradburn, N., 328

Bradley, L., 365, 367, 400, 420, 422

Braet, C., 465

Brage, N., 212

Brage, S., 212, 213, 217

Brähler, E., 5, 131

Brambilla, P., 492t–495t, 502

Bramson, R., 14

Brand, N., 142

Brand-Miller, J. C., 297, 449

Brandsma, J., 20

Branehog, I., 41

Brannick, M. T., 116t–125t, 127

Brantsaeter, A. L., 274

Bratteby, L. E., 273

Bravata, E. A., 15

Bray, G. A., 447, 540

Bray, M. S., 212

Brazier, J. E., 40

Bredbacka, S., 537

Brehm, M. A., 537

Brelsford, T. N., 359, 360, 431, 433

Brenn, T., 187, 262

Bresnan, J., 85

Breteler, M. H. M., 148

Breteler, R., 358

Brewerton, T., 464, 468

Brewerton, T. D., 116t–125t, 463

Bridgwater, C. A., 450

Brink, P. J., 154

Brinkmann, G., 516

Brinkworth, G. D., 492t–495t, 507

Brisko, N., 539

Broberg, A. G., 376

Brochu, P. M., 96, 102t–105t

Broeckmann, P., 140

Brolin, R. E., 365, 367, 400, 420, 422
Broocks, A., 193t–196t
Brook, C. G. D., 503
Brook, R. H., 34
Brookhart, A., 43t–51t, 53
Brookings, J. B., 417, 419
Brooks, W. B., 41
Brown, A. L., 237
Brown, C. C., 262
Brown, G., 15
Brown, G. K., 15, 67
Brown, I., 80, 108
Brown, K. H., 483, 492t–495t, 496, 507
Brown, M., 80, 86, 88
Brown, T., 66
Brown, T. A., 116t–125t, 130
Brown, W. J., 36, 229, 230
Brownbill, R. A., 221
Brownell, K. D., 2, 79, 80, 86, 87, 93, 96, 99, 100, 101,
    102t–105t, 106nn1–2,4, 107n15
Brozek, J., 3, 143, 485, 485t, 502
BRS (Body Rating Scale), 467–468, 632
Brubaker, P. H., 532
Bruch, H., 1
Brug, J., 237
Brun, T., 545
Brunner, E. J., 269
Brunstrom, J. M., 291, 304
Brunswik, E., 295
Bryant, J. L., 448, 449
Bryant, M., 265
Bryant, R. A., 156
Bryant-Waugh, R. J., 128
Brylinsky, J. A., 84
Bryson, S., 168
Bryson, S. W., 363
Bubb-Lewis, C., 86t, 90, 95t, 569, 571
Buckley, J. D., 492t–495t, 507
Buddeberg, C., 356
Bueno-De-Mesquita, H. B., 221
Bueno-de-Mesquita, H. B., 221
Built environment
    conceptualization of, 230–232
    described, 230
    districts, 231, 232, 233f, 234f
    edges, 231, 234
    future directions for measurement of, 236–237
    GIS model and, 232
    landmarks measurements and, 231, 232–234
    nodes, 231, 232–234
    paths, 231, 232, 234
    physical activity and exercise, and effects of, 230, 231f
    urban fabric and sprawl, and measurement of,
        235–236, 236f
    urban indices, and measurement of, 236

Bulik, C., 161, 163, 175
Bulik, C. M., 19
Bulimia Investigatory Test, Edinburgh
    availability of, 438–439
    described, 436, 437t–438t
    norms for, 437t–438t, 438
    questionnaire, 586–589
    reliability of, 436, 437t–438t
    special issues/considerations/pros and cons for, 439
    validity of, 436–437, 437t–438t
Bulimia nervosa. *See also* Binge eating scale; Binge
        Eating Scale Questionnaire; Bulimia
        Investigatory Test; Bulimia Test–Revised;
        Structured Interview for Anorexic and Bulimic
        Disorders
    defined, 347–348
    purging and, 347, 350
    RAB-R and, 376
Bulimia Scale–Eating Disorders Inventory
    availability of, 359
    construct validity of, 357–358
    criterion validity of, 358
    described, 357
    norms for, 359
    reliability of, 357
    sensitivity to change and, 358–359
    validity of, 357–358
Bulimia Test–Revised
    availability of, 433
    construct validity of, 360
    criterion validity of, 360
    described, 359, 431
    norms for, 360–361, 432t–433t, 433
    questionnaire, 589–594
    reliability of, 359–360, 361t, 431, 432t–433t
    special issues/considerations/pros and cons for,
        433–434
    validity of, 360, 431, 432t–433t, 433
BULIT-R. *See* Bulimia Test–Revised
Bullinger, M., 60
Buono, M. J., 210
Burastero, S., 492t–495t, 506
Burge, M. R., 205
Burke, P. J., 84
Burke, R. K., 543
Burley, V., 294
Burley, V. J., 306, 308
Burns, A. A., 290
Burns, D., 517
Burns, T. L., 230
Burwinkle, T. M., 60, 61
Bush, J. W., 42
Bushnell, D. M., 43t–51t, 58
Buskirk, E. R., 545
Bussolotti, D., 438

Butcher, J. N., 4, 5, 5t–7t, 8, 9
Butler, B. A., 530
Butler, G., 43t–51t
Butler, J. C., 89
Butryn, M., 141, 143, 178
Butryn, M. L., 139, 143, 157, 317
Butte, N. F., 212, 213, 538
Butterworth, D. E., 20
Buxton, B. F., 510
Buys, M., 41
Buysse, D. J., 226
Byers, T., 257
Byrant-Waugh, R., 377
Byrne, B. M., 88
Byrne, T. K., 55
Byrnes, J. P., 4

Cabral, K., 128
Cafri, G., 115, 116t–125t, 126, 131
Cahill, S., 15
Cain, M., 376
Calam, R., 438
Calcagno Mde., L., 500
Calder, S. J., 40, 41
Calfas, K. J., 212, 228
Calle, E. E., 230
Callewaert, I., 3
Calnan, A., 116t–125t
Calogero, R. M., 129
Calorimeter techniques, and field setting for energy expenditure measurement, 532
Calorimetry, 531
Camara, W. J., 8
Cameron, C., 221
Camey, S., 419
Campbell, D. T., xii
Campbell, M., 371, 372, 373
Campbell, W. W., 221
Candy, C. M., 469
Cani, P. D., 290
Caniato, D., 52
Cantwell, M. M., 260
Cardello, A., 297
Cardello, A. V., 305
Carels, R. A., 20
Carleton, R. A., 221
Carlson, D., 210
Carlsson, A. M., 11, 12, 13
Carmichael, A. R., 38
Carnell, S., 449
Carol, B., 228
Carpenter, J. S., 193t–196t
Carpenter, M. R., 20
Carriquiry, A. L., 261
Carr-Nangle, R. E., 369

CARS (Children's Activity Rating Scale), 201–202
Carskadon, M. A., 224, 226
Carter, J. C., 364, 367, 420, 423
Carter, P. I., 465
Carter, W. B., 41
Cartoon faces assessment in laboratory, and eating and weight-related problems in children, 456–457, 456f, 457f
Cartoon figures for child-reported hunger and satiety assessment in laboratory, and eating and weight-related problems in children, 451, 451f
Cash, T. F., 86t, 90, 91, 95t, 115, 116t–125t, 126, 127, 128, 130, 131, 569, 571
Casillas, A., 9
Casper, R. C., 10
Caspersen, C. J., 221
Casperson, C. J., 189, 215
Cassidy, J. F., 2
Cassin, S. E., 2, 3
Cassisi, J. E., 11
Castro, J., 66, 419, 466
Caswell, N., 173
Caterson, I. D., 79
Cattarin, J., 116t–125t
Cattell, R. B., 17
CBIS (Children's Body Image Scale), 468, 633
CEBI (Children's Eating Behavior Inventory), 466–467, 629–631
Cecil, J. E., 316
Ceesay, S. M., 542
Celio, A. A., 351, 352, 365, 367, 370, 423
Cella, D. F., 33
Cesena, J., 466
Chabrol, H., 129
Chaiken, S., 80
Chambers, C. T., 451, 454
Chambliss, H., 80
Chambliss, H. O., 80, 91, 99, 101, 102t–105t, 107n15
Champagne, C. M., 447
Chan, C. B., 208–209
Chan, D., 11, 542
Chan, H., 226
Chan, K. L., 542
Chandon, P., 327, 332, 333, 339, 340
Chandu, V., 492t–495t, 506
Chang, K. S., 535
Chapman, I., 302
Charbonnier, A., 540
Charles, G., 16
Charter, R. A., 20
Chasan-Taber, L., 216, 221
Chasan-Taber, S., 216, 221
Chatr-Aryamontri, B., 536
Chatterton, B. E., 485t, 486
Chaumeton, N. R., 208

ChEAT (Children's Eating Attitudes Test), 466, 628
Chen, D. D. T., 236
Chen, E. Y., 80, 86, 88
Chen, K. Y., 228, 546
Chen, Z., 513
Cheney, M. M., 327
Chernyak, Y., 141
Cheskin, L. J., 33
Cheung, F. M., 4
Child Health Questionnaire, 59–60
Children. *See also* Adolescents
    ACS, and measurement of explicit anti-fat
        attitudes of, 85
    BMI and, 496–497
    CHQ, and HRQOL assessment of, 60
    descriptors for adjectival and semantic differential
        explicit anti-fat attitudes of, 84, 565
    disease-specific instruments for obesity HRQOL
        assessment of, 62
    food intake measurement in free-living
        populations and, 272–273
    friendship measures, and measurement of explicit
        anti-fat attitudes of, 85–86
    IWQOL-Kids and, 54–56, 62, 557, 563
    KINDL, and HRQOL assessment of, 60
    measurement of and measurement of explicit
        anti-fat attitudes of, 81–86
    obesity generic instruments for HRQOL
        assessment of, 59–62
    pedometers, and applications for, 209
    PedsQL, and HRQOL assessment of, 60–62
    ranking tasks, and measurement of explicit anti-fat
        attitudes of, 81–83
Children's Activity Rating Scale, 201–202
Children's Body Image Scale, 468, 633
Children's eating and weight-related problems. *See*
    Eating and weight-related problems in
    children
Children's Eating Attitudes Test, 466, 628
Children's Eating Behavior Inventory, 466–467,
    629–631
Children's Physical Activity Form, 201
Child-reported food preferences and palatability
    assessment in laboratory
    cartoon faces for, 456–457, 457f
    described, 456
    ordinal measures for, 456–458
    questionnaires for, 458
    visual analog scales for, 457, 458f
Child-reported hunger and satiety assessment in
    laboratory, 454f, 455f. *See also* Ordinal scale
    measures
    continuous measures for, 454–456, 454f, 455f
    described, 451
    silhouettes for, 453–454, 453f

Childress, A. C., 116t–125t, 463, 464, 468
Chiu, V., 221
Choca, J. P., 20, 21
Choi, J. M., 502
Choi, P., 128
Chondros, P., 449
Choudry, I. Y., 419
Chouinard, L. E., 484
Chow, P., 106n4
CHQ (Child Health Questionnaire), 59–60
Christ, C. B., 486
Christensen, N. J., 540
Christenson, G. M., 189
Christiansen, C., 492t–495t
Christie, C., 107n13
Christie, M., 376
Chronister, K. M., 129
Chu, E. Y., 81
Chumlea, W. C., 486, 496, 505
Ciampi, A., 256
Cieslik, C. J., 201
Cifani, S., 36
Circumference measurements
    accuracy and validity of, 502
    availability and cost of, 502
    described, 498–500, 501f
    norms for, 502
    reliability of, 500
Clark, E., 208
Clark, L. A., 9, 18
Clarke, K. K., 208
Cleary, P. A., 17, 430
Clement, P. F., 354, 355, 356, 360
Clemow, L., 256
Clendenen, V., 329
Cleven, A., 149t–151t, 159, 171t, 176
Clifton, P. M., 492t–495t, 507
Clinton, D., 376
Clocksin, B. D., 202
Cloninger, C. R., 5, 5t–7t, 13
Closed circuit system, 540–541
Cochran, W. J., 492t–495t
Cohane, G., 116t–125t, 126
Cohen, D. A., 203, 205t–206t, 230
Cohen, H., 419
Cohen, J., 41
Cohn, S. H., 486, 492t–495t, 496, 515
Coin, A., 484
Coker, S., 175
Colditz, A. M., 463
Colditz, G. A., 459
Cole, S., 145t–146t, 147, 152
Cole, T. J., 256, 461, 497, 500, 535, 541
Coleman, K. J., 193t–196t, 202, 205t–206t
Coll, M., 312

Collette, H. J., 221
Collins, L. M., 238, 239
Collins, M. S., 468, 634
Colliver, J. A., 492t–495t
Comer, R. J., 1
Computerized tomography, 517
Cone, J., 50
Confinement systems, 540
Connelly, D. M., 532
Consolazio, C. F., 532
Conway, J. M., 221, 542, 544
Conway, T. L., 193t–196t, 203, 205t–206t
Cooke, L., 449
"Cool data," and food intake field studies
    measurement, 327–328, 343
Cooling, J., 300
Cooper, M., 544
Cooper, M. J., 116t–125t, 127
Cooper, P. J., 2, 116t–125t, 127, 128, 379, 398
Cooper, Z., 116t–125t, 127, 379, 397, 398, 401
Copinschi, G., 223
Corbett, W. T., 493
Corbin, C. B., 200
Corcos, M., 2
Cordle, C., 376
Corey-Lisle, P., 54
Corica, F., 39
Cornelissen, P., 82
Cornell, J., 65
Cornish, B. H., 506
Corrigan, S. A., 153, 158, 174
Corruble, E., 16
Corte, C. M., 377, 378, 387
Coscina, D. V., 466
Costa, P. T., 5t–7t, 158
Cotton, J. R., 291, 293, 308
Cotton, M., 411, 413, 414
Coufopoulos, A. M., 273
Counte, M. A., 33
Coutinho, W., 351
Covents, M., 261
Covi, L., 15
Coward, W. A., 256, 459, 541
Cradock, A. L., 217
Craig, C. L., 193t–196t, 221, 239
Craig, D. L., 227
Craig, K. D., 451
Craig, R. J., 20
Craig, S. E., 21
Cramer, P., 83, 86
Cramer, S. R., 20
Crandall, C. S., 80, 85, 85t, 86t, 88, 89, 90, 94, 95t,
    106n6, 567, 568
Cravero, J. P., 451
Crerand, C. E., 106n4

Crncevic-Orlic, Z., 221
Crocker, J., 89, 567, 568
Crocker, L., 148
Crosby, R. D., 43t–51t, 54, 55
Crossan, S., 116t–125t
Crouter, S. E., 207, 209, 546
Crow, S., 401
Crow, S. G., 398, 400
Crow, S. J., 56, 351, 367, 377, 400, 423
Crowne, D. P., xi, xii, 157
Crowther, J. H., 363, 420, 422
Crusco, A. H., 153
Cruz, M. L., 498
Crystal, S. R., 304
Cuddihy, T. F., 191
Cullen, K. W., 458
Culture, and personality and psychopathology
    assessment, 4
Cumella, E. J., 10, 424, 430
Cummings, S. R., 270
Cummings, T., 462
Cunningham, J. J., 534
Cunningham, W. A., 96, 107n14
Curb, J. D., 265
Cureton, A. L., 221
Curnow, J. S., 212
Custer, W. F., 20
Cutting, T. M., 449
Cuzzolaro, M., 116t–125t, 127, 419, 439
Cyarto, E. V., 209
Cyr, H., 459
Cyr, H. N., 155, 273, 459
Cyr, J. J., 17
Czerwinski, S. A., 503

Daanen, H., 509
Dahl, R. E., 224
Dahlkoetter, J., 450
Dahlstrom, W. G., 5t–7t, 8, 10
Dale, D., 200
Dallosso, H. M., 538
Dalton, M., 500
Damask, M. C., 538
Dan, A., 221
Dan, P. L., 163
Dana, R. H., 4
Danforth, E., 541
Danforth, E., Jr., 529
Daniels, J., 537
Daniels, S. R., 61, 419, 466
Danielsson, A., 1
Darby, L., 20
Daston, S., 350, 353, 423
Daun, H., 449
Dauncey, M. J., 535, 542

Davies, A. R., 35
Davies, D., 376
Davies, P. S., 459
Davis, C. J., 381
Davis, J. A., 538
Davis, K., 430
Davis, M. P., 307, 539
Davis, S. E., 192
Davis, T. L., 401
Davis, W. N., 129
Davis-Coelho, B., 79
Davis-Coelho, K., 79
Davison, K. K., 86t, 93, 94, 142, 449
Dawson, B., 450, 539, 543
Dawson-Hughes, B., 513
De Abajo, S., 221
DeBacker, G., 221
De Benoist, B., 545
DEBQ. See Dutch Eating Behavior Questionnaire
De Bruin, A. F., 41
De Castro, J., 155, 156, 167, 294, 296
De Castro, J. M., 304, 331
Dechert, R., 540
Deckelbaum, R. J., 230
De Coppi, M., 465
DeCourville, N., 145t–146t, 147, 149t–151t
Defares, P. B., 138, 149t–151t, 171t, 172, 173, 174
De Graaf, C., 291, 292, 307, 449
De Graaf, K., 300
De Graf, C., 29
De Graff, C., 292
De Groot, G., 536
De Guise, J., 517
De Jong, L. S., 291
De Jonge, L., 540
Dekker, L., 492t–495t, 510
Delahunty, M. J., 3
Delaney, H. D., 147
DeLany, J. P., 447
Delargy, H. J., 298, 299, 300, 302
De la Rie, S. M., 63
De Lauzon-Guillain, B., 166
De Leeuw, I., 492t–495t, 506
Dell'Olio, J., 20
De Lorenzo, A., 539
Delpeuch, F., 483
Delzenne, N. M., 290
DeMaio, T. J., 261, 461
De Man Lapidoth, J., 374
Demeke, T., 545
Dement, W., 223
Demerath, E. W., 492, 508
De Mey, H., 21
Dempster, P., 308, 509
Denmeade, S., 258t–259t

Dennis, B., 261
Denyes, M. J., 451
De Paz, J. A., 221
Deriaz, O., 529
Derksen, J., 21
Derogatis, L. R., 5t–7t, 15, 16, 17, 24, 386, 410, 430
Descriptors for adjectival and semantic differential anti-fat measurement, 84, 565
Desor, J. A., 138, 148
Despres, J. P., 529
Deurenberg, P., 173, 221, 483, 484, 486, 492t–495t, 504, 506
De Veber, L. L., 454
Devine, E. B., 227
Devlin, M., 348, 352, 369
Devlin, M. J., 364, 367, 423
DeVries, H. A., 543
De Wijk, R. A., 292
DeWinstanley, P. A., 377, 387
De Witte, L. P., 41
Deysher, M., 307, 449
De Zwaan, M., 38, 55
De Zwann, M., 370
DH (diet history), 259–260
DHHS (U.S. Department of Health and Human Services), 188, 189, 191, 202
Diabetes Prevention Program Research Group, 187, 215
Diagnostic and Statistical Manual of Mental Disorders
    BED and, 348, 349
    BN and, 349
    purging and, 350
Diederiks, J. P., 41
Dietary assessment methods
    checklists and, 261–262, 263f, 264f
    described, 257, 258f–259f, 258t–259t, 262, 265
    DH and, 259–260
    FFQs and, 257, 259
    food balance data and, 262
    food records and, 260
    screeners and, 261–262, 263f, 264f
    24HR and, 260–261
Dietary Intent Scale, 465, 626
Diethelm, R., 99, 546
Diet history (DH), 259–260
Dietz, W. H., 155, 273, 459, 482, 496, 497, 500, 512
Di Francesco, V., 54
Di Lieto, A., 438
Dilmanian, F. A., 515
Di Marzo, V., 317
DiMeglio, D. P., 291
Dinello, F. A., 3
Dioum, A., 483
Dipietro, L., 221

Direct calorimetry
  availability and costs of, 535
  described, 534
  norms for, 535
  reliability of, 535
  special issues/considerations/pros and cons for, 535
  validity of, 535
Direct objective physical activity and exercise
    measures. *See also* Accelerometers; Pedometers
  described, 204
Direct observation for physical activity and exercise
    measures
  challenges and, 199–200
  direct observation for, 198t
  instruments for, 192, 193t–196t, 198t
  monitoring trail traffic in Indiana and, 199
  multiple, 193t–196t
  observation methods for, 197, 199
  operational logistics and, 199–200
  physical activity and exercise measures, 197, 198t
  problems and, 199–200
  technologically based challenges in, 197, 200
Direct observation techniques for physical activity
    and exercise measures
  CARS and, 201–202
  CPAF and, 201
  limitations of, 204
  SOFIT and, 200–201, 202
  SOPARC and, 203
  SOPLAY and, 201–202, 203
  validation of, 203–204, 205t–206t
DIS (Dietary Intent Scale), 465, 626
Disease-specific HRQOL assessments for eating
    disorders
  described, 64, 67
  EDQLS and, 65
  EDQOL and, 64
  HeRQoLED and, 65–66
  QOLED and, 66–67
Diseker, R. A., 493
Dittmar, M., 37, 40
Divine, G. W., 41
Dixon, J. B., 39
Dixon, M. E., 39
Doak, C. M., 79
Dobbelsteyn, C. J., 500
Dobratz, J. R., 539
Dobrosielski, D. A., 532
Dobson, A. J., 36
Dodd, K. W., 259, 261
Dodrill, C. B., 19
Doebbeling, B. N., 9
Dohrenwend, B. P., 387, 410
Dolan, B., 354, 355, 356
Dolivo, M., 534

Doll, H. A., 40
Dolls with attached stomachs for laboratory
    child-reported hunger and satiety assessment,
    451–453, 452f
Domel, S. B., 458
Dongelmans, P. C., 221
Donnelly, J. E., 256, 544
Donnelly, J. M., 467, 632
Dornbusch, S. M., 81, 82
Dorr, D., 20
Dorsch, K. D., 131
Doubly labeled water, and energy expenditure
    measurement, 531, 541–542
Doucet, E., 300
Douglas, C. G., 536
Douros, I., 492t–495t, 510
Dow, S., 327
Dowda, M., 193t–196t, 216, 239
Drab, D. L., 116t–125t
Drabman, R. S., 450
Drapeau, V., 297, 300, 302, 316
Draper, E., 364
Drewnowski, A., 138, 148, 152, 155, 384
Driscoll, P., 461
Droppleman, L. F., 5t–7t, 19
DSM-IV. See Diagnostic and Statistical Manual of
    Mental Disorders
Dual energy X-Ray absorptiometry
  accuracy and validity of, 513
  availability and costs of, 514
  described, 513
  norms for, 513, 514f
  reliability of, 513
Duan, X., 502
Dubale, G. M., 80
Duchmann, E. G., 434
Dudeck, U., 419
Duffield, R., 539
Dufour, D. L., 545
Duijsens, I. J., 14
Duncan, S. C., 208
Duncan, T. E., 208
Dunn, M. E., 116t–125t
Dunn, S. M., 156
Dupertuis, C. W., 509
Duran, C., 5
Duret, C., 16
Durff, A. C., 447
Durnin, J. V., 484, 503
Dutch Eating Behavior Questionnaire
  availability of, 174
  construct validity of, 172–175
  convergent validity of, 172–175
  described, 169–170
  discriminant validity of, 172–175

eating disorders and psychopathology and, 174
factorial composition and, 172
factor stability and, 172
internal consistency and, 170
naturalistic food consumption and, 173
norms for, 170
predictions of laboratory behavior and, 173–174
questionnaire measures for eating-related problems
    in children and, 464–465
readability of, 174
relationships among restraint scales and,
    175–177, 176t
reliability of, 170–172, 171t
sample and, 170
scales and, 175
susceptibility to response sets and, 174
test-pretest and, 172
validity of, 172
weight and obesity status and, 173
Duval, K., 35, 58
Dworkin, R. J., 201
DXA. *See* Dual energy X-Ray absorptiometry
Dye, L., 284
Dykens, E. M., 116t–125t, 368
Dymek, M. P., 56
Dyr, H. N., 155, 273, 459
Dzumbira, T. M., 545

Eagly, A. H., 80
Earlywine, M., 401
EARS (Electronic Appetite Rating System) studies,
    299–300, 299f, 302
EAT. *See* Eating Attitudes Test
EAT-26. *See* Eating Attitudes Test-26
EAT-40 (Eating Attitudes Test-40), 372, 465–466
Eating and weight-related problems in children
    measurement in laboratory. *See also* Child-
    reported food preferences and palatability
    assessment; Child-reported hunger and satiety
    assessment; Food records for eating in free-living
    environment assessment; Weight-related
    problems in children assessment
analog scale device assessment and, 455–456, 455f
BATMAN and, 450
BE and, 636
behavior assessment of eating-behavior and, 450
BET and, 450
BIS and, 635
cartoon faces assessment and, 456–457, 456f, 457f
cartoon figures for child-reported hunger and
    satiety assessment and, 451, 451f
CBIS and, 633
CEBI and, 629–631
ChEAT and, 628
described, 458–459

dietary recalls, and eating in free-living
    environment assessment of, 461–462
dietary recalls and, 461–463
DIS and, 626
dolls with attached stomachs for child-reported
    hunger and satiety assessment and,
    451–453, 452f
EAT-26 and, 594–596
eating behavior assessment and, 448–450, 449t
FFQs and, 462–463
FJV Preference Questionnaire and, 458
food records and, 460–463, 460t
GEMS and, 458
GEMS Beverage Preferences Questionnaire and,
    458, 622
GEMS Fruit, Juice, and Vegetable Preference
    Questionnaire and, 458, 623–624
KEDS and, 625
ordinal scale measures for child-reported food
    preferences and palatability assessment and,
    456–458, 456f, 457f, 458f
ordinal scale measures for child-reported hunger
    and satiety assessment and, 451–453,
    451f, 452f
questionnaires for assessment and, 458
silhouettes for child-reported hunger and satiety
    assessment and, 453–454, 453f
summary of, 447–448, 469–470
visual analog scales assessment and, 454–455, 454f
Eating Attitudes Test
availability of, 419
described, 416–417
norms for, 417, 418t–419t
questionnaire measures for eating-related problems
    in children and, 465–466
reliability of, 417, 418t–419t
special issues/considerations/pros and cons for, 419
validity of, 417, 418t–419t
Eating Attitudes Test-26
availability of, 419
described, 416–417
norms for, 417, 418t–419t
questionnaire measures for eating-related problems
    in children and, 466, 594–596
reliability of, 417, 418t–419t
special issues/considerations/pros and cons for, 419
validity of, 417, 418t–419t
Eating Attitudes Test-40, 372, 375, 419t, 432t,
    465–466
Eating Disorder Diagnostic Scale
availability of, 363, 416
criterion validity of, 362
described, 361–363, 414
norms for, 363
questionnaire, 581–582

reliability of, 362, 414, 415t–416t, 416
special issues/considerations/pros and cons for, 416
validity of, 415t–416t, 416
Eating disorder disease-specific instruments for
    HRQOL assessment. *See also* Disease-specific
    HRQOL assessments for eating disorders
described, 64
EDQLS and, 65
EDQOL and, 64, 560–561
HeRQoLED and, 65–66
QOLED and, 66–67
summary of, 67
Eating-disordered thoughts, feelings, and behaviors.
    See also Interviews for eating-disordered
    thoughts, feelings, and behaviors
future directions for, 439
interviews and, 399t, 400t
summary of, 397, 439
Eating Disorder Examination
availability of, 379, 401
binge eating size and, 348–349
concurrent validity of, 377–378
criterion validity of, 377–378
described, 376–377, 397–398
interrater reliability of, 377
norms for, 379, 399t–400t, 401
predictive validity of, 378, 379t
reliability of, 377, 398, 399t–400t
sensitivity to change and, 379
special issues/considerations/pros and cons
    for, 401
stability of, 377
validity of, 398, 399t–400t, 400–401
Eating Disorder Examination-Questionnaire
availability of, 366, 367t, 423
criterion validity of, 364–366
described, 363, 419–420
norms for, 366, 367t, 421t–422t, 423
predictive validity of, 365–366
reliability of, 363–364, 420, 421t–422t
sensitivity to change and, 366
validity of, 420, 421t–422t, 423
Eating Disorder Inventory
availability of, 430
described, 423–424 *See also* Bulimia Scale–Eating
    Disorders Inventory
reliability of, 424, 425t–429t, 430
special issues/considerations/pros and cons for,
    430–431
validity of, 425t–429t, 430
Eating Disorder Inventory-2, 65, 424, 467
Eating Disorder Inventory-3, 357–359, 424,
    430–431
Eating Disorder
    Inventory–C, 467

Eating Disorder Quality of Life, 64, 560–561
Eating disorders. *See also* Anorexia nervosa;
    Binge-eating disorder; Bulimia nervosa;
    Self-report questionnaires
described, 347, 387, 389
generic instruments for HRQOL assessment of, 63
psychopathology assessment and, 168
purging and, 347, 350
Eating Disorders Quality of Life Scale, 65
Eating-related problems, 463. *See also* Questionnaire
    measures for eating-related problems
Eating Symptoms Inventory, 366
Eberenz, K. P., 8
Ebert, L., 448
Eck, L. H., 447
Eckerson, J. M., 492t–495t
EDDS. *See* Eating Disorder Diagnostic Scale
EDE. *See* Eating Disorder Examination
Edelmann, R., 145t–146t, 147, 152
Edelmann, R. J., 152
EDE-Q. *See* Eating Disorder Examination
EDI. *See* Bulimia Scale–Eating Disorders Inventory;
    Eating Disorder Inventory
EDI-2 (Eating Disorder Inventory-2), 65, 424, 467
EDI-3 (Eating Disorder Inventory-3), 357–359, 424,
    430–431
EDI-BD (Body Dissatisfaction Scale of the Eating
    Disorder Inventory), 469
EDI-C (Eating Disorder Inventory–C), 467
Edlund, B., 129, 467
Edman, G., 5t–7t
Edman, J., 90
Edmundson, H. M., 545
EDNOS (eating disorder not otherwise specified), 348
EDQLS (Eating Disorders Quality of Life Scale), 65
EDQOL (Eating Disorder Quality of Life), 64, 560–561
Edwards, A. L., 157
Edwards, S., 116t–125t, 208
Edwards-Leeper, L., 84
EES-C (Emotional Eating Scale Adapted for Children
    and Adolescents), 465, 626–627
Egger, J., 21
Egle, U. T., 37
Egri, G., 387, 410
Eiben, G., 259, 270
Einhorn, A. M., 414
Eipe, A., 15
Eisenmann, J. C., 539
Eisinga, R., 142
Ekelund, U., 213, 217
Eklund, K., 467
Ekman, S., 312, 313, 454
Ekstrand, M. L., 158, 174
Elal, G., 419
Elder, J. P., 202

Elder, K. A., 363, 370, 377, 401, 420, 423

Elderly population, pedometer applications for, 209

Electronic Appetite Rating System studies, 299–300, 299f, 302

Elfhag, K., 11, 12, 13, 312, 313, 315

Elia, M., 492t–495t, 510, 513

Ellenberg, D., 116t–125t

Elley, C. R., 221

Elliman, T. D., 302

Ellis, K. J., 486, 492t–495t, 496

Elmore, D., 294, 296

Elosua, R., 221

Emanual, I., 509

Emery, G., 64

Emery, J., 82

Emery, R. W., 41

Emmett, P., 274

Emotional Eating Scale Adapted for Children and Adolescents, 465, 626–627

Emurian, C., 294

Energy expenditure measurement. *See also* Assessment issues in energy expenditure measurement; Direct calorimetry; Field setting for energy expenditure measurement; Indirect calorimetry; Noncalorimeter techniques; Open-circuit indirect calorimetry; Physiological measurements; Physiological observations

   calorimetry and, 531

   closed circuit system and, 540–541

   components of energy expenditure and, 529–530

   confinement systems and, 540

   direct calorimetry and, 534–535

   doubly labeled water and, 531, 541–542

   expiratory open-circuit indirect calorimetry and, 539

   future directions for, 547

   historical background of, 529

   integrated EMG and, 543–544

   isotope dilution and, 541–542

   open-circuit indirect calorimetry and, 537–539

   physiological observations and, 544–546

   population assessment and, 532–534, 533t

   pulmonary ventilation volume and, 543

   review of, 534

   sample analysis interval and, 531–532

   summary of, 529–530, 547

   thermal imaging and, 544

   total collection systems and, 536–537

   ventilated open-circuit indirect calorimetry and, 538–539

Engel, S. G., 54, 55

Engell, D., 329, 449

Engels, R. C., 464

Engels, R. C. M. E., 142, 148, 171t, 176

Engelsen, B. K., 363

Enghardt, H., 273

Engle, E. K., 116t–125t, 131

Engler, L. B., 369

Engstrom, I., 129

Engström, I., 467

Epkins, C. C., 151, 155

Eppers, K., 466

Eppers-Reynolds, K., 466

Eppley Institute for Parks and Public Lands, 197

Epstein, L. H., 293, 309, 449

Erbaugh, J., 386, 410

Erdberg, P., 12

Erickson, C. J., 454

Erickson, J. B., 216, 221

Erni, T., 3

Ernst, N., 261

Erskine, B., 332

ESI (Eating Symptoms Inventory), 366

Esplen, M. J., 358

Essink-Bot, M. L., 35, 40

Ethnicity

   human body composition assessment and, 483–484

   personality and psychopathology assessment and, 4

Eurelings-Bontekoe, E. H. M., 14

Evans, C., 212

Evans, G. W., 329

Evans, W. J., 221, 484

Evensen, D., 265

Evers, W., 228

Ewing, R., 230, 236

Exner, J. E., Jr., 11, 12

Expert Panel on the Identification, Evaluation and Treatment of Overweight in Adults, 496

Expiratory open-circuit indirect calorimetry, 539

Explicit anti-fat attitudes of adolescents and adults

   adjectival evaluations, and measurement of, 83–85, 565

   AFA, and measurement of, 88–90, 106–107nn6–7, 567–568

   AFAS, and measurement of, 90–91, 568

   AFAT, and measurement of, 91–92, 569–571

   ATOP, and measurement of, 92–94, 107nn8–9, 571–572

   described, 86, 86t

   F scale, and measurement of, 87, 566

   FSQ, and measurement of, 94

   measurement of, 86–96, 95t, 106n4

   ranking tasks, and measurement of, 87–88, 106n3

   semantic differential measures of, 86–87, 106n5

Explicit anti-fat attitudes of children

   ACS, and measurement of, 85

   descriptors for adjectival and semantic differential anti-fat measurement and, 84, 565

   friendship measures, and measurement of, 85–86

   measurement of, 81–86

   ranking tasks, and measurement of, 81–83

Faber, P., 535

Fabrigar, L. R., 88

Factoral method, and physiological observations, 545–546

Faerstein, E., 42

Fairburn, C., 63, 175, 358, 363, 364, 401, 411, 419, 420, 422

Fairburn, C. G., 3, 16, 17, 63, 116t–125t, 127, 143, 175, 348, 358, 363, 364, 366, 367, 379, 397, 398, 400, 401, 411, 419, 420, 422, 423

Fairchild, K., 99, 102t–105t

Fairweather, S. C., 200, 212, 213

Faith, M. S., 81, 257, 449, 453, 453f

Falcone, A. R., 52

Falconi, C., 413

Falk, D. B., 538

Fallon, J. A., 193t–196t, 202

Fallowfield, L., 35

Falls, H. B., 189

Fan, H., 273

Fanciullo, G. J., 451

FAO/WHO Ad Hoc Committee of Experts, 532

Farewell, K., 61

Farmakalidis, E., 302

Farmer, J., 156, 356

Fassino, S., 4, 14

Fat Stereotypes Questionnaire, 94

Faulkner, G. E., 229

Faupel-Badger, J. M., 274

Favre, R., 534

Favretti, F., 52

Fayers, P. M., 34, 35

Feary, R., 438

Fee, V. E., 469

Feen, B. G., 485, 485t

Feeny, D. H., 33

Feighner, J. P., 416

Fein, M., 563

Feinberg, J., 99, 102t–105t

Feinstein, A. R., 35

Fenton, T. W., 543

Fercho, M. C., 8

Ferguson, G. A., 164

Ferguson, K. J., 154

Fernandez, S., 431

Fernández-Aranda, F., 4

Ferrari, P., 256, 259

Ferrier, A. G., 417, 419

Ferro-Luzzi, A., 545

FFQs (food frequency questionnaires), 257, 259, 462–463

FFQs, and free-living environment assessment of, 462–463

Fichter, M., 17

Fichter, M. M., 3, 128, 358, 384, 385, 386, 387, 389, 398, 404, 405, 410

Ficker, J. L., 221

Fidanza, F., 487

Fiedler, K., 107nn10,13

Fields, D. A., 508

Field setting for energy expenditure measurement. See also Noncalorimeter techniques calorimeter techniques and, 532

Field studies for food intake measurement. See Food intake field studies measurement

Figure drawings, and weight-related problems in children assessment, 468, 634

Fikkan, J., 80

Filiberti, A., 36

Finch, A., 451

Finch, J. F., 88

Fine, J. T., 40

Finer, N., 56

Finlayson, G. S., 309, 310, 311

Finley, C. E., 80, 102t–105t

Finn, K. J., 200, 201, 213

Fiorito, L. M., 447, 461, 462

First, M. B., 5t–7t, 8, 353, 362, 383, 397

Fischler, C., 327

Fischman, M., 294

Fishbein, H. D., 106–107n7

Fisher, D. C., 41

Fisher, E., 116t–125t, 129

Fisher, J. O., 142, 327, 448, 449, 451, 451f, 456, 456f

Fisher, M., 141, 362, 416, 464

Fiske, D. W., xii

Fitzpatrick, R., 40

Flakoll, P. J., 492

Flegal, K. M., 497, 500

Fleming, E. C., 116t–125t, 128, 130

Flexible total collection systems, 536–537

Flier, J. S., 286

Fliess, J. L., 377

Flint, A., 300

Flood, D., 145, 147, 149t–151t, 159

Flowerdew, G., 500

Flynn, M. A., 484

Fogg, B. J., 228

Folkard, S., 298

Folope, V., 53

Foltin, R., 294

Fomon, S. J., 483

Fontaine, K., 328

Fontaine, K. R., 33, 34, 35, 36, 37, 40, 68

Fontenelle, L. F., 15

Food frequency questionnaires, 257, 259, 462–463

Food intake field studies measurement in free-living populations. See also Intake field studies; Intake

measure selection; Intake volume per occasion measures; Nonusers, screening and segmenting
analysis of, 338
"cool data" and, 327–328, 343
framework for, 329, 340t
importance of, 328
summary of, 327–328, 343
Food intake measurement in free-living populations. *See also* Dietary assessment methods; Obesity-related bias in free-living populations
adolescent populations and, 272–273
bias in case control studies and, 272
children and, 272–273
described, 274–275, 283
dietary assessment methods and, 263f
foods and eating patterns analysis and, 271–272
international studies on underreporting and, 273
intervention population and, 274
obesity-related bias studies and, 268f, 269f
OPEN Study and, 268f, 269f
pregnant population and, 273–274
selective underreporting and, 256
special populations and, 272–274
summary of, 255–257
underreporting and, 256–257
underreporting bias and obesity in, 255–256
Food intake measurement in laboratory. *See also* Appetite studies; Automated food measuring systems; Subjective measures of appetite; Visual analog scale technique
advantages of subjective measures of appetite and, 302
applications for, 316
assessment of sensory-specific effects in different groups and, 307
automated food measuring systems and, 314f, 316f
described, 315–317
EARS studies and, 299–300, 299f, 302
experimental designs and, 290–296
familiar food use in, 296
food intake laboratory described, 289–290, 289f
food selection measurement and, 307–311, 309t, 310t, 311f, 311t, 312f
fundamental assessment issues and, 304–305
future directions for, 315–317
hedonic processes and, 317
homeostatic principles and, 317
innovation and, 316–317
justification for, 315–316
learning with manipulated diets, and role in, 295–296
manipulating whole diet and, 294–295
modifications of basic design and, 294

Food records for eating in free-living environment assessment
24HR and, 258t–259t, 260–261, 460t, 462
described, 459–461, 460t
dietary assessment methods and, 260
eating and weight-related problems in children and, 460–463, 460t
FFQs and, 462–463
Foods and eating patterns analysis in free-living populations, 271–272
Food selection measurement, and food intake measurement in laboratory, 307–311, 309t, 310t, 311f, 311t, 312f
Forbes, G., 481
Ford, E. S., 262
Ford, K., 354, 355, 356
Ford, L. E., 529
Formica, C., 513
Forrest, L., 129
Forrester, T., 273
Forsum, E., 544
Foss, O., 537
Fossel, A. H., 39
Foster, G. D., 10, 80, 86, 165, 166, 178, 351
Foster, R., 306
Foster, R. C., 546
Foster, S. L., 50
Four-compartment model, 485t, 486
Fournier, G., 529
Fowler, B., 116t–125t
Fox, D. T., 450
Fox, S., 193t–196t, 202, 205t–206t
Frampton, I., 377
Francis, L. A., 449
Franciscy, D. M., 53
Franckowiak, S. C., 37
Frank, G. C., 261, 273
Frank, L. D., 230, 235
Frankenburg, F. R., 383, 384
Franklin, R. D., 159, 169, 174, 464
Franks, P. W., 217
Fraser, G. E., 221
Fredrickson, B. L., 116t–125t, 129
Freedman, D. S., 259, 260, 497
Freedson, P., 191, 216
Freedson, P. S., 203, 208, 213, 215t, 216, 221, 546
Free-living population food intake measurement. *See* Food intake field studies measurement in free-living populations; Food intake measurement in free-living populations
Freeman, C. P., 360, 372, 375, 376, 436, 438
Freitas, S. R., 351, 353, 384
Frelut, M. L., 79
French, S. A., 142, 145t–146t, 147, 156, 162, 167, 174, 328, 401, 439

French, S. J., 293, 314
Freudenheim, J., 259
Frezza, M., 465
Friedenreich, C. M., 187, 272
Friedman, K. E., 55, 80, 93, 106n2
Friedman, L. N., 328
Friedman, M. A., 2, 433
Friedman, W. J., 377, 387
Friis, R., 230
Frijters, J. E., 138, 149t–151t, 171t, 172, 174, 465
Frijters, J. E. R., 169, 173, 174
Frisch, M. B., 65
Froberg, K., 212, 217
Froelicher, V., 532
Frost, R. O., 148, 152, 153
F scale, 87, 566
FSQ (Fat Stereotypes Questionnaire), 94
Fudge, H., 3
Fuenekes, G. I., 29
Fujii, M., 492t–495t, 502
Fujioka, K., 53
Fuller, A., 498
Fuller, L., 85
Fuller, N. J., 492t–495t, 510
Fullerton, G., 61
Furr, R. M., x

Gaard, M., 187
Gadde, K. M., 53
Gaertner, S. L., 96
Gaffney, R. D., 485t, 486
Gaines, J. M., 208
Galer-Unti, R. A., 431
Gallagher, D., 492, 496, 497, 516, 517
Gallop, R. M., 358
Galloway, A. T., 449
Galloway, D. J., 53
Galster, G., 236
Gamble, C., 372, 373
Gandek, B., 33, 63
Ganiats, T. G., 42
Ganley, R. M., 162t, 163
Gapinski, K. D., 80, 87, 99, 101, 102t–105t, 106n4
Garaulet, M., 447
Garb, H. N., 11, 12
Garber, L., 335
Garby, L., 535
Garcia-Campayo, J., 411, 413
García-García, E., 430
Gardner, R., 115
Garfinkel, P. E., 116t–125t, 127, 156, 168, 358, 368, 375, 381, 416, 417, 419, 465, 466
Garg, A., 517
Garn, S. M., 498
Garner, D., 358, 359

Garner, D. M., 2, 65, 67, 126, 127, 143, 156, 168, 349, 357, 358, 368, 369, 374, 375, 381, 386, 410, 416, 417, 419, 423, 424, 430, 431, 465, 466, 467, 469
Garratt, A. M., 39
Garren, M. J., 53
Garrow, J. S., 535
Gartner, A., 483
Gashetewa, C., 205
Gass, C. S., 11
Gaston, M. F., 8
Gately, P. J., 300
Gater, R. A., 41
Gawronski, B., 81, 99
Gayton, W. F., 151, 158
Gee, A., 15
Geenen, R., 142
Geier, A. B., 93, 102t–105t
Geissler, C. A., 545
Geliebter, A., 303
GEMS (Girls Health Enrichment Multisite Studies), 458
GEMS Fruit, Juice, and Vegetable (FJV) Preference Questionnaire, 458
Gender
    Herman and Polivy's Restraint Scale and, 147
    personality and psychopathology assessment and, 4–5
General Health Questionnaire (GHQ), 41–42
Generic assessment instruments
    adolescents, and obesity, 59–62
    children, and obesity, 59–62
    CHQ, and children's HRQOL, 59–60
    eating disorder, 63
    KINDL, and children's HRQOL, 60
    web sites for, 564
Generic HRQOL assessment instruments
    described, 35–36
    SF-36 and, 35–36
Geographic information system (GIS) model, 232
George, J. D., 221
Gerace, L., 496
Gerard, E. L., 494, 517
Gerrard, M., 116t–125t, 368
Geye, M., 5
Ghaderi, A., 374, 375, 420
Giacomelli, A. M., 449
Gibbon, M., 5t–7t, 8, 353, 362, 383, 397
Gibbons, M., 493
Gibson, R. S., 164, 257
Giesen, J. C. A. H., 309
Gila, A., 466
Gilbertson, H. R., 449
Gill, T. M., 35
Gill, T. P., 79
Gilson, B. S., 41

Ginde, S. R., 492, 508
Ginis, K. A. M., 86, 87
Ginsburg, H., 454
Giovannucci, E., 272
Gipson, M. T., 128
Girls Health Enrichment Multisite Studies, 458
Glades, M. A., 1
Gladis, M. M., 351, 352, 370
Glanz, K., 265
Glaser, D., 303
Glassman, A. H., 1
Gleaves, D. H., 8, 116t–125t, 128, 140, 361, 379, 381, 401, 404, 434, 436
Gleghorn, A., 221
Gleghorn, A. A., 116t–125t
Glenn, C. V., 106n4
Gleser, G. C., 496
GLP (good laboratory practice), 286, 288–289
Godin, G., 193t–196t
Godt, K., 2
Goekoop, J. G., 14
Going, S., 484, 508
Going, S. B., 494, 504, 508
Gold, B. C., 265
Goldberg, D. P., 41
Goldberg, G. R., 269, 513
Goldberg, L. R., 64
Goldfarb, L. A., 116t–125t, 368
Goldfein, J. A., 364, 365, 366, 367, 423
Goldfield, S. R., 221
Goldring, R. M., 538
Goldstein, G. L., 449
Goldstein, S. E., 84
Golinelli, D., 203, 205t–206t
Gomez, T. D., 492t–495t
Góngora, V., 21
Gonzales, P. M., 107n13
Gonzalez, C., 11
Gonzalez, E. C., 193t–196t, 202, 205t–206t
Gonzalez, N., 63
Good laboratory practice, 286, 288–289
Goodman, N., 81, 82
Goodpaster, B. H., 517
Goodwin, R. D., 4
Goold, K. W., 94
Goran, M. I., 187, 212, 217, 461, 462, 463, 498, 508, 512, 541
Gorber, B., 498
Gorber, S. C., 498
Goreczny, A. J., 381
Goris, A. H. C., 266
Gormally, J., 350, 351, 353, 354, 423
Gorman, B. S., 142, 145t–146t, 147, 149t–151t, 164, 172, 464
Gorusch, R., 5t–7t, 67

Götestam, K. G., 374
Gotfredsen, A., 492t–495t
Gotlib, I. H., 4
Gottdiener, C., 3
Gottfried, A. E., 5
Gottfried, A. W., 5
Gottheil, N., 419
Gottlieb, D. G., 223
Gould, J. C., 53
Government Office for Science, 79
Gower, B. A., 221, 508
Grace, P. S., 141, 187
Graham, J. R., 5t–7t, 8, 9
Grambsch, V., 261
Grande, F., 485, 485t
Grant, J. P., 55, 56
Grant, S., 200, 215
Grasso, K., 116t–125t
Graubard, I., 257
Grave, R. D., 14
Graves, J., 493, 507
Graves, N. S., 16
Gray, J. J., 116t–125t, 126, 131
Gray, R. W., 293, 300, 312, 314, 315
Greaves, K., 193t–196t, 200, 205t–206t
Green, B. A., 16
Green, D., 539
Green, J., 227
Green, S. M., 302
Greenberg, R. P., 2, 11, 12
Greenleaf, C., 80, 90, 94, 96, 106n5
Greeno, C. G., 9, 351
Greenwald, A. G., 96, 97, 98, 99, 101
Gregg, E. K., 145t–146t
Gregg, E. W., 22
Gregg, P. J., 40
Gregory, I., 459
Greil, H., 483
Greve, J. W., 40
Griffiths, R. A., 145, 156
Grilo, C. M., 364, 365, 367, 377, 380, 398, 400, 401, 420, 423
Grimm-Thomas, K., 449
Groepenhof, H., 537
Groer, M., 204
Groessl, E. J., 42
Gronnerod, C., 11
Gross, J., 417
Gross, L. S., 262
Grossman, P., 237
Groth-Marnat, G., 4, 17
Grover, V. P., 99, 101, 102t–105t
Gruber, A., 128
Gruber, A. J., 116t–125t, 126
Grundy, S. M., 517

Grzeskiewicz, C., 116t–125t
Gschwender, T., 99
Gu, D., 502
Guarda, A. S., 116t–125t, 129
Guardo, R., 517
Gudex, C., 41
Guedes, D. P., 494, 508
Guelfi, J. D., 16
Guenther, P. M., 261, 461
Guillen, C. P., 484
Guimera, E., 66, 419
Gulab, N. A., 15
Gullion, C. M., 16
Guo, S. S., 496
Gupta, N. K., 226
Guss, J. L., 313, 314, 315
Gutiérrez, F., 14
Gutniak, M., 312
Guvakov, D., 536
Guyatt, G. H., 33, 35

Haarbo, J., 492t–495t
Haas, J. D., 542
Haber, G. B., 392
Habicht, J. P., 492t–495t
Hackett, A., 273
Hackett, R., 332
Haddock, G., 86
Hagglof, B., 129
Hägglöf, B., 467
Hague, A. L., 93
Hajduk, C. L., 462
Hakim, Z., 227
Halford, J. C. G., 312, 313, 315
Hall, A., 357, 360, 431, 433
Hall, C. B., 506
Hall, J. R. H., 192
Hall, M. C., 504
Hallen, J., 537
Hallmans, G., 259
Hallowell, P. T., 38
Halmi, K., 400
Halmi, K. A., 414
Ham, S. A., 208, 222
Hambleton, R. K., 164
Hamilton, M., 5t–7t
Hamilton, M. A., 43t–51t, 53
Hammer, D., 450
Hammer, L., 156
Hammer, L. D., 483
Hammersley, R., 20
Han, T. S., 36
Han, Y., 197
Handel, R. W., 16

Hander, E. H., 540
Handy, S. L., 230
Hanson, C. L., 447
Hanson, J., 493
Harada, N. D., 221
Harbron, C., 294
Harbron, C. G., 294, 296, 300
Hardt, J., 37
Hardy, L. L., 229, 230
Harlaar, J., 537
Haroian, J., 12
Harper, W. M., 40
Harrell, T. H., 8
Harrington, R., 3
Harris, D., 61
Harris, J., 459
Harris, R., 80
Harris, W. J., 35
Harrison, G. G., 273
Harrison, J. E., 492t–495t
Harrison, K., 129
Harsha, D. W., 447
Hart, K. J., 8
Hartini, T. N., 273
Hartley, G. G., 54
Hartman, A. M., 259, 261
Hartman, T. J., 221
Hartwell, S. L., 42
Harvey, E. L., 79, 92, 93, 96
Harvey, P., 116t–125t, 127
Harvey, P. D., 156
Harvey-Berino, J., 265
Haschke, F., 483
Haskell, W. L., 190, 221, 545
Hassager, C., 492t–495t
Hastorf, A. H., 81, 82
Hathaway, S. R., 5t–7t, 8
Hauben, C., 21
Hauri, P. J., 227
Hauser, R., 356
Hautvast, J. G., 483
Havermans, R. C., 309
Hawilo, M. E., 303
Hawkins, R. C., 354, 355, 356–357, 360
Hawthorne, V. M., 498
Hay, P., 83
Hay, P. J., 63, 363, 420, 422
Haydel, K. F., 156
Hays, N., 162, 166
Hays, R. D., 35
Hayton, J. C., 88
Hayward, C., 156
He, J., 502, 517
He, Q., 483, 496

Head, S., 43t–51t, 53
Health-related quality of life assessment. *See also*
    Obesity-specific HRQOL instruments
  adolescents, and obesity disease-specific
      instruments for, 62
  adolescents, and obesity generic instruments for,
      59–62
  BQL Questionnaire and, 561–563
  childhood, and obesity disease-specific instruments
      for, 62
  childhood, and obesity generic instruments for,
      59–62
  CHQ and, 59–60
  described, 33–34, 67–69
  eating disorder disease-specific instruments for,
      64–68
  eating disorder generic instruments for, 63
  EDQLS and, 65
  EDQOL and, 64, 560–561
  generic instruments for, 35–36
  generic versus disease-specific measures and, 35
  GHQ and, 41–42
  HeRQoLED and, 65–66
  introduction to measurement of, 35
  IWQOL-Kids and, 62, 563
  KINDL and, 60
  limitations of, 68–69
  MA II and, 52, 558
  M.A QoL QII scoring key and, 559
  NHP and, 40–41
  obesity-specific instruments for, 43t–51t
  OWLQOL and, 58, 555
  PedsQL and, 60–62
  QOLED and, 66–67
  QWB and, 42
  reasons for measuring, 34–35
  SF-36 HRQOL assessment in obese populations
      and, 36–37
  SF-36 in weight loss intervention studies and,
      37–42
  SIP and, 41
  techniques for, 35–67
  web sites for generic measures of, 564
  WRSM and, 58, 556
Health-Related Quality of Life in Eating Disorders,
    65–66
Health-Related Quality of Life in Eating Disorders
    (HeRQoLED), 65–66
Hearn, M., 454
Heaslip, S., 80
Heath, E. M., 193t–196t, 202, 205t–206t
Heatherton, T. F., 4, 139, 141, 144, 152, 154, 156, 157,
    159, 357
Heaton, K. W., 392

Hebebrand, J., 405
Hebert, J., 256
Hebl, M. R., 80, 130
Hedeker, D., 10
Hedger, K. M., 127
Heerlein, A. S., 15
Heinberg, L. J., 116t–125t, 126, 129
Heini, A. F., 262
Heintz, A., 37
Heitmann, B., 256, 262, 275
Heitmann, B. L., 256, 258t–259t, 260, 266, 272, 275,
    447, 492t–495t
Helbok, C., 433
Hell, E., 52
Heller, M., 516
Hellström, P. M., 312
Helmes, E., 9, 10
Henderson, B. E., 187
Henderson, M., 360, 372, 375, 376, 436, 438
Hendy, H. M., 449
Henning, B., 540
Hennings, S. J., 542
Henrich, G., 60
Henry, C. J., 449
Henry, C. J. K., 304
Henschel, A., 3, 143
Henson, D. A., 20
Hentinen, M., 40, 41
Hergenroeder, A. C., 492t–495t
Herman, C. P., 80, 102t–105t, 137, 138, 139, 140, 141,
    142, 143, 144, 148, 149t–151t, 151, 152, 158, 159,
    160, 171t, 176, 178, 329, 332, 465
Herman and Polivy's Restraint Scale
  age, and norms in, 147
  construct validity of, 154–159
  content validity of, 151–152
  convergent validity of, 154–159
  described, 143–144
  discriminant validity of, 154–159
  eating disorders and psychopathology and,
      156–157
  factorial composition in primarily normal-weight
      samples and, 152–153
  factorial composition in samples with significant
      proportion of overweight participants and, 153
  factor stability and, 153–154
  gender, and norms in, 147
  internal consistency and, 148
  naturalistic food consumption and, 155–156
  norms for, 144–147, 145t–146t
  predictions of laboratory behavior and, 158–159
  readability of, 159
  reliability of, 148
  sample and, 144

susceptibility to response sets and, 157–158
test-retest reliability of, 148
validity of, 148–154, 150t–151t
weight and obesity status and, 154–155
Herpertz, S., 128, 384, 389, 404
Herpertz-Dahlmann, B., 128, 384, 389, 404, 405
Herschbach, P., 60
Hersen, M., 18
Hertzberg, H. T., 509
Heshka, S., 56, 256
Hesketh, K., 59, 61
Hesketh, K. D., 59
Hessel, A., 5
Hester, J., 300
Hetherington, E. M., 454
Hetherington, M., 290, 306, 307, 454
Hetherington, M. M., 99, 102t–105t, 173, 290, 304,
    306, 307
Heun, R., 4
Hevesy, G., 512
Hewes, H., 205
Heymsfield, S., 482, 486
Heymsfield, S. B., 256, 484, 485, 486, 492, 492t–495t,
    496, 497, 498, 504t–505t, 513, 515
Heyward, V. H., 189, 483
Hibscher, J. A., 151, 160
Hicken, M., 85
Hickey, J. S., 450
Hieggelke, J. B., 337
Higgins, P. B., 508
Hildebrandt, T., 116t–125t, 126
Hill, A. J., 79, 92, 93, 169, 175, 285, 309, 311, 315, 364
Hill, J., 3
Hill, J. O., 530, 538, 544
Hill, K., 13
Hill, K. K., 359, 431, 467
Hillard, M. C., 12
Hillman, K. H., 449
Hirschler, V., 498
Hise, M. E., 256
Hjortland, M., 261
Ho, E. Y., 542
Hoch, S. J., 327
Hodges, E. L., 116t–125t, 463
Hodges, W. F., 17
Hoek, H. W., vii, 3
Hoelscher, D. M., 447, 460t
Hofer, E., 512
Hoffart, A., 4
Hofmann, W., 99
Hofstetter, C. R., 221
Hohagen, F., 193t–196t
Hohlstein, L., 162t, 163
Holden, R. R., xii
Holm, K., 221

Holmbeck, G. N., 116t–125t
Holmberg, L., 272
Holmgren, S., 350
Holt, S. H., 297, 302
Holterman, A. X., 61
Holtkamp, K., 405
Holub, S. C., 84
Honaker, L., 8
Hooper, M. M., 38
Hopkins, C., 91, 116t–125t, 131
Hopper, R. T., 543
Horber, F. F., 52
Horcajo, M. J., 63
Horchner, R., 38
Horgan, G. W., 300
Horlick, M., 496
Hormonal dysregulation, and sleep
    measurement, 224
Horner, N. K., 462
Horsemans, Y., 290
Horst, P., 164
Horton, E. S., 530
Horvath, P., 10
Hould, F. S., 35
Housh, T. J., 492t–495t
Houtkooper, L. B., 504
Hovell, M. F., 221
Howard, A. B., 265
Howard, B. V., 274
Howard, K., 143, 149t–151t
Howarth, N. C., 462
Howe, G. R., 272
Howley, E. T., 537
Høyer, G., 262
Hoyle, R. H., 154, 164
Hoyt, M., 193t–196t, 200, 205t–206t
Hoyt, W. I., 81
Hrabosky, J. I., 116t–125t, 127, 131
HRQOL. *See* Health-related quality of life assessment
Hsieh, C. -C., 274
Huang, H., 192
Huang, T. T., 462
Huang, Y. C., 483
Hubbard, F. A., 354
Hubel, R., 313, 315
Hubert, P., 300
Hubley, A. M., 90
Hudson, J., 128
Hudson, J. I., 1
Hudson, W. W., 96
Huecking, K., 187
Huggins, R. A., 506
Hughes, A. R., 61
Hughes, D. A., 300
Hulshof, T., 292

Hultén, B., 256

Human body composition assessment. *See also* Air
displacement plethysmography; Bioelectrical
impedance analysis; Body mass index;
Circumference measurements; Dual energy
X-Ray absorptiometry; Hydrodensitometry;
Imaging techniques; In vivo neutron activation
analysis and whole-body counting; Skinfold
thickness measurement; Three-dimensional
photonic scanning; Tracer dilution techniques
ADP and, 508–509
aging and, 484
anthropometry and, 487
assumptions and, 482–484
BCM and, 515
BIA and, 483t, 505–507
body fat values and, 483t, 505–507
body weight and, 487
clinical practice and, 482
CT and, 517
DXA and, 483t, 513–514, 514f
ethnicity and, 483
five-level model and, 486–487
4C model and, 485t, 486
future directions of, 517–518
historical background for, 482
imaging techniques and, 515–517, 516f
models for, 484–487
obesity and, 484
phenotyping and, 481
population being assessed and, 482–484
race/ethnicity and, 483–484
sex and, 483, 483t
special populations and, 484
stature and, 487
summary of, 481, 517–518
3C model and, 485t, 486
3-DPS and, 483t, 509–512, 510f, 511f
tracer dilution techniques and, 512
2C models and, 485–486, 485t
UWW and, 507–508
in vivo neutron activation analysis and
whole-body counting and, 483t, 490t,
514–515, 514f
Hummel, R. M., 359, 431, 433
Hunger. *See also* Food intake measurement in
laboratory
cartoon figures for laboratory child-reported
hunger in, 451, 451f
child-reported laboratory, 451–456, 454f, 455f
child-reported laboratory assessment of, 451–453,
451f, 452f
continuous measures in laboratory for
child-reported hunger and satiety assessment
and, 454–456, 454f, 455f

dolls with attached stomachs for laboratory child-
reported hunger and satiety assessment and,
451–453, 452f
hedonic, 317
ordinal scale measures for laboratory
child-reported hunger and satiety assessment
and, 451–453, 451f, 452f
principles and concepts about, 285
silhouettes for laboratory child-reported hunger
and satiety assessment and, 453–454, 453f
Hunt, S. M., 40, 63
Hunter, D. J., 270
Hunter, G. R., 221, 508
Hunter, J. A., 80, 102t–105t
Hunter, W., 192
Huntjens, L., 307
Huot, A., 538
Hurling, R., 237
Huynh, T. N., 208
Hyde, J. S., 116t–125t, 129
Hydrodensitometry
accuracy and validity of, 507
availability and costs of, 508
described, 507
norms for, 508
reliability of, 507–508
Hyer, L., 20
Hyland, M. E., 163
Hyler, S. E., 163t

Iacono, W. G., 467, 632
Iacopino, L., 539
IAT (Implicit Association Test), 97–106, 99f, 100f,
102t–105t, 107n10, 107nn11–16
Ibanez, J., 537
Iber, C., 225
IDED-IV. *See* Interview for Diagnosis of Eating
Disorders-IV
Iglowstein, I., 224
Ilich, J. Z., 221
Illing, V., 357, 422, 423
Illner, K., 516
Imaging techniques
CT and, 517
described, 515–516
MRI and, 516, 516f
Impact of Weight on Quality of Life, 53–54
Impact of Weight on Quality of Life–Kids,
62, 563
Impact of Weight on Quality of Life–Lite,
54–56, 557
Implicit anti-fat attitude measurement
described, 96
IAT and, 97–106, 99f, 100f, 102t–105t, 107n10,
107nn11–16

implicit measures and, 96–106, 99f, 100f, 102t–105t, 107nn11–16
  Lexical Decision Task and, 96–97
Implicit Association Test, 97–106, 99f, 100f, 102t–105t, 107n10, 107nn11–16
Inactivity, 229–230
Indirect calorimetry, 534, 536. *See also* Total collection systems
Inge, T. H., 61
Inglis, H., 536
Ingwersen, L., 267
Ingwersen, L. A., 261, 461
Inman, J. J., 328, 334, 342
Institute of Medicine, 219
Intake field studies
  boundary conditions, and increasing effective size of, 332–334
  described, 329–330, 330f, 331f
  intake floors and ceiling and, 334
  intake process models, and reduction of systematic variance in, 331–332, 333f
  intake-prone populations and, 333–334
Intake measure selection
  acquisition measures and, 335
  described, 334–335, 335f
  intake intentions measurement and, 335–336
  intake recall measures and, 336–337
  postintake measures and, 336–337
  preintake measures and, 335–337
  residual and inferential measures of intake and, 337
  scenario-based methods of measuring intake and, 337–338
Intake of food field studies measurement. *See* Food intake field studies measurement; Food intake measurement in free-living populations
Intake volume per occasion measures
  accounting for satiation and, 342
  actual versus inferred intake and, 341
  counting versus weighing and, 341–342
  described, 341
  identification of appropriate level of analysis and, 342–343
Integrated EMG, and energy expenditure measurement, 543–544
International studies on underreporting, and food intake measurement in free-living populations, 273
Intervention population
  food intake measurement in free-living, 274
  technological innovations for physical activity and exercise measures and, 238–239
Interview for Diagnosis of Eating Disorders-IV
  availability of, 381, 402
  construct validity of, 380–381
  content validity of, 380–381

criterion validity of, 381
described, 379–380, 401–402
norms for, 402
questionnaire, 596–617, 617f
reliability of, 380, 402, 403t–404t
special issues/considerations/pros and cons for, 402, 404
validity of, 402, 403t–404t
Interviews for eating-disordered thoughts, feelings, and behaviors. *See* Bulimia Test–Revised; Eating Attitudes Test; Eating Attitudes Test-26; Eating Disorder Examination; Eating Disorder Examination-Questionnaire; Eating Disorder Inventory; Interview for Diagnosis of Eating Disorders-IV; Multifactorial Assessment of Eating Disorder Symptoms; Structured Interview for Anorexic and Bulimic Disorders
Intille, S. S., 237
In vivo neutron activation analysis and whole-body counting
  availability and costs of, 515
  described, 514–515, 514f
  norms for, 515
  reliability of, 515
  Whole-Body 40K Counting Technique and, 515
Irie, M., 42
Irvine, S. H., 163
Irving, L. M., 84
Irwin, M. L., 221, 544
Isaksson, B., 256
Isbell, T. R., 142
Isotope dilution, and energy expenditure measurement, 531, 541–542
Israel, R. G., 494
Ito, T. A., 145t–146t, 149t–151t
Iwane, M., 204
Iwaoka, H., 492
IWQOL-Kids (Impact of Weight on Quality of Life–Kids), 62, 563
IWQOL-Lite (Impact of Weight on Quality of Life–Lite), 54–56, 557
Iynegar, S. S., 327

Jaccard, J., 107n13
Jackman, L. P., 439, 467
Jackson, A. S., 493, 507
Jackson, C., 41, 42
Jackson, K., 221
Jackson, R. J., 230
Jackson, S. R., 439, 467
Jacobi, L., 86t, 90, 95t, 569, 571
Jacobs, D. R., 221
Jacobs, D. R., Jr., 221, 544
Jacobsen, D. J., 256, 544
Jacobsen, S., 535

Jadzinsky, M., 500
Jaffe, K., 106–107n7, 106n4
Jagger, C., 40
Jago, R., 230
Jakatdar, T. A., 116t–125t, 131
Jakicic, J. M., 530
James, P. T., 79
James, W. P., 538, 542
Janney, C. A., 221
Jannsen, I., 517
Jansen, A., 148, 174, 178, 309
Janssen, I., 498
Janssen, J. D., 546
Janssens, J. M., 464
Janz, K. F., 191, 213, 230
Jaramillo, S. J., 457
Jarcho, H. D., 116t–125t, 126
Jarrell, M. P., 116t–125t, 463, 464, 468
Jarrett, R. B., 16
Jarvie, G. J., 450
Jass, J., 313
Jeammet, P., 2
Jean-Mary, J., 265
Jebb, S. A., 513
Jee, S. H., 222
Jeffery, R. W., 142, 145t–146t, 162, 167, 174, 328
Jeffrey, D. B., 450
Jeffrey, R. W., 79
Jellar, C. C., 420
Jenkins, J. T., 53
Jenkinson, C., 40
Jenni, O. G., 224
Jennings, G., 513
Jensen, B. E., 417
Jensen, C. L., 538
Jensen, M. D., 538
Jequier, E., 99, 534, 538, 546
Jette, A. M., 221
Jette, M., 536
Jeyaram, S., 80, 102t–105t
Jia, H., 40
Jimenez, M., 439
Jiménez-Murcia, S., 4
Joanes, D., 302
Joffres, M. R., 500
Johansen, O., 535
Johansson, A. J., 493
Johansson, G., 256, 259
Johansson, I., 259
Johns, M. W., 193t–196t, 227
Johnson, C. L., 466
Johnson, D. T., 17
Johnson, F., 174
Johnson, G. O., 492t–495t
Johnson, M. S., 189

Johnson, N. J., 226
Johnson, P. E., 493, 512
Johnson, R. K., 212, 265, 461, 462, 463
Johnson, R. L., 116t–125t
Johnson, S. L., 256, 448, 449, 451
Johnson, W. G., 149, 153, 158, 369
Johnston, C., 454
Johnston, D., 38
Johnstone, A. M., 294, 300
Joiner, G. W., 433
Joiner, T. E., Jr., 4, 357
Jolliffe, D., 79
Joly, E., 290
Jonas, J. M., 1
Jonat, L. M., 433
Jones, A., 116t–125t
Jones, D. I., 212
Jones, M. B., 449
Jones, S., 213
Jonsdottir, S. M., 431
Jordan, H. A., 313, 315
Jordan, J. S., 41
Jorgensen, T., 221
Joseph, A., 230
Joseph, N. T., 543
Judd, C. M., 96
Judd, J., 221
Junghanns, K., 193t–196t
Junker, M., 354

Kaaks, R., 230, 256
Kabacoff, R. I., 18
Kabnick, K., 327
Kaemmer, B., 5t–7t, 8
Kahaly, G. J., 37
Kahl, M. J., 484
Kahn, B. E., 327, 342
Kalarachian, M. A., 365, 367, 400, 420, 422
Kales, A., 224
Kalfarentzos, F., 52
Kalinsky, L. B., 142, 145t–146t
Kalkwarf, H. J., 291, 542
Kamenetz, C., 364, 367, 423
Kameoka, V. A., 18
Kantz, M. E., 35
Kaplan, D., 312
Kaplan, R. M., 42, 193t–196t
Karabulut, M., 207, 209, 546
Karlsson, J., 41, 43t–51t, 56, 57, 161
Karvonen, M. J., 487
Kashima, A., 116t–125t, 129
Kashiwazaki, H., 542
Kashubeck, S., 433
Kaskoun, M. C., 463
Katch, V. L., 536

Katula, J., 221
Katz, D., 128
Katz, J., 4
Katz, J. N., 39, 41
Katz, R., 2
Katz, R. C., 128
Katzmarzyk, P. T., 545
Kaukua, J., 38, 57
Kawachi, S., 537
Kaye, W. H., 9, 19
Kechagias, I., 52
KEDS Body Image Silhouettes, 468–469, 635
Keel, P., 99, 102t–105t
Keel, P. K., 80, 84, 357, 401, 419, 565
Keery, H., 116t–125t, 129
Kees, M., 148, 176t
Keeser, W., 358, 405
Keeton, P., 116t–125t, 127
Kehagias, I., 52
Kehayias, J. J., 513
Keilen, M., 63
Keizer, H. A., 537
Kelder, P. H., 38
Keller, K. L., 449, 455f
Keller, S. D., 40
Kelley, D. E., 517
Kelly, L. A., 200, 213
Kelly, W. G., 492t–495t, 512
Keltikangas-Jarvinen, L., 13
Kely, T., 294
Kempen, K. P., 145t–146t, 167
Kemper, H. C., 200, 215t, 221
Kenardy, J., 465
Kendall, A., 291, 294, 296
Kendrick, Z. V., 492t–495t
Kennedy, J. M., 449
Kennedy, S., 358
Kennedy, S. H., 2
Kenny, D. A., 329
Kenrick, J., 376
Kent, K. M., 449
Kent, R. J., 327
Kermanshah, M., 453, 453f
Kerr-Almeida, N., 10
Kerse, N. M., 221
Kester, A. D., 537
Keys, A., 3, 143, 485, 485t, 487
Khan, S. R., 98
Khosla, T., 487
Kickham, K., 151, 158
Kid's Eating Disorders Survey
    BIS and, 468–469, 635
    described, 463–464, 625
Killen, J. D., 156

Killingsworth, R., 230
Killingsworth, R. E., 230
Kim, J., 4, 337
Kim, Y. S., 502
Kimura, N., 487
Kind, P., 41
Kinder, B. N., 116t–125t
KINDL, 60
Kinematic measurements, and physiological
    observations, 546
King, A. C., 221, 228
King, E. B., 130
King, G. A., 215t, 537
King, L. E., 192
King, N., 300
King, N. A., 298, 300, 309
Kinney, J. M., 538
Kinzl, J. F., 52
Kipnis, V., 270, 275
Kirk, A. A., 369
Kirk, B., 537
Kirk, S. F. L., 93
Kirk, T. R., 290
Kirkbride, A., 130
Kirkpatrick, S. W., 83
Kirschenbaum, D. S., 354, 356
Kirshenbaum, D. S., 260
Kissileff, H., 290, 292, 301, 315
Kissileff, H. R., 304, 306, 313, 314, 315, 448, 453, 453f
Kjelsås, E., 374
Klaczynski, P. A., 94, 106n4
Klaghofer, R., 356
Kleifield, E., 140
Klein, S., 5, 500
Kleitman, N., 223
Klem, M. L., 145t–146t, 147, 148, 149t–151t, 151, 152, 155
Klesges, L. M., 142, 151, 155, 212, 294, 458
Klesges, R. C., 142, 145t–146t, 147, 148, 149t–151t, 151, 152, 155, 212, 294, 328, 447, 450
Kline, G. M., 221
Kline, P., x
Klinger, W. R., 8, 10
Klingsberg, G., 306, 314, 448
Klump, K. L., 3, 14
Knerr, A. N., 492t–495t
Knott, C. B., 451
Knotter, A., 129
Knous, J. L., 492t–495t, 497
Knuiman-Hijl, W. F. H., 174
Knutsen, S. F., 221
Knutson, K. L., 227
Ko, C., 419
Kochersberger, G., 212

Kochtitzky, C., 230
Koerner, J., 171t, 172, 419, 464
Kohl, H. W., 212
Kohl, H. W., III, 221
Kohl, I. H. W., 222
Kohlmeier, L., 260
Kohrt, W. M., 213, 517
Kok, F. J., 449, 492t–495t
Kolar, A. S., 260
Koletzko, B., 224
Kolotkin, R. L., 35, 37, 43t–51t, 53, 54, 55, 56, 62
Komiya, S., 482
Konik, J., 87
Kono, M., 419
Konradi, D. B., 221
Koop, P. M., 154
Kopec-Schrader, E. M., 376
Korn, S. J., 84
Korolija, D., 58
Kortner, B., 52
Kosinski, M., 40, 63
Kosloski, K. D., 43t–51t, 54
Koslowsky, M., 417, 419
Kotler, D. P., 492t–495t, 498, 506
Kotthaus, B. C., 149t–151t, 156, 162t, 171t, 176t
Kovera, A. J., 496
Kowalski, R., 1
Kozee, H. B., 130
Kozin, F., 42
Kraak, V. I., 187
Krabbe, P. F., 35
Kraemer, H., 379
Kraemer, H. C., 400
Krahn, D. D., 384
Kraig, K. A., 80, 84, 565
Kral, J. G., 33, 34
Kral, T. V. E., 138, 142, 257, 272
Kramer, F. M., 297
Kraus, A., 15
Krause, G., 484
Krebs-Smith, S. M., 257
Krefetz, D. G., 15
Kressel, S., 41
Krieg, J. C., 354
Krishna, A., 328, 332
Krishnan, K. R., 53
Kriska, A. M., 193t–196t, 221
Kroeze, W., 237, 238
Kroll, L., 162t, 163
Kromhout, D., 221
Kronenberg, F., 229
Kronenfeld, J. J., 212
Kruskall, L. J., 221
Kubacki, S. R., 12

Kuchibhatla, M. N., 212
Kuhlmann, H. W., 52
Kuhnert, M. E., 116t–125t
Kuipers, H., 537
Kuldau, J. M., 175
Kuleshnyk, I., 332
Kullberg, J., 498
Kumanyika, S., 79
Kump, K., 193t–196t, 338
Kupfer, D. J., 226
Kurpad, A. V., 541
Kurth, C. L., 384
Kurtin, P. S., 60
Kushida, C. A., 226
Kushner, R. F., 35, 498, 512
Kutlesic, V., 128, 379, 380, 381, 401, 402, 404
Kyere, K., 493

Laberg, J. C., 363
Laboratory measurement for eating and weight-
    related problems in children. *See* Eating and
    weight-related problems in children
    measurement in laboratory
Lacey, H., 411, 413
LaComb, R., 261
Ladetto, Q., 545
Laessle, R. G., 149t–151t, 156, 162t, 169, 171t, 173,
    176t, 177, 312, 313, 359
Lafay, L., 258
Laforgia, J., 486
Lagiou, P., 274
Lagman, R., 307
Lahteenmaki, L., 167
Lake, K. D., 41
Lake, L., 149, 153
Laliberte, M., 417, 419
Lam, E. T. C., 417
Lambers, A. C., 291
Lambert, N., 265
Lammert, O., 535
LaMonte, M., 222
Lamparski, D. M., 350
Lancaster, K. L., 38
Landahl, S., 258, 260
Landgraf, J., 59
Lane, K. A., 98
Lang, T., 356
Langenbucher, J., 116t–125t, 126
Lanningham-Foster, L., 230
Lanningham-Foster, L. M., 229
LaPorte, R. E., 221
Lappalainen, R., 290, 449
Largo, R. H., 224
Larriba, R., 221

Larsen, J. K., 142, 171t, 176, 351
Larson, K., 237, 492t–495t
Larson, M. G., 39
Lartamo, S., 314
Lasater, T. M., 221
Las Hayas, C., 65
Lask, B., 371, 377
Lask, B. D., 128
Latner, J. D., 80, 82, 84, 86, 88
Lattimore, P., 173
Lau, A. S., 129
Lauderdale, D. S., 227
Launder, C., 116t–125t
Lawless, H. T., 332
Lawrence, B., 371
Lawrence, C., 116t–125t
Lawton, C., 294, 296
Lawton, C. L., 291, 298, 308
Le, H., 99
Leahy, K. E., 449
Lean, M. E., 36
Leary, M. R., 86, 87
Leathwood, P., 297
Le Carvennec, M., 492t–495t
Lechner, H., 43t–51t, 52, 559
Lecrubier, Y., 382
Lee, C. C., 542
Lee, H., 230
Lee, J. W., 20
Lee, M. D., 314
Lee, S. M., 207
Lee, Y., 449
Leenen, R., 483, 504
Lefevre, J., 221
Leger, L., 517
Legrand, J. M., 16
Le Grange, D., 56, 420
Lehrke, S., 313
Leichner, P., 419
Leichtman, M., 12
Leitenberg, H., 398, 400, 417
Leiter, L. A., 454
Le Magnen, J., 304, 313
Le Masurier, G. C., 207
Lemm, K. M., 97, 98
Lemmel, G., 11
Lemnitzer, N. B., 450
Lensegrav, T. L., 193t–196t, 202
Leon, A. S., 221
Leon, I., 5
Leonard, C. E., 17
Leonard, W. R., 498, 545
LePen, C., 36, 39, 43t–51t
Lepore, S. J., 329

Lepper, M. R., 327
Leproult, R., 223
Lerner, R. M., 84
Lernfelt, B., 258, 260
Lescelleur, O., 35, 58
Lester, R., 433
Letizia, K. A., 10
Leung, N., 438
Levenhagen, D. K., 493, 505
Levin, B., 430
Levine, A. S., 141, 143, 178
Levine, D. W., 193t–196t, 226
Levine, J. A., 229, 230, 530, 538, 539, 544, 546
Levine, M. P., 129
Levitsky, D., 327
Levitsky, D. A., 291
Levitsky, K., 35
Levitsky, L., 270
Levy, E., 36, 43t–51t
Levy, S. M., 230
Lewis, M. A., 193t–196t, 226
Lewis, R. J., 86t, 90, 91, 95t, 116t–125t, 127, 569, 571
Lexical Decision Task, 96–97
Li, H., 54
Li, L., 213, 215t, 262
Liang, M. H., 39
Lichtermann, D., 4
Lichtman, S., 486, 504t–505t
Lichtman, S. W., 155, 156, 462
Licinio, J., 15
Liddell, H. G., 347
Liem, D. G., 449
Lilenfeld, L. R. R., 2
Lilienfeld, S. O., 11, 12
Liljequist, L., 9
Limbers, C. A., 60
Lin, B. -H., 462
Lin, D. H. Y., 496
Lin, J., 130
Lind, B. K., 225
Lindberg, S. M., 116t–125t, 129
Lindel, B., 312, 314
Linder, L. W., 342
Lindgren, A. C., 312
Lindquist, C. H., 187, 462
Lindroos, A. K., 256, 258t–259t, 266, 270, 275
Lindsey, C., 221
Lindsey, G., 197, 199
Lindsey, S., 101
Lindsted, K. D., 221
Lindström, M., 430
Lipman, R. S., 15
Lissner, L., 256, 258t–259t, 260, 262, 266, 268, 270, 275, 291, 447

Littman, A. J., 221
Liu, K., 260
Liu, S., 262
Liu, Y., 449
Livingstone, M. B., 155, 273, 447, 458, 459, 462
Lloyd, D. G., 543
Lluch, A., 298, 300
Lobstein, T., 79
Locard, E., 224
Lock, J., 363
Loeb, K., 366
Loeb, K. L., 4
Loewen, R., 449
Lof, M., 544
Lofgren, R., 540
Lohman, T., 484
Lohman, T. G., 485, 487, 492t–495t, 494, 498, 504,
    508, 513
Loiseau, A., 538
Loken, E., 462
Longobardi, N., 438
Loos, F., 36
Lopes, C. S., 42, 351
Lopez, E., 130
Lopez, M. N., 20
Lopez, R., 230
López-Albarenga, J. C., 430
Lopez-Zetina, J., 230
Lore, R., 3
Lorr, M., 5t–7t, 19
Loukidi, A., 52
Lovell, N., 66
Lovibond, P. F., 18
Lovibond, S. H., 18
Lowe, M., 168
Lowe, M. R., 138, 139, 140, 141, 142, 143, 148, 152,
    153, 155, 158, 159, 169, 178, 317, 464
Lowe, R., 487
Lowik, M. R., 492t–495t
Loyden, J., 85
Lozano, C., 377, 401
Lozano-Blanco, C., 377, 398, 400
Lu, J. F., 35
Lubetkin, E. I., 40
Lucas, F., 304
Luce, K. H., 363, 420, 422
Luchetta, T., 19
Lucio, E., 5
Luck, A. J., 411, 413, 414
Ludwig, D. S., 454
Luis, C. A., 11
Lukajic, O., 207
Lukaski, H. C., 493, 506, 512
Lukkarinen, H., 40, 41

Lum, L., 536
Lum, S. K., 129
Lumeng, J. C., 449
Lund, E., 187
Lundgren, J., 116t–125t
Lundquist, S., 312
Luschene, R., 5t–7t, 67
Luscombe, G., 66
Lutfi, R. E., 39
Lybanon-Daigle, V., 357, 422, 423
Lyle, R. M., 431
Lynch, J., 129
Lynch, K., 231, 232, 235
Lynch, W., 466
Lynch, W. C., 466
Lyon, B. L., 221
Lyons, J., 411, 413
Lysen, V. C., 187

Ma, G. S., 492t–495t, 509
Ma, R., 486
Maccalini, G., 500
MacCallum, R. C., 88
Macdiarmid, H. I., 291
Macera, C. A., 212
Macfarlane, D. J., 191, 536, 542
Machin, D., 34, 35
Maciejewski, M. L., 40, 68
Mack, D., 137, 144
MacKay, S. J., 538
MacLean, D. R., 500
Maddi, S. R., 2
MAEDS. *See* Multifactorial Assessment of Eating
    Disorder Symptoms
Maes, L., 261
Maes, M., 438
Maffeis, C., 542
Maggs, C., 273
Magnetic Resonance Imaging, 516
Magson, L. D., 315
Mahabir, S., 544
Mahan, J. M., 149, 153
Mahar, M. T., 493, 507
Maher, E., 61
Maier, W., 4
MA II (Moorehead-Ardelt Quality of Life
    Questionnaire II), 52, 558
Maiolo, C., 539
Maire, B., 483
Maj, M., 438
Makan, T., 530
Makela, J., 53
Malcarne, V. L., 431
Maldonado, A. J., 354

Malhotra, M. S., 543
Malina, R. M., 483, 496
Malkoff, S. B., 20
Maller, O., 305
Malone, M., 351, 353
Maloney, K. C., 400, 439
Maloney, M. J., 419, 466, 467
Malouff, J. M., 19
Manchester, D. S., 80
Manke, F., 3, 10
Mann, B., 438
Mann, T., 158
Mannucci, E., 43t–51t, 439
Manson, J. E., 274, 328
M.A QoL QII scoring key, 559
M.A QoL QII scoring key, and HRQOL assessment, 559
Mara, O., 294
Marano, G., 116t–125t, 127
Marceau, P., 35, 58
Marceau, S., 35
Marchesini, G., 37
Marcus, M. D., 350, 351, 354, 369
Mari, J. J., 419
Marino, V., 56
Mark, M., 430, 431
Marks, G. C., 492t–495t
Marlowe, D., xi, xii, 157
Marmot, M. G., 269
Marquez, S., 221
Mars, M., 292, 449
Marse, P., 537
Marsh, G. M., 21
Marshall, S. J., 193t–196t, 203, 205t–206t, 229
Marsland, L., 464
Martens, M. P., 417, 419
Martikainen, T., 52
Martin, C. K., 368, 434, 436
Martin, D. P., 41
Martin, G. S., 258t–259t
Martin, S. B., 80
Martin, W. M., 484
Martinez, E., 362, 416
Martinez, R., 88
Martins, Y., 130
Martinsen, E. W., 4
Martorell, R., 498
Maruish, M. E., 16
Masala, S., 539
Masheb, R. M., 364, 367, 377, 398, 400, 423
Mason, A. D., Jr., 540
Masse, L. C., 217
Mathias, S., 43t–51t
Matisoo-Smith, E., 449

Matos, M. I. R., 2, 18
Mattes, R. D., 291
Matthews, C. E., 208
Matthews, D. E., 221
Matthys, C., 261
Mattias, I., 317
Matz, P. A., 9
Maurer, J., 156, 168, 256, 257
Maurovich-Horvat, P., 493, 502
Maxwell, S. E., 147
Mayclin, P., 492t–495t
Maycock, B., 169
Mayer, C., 290
Mayville, S., 128
Mayville, S. B., 116t–125t
Mazariegos, M., 484, 496
Mazel, R. M., 35
Mazess, R. B., 493
Mazlan, N., 290
Mazure, C. M., 414
Mazzeo, S., 161, 163, 175
McArthur, L. H., 106n4
McAuley, E., 221
McCabe, M. P., 359
McCaffrey, R. J., 9
McCarthy, D., 162t, 163
McCarthy, D. M., 359, 431, 467
McClough, J. F., 10
McConaha, C. W., 19
McConnell, E., 212
McCrae, R. R., 5t–7t, 158
McCreary, D. R., 131
McCrory, M., 162, 166, 462
McCrory, M. A., 462, 492t–495t, 508
McCullough, M. L., 271
McDermott, T., 307, 454
McDermott, T. M., 307, 454
McDevitt, R., 290
McDonald, R. P., 164
McDougall, P., 417, 419
McDowell, A. J., 149t–151t, 163
McDowell, C. J., II, 11
McDuffie, J., 260
McEwen, J., 40
McGhee, D. E., 97
McGrath, P. A., 454
McGrath, R. E., 11, 454
McGuire, J. B., 419, 466
McHenry, K., 270
McHorney, C. A., 35, 36
McHugo, G. J., 451
McIntosh, J. A., 451
McKenna, S. P., 40
McKenna-Foley, J. M., 17

McKenzie, T. L., 193t–196t, 202, 203, 205t–206t
McKinlay, J. B., 221
McKinley, J. C., 5t–7t, 8
McKinley, N. M., 116t–125t, 129
The McKnight Investigators, 464
McKnight Risk Factor Survey III, 464
McLaughlin, J. E., 537, 539
McLaughlin, J. P., 96
McLean, J. A., 529, 536, 537, 540, 543
McLellarn, R. W., 450
McLeod, H. A., 80
McMahon, R. L., 56
MCMI-III. *See* Millon Clinical Multiaxial Inventory–
    Third Edition inventory
McNair, D. M., 5t–7t, 19
McNaughton, L. R., 539
McNeill, K. G., 492t–495t
McNulty, J. L., 9
McPhee, L., 448, 449
McPhee, L. S., 448, 449
McPherson, R. S., 447, 459, 460t, 462
McPhie, L., 430
McQuaid, J., 431
McSwegin, P., 189
McTiernan, A., 187, 215
McVey, G., 2
Mead, N., 52
Meagher, M. W., 14
Measurement issues and techniques
    BMI and, vii
    classic test theory and, x–xi
    construct validity of, xi–xii
    convergent validity of, xii
    described, x, xiii
    discriminant validity of, xii
    factor structure and, xi
    high-quality assessment measures and, vii–viii
    internal consistency and, xi
    interrater reliability of, xi
    journals on, vii
    norm referencing for tests and, xiii
    predictive validity of, xii
    reliability of, x–xi
    statistics, vii
    susceptibility to dissimulation testing and, xii
    test-retest reliability of, xi
    validity of, xi–xii
Measuring attitudes about obese people. *See* Anti-fat
    attitude measurement
Meengs, J. S., 306
Meininger, J. C., 226
Meiselman, H. L., 327
Melanson, E. L., 203, 208, 209, 213, 215t, 546
Melanson, E. L., Jr., 203, 213, 215t, 546

Melanson, K. J., 20
Melbye, M., 274
Melchiorri, G., 539
Mellon, M. W., 145t–146t, 147, 148, 149t–151t, 155
Melnyk, S. E., 116t–125t, 127, 131
Mendel, C. M., 37
Mendelsohn, F. S., 387, 410
Mendelsohn, M. E., 532
Mendelson, J. M., 410
Mendelson, M., 386, 410
Mendelson, M. J., 116t–125t
Mendez, M., 260
Mendez, M. A., 273
Mendlowicz, M. V., 15
Mennella, J. A., 449
Merminod, B., 545
Mernagh, J. R., 492t–495t
Merom, D., 208
Merrill, E. P., 297
Mertes, J. D., 192
Messick, S., 138, 141, 149t–151t, 159, 160, 161, 162,
    162t, 163, 165, 375, 386, 410, 416
Messner, C., 107n10
Metcalf, B. S., 212
Meter, K., 35
Metter, E. J., 208
Metzdorff, M., 138
Meyer, C., 438
Meyer, D. E., 96
Meyer, G. J., 11, 12, 438
Meyer, I. H., 80
Meyer, J. -E., 312, 313, 315
Meyer, R. J., 328
Meyers, A., 312
Michielutte, R., 493
Mickelsen, O., 3, 143
Mickley, D., 366
Midthune, D., 262
Miettunen, J., 5
Mihalko, S. L., 221
Mihura, J. L., 11
Mikkelsen, T. B., 274
Mikulka, P. J., 116t–125t, 130
Miles, C. W., 542
Miller, A. B., 272
Miller, D. C., 4
Miller, D. J., 221
Miller, H. S., 532
Miller, J., 12, 466
Miller, J. A. A., 496
Miller, J. C., 302
Miller, J. L., 417, 419
Miller, K. A., 52
Miller, K. B., 375, 385

Miller, M., 260
Miller, R., 229
Miller, Y. D., 229
Millon, T., 5t–7t, 20, 21, 430
Millon Clinical Multiaxial Inventory–Third Edition
    inventory
    availability, 21
    limitations, 20
    norms, 19
    overview, 20
    reliability of, 19
    research applications, 20
    validity, 19
Mills, A., 459
Mills, J. K., 17
Mills, J. S., 364, 367, 420, 423
Milnes, S., 401
Milos, G., 4
Minges, J. R., 4
MINI. *See* Mini International Neuropsychiatric
    Interview
Mini International Neuropsychiatric Interview
    availability of, 382
    construct validity of, 382
    criterion validity of, 382
    described, 381–382
    interrater reliability of, 382
    reliability of, 382
    stability of, 382
MINI-Kid. *See* Mini International Neuropsychiatric
    Interview
MINI-Plus. *See* Mini International Neuropsychiatric
    Interview
Minnesota Multiphasic Personality Inventory–Second
    Edition
    availability, 9–10
    limitations, 10
    MMPI-2 short form, 10–11
    norms, 9
    overview, 8–9
    reliability of, 9
    research applications, 10
    validity, 9
Minten, V. K., 492t–495t
Mintz, L. B., 359, 361, 411, 417, 419, 431, 433
Miotto, P., 465
Mirch, M. C., 307
Mishra, G., 36
Misra, A., 502
Mitchell, C. J., 300
Mitchell, D. C., 447, 459, 461, 462
Mitchell, J., 351, 367, 423, 438, 542
Mitchell, J. E., 55, 370, 400, 401
Mitchell, J. P., 99, 102t–105t

Mittelstaedt, R., 80
Miyatake, N., 492t–495t, 502
Mizes, J. S., 19, 433
Mlynarski, L., 85
MMPI-2. *See* Minnesota Multiphasic Personality
    Inventory–Second Edition
Mobini, S., 302
Mock, J., 386, 410
Modak, P., 53
Modestin, J., 3
Modi, A. C., 61
Moe, P. W., 221
Moher, D., 498
Mole, P. A., 492t–495t
Molinari, L., 224
Moller, A. C., 291
Mond, J., 63
Mond, J. M., 63, 363, 365, 420, 422
MONICA-Denmark study, 266
Monk, T. H., 226, 227
Monroe, D., 80
Monteleone, P., 438
Montgomery, P., 227
Montoye, H. J., 200, 204, 212, 215t, 221
Mook, D. G., 200
Moon, J. K., 538
Moon, R. D., 313
Moore, F. D., 515
Moore, J. B., 204, 209
Moore, J. C., 84
Moore, M. C., 261
Moore, T. R., 15
Moorehead, M. K., 43t–51t, 52, 559
Moorehead-Ardelt Quality of Life Questionnaire II,
    52, 558
Morabia, A., 79
Moran, T., 294
Mordant, A., 169
Moreira, R. O., 15
Morey, L., 5t–7t, 430
Morgan, C. D., 20
Morgan, C. G., 212
Morgan, J. F., 411, 413, 414
Morgan, S. B., 83
Morgenthaler, T., 225, 226
Morley, J. E., 484
Morris, D., 517
Morris, J. A., 461
Morris, J. R., 41
Morrison, M. A., 91, 96, 102t–105t, 116t–125t, 131
Morrison, T. G., 80, 86t, 89, 90, 91, 94, 95t,
    106–107n7, 116t–125t, 131, 568
Morrow, J. R., 80
Morrow, J. R., Jr., 212

Morrow, J. R. J., 189
Morton, G. J., 286
Mosconi, P., 36
Moscovitch, M., 327
Moshfegh, A. M., 261
Moskowitz, R. W., 38
Moss, R. A., 465
Mossman, D., 16
Moss-Racusin, C. A., 107n9
Motion studies, and physiological observations, 544–545
Mott, J. W., 484
Mowen, A. J., 230
Moya, T. R., 438
Moylan, J., 265
MRFS-III (McKnight Risk Factor Survey III), 464
MRI (Magnetic Resonance Imaging), 516
Muck, R., 433
Mudge, B. O., 451
Mudry, J. J., 94
Mueller, J. K., 227
Mueller, W., 226
Mueller, W. H., 492t–495t
Muhlheim, L. S., 256, 266
Muir, J., 498
Muir, S. L., 173
Mukherjee, D., 492t–495t
Mulholland, A. M., 411
Müller, A., 312, 314
Müller, M. J., 516
Multifactorial Assessment of Eating Disorder Symptoms
  availability of, 369
  construct validity of, 368
  criterion validity of, 368
  described, 367, 434
  discriminant validity of, 368–369
  norms for, 369, 434, 435t–436t
  predictive validity of, 368
  questionnaire, 617–621
  reliability of, 367–368, 434, 435t–436t
  special issues/considerations/pros and cons for, 434
  validity of, 434, 435t–436t
Mumford, D. B., 419
Mummery, K., 230
Munch, A. K., 140
Murgatroyd, P., 294
Murgatroyd, P. R., 535
Muro, M., 536
Murphy, D., 392
Murphy, S., 265
Murphy, S. A., 238
Murphy-Eberenz, K. P., 128, 140, 379, 401, 404
Murzi, E., 305

Musante, G. J., 55
Musher-Eizenman, D. R., 84, 85, 86
Mussap, A. J., 15
Must, A., 229, 459
Mustajoki, P., 57
Myers, A., 106n2
Myers, A. M., 209, 228
Myers, J., 532
Myers, J. A., 53

Nadel, E. R., 221
Nader, P. R., 193t–196t, 202, 203
Nagata, A., 536
Nair, K. S., 512, 541
Nairn, K., 384
Nakao, T., 482
Nangle, D. W., 369, 370
Nasca, P. C., 216, 221
Näslund, E., 300, 312, 313, 315
Nasser, M., 419
Nathan, J. S., 8
National Research Council, 231
National Sleep Foundation, 224
Naughton, D., 259
Nawyn, J., 237
Neale, B., 161
Nebeling, L., 229
Neelon, F. A., 41
Neiderman, M., 371
Nelson, J. A., 210
Nelson, M., 221, 270, 271, 461
Nelson, R. A., 544
Nelson, S. E., 483
Nelson, W., 8
Nelson, W. M., III, 8
Nemeroff, C., 116t–125t, 129
Netemeyer, R., 116t–125t, 127
Netemeyer, S., 450, 463
Neuhouser, M., 274
Neumärker, K. J., 419
Neumärker, U., 419
Neven, K., 56
Nevonen, L., 376, 430, 431
Newby, P. K., 271, 272
Newman, A., 417
Newson, L., 305
Nezworski, M., 11, 12
Nezworski, M. T., 11
Nguyen, M. H., 37
Nguyen, N. T., 38, 52, 53
Nguyen, T., 540
NHP (Nottingham Health Profile), 40–41
Nichols, J. F., 212
Nicholson, J. C., 492t–495t

Nickols-Richardson, S., 166, 167

Nicol, S., 54

Nicoll, G. L., 230

Nicolson, N. A., 169

Nieman, D. C., 20, 116t–125t, 537

Niero, M., 43t–51t, 58

Nilssen, O., 262

Nilsson, A., 213, 216

Ni Mhurchu, C., 37

Nisbett, R. E., 138, 143

Noakes, M., 492t–495t, 507

Noll, S. M., 116t–125t, 129

Nolph, G. B., 484

Noma, S., 411, 413

Nonaka, K., 492t–495t, 502

Noncalorimeter techniques
  described, 541
  field setting for energy expenditure measurement
    and, 533–534
  isotope dilution, "doubly labeled water" and,
    541–542
  summary of, 534

Nonusers, screening and segmenting
  accounting for usage facilitators and, 339–340, 340t
  comparative versus absolute measures of usage
    frequency and, 340–341
  described of, 338–339
  identification of broad intake intervals and, 339
  specification of intake situations and usage
    occasions for, 339
  user frequency measurement and, 339–341

Noor, M. I., 545

Noordenbos, G., 63

Norlander, O., 537

Norman, A., 221

Norman, G. J., 229, 237, 239

Norman, S., 52

Norms
  DEBQ and, 170
  Herman and Polivy's Restraint Scale and, 144–147,
    145t–146t
  personality and psychopathology assessment and,
    2, 5
  Stunkard and Messick's TFEQ-R Scale and, 161

Norring, C., 350, 357, 374, 376

Norris, M. P., 14

North, J., 292

Norton, A. C., 538

Norton, G. N. M., 305, 306

Nosek, B. A., 98, 99, 102t–105t

Nottingham Health Profile, 40–41

Novitsky, S., 536

Nulicek, D. N., 484

Nunally, J. C., 377

Nunes, M. A., 419

Nuñez, C., 506, 508

Nurse, R. J., 449

Nyboer, J., 505

Nyenhuis, D. L., 19

Nysse, L. J., 230

Oates-Johnson, T., 145t–146t, 147, 149t–151t

Oberlander, S., 87

Oberrieder, H., 80

Oberson, B., 3

Obese populations. *See also* Food intake
    measurement in free-living populations
  pedometer applications for, 208–209
  SF-36 HRQOL assessment in, 36–37

Obesity. *See also* Obesity and relevant analytical
    issues; Obesity-specific HRQOL instruments
  defined, 79
  obesity-related bias studies and, 268f, 269f
  passive obesity and, 79
  sleep measurement, and risk factors for, 224, 225
  underreporting bias and, 255–256

Obesity and relevant analytical issues
  energy adjustment for underreporting bias and,
    267–270
  portion size issues and, 270–271, 271f

Obesity and Weight Loss Quality of Life
    Questionnaire, 58, 555

Obesity-related bias in free-living populations
  described, 266
  MONICA-Denmark study and, 266
  OPEN Study and, 267
  Swedish obese subjects study and, 266

Obesity-Related Psychosocial Problems, 56–57, 556

Obesity-specific HRQOL instruments
  BAROS and, 42, 52–53
  described, 42, 43t–51t, 57–59
  IWQOL and, 53–54
  IWQOL-Lite and, 54–56, 557
  OP Scale and, 56–57, 556

O'Brian, K. S., 102t–105t

O'Brien, B., 40

O'Brien, K. M., 2, 3

O'Brien, K. S., 80, 90, 99, 101, 106

O'Brien, P. E., 39

O'Bryan, M., 106–107n7

Observing Protein and Energy Nutrition Study, 267,
    268f, 269f

Ochoa, P., 221

Ocke, M. C., 221

Ockene, I. S., 256

Ockene, J. K., 256

Ocker, L. B., 417

O'Connor, M. E., 401

O'Connor, W. E., 80, 86t, 89, 90, 94, 95t,
    106–107n7, 568

Ode, J. J., 492t–495t, 497
O'Doherty, J., 303, 305
Oetting, M., 138
Offer, D., 116t–125t, 126
Ogden, C. L., vii
Ogden, J., 80, 172, 173
O'Halloran, M. S., 411, 417, 419
O'Hara, N., 200, 201, 203, 204
O'Hara, N. M., 205t–206t
Ojerholm, A. J., 91
Okamoto, A., 116t–125t, 129
Olinto, M. T. A., 419
Olivardia, R., 128
Oliveira, B., 228
Oliver, A., 300
Oliveria, S. A., 221
Olmstead, M. P., 67
Olmsted, M., 358
Olmsted, M. P., 357, 358, 375, 410, 417, 465, 466, 467
Olsen, J., 274
Olsen, S. F., 274
Olson, R., 20
Oman, C., 332
O'Neil, P. M., 55, 170
Open-circuit indirect calorimetry
    described, 537–538
    ventilated, 538–539
Openshaw, C., 371, 372
OPEN (Observing Protein and Energy Nutrition)
    Study, 267, 268f, 269f
Opper, S., 454
OP Scale (Obesity-Related Psychosocial Problems),
    56–57, 556
O'Rahilly, S., 56
Ordinal scale measures
    child-reported food preferences and palatability
        assessment in laboratory and, 456–458, 456f,
        457f, 458f
    child-reported hunger and satiety assessment in
        laboratory and, 451–453, 451f, 452f
Ordman, A. M., 354, 356
O'Reilly, J., 87
O'Reilly, L. M., 294, 296
Oreland, L., 5t–7t
Orenstein, M. R., 187
Oria, H., 43t–51t, 52
Oria, H. E., 43t–51t, 52, 559
Orlandi, E., 439
Orlet Fisher, J., 449
Ortega, A., 9
Ortega, D. F., 354, 356
Ortiz, O., 496
Osler, M., 256, 272, 274
Osterhaus, J. T., 33
Ostfeld, A. M., 221

Ostrove, S. M., 492t–495t
Ouwens, M., 149t–151t, 159, 165, 169, 171t, 173, 176t
Ouwens, M. A., 148
Overduin, J., 148
Overend, T. J., 532
Owen, C., 63, 363, 420, 422
Owen, N., 230
Owen, O. E., 492t–495t
OWLQOL (Obesity and Weight Loss Quality of Life
    Questionnaire), 58, 555
Ozer, S., 148, 176t

Paavonen, E. J., 467
Pace, L. M., 256
Pace, T. M., 4
Pacy, P., 535
Padierna, A., 63
Paffenbarger, R. S., Jr., 212, 221
Paganini-Hill, A., 187
Paice, N., 438
Painter, J. E., 292, 337, 340
Palav, A., 9
Palmer, R., 348, 376
Paluch, R., 449
Pambianco, G., 546
Pangrazi, R. P., 209
Papa, A., 413
Papathakis, P. C., 492t–495t, 507
Papp, E., 40
Paquet, E., 509
Parcel, G., 205t–206t
Parides, M. K., 366
Park, B., 96
Park, H. S., 502
Park, J. Y., 502
Park, S., 327
Parke, R. D., 454
Parker, S. C., 411, 413, 414
Parmentier, A., 19
Parnell, T., 8
Parr, R. M., 515
Passi, V. A., 363
Passive obesity, 79
Pate, R. R., 188, 189, 191, 193t–196t, 200, 203, 208,
    210, 216, 219, 239
Patel, A., 187
Patel, S. R., 223
Paterniti, S., 2
Pateyjohns, I. R., 492t–495t, 507
Paton, J. Y., 200, 215
Patrick, D. L., 33, 40, 43t–51t, 58
Patrick, K., 228, 237
Patterson, T. L., 193t–196t, 202, 203
Patton, M. M., 208
Paulosky, C. A., 397, 401, 419, 431, 439

Paulson-Karlsson, G., 430
Pavlidis, I., 544
Paxton, S. J., 116t–125t, 173, 174, 468
Payne, C. R., 327
Payton, J. Y., 200
Pbert, L., 256
Peacock, E., 17
Pediatric Quality of Life Inventory, 60–62
Pedometers
    children, and applications for, 209
    described, 204, 207, 209
    elderly, and applications for, 209
    field studies, and applications for, 208
    internal mechanisms, and features of, 204, 207
    overweight and obese populations, and
        applications for, 208–209
    step count as an indicator of physical activity, and
        use of, 207–208
PedsQL (Pediatric Quality of Life Inventory), 60–62
Peeters, P. H., 221
Pekkarinen, T., 38, 57
Pelchat, M. L., 449
Pelletier, C., 332
Pendall, R., 236
Pendleton, R., 55
Penev, P., 223
Penny, H., 86
Penpraze, V., 215, 216
Pepino, M. Y., 449
Peppler, W. W., 493
Perez, A., 356
Perez-Lopez, M. S., 91
Perkins, S., 438
Perks, S. M., 463
Perlman, B., 9
Perloff, B., 267
Perloff, P., 261
Perreault, M., 419
Perry, L., 411, 413, 414
Perry, W., 12
Personality and psychopathology assessment. *See also*
    Beck Depression Inventory–II inventory; Millon
    Clinical Multiaxial Inventory–Third Edition
    inventory; Minnesota Multiphasic Personality
    Inventory–Second Edition; Profile of Mood
    States inventory; Psychopathology instruments;
    Rorschach inventory; State-Trait Anxiety
    inventory; Symptoms Checklist 90 Revised
    inventory; Temperament and Character
    inventory
    cause and effect issues and, 2–3
    culture and, 4
    ethnicity and, 4
    fundamental issues for, 2–4
    gender and, 4–5
    instruments overview for, 5, 5t–7t, 8
    mental state versus personality trait and, 3
    norms for, 2, 5
    personality defined, 1
    personality instruments for, 8–14
    population issues and, 4–8
    race and, 4
    self-report inventories versus diagnostic interviews
        and, 3–4
    summary of, 1–2, 21–22
Persson, V., 273
Peshock, R. M., 517
Pete, E., 327
Peters, J. C., 449
Petersen, A. C., 116t–125t, 126
Petersen, S. E. K., 40
Peterson, C. B., 375, 377, 385, 398, 400, 420, 422
Peterson, M. J., 503
Peterson, P., 450
Petocz, P., 302
Petrella, R. J., 532
Petrie, T. A., 116t–125t, 127, 431, 433
Petrilli, A., 419
Petroni, M. L., 508
Pettigrew, T. F., 80
Peveler, R. C., 3, 16, 17
Pfeiffer, K. A., 216
Phelan, S., 58, 68
Pheley, A. M., 212
Philippaerts, R. M., 221
Phillips, C. B., 39
Phillips, K., 128
Phillips, K. A., 116t–125t, 128, 131
Phillips, R. A., 496
Phillips, W. T., 532
Physical activity and exercise measures. *See also* Built
    environment; Direct objective physical activity
    and exercise measures; Direct observation for
    physical activity and exercise measures; Self-
    report of physical activity and exercise measures;
    Sleep measurement; Technological innovations
    for physical activity and exercise measures
    accelerometers and, 210–217, 214t, 215t
    budgetary considerations domain of, 191
    constraints of, 190–192
    domains of measurement and, 190
    instruments for, 197
    modalities for, 189–192
    monitoring trail traffic in Indiana and, 197
    multiple measures of, 192
    physical activity defined, 188
    physical activity recommendations domain of,
        191–192

physical fitness measures and, 188
reasons for, 187–188
recommendations for, 191–192
research hypothesis and physical activity domains
of interest and, 190–191
sedentariness, and measuring lack of,
229–230
sleep, and relevance of, 223–224
special population domain of, 191
summary of, 188–189, 239–240
target population domain of, 191
time constraints domain of, 192
Physiological measurements, and energy expenditure
measurement
heart rate monitoring and, 542–543
integrated EMG and, 543–544
pulmonary ventilation volume and, 543
thermal imaging and, 544
Physiological observations
activity logs and, 545–546
activity recall and, 544–545
factoral method and, 545–546
kinematic measurements and, 546
motion studies and, 544–545
time studies and, 544–545
Piccinini, L., 532
Pick, T., 11
Picot, A. K., 2
Piec, G., 52
Pieper, C., 212
Piers, L. S., 530
Pierson, R. N., 494
Pierson, R. N., Jr., 484, 486, 492t–495t, 496, 504t–
505t, 506, 512
Pietrobelli, A., 257, 481, 506, 513
Pike, K. M., 4, 366, 376
Pinhas-Hamiel, O., 71
Pinnington, H. C., 539, 543
Pirke, K., 169
Pirke, K. M., 149t–151t, 156, 162t,
171t, 176t
Pirok, E., 448, 449
Pivarnik, J. M., 212, 213, 492t–495t, 497
Plank, L. D., 492t–495t, 506
Plante, T. G., 2
Plat, L., 223
Platte, P., 169, 178
Pliner, P., 332, 449
Pliner, P. L., 327
Plummer, M., 256
Pober, D., 191
Poehlman, E. T., 221, 541
Poivre, R., 538
Polinko, N. K., 87

Polivy, J., 67, 80, 102t–105t, 137, 138, 139, 140, 141,
142, 143, 144, 148, 149t–151t, 152, 156, 157, 158,
159, 178, 329, 332, 410, 465, 467
Pollard, W. E., 41
Pollet, P., 297
Pollice, C., 9
Pollock, M. L., 493, 507
Pols, M. A., 95, 221
Polysomnography method, 225–226
Pomhoff, I., 563
POMS. *See* Profile of Mood States inventory
Pook, M., 131
Pope, H., 128
Pope, H. G., 116t–125t, 126
Pope, H. G., Jr., 1
Pope, R. P., 193t–196t, 202, 205t–206t
Popkin, B. M., 79
Popovich, P. M., 87
Poppitt, A. M., 256
Poppitt, S., 256, 266
Population. *See also* Adolescents; Adults; Children;
Elderly population; Food intake field studies
measurement in free-living populations; Food
intake measurement in free-living populations;
Gender; Race; Special populations
gender, and personality and psychopathology
assessment of, 4–5
human body composition assessment by sex and,
483, 483t
physical activity and exercise measures, and
target, 191
SF-36 HRQOL assessment, and obese, 36–37
Population assessment
energy expenditure measurement and,
532–534, 533t
field setting for energy expenditure measurement
and, 532
laboratory setting for energy expenditure
measurement and, 532
Porter, J., 469
Portion size issues, 270–271, 271f
Potischman, N., 259, 274
Potter, J., 187
Pouliot, M. C., 498
Powell, A. L., 116t–125t
Powell, K. E., 189, 230
Powell, S. M., 212
Power, K., 371, 373
Powers, P. S., 116t–125t, 356
Prange, M., 116t–125t
Pregnant population, and food intake measurement
in free-living, 273–274
Prentice, A., 290, 294
Prentice, A. M., 155, 156, 256

Prentice, R. L., 274
Presnell, K., 140, 142, 178
Preti, A., 465
Primavera, L. H., 142, 147, 149t–151t
Prochaska, J. J., 228
Profile of Mood States inventory
    availability, 19–20
    limitations, 20
    norms, 19
    overview, 19
    reliability of, 19
    research applications, 20
    validity, 19
Proter, E. L., 314
Prothro, J. W., 496
Prussin, R. A., 156
Pruzinsky, T., 115
Pryor, T., 8, 10
Przybeck, T. R., 5, 5t–7t, 13
Psychopathology assessment. *See also* Personality and
        psychopathology assessment
    eating disorders and, 168
    psychopathology defined, 1
Psychopathology instruments. *See also* Millon Clinical
        Multiaxial Inventory–Third Edition inventory;
        State-Trait Anxiety inventory; Symptoms
        Checklist 90 Revised inventory
    BDI-II inventory and, 15
    psychopathology assessment and, 5, 5t–7t, 8
Pudel, V., 138, 140, 160, 166, 169, 175, 312, 313, 315
Puente, A. E., 8
Puentes-Neuman, G., 419
Puhl, J., 193t–196t, 200, 201, 202, 204, 205t–206t
Puhl, R. M., 79, 80, 93, 106nn1–2,4, 107n9
Pulmonary ventilation volume, and energy
        expenditure measurement, 543
Purging, 347, 350. *See also* Anorexia nervosa;
        Bulimia nervosa
    described, 387, 389
Puttonen, S., 13
Puyau, M. R., 213, 216
Puzziferri, N., 53

QEWP-R. *See* Questionnaire of Eating and Weight
        Patterns–Revised
QOLED (Quality of Life for Eating Disorders),
        66–67
Quaade, F., 496
Quadflieg, N., 3, 128, 384, 385, 386, 387, 389, 398,
        404, 405, 410
Quality of Life for Eating Disorders, 66–67
Quality of Well-Being Scale, 42
Quan, S. F., 227
Quatman, G., 8

Questionnaire measures for eating-related problems in
        children. *See also* Kid's Eating Disorders Survey
    CEBI and, 466–467
    ChEAT and, 466
    DEBQ and, 464–465
    DIS and, 465, 626
    EAT-26 and, 466, 594–596
    EAT-40 and, 465–466
    EAT and, 465–466
    EES-C and, 465, 626–627
    MFRS-III and, 464
    MRFS-III and, 464
Questionnaire of Eating and Weight Patterns–Revised
    availability of, 370
    concurrent validity of, 370
    criterion validity of, 370
    described, 369
    predictive validity of, 370
    questionnaire, 573–580
    validity of, 369–370
Quetelet, L. A. J., 487
Quinn, D. M., 89, 567, 568
Quintana, J. M., 63
QWB (Quality of Well-Being Scale), 42

Raben, A., 291, 300, 540
RAB-R (Rating of Anorexia and Bulimia Interview–
        Revised), 376
Race
    human body composition assessment and, 483–484
    personality and psychopathology assessment and, 4
Rachlinski, J., 294
Radley, D., 492t–495t
Rafamanantantsoa, H. H., 542
Ragazzoni, P., 10
Raghubir, P., 328, 332
Raich, R., 129
Rajaram, S., 327
Ramaswamy, S. S., 543
Ramerth, W., 19
Ramirez, E., 116t–125t
Rammohan, M., 494
Rand, C. S., 175
Ranieri, W., 14
Raper, N., 267
Rapoport, D. M., 538
Rardin, D., 350, 353, 423
Rasinski, K. A., 222
Rasmussen, F., 161
Rathner, G., 357, 358
Rating of Anorexia and Bulimia Interview–
        Revised, 376
Raudenbush, B., 449
Raudenbush, S., 230

Rauh, M. J., 221
Raurich, J. M., 537
Rauter, U. K., 17
Ravaja, N., 13
Ravelli, A. C., 221
Ravens-Sieberer, U., 60
Ravussin, E., 99, 492t–495t, 529, 530, 546
Rawlins, M., 80, 102t–105t
Ray, M. L., 335, 339
Raynor, H. A., 293
Reas, D. L., 116t–125t, 127, 434
Rechtschaffen, A., 224
Reddon, J. R., 9, 10
Redegeld, M., 60
Redwine, B. A., 204
Reed, A. E., 369
Reed, D. L., 116t–125t, 127
Reed, D. R., 449
Reed, G. W., 530, 538
Reeves, M. J., 492t–495t, 497
Regan, P. C., 106n5
Reid, C. A., 300
Reid, F., 411, 413
Reid, M., 20
Reilly, J. J., 61, 200, 215, 216, 229
Reilly, T., 529
Reina, J. C., 545
Reinhardt, S., 82
Reiter, J., 116t–125t, 128, 131
Rejeski, W. J., 15
Rennie, K. L., 542
Renninger, L., 85
Resch, M., 439
Resnicow, K., 221
Restrained eating measures. *See also* Herman and
    Polivy's Restraint Scale
    definition and conceptualization of restrained
        eating and, 139–143
    Dutch Eating Behavior Questionnaire and, 169–
        177, 171t, 176t
    eating in absence of hunger and, 142, 160
    future research directions for, 177–178
    history of, 137–138
    meaning of restrained eating and, 139–140
    Stunkard and Messick's TFEQ-R scale and, 138,
        150t, 151t, 159–169, 162t
    summary of, 137, 140–143
Restraint scales. *See also* Herman and Polivy's
    Restraint Scale
    DEBQ, and relationships among, 175–177, 176t
    historical background of, 137–138
    measurements made with, 140–143
Retzlaff, P. J., 65
Reutzel, T. J., 41

Reveillere, C., 11
Revicki, D. A., 494
Reynolds, C. F., III, 226
Reynolds, K., 217, 502
Reynolds, K. D., 187
Rguibi, M., 130
Rhea, D. J., 80
Rhyne, M., 466
Riboli, E., 256
Ricca, V., 351, 352, 438
Ricciardelli, L., 150, 162, 163, 165, 168
Richard, D., 308
Richards, S. S., 448, 449
Richards, W. O., 39
Richardson, M. T., 221
Richardson, S. A., 81, 82
Richter, P., 15
Rickels, K., 15, 386, 410
Ricklin, T., 52
Riddoch, C. J., 217
Rieder, R. O., 163t
Rief, W., 17
Rieger, E., 56
Riemann, D., 193t–196t
Rietjens, G. J., 537, 539
Rigid total collection systems, 536
Riley, R. E., 545
Riley, W. T., 265
Rippe, J. M., 37
Rips, L. J., 222
Rising, R., 492t–495t
Riskey, D., 138, 148
Riskind, J. H., 15
Rissanen, A., 34
Rissanen, A. M., 38
Ritchey, P. N., 106–107n7
Ritenbaugh, C., 79
Ritz, P., 300
Riva, G., 10
Rizvi, S. L., 357, 361, 377, 398, 400, 414, 416
Ro, O., 4, 17
Roach, R. C., 542
Roberti, J. W., 15
Roberts, S., 162, 166, 462, 539
Roberts, S. B., 462, 541
Robertson, D., 376
Robertson, H. D., 192
Robertson, K., 294
Robertson, R., 546
Robertson, R. J., 530
Robinette, K. M., 509
Robinson, B. E., 86, 87
Robinson, E., 221
Robinson, P., 411, 413

Robinson, T. E., 303
Robinson, T. M., 293, 314, 315
Robinson, T. N., 229, 449
Robson, P. J., 273, 447, 458
Roby, J. J., 210
Roche, A. F., 492t–495t, 498, 505
Rock, A. F., 386, 410
Rockert, W., 466
Rockett, H. R., 459, 463
Rodefer, J. S., 449
Rodgers, B., 63, 363, 420, 422
Rodin, J., 1, 2, 138, 140, 292, 448
Rodriguez, D. A., 237
Roe, D. A., 291, 542
Roe, L. S., 306, 449
Roehrig, H. R., 61
Roehrig, M., 116t–125t, 129
Roemmich, J. N., 449
Roeykens, J., 221
Roger, D., 175
Rogers, E., 505
Rogers, H. J., 164
Rogers, I., 274
Rogers, P. J., 169, 175, 285, 296, 297, 300, 311, 312, 313
Rogers, R. L., 431, 433
Rohde, P., 142
Rohles, F. H., Jr., 3
Rojdev, R., 8
Roll, S., 116t–125t
Rolland, V., 540
Rolland-Cachera, M. F., 496
Rollins, N. C., 492t–495t, 507
Rolls, B., 294
Rolls, B. J., 205, 284, 303, 305, 306, 307, 327, 329, 331, 449, 454
Rolls, E. T., 303, 305, 306
Rolls, J. H., 306
Rolls, L., 449
Romano, S. J., 414
Romero, N., 449
Rookus, M. A., 187
Roose, S. P., 1
Roosen, R. G. F. M., 174
Rooth, P., 312, 313, 315
Rorschach, H., 5t–7t, 11
Rorschach inventory
    availability, 12
    limitations, 12
    norms, 12
    overview, 11
    reliability of, 11–12
    research applications, 12–13
    validity, 11

Rose, K. S., 116t–125t, 127
Rosemurgy, A., 356
Rosen, J. C., 106n2, 116t–125t, 127, 128, 131, 398, 400, 417
Rosen, L. W., 349
Rosenbaum, P. L., 466
Rosenbaum, S. H., 538
Rosenbloom, C. A., 496
Rosenvinge, J. H., 4, 358
Rosewall, J. K., 82, 84, 88
Rosner, B., 275
Ross, A. G., 545
Ross, J. K., 106n4
Ross, R., 193t–196t, 239, 498, 516, 517
Ross, R. K., 187
Rosser, R., 42
Rossi, G., 21
Rossi, M., 465
Rossiter, E. M., 348, 349
Rossner, J., 260
Rossner, S., 11, 12, 13
Rössner, S., 312, 313, 315, 454
Rotenberg, K. J., 145, 147, 149t–151t, 159
Roth, D. A., 15
Roth, D. L., 256
Rothblum, E., 80
Rothblum, E. D., 85, 91
Rothenberg, B. M., 42
Rothenberg, E., 258, 260
Rothman, M., 43t–51t, 58
Roubenoff, R., 162, 166, 513
Rousseau, A., 129
Rowan, E. T., 91, 116t–125t, 131
Rowe, E. A., 205, 303, 305
Rowe, P., 193t–196t, 202, 205t–206t
Rowland, C. V., Jr., 3
Rowlands, A. V., 212
Royce, J., 82
Rozin, P., 327, 448
RS. *See* Restraint scales
Rubchinskaya, E., 197
Ruderman, A. J., 141, 152, 153, 155, 158, 160, 187
Rudman, L. A., 99, 102t–105t
Ruggiata, R., 36
Rumpler, W. V., 542
Rumpold, G., 357, 358
Rush, A. J., 16, 64
Rush, E. C., 492t–495t, 506
Russ, J., 212
Russell, C. J., 419
Russell, G., 139, 143
Russell, G. F. M., 348
Russell, I. T., 39

Russell, J., 66
Russell, K. G., 258t–259t
Russell, S. J., 221
Russell-Aulet, M., 492t–495t
Ruta, D. A., 39
Rutter, M., 3
Ryan, L. M., 300
Rychlak, J. F., 5
Ryden, A., 5, 43t–51t
Rydén, O., 1
Ryu, H. R., 431

Saad, F. G., 449
Sacco, W. P., 116t–125t, 127
Sadeh, A., 225, 226
Sadik, C., 1
Saelens, B. E., 309
Safer, D., 168
Safer, D. L., 139
Salamero, M., 66, 419
Salamone, L. M., 513
Salehi, M., 85
Salinsky, M. C., 19
Sallis, J. F., 189, 193t–196t, 202, 203, 205t–206t, 208, 210, 212, 213, 221, 228, 230
Salmon, L., 59
Salmon, L. A., 59
Salorio, P., 11
Saltzberg, E., 116t–125t, 127
Salvy, S. J., 449
Sample analysis interval, and energy expenditure, 531–532
Samsa, G. P., 37, 53
Samuelson, G., 273
Sanchez-Santos, R., 42
Sanders, D. M., 83
Sanders, R. D., 16
Sandhagen, B., 273
Sane, T., 57
Santos, M., 116t–125t, 128
Santos, M. T., 116t–125t
Saravis, S., 454
Sardinha, L. B., 494, 508
Sargent, R. G., 106n4
Saris, W. H., 145t–146t, 167, 200, 215t, 227
Saris, W. H. M., 221
Sarkin, J. A., 212
Sarlio-Lahteenkorva, S., 34
Sarwer, D. B., 142
Sasse, D. K., 116t–125t, 131
Satiation. *See also* Food intake measurement in laboratory
    AUC, and quantifying, 301
    child-reported laboratory assessment of, 451–453

intake volume per occasion measures, and accounting for, 342
    intra- and intermeal changes, and quantifying, 300–301
    principles and concepts about, 285
    quantifying, 300–302
    quantifying satiety and, 300–302, 303f
    recovery or rate of return of hunger, and quantifying, 301, 301f
    SQ and, 301–302
    VAS technique and quantifying, 300–302, 303f
Satiety assessment
    cartoon figures for laboratory child-reported satiation and, 451, 451f
    child-reported laboratory satiation and, 451–456
    child-reported satiation, and laboratory, 451–453
    continuous measures in laboratory for child-reported satiation and, 454–456, 454f, 455f
    dolls with attached stomachs for laboratory child-reported satiation and, 451–453, 452f
    food intake measurement in laboratory and, 290–292
    ordinal scale measures for laboratory child-reported satiation and, 451–453, 451f, 452f
    preload type design, and procedures for, 292–294
    preload type design, and procedures for satiety assessment and, 292–294
    principles and concepts for, 284–286, 286f–288f
    procedure and description of subjective measures of appetite and, 297–298, 297f
    procedures for, 290–292
    quality control for, 286–289, 288f, 317
    quantifying satiation and satiety for, 300–302, 303f
    reliability of VAS and, 300
    satiety assessment and, 290–292
    sensory aspects of appetite measurement and, 303–307
    silhouettes for laboratory child-reported satiation and, 453–454, 453f
    SQ and, 301–302, 303f
    subjective measures of appetite and, 297f, 299f
    UEM and, 306–307, 313–315, 314f, 316f
    VAS technique and, 297f, 299f, 300–302, 303f
Satiety quotient, 301–302, 303f
Sattler, D. N., 98
Saucier, D. M., 131
Sauer, H., 15
Sauerland, S., 563
Sauerwald, T., 224
Saville, A., 536
Savitz, K. L., 16
Saylor, C. F., 451
Scaccini, C., 545
Scagliusi, F. B., 145t–146t, 148, 149t–151t, 155, 156

Scanlon, K., 447, 460t
Scanlon, K. S., 459
Scarpello, V., 88
Schacher, R., 454
Schachter, S., 138, 327, 328, 448
Schaefer, S., 85
Schafer, W. D., 4
Schall, J., 448
Schalling, D., 5t–7t
Schatzkin, A., 257, 261
Scheier, I. H., 17
Scheltema, K. E., 86
Schey, H. M., 493
Schiele, B. C., 3
Schilling, P. E., 261
Schippers, G., 149t–151t, 159, 171t, 176
Schirmer, H., 262
Schleusner, S. J., 538
Schlundt, D. G., 116t–125t, 126, 128, 153
Schmatz, C., 496
Schmid, T., 230
Schmidt, L. A., 417, 419
Schmidt, M. D., 216, 217
Schmidt, U., 63
Schmitt, M., 99
Schmitz, K. H., 532
Schmoll, K., 87
Schmölz, U., 354
Schneider, B., 208
Schneider, P. A., 411
Schneider, P. L., 207, 208, 209, 546
Schoeller, D. A., 155, 256, 273, 459, 492t–495t, 498, 512, 541
Schoemaker, C., 358
Schoenberg, M. R., 20
Schok, M., 38
Scholz, G. H., 56
Schooler, T. Y., 101
Schrauwen, P., 540
Schreurs, A. W., 536
Schuit, A. J., 221
Schuldheisz, J., 193t–196t, 202, 205t–206t
Schuldheisz, J. M., 202
Schulenberg, J. E., 116t–125t, 126
Schuler, P. B., 221
Schuler, R., 116t–125t
Schulman, R. G., 116t–125t
Schulsinger, F., 116t–125t, 464
Schultz, A. B., 496
Schultz, C. G., 485t, 486
Schumacher, J., 5
Schuppenies, A., 15
Schutte, N. S., 19
Schutz, H., 297

Schutz, H. K., 173
Schutz, Y., 99, 538, 545, 546
Schvaneveldt, R. W., 96
Schwartz, J. L. K., 97
Schwartz, J. P., 116t–125t
Schwartz, M. B., 80, 87, 93, 99, 101, 102t–105t, 106n4, 107n9, 364, 367, 400, 420, 422
Schwartz, M. W., 286
Schwerdtfeger, H., 83
Schwimmer, J. B., 61
SCID for DSM-IV. *See* Structured Clinical Interview for DSM-IV Axis I Disorders
SCL-90-R. *See* Symptoms Checklist 90 Revised inventory
Sclafani, A., 304
The SCOFF
    described, 411, 621
    norms for, 412t–413t, 414
    reliability of, 411, 412t–413t
    special issues/considerations/pros and cons for, 414
    validity of, 411, 412t–413t, 414
Scott, B., 374, 375, 420
Scott, C. B., 547
Scott, R., 347
Scott, R. L., 10
Scruggs, P. W., 202, 208
Seale, J. L., 542, 544
Sedentariness, 229–230
SEDS. *See* Stirling Eating Disorder Scales
SEDs. *See* Survey for Eating Disorders
Segal, D. L., 18
Segal, K. R., 536
Sehgal, A., 203, 205t–206t
Seicean, A., 224
Seid, M., 60
Seidel, R., 417
Seidell, J., 504
Seidell, J. C., 36
Seifer, R., 224
Seitz, B. A., 38
Sekine, M., 224
Self-report of physical activity and exercise measures
    criteria for selection of, 222–223
    described, 217, 218, 218t, 220f
    walking and bicycling case study and, 219, 221–222
Self-report questionnaires for binge eating and purging. *See also* Binge eating scale; Binge Eating Scale Questionnaire; Bulimia Scale–Eating Disorders Inventory; Bulimia Test–Revised; Eating Disorder Diagnostic Scale; Eating Disorder Examination; Eating Disorder Examination-Questionnaire; Interview for Diagnosis of Eating Disorders-IV; Mini International Neuropsychiatric Interview;

Multifactorial Assessment of Eating Disorder Symptoms; Questionnaire of Eating and Weight Patterns–Revised; Stirling Eating Disorder Scales; Structured Clinical Interview for DSM-IV Axis I Disorders; Structured Interview for Anorexic and Bulimic Disorders; Survey for Eating Disorders
    described, 350
    ESI and, 366
    self-report measures and, 375–376
Self-report questionnaires for eating-disordered thoughts, feelings, and behaviors. *See* Eating Disorder Diagnostic Scale; The SCOFF
Sellbom, M., 9
Sellinger, A., 485t, 486
Sempolska, K., 497
Sen Gupta, J., 543
Sensory aspects of appetite measurement
    assessment of sensory-specific effects in different groups and, 307
    described, 303–304
    description of methods for, 305–307
    fundamental assessment issues and, 304–305
Sepp, A., 300
Serdula, M. K., 459, 462
Serfass, R., 221
Serpell, L., 371
Seruda, M. I., 447, 460t
Sexton, H., 4
SF-36. *See* Short Form 36
Shadish, W., 152
Shadrick, D., 539
Shafer, C. L., 349
Shaffer, T. W., 12
Sharkey, K. M., 226
Shaw, B. F., 64
Shaw, H., 116t–125t, 129, 142
Sheehan, D. V., 381, 382
Sheehy, M. J., 417, 419
Sheeran, P., 80
Shen, W., 481, 482, 517
Sheng, H. P., 506
Shephard, R. J., 193t–196t
Sherbourne, C. D., 35
Sherman, D. K., 467, 468, 632
Sherman, J. W., 97
Sherman, R., 539
Sherrodd, J., 466
Shetty, P. S., 530, 541
Shide, D. J., 284
Shields, C., 327
Shiffman, S., 229, 439
Shisslak, C. M., 464
Shoba, B. C., 448, 449

Shore, R., 469
Short Form 36
    described, 39–40
    generic HRQOL instruments and, 35–36
    GHQ and, 41–42
    NHP and, 40–41
    obese population HRQOL assessment and, 36–37
    obese population seeking weight loss, and HRQOL, 37
    QWB and, 42
    SIP and, 41
    weight loss intervention studies, and HRQOL assessment, 37–42
Shroff, H., 116t–125t, 129, 385
Shrout, P. E., 377, 387, 410
Shuran, M., 544
SIAB-EX. *See* Structured Interview for Anorexic and Bulimic Disorders
Sichieri, R., 42
Sickness Impact Profile (SIP), 41
Siconolfi, S. F., 221
Siders, W., 506
Sidhu, S., 80
Sidman, C. L., 208
Sieber, W. J., 42
Siervo, M., 413
Siervogel, R. M., 492t–495t, 503
Silberhumer, G. R., 53
Silberstein, L. R., 140
Silhouettes for child-reported hunger and satiety assessment in laboratory, 453–454, 453f
Silver, A. J., 484
Silverstone, J. T., 296
Simmonds, M., 82, 84
Simmonds, M. B., 82, 84, 88
Simmons, A. M., 401, 417, 419
Simmons, J. R., 359, 431, 467
Simms, L. J., 9
Simonite, V., 449
Simons-Morton, B. G., 205t–206t
Simpson, S. J., 305
Singh, P. N., 221
SIP (Sickness Impact Profile), 41
Siperstein, G. N., 83
Sirard, J., 193t–196t, 239
Sirard, J. R., 188, 189, 200, 203, 210, 213, 215t, 216, 219
Siri, W. E., 485t, 486, 502
Sirikul, B., 221
SISDCA–Study Group on Psychometrics, 439
Sjostrom, L., 540
Sjöström, L., 41, 43t–51t, 56, 256, 258t–259t, 266, 275
Sjöström, L. V., 34
Sjöström, M., 213, 217

Skinfold thickness measurement
  accuracy and validity of, 505
  availability and costs of, 505
  described, 502–505, 503t–504t
  norms for, 505
  reliability of, 505
Skogar, S., 312
Skorjanec, B., 52
Skrondal, A., 17
Skroubis, G., 52
Slade, P., 12, 419, 466
Slate, S., 187
Slater, A., 129
Slattery, M. L., 187
Slaughter, M. H., 486, 503, 505
Slawik, H., 56
Slawinski, J. S., 532
Sleep measurement
  actigraphy method for, 226–227
  activity, and relevance for, 223–224
  declines in sleep and, 224–225
  described, 229
  historical background for, 223
  hormonal dysregulation and, 224
  hunger and, 224
  methods for, 225–227
  obesity risk factors and, 224, 225
  polysomnography method for, 225–226
  questionnaires and, 227–229
Slimani, N., 221, 261
Sloan, D. M., 433
Sloan, J. H., 543
Sloore, H., 21
Smalley, K. J., 492t–495t
Smari, J., 431
Smead, V. S., 175
Smeets, A. J., 303, 306
Smiciklas-Wright, H., 447, 459, 461, 462, 463
Smith, B. L., 11
Smith, C. A., 87
Smith, D., 398, 400
Smith, D. A., 485t, 486
Smith, F. C., 298
Smith, G., 162t, 163
Smith, G. P., 304
Smith, G. T., 145t–146t, 147, 154, 162t, 164, 359, 431, 433, 467
Smith, J. A., 449
Smith, J. E., 12
Smith, K. S., 41
Smith, K. W., 221
Smith, M., 156, 356
Smith, M. C., 156, 356, 431
Smith, S. R., 540

Smith, W., 535
Smolak, L., 116t–125t, 129
Snel, P., 227
Snellen, J. W., 535
Snoek, H. M., 307, 464
Snook, J. T., 545
Snow, K., 63
Snow, R. C., 221
Snyder, C. R., 256
Snyder, W. S., 482, 516
Soares, M. J., 530
Sobal, J., 328
Soeters, P. B., 40
SOFIT (System for Observing Fitness Instruction Time), 202
Song, M. Y., 516
Sonko, B. J., 544
SOPARC (System for Observing Play and Recreation in Communities), 203
Sopher, A., 481
SOPLAY (System for Observing Play and Leisure Activity in Youth), 203
SOPs (standard operating procedures), 286, 288
Sorensen, T., 116t–125t
Sørensen, T., 464
Sørensen, T. I., 272, 274
Sorkin, B., 538
Soulikia, K., 52
Spangler, D. L., 116t–125t
Spangler, E., 208–209
Spanier, P. A., 229
Speakman, J. R., 512
Special populations. *See also* Population
  adolescent populations, and food intake measurement in free-living, 272–273
  bias in case control studies in food intake measurement in free-living populations and, 272
  children, and food intake measurement in free-living, 272–273
  food intake measurement in free-living, 272–274
  human body composition assessment and, 484
  international studies on food intake measurement in free-living, 273
  intervention population, and food intake measurement in free-living, 274
  physical activity and exercise measure and, 191
  pregnant population, and food intake measurement in free-living, 273–274
Specker, B., 200, 201, 213
Spencer, C. P., 152
Speranza, M., 2
Spermon, T., 14
Spiegel, K., 223

Spiegelman, D., 275
Spielberger, C., 5t–7t, 67
Spielberger, C. D., 17, 18, 20, 438
Spilker, B., 40, 42
Spillane, N. S., 145t–146t, 147, 162t, 431, 433
Spilsbury, J. C., 193t–196t, 224, 227, 238
Spindler, A., 4
Spinhoven, P., 14
Spinnler, G., 534, 535
Spitzer, L., 292
Spitzer, R. L., 5t–7t, 8, 347, 348, 352, 353, 356, 362,
    369, 383, 397
Springer, D. W., 96
Spungen, A. M., 484
Spurr, G. B., 545
Spurrell, E. B., 364, 367, 400, 420, 422
SQ (satiety quotient), 301–302, 303f
Srebnik, D., 116t–125t, 127
Srinivasagam, N. M., 2
Stack, J., 364
Staffieri, J. R., 83, 84, 565
Stafleu, A., 291
Stager, S. F., 84
Stallberg-White, C., 449
Stallings, V. A., 187
Stallone, D. D., 269
Standard operating procedures, 286, 288
Stanford, E. A., 451
Stanley, M. A., 18, 116t–125t
Starling, J. R., 53
Starling, R. D., 221
Staten, L. K., 193t–196t, 221, 238
Staten, M. A., 517
State-Trait Anxiety inventory
    availability, 18
    limitations, 18
    norms, 18
    overview, 17–18
    reliability of, 18
    research applications, 18–19
    validity, 18
Stature, body weight, and body mass index
    accuracy and validity of, 497
    considerations for, 497–498
    reliability of, 497
Stature, description of, 487, 488t–489t, 489, 490t–
    495t, 496–497, 496t, 497t, 498f
Staveren, W. A., 173
Steen, B., 258, 260
Steer, R. A., 14, 15, 67
Steffen, R., 52
Steiger, H., 419
Steijaert, M., 492t–495t, 506
Stein, D., 19

Stein, D. M., 147
Stein, K. E., 127
Stein, K. F., 377, 378, 387
Stein, R. I., 56
Steinberg, L., 448, 449
Steinbrook, R., 36
Steiner, J. E., 303, 304
Steinfeldt, L., 267
Steinhausen, H. C., 417, 419
Steinmann, L., 449
Steinwert, T., 83, 86
Stejskal, W. J., 11, 12
Stel, V. S., 221
Stellar, E., 313
Stellato, T. A., 38
Stephen, J. R., 299
Stephen, M. A., 545
Sternfeld, B., 221
Stevens, F., 41
Stevens, J., 265, 328
Stevens, N. H., 260
Stevens, R., 424
Stevens, V. J., 260
Stevenson, R. J., 302
Stewart, A. L., 34, 35, 221
Stewart-Brown, S. L., 40
Stice, E., 116t–125t, 129, 140, 141, 142, 148, 156, 157,
    176t, 178, 357, 361, 362, 414, 416, 464, 465, 626
Stillman, R. J., 486
Stirling Eating Disorder Scales
    availability of, 374
    construct validity of, 372
    criterion validity of, 372–373
    described, 371, 373t
    internal consistency of, 371–372
    norms for, 373, 373t
    predictive validity of, 373
    reliability of, 371–372
    validity of, 372
Stitt, P. A., 297
Stock, M. J., 540
Stolarczyk, L. M., 483
Stone, A., 229, 439
St-Onge, M. P., 482
Storch, E. A., 15
Storch, J. B., 15
Stores, G., 227
Story, M., 328
Storzbach, D., 19
Stout, A. L., 55
St-Pierre, S., 300
Strahan, E. J., 88
Strain, J. J., 155
Strath, S. J., 204, 209

Stratton, R. J., 296, 299, 300
Strecher, V., 238
Streiner, D. L., 91, 466
Streit, K. J., 260
Striegel-Moore, R., 1
Striegel-Moore, R. H., 140
Stroebe, W., 142
Stroebele, N., 304
Structured Clinical Interview for DSM-IV Axis I
    Disorders
  availability of, 384
  concurrent validity of, 384
  criterion validity of, 384
  described, 383
  reliability of, 383–384
Structured Interview for Anorexic and Bulimic
    Disorders. *See also* Eating Disorder Examination
  availability of, 387, 410
  concurrent validity of, 386
  construct validity of, 386
  criterion validity of, 386–387
  described, 384–385, 404–405, 406t–409t
  discriminant validity of, 386–387
  interior reliability of, 385
  norms for, 387, 388t–389t, 406t–409t, 410
  reliability of, 385, 405, 406t–409t
  special issues/considerations/pros and cons for, 410
  validity of, 386, 405
Strupp, B. J., 291
Strycker, L. A., 208
Stubbs, R. J., 290, 294, 295, 296, 298, 299, 300
Stucki, A., 34, 58, 68
Stumpf, R. E., 2, 3, 4, 5
Stunkard, A., 34, 166, 312
Stunkard, A. J., 1, 80, 82, 116t–125t, 138, 141, 149t–
    151t, 159, 160, 161, 162, 162t, 163, 165, 178, 296,
    313, 348, 375, 386, 410, 416, 448, 464, 468
Stunkard and Messick's TFEQ-R Scale
  availability of, 169
  constant validity of, 163–164
  construct validity, 165–169
  convergent validity of, 165–169
  described, 159–161
  discriminant validity of, 165–169
  eating disorders and psychopathology and, 168
  factor stability and, 164
  hunger and, 160, 165, 166
  internal consistency and, 161
  naturalistic food consumption and, 167–168
  norms for, 161
  predictions of laboratory behavior and, 169
  readability of, 169
  relationship among TFEQ scales and, 164
  reliability of, 161–163, 162t

sample and, 161
susceptibility to response sets and, 168–169
test-pretest and, 161, 163
validity of, 163–165
weight and obesity status and, 164–167
Stupnicki, R., 497
Sturgeon, S. R., 187
Subar, A. F., 257, 258, 259, 261, 262, 267, 275
Subjective measures, for body image assessment,
    126–127
Subjective measures of appetite. *See also* Visual analog
  advantages of, 302, 303f
  advantages of subjective measures of appetite
      and, 302
  described, 296–297
  EARS studies and, 299–300, 299f
  procedure and description for, 297–298, 297f
  procedure and description of, 297–298, 297f
  quantifying satiation and satiety for, 299f,
      300–302, 303f
  reliability of VAS and, 300
  VAS recent developments and, 298–299, 299f
Suda, Y., 536
Sudman, S., 328, 343
Sue-Ling, H. M., 38
Suitor, C. W., 187
Suleiman, S., 221
Sullivan, D. K., 256
Sullivan, L., 41
Sullivan, L. G., 33
Sullivan, M., 33, 34, 41, 43t–51t, 56, 57, 532
Sullivan, M. B., 34
Sullivan, S., 5, 14, 449
Sullivan, S. A., 457
Sultan, S., 11
Summerbell, C. D., 93
Summerfeldt, L. J., 381, 383
Sun, M., 538
Sun, S. S., 504t–505t
Sunday, S. R., 384, 414
Survey for Eating Disorders
  availability of, 375
  concurrent validity of, 374
  criterion validity of, 374
  described, 374
  predictive validity of, 374–375
  reliability of, 374
Svendsen, O. L., 492t–495t
Svrakic, D. M., 5t–7t, 13
Swain, R. M., 178
Swami, V., 82
Swaminathan, H., 164
Swann, D., 256
Swanson, D. W., 3

Swanson, J., 54
Swartz, A. M., 204, 209
Sweeney, K., 303
Swenson, A. M., 212
Swett, C. P., 17
Swinburn, B., 221, 492t–495t
Swinson, R. P., 18
Symes, T., 304
Symptoms Checklist 90 Revised inventory
    availability, 17, 18
    limitations, 17, 18
    norms, 16, 16t, 18
    overview, 15–16
    reliability of, 16, 18
    research applications, 17, 18–19
    validity, 16, 18
Sysko, R., 366, 423
System for Observing Fitness Instruction
    Time, 202
System for Observing Play and Leisure Activity in
    Youth, 203
System for Observing Play and Recreation in
    Communities, 203
Szatmari, P., 467
Szymanski, M. L., 116t–125t, 127

Taffese, S., 545
Taft, C., 41, 43t–51t, 56
Tagliabue, A., 300
Takeuchi, N., 536
Talbot, L. A., 208
Talbot, P., 376
Tanaka-Matsumi, J., 18
Tanofsky-Kraff, M., 465
Tantleff, S., 116t–125t, 129
Tantleff-Dunn, S., 116t–125t, 126
Tapsell, L. C., 258t–259t
Tasali, E., 223
Tasca, G. A., 357, 358, 375, 422, 423, 424, 430
Task Force on Statistical Inference, 389
Tate, D., 150, 162, 168
Tay, J., 539
Taylor, C. B., 156
Taylor, C. L., 128
Taylor, H. L., 3, 143, 221, 487
Taylor, J. A., 17, 18
Taylor, L. H., 191
Taylor, M. J., 116t–125t, 127, 398
Taylor, P., 512
Taylor, P. R., 221
Taylor, W. C., 208
TCI. *See* Temperament and Character inventory
Teachman, B. A., 80, 86, 87, 96, 99, 100, 101,
    102t–105t, 106, 107, 107nn11–12,15–16

Technological innovations for physical activity and
    exercise measures
    described, 237–238
    introduction to, 237
    physical activity interventions and,
        238–239
Teff, K. L., 304
Teixeira, P. J., 494, 508
Tekcan, A., 419
Telch, C. F., 361, 414, 416
Tellegen, A., 5t–7t, 8, 9
Temperament and Character inventory
    availability, 14
    limitations, 14
    norms, 13
    overview, 13
    reliability of, 13
    research applications, 14
    validity, 13
Temple, J. L., 449
Ten Hoor, F., 159
Tepper, B. J., 449
Terrien, A., 19
Terrier, P., 545, 546
Terry, K., 327
Tetlock, P. E., 107n13
Thacker, C., 163
Thaete, F. L., 517
Thaw, J. M., 368, 434, 436
Thelen, M. H., 156, 168, 356, 358, 359, 360, 361,
    431, 433
Thermal imaging, and energy expenditure
    measurement, 544
Tholin, S., 161
Thomas, B. J., 506
Thomas, J. G., 139
Thompson, D. L., 209
Thompson, F. E., 257, 259, 262, 270
Thompson, J. K., 115, 116t–125t, 126, 127, 129, 130,
    131, 417, 469
Thompson, L., 360, 431, 433
Thompson, M. A., 116t–125t, 126, 131
Thompson, R. W., 208, 213
Thompson, S. H., 106n4
Thomson, E. S., 545
Thorburn, A. W., 449
Thornorsteinsdottir, G., 431
Thornton, J., 313, 492t–495t
Thorogood, M., 498
Thorpe, S. J., 305
Thorwart, M. L., 284
Three-compartment (3C) model, 485t, 486
Three-dimensional photonic scanning
    accuracy and validity of, 511–512

availability and costs of, 512
described, 509–510, 510f, 511f
norms for, 512
reliability of, 511
Thune, I., 187, 215
Thurfjell, B., 129, 467
Tiggeman, M., 129
Tiggemann, M., 81, 83, 85, 86, 106n3, 129, 130, 144, 155
Tijhuis, M. A., 36
Tikotzky, L., 225
Tilgner, L., 116t–125t
Tillotson, J., 261
Time studies, and physiological observations, 544–545
Timmerman, G. M., 145t–146t, 351
Tissot, J., 536
Tissot, S., 537
Titi, M., 53
Tobac, A., 21
Tobey, L., 85
Tobin, G., 529, 536, 537, 540
Togo, P., 272
Tolonen, P., 52, 53
Tomita, T., 14
Tomlinson, K. L., 359, 431, 467
Tonstad, S., 221
Toobert, D. J., 208
Tooze, J. A., 256, 258t–259t, 261, 267, 462
Torgerson, J. S., 43t–51t, 56
Toro, J., 66, 419, 466
Torquati, A., 39
Tortorella, A., 438
Toschke, A. M., 224
Total collection systems
availability and costs of, 537
flexible, 536–537
norms for, 537
reliability of, 537
rigid, 536
special issues/considerations/pros and cons for, 537
Totterdell, P., 298
Totty, W. G., 517
Toubro, S., 540
Tourangeau, R., 222
Touyz, S. W., 156, 376
Tovée, M. J., 82
Townsend, R. J., 33
Tozzi, F., 163, 175
Tracer dilution techniques
accuracy and validity of, 512
availability and costs of, 512
described, 512
norms for, 512

practical considerations for, 512
reliability of, 512
Trafimow, D., 80
Treasure, J., 63
Treasure, T., 63
Treleaven, P., 510
Tremblay, A., 294, 295, 296, 308, 529
Tremblay, M., 498
Triaxial accelerometers, 211
Trichopoulos, D., 221
Tripp, M. M., 116t–125t, 127
Troiano, R. P., 191, 217
Troisi, R., 274
Troop, N. A., 15
Troped, P. J., 237
Tropp, L. R., 80
Trost, S., 193t–196t, 239
Trost, S. G., 208, 212, 213, 215, 216, 230
Trotter, M., 496
Troutman, S. J., Jr., 535
Truby, H., 468
True, S., 300
Tse, C. T. J., 43t–51t, 53
Tsepas, S., 230
Tucker, K. L., 271, 272
Tucker, L. R., 153
Tudor-Locke, C., 204, 207, 208, 209, 228
Tuero, C., 221
Tuinebreijer, M. W., 38
Tuomisto, M. T., 290
Tuomisto, T., 290
Tuorila, H., 167
Turconi, G., 270
Turnbull, B., 449
Turnbull, J. D., 80, 83
Turner, H., 116t–125t, 127
Tuschen-Caffier, B., 131
Tuschl, R. J., 149t–151t, 156, 162t, 169, 171t, 176t
Tuthill, A., 56
24-hour recall, 260–261
Two-compartment (2C) models, 485–486, 485t
Tybor, D. J., 229
Tylka, T. L., 130
Tynelius, P., 161
Tzen, K. Y., 492t–495t
Tzischinsky, O., 224

UEM (Universal Eating Monitor), 306–307, 313–315, 314f, 316f
Uhl, H., 312, 314
Uhlenhuth, E. H., 15
Ujiie, T., 419
Ulbrecht, J. S., 284
Ulrich, C., 187

Underreporting
energy adjustment for bias in, 267–270, 268f, 269f
food intake measurement in free-living
populations and, 256–257
international studies on food intake measurement
in free-living populations and, 273
Uniaxial accelerometers, 210
Universal Eating Monitor, 306–307, 313–315,
314f, 316f
Urbina, S., 64
Ureda, J. R., 493
Urland, G. R., 145t–146t, 149t–151t
Urlando, A., 509
U.S. Department of Agriculture (USDA), 191,
261, 273
U.S. Department of Health and Human Services, 188,
189, 191, 202
U.S. Department of Transportation, 197
Utter, A. C., 20
UWW (underwater weighing). *See*
Hydrodensitometry

Vacc, N. A., 466
Vagenas, K., 52
Vaillancourt, T., 417, 419
Valcour, J., 208–209
Validation and calibration of techniques for
assessment issues in energy expenditure
measurement, 531
Valtolina, G., 10
Van Cauter, E., 223
Van Citters, G., 187
Vandegrift, D., 230
Van den Berg, P., 116t–125t, 129
Van den Brande, I., 21
Van der Kooy, K., 483
Vanderkooy, K., 504
Van der Kooy, K., 187
Van der Mars, H., 193t–196t, 202, 205t–206t
Van der Staak, C., 21, 358
Van der Staak, C. F., 149t–151t, 159, 171t, 176t
Van der Ster Wallin, G., 350
Vander Wal, J. S., 359, 361, 431, 433
Van Doornen, L. J. P., 142
Van Furth, E., 3
Van Furth, E. F., 63
Van Gaal, L., 492t–495t, 506
Van Gemert, L. J., 307
Van Gemert, W. G., 40
Van Hasselt, V. B., 18
Van Hoeken, D., vii
Van Horn, L., 274
Van Ingen Schenau, G. J., 536
Van Itallie, T. B., 306, 314

VanItallie, T. B., 328
Van Itallie, T. B., 448, 492t–495t
Van Ittersum, K., 330
Van Leeuwe, J. F. J., 171t, 176
Van Leeuwen, F. E., 187
Van Loan, M., 492t–495t
Van Loan, M. D., 492t–495t, 507
Van Marken Lichtenbelt, W. D., 540
Vannotti, A., 534
Van Ramshorst, B., 142
Van Staveren, W., 148
Van Staveren, W. A., 29, 221, 465
Van Strien, T., 138, 141, 142, 148, 149t–151t, 154, 159,
169, 171t, 172, 173, 174, 176, 176t, 464, 465
Van Waesberghe, F., 227
Vara, L., 398, 400
Vara, L. S., 449
Varni, J. W., 60, 61
Vartanian, L. R., 80, 96, 99, 102t–105t, 141
Vartsky, D., 492t–495t
VAS. *See* Visual analog scale technique
Vasilaras, T. H., 291, 540
Vassend, O., 17
Vaswani, A. N., 486, 492t–495t, 496
Vázquez-Velásquez, V., 430
Veggi, A. B., 42
Velicer, W. F., 164
Vella, C. A., 205
Venkataraman, P. S., 492t–495t
Venkataraman, S. T., 536
Ventilated open-circuit indirect calorimetry,
538–539
Ventura, A. K., 447, 461, 462
Verboeket–van de Venne, W. P., 546
Verbraak, M., 358
Verduin, M., 546
Vereecken, C. A., 261, 265, 273
Verloop, J., 187
Veron-Guidry, S., 126
Verschell, M. S., 11
Vescovi, J. D., 508
Vetrone, G., 116t–125t, 127
Victorzon, M., 52, 53
Villanueva, M., 65
Villarruel, A. M., 451
Vincent, M. A., 359
Vincent, N. K., 2, 3
Vincent, S. D., 208
Visser, M., 485
Visual analog scale technique
advantages and wider implications of, 302
described, 296–297, 297f
eating and weight-related problems in children
and, 454–455, 454f

procedure and description of, 297–298, 297f
quantifying satiation and satiety and, 300–302, 303f
recent developments of, 298–300, 299f
reliability of, 300
sensitivity of, 300
validity of, 300
Vitousek, K. M., 2, 3, 4, 5, 10
Vogt, R. A., 178, 351
Vohra, F. A., 213
Vollrath, M., 419
Volz, P. A., 492t–495t
Von Kries, R., 224
Von Ranson, K. M., 2, 3
Voorrips, L. E., 221
Voss, L. D., 212
Votaw, M. C., 200
Voudouris, N., 171t, 172, 419, 464

Wadden, T., 347, 348, 356, 369
Wadden, T. A., 1, 10, 58, 68, 99, 102t–105t, 142, 143,
    157, 178, 351
Wade, S., 483
Wade, T. J., 85
Wagner, A., 19
Wagner, H. R., II, 53
Wahl, P. W., 225
Wahter, M., 256
Wake, M., 59, 61
Waki, M., 483, 506
Wales, J., 294
Walker, H. C., 302
Walker, M., 83
Walker, R., 80, 187
Walker, S. R., 42
Wall, A. D., 10
Wallace, A., 9
Wallace, J. M., 447
Wallace, J. P., 42
Waller, G., 12, 371, 372, 375, 438, 466
Wallis, D. J., 173
Walsh, B. T., 1, 4, 351, 366, 367, 379, 423
Walsh, D., 307, 532
Walsh, J. A., 450
Walsh, M. C., 221
Walsh, R. A., 12
Walsh, T. B., 366
Waltz, J., 79
Wan, G. J., 33
Wang, J., 483, 484, 486, 492t–495t, 500, 504t–505t,
    506, 510, 511, 512
Wang, M. Q., 221
Wang, S. S., 99, 101, 102t–105t
Wang, Z., 482, 486, 513
Wang, Z. M., 486, 492t–495t, 515

Wansink, B., 292, 327, 328, 329, 330, 332, 333, 334,
    335, 337, 339, 340, 342, 343
Waranch, H. R., 354
Warbasse, R. E., 81
Ward, A., 158
Ward, C., 410
Ward, C. H., 386, 410
Ward, D., 265
Ward, G. M., 495
Ward, L. C., 506
Wardle, J., 145t–146t, 171t, 172, 173, 174,
    449, 464
Ware, J., 63, 64
Ware, J., Jr., 35, 40, 63, 66, 67
Ware, J. E., 35, 59
Ware, J. E., Jr., 33, 35
Wareham, N. J., 221, 542
Warren, J. M., 449
Warwick, P. M., 545
Washburn, R. A., 200, 215t, 221, 544
Waters, E., 59, 61
Waters, E. B., 59
Watkins, B., 377
Watkins, D., 88
Watkins, P. C., 116t–125t, 128
Watson, D., 9, 18
Watson, D. L., 202
Watson, K., 230
Waugh, B. A., 331
Waxman, S., 116t–125t
Weaver, C., 175
Webb, P., 529, 535, 542, 545
Weber, M., 430
Webster, J. D., 535
Wedderkopp, N., 212, 217
Weenen, H., 291, 307
Wegener, D. T., 88
Weight loss, and SF-36, 36–37
Weight loss intervention studies
    GHQ and, 41–42
    NHP and, 40–41
    OWLQOL and, 58, 555
    QWB and, 42
    SF-36 and, 37–42
    SIP and, 41
Weight-related problems in children assessment
    BE and, 469
    BESAA and, 469
    BRS and, 467–468, 632
    CBIS and, 468
    described, 467
    EDI-2 and, 467
    EDI-BD and, 469
    EDI-C and, 467

figure drawings and, 468, 634
  KEDS BIS and, 468–469, 635
Weight-Related Symptom Measure, 58, 556
Weiller, K., 80, 90, 96
Weiner, I. B., 11
Weiner, R. A., 563
Weiner, S., 43t–51t, 563
Weingarten, H. P., 334
Weinsier, R. L., 262
Weir, J. B., 534, 538
Weismayer, C., 272
Weiss, D. J., 64
Weiss, T. W., 221
Weissman, C., 239, 538
Weissman, M. M., 64
Welch, G., 357, 360, 431, 433
Welham, W. C., 485, 485t
Welk, G., 190
Welk, G. J., 189, 200, 204, 213, 216
Wells, J. C., 492t–495t, 510
Welsh, G., 535
Welsh, S., 539
Weltzin, T. E., 9, 19
Wendel-Vos, G. C. W., 221
Wendt, S., 116t–125t, 127, 398, 400
Weng, L.-J., 94
Wentzlaff, T. H., 314, 315
Werkman, A., 237
Werle, C., 330
Werner, J., 15
Wertheim, E., 116t–125t, 129, 171t, 172, 419, 464
Wertheim, E. H., 173
Werther, G. A., 449
West, S. G., 88
Westen, D., 1
Westenhoefer, J., 140, 162t, 163, 164, 166, 168, 178
Westerbeek, A., 449
Westerterp, K., 213, 217, 529
Westerterp, K. R., 169, 221, 266, 540, 546
Westerterp, M. S., 169
Westerterp-Plantenga, M. S., 145t–146t, 159, 167, 169, 266, 292, 303, 306, 312, 313, 314, 315
Westman, E. C., 56
Westrate, J. A., 293
Weststrate, J., 504
Wetzel, R. D., 5t–7t, 13
Whisenhunt, B. L., 116t–125t, 127
Whisman, M. A., 433
Whitaker, A., 366
White, A., 459
White, A. A., 93
White, D. R., 116t–125t
White, M. A., 55, 116t–125t
White, W. C., 348

Whitlow, J. W., 139
Whitney, C. W., 225
Whittaker, A., 200
WHO (World Health Organization), 33, 79, 382
Whole-Body 40K Counting Technique, 515
Whybrow, S., 290, 299, 300
Wiederman, M. W., 8, 10
Wiegand, M., 354
Wieland, W. F., 313
Wiepkema, P. R., 304
Wiggs, L., 227
Wijndaele, K., 16
Wikman, A., 259
Wilbur, J., 221
Wildman, R. P., 502
Wilfley, D. E., 56, 351, 364, 367, 378, 379, 400, 420, 422, 423, 431
Wilk, J. E., 10
Wilkin, T. J., 212
Wilkinson, J. Y., 149t–151t, 163
Wilkinson, L., 163, 389
Wilks, R., 273
Willett, W., 257, 259, 270
Willett, W. C., 271, 275
Williams, A., 152, 153
Williams, C. L., 230
Williams, D., 484
Williams, E., 116t–125t, 128
Williams, G. -J., 371, 372, 373, 375
Williams, G. R., 35, 37, 43t–51t, 54, 55
Williams, J., 40, 61
Williams, J. B., 5t–7t, 8, 362
Williams, J. B. W., 353, 383, 397
Williams, R., 150, 162, 163, 165, 168
Williamson, D., 450, 463
Williamson, D. A., 116t–125t, 126, 128, 140, 145t–146t, 155, 166, 314, 361, 368, 379, 381, 401, 404, 434, 436, 439, 466, 467
Williamson, D. F., 40
Williamson, S., 203, 205t–206t
Willmuth, M. E., 417
Wilmore, J. H., 538
Wilson, A. J., 156
Wilson, B. S., 205t–206t
Wilson, D. K., 42
Wilson, D. M., 156
Wilson, G. T., 4, 80, 364, 365, 367, 379, 398, 400, 420, 422, 423
Wilson, J., 197
Wilson, J. F., 417, 419
Wilson, L. M., 3
Wilson, S. A., 540
Wilson, S. E., 53
Wilson, T. D., 101

Wilson-Barrett, E., 83
Wing, R. R., 142, 145t–146t, 162, 167, 350, 351, 530, 546
Wingard, D. L., 223
Wingate, B. J., 351
Winkvist, A., 273
Wisbey, J., 227
Withers, R. T., 485t, 486
Wittenbrink, B., 96, 97
Wohl, J., 4
Wolf, A. M., 52, 222, 463
Wolfe, B. M., 53
Wolfson, A. R., 193t–196t, 224, 227
Wolk, A., 221, 272
Wolterink, S., 449
Womersley, J., 484, 503
Wonderlich, S., 156, 356
Wong, M. L., 15
Wong, P., 539
Wong, W. W., 212, 512
Wood, A., 12, 466
Wood, J. M., 11, 12
Wood, K., 213
Wood, K. C., 469
Wood, M., 154
Workman, D. E., 11
World Health Organization, 33, 79, 382
Worobey, J., 106–107n7, 106n4
Wouters, L., 159
Wright, M., 59
Wright, M. J., 300
WRSM (Weight-Related Symptom Measure), 58, 556
Wu, A. H., 187
Wu, C., 492t–495t
Wu, H. C., 221
Wurmser, H., 224
Wurtman, J. J., 308
Wurtman, R. J., 308
Wynter, S., 273

Xu, J., 80

Yamamiya, Y., 129
Yamamoto, C., 19
Yamashita, T., 116t–125t, 129
Yancey, A. K., 116t–125t, 229

Yang, J., 197
Yanover, T., 115
Yanovski, S., 347, 348, 356, 369, 423
Yanovski, S. Z., 369
Yasumura, S., 486, 492t–495t, 496
Yates, A., 90
Yavuszen, T., 307
Yaxley, S., 305
Yeomans, M. R., 293, 300, 302, 304, 306, 312, 313, 314, 315
Yngve, A., 213, 217
Yoes, M. E., 64
Yoked, T., 230
Yon, B. A., 265
Yore, M. M., 222
Yoshida, T., 536
Youn, T., 327
Young, B. A., 543
Young, D. R., 222
Younger, J. C., 332
Youssef, G., 8
Yuen, K., 486, 492t–495t, 496
Yuker, H. E., 81, 86t, 92, 95
Yun, Y. S., 502
Yurgelun-Todd, D., 1

Zabinski, M. F., 228, 237
Zanarini, M. C., 383, 384
Zavaleta, A. N., 496
Zebb, B. J., 18
Zebley, S. P., 313
Zeller, M., 61, 62
Zeller, M. H., 61
Zhang, J. J., 417
Ziebland, S., 498
Ziegler, E. E., 483
Zijlstra, N., 292
Zimring, C., 230
Ziuraitis, J. R., 532
Zlot, A., 230
Zlotkin, S., 454
Zucker, N. L., 434
Zumbo, B. D., 90
Zung, W. W., 5t–7t, 18
Zwick, W. R., 164

About the Editors

David B. Allison received his PhD from Hofstra University in 1990. He then completed a postdoctoral fellowship at the Johns Hopkins University School of Medicine and a second postdoctoral fellowship at the NIH-funded New York Obesity Research Center at St. Luke's/Roosevelt Hospital Center. He was a research scientist at the NY Obesity Research Center and Associate Professor of Medical Psychology at Columbia University College of Physicians and Surgeons until 2001. In 2001, he joined the faculty of the University of Alabama at Birmingham, where he is currently Professor of Biostatistics, Head of the Section on Statistical Genetics, and Director of the NIH-funded Clinical Nutrition Research Center. He has authored over 300 scientific publications and edited five books. He has won several awards, including the 2002 Lilly Scientific Achievement Award from The Obesity Society, the 2002 Andre Mayer Award from the International Association for the Study of Obesity, the American Society of Nutrition's 2009 Centrum Center for Nutrition Science Award given in recognition of recent investigative contributions of significance to the basic understanding of human nutrition, and the National Science Foundation Administered 2006 Presidential Award for Excellence in Science, Mathematics, and Engineering Mentoring (PAESMEM). He was elected as a Fellow of the American Statistical Association in 2007 and the American Psychological Association in 2008, holds several NIH and NSF grants, and has been a member of the Board of Trustees for the International Life Science Institute, North America, since 2002. He serves or has served on the editorial boards of *Behavior Genetics; Computational Statistics and Data Analysis; Human Heredity; International Journal of Eating Disorders; International Journal of Obesity; Nutrition Today; Obesity Reviews; Obesity; Public Library of Science (PLOS) Genetics;* and *Surgery for Obesity and Related Diseases (SOARD)*. Dr. Allison's research interests include obesity, quantitative genetics, clinical trials, and statistical and research methodology. He also serves as a frequent consultant and expert witness in the legal setting.

Monica L. Baskin received her PhD in Counseling Psychology in 1999 from Georgia State University. She then completed a postdoctoral fellowship at Emory University School of Medicine. After completion of her postdoctoral fellowship, she was a research project director and later a Research Assistant Professor in the Department of Behavioral Science and Health Education in the Rollins School of Public Health at Emory University. In 2003, Dr. Baskin joined the faculty of the

University of Alabama at Birmingham where she holds a primary appointment as an Assistant Professor in the Department of Health Behavior in the UAB School of Public Health and a secondary appointment in the Department of Nutrition Sciences in the UAB School of Health Professions. She is an Associate Scientist for the UAB Clinical Nutrition Research Center (CNRC) and the UAB Minority Health and Research Center (MHRC) and a Scientist in the UAB Diabetes Research and Training Center (DRTC). She is also a member of the UAB Psychology Internship Training Consortium faculty. Dr. Baskin has been the recipient of numerous honors and awards, including the American Psychological Association (APA) Minority Fellowship (1997–1999), the National Institutes of Health/National Center on Minority Health and Health Disparities Scholar Award (2002–2004), the UAB Clinical Nutrition Research Center Named New Investigator Award (2005–2006), and a 2007 finalist for the International Life Science Institute (ILSI), North American Future Leaders Award. She has been a licensed professional psychologist since 2000 and has extensive training and experience in pediatric psychology. Her research focuses primarily on childhood obesity prevention. She has led multiple funded research projects focusing on individual, family, and environmental factors associated with healthy eating, physical activity, and/or obesity and has published in the areas of obesity, culturally competent interventions, health promotion programs in Black churches, and motivational interviewing (MI). She serves on the journal review board of the *American Journal of Health Behavior* and is an ad hoc reviewer for numerous journals, including *Health Psychology, Journal of Clinical Child Psychology, Obesity Research, Obesity Reviews, American Journal of Clinical Nutrition,* and *International Journal of Eating Disorders.* In addition, Dr. Baskin has frequently served on special emphasis panels reviewing the scientific merit of obesity-related grants for the National Institutes of Health, the Centers for Disease Control and Prevention, the Health Resources and Services Administration, and the Robert Wood Johnson Foundation.

About the Contributors

Drew Anderson, PhD, is Associate Professor of Psychology at the University at Albany, State University of New York. He received his PhD in clinical psychology from Louisiana State University. His research interests center broadly on eating and eating-related constructs, and he has conducted research related to eating disorders, obesity, and body image disturbance. He has a particular interest in the assessment of eating and related behaviors.

Audie A. Atienza, PhD, is a Behavioral Scientist/Program Director at the National Cancer Institute (NCI), Division of Cancer Control and Population Sciences, Behavioral Research Program, Health Promotion Research Branch. He received his bachelor's degree from the University of California at San Diego in 1991 and obtained his doctorate in Clinical Psychology from Kent State University in 1998. He completed a clinical psychology internship at the Palo Alto Veterans Administration Health Care System as part of his doctoral training. Prior to coming to the NCI, he was a postdoctoral Fellow at the Stanford University School of Medicine, Stanford Prevention Research Center (formerly the Center for Research in Disease Prevention). His research interests include health promotion/disease prevention, ethnic minority health, health disparities, psychosocial aspects of health, health and aging, community health, and real-time data capture (e.g., ecological momentary assessment) in health research using innovative technology.

David Berrigan, PhD, is a biologist in the Applied Research Program of the National Cancer Institute's Division of Cancer Control and Population Sciences. His research and administrative responsibilities currently focus on environmental determinants of energy balance behavior, physiological consequences of exercise, surveillance of walking and its correlates, and biomarker-based links between energy balance and carcinogenesis. He received his PhD. in Evolutionary Biology from the University of Utah and his MPH from UC Berkeley. He carried out postdoctoral research on evolutionary physiology of ectotherm responses to temperature at the University of Washington and La Trobe University in Melbourne, Australia, and spent 4 years as a Cancer Prevention Fellow at NCI.

Hany Bissada, MD, is Associate Professor in Psychiatry at the University of Ottawa and is Director of the Regional Centre for the Treatment of Eating Disorders at The Ottawa Hospital. He recently completed a randomized control trial of olanzapine in the treatment of anorexia nervosa, published in the *American Journal of Psychiatry* in 2008.

John Blundell currently holds a personal chair in psychobiology at the University of Leeds. He was trained in neuroscience at the Institute of Neurology in London and has been active in research on the mechanisms of human appetite control for about 25 years. One landmark paper from the early years on the role of serotonin on feeding has since become an ISI citation classic. Fifteen years ago, the Human Appetite Research Unit was established at Leeds University. The purpose of this unit is the investigation of mechanisms underlying the control of human appetite. Investigations are supported by EU Framework 5 (Resistance and Susceptibility to weight gain in Europe) and 6 (DIOGENES), research councils (BBSRC, MRC-case), and industrial sponsors. The major focus of current research is on the individual variability in the human appetite response and the identification of phenotypes—susceptible or resistant—in the face of overconsumption or exercise-induced energy deficit.

Rachel M. Calogero is currently a Lecturer in the Department of Psychology at the University of Kent in Canterbury. The focus of her PhD thesis was the development and validation of an implicit lexical measure of close-mindedness. Her diverse research areas include motivated social cognition, antecedents and consequences of self-objectification processes, resistance to change, and the prevention of body image and eating problems. She has presented her research regularly at international conferences for the past 7 years and continues to publish her research in a variety of scholarly journals. She has developed and is actively involved in several cross-cultural collaborations related to her research areas.

Chi A. Chan, BA, is Assistant Researcher at Temple University's Center for Obesity Research and Education. She obtained her bachelor's degree in psychology with a specialization in neuroscience from Temple University. Her current research interests include obesity and healthy weight management, as well as associations between neuroanatomy, neurophysiology, and behavior.

Kees de Graaf is Professor with respect to Eating Behavior in Wageningen. He did his PhD on psychophysical studies of mixtures of tastants. Since 1989, he has been a staff member at the division of Human Nutrition in Wageningen. In 1997, he had a sabbatical leave focused on food acceptability at the Behavioral Science section of the U.S. Army research center in Natick, Massachusetts. From 2000 to 2004, he worked as an adviser at TNO–Quality of Life on a project focused on biomarkers of satiety. Research interests are the regulation of food intake and food choice, particularly in relation to sensory, psychological, and physiological factors.

Kyle P. De Young, MA, is a graduate student at the University at Albany, State University of New York. His research interests include course and outcome, exercise behavior, and assessment in eating disorders.

Natasha Demidenko, PhD, is a Clinical Psychologist at the Regional Centre for the Treatment of Eating Disorders at the The Ottawa Hospital. She is involved in a clinical trial of group psychotherapy for binge-eating disorder. Other research interests include attachment, sexual abuse trauma, and depression.

Donna Dueker, MPH, is a PhD candidate in epidemiology at the Keck School of Medicine University of Southern California. She received her MPH from the

University of Southern California and a BA in Biology from Pomona College. Her current research examines new methodologies for assessing environmental exposures.

Myles S. Faith is Assistant Professor of Psychology in Psychiatry at the University of Pennsylvania School of Medicine. His research focuses on the development of child food preferences, eating styles, and body weight. With his colleagues, Dr. Faith studies the interplay of genetic and environmental influences on child eating patterns, parent-child feeding dynamics, and the measurement of child appetite and satiety. He tests interventions to help treat and/or prevent obesity in children. He holds grants from the National Institutes of Health to study these issues. He is active in different professional organizations concerning child health, development, and obesity and is past Chair of the "Pediatric Obesity Interest Group" for The Obesity Society (TOS).

Graham Finlayson is a biological psychologist and lecturer in the Institute of Psychological Sciences at the University of Leeds. His research is concerned with the hedonic and homeostatic systems that underpin human appetite control. His current research interests focus on the characterization and experimental assessment of liking and wanting for food. During his PhD studies, Graham developed a laboratory-based procedure to assess dissociations between implicit and explicit liking and wanting in relation to food preference. Subsequently, the procedure has been applied to distinguish the effect of sensory and metabolic satiety on liking and wanting, investigate the acute and postingestive influence of taste and macronutrient properties, and assess the consequences of an energy deficit (effect of exercise) on liking, wanting, and subsequent energy intake. A more recent strategy for the tool has been to characterize susceptible "phenotypes" of scientific interest based on binge-eating tendencies and compensatory responses to exercise.

Kevin R. Fontaine is a health psychologist and faculty member in the Division of Rheumatology at Johns Hopkins University. His research interests include (1) the physical and emotional consequences of chronic diseases such as obesity and arthritis; (2) the association between obesity, body composition, and mortality; and (3) the effect of lifestyle modification interventions on quality of life in persons with arthritis and fibromyalgia. The author of over 70 publications, his work has been supported by the Arthritis Foundation, the American College of Rheumatology, and the National Institutes of Health.

Gary D. Foster, PhD, is Professor of Medicine and Public Health and Director of the Center for Obesity Research and Education at Temple University. His research interests include the behavioral and metabolic aspects of obesity. He studies a variety of treatment approaches, including behavior therapy, pharmacotherapy, and surgery. His current research studies include the effects of weight loss on sleep apnea, the safety and efficacy of low- and high-carbohydrate diets, and the prevention of obesity and diabetes in school settings. Dr. Foster has been a frequent presenter at national and international scientific meetings. He also has considerable clinical experience treating overweight patients in individual and group therapy for over 20 years.

Dympna Gallagher is Associate Professor of Nutritional Medicine at Columbia University and is Director of the Human Phenotyping Core Laboratory of the New

York Obesity Research Center, St. Luke's-Roosevelt Hospital. She has wide expertise in the area of body composition methodology and its application in clinical studies involving obesity, weight loss, and growth. Dr. Gallagher's recently completed and ongoing NIH-funded projects include investigating variations in resting energy expenditure with age and across race groups, body composition changes using whole-body magnetic resonance imaging (MRI) in type 2 diabetic adults with weight loss, in children as they advance through puberty, and in the morbidly obese before and after bariatric surgery. She serves as a mentor to many foreign postdoctoral fellows receiving training in body composition assessment, serves as a consultant on body composition measurement-related issues, and publishes scholarly articles relating to body composition assessment, adipose tissue distribution and depots, obesity and weight loss, and resting metabolic rate.

Steffany Haaz, MFA, is a doctoral candidate in the Johns Hopkins School of Public Health, studying individual and societal factors that influence health behaviors, such as diet, physical activity, and stress management. She is a Registered Yoga Teacher and is currently supported by the NIH National Center for Complementary and Alternative Medicine (NCCAM) and the Arthritis Foundation to assess the effects of yoga on quality of life for patients with rheumatoid and osteoarthritis. Her primary interests lie in the biopsychosocial mechanisms by which interventions affect quality of life.

Jason C. G. Halford performed his undergraduate and postgraduate work in Leeds with Professor John Blundell in the late 1980s and early 1990s. His research then focused on the role of serotonin in satiety and the use of feeding behavior to screen antiobesity drugs. Some of this included early work on sibutramine. He has been involved in the behavioral assessment of potential antiobesity drugs in preclinical models and humans ever since, including recent work on rimonabant. Over the past 10 years, his research has focused on drug-induced weight gain, the effects of nutrients and fiber on appetite and hormone release, the effects of stress on eating behavior, and lean-obese differences in the expression of appetite. More recently, he has focused on the effects of branding and food promotion on children's food preferences and diet. He is currently a reader in appetite and obesity at the University of Liverpool and Director of the Human Ingestive Behaviour laboratory.

Ann M. Harris works with Dr. James Levine at the Mayo Clinic.

Marion Hetherington is Professor of Biopsychology at Glasgow Caledonian University. She received her D.Phil in Experimental Psychology from the University of Oxford and then completed a postdoctoral fellowship at the Johns Hopkins University School of Medicine. This was followed by a Fogarty International Fellowship at the National Institutes of Health. She returned to the United Kingdom in 1990 working at the Universities of Dundee and Liverpool. She has spent 25 years in the field of ingestive behavior, specifically investigating mechanisms of satiety and characterizing individual differences in susceptibility to overweight and obesity. Marion has recently been appointed to a research chair of Biopsychology at the University of Leeds.

Melinda L. Irwin, PhD, is Associate Professor in the Department of Epidemiology and Public Health at Yale School of Medicine. She is an expert in the design and conduct of randomized controlled exercise trials and population-based prospective cohort studies in women with and without breast cancer. She has published numerous papers in peer-reviewed journals on the effect of exercise on breast cancer biomarkers, influence of physical activity on obesity, and physical activity measurement issues. She also has considerable experience with the development and validation of physical activity surveys and objective measures of physical activity such as motion sensors and cardiorespiratory fitness.

Fahad Javed, MD, was a Research Fellow at the New York Obesity Research Center, St. Luke's–Roosevelt Hospital prior to joining the internal medicine residency program (June 2008) where he is currently a resident. He participated in research projects related to studies of human body composition and metabolic bone disease, as well as various weight loss studies within the Clinical Pharmacology Program during his research fellowship.

Michael Jerrett, PhD, is Associate Professor in the Division of Environmental Health Science, School of Public Health, University of California, Berkeley. Building on expertise in Health Geography, Geographic Information Science, and Spatial Analysis, Dr. Jerrett assesses the role of the built environment on numerous health risks and outcomes. His topical areas of focus are (a) air pollution exposure modeling and health effects assessment, (b) obesity and the built environment (i.e., how the built landscape influences physical activity and food intake), and (c) the social distribution of environmental exposures. He has published some of the most widely cited studies on air pollution health effects, social susceptibility, and environmental inequality. His research spans the United States, Canada, Mexico, China, and parts of Europe. He has principal investigator (PI) and co-PI grants from the U.S. National Institute of Environmental Health Science, the U.S. National Cancer Institute, the U.S. Environmental Protection Agency, the Health Effects Institute, the Canadian Institutes of Health Research, the California Air Resources Board, and the Robert Wood Johnson Foundation. In 2004, he was selected as the Dangermond Endowed Speaker in Geographic Information Science.

Louise A. Kelly holds an assistant professorship in the Department of Exercise Science and Sports Medicine at California Lutheran University. In 2005, she earned her PhD in Pediatric Exercise Science from the University of Glasgow, Scotland. She subsequently completed a 3-year postdoctoral fellowship in Preventive Medicine at the University of Southern California. She has conducted research on the etiology, prevention, and treatment of pediatric obesity, using her expertise in methodologies such as accelerometers, indirect calorimeters, and doubly labeled water. Her research is currently focused on the role of exercise in the prevention and treatment of obesity-related pediatric cancers.

Neil King is currently Associate Professor in the School of Human Movement Studies at Queensland University of Technology in Brisbane. Neil has a BSc degree in Sports Science and Chemistry and an MSc in Human Nutrition. In 1994, he was awarded his PhD on "The Relationship Between Exercise and Appetite" from the Institute of Psychological Sciences at the University of Leeds. His areas of expertise and research interests are concerned with the relationships among physical activity, appetite regulation, and weight management. He has published extensively in this field and is recognized internationally as a key researcher in the understanding of the behavioral aspects of weight management. He is particularly interested in the individual variability in compensatory responses to exercise and dietary interventions.

Ronette "Ronnie" L. Kolotkin, PhD, is a clinical psychologist, researcher, and consultant who specializes in the treatment of obesity and the study of quality of life in obesity. She received her PhD in Clinical Psychology from University of Minnesota. Dr. Kolotkin is currently a Consulting Associate Professor at Duke University in the Department of Community and Family Medicine. From 1984 to 1999, she served as the Director of the Behavioral Health Program at Duke University's Diet and Fitness Center. In 1999, she began a consulting company, Obesity and Quality of Life Consulting. She is the primary developer of the Impact of Weight on Quality of Life questionnaire for adults (IWQOL-Lite), as well as the IWQOL-Kids for adolescents. She has published numerous scientific articles about obesity and is the coauthor of a book titled *Duke University Medical Center Book of Diet and Fitness.*

Tanja V. E. Kral, PhD, is Assistant Professor of Nutrition in the Department of Psychiatry at the University of Pennsylvania School of Medicine. She received her PhD in Nutritional Sciences from The Pennsylvania State University in 2003. Her research interests focus on the study of human ingestive behavior in children and adults. In particular, she is interested in characterizing differences in eating behaviors of individuals with a different familial predisposition to obesity and of different weight status and in identifying factors that promote increased energy intake.

Valerie Krysanski, PhD, is a Clinical Professor in Psychology at the University of Ottawa and a Clinical Psychologist at the Regional Centre for the Treatment of Eating Disorders at the Ottawa Hospital. She is a coinvestigator in a clinical trial of group psychotherapy for binge-eating disorder. Her other research interests include program evaluation, psychotherapy outcome research, anxiety sensitivity, attachment, and sexual abuse in eating disorders.

James A. Levine is Professor of Medicine, Physiology, and Bioengineering and the Richard Emslander Chair of Nutrition and Metabolism at the Mayo Clinic in Rochester, Minnesota. He is a renowned expert in obesity. His research has focused on understanding nonexercise activity thermogenesis (NEAT), obesity, and body weight regulation. He has published articles in the most prestigious scientific journals, including *Science, Nature, New England Journal of Medicine,* and *Lancet.* He has served as a scientific adviser to the U.S. government, United Nations, and the government of the People's Republic of China as well as other countries.

Lauren Lissner's major research areas are obesity and nutritional epidemiology. She did her graduate studies at the UCLA School of Public Health and the Department of Human Nutrition at Cornell University, followed by postdoctoral work with the Obesity Research Group at The University of Pennsylvania. During this period, her research focused on energy balance and weight regulation issues, ranging from the role of dietary fat to weight cycling. Since 1989, she has been living and working in

Göteborg, Sweden. In Sweden, she has been directing research in several population-based studies from Göteborg, including the Prospective Population Study of Women in Gothenburg, the InterGene Program, the Geriatric and Gerontological Population Studies in Gothenburg, and recently the Childhood Obesity Project in Västra Götaland. Since 2000, she has been an adjunct professor at the Nordic School of Public Health and is currently Professor of Epidemiology at the Department of Public Health and Community Medicine, Sahlgrenska Academy at Göteborg University.

Greg Lindsey, PhD, is Associate Dean of the Hubert H. Humphrey Institute of Public Affairs at the University of Minnesota. He specializes in environmental planning, policy, and management. His current projects involve analyses of activity patterns on urban greenways and studies of the effects of greenways in urban communities. Dr. Lindsey earned his doctorate and a master's degree from the Department of Geography and Environmental Engineering at the Johns Hopkins University. He also received a master's degree in geography and environmental studies from Northeastern Illinois University. His bachelor's degree is in urban planning from the University of Illinois. He has published articles in the *Journal of the American Planning Association, Journal of Environmental Planning and Management, Journal of Physical Activity and Health, Professional Geographer, Journal of Recreation and Park Administration, Landscape and Urban Planning,* and *Journal of Urban Design.*

Michael R. Lowe, PhD, is Professor of Clinical Psychology at Drexel University and Senior Research Consultant at the Renfrew Center for eating disorders. His research contributions include (1) the development of the three-factor model of dieting, (2) a new model of the role of both current dieting and weight suppression in bulimia nervosa, (3) the application of nutritional research to the prevention of weight gain and regain, (4) the use of functional MRI (fMRI) and electroencephalography (EEG) to better understand neurophysiological correlates of obesity-proneness, and (5) the development of the Power of Food Scale to assess "hedonic hunger." He has been the recipient of six NIH grants in the past 10 years. He is on the Scientific Advisory Board of Weight Watchers, is a consultant to Pfizer, and is currently an editorial board member (and formerly an Associate Editor) for the *Journal of Abnormal Psychology.*

Rob McConnell, PhD, is Professor of Preventive Medicine at the University of Southern California. His research interests include the determinants of physical activity and obesity in children and the epidemiology of childhood respiratory disease, especially its relationship to air pollution. He has several NIH grants to examine these research questions and is the Deputy Director of the Southern California Children's Environmental Health Center at USC and UCLA. He has also worked extensively in Latin America and the Caribbean and is a former director of the World Health Organization's Center for Human Ecology and Health.

Melissa A. Napolitano, PhD, is Associate Professor in the Departments of Kinesiology and Public Health and Research Scientist at the Center for Obesity Research and Education at Temple University. Her research interests are related to the prevention of weight gain (e.g., following smoking cessation), physical activity adoption and maintenance, and using the Internet for delivering health behavior change interventions with a particular focus on women's health. She has given lectures both nationally and internationally on these topics. Dr. Napolitano has authored or coauthored more than 30 publications and more than 65 conference presentations. As a principal investigator or coinvestigator, she has secured extramural funding from small foundation sources, as well as the National Institutes of Health, the American Heart Association, and the Robert Wood Johnson Foundation. Dr. Napolitano also directs the clinical weight loss services at the Center for Obesity Research and Education, where she supervises clinical psychology interns and postdoctoral fellows.

Todd G. Morrison, PhD, is an associate professor in the Applied Social Psychology programme at the University of Saskatchewan. His research interests include male body image (in particular, the drive for muscularity), gay and lesbian psychology, and scale development. He is the author/coauthor of publications that have appeared in various peer-reviewed journals, including *Body Image, Journal of Men's Studies, European Journal of Psychological Assessment, Psychology of Men and Masculinity, Journal of Cross-cultural Psychology,* and the *International Journal of Sexual Health.* He also is the editor/co-editor of several books including *Psychology of Modern Prejudice* and *Male Sex Work: A Business Doing Pleasure* and serves on the editorial boards of *The Journal of Social Psychology* and *Journal of Homosexuality.*

Angelo Pietrobelli, MD, is a pediatric endocrinologist who worked with Dr. S. B. Heymsfield at the New York Obesity Research Center, Columbia University, New York. Currently, he is Senior Staff Physician at the Pediatric Unit, Verona University Medical School, Verona, Italy. His research is mainly focused on pediatric body composition as well as the prevention and treatment of pediatric obesity. He is the Pediatric Associate Editor of the *International Journal of Obesity,* Associate Editor of the *International Journal of Body Composition Research,* and the Associate Editor of the *International Journal of Pediatric Obesity.*

Nancy Potischman, PhD, is a nutritional epidemiologist in the Applied Research Program in the Division of Cancer Control and Population Sciences at the National Cancer Institute. Her primary research efforts focus on biomarkers of nutritional status and hormonal factors related to cancer. Nutritional exposures cover a range dietary instruments, biomarkers, and anthropometric indices. She has conducted methodologic work to assess laboratory performance and to improve dietary assessment methods. Methodologic work has included comparing estimates from commonly used dietary questionnaires to serologic measures, as well as applications of new techniques to minimize measurement errors. Current work involves development of questionnaires for pregnant and lactating women, addressing diet in children, assessing diet in the distant past, and development of an automated self-administered 24-hour recall instrument. Another area of interest involves evaluation of early life factors and risk factors across the life span, in relation to each other and in relation to cancer risk in adulthood.

Susan Redline, MD, MPH, is Professor of Medicine, Epidemiology and Biostatistics, and Pediatrics; Academic Program Director of the Center for Clinical Investigation at Case Western Reserve University School of Medicine; and Director of University Hospitals Sleep Disorders Center. Her research focuses on the epidemiology of sleep disorders in both children and adults, including the relationships of sleep disorders with other health outcomes (diabetes, obesity, cardiovascular disease, and behavioral morbidity) and the genetic and environmental etiologies of these disorders.

Sarah Roddy, BA (1st class honors), is currently completing her PhD in Experimental Psychology at the National University of Ireland, Galway. Her research interests include the implicit assessment of antifat attitudes, body image, and contextual behavior science.

Selena Nguyen-Rodriguez, MPH, PhD, is a Postdoctoral Research Associate at USC's Institute for Health Promotion and Disease Prevention Research. She currently is involved in research that assesses psychosocial and physiological determinants of physical activity in minority girls. Her main research interests revolve around stress and other psychological correlates of health behaviors. She is also interested in other health psychology issues, specifically the impact of psychological health/well-being on chronic disease management and survival.

Travis A. Ryan, BA, Higher Diploma in Arts (Psychology), is a PhD student at the National University of Ireland, Galway. His current research interests include the sociocultural and social comparative underpinnings of male body image and student attitudes toward people with communication disabilities. He is coauthor of a study scheduled for publication in the *Journal of Homosexuality* and held a Visiting Scholar appointment at the University of California (2007–2008).

Donna Spruijt-Metz, MFA, PhD, is Associate Professor of Research in the Department of Preventive Medicine, Keck School of Medicine, University of Southern California. Building on deeply transdisciplinary approaches to minority adolescent and child health, her research focuses on physical activity, diet, obesity, and their relationships to cancer. Research topics include (a) acute effects of specific nutrients on behavior; (b) biological, cultural, environmental, and psychosocial determinants of physical activity and exercise in minority youth; (c) neural correlates of appetite using fMRI; (d) mind-body intervention modalities to help overweight minority youth overcome stress, control caloric intake, and increase physical activity levels; and (e) testing and development of total body biosensing modalities in minority youth.

Hemal P. Shroff, PhD, is Assistant Professor in the School of Health Systems Studies at the Tata Institute of Social Sciences, Mumbai, India. She received her doctoral degree in clinical psychology from the University of South Florida and her internship training was at the Long Island Jewish Medical Center. She also completed a postdoctoral fellowship in eating disorders at the University of North Carolina. She has published several articles and a chapter in the fields of body image and eating disorders and is a reviewer for the journal *Body Image.* Currently, she is doing research on the impact of psychological and social factors on child nutrition in India.

James Stubbs is a Slimming World's Research Specialist. He received his PhD from Cambridge University. He then progressed to a Glaxo Junior Research Fellowship, which he resigned in 1993 to join the Rowett Research Institute. He was a Principle Scientific Officer at Rowett and has over 15 years experience in designing, coordinating, and writing up large-scale human trials and interventions concerned with weight control and obesity. He has organized numerous scientific meetings and symposia for The Nutrition Society and is well versed in delivering contract research to government agencies and industry alike. He has now conducted over 50 studies on aspects of feeding behavior, appetite control, diet composition, and energy balance. Initial work focused on testing models of human intake regulation. Dr. Stubbs joined Slimming World as its Research Specialist to focus more on the development of applied solutions to weight control among consumers.

Giorgio A. Tasca, PhD, is Associate Professor in Psychiatry and Clinical Professor in Psychology at the University of Ottawa. He is also the Director of Research at the Regional Centre for the Treatment of Eating Disorders at The Ottawa Hospital. Aside from his interests in psychometrics, he has also conducted randomized clinical trials of group psychotherapy for binge-eating disorder and of olanzapine in the treatment of anorexia nervosa, the latter published in the *American Journal of Psychiatry* in 2008.

Zaria Tatalovich, PhD, is Research Assistant Professor of Geography at the University of Southern California, where she collaborates on a number of research projects that combine geographic information science (GIS) and risk assessment, teaches a course on principles of geographic information science, and chairs graduate student progress report meetings. Her research is focused on GIS model development and assessment in the health and hazards contexts; specifically, it examines how we can model the risks associated with natural hazards and adverse environmental conditions, given the measurement network, geospatial technology, and methods available to us. These efforts are part of larger collaborative initiative to improve our understanding of the environmental and social components of risk.

J. Graham Thomas, MS, is a doctoral student in Clinical Psychology at Drexel University, where he studies the assessment and treatment of obesity and eating disorders with Michael R. Lowe, PhD. He anticipates obtaining his PhD in 2009 upon completion of the Obesity Clinical-Research internship at Brown University, where he studies behavioral interventions for weight loss and long-term weight maintenance with Rena R. Wing, PhD. His research interests include (1) the application of technological innovations such as ecological momentary assessment (EMA) for the measurement and treatment of obesity and eating disorders, (2) the effect of environmental influences on weight regulation, (3) the relationship between weight change and eating-disordered symptoms, and (4) the use of advanced statistical techniques to better understand disease processes and treatment response.

J. Kevin Thompson, PhD, received his doctoral training at the University of Georgia, where he obtained his PhD in 1982. He has been at the University of South Florida since 1985 and is Professor in the Department of Psychology. He has authored, coauthored, or edited five books in the area of body image, eating disorders, and obesity (*Body Image Disturbance: Assessment and Treatment,* 1990; *Body Image, Eating Disorders, and Obesity: An Integrative Guide for Assessment and Treatment,* 1996; *Exacting Beauty: Theory Assessment and Treatment of Body Image Disturbance,* 1999; *Body Image, Eating Disorders and Obesity in Youth,* 2001, 2009; *The Muscular Ideal,* 2007). He has been on the editorial board of the *International Journal of Eating Disorders* since 1990.

D. Catherine Walker, MA, is a graduate student at the University at Albany, State University of New York. Her research interests are in body checking and avoidance behaviors in men and women suffering from eating disorders and body image dissatisfaction, as well as the application of exposure and response prevention techniques in eating disorder and body image treatments.

Brian Wansink is the John Dyson Professor of Consumer Behavior at Cornell University, where he directs the Cornell Food and Brand Lab. He is author of over 100 academic articles and books, including the best-selling *Mindless Eating: Why We Eat More Than We Think* (2006) along with *Marketing Nutrition* (2005), *Asking Questions* (2004), and *Consumer Panels* (2002). From 2007 to 2009, he was granted a leave of absence from Cornell to accept a presidential appointment as Executive Director of USDA's Center for Nutrition Policy and Promotion, the federal agency in charge of developing 2010 Dietary Guidelines and promoting the Food Guide Pyramid (MyPyramid.gov). His award-winning academic research on food psychology and behavior change has been published in the world's top marketing, medical, and nutrition journals. It contributed to the introduction of smaller " 100-calorie" packages (to prevent overeating), the use of taller glasses in some bars (to prevent the overpouring of alcohol), and the use of elaborate names and mouth-watering descriptions on some chain restaurant menus (to improve enjoyment of the food).

Jennifer Wolch, PhD, is Professor of Geography and Urban Planning and Director of the Center for Sustainable Cities at the University of Southern California. Her research investigates urban poverty and homelessness, metropolitan sprawl, parks and public health, and environmental justice. Her books include *Landscapes of Despair: From Deinstitutionalization to Homelessness* (1986) and *Malign Neglect: Homelessness in an American City* (1993; both with Michael Dear), and *Up Against the Sprawl: Public Policy and the Making of Southern California* (2004, edited with Manuel Pastor Jr. and Peter Dreier). She is a past recipient of fellowships or awards from the Guggenheim Foundation, Center for Advanced Study in the Behavioral Sciences, and the Association of American Geographers.

Supporting researchers for more than 40 years

Research methods have always been at the core of SAGE's publishing program. Founder Sara Miller McCune published SAGE's first methods book, *Public Policy Evaluation*, in 1970. Soon after, she launched the *Quantitative Applications in the Social Sciences* series—affectionately known as the "little green books."

Always at the forefront of developing and supporting new approaches in methods, SAGE published early groundbreaking texts and journals in the fields of qualitative methods and evaluation.

Today, more than 40 years and two million little green books later, SAGE continues to push the boundaries with a growing list of more than 1,200 research methods books, journals, and reference works across the social, behavioral, and health sciences. Its imprints—Pine Forge Press, home of innovative textbooks in sociology, and Corwin, publisher of PreK–12 resources for teachers and administrators—broaden SAGE's range of offerings in methods. SAGE further extended its impact in 2008 when it acquired CQ Press and its best-selling and highly respected political science research methods list.

From qualitative, quantitative, and mixed methods to evaluation, SAGE is the essential resource for academics and practitioners looking for the latest methods by leading scholars.

For more information, visit **www.sagepub.com**.

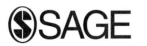

Supporting researchers
for more than 40 years